D1171614

Current Therapy in

EQUINE
REPRODUCTION

Current Therapy in

EQUINE
REPRODUCTION

Juan C. Samper, DVM, MS, PhD, DACT
JS Equine Service
Langley, British Columbia
Canada

Jonathan F. Pycock, BVetMed, PhD, DESM, MRCVS
Messenger Farm, Ryton
Malton, North Yorkshire
United Kingdom

Angus O. McKinnon, BVSc, MSc
Goulburn Valley Equine Hospital
Congupna, Victoria
Australia

SAUNDERS

ELSEVIER

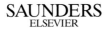

SAUNDERS
ELSEVIER

11830 Westline Industrial Drive
St. Louis, Missouri 63146

CURRENT THERAPY IN EQUINE REPRODUCTION   ISBN 13: 978-0-7216-0252-3
ISBN 10: 0-7216-0252-5

Copyright © 2007 by Saunders, an imprint of Elsevier Inc.

All rights reserved. No part of this publication may be reproduced or transmitted in any form or by any means, electronic or mechanical, including photocopying, recording, or any information storage and retrieval system, without permission in writing from the publisher. Permissions may be sought directly from Elsevier's Health Sciences Rights Department in Philadelphia, PA, USA: phone: (+1) 215 239 3804, fax: (+1) 215 239 3805, e-mail: healthpermissions@elsevier.com. You may also complete your request on-line via the Elsevier homepage (http://www.elsevier.com), by selecting "Customer Support" and then "Obtaining Permissions."

Notice

Knowledge and best practice in this field are constantly changing. As new research and experience broaden our knowledge, changes in practice, treatment and drug therapy may become necessary or appropriate. Readers are advised to check the most current information provided (i) on procedures featured or (ii) by the manufacturer of each product to be administered, to verify the recommended dose or formula, the method and duration of administration, and contraindications. It is the responsibility of the practitioner, relying on their own experience and knowledge of the patient, to make diagnoses, to determine dosages and the best treatment for each individual patient, and to take all appropriate safety precautions. To the fullest extent of the law, neither the Publisher nor the Editors assumes any liability for any injury and/or damage to persons or property arising out or related to any use of the material contained in this book.

ISBN 13: 978-0-7216-0252-3
ISBN 10: 0-7216-0252-5

Publishing Director: Linda Duncan
Senior Editor: Penny Rudolph
Managing Editor: Jolynn Gower
Publishing Services Manager: Patricia Tannian
Project Manager: John Casey
Designer: Jyotika Shroff

Printed in United States of America

Last digit is the print number: 9 8 7 6 5 4 3 2 1

Working together to grow
libraries in developing countries

www.elsevier.com | www.bookaid.org | www.sabre.org

ELSEVIER   BOOK AID International   Sabre Foundation

Contributors

Gregg P. Adams, DVM, MS, PhD, DACT

Professor, Veterinary Biomedical Sciences
Western College of Veterinary Medicine
University of Saskatchewan
Saskatoon, Saskatchewan
Canada

Beth A. Albrecht, DVM

Department of Clinical Sciences
Kansas State University
Manhattan, Kansas

Mimi Arighi, DVM, MSc, DACVS

Director, Veterinary Teaching Hospital
School of Veterinary Medicine
Purdue University
West Lafayette, Indiana

Scott D. Bennett, DVM

Equine Services Clinic
Simpsonville, Kentucky

Don R. Bergfelt, MS, PhD

Honorary Fellow, School of Veterinary Medicine
Animal Health and Biomedical Sciences
University of Wisconsin
Madison, Wisconsin
Scientist/Biologist
Office of Science Coordination and Policy
Environmental Protection Agency
Washington, DC

Terry L. Blanchard, DVM, MS, DACT

Hill 'N Dale Farm
Lexington, Kentucky

Etta Agan Bradecamp, DVM, DACT, ABVP

Old Waterloo Equine Clinic
Warrenton, Virginia

Theresa Burns, DVM, MSc

Abbotsford, British Columbia
Canada

Claire Card, DVM, PhD, DACT

Professor, Department of Large Animal Clinical Sciences
Western College of Veterinary Medicine
University of Saskatchewan
Saskatoon, Saskatchewan
Canada

Jacqueline M. Cardwell, MA, VetMB, MRCVS

Epidemiology Unit, Centre for Preventive
  Medicine
Animal Health Trust
Newmarket, Suffolk
UK

Elaine M. Carnevale, DVM, MS, PhD

Assistant Professor, Biomedical Sciences
Colorado State University
Fort Collins, Colorado

Javier Castillo-Olivares, LV, MSc, PhD, MRCVS

Veterinary Virologist
Urology Department
Animal Health Trust
UK

Robert C. Causey, DVM, PhD, DACT

Assistant Professor, Animal and Veterinary Sciences
University of Maine
Orono, Maine

Tracey S. Chenier, DVM, DVSc, DACT

Assistant Professor, Large Animal Theriogenology
Department of Population Medicine
Ontario Veterinary College
University of Guelph
Guelph, Ontario
Canada

H. Steve Conboy, DVM

Equine Practice
Lexington, Kentucky

John J. Dascanio, VMD, DACT, DABVP

Associate Professor, Large Animal Clinical Sciences
Virginia-Maryland Regional College of Veterinary
  Medicine
Virginia Polytechnic Institute and State University
Blacksburg, Virginia

Robert Douglas, PhD

BET Labs
Lexington, Kentucky

Rolf M. Embertson, DVM, DACVS

Rood & Riddle Equine Hospital
Lexington, Kentucky

Andrés J. Estrada, DVM

Resident, Equine Theriogenology
Department of Clinical Sciences
Veterinary Medical Teaching Hospital
Kansas State University
Manhattan, Kansas

Nathalie F. Faber, MV, MS

University of California
Davis, California

Grant S. Frazer, BVSc, MS, MBA, DACT

Assistant Professor, Large Animal Theriogenology
College of Veterinary Medicine
The Ohio State University
Columbus, Ohio

Earl M. Gaughan, DVM, DACVS

Professor, Clinical Sciences
Veterinary Medical Teaching Hospital
Auburn University
Auburn, Alabama

James K. Graham, PhD

Associate Professor, Department of Biomedical Sciences
Colorado State University
Fort Collins, Colorado

Justin T. Hayna, DVM, DACT

Director of Equine Reproduction
Minitube of America
Verona, Wisconsin

Cortney E. Henderson, DVM, MS

Harris Equine Hospital
Whitesboro, Texas

Katrin Hinrichs, DVM, PhD, DACT

Professor and Link Chair in Mare Reproductive
    Studies
Veterinary Physiology and Pharmacology
College of Veterinary Medicine
Texas A&M University
College Station, Texas

Richard D. Holder, DVM

Hagyard-Davidson-McGee Associates, PSC
Lexington, Kentucky

G. Reed Holyoak, DVM, PhD, DACT

Associate Professor, College of Veterinary Medicine
Oklahoma State University
Stillwater, Oklahoma

John P. Hurtgen, DVM, MS, PhD, DACT

Owner, NANDI Veterinary Associates
New Freedom, Pennsylvania

Vivienne Irwin, BVSc (Hons)

Regulatory Associate
Parnell Laboratories Pty. Ltd.
Alexandria, New South Wales
Australia

Terttu Katila, DVM, MS, PhD

Professor, Animal Reproduction
Department of Clinical Veterinary Sciences
University of Helsinki
Finland

Teri L. Lear, MS, PhD

Research Associate Professor
Maxwell H. Gluck Equine Research Center
Veterinary Science Department
University of Kentucky
Lexington, Kentucky

Michelle M. LeBlanc, DVM, DACT

Rood & Riddle Equine Hospital
Lexington, Kentucky

William B. Ley, DVM, MS, DACT

Regional Equine Associates Central Hospital
Millwood, Virginia

Margo L. Macpherson, DVM, MS, DACT

Associate Professor, Reproduction
Large Animal Clinical Sciences
University of Florida
Gainesville, Florida

Phil Matthews, DVM

Peterson & Smith Equine Hospital
Ocala, Florida

Patrick M. McCue, DVM, PhD, DACT

Associate Professor, Department of Clinical Sciences
Colorado State University
Fort Collins, Colorado

Elizabeth S. Metcalf, MS, DVM, DACT

CEO
Honahlee, PC
Sherwood, Oregon

Stuart A. Meyers, DVM, PhD, DVM

Assistant Professor
Anatomy, Physiology, and Cell Biology
College of Veterinary Medicine
University of California
Davis, California

Corey D. Miller, DVM, MS, DACT

Co-Founder and Head of Reproduction
Equine Medical Center of Ocala
Ocala, Florida

Lee Morris

The University of Sydney
Narellan, New South Whales
Australia

John R. Newcombe

Warren House Equine Infertility Clinic
Warren House Farm
Brownhills, Walsall
UK

Gary J. Nie, DVM, MS, PhD, DACT, DABVP, DACVIM

World Wide Veterinary Consultants, LLC
Springfield, Missouri

Reginald R. Pascoe, BVSc, MVSc, DVSc, FRCVS, FACVSc

Professor (Retired), Veterinary Science
University of Queensland
Veterinary School
Queensland
Australia

Virginia B. Reef, DVM, DACVIM

Mark Whittier and Lila Griswold Allam Professor of
   Medicine
Clinical Studies
New Bolton Center
University of Pennsylvania
Kennet Square, Pennsylvania

Sidney Ricketts, LVO, BSc, BVSc, DESM, DECEIM, FRCPath, FRCVS

Rossdale & Partners
Beaufort Cottage Stables
Newmarket, Suffolk
UK

W. Thomas Riddle, DVM

Partner, Rood & Riddle Equine Hospital
Lexington, Kentucky

Janet F. Roser, MS, PhD

Professor, Department of Animal Science
University of California
Davis, California

Patricia L. Sertich, VMD, MS, DACT

Associate Professor, Clinical Studies
New Bolton Center
University of Pennsylvania
Kennzate Square, Pennsylvania

Sherman J. Silber, MD

Infertility Center of St. Louis
St. Luke's Hospital
St. Louis, Missouri

Edward L. Squires, BS, MS, PhD, DACT (Hon)

Professor, Department of Biomedical Sciences
Animal Reproduction and Biotechnology Laboratory
Colorado State University
Fort Collins, Colorado

Melinda Story, DVM

Kansas State University
Manhattan, Kansas

Ahmed Tibary, DMV, PhD, DACT

Associate Professor, Theriogenology
Department of Veterinary Clinical Sciences
Washington State University
Pullman, Washington

Mats H. T. Troedsson, DVM, PhD, DACT

Professor, Large Animal Clinical Sciences
College of Veterinary Medicine
University of Florida
Gainesville, Florida

Alan O. Trounson, MD

Professor
Monash Immunology and Stem Cell Laboratories
Monash University
Melbourne
Australia

Regina M. O. Turner, VMD, PhD, DACT

Assistant Professor, Large Animal Reproduction
Department of Clinical Studies
New Bolton Center
University of Pennsylvania
Kennett Square, Pennsylvania

Philip D. van Harreveld, DVM, MS, DACVS

Owner, Vermont Large Animal Clinic
Milton, Vermont

Dirk K. Vanderwall, DVM, PhD, DACT

Assistant Professor, Animal and Veterinary Science
University of Idaho
Moscow, Idaho

James R. Vasey, BVSc, DVS, FACVSc

Director
Goulburn Valley Equine Hospital
Congupna, Victoria
Australia

James L. N. Wood, BSc, BVetMedMSc, PhD, DLSHTM, DECVPH, MRCVS

Director, Cambridge Infectious Diseases Consortium
Department of Veterinary Medicine
University of Cambridge
Cambridge
UK

Walter W. Zent, DVM

President, Society of Theriogenology, KAEP, AAEP,
   AVMA
Hagyard Equine Medical Institute
Lexington, Kentucky

Preface

Our purpose in creating *Current Therapy in Equine Reproduction* is to provide practicing veterinarians, veterinary students, and equine breeding managers with a succinct and contemporary source of information regarding the equine reproductive process. As implied by the words "current therapy," this text offers the most up-to-date information on diagnosis and management of all facets of horse breeding.

We cannot stress how important proper breeding management is to ensure the success of a breeding operation. Managing the reproduction problems of mares and stallions properly can and will enhance their fertility, whereas mismanagement can reduce fertility even in normal mares and stallions.

The book is divided into eight sections, but basically covers the mare and the stallion and problems with each. Section I covers the normal reproductive system of the mare, and Section II addresses female reproductive problems. Sections III and IV focus on the stallion with normal reproductive system and then reproductive problems. Section V is all about semen collection and evaluation, and Section VI moves into the topic of assisted reproductive techniques. Section VII is devoted to successful breeding strategies for the pregnant mare. The last section wraps up with a discussion of the postpartum breeding mare and any problems or complications that might arise.

Our philosophy in compiling the outline for this text was to address recent changes that have occurred in equine reproduction, specifically those that have not been adequately addressed in comparable texts to date. Let us turn the page and see if we have met those objectives.

Juan C. Samper
Jonathan F. Pycock
Angus O. McKinnon

Acknowledgments

When asked by Juan and Jon to join them in editing this *Current Therapy* I accepted without much thought. The chance to work with authors, learn from reading and editing their manuscripts, and to publish a book with editors who were employed in private practice was a temptation too much to deny. Apart from the edification, it emphasized to me that specialization in private practice was so well accepted that authors and editors need not be restricted solely to those institutions of higher learning.

The *conception* and *gestation* of this *Current Therapy* was clearly Juan's domain. He decided on the necessity of this, *his progeny* to be introduced. He provided *the gametes* with the outline and list of authors and Jon and I were co-opted for the *fertilization* process. Early in gestation a problem with this *pregnancy* was identified wherein, after narrowly avoiding *early embryonic death*, it began to look like *elective termination or even abortion* was a possibility. After identifying and rectifying the problems and deficiencies, the gestation then became somewhat *prolonged*.

At last, successful delivery!

Angus O. McKinnon

We all owe a great deal to Jolynn Gower who was our managing editor from Elsevier. How she handled the difficulties of delinquent authors and editors with such level-headed aplomb was a surprise and an inspiration to us all. The only reason the project eventually came together was through her untiring efforts to keep us all on track.

Juan C. Samper
Jonathan F. Pycock
Angus O. McKinnon

Contents

SECTION III   THE NORMAL MALE REPRODUCTIVE SYSTEM

SECTION IV   MALE REPRODUCTIVE PROBLEMS: DIAGNOSIS AND MANAGEMENT

SECTION I

The Normal Female Reproductive System

CHAPTER 1

Ovulation and Corpus Luteum Development

DON R. BERGFELT
GREGG P. ADAMS

The events of ovulation and subsequent formation of the corpus luteum involve systemic and local hormones that signal cellular degeneration and morphogenesis of theca, granulosa, and other associated cells of the preovulatory follicle. Specific cellular aspects of the ovulatory and tissue remodeling processes associated with luteogenesis have been reviewed elsewhere for the mare[1,2] and other species[3] and will not be discussed herein. Instead, the gross morphologic and physiologic relationships associated with development of the primary follicular wave that leads to ovulation and subsequent formation of the equine corpus luteum, especially during the estrous cycle, will be the primary focus of this chapter. A brief discussion will address the formation of supplemental corpora lutea from ovulatory and anovulatory follicles during early pregnancy in the mare.

Undoubtedly, ultrasound imaging has played a major role in advancing our understanding of ovulation and luteal gland development and is an invaluable diagnostic and prognostic tool for evaluating these events in the mare. Ultrasonographic methods for examining ovarian morphology have been documented in other reviews[4,5]; therefore the applications and not the technique will be emphasized in this review. The technique of gathering ultrasonographic information will be discussed in more detail only in situations where morphologic characteristics can be used as a measure of physiologic status. We believe that comprehension of the fundamental structural and functional relationships associated with follicular and luteal development will allow the practitioner to diagnose the imminence and occurrence of ovulation and subsequent integrity of the developing corpus luteum to within hours. Quantitative changes in the brightness and darkness of the ultrasonographic gray-scale image (i.e., echogenicity) of the preovulatory follicle, ovulation

site, and corpus luteum will be presented as a diagnostic and prognostic aid to allow the practitioner to assess cellular and tissue attributes in real time.

Many of the results presented herein comprise averages obtained from numerous mares under experimental conditions and may not necessarily reflect what is observed under clinical or field conditions in individual animals. The mean results, which are often encompassed by an indicator of population variance (i.e., standard error of the mean, SEM), are intended to serve as a guide that can be used to estimate or predict a particular outcome in an individual mare.

THE OVULATORY FOLLICULAR WAVE

The primary follicular wave of the estrous cycle is a major wave, characterized by a dominant ovulatory follicle and several subordinate follicles.[1,2,4-8] A group of 7 to 11 growing follicles greater than 5 mm can be detected ultrasonically at about midcycle of a 22- to 24-day estrous cycle. To distinguish between growing and regressing follicles of the ovulatory wave, more than one ultrasound examination is necessary, especially because atretic follicles of a proceeding minor or major wave may linger and confuse the identity of newly emerging follicles. In regard to the latter, follicular wave dynamics have been critically studied by ablating all follicles greater than 5 mm using ultrasound-guided transvaginal follicle aspiration and inducing luteal regression with prostaglandin-$F_{2\alpha}$ ($PGF_{2\alpha}$) at 10 days after ovulation. As a result, evaluation of the ovulatory wave can be done with respect to a relatively homogenous population of growing follicles because the population of regressing follicles was removed. The mean diameter profiles of newly emerging follicles and corresponding concentration profiles of systemic hormones of an ablation-induced wave have been compiled from several studies[9] and are presented in Figure 1-1 to assist in the following discussion. At the time of wave emergence, the largest follicle usually has a 2- to 3-mm size advantage (approximately 1 day of growth) over other smaller follicles of the wave (see Figure 1-1, *A*). During the common growth phase, the largest follicle is referred to as the future dominant follicle and the others as future subordinate follicles, because the hierarchal position is often maintained after emergence. Endowed with granulosa cell follicle-stimulating hormone (FSH) receptors, antral follicles of the ovulatory wave develop in response to an increase in circulating concentration of FSH. When the future dominant follicle reaches about 13 mm, peak concentration of the wave-inducing FSH surge is attained and the decreasing portion of the surge begins (see Figure 1-1, *B*). Concomitantly, circulating concentrations of progesterone are decreasing, while inhibin and luteinizing hormone (LH) are increasing (see Figure 1-1, *B* and *C*). The opposing changes in concentrations of FSH and LH during late diestrus/early estrus are attributable, in part, to increasing concentrations of inhibin emanating from the growing follicles of the preovulatory wave and decreasing concentrations of progesterone as a result of a regressing corpus luteum, respectively. During the early stages of this hormonal exchange, the future dominant and subordinate follicles continue growth at a relatively parallel rate (2 to 3 mm/day) until the future dominant follicle reaches 20 to 25 mm at early estrus (Figure 1-1, *A*). Thereafter, growth of the dominant follicle proceeds unabated, and the remaining subordinate follicles cease growth and eventually regress. The change in growth rates between the dominant and subordinate follicles beginning at the start of the dominance phase is a key event during selection of the ovulatory follicle, and has been termed follicle deviation.[6-8] The mechanism associated with follicle selection is not known but appears to involve a developmental advantage of one follicle over another such that the future dominant follicle has an increased capacity for estradiol production, sensitivity to FSH, and specificity to respond to LH through the induction of granulosa cell LH receptors. It appears that subordinate follicles are insensitive to low systemic concentrations of FSH and are not endowed with an abundance of granulosa cell LH receptors. Hence, subordinate follicles regress because of an insufficient ability to respond to subthreshold concentrations of gonadotropins. As reviewed,[6] recent studies have shown that intrafollicular concentrations of estradiol, IGF-1, inhibin-A and activin-A increase differentially in the future dominant and subordinate follicles before the beginning of deviation and, therefore, may act as modulators for differentially enhancing the FSH and LH responsiveness of the future dominant follicle. Nonetheless, the developmental disadvantage of subordinate follicles can be circumvented by artificially elevating gonadotropin concentrations before follicle dominance has been established. This is the basis of treatments designed to induce multiple dominant follicles and ovulations using gonadotropin preparations.

Continued suppression of FSH during the dominance phase has been attributed to the synergistic effect of

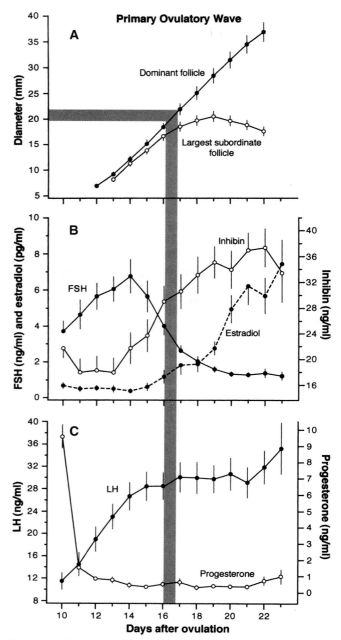

Figure 1-1 Mean (±SEM) follicle diameters and circulating concentrations of hormones associated with development of the primary ovulatory wave are depicted. The data were compiled from several studies[9] involving ablation of all follicles greater than 5 mm using ultrasound-guided transvaginal follicle aspiration and induction of luteal regression with prostaglandin-F$_{2\alpha}$ (PGF$_{2\alpha}$) at 10 days after ovulation in 16 mares. The departure in growth rates between the two largest follicles (follicle deviation) beginning on day 16 when the largest follicle reaches approximately 22.5 mm, on average, represents a key component of the follicle selection phenomenon.[6-8] *SEM,* Standard error of the mean; *FSH,* follicle-stimulating hormone; *LH,* luteinizing hormone.

inhibin and estradiol. The increase in circulating concentrations of both hormones primarily originate from the developing dominant or ovulatory follicle (see Figure 1-1, *B*). Apart from its FSH-suppressive effects, high concentrations of estradiol, in the absence of progesterone, appear to exert a stimulatory effect on circulating concentrations of LH.[1,2] High concentrations of LH during the latter part of estrus are necessary for continued growth of the dominant follicle, as well as for signaling and preparing the follicle and its contents for ovulation.

OVULATION

Ovulation is a complex process involving a sequence of events[1,2] that leads to rupture of a dominant follicle (>30 mm) at the ovulation fossa and the extrusion of follicular fluid, granulosa cells, and the cumulus/oocyte complex. The authors are not aware of any documentation describing ovulation occurring at a site other than the fossa in the equine species. For simplification, spontaneous ovulation occurs as a result of the dominant follicle responding to a rise in circulating concentrations of LH. Under normal physiologic conditions, failure of ovulation of a large dominant follicle may be attributable to inadequate levels of LH or perhaps to an insufficient number of LH receptors (e.g., during early spring and late fall transitional periods, and during diestrus and early pregnancy). Ovulation may be induced artificially or hastened during the transitional and breeding seasons by exogenous LH-like preparations (e.g., human chorionic gonadotropin [hCG]) or LH-releasing preparations (e.g., gonadotropin-releasing hormone [GnRH]) as discussed in Chapter 12 and other reviews.[1,2,10,11]

Ultrasonographic characteristics associated with impending ovulation of a dominant follicle appear similar whether ovulation is spontaneous or artificially induced. Multiple primary ovulations (synchronous or asynchronous ovulations during estrus) and secondary ovulations (ovulations during diestrus) are considered ovarian irregularities and are discussed in detail in Chapter 13. The following discussion will focus on the characteristics of a single, spontaneous ovulation in association with estrus.

Impending Ovulation

Breeding close to the time of ovulation is an important issue for horse registries that allow only natural mating, for clinics and farms that use cooled or frozen semen, and in instances in which semen quality or quantity is limited as a result of stallion age or morbidity. Ultrasonographic characteristics of the preovulatory follicle have been documented and reviewed.[4,5] Figure 1-2 was selected from a later study[12] to illustrate changes in the ultrasonographic characteristics of the dominant follicle before ovulation.

Follicle size alone has been the most common and simplest criterion to estimate the time of ovulation. A relatively accurate assessment of size, especially when the follicle has lost its spherical shape, is determined by calculating the average of two lines of measurement from a frozen ultrasound image.[4,5,13] Briefly, a line is drawn from border to border of the greatest antral area using the electronic calipers of the ultrasound machine, and a second line is drawn from border to border approximately perpendicular to the first line. Some ultrasound machines have the capability of freezing two different images of the preovulatory follicle side by side. By comparing the quality and area of the two images, the most desirable image may be selected for evaluation.

The mean maximum diameter of the ovulatory follicle is usually between 40 to 45 mm in riding-type mares (Quarter Horse, Arabian, and Thoroughbred),[4] but the range can be much greater (e.g., 30 to 70 mm). Maximum follicle diameter can be affected by season (5 to 8 mm larger in the spring versus the summer or fall), breed (approximately 3 mm difference among riding-type mares, 5 mm smaller in miniature, and 10 mm larger in draft mares versus riding-type mares), and multiple ovulations (approximately 4 to 9 mm smaller in double versus single ovulations).[4] The effect of animal age on maximum diameter of the ovulatory follicle is equivocal,

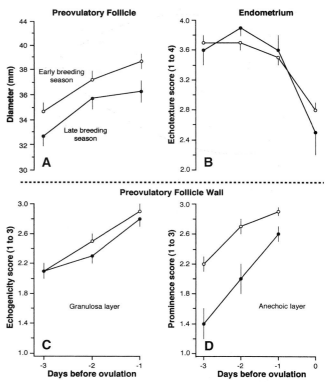

Figure 1-2 Mean (±SEM) ultrasonographic changes in diameter (**A**) and wall (**C, D**) of preovulatory follicles and endometrial echotexture (**B**) 3 days before ovulation during the early breeding season in 32 mares and during the late breeding season in 14 mares as previously reported.[12] Follicle growth rate, granulosa layer echogenicity, and endometrial echotexture were not significantly affected by season, but diameter and prominence of the anechoic layer were significantly smaller and less obvious later in the season. Mean follicle diameter and granulosa layer echogenicity and anechoic layer prominence scores were reached the day before ovulation, whereas mean endometrial echotexture scores were reached 2 or 3 days before ovulation. *SEM*, Standard error of the mean.

and the influence of nutrition and parity has apparently not been critically examined. In a study of 181 single ovulations involving riding-type horse mares, none of the follicles ovulated before reaching 35 mm.[1] Based on ultrasound examinations done at 24-hour intervals, ovulation occurred a mean of 4.2 days after the dominant follicle first attained 35 mm.[1]

The mean diameter of the dominant follicle did not change significantly during the 48 hours before ovulation As reviewed,[2] and, as illustrated, the rate of growth of the preovulatory follicle slowed 24 hours before ovulation (see Figure 1-2, A). Hence, the maximum ovulatory diameter is not necessarily attained on the day before ovulation; maximum diameter may be attained a day or two earlier. This characteristic was more prominent later than earlier in the breeding season.

If natural mating or artificial insemination with fresh semen is being considered, then daily or every-other-day examinations may be sufficient to estimate ovulation based on size alone. However, insemination is recommended within 12 hours of ovulation (before or after) when using cooled semen, and preferably within 6 hours of ovulation if frozen semen is used.[2,10,11] Under these conditions, it may be necessary to shorten the interval between ultrasound examinations and to consider additional criteria to estimate the time to ovulation.

Changes in follicle shape and tone, follicle wall echogenicity (i.e., degree of brightness/darkness of the ultrasound image) and endometrial echotexture (i.e., degree of homogeneity/heterogeneity of the ultrasound image), and sensitivity of the mare to ovarian palpation are additional diagnostic aids that can help to more accurately estimate ovulation to within hours. The change in endometrial echotexture (Figure 1-3) from relatively homogenous during diestrus to relatively heterogeneous during estrus is attributable to an increase in edema of the endometrial folds as a result of the high estrogen:progesterone ratio during estrus.[4,5] Changes in endometrial echotexture closely parallel sexual behavior in the mare (e.g., urination, vulvar wink, tail raising, squatting)[2] and can be very useful in determining the time to ovulation. The mean duration of estrus during the ovulatory season is 5 to 7 days, but the majority of ovulations (69% to 78%) occur during the last 2 days of estrus, and 10% to 14% occur after the end of estrus.[1,2] On average, the degree of endometrial heterogeneity peaks 24 to 48 hours before ovulation and decreases thereafter (see Figure 1-2, B). The change in endometrial echotexture from less estrus-like (see Figure 1-3, A) to more diestrus-like (see Figure 1-3, B) corresponds to the decline in circulating concentrations of estradiol that begins to occur about 1 day before ovulation.[1] Typical and atypical characteristics of the uterus during various reproductive states are discussed in more detail in Chapter 5 and other reviews.[2,11,14]

An increase in the thickness of the follicle wall (i.e., theca layer, basal lamina, and granulosa layer) preceding ovulation has been used as an indicator of impending ovulation.[2,4,5] However, in a more critical study,[12] ultrasonographic artifacts (e.g., refractory shadows and reverberations) often obscured identification of the antral and stromal borders of the wall. Perhaps a more useful indicator of impending ovulation is the granulosa cell layer

Endometrium

Estrus-like   **Dietrus-like**

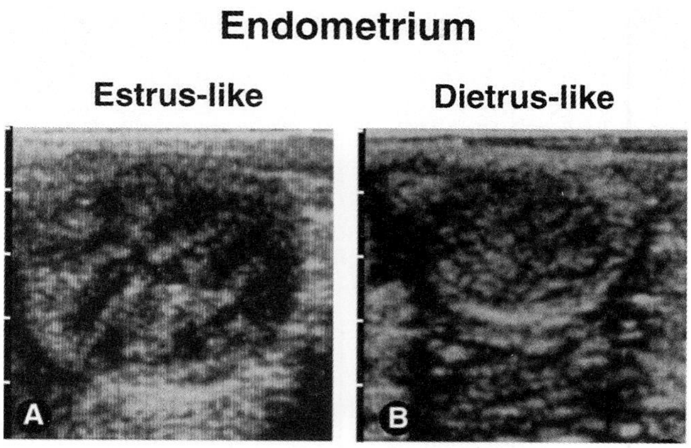

Figure 1-3 Ultrasonograms depicting the cross section of a uterine horn during estrus (**A**) and diestrus (**B**). Note the heterogeneity of the endometrium associated with an estrus-like uterus reflecting an echotexture score of 3 or greater. Conversely, note the homogeneity of the endometrium associated with a diestrus-like uterus reflecting an echotexture score of 2 or less.

alone, which is readily identified by a distinct demarcation between the echoic outer border (basal lamina) and the anechoic inner border (follicular fluid) of the follicle wall (Figure 1-4). Another indicator of impending ovulation may be the appearance of an anechoic layer peripheral to the granulosa layer (Figure 1-4, C and F). Based on daily scanning, mean echogenicity scores of the granulosa layer and prominence of the anechoic layer progressively increased and reached maximal values 24 hours before ovulation (see Figure 1-2, C and D). Prominence of the anechoic layer was more noticeable early in the breeding season than later (see Figure 1-2, D, and Figure 1-4, C and F). Histologic characteristics of the preovulatory follicle led to the interpretation that the increase in echogenicity of the granulosa layer may be due to the increase in the size and number of granulosa cells and that the increase in prominence of the anechoic layer may be due to the increase in size and tortuosity of blood vessels in the theca interna and edema in the theca interna and externa.[15] Similar histologic attributes of the preovulatory follicle have been identified in response to hCG.[16] In this regard, an anechoic layer in the follicle wall of women has been referred to as a double-contour and reportedly occurs within 8 hours of the LH surge or within a few hours before ovulation.[17]

Approximately 12 hours before ovulation, 90% of the dominant follicles become softer or less turgid, 89% change shape from spherical to nonspherical, and mares are more prone to become agitated during palpation of the ovary containing the preovulatory follicle.[1,2] Softness of the preovulatory follicle and ovarian sensitivity to manipulation presumably reflect the enzymatic degradation and inflammation that are associated with the ovulatory process. Investigation of a more objective method of determining softening of the preovulatory follicle using transrectal tonometric measurements has been reported.[18] A drop in follicular pressure combined with separation of the follicular wall as assessed by ultrasound

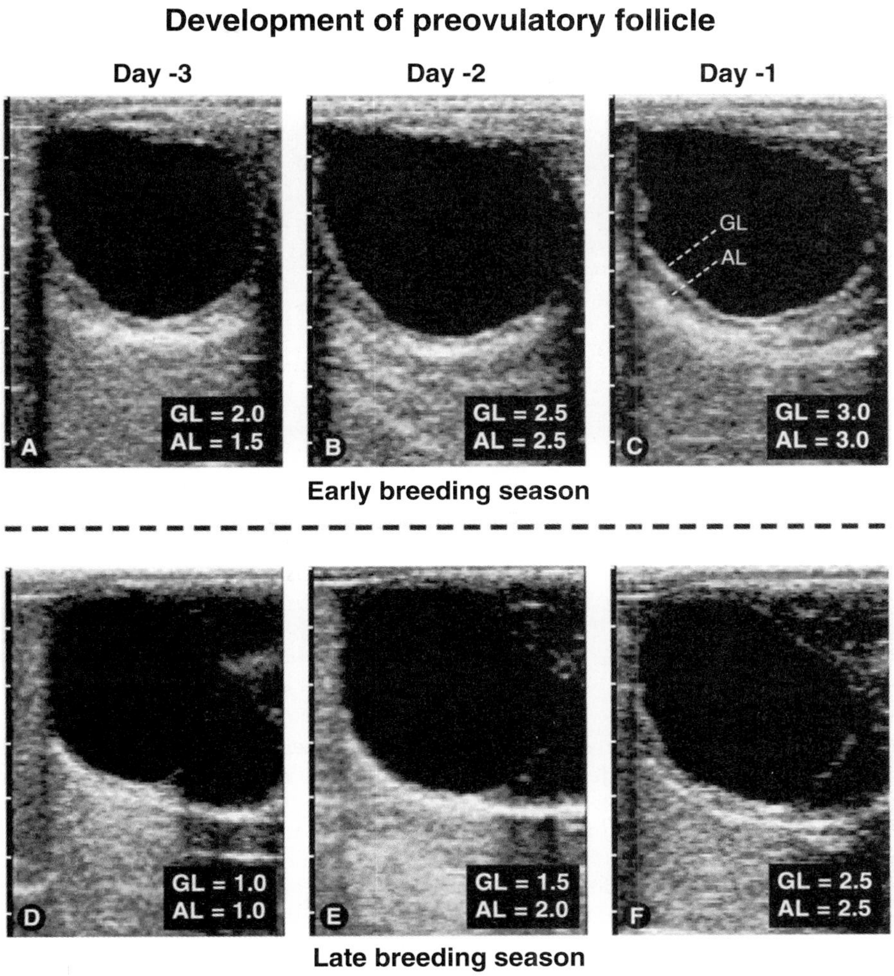

Development of preovulatory follicle

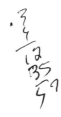

Day -3	Day -2	Day -1
GL = 2.0 AL = 1.5 A	GL = 2.5 AL = 2.5 B	GL AL GL = 3.0 AL = 3.0 C

Early breeding season

GL = 1.0 AL = 1.0 D	GL = 1.5 AL = 2.0 E	GL = 2.5 AL = 2.5 F

Late breeding season

Figure 1-4 Sequential ultrasongrams taken during development of preovulatory follicles 3 days before ovulation in a mare during the early breeding season (**A** to **C**) and a mare during the late breeding season (**D** to **F**), as previously reported.[12] Regardless of season, the granulosa layer *(GL)* became more echogenic and the anechoic layer *(AL)* became more prominent and involved more of the circumference of the follicle. As ovulation approached, score values for echogenicity and prominence increased (see Figure 1-2, *C* and *D*).

image analysis may eventually prove to be a more reliable method to predict the timing of spontaneous and induced ovulations. Other characteristics of impending ovulation, such as echogenic material in the follicular fluid and electrical resistance of vaginal mucus, have also been evaluated, but the diagnostic value of these changes is limited by the rarity of the event or inconsistency in the results, respectively.[2]

In the near future, color-flow Doppler ultrasonography will permit direct, real-time assessment of the degree of vascularization of the ovulatory follicle in the mare, as it has in women.[17] In a recent review,[19] the principles, techniques, and potential of Doppler ultrasound were presented with respect to equine reproduction. It is expected that the differential changes in vascular perfusion of a dominant-sized follicle can be quantitated by the number of colored pixels in an image so that follicle status (anovulatory or ovulatory) can be assessed and time to ovulation predicted.

In conclusion, the predictive accuracy of the imminence of ovulation may be enhanced by integrating the results obtained by ultrasonographic imaging and palpation of the reproductive tract, as well as by assessing behavior. Some or all of the characteristics described above may be used to estimate ovulation to within 24

hours. To ensure inseminating within 12 hours after ovulation, especially when using cooled or frozen semen or semen of limited quality or quantity, less than 12-hour intervals between examinations may be necessary.

Follicle Rupture and Evacuation

Detecting ovulation of a dominant follicle involves diagnosing the sudden disappearance of a large follicle that was present at a previous examination. The time of ovulation is commonly used as a reference for the purpose of communicating the time of other reproductive events or treatments after ovulation and, therefore, is often designated day 0. Follicle rupture and the extrusion of follicular fluid during ovulation in the mare is a dynamic event that has been well described in several reviews.[1,2,4,5] Figure 1-5 is presented from an original study[20] to illustrate some prominent aspects of follicle rupture and evacuation.

Ovulation has been characterized by a break or rupture in the follicle wall, resulting in a decrease in size of the antrum and collection of follicular fluid in the ovarian bursa or surrounding area (Figure 1-5). In about 50% of ovulations, evacuation of follicular fluid from the dominant follicle is an abrupt process ranging from 5 to 90 seconds, with approximately 15% of the initial fluid

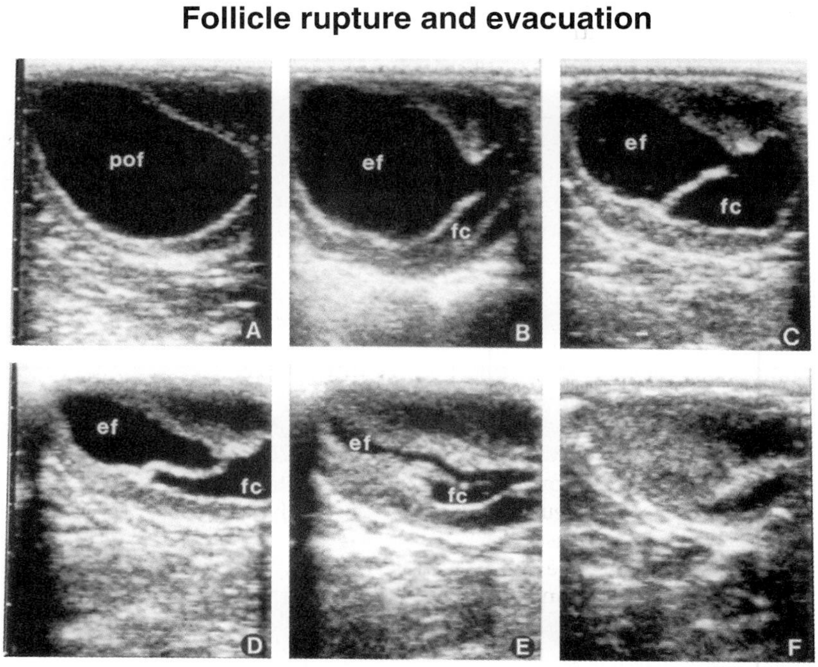

Figure 1-5   Sequential ultrasonograms taken during the beginning of follicle rupture (**A**) and follicular fluid evacuation (**B** to **E**) showing the accumulation of fluid *(fc)* apparently outside the evacuating follicle in the area of the ovulation fossa.[20] **A,** Preovulatory follicle *(pof)* approximately 5 minutes before rupture of the follicle wall. **B,** Evacuating follicle *(ef)* shortly after rupture of the follicle wall. **C** to **E,** Evacuating follicle taken 37 minutes, 60 minutes, and 60 minutes and 15 seconds after image **B.** Note that the fluid accumulation in the area of the ovulation fossa is continuous with the antral fluid through a distinct rent in the follicle wall. The accumulation of extrafollicular fluid increased (**B** and **C**) and then decreased (**D** and **E**) in size as evacuation progressed. Extrafollicular fluid was undetectable after approximately 65 minutes relative to image **B,** corresponding with the elimination of intrafollicular fluid (**F**).

Follicle rupture and evacuation

remaining in the antrum. In the other 50%, release of follicular fluid is a slow and gradual process taking 6 to 7 minutes to evacuate all but 4% to 17% of the initial volume. Complete loss of detectable fluid from the antrum and the extraovarian space may take 30 minutes or as long as 5 to 20 hours.[2,20] In some instances, residual antral fluid may not be lost before blood or transudate begins to collect within the antral cavity. The follicular fluid remaining in the antrum and the escaped fluid in the surrounding area at the time of ovulation may easily be mistaken as separate follicles, particularly if the imminence of ovulation is not known (Figure 1-5, *C*). Ovulation may be confirmed quickly by reexamination several minutes later and by observing a progressive loss of fluid in both the follicle and the surrounding area (Figure 1-5, *D* to *F*). Recognizing ovulation in progress may be more difficult in older mares because of atypical ovulations.[2] Highly irregular, semievacuated, and numerous echogenic particles are atypical characteristics of the ovulating follicle[4] observed more often in 20-year-old mares (16%) than in 15- to 19-year-olds (8%), and 5- to 7-year-olds (0.02%). Regardless of whether follicle rupture and follicular fluid evacuation are characterized as typical or atypical, ovulation can be confirmed by detecting a corpus luteum upon reexamination at a later date.

Ovulation Site

Rectal palpation and ultrasonography are often used together to diagnose ovulation, and the efficacy of each has been compared.[2] Based on assessment at 12-hour intervals, palpation and ultrasonography were nearly the same (94%) in detecting single ovulations. However, with the palpation technique, ovulation was occasionally detected later (i.e., 36 hours after ultrasonographic detection) or not at all, and none of the double ovulations (9%)

detected by ultrasonography were detected by palpation. Detection of ovulation based on palpation alone is even more difficult if more than 24 hours has elapsed between examinations. As discussed in the next section, the antrum of the ruptured follicle may rapidly refill with blood and transudate, forming a corpus hemorrhagicum, and be palpably indistinguishable from a preovulatory follicle or a hemorrhagic anovulatory follicle. Ultrasonography therefore is a superior method for detecting a recent ovulation and especially for detecting double ovulations, which may pose a challenge for the management of twins as discussed in Chapter 54 and other reviews.[1,2,4,10,11]

Ultrasonographic detection of a recent ovulation is characterized by a highly echogenic area at the site of the previous dominant follicle (see Figure 1-5, *F*, and Figure 1-6, *A*). The collapse and apposition of the follicle walls following evacuation of a majority or all of the follicular fluid results in an area of hyperechogenicity in 88% of ovulations on day 0. Moreover, ultrasonographic assessment of the site of ovulation can provide morphologic information that can be used to estimate the number of hours after ovulation. Because postovulation insemination is recommended[10] within 12 hours after ovulation (or within 6 hours if frozen semen is used) to achieve a pregnancy/embryo loss rate similar to preovulatory insemination, accurate detection and assessment of the ovulatory site is imperative. Recently[21] the change in echogenicity of the ovulatory site was evaluated at 2-hour intervals for 14 hours postovulation. Gray-scale pixel intensity (i.e., echogenicity) of selected segments of the ovulatory site was assessed by computer-assisted image analysis. On average, tissue echogenicity decreased significantly by 4 hours and then increased significantly by 8 hours after ovulation; the lowest mean values were at 2 to 4 hours postovulation. Although pregnancy rates were not evaluated, it was concluded that computer-assisted image analysis may assist the practitioner in determining if ovulation has occurred within the recommended time to initiate postovulatory insemination.

CORPUS LUTEUM DEVELOPMENT

The ovulation fossa is the result of a unique structural rearrangement of the equine ovary that is established before puberty.[1] As the cortex or germinal zone is invaginated into the medulla or vascular zone, the two poles of the ovary are drawn toward one another to give the ovary its kidney-bean shape and form the ovulation fossa. Unlike the corpus luteum in other domestic species (e.g., bovine, ovine), the equine luteal gland is fully contained within the ovarian stroma. The ovulation papilla of the newly forming corpus luteum may be seen on gross inspection in the area of the fossa; however, it typically does not project from the surface of the ovary. In this regard, digital assessment of the corpus luteum is difficult and highly subjective. Alternatively, ultrasonographic imaging provides an immediate and objective evaluation of the luteal gland.

The intimate relationship between follicle granulosa and theca cells provides the foundation for steroidogenesis in the ovary. Concurrent with and subsequent to ovulation, granulosa cells undergo biochemical and morphologic changes (luteinization). For simplification, luteinization involves morphogenesis of estrogen-secreting granulosa cells to progesterone-secreting luteal cells in association with intensive neovascularization. Histologic characteristics of the equine corpus luteum[1,2] and ultrasonographic characteristics[4,5] have been reviewed. This section will focus on the gross ultrasonographic morphology (e.g., diameter, echogenicity, and vascularity) of the primary corpus luteum and related physiology (e.g., progesterone production) during the estrous cycle and early pregnancy.

Terminology

Inconsistent use of terms associated with the equine corpus luteum has resulted in a semantic quagmire[22] and considerable confusion about normal and aberrant luteal function. Suggested terminology to effectively communicate typical and atypical aspects of luteal gland development is summarized in Table 1-1. A primary corpus luteum results from ovulation of a dominant follicle of a primary follicular wave at or near the end of estrus when estrogen prevails (i.e., single or double ovulation), whereas a secondary corpus luteum results from ovulation of a dominant follicle of a secondary wave during diestrus or pregnancy when progesterone prevails. Primary and secondary corpora lutea that develop with a fluid-filled cavity are referred to as corpora hemorrhagica. Accessory corpora lutea result from luteinization of anovulatory follicles during early pregnancy. Both secondary and accessory corpora lutea are referred to as supplemental corpora lutea. A regressed luteal gland, regardless of origin, is referred to as a corpus albicans.

Abbreviated and prolonged luteal function is often associated with a uteropathic condition.[1,2,11,22] Premature release of $PGF_{2\alpha}$ associated with endometritis has resulted in early regression of the corpus luteum and shorter interovulatory intervals (e.g., 13 to 19 days). Conversely, conditions associated with more severe endometrial damage (e.g., pyometra and mucometra) have been associated with impaired endometrial $PGF_{2\alpha}$ production. Chronic pyometra with extensive loss of endometrial epithelium has been related to prolonged luteal function and longer interovulatory intervals (29 to 75 days). Prolonged luteal function has also been associated with ovarian irregularities (e.g., secondary or diestrus ovulations and corpora hemorrhage). Altered luteal function, unassociated with uterine abnormalities, has also been described (e.g., abbreviated luteal function following GnRH-induced ovulation during the midanovulatory season).[23]

The term *pseudopregnancy* was initially used to describe a prolonged interestrus interval in nonpregnant mares, especially if early embryo loss was suspected.[1] With the advent of ultrasonography, pseudopregnancy has been more strictly defined as a prolonged interval from one ovulation to the next that occurs in association with luteal persistence and tense uterine tone following embryo loss.[22] The critical period during which the embryo must be present to block luteolysis is approximately 11 to 16 days post ovulation; embryo loss after the critical period results in a prolonged interval to ovulation

Table　1-1

Luteal Gland Terminology Used During the Estrous Cycle and Early Pregnancy

Luteal Structure	Definition
Primary corpora lutea	Result from single or multiple ovulations during the follicular phase (*estrogen dominance*)
Secondary corpora lutea	Result from ovulations during the luteal phase (diestrus ovulation; >2 days from the primary ovulation) or early pregnancy (*progesterone dominance*)
Accessory corpora lutea	Result from luteinization of anovulatory follicles during early pregnancy
Supplemental corpora lutea	Includes secondary and accessory corpora lutea that develop during early pregnancy
Corpora hemorrhagica	Primary or secondary corpora lutea that develop an intraluteal fluid-filled cavity subsequent to ovulation
Corpora albicantia	Regressed corpora lutea

Modified from Ginther OJ: Reproductive Biology of the Mare: Basic and Applied Aspects, 2nd edition, Cross Plains, Wis, Equiservices, 1992.

Site of ovulation

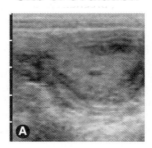

Development of primary corpus luteum

| Early diestrus | Mid-diestrus | Late diestrus |

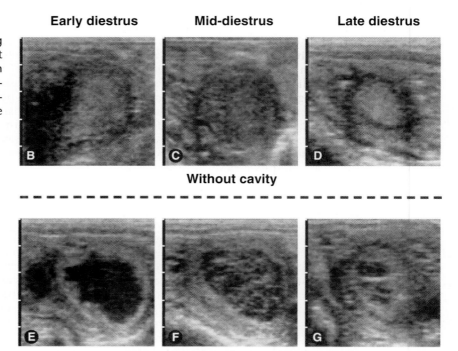

Without cavity

With cavity (corpus hemorrhagicum)

Figure 1-6 Ultrasonograms depicting the site of ovulation (**A**) and development of the primary corpus luteum without an intraluteal cavity (**B** to **D**) and with an intraluteal fluid-filled cavity (corpus hemorrhagicum, **E** to **G**) during various stages of the luteal phase.[24]

(luteal persistence). Uterine tone during early pregnancy is much greater than during diestrus. In this regard, if embryo loss occurs after maximal uterine tone has been achieved, uterine turgidity is maintained. Historically, considerable confusion has resulted from the use of the term *pseudopregnancy*, and therefore it is appropriate to emphasize the importance of a more strict definition that includes (1) a prolonged interovulatory interval, (2) tense uterine tone, and (3) confirmed embryonic loss. Idiopathic persistence of the corpus luteum may be used to describe prolonged interestrus or interovulatory intervals in nonbred and nonpregnant mares if the origin of persistence is unknown.

Form and Function of the Corpus Luteum During the Estrous Cycle

Formation of the primary corpus luteum after ovulation does not necessarily result in a single uniform morphology (Figure 1-6). Following the loss of follicular fluid during the ovulatory process, 30% to 50% of corpora lutea develop uniformly, without forming an intraluteal cavity (Figure 1-6, *B* to *D*). Alternatively, 50% to 70% of luteal glands accumulate fluid within the antral cavity and form a corpus hemorrhagicum (Figure 1-6, *E* to *G*). The cavity begins to fill with blood and transudate within 24 hours of follicular fluid evacuation, even if the original fluid was not totally evacuated, reaching a maximal size approximately 3 days later. A corpus hemorrhagicum is not considered a pathologic condition and is first evident on day 0 (28%), on day 1 (62%), on day 2 (6%), or on day 3 (4%). The ratio of luteal to nonluteal tissue of a newly formed corpus hemorrhagicum is minimal during early diestrus (Figure 1-6, *E*) and maximal during mid-diestrus (Figure 1-6, *F*). Throughout development, the fluid-filled cavity of a corpus hemorrhagicum gradually decreases as a result of production and organization of connective tissue associated with the clotting process.

The cavity may still be identified even during late diestrus (Figure 1-6, *G*). However, during pregnancy, luteal glands that initially formed an intraluteal cavity may later become relatively uniform and resemble a corpus luteum that developed without a cavity. Nevertheless, the ratio of luteal to nonluteal tissue, especially during the estrous cycle, can be used to estimate the age of the corpus luteum.[4,24] The formation of a corpus hemorrhagicum appears to be a random event; repeatable luteal morphology was not detected within mares from one ovulation to the next, and luteal glands within mares with double ovulations were as likely to be similar as dissimilar. Furthermore, the length of an interovulatory interval is similar whether the corpus luteum develops with or without an intraluteal cavity.[1,4,24]

Ultrasonographic measurement of the corpus luteum[4,24] is first accomplished by identifying the relatively hypoechogenic (darker) tissue of the corpus luteum from the more echogenic connective tissue of the ovarian stroma (see Figure 1-6). Although the corpus luteum may appear mushroomlike or gourdlike in shape with an irregular boundary, the ultrasonographic image is frozen at the maximal cross-sectional area. The diameter of the corpus luteum is determined by calculating the average of perpendicular lines of measurement, similar to that described for nonspherical preovulatory follicles. To calculate luteal tissue area for a corpus hemorrhagicum, the area of the intraluteal cavity may be subtracted from the overall area. Despite a larger overall diameter for a corpus hemorrhagicum, the absolute luteal tissue area is not different between the two luteal morphologies. The daily diameter profile of the primary corpus luteum is shown in Figure 1-7, *A*.

The echogenicity of the corpus luteum may be determined by assigning a gray-scale score to the luteal portion of the gland. Lower scores represent darker, less echogenic tissue, and higher scores represent lighter, more echogenic tissue. The reliability of the subjective nature of visually scoring the echogenicity of luteal tissue has been verified using a more objective image analysis approach.[4] Determination of the hourly changes in luteal tissue echogenicity by visual assessment concomitantly with computer-assisted image analysis indicated close parallelism between the two approaches. Daily changes in luteal tissue echogenicity of the primary corpus luteum throughout the luteal phase is shown in Figure 1-7, *B*. Apart from the transient decrease in echogenicity at the ovulation site immediately following follicular fluid evacuation as reported in a separate study,[21] mean echogenicity scores increased, reaching maximal values 24 to 48 hours after ovulation. Thereafter, mean values progressively decreased to relatively low values by 9 days after ovulation. The similarity in the results between the subjective and objective approaches[4] is encouraging for the practitioner who may choose to use visual gray-scale scoring as a diagnostic tool for assessing luteal gland development.

Alternatively, current computer technology offers the practitioner the opportunity of gathering image data in the field.[13,25] Images may be recorded to high-resolution videotape and digitally captured to a computer in the field or at the clinic. Disadvantages of the analog (tape)

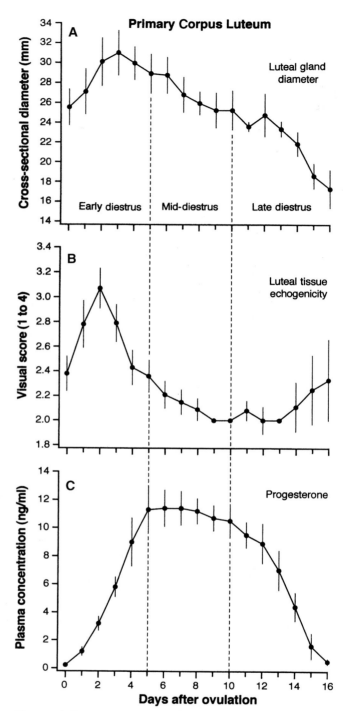

Figure 1-7   Mean (±SEM) diameter of the primary corpus luteum (**A**), luteal tissue echogenicity (**B**), and circulating concentrations of progesterone (**C**) are depicted during various stages of the luteal phase in 13 mares. The daily changes illustrate the temporality between the structural (luteal gland diameter and tissue echogenicity) and functional (progesterone production) aspects of the corpus luteum associated with maturation (early to mid-diestrus) and regression (late diestrus). *SEM,* Standard error of the mean.

to digital (computer) conversion, however, are the loss of quality of the original image and the necessity of several valuable pieces of equipment. More recent ultrasound machines, however, are equipped with the capability to store and download images directly to a computer either in the field or at the clinic.[25] Hence less equipment is involved, and the quality of the original image is conserved for a more accurate evaluation of gray-scale pixel intensity by the computer software; Internet connections make it possible to relay images to a remote service provider for image analysis.[25] Although this method provides more objective, quantitative evaluation, the practitioner is still responsible for selecting and delineating the areas of the luteal gland to be analyzed (i.e., the analysis is only as good as the data).

The potential of color-flow Doppler for evaluating the vascular dynamics associated with large animal reproduction was first documented in 1997,[24,26] when the blood flow in the endometrium, conceptus, and primary corpus luteum was demonstrated in a pregnant mare. A more recent review[19] further promotes the value of this emerging technology in equine reproduction. The ratio of systolic-to-diastolic blood flow, as measured by the amplitude of the waveforms from the spectral Doppler trace patterns, may be used to estimate resistance to flow. In women, the resistance to blood flow was relatively low during luteal maturation and increased during luteal regression.[17] Only recently has an attempt been made to use color-flow Doppler ultrasonography to quantitate blood flow during development of the primary corpus luteum in the mare (Figure 1-8).[27] Ultrasound examinations were done daily or every other day from ovulation to 15 days after ovulation in six mares. An image of the corpus luteum was frozen when the number of colored pixels associated with the luteal gland appeared maximal, downloaded to a laptop computer, and assessed by computer-assisted analysis of pixel intensity. Mean number of colored pixels/luteal gland image (i.e., vascularity) was low on the day of ovulation, increased to maximal values 5 days post ovulation, and decreased between 7 and 15 days after ovulation in association with luteal regression (Figure 1-8, *B*).

Several reviews[1,2,4,5] and recent studies[15,16] together provide evidence that changes in the ultrasonographic morphology of the corpus luteum are reflective of the ultrastructural changes associated with functional development of the corpus luteum. This relationship should provide the practitioner with a better understanding of the value of ultrasonography for evaluating the integrity of the luteal gland when diagnosing ovulation and for making a prognosis of its future development.

The temporal relationships between the morphologic and physiologic aspects of the primary corpus luteum are presented in Figures 1-7 and 1-8. After ovulation, functional maturation of the primary corpus luteum during early diestrus is indicated by a progressive increase in circulating concentrations of progesterone that relates structurally to an increase in luteal diameter (Figure 1-7, *A* and *C*) or area (Figure 1-8, *A* and *C*) and vascularity (Figure 1-8, *B* and *C*) and a decrease in echogenicity (Figure 1-7, *B* and *C*), which may also be considered to reflect vascular changes. By days 5 to 7, maximal concentrations of pro-

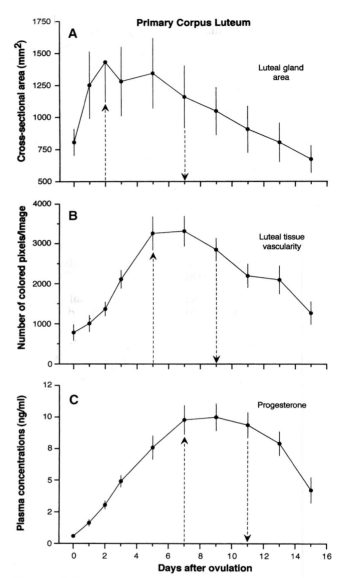

Figure 1-8 Mean (±SEM) area of the primary corpus luteum (**A**), luteal tissue vascularity (**B**), and circulating concentrations of progesterone (**C**) are depicted during various stages of the luteal phase in six mares as previously reported.[27] The degree of vascularity was determined by the number of colored pixels per luteal image using color-flow Doppler ultrasonography. The daily changes illustrate the temporality between the structural (luteal gland area and vascularity) and functional (progesterone production) aspects of the corpus luteum. Placement of the arrows in an upward direction illustrates that mean maximal luteal area precedes mean maximal vascularity, which precedes mean maximal progesterone concentrations at maturation (mid-diestrus), whereas placement of the arrows in a downward direction associated with the first apparent mean decrease in luteal area, vascularity, and progesterone illustrates that the same relational sequence occurs during regression. *SEM,* Standard error of the mean.

gesterone during mid-diestrus correspond to maximal or intermediate luteal diameter or area, maximal vascularity, and minimal echogenicity. After day 9, functional regression of the corpus luteum during late diestrus is indicated by a progressive decrease in progesterone that relates structurally to a decrease in luteal diameter or area and vascularity and an increase in echogenicity. Temporally the structural changes of the luteal gland precede functional changes during maturation as well as regression (see Figure 1-8). Thus assessment of luteal gland development may begin with a morphologic evaluation (i.e., diameter or area, echogenicity, and vascularity), and, if structural characteristics atypical of the expected stage of luteal gland development are suspected, a more definitive physiologic assessment may be done by drawing a blood sample for progesterone analysis.

Form and Function of the Corpus Luteum During Early Pregnancy

An ovarian source of progesterone is essential for maintenance of pregnancy until approximately days 50 to 70; thereafter the fetal-placental unit begins producing sufficient progestogens to support pregnancy.[1,2] Progesterone from the primary corpus luteum is needed for physical embryo-uterine interactions (i.e., embryo mobility, fixation, and orientation) and uterine secretions, whereas the functional role of supplemental corpora lutea that begin to form in most mares around day 40 is not clearly understood. Pregnancy maintenance and the role of progesterone are not the focus of this section but are discussed in Chapter 52 and other reviews.[1,2,11,14]

The use of ultrasonography to study luteal development during pregnancy has received limited attention. In a study done under laboratory conditions,[24] daily changes in diameter of the primary corpus luteum, luteal tissue echogenicity, and circulating concentrations of progesterone were similar between nonpregnant and pregnant mares from days 0 to 13 (Figure 1-9); thereafter profiles differed as a result of regression of the primary corpus luteum in nonpregnant mares. In a study done under field conditions,[28] the area of the primary corpus luteum was measured and expressed as a volume ratio of measurements taken 1 or 2 days and 8 or 9 days after ovulation. A blood sample was collected on days 8 or 9 for progesterone analysis, and pregnancy status was evaluated on day 17. Averaged over 51 pregnant mares, the mean luteal volume ratio and progesterone concentration was higher on days 8 to 9 compared with nonpregnant mares. In nonpregnant mares, luteal area decreased by mid-diestrus compared to maintained values in pregnant mares. Differentiating pregnant from nonpregnant mares based on diameter versus area of the primary corpus luteum apparently occurred later in the former study at late diestrus (approximately day 13) compared to mid-diestrus (days 8 to 9) in the latter study. Perhaps quantitating the change in luteal tissue area as a volume ratio versus diameter is a more sensitive measure of luteal function.[29] Regardless, these studies document the utility of ultrasonography as a tool to aid the practitioner in the diagnosis of luteal gland development associated with

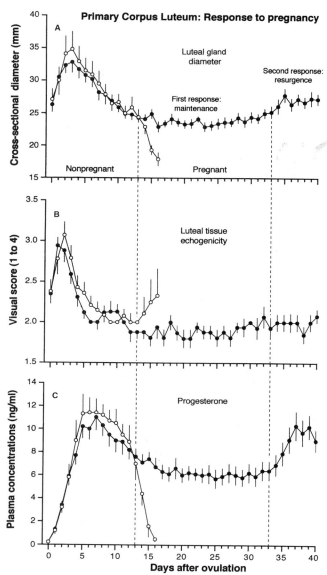

Figure 1-9   Mean (±SEM) diameter of the primary corpus luteum (**A**), luteal tissue echogenicity (**B**), and circulating concentrations of progesterone (**C**) are depicted for 13 nonpregnant mares during the luteal phase and 15 pregnant mares during early gestation.[24] The first luteal response to pregnancy occurred on day 14 or 15 as indicated by a departure in the mean values associated with luteal gland diameter, echogenicity, and progesterone between nonpregnant and pregnant mares. The second luteal response to pregnancy occurred after day 30 as indicated by a resurgence in the mean values associated with diameter and progesterone concentrations. *SEM,* Standard error of the mean.

pregnancy. Maintenance of the primary corpus luteum after the expected time of luteal regression in nonpregnant mares represents the first luteal response to pregnancy (see Figure 1-9).[1,24]

Resurgence of the primary corpus luteum in pregnant mares occurs between days 30 and 35 and represents the second luteal response to pregnancy (see Figure 1-9).[1] It was hypothesized that this resurgence is in response to the release of equine chorionic gonadotropin (eCG) into the circulation. On the first day that systemic eCG concentrations were detected (mean, day 35), systemic progesterone concentrations began to increase and were significantly elevated 2 days later. A corresponding increase in the size of the primary corpus luteum, but not luteal tissue echogenicity, paralleled the increase in progesterone. The observed resurgence in progesterone was not confounded by the contribution from supplemental luteal glands because secondary and accessory corpora lutea were not detected until after day 40. The hypothesis for resurgence of the primary corpus luteum was further supported by comparing pregnant mares and mares with embryo loss in which the primary corpus luteum was maintained.[30] Both the size of the corpus luteum and circulating concentrations of progesterone were greater on day 36 in mares that maintained pregnancy than in mares with embryo loss. Because embryo loss occurred before endometrial cup formation, the primary corpus luteum did not resurge but gradually regressed in the absence of eCG.

Formation of supplemental luteal glands occurs during eCG production and represents the third luteal response to pregnancy.[1,24] The development of major follicular waves composed of dominant follicles (>30 mm) during early pregnancy is closely associated with the formation of supplemental corpora lutea and varies greatly within and among mares.[31] The initial formation of supplemental corpora lutea results from luteinization of dominant ovulatory follicles referred to as secondary corpora lutea and later from luteinization of unovulated dominant follicles referred to as accessory corpora lutea.[1] The role of supplemental corpora lutea in maintaining pregnancy before a placental source of progesterone has been established has not been critically studied. For instance, it is not unusual to find mares at 60 to 160 days of pregnancy without supplemental corpora lutea, especially if they were bred late in the season. Depressed follicular development that occurs during the fall transition may suppress the development of supplemental corpora in late-bred mares.

The ratio of FSH-like to LH-like activity of eCG is thought to play a role in determining whether supplemental corpora lutea result from ovulation or anovulation.[1,2] Equine CG is not only involved in the formation of supplemental corpora lutea, but also assists in maintaining their steroidogenic function. Ultrasonographically, it appears that secondary corpora lutea go through a developmental stage similar to that of the primary corpus luteum (see Figure 1-6). Subsequent to ovulation, secondary corpora lutea are uniform, whereas others form intraluteal cavities (corpora hemorrhagica) of various sizes and shapes. Because accessory corpora lutea develop from unovulated follicles, they inherently have a relatively uniform intraluteal cavity and follow a developmental pattern similar to that of hemorrhagic anovulatory follicles discussed in Chapter 12 and other reviews.[1,2,4,24] Typically the fetal-placental unit begins to produce progesterone by 50 to 70 days of gestation, and the primary and supplemental corpora lutea regress 180 to 200 days of gestation.

SUMMARY

Gathering and integrating data obtained from ultrasonographic imaging and palpation of the reproductive tract, as well as mare behavior, can aid in predicting ovulation to within hours, which is critical when considering insemination with cooled or frozen semen or semen of reduced quantity or quality. In addition to visual assessment of ultrasonographic images, a more objective evaluation can be done using computer-assisted image analysis. Ultrasonographic data can be readily captured to a computer and immediately evaluated in the field or at the clinic after the electronic transfer of data. Critical evaluation of the site of ovulation and the developing corpus luteum may aid the practitioner in estimating the time that has elapsed since the follicle ruptured and collapsed, especially if impending ovulation was not known, and allow an immediate diagnosis of the functional status of the luteal gland and perhaps prognosis of its future development. Traditional as well as new, nontraditional methods of assessing ovarian function are available to be used together to optimize current breeding management practices.

References

1. Ginther OJ: Reproductive Biology of the Mare: Basic and Applied Aspects, 2nd ed., Cross Plains, WI, Equiservices Publishing, 1992.
2. McKinnon AO, Voss JL: Equine Reproduction, Philadelphia, Lea & Febiger, 1993.
3. Niswender GD, Juengel JL, Silva PJ, et al: Mechanisms controlling the function and life span of the corpus luteum. Physiol Rev 2000; 80:1-29.
4. Ginther OJ: Ultrasonic Imaging and Animal Reproduction: Horses. Book 2. Cross Plains, WI, Equiservices Publishing, 1995.
5. Rantanan NW, McKinnon AO: Equine Diagnostic Ultrasonography, Baltimore, Williams & Wilkins, 1998.
6. Ginther OJ, Beg MA, Gastal MO, Gastal EL: Follicle dynamics and selection in mares. Anim Reprod 2004; 1:45-63.
7. Ginther OJ, Bergfelt DR, Donadeu FX: Follicular waves and selection of follicles in mares, Proceedings of the 5th International Symposium on Equine Embryo Transfer, Monograph 2001; 3:15-18.
8. Ginther OJ, Beg MA, Donadeu FX, Bergfelt DR: Mechanism of follicle deviation in monovular farm species. Anim Reprod Sci 2003; 78:239-257.
9. Bergfelt DR, Gastal EL, Ginther OJ: Response of estradiol and inhibin to experimentally reduced luteinizing hormone during follicle deviation in mares. Biol Reprod 2001; 65:426-432.
10. Samper JC: Equine Breeding Management and Artificial Insemination, Philadelphia, WB Saunders, 2000.
11. Threlfall WR: Equine Theriogenology. In Youngquist RS (ed): Current Therapy in Large Animal Theriogenology, Philadelphia, WB Saunders, 1997.
12. Gastal EL, Gastal MO, Ginther OJ: The suitability of echotexture characteristics of the follicular wall for identifying the optimal breeding day in mares. Theriogenology 1998; 50:1025-1038.
13. Ginther OJ: Ultrasonic Imaging and Animal Reproduction: Fundamentals, Book 1, Cross Plains, WI, Equiservices Publishing, 1995.
14. Troedsson HT: Reproduction. In Robinson NE (ed): Current Therapy in Equine Medicine, Philadelphia, WB Saunders, 1997.

15. Watson ED, Al-zi'abi MO: Characterization of morphology and angiogenesis in follicles of mares during the spring transition and breeding season, Reproduction 2002; 124:227-234.

16. Kerban A, Dore M, Sirois J: Characterization of cellular and vascular changes in equine follicles during hCG-induced ovulation. J Reprod Fertil 1999; 117:115-123.

17. Jaffe R, Pierson RA, Abramowicz JS: Imaging in Infertility and Reproductive Endocrinology, Philadelphia, JB Lippincott, 1994.

18. Bragg N, Pierson RA, Buss DG, Card CE: Transrectal tonometric measurement of follicular softening and computer assisted ultrasound image analysis of follicular wall echotexture during estrus in mares. Proceedings of the 47th Annual Convention of American Association of Equine Practitioners 2001;242-245.

19. Ginther OJ, Utt MD: Doppler ultrasound in equine reproduction: principles, techniques and potential. J Equine Vet Sci 2004; 24:516-526.

20. Townson DH, Ginther, OJ: Ultrasonic characterization of follicular evacuation during ovulation and fate of the discharged follicular fluid in mares. Anim Reprod Sci 1989; 20:131-141.

21. Carnevale EM, Checura CM, Coutinho da Silva MA, et al: Use of computer-assisted image analysis to determine the interval before and after ovulation, Proceedings of the 48th Annual Convention of American Association of Equine Practitioners 2002; 48-50.

22. Ginther OJ: Prolonged luteal activity in mares: a semantic quagmire. Equine Vet J 1990; 22:152-156.

23. Bergfelt DR, Ginther OJ: Embryo loss following GnRH-induced ovulation in anovulatory mares. Theriogenology 1992; 38:33-43.

24. Pierson RA, Adams GP: Computer-assisted image analysis, diagnostic ultrasonography, and ovulation induction: strange bedfellows. Theriogenology 1995; 42:105-112.

25. Bergfelt DR, Pierson RA, Adams GP: Form and function of the corpus luteum. In Rantanan NW, McKinnon AO (eds): Equine Diagnosic Ultrasonography, Baltimore, Williams & Wilkins, 1998.

26. Bergfelt DR, Adams GP, Pierson RA: Pregnancy. In Rantanan NW, McKinnon AO (eds): Equine Diagnostic Ultrasonography, Baltimore, Williams & Wilkins, 1998.

27. Bollwein H, Mayer R, Weber F, Stolla R: Luteal blood flow during the estrous cycle in mares. Theriogenology 2002; 65:2043-2051.

28. Sevinga M, Schukken YH, Hesselink JW, Jonker FH: Relationship between ultrasonic characteristics of the corpus luteum, plasma progesterone concentration and early pregnancy diagnosis in Friesian mares. Theriogenology 1999; 52:585-592.

29. Lofstedt RM, Ireland WP: Measuring sphere-like structures using transtrectal ultrasonography. Vet Radiol Ultrasound 2000; 41:178-180.

30. Bergfelt DR, Woods JA, Ginther OJ: Role of the embryonic vesicle and progesterone in embryonic loss in mares. J Reprod Fertil 1992; 95:339-347.

31. Bergfelt DR, Ginther OJ: Relationships between FSH surges and follicular waves during early pregnancy in mares. J Equine Vet Sci 1992; 12:274-279.

CHAPTER 2

The Follicle: Practical Aspects of Follicle Control

JOHN R. NEWCOMBE

Much time spent in stud medicine is in the practice of follicle palpation and ultrasonography with the object of predicting ovulation. Accuracy in this skill allows the veterinarian to advise the stud manager regarding key reproductive strategies:

- When not to mate the mare
- When the mare will need re-examination
- When to mate the mare
- When the mare may need mating again
- When the mare has ovulated (precluding mating)

Prediction of ovulation probably is the most difficult of all skills in this field, and no honest practitioner will deny that mistakes are made. An experienced stud manager will accept this uncertainty—a tradeoff between being overcautious and mating mares too early, so that a significant proportion need mating more than once per estrous cycle, and being overconfident, so that some mares have ovulated before being mated.

As a general rule, because enough sperm normally live for at least 3 days or even longer after natural mating,[1,2] it is not necessary to mate mares more than once every 3 or possibly 4 days. In normal healthy mares, those not susceptible to mating-induced endometritis (MIE), mating up to 12 hours after ovulation may achieve good pregnancy rates.[3] By contrast, it is contraindicated to mate susceptible mares more than once per normal-length estrus, especially close to ovulation.

Obviously, the more frequent the examination, the more accurate the prediction of ovulation should be. The use of ovulation-advancing drugs has simplified this procedure. In typical reports from the literature, when the dominant follicle reaches 35 mm in diameter, human chorionic gonadotropin (hCG) or gonadotropin-releasing hormone (GnRH) analogue is given, and ovulation is guaranteed to follow in 36 to 48 hours. What is never reported is the occurrence of ovulation in mares within 24 hours (because it was going to occur anyway), or recent ovulation from follicles smaller than 35 mm preceding the administration of "induction agents." Most reports suggest a response rate of less than 90% to hCG, and this can only be the result of administration too early. If all mares were treated in the 48 hours before ovulation, then the response would be 100%! Thus, even with the use of these drugs, total accuracy is not possible.

OVARIAN PALPATION

With the increasing use of ultrasonography, the art of ovarian palpation is becoming neglected. To be an effective diagnostician using this modality, the practitioner will need to perform many more examinations by palpation than are required with the use of ultrasonography. The value of palpation, however, should not be underestimated. Assessment of the texture of follicles, important in the prediction of ovulation, cannot be performed with ultrasonography. Fresh ovulations that are barely visible, and would certainly have been missed with ultrasound examination, may be detected or at least suspected on palpation. Very small anestrous or hypoplastic ovaries, which may not be found with ultrasonography alone, can be detected by palpation. Sometimes a large "follicle" is visualized with ultrasound that was not palpated in the ovary. Returning to palpation confirms the absence of any large follicle but may reveal the presence of a large soft structure adjacent to the ovary, such as a para-ovarian cyst.

The position of the whole uterus will have a major influence on the location of the ovaries. Uterine position may be quite variable. In young mares, for example, the uterus may lie predominantly within the pelvic cavity; during pregnancy and post partum, it may tip forward and downward, with the cervix lying on the pelvic brim. Although the ovaries of the mare are situated just beyond the tip of the uterine horns, their position is extremely variable. Each ovary lies on the free edge of the broad ligament and is loosely attached to the body wall by the mesovarium and to the uterine horn by the ovarian ligament. The laxity of these two attachments allows the ovary to rotate or to lie under the broad ligament. An experienced practitioner, given the cooperation of the mare, can manually rotate the ovary both along and around its axis by at least 180 degrees. In order to palpate all surfaces of the ovary with the most sensitive parts of the fingers, it is necessary to learn to manipulate the ovary.

On occasion, both the ovary and part of the kidney may be visualized together on ultrasonography. In other instances, the ovary may be situated on the midline, anterior to the uterine bifurcation. Not infrequently an ovary can be found only by running the examiner's fingers along the anterior edge of the uterine horn to the tip;

then, by pulling the tip backward, the ovary can be dragged into a more posterior position, under some tension between the tip of the horn and the body wall. In still other instances, it may be found lateral but posterior to the tip of the horn.

Some left-handed practitioners find the left ovary difficult to palpate, whereas others find the right difficult, and vice versa. No apparent advantage is associated with the use of either hand. Whichever feels more comfortable generally is the best. Some authorities argue for a bilateral ability, but then each hand will acquire only half the experience, and changing hands is both awkward and time-consuming. To be ambidextrous, however, is advantageous when the examination area is suitable for only the left-handed (or right-handed) or when a hand becomes injured. On balance, it may be better to give one hand all of the available experience.

The ovarian examination should begin with a total evacuation of the rectum, which may necessitate several entries. The presence of even small pieces of feces, when encountered by the hand and fingers, makes it difficult for the brain to "focus" on the structures being palpated. For the less experienced, it may be best to first identify the uterine bifurcation and then extend the examination up to the tip of the horn and "look around" from this point in every direction. The ovary normally is found anterolaterally, but not always.

The examiner may not know what size structure to feel for. The deep anestrous ovary of a young mare may be less than 4 cm long, whereas at times the ovary with a number of large follicles can be greater than 10 cm. If the ovary cannot be found, then maneuvers to pull it into a more posterior position, as already described, may be necessary. Even if palpation of the ovary is not the object of the examination, ascertaining its position manually may save time looking for it with ultrasonography. When the ovary lies underneath the broad ligament, the examiner must "flip" it back up with the middle finger in order to palpate it effectively. Occasionally, gaseous intestines seem to prevent access to the ovary, and on rare occasions, even the experienced practitioner cannot find an ovary. Absence of an ovary usually is the result of a previous ovariectomy, but one case of agenesis has been reported.[4]

ESTIMATION OF FOLLICULAR MATURITY AND PREDICTION OF OVULATION

Cyclic mares may be presented for examination either on arrival at the stud farm, at the end of diestrus (for pregnancy diagnosis), at a predetermined time after luteal regression (e.g., day 16), at the first signs of estrus, or already several days into estrus. The veterinarian is expected to be able to estimate the stage of the cycle and, by examining the dominant follicle, predict when ovulation may occur.

Palpation

Before the use of ultrasonography, palpation of the follicle was the most reliable method of predicting ovulation. Not only can its diameter be estimated with some accuracy, but also its turgidity (hardness/softening) and its

prominence within the ovary can be assessed. The value of diameter already has been discussed; however, some practitioners agree to a phenomenon whereby the diameter can be assessed with more accuracy nearer to ovulation. When followed serially with palpation and ultrasonography, the follicle appears to grow more rapidly with palpation. A large follicle apparent on ultrasonography but located deep within the stroma may palpate as smaller and much less prominent. Ultrasonography may suggest ovulation within 2 days, yet palpation suggests 3 to 4 days and frequently is more accurate. This may be explained by an increase in the area of palpable follicle surface. Although the follicle eventually ovulates from the ovulation fossa at the hilus of the ovary, the follicle bulges from surfaces away from the fossa and communicates with the fossa only immediately before and during ovulation. The experienced practitioner may well prefer to rely on palpation than on ultrasonography.

Occasionally but not invariably, the follicle appears to be painful when palpated. This symptom when present is a good predictor of imminent ovulation. It must not, however, be confused with the tenderness of a fresh ovulation. When this area is particularly tender, maneuvers to distinguish between the two may be unrewarding, difficult, and even dangerous.

Turgidity

A great deal of emphasis is placed on the turgidity of the follicle. Smaller follicles are relatively hard and exhibit less preovulatory softening than that found with larger follicles. With examination every 48 hours, no detectable softening of smaller follicles may be found. Larger follicles appear to be more turgid than hard and may not exhibit any softening. Distinct and reliable softening normally only occurs in the immediate preovulatory period, which may be as much as 24 hours before ovulation but more frequently is only a few hours before ovulation.

Larger follicles may undergo some degree of softening several days before ovulation, but such changes also may be detected in those follicles that are undergoing regression. This distinction presents a challenge during the transitional phase; therefore, other features such as development and regression of endometrial edema and the growth pattern of the follicle should be taken into account in deciding whether to mate a mare found to have follicular softening.

Ginther (1986) concluded that softening was not a reliable feature.[5] Unless mares are examined at least every 12 hours, this phase may well be missed. It is therefore inadvisable to wait for softening before mating.

Ultrasound Changes

The ultrasound changes seen in the preovulatory follicle are described in Chapter 1. The preeminent feature is loss of the spherical shape of the follicle. Pressure from the transducer applied in attempts to produce a good ultrasonographic image will flatten the softening follicle. When a follicle can be flattened so that the transverse measurement is greater than twice that of its depth, ovulation is imminent. Once the outline is irregular, ovulation is invariably very close, and when invaginations of the wall begin to form compartments within the follicle, ovulation is beginning.[6]

Occasionally a follicle is seen apparently during collapse, but the stage does not progress and about 25% to 50% of the fluid is retained. This is followed within 24 hours by influx of fluid, presumably blood, into the antrum, with partial or complete refilling of the follicle. The new structure luteinizes to form an apparently normal and functional corpus luteum; in my experience, however, pregnancy has never resulted from such "partial follicular collapse."

The value of ultrasonography cannot be overemphasized in mares in which palpation is difficult and in those in which (1) more than one follicle is present in the same ovary, (2) a very soft follicle appears to be a fresh ovulation, or (3) a corpus luteum is palpated as a follicle. Instances of follicular hemorrhage without collapse, referred to in human medicine as "luteinized unruptured follicle syndrome," could only be suspected before the advent of ultrasonography.[7]

Follicular Diameter

In estimating follicular diameter, previous knowledge of the individual mare is invaluable. Some mares regularly ovulate when follicular size greater than 50 mm is reached, whereas others rarely ovulate when follicular size is greater than 30 mm. Typically, ovulation occurs when the follicle approaches 40 mm or greater in diameter. In considering diameter, allowance should be made for time of year (follicular size is 5 to 8 mm larger in spring than in summer),[5,8] breed (Shire horses and other Draft breeds ovulate at follicular sizes of 40 to 75 mm),[8] and whether single or multiple follicles are ovulated. With twin follicles, follicular size at ovulation is approximately 3 mm less than for a single follicle in the same mare at the same time of year. With multiple follicles, ovulation of follicles of even smaller diameters (<25 mm) is possible.

An asynchronous twin follicle frequently will undergo ovulation when it is smaller than the first by greater than 5 mm. This potential difference is important to appreciate in considering the possibility of twin conception. For example, in a mare mated 24 hours before the ovulation of a 40-mm follicle, a second (developing) 25-mm follicle may be present at the time of ovulation. This follicle, especially if hCG or deslorelin has been used, may undergo ovulation within 48 hours, so that sperm need to survive only 3 days for the mare to conceive twins. Twins can easily be missed when only a single ovulation has been suspected and only a single vesicle is visible 14 to 15 days after the first ovulation. In evaluating the mare for pregnancy at this stage, it is always advisable to examine both ovaries for corpora lutea.[9] If the presence of more than one corpus luteum is suspected, a multiple pregnancy should be assumed, unless the younger corpus luteum is obviously only a few days old.

Day of Cycle

Knowledge of the time of the previous ovulation is advantageous. Not that all mares can be relied on to cycle on a period of 21 days. In early season, the normal cycle may well be nearer to 25 days, whereas in summer it can be as short as 17 to 18 days. Knowledge of previous cycle length is of great help, particularly in old mares, which tend to have longer cycles. When the mare is presented early enough, the development of the dominant follicle can be monitored over several days. If, however, the mare is first presented with a 40-mm follicle, a critical decision has to be made about whether this follicle is close to ovulation, will take another 2 to 3 days to undergo ovulation, or will regress. In a mare presented with such a follicle 16 days after the previous ovulation, it is more likely to be a diestrous follicle that will regress. If the clinical presentation is at 19 days after the last ovulation and no other follicle also is present, a reasonable assumption is that ovulation is imminent, but this either could occur very soon (with a 19-day cycle) or, in some animals and in some breeds, could take another 4 days until a follicular size of 55 mm is attained.

Rate of Follicular Growth

Follicles that grow rapidly are the most likely to undergo ovulation. Pierson and Ginther[10] suggested a daily increase of 2.7 mm, but in my experience, growth rates may range from 2 mm up to 5 mm per day, or possibly no further growth may occur in the 3 to 4 days preceding ovulation.[8] Some studies have shown that impaired fertility in old mares is associated with a slow follicular growth rate.

MULTIPLE FOLLICLES

Data from our clinic confirm other reports of the high incidence of the development of multiple ovulatory follicles, which ranged from 22% of estrous periods in 2- to 4-year-old mares to 51% in 17- to 19-year-old mares. Triple ovulations similarly peaked at a mean of 4.8% in 15- to 18-year-old mares. Other data also suggest a higher incidence in summer months.

The incidence of multiple ovulation is highest in Thoroughbreds and Thoroughbred crossbreds,[11] but similar in Warmbloods and Irish Draughts, less in Arabs and other draughts, low in ponies, and almost zero in native ponies. This is a curious development in an animal whose ancestors certainly would have had a very low incidence of 'twin' ovulation, because natural selection would have ensured that the birth of twins would have been self-limiting.

As has been described elsewhere, several follicles develop in late diestrus, but at some stage in early to midestrus, growth of the dominant follicle accelerates while the others begin to regress. Not uncommonly, more than one follicle continues to develop. These may be of approximately equal size, in which case they ovulate relatively synchronously. As another possibility, one may be considerably smaller and will undergo ovulation asynchronously, often as much as 3 days after the first. When two follicles continue to develop from mid-estrus, it is unusual for one to regress, although occasionally one will hemorrhage. Follicles as small as 20 mm that are present at the time of ovulation may still continue to develop and undergo ovulation as a diestrous event, several days later (see subsequent section on diestrous follicles).

Triple ovulations, although rare in younger mares (0.3% of 2-year-olds), become more common with maturity, as do double ovulations. The incidence of triplet pregnancies is approximately 1%; some appear to originate from twin ovulations.[12] Quadruple ovulations are seen occasionally, but quadruplet pregnancies are very rare.

The tendency to multiple ovulation is influenced by breed, season, and age but also is known to run in families. Some mares repeatedly experience twin ovulations and are as likely to have a triple as a single ovulation. Younger mares have a higher percentage of twin conceptions because although older mares have more twin ovulations, they are increasingly likely to conceive a single embryo as they age. The incidence also varies between stud farms, which suggests the possibility of a management factor.[11]

Before the use of ultrasonography enabled the relatively successful elimination of one twin at an early stage, strategies were proposed to avoid twin conception. Little can be done to prevent the development of more than one follicle (other than ultrasonographically guided follicle ablation). Mares with a propensity for twin ovulation could be put onto a very restricted diet for 10 days before ovulation, but the success of this treatment has not been evaluated.

Where two follicles of different sizes are developing and asynchronous ovulations can be anticipated, then it is possible to consider mating more than 24 hours after the first ovulation but in time for the second. Ginther, however, reported that this strategy actually decreased the overall pregnancy rates per cycle and did not reduce the percentage of twin pregnancies detected.[13] Since the development of "crushing" one of the conceptions at 14 to 16 days, there is no need to follow any of these strategies.

DIESTROUS FOLLICLES

It is not uncommon on first examining a mare to find a large follicle, leading to the assumption that she is in estrus. Concomitant absence of endometrial edema and presence of a firm, closed cervix will refute this assumption, however. Teasing should be performed to confirm that the mare is in fact not in estrus. A further examination of the ovaries reveals what appears to be a functional corpus luteum. Such a follicle is a *diestrous follicle*. If the corpus luteum is relatively recent, the follicle may have developed during the previous estrus and continued to grow after ovulation. If the corpus luteum is mature, the follicle has developed during diestrus from a follicular wave that began soon after ovulation (see Chapter 1).

A majority of diestrous follicles regress, but some will undergo ovulation. Although this ovulation typically occurs during the first 8 days of diestrus, it can occur at any stage. The incidence of follicles found to be still developing in late diestrus (excluding asynchronous twin ovulations up to 72 hours apart) has been reported to be 8.1%.[14] It cannot be overemphasized that in the absence

of a teaser, the finding of a large follicle in a mare does not constitute firm evidence of estrus.

INDUCTION OF OVULATION

Induction is really the wrong term in the context of ovulation because in most instances the follicle will undergo ovulation spontaneously within the next 2 to 4 days. The "ovulation induction" agents hCG and GnRH are more properly said to *advance* ovulation.

As previously discussed, even with experience, it is not possible to accurately predict ovulation with a high degree of confidence. In most instances, however, on the basis of not only follicular diameter but the various other parameters already discussed, it is possible to predict when a follicle is 1 to 4 days from ovulation. Use of an ovulation-advancing hormone normally will ensure that ovulation occurs within a window of 48 hours. In most instances, apart from those in which the follicle was destined to undergo ovulation within 36 hours, ovulation will occur 36 to 48 hours after injection. This interval may be longer in spring than in summer.[15]

Human CG is a gonadotropin extracted from the urine of pregnant women and marketed in freeze-dried ampules of 1,500 to 10,000 units (U). In many reports, the dose rate has varied, ranging from 1,000 to 5,000 U given intravenously, intramuscularly or subcutaneously. In my experience, no advantage is associated with use of any specific route. Many practitioners use a 1,500-U dose, although a lower dose (750 U) may be as effective later in the breeding season. In one series, success rates for both doses were identical, with 92.5% of all single follicles undergoing ovulation within 48 hours of treatment. With multiple follicles, ovulation occurred less frequently within 48 hours at all dose rates because in approximately 50% of instances, the smaller twin follicle was too immature to respond. With multiple follicles, ovulation occurred more frequently within 96 hours after 750 U (91.6%) than after 1,500 U (88.2%), as also found with single follicles (97.3% versus 96.2%), showing no advantage in using the higher dose.

A surprising proportion of mares mated 4 and 5 days before ovulation become pregnant. Those mares that have not been mated but are found to have ovulated are assessed for susceptibility to endometritis. If the ovulation appears to be recent, as indicated by an ill-defined area of increased echogenicity on ultrasonography (Fig. 2-1), mating should be considered.[6,8] If a corpus luteum is beginning to form (a soft structure on palpation and an echodense area or defined structure on ultrasonography), a mating should not be considered. The fact that a mare is still in good standing estrus should not be taken as evidence of recent ovulation, because some mares will be in estrus for 48 hours or longer after ovulation.[16]

There is another situation in which mating may be considered after ovulation. Provided that the mare is not considered susceptible to PME, and although she may have ovulated more than 12 to 16 hours earlier, if a second follicle is still developing, a successful pregnancy may result. In such a situation, extra regard should be taken to prevent PME, and the possibility of twin

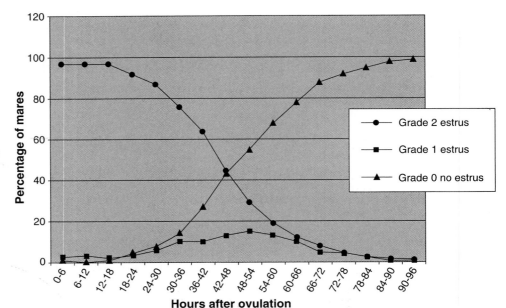

Figure 2-1 Persistence of estrus after ovulation.

embryos should be kept in mind. Pregnancies may result from matings as long as 24 hours after ovulation.

In a management regimen of veterinary visits to the stud farm only every third or fourth day, the dominant follicle must be assessed and a decision made:

- Is there a possibility that this follicle will ovulate within 24 hours? If so, then mate the mare within 18 hours and give hCG (as insurance).
- Will the follicle definitely last until the next visit? Do nothing until the next visit.
- Will the follicle possibly ovulate before the next visit? Then mate the mare in 2 days' time and perhaps also give hCG.
- Is the follicle likely to ovulate in more than 24 hours but probably before the next visit? Then mate her tomorrow and give hCG at the same time.
- Is this follicle likely to regress? Then evaluate the next largest follicle.

It is assumed that at each examination the veterinarian will identify and preferably record the size, side, and even the site of all multiple follicles that may possibly go on to ovulate—normally, all follicles greater than 25 mm in diameter. Such follicles should be evaluated at each examination, preferably until either ovulation has occurred or the follicle has hemorrhaged or begun to regress. Follicles that are still growing at the time of the last examination may undergo ovulation; therefore, an estimation of the difference in age of the two possible pregnancies should be made.

The accurate detection of twin or multiple ovulations is essential for the diagnosis of multiple pregnancy and for the successful elimination of excess embryos. Accurate knowledge of the time of each ovulation allows for strategic early pregnancy examination. Accurate aging of the embryos enables detection of normal pregnancies and recognition of small for age embryos. Twin reduction is discussed elsewhere, but it is emphasized here that a high foaling rate after twin reduction cannot be achieved without a good knowledge of the time of all ovulations.

SEASONAL (WINTER) ANESTRUS

Many mares cease cyclic activity in the winter. The last ovulation before a period of anestrus may vary from August to January or even February.[17,18] Reported percentages of non-Thoroughbred mares in anestrus on the first day of October, November, December, and January were 7%, 16%, 36%, and 69%, respectively.[19] In a Thoroughbred population, however, only 0%, 7%, and 17% of mares were in diestrus in January, February, and March, respectively.[19] By contrast, Hughes and others[20] in California found 64% remaining cyclic throughout the winter.

Mares do not have a clearly defined transitional period before anestrus.[18] Only a third of mares grew a nonovulatory follicle larger than 30 mm, whereas a third did not grow a follicle larger than 20 mm. No mare had more than one follicular wave after the last ovulation. Nequin and co-workers[21] describe a period of lower progesterone, estrogen, and luteinizing hormone preceding the last ovulation, but both they and Snyder and colleagues[22] describe a single follicular wave in most mares in which follicle size reached greater than 30 mm. Nunes and associates,[23] however, found that a dominant follicle developed during the transitional phase in only 43%.

Cessation of activity is influenced by decreasing day length and also by various levels of stress. Young, lactating mares losing body condition become anestrous before those that are mature, nonlactating, housed, and maintaining body condition. Individual mare factors also are important, and some animals consistently cycle all winter provided that they are relatively stress free and well fed.

Winter Anestrus

The seasonal period of anestrus can vary, ranging from 3 to 8 months. During this time the ovaries may become almost totally quiescent as a result of absence of GnRH output. Growth and regression of follicles greater than 10 mm continue independent of GnRH. Other mares may have very "shallow" waves of follicles growing from 15 to 20 mm for most of the period until near to ovulation. A few, probably only those that are housed and well fed, have continuous ovarian activity and estrous behavior with follicles greater than 25 mm but without ovulation.

Numerous studies have shown that resumption of cyclic activity is largely dependent on increasing day length and was first described by Burkhard.[24] The first ovulation of the new breeding season occurs within a more limited time period than that observed for the last ovulation. Depending on management, latitude, and breed, mean ovulation dates for groups of mares vary by as much as a month from late April to late May.[13] In one series, the mean date of ovulation in housed Thoroughbred mares was April 24th. Occasional animals will ovulate in March or as late as June.[25] Ponies appear to ovulate later than horses.[13]

The first ovulation of the year is the most difficult to predict. Mares may develop nonovulatory follicles greater than 30 mm and not infrequently greater than 40 mm, which may or may not be responsive to hCG or deslorelin (Ovuplant). Response to ovulatory stimulants is more likely to be successful when the follicle is still growing or has only just stopped growing. Follicles that are static or in regression are unlikely to respond to stimulation. Use of the endometrial edema pattern can help to identify those follicles that may undergo ovulation. When rapid growth of a follicle is accompanied by an increasing level of edema, ovulation is more likely. If edema has disappeared for more than 2 days or has never been present, the follicle is more likely to regress. Occasional mares, however, will ovulate after either a period of anestrus or diestrus without significant edema, and absence of edema should therefore not be taken as a guarantee of nonovulation in the presence of other, more positive signs.

Not all mares have a defined transitional phase. Some have several follicles fluctuating in size between 20 and 25 mm, without an obvious follicular wave. Then one of these follicles may suddenly grow to ovulatory size within a few days. A few mares remain in deep anestrus with no follicles larger than 20 mm until one follicle, without warning, grows to ovulatory size within 10 days.

Hastening the Transition

Because mares arrive at the stud farm in anestrus but not having been previously treated with increased day length, the problems of the transitional period are best overcome by the use of intravaginal progesterone-releasing devices[26-29] or of oral progestagens.[30,31] These will regularize the first estrus without the need for multiple matings and also advance the first ovulation in some mares. After the withdrawal of such therapy, follicular development should be rapid and ovulation more reliable.

Three types of progesterone-releasing intravaginal devices are available: PRID, CIDR-B, and CuMate. These contain either 1.55 g or 1.9 g of progesterone, which is released and absorbed through the vaginal wall, giving initial peripheral progesterone concentrations of 3 to 5 ng/ml, decreasing to approximately 1.5 to 2 ng/ml after 10 days. Alternatively, the orally active synthetic progestagen altrenogest (Regumate) may be fed for approximately 10 days. The difference between the two methods is that in most mares after 10 days of altrenogest, most follicular activity is suppressed and ovulation occurs 9 to 12 days after cessation of treatment. Using progesterone, the dominant follicle present at the time of insertion regresses, but in response to the falling levels of progesterone, a new follicle develops and after 10 days of treatment may be as large as 35 mm. It also is suspected that in the transitional phase, progesterone itself is folliculogenic. When the device is removed, the mare comes rapidly into estrus and ovulates within 4 to 8 days. Use of hCG or deslorelin will advance ovulation by 1 or 2 days and also will reduce the percentage of mares that fail to ovulate. The pregnancy rate may be decreased, however, in mares that ovulate less than 6 days after removal of the device. Although no trial has been done to compare progesterone with altrenogest treatment, it is thought that ovulation can be further advanced with progesterone, but the method needs closer control by a more experienced clinician.

All of the intravaginal devices cause some degree of vaginitis; usually *Streptococcus equi* var. *zooepidemicus* is the causative organism. The amount of discharge varies between mares and between devices. It has been shown that the infection is limited to the vagina and clears spontaneously, the discharge ceasing within 24 hours of removal. They can be safely inserted into pregnant mares, and once one gave birth to "twins": a foal and a PRID!

Up to 5% of mares attempt to expel the devices by straining, but this has been largely overcome by the design of the CuMate.

All acyclic mares arriving up to about the middle of April will benefit from exposure to increased day length, although this benefit is minimal from April onward. Mares that appear to be in deep anestrus on arrival should be monitored weekly until the onset of increased ovarian activity. For example, in mares initially found to have 5- to 15-mm follicles, change in follicular diameter up to 25 mm may be noted, or in mares with initial follicular sizes of 20 to 25 mm, development of follicles larger than 30 mm may occur. Progesterone/progestagen treatment started at this stage will be highly effective in causing estrus and ovulation. If such treatment is started too early in the transition phase, then only an anovulatory follicle may develop. If it is started later, then an ovulatory-size follicle may develop within the 10 days of treatment. To avoid this, mares with progesterone devices should be examined 6 to 8 days after insertion to identify any rapidly developing follicle, so that the device may be removed earlier.

If treatment is started while mares are still in deep anestrus, no follicular response at all may occur. However, by mid-March onward, or earlier in those mares that have been exposed to 4 to 5 weeks of increased day length, some will respond (with estrus and ovulation) although they demonstrated little or no ovarian activity at the start of treatment. If treatment is started in mares that are due to ovulate within 6 to 7 days, ovulation will not be postponed, but of course the mare will not show estrus.

Silent Heat

Mares that on examination appear to be in physiologic estrus, but do not respond with any positive signs of heat when teased and reject natural mating, are said to be in "silent heat." This condition is diagnosed by a relatively relaxed and possibly an edematous external cervix, ultrasonic evidence of a mature follicle, no apparent functional corpus luteum, and typically some endometrial edema. It is confirmed by a peripheral progesterone concentration of less than 0.5 ng/ml and eventual ovulation of the follicle. Mares inseminated with viable sperm seem to have normal or at least acceptable pregnancy rates, which suggests that the problem is purely a psychological one.

Estrous behavior most often is described as the behavior of a mare toward a teaser stallion. In fact, however, some mares will "show" to other mares, to geldings, or even to their owner but may be reluctant to show to the teaser. Others will show only to a mature stallion, which may have to be noisy and aggressive or, alternatively, may have to be relatively quiet and "gently persuasive."

For a firm diagnosis of silent heat, every possible combination of factors in teasing must be tried, including different stallions, different surroundings, teasing only nose to nose, teasing only the hindquarters, with or without a twitch, and so on. Even then, some mares show no signs until the stallion is about to mount and at the last minute are suddenly in good estrus. The important question in the end is whether the mare will stand to be mated. If she will, even in the absence of all other signs of estrus, then she is not in silent heat. Conversely, it should be pointed out that occasionally a mare that is diestrous or even pregnant will stand to be mated, possibly with a minimum of restraint. Would such a mare stand, however, if she were running out with the stallion?

A host of "ad hoc" instances of unusual behavior have been described. I have observed mares that regularly show no estrus until at or just after ovulation, others that are in estrus in the evenings but not in the mornings when being turned out, some that show well to one stallion but completely reject another, and miniature Shetlands that won't show to an Irish Draught. If mares are teased regularly but gently with the same stallion in familiar surroundings from the end of diestrus, in my experience all mares in true physiologic estrus will show at least some positive behavioral signs.

Mares with a foal at foot often are difficult to tease, particularly at the "foal heat." It may be necessary to leave the foal in the stable, even out of the mare's earshot, before she will concentrate on the stallion. Others will not relax unless the foal is held right in front of them. Use of a twitch usually will suffice to keep the attention of a "foal-proud" mare on mating.

Estrus is not necessarily expressed immediately after luteal regression. Some mares have long estrous periods—they begin to show heat as early as 15 or 16 days after ovulation. Others may not be in estrus until 1 or 2 days before ovulation. If the follicular phase is foreshortened by the ovulation of a large follicle that has developed during diestrus, then some mares may not have time to come into estrus before they ovulate. Years ago, when it was not routine to manually examine mares for pregnancy until after 21 days when they had failed to return to estrus, although some nonpregnant mares were in prolonged diestrus or had experienced embryonic resorption, a majority were found to be in early luteal phase. This could only have been due to inadequate teasing methods.

Occasionally, mares show some but not all the clinical signs of estrus. Cervical relaxation may be minimal, and only slight or transient endometrial edema is seen; and although a follicle continues to grow normally and undergoes ovulation, the other clinical and behavioral signs are reflective of diestrus as much as estrus. In at least some cases, peripheral progesterone concentrations either remain at a level sufficient to block normal estrous behavior (e.g., 0.5 to 1.0 ng/ml) or fall initially to non–luteal phase levels but, during the follicular phase, rise back above the behavior cutoff value. These are spontaneously occurring cases of partial luteal regression, a condition that more frequently is seen after subluteolytic doses of exogenous prostaglandin.

References

1. Woods J, Bergfelt DR, Ginther OJ: Effects of time of insemination relative to ovulation on pregnancy rate and embryonic loss rate in mares. Equine Vet J 1990; 22;410-415.
2. Newcombe JR: The effect of interval from mating to ovulation on pregnancy rate and pregnancy loss rate. Proceedings of the 40th Congress of the British Equine Veterinary Association, 2001.
3. Newcombe JR: High pregnancy rate to post-ovulatory mating and insemination. Proceedings of the British Equine Veterinary Association Meeting on Artificial Insemination, Whitchurch, UK, 2003.
4. Newcombe JR: Uterus unicornis in two mares. Vet Rec 1997b; 141:21.
5. Ginther OJ: Ultrasonic Imaging and Reproductive Events in the Mare. Cross Plains, WI, Equiservices, 1986.
6. Newcombe JR: Ultrasonography of ovulation and development of the corpus luteum in the mare. Equine Vet Educ 1996b; 8:47-58.
7. Newcombe JR: Investigation of equine ovarian cyclical changes by ultrasound scanning and rectal palpation. Br J Radiol 1987; 60:628.
8. Newcombe JR: Ovulation and formation of the corpus luteum. J Equine Vet Sci 1996a; 16:48-52.
9. Newcombe JR: Identification of the corpus luteum in early pregnancy in the mare using ultrasound. J Equine Vet Sci 1994; 14:655-657.
10. Pierson RA, Ginther OJ: Ultrasonic evaluation of the pre-ovulatory follicle in the mare. Theriogenology 1985; 24:359-368.
11. Newcombe JR: Incidence of multiple ovulation and multiple pregnancy in the mare. Vet Rec 1995; 137:121-123.
12. Newcombe JR: The probable identification of monozygous twin embryos in the mare. J Equine Vet Sci 2000b; 20: 269-274.

13. Ginther OJ: Reproductive Biology of the Mare. Cross Plains, WI, Equiservices, p 111, 1992.
14. Newcombe JR: The incidence of ovulation during the luteal phase from day 4 to day 20 in pregnant and non-pregnant mares. J Equine Vet Sci 1997a; 17:120-122.
15. Sieme H, Scafer T, Stout TAE et al: The effects of different insemination regimes on fertility in mare. Theriogenology 2003; 60:1153-1164.
16. Newcombe JR: Persistence of oestrous behaviour after ovulation and its relationship to the activity of the corpus luteum in the preceding dioestrus period. Proceedings of the 37th Congress of the British Equine Veterinary Association, 1998a.
17. Ginther OJ: Occurrence of anoestrus, oestrus, dioestrus and ovulation over a 12 month period in mares. Am J Vet Res 1974; 35:1173-1179.
18. Newcombe JR: The transition from cyclicity to anoestrum in mares. J Equine Vet Sci 2000a; 20:307-309.
19. Newcombe JR: Seasonal influence on ovarian activity: winter anoestrus and transition to cyclic activity. J Equine Vet Sci 1998b; 18:354-357.
20. Hughes JP, Stabenfeldt GH, Kennedy PC: The oestrous cycle and selected functional and pathological ovarian abnormalities in the mare. Vet Clin NorthAm 1980; 2:225-239.
21. Nequin LG, King SS, Roser JF et al: Uncoupling of the equine reproductive axes during transition into anoestrus. J Reprod Fertil Suppl 2000; 56:153-161.
22. Snyder DA, Turner DD, Miller KF et al: Follicular and gonadotrophic changes during transition from ovulatory to anovulatory seasons. J Reprod Fertil Suppl 1979; 27:95-101.
23. Nunes MM, Gastal EL, Gastal MO et al: Follicle and gonadotropin relationships during the beginning of the anovulatory season in mares. Anim Reprod 2005; 2:41-49.
24. Burkhard J: Transition from anoestrus in the mare and the effects of artificial lighting. J Agr Sci 1946; 37:64-68.
25. Katila T, Koskinen E: Onset of luteal activity in different types of mares after winter anoestrus. J Reprod Fertil Suppl 1991; 44:678-679.
26. Newcombe JR, Wilson MC: The use of progesterone releasing intravaginal devices to induce seasonally anoestrous Standardbred mares in Australia. Equine Pract 1997; 19:13-21.
27. Newcombe JR: Field observations on the use of a progesterone releasing intravaginal device to induce oestrus and ovulation in seasonally anoestrous mares. J Equine Vet Sci 2002; 22:378-382.
28. Newcombe JR, Handler J, Klug E et al: Treatment of transition phase mares with progesterone intravaginally and with deslorelin or hCG to assist ovulations. J Equine Vet Sci 2002; 22:57-64.
29. Foglia RA, McCue PM, Squires EL, Jochle W: Stimulation of follicular development in transitional mares using a progesterone vaginal insert (CIDR-B). Proceedings of the Annual Conference of the Society for Theriogenology/American College of Theriogenologists, p 33, 1999.
30. Webel SK, Squires EL: Control of the oestrous cycle in mares with altrenogest. J Reprod Fertil Suppl 1982; 32:193-198.
31. Squires EL, Heesemann CP, Webel SK et al: Relationship of altrenogest to ovarian activity, hormone concentrations and fertility of mares. J Anim Sci 1983; 56:901-910.

Suggested Reading

Newcombe JR: Follicular luteinisation without ovulation. The W. "Ed" Allen Memorial Lecture BEVA Meeting, Bristol, March 1993.

CHAPTER 3
Estrous Synchronization

ETTA AGAN BRADECAMP

As a prelude to this chapter, it is necessary to make a few comments about estrous synchronization as it pertains to the mare and how this varies from estrous synchronization in the cow. Practitioners who are familiar with estrous synchronization in cattle and the number of different synchronization programs available must realize that estrous synchronization in the mare is much more relative and does not yield as reliable results as estrous synchronization in cattle. In the bovine industry a large number of cows can be synchronized to reliably display estrus and ovulate within a narrow window of time, and there are several programs described to achieve the desired results. Unfortunately, the mare's reproductive cycle does not lend itself to such a tight synchronization among a group of mares, and currently there is only one protocol that consistently provides reliable results. The length of estrus in the mare is 5 to 7 days, and the time of ovulation relative to the end of estrus varies with ovulation occurring on the last 2 days of estrus in 69% of mares and after the end of estrus in 14% of mares.[1] These factors make the development of a synchronization program that allows for a single breeding at a predetermined time difficult.

In equine reproduction the most common use of estrous synchronization is in embryo transfer programs. If a large recipient herd providing mares that have ovulated in synchrony with the donor is not available, then a small group of recipient mares must be synchronized with the donor mare. To be suitable recipients, these mares must ovulate from 1 day before to 3 days after the date of ovulation of the donor mare. There is even one report in the literature that recipient mares that ovulated up to 5 days after the donor have been used successfully in a large embryo transfer program.[2]

A second less common use of estrous synchronization in the mare is to synchronize a group of mares for breeding due to limited availability of a stallion, for example due to a show schedule.

In addition to synchronization of estrus in a group of mares, pharmacologic agents can be used to induce ovulation to allow for the synchronization of ovulation. When breeding with both frozen and cooled shipped semen it is often desirable to use only one dose of semen, and therefore it is essential that the ovulation be synchronized within 36 to 48 hours of breeding. This is also important where natural service of mares is performed and the stallion has a full book of mares, thereby limiting the number of times a mare can be bred during a cycle.

There are four basic methods used to achieve estrous synchronization in the mare: termination of the luteal phase, lengthening of the luteal phase, induction of ovulation, and inhibition of the follicular phase. The pharmacologic agents most commonly used to accomplish these methods are prostaglandins, progestins, human chorionic gonadotropin (hCG) (Chorulon, Intervet Inc., Millsboro, Del.) or deslorelin acetate (Ovuplant, Peptech Limited, NSW, Australia), and estradiol-17β. The most reliable and successful estrous synchronization programs are achieved when a combination of these methods and pharmacologic agents are used.

Prostaglandin $F_{2\alpha}$ ($PGF_{2\alpha}$) is used to terminate the luteal phase by causing lysis of the corpus luteum (CL), thereby allowing the return to estrus. The most common prostaglandins used are dinoprost (Lutalyse, Pfizer, New York) and cloprostenol (Estrumate, Schering-Plough Animal Health Corporation, Union, N.J.). Dinoprost is a naturally occurring $PGF_{2\alpha}$, and cloprostenol is a synthetic prostaglandin analogue. For prostaglandins to effectively terminate the luteal phase a mature CL must be present that is responsive to prostaglandin. The equine CL exhibits incomplete sensitivity to $PGF_{2\alpha}$ until approximately day 5 postovulation in most mares.[3] The standard recommended dose of dinoprost is 9 µg/kg (5 to 10 mg per 1000 lb/454 kg horse). The recommended dose of cloprostenol is 250 µg per 1000 lb/454 kg horse (0.55 µg/kg). More recent research has shown that much lower doses of prostaglandin are just as effective at lysing the CL with fewer negative side effects. Douglas and Ginther demonstrated that doses of prostaglandin as low as 1.25 mg were as effective at inducing luteolysis as more standard doses.[4] Nie et al showed that a microdose of cloprostenol (25 µg) was just as effective at lysing the equine CL as the larger standard dose.[5]

On average, mares return to estrus 5 to 7 days after administration of prostaglandin in the presence of a mature CL, and ovulation occurs 9 to 11 days after administration. However, because the follicular phase plays a greater role in controlling the total length of the estrous cycle in the mare, the length of time from administration of prostaglandin to onset of estrus and ovulation can be quite variable depending on the size and status of follicles present on the ovaries at the time of administration. The time of ovulation after $PGF_{2\alpha}$-induced estrus may vary as much as 2 to 15 days post treatment.[6] If prostaglandin is administered when there is a large follicle present, the mare may return to estrus and ovulate in 2 to 3 days. Some of these mares never develop overt signs of standing heat, endometrial folds, or relaxation of the cervix before ovulation. If a large follicle destined for atresia is present on the ovary at the time of prostaglandin administration, the follicle may not ovulate and instead regress as a new wave of follicles develops.[7]

In cattle the administration of two doses of prostaglandin 11 to 12 days apart results in approximately 80% exhibiting estrus within 2 to 5 days after the second injection. Although the administration of two doses of prostaglandin 14 days apart has been described in the literature as a protocol for estrous synchronization in mares, it is not a very reliable method of ensuring that a recipient mare will be synchronized with a donor.[6] Research has shown that after two injections of prostaglandin, on average ovulation occurs between 7 and 10 days after the second injection,[6,8,9] with ovulation potentially occurring anywhere between 0 and 17 days.[8,9] In a review of the literature it was stated that when this protocol was administered, one would need to treat at least 10 recipient mares to have an 80% chance that at least 1 recipient would ovulate within 24 hours of the donor.[10] Obviously, this is not ideal, especially when in most small embryo transfer programs there are only a few mares available to be used as recipients. Due to the large variation in time of ovulation from administration of prostaglandin, it is not very useful when used alone in the synchronization of estrous cycles in mares. However, if examination via transrectal ultrasonography is performed first to eliminate those mares that will not respond appropriately to the administration of prostaglandin, tightening of date of ovulation can be achieved with this protocol.

Exogenous progestins are commonly used in estrous synchronization programs to lengthen the luteal phase. The two most common forms of progestins used are progesterone in oil and altrenogest (allyl trenbolone, Regumate, Intervet Inc., Millsboro, Del.), a synthetic progestin. Progesterone or a synthetic progestin administered alone or in combination with estradiol-17β will effectively lengthen the luteal phase indefinitely until their administration is discontinued. Progesterone has an inhibitory effect on LH release from the anterior pituitary; therefore the rationale is if it is administered for a long enough period of time (15 to 18 days), the CL will regress and the only source of progesterone to suppress estrus is the exogenous progesterone. However, even the endogenous level of progesterone present during the midluteal phase is not sufficient to suppress gonadotropin release, follicular development, and ovulation.[11] Studies have also shown that the synthetic progestin, altrenogest, administered at 0.044 mg/kg orally once a day fails to suppress follicular development.[12] When using progestins for estrous synchronization it is recommended that either altrenogest (0.044 mg/kg PO q24h) or progesterone in oil (150 mg/day IM) be administered for 10 days combined with the administration of $PGF_{2\alpha}$ on the last day of progestin therapy to lyse any CLs present.

To improve estrous synchronization in randomly cycling mares, a combination of progesterone and estrogen, rather than progesterone alone, is administered. The combined effect of the two hormones provides a more profound negative feedback on gonadotropin release than does progesterone alone, which results in a more uniform inhibition of follicular development. When the exogenous progesterone/estrogen therapy is discontinued, there is less diversity in follicular maturation and the date ovulation occurs can be more closely synchronized. The recommended protocol involves intramuscular injections of progesterone (150 mg) combined with estradiol-17β (10 mg) in oil for 10 consecutive days with a single injection of $PGF_{2\alpha}$ administered on the tenth day of treatment. To further tighten the synchronization of ovulation, hCG (5 IU/kg IV) or deslorelin acetate is administered when a 35-mm follicle is present. With this protocol, greater than 70% of mares ovulate between 10 and 12 days after the last steroid injection with a range of ovulations occurring from 8 to 17 days. Currently, there is no commercial preparation containing progesterone and estradiol-17β combined; therefore this formulation must be ordered from a compounding pharmacy.[13]

Induction of ovulation is also an important part of an estrous synchronization program. The two most common pharmacologic agents used to induce ovulation are hCG and deslorelin acetate. Human chorionic gonadotropin is a protein consisting of two peptide chains that, although chemically different from pituitary luteinizing hormone (LH), has primarily luteinizing-like activity. hCG is produced by cytotrophoblasts of the chorionic villi of the human placenta and appears in the urine of pregnant women a few weeks after conception.

Deslorelin acetate is a potent synthetic gonadotropin-releasing hormone (GnRH) analogue. Deslorelin is a small peptide that is administered subcutaneously in the form of an implant (Ovuplant) containing 2.1 mg of the active ingredient. The advantage to using deslorelin over hCG to induce ovulation is that its smaller molecular weight makes it less antigenic, thereby reducing the chance that antibodies will be developed against it after multiple administrations in a season. However, it must be noted that administration of deslorelin implants in a small percentage of mares does result in a prolonged interovulatory interval due to down-regulation of the pituitary by the continued release of deslorelin from the implant after ovulation has occurred.[14-16] This down-regulation is most pronounced when prostaglandins are administered early in diestrus after the administration of deslorelin, compared with mares that are allowed to return to estrus naturally. This side effect can be avoided by removing the implant after ovulation has occurred.[16] Currently, Ovuplant is not available in the United States; however, an injectable formulation of deslorelin, BioRelease Deslorelin Injection (BET Pharm, Lexington, Ky.), has become available. This deslorelin product is administered intramuscularly at the recommended dose of 1.5 mg when a 35-mm or greater follicle is present and the mare is in estrus. Based on the results of recent research, this injectable formulation of deslorelin does not cause the prolonged interovulatory interval seen with the administration of deslorelin implants.[17] Administration of hCG when a 35-mm or greater diameter follicle is present in an estrual mare results in ovulation in 36 ± 4 hours and deslorelin acetate administration with the presence of a 35-mm or greater follicle in an estrual mare results in ovulation in 41 ± 3 hours.[18]

hCG and deslorelin are most commonly used to induce ovulation to occur within 48 hours post breeding.

In addition to their application in programs using fresh and cooled semen, these pharmacologic agents are used extensively in frozen semen programs. Due to the decreased longevity of frozen semen, insemination must occur within the time frame of 12 hours before to 6 hours after ovulation. If two doses of semen are available, a timed insemination program can be used. In this program, once a 35-mm follicle is detected in an estrual mare, deslorelin is administered at 7 PM that day. The mare is then examined via transrectal ultrasonography and inseminated at 24 and 41 hours. If hCG is used, then the second dose is inseminated at hCG + 36 hours. If only one dose of semen is available, the same basic plan is followed, except the mare is not inseminated at the 24-hour examination and is then examined via transrectal ultrasonography every 6 hours until ovulation is detected. Once ovulation is detected, the mare is inseminated.

In addition to the pharmacologic agents previously described, there are other products and estrous synchronization programs described in the literature that warrant discussion. Numerous reports in the literature discuss the use of an intravaginal progesterone-releasing device originally designed for cattle (CIDR-B) in mares to synchronize estrus. These devices have been used with and without the administration of estradiol (10 mg, IM or intravaginal) on the day of CIDR-B placement. Results of these studies were similar to those with progesterone in oil or Regumate. Without the addition of the estradiol, CIDR-B administration resulted in synchronization of estrus but not of ovulations.[19-21] The CIDR was first produced in New Zealand and was approved in May 2002 for use in the United States, where it is marketed under the name Eazi-Breed CIDR Cattle Insert (Pharmacia Animal Health, Kalamazoo, Mich.) and contains 1.38 g of progesterone. In Canada this product contains 1.9 g of progesterone. These products are not labeled for use in horses. A similar intravaginal progesterone-releasing device designed for mares, Cue-Mare (Duirs PfarmAg, Hamilton, New Zealand), has been described for the use of estrous synchronization in transitional mares.[22] After a 10-day application of the Cue-Mare in 38 transitional mares, all of the mares exhibited signs of estrus 3 days following removal of the devices. Further research is needed to determine the value of this product in estrous synchronization programs.[22] One advantage to intravaginal progesterone-releasing devices is that they do not require the labor associated with daily administration of progesterone in oil or Regumate. However, mild to moderate vaginitis is observed in most mares that have an intravaginal device administered.

The use of ultrasound-guided transvaginal follicle ablation for synchronizing ovarian function in the mare has been described. In one study, on day 0 all follicles greater than or equal to 10 mm were ablated via ultrasound-guided transvaginal follicular aspiration. Four days later two doses of cloprostenol (250 μg IM) were given 12 hours apart followed by hCG administration 6 days after that. Results of this study showed that 96% (22/23) mares ovulated within 48 hours of hCG treatment. Compared with conventional steroid regimens where the interval from beginning of treatment to ovulation can be up to 20 to 25 days with[23] or without[24] hCG administration,

this protocol represents an approximate 50% reduction in the interval from follicle ablation to ovulation. In addition, use of this procedure avoids the labor associated with administration of steroids daily. However, more research is needed to assess the effects of this procedure on pregnancy rates and its practicality in a practice setting.[25]

As mentioned previously, one of the most common uses of estrous synchronization is in an embryo transfer program. To achieve the best results, at least three recipient mares should be synchronized with the donor mare. Administration of a progestin or progesterone/estradiol combination should be in the donor and recipients at the same time. Discontinuation of the progestin therapy and administration of prostaglandin should also occur on the same day among all of the mares. Realizing that it is ideal for the recipient to ovulate from 1 day before to 3 days after the donor, hCG or deslorelin should be administered to induce ovulations to occur preferably 1 to 3 days after the donor. It is important to realize that all of the recipients may not synchronize with the donor, nor may they be ideal recipients at the time of transfer due to presence of uterine fluid or edema, poor cervical tone, or inadequate CL formation. For this reason, it is important to synchronize at least three recipients with each donor to maximize the chances of having a suitable recipient at the time of transfer.

Synchronization of estrus and, more importantly, ovulation plays an important role in equine breeding management programs. The use of a combination of pharmacologic agents, most commonly progesterone and estradiol-17β, followed by the administration of $PGF_{2\alpha}$ and hCG or deslorelin, yields the most reliable results. However, there is ongoing research in this field, and current knowledge of the latest results will afford the veterinarian the best options when developing an estrous synchronization program.

References

1. Ginther OJ: Reproductive Biology of the Mare: Basic and Applied Aspects, 2nd edition, pp 173-232, Cross Plains, Wis, Equiservices, 1993.
2. Foss R, Wirth N, Schiltz P et al: Nonsurgical embryo transfer in a private practice (1998). Proceedings of the 45th Annual Convention of the American Association of Equine Practitioners, pp 210-212, 1999.
3. Allen WR, Rowson LEA: Control of the mare's oestrous cycle by prostaglandins. J Reprod Fertil 1973; 33:539-543.
4. Douglas RH, Ginther OJ: Route of prostaglandin F₂a injection and luteolysis in mares. Proc Soc Biol Med 1975; 148:263-269.
5. Nie GJ, Goodin AN, Braden TD et al: Luteal and clinical response following administration of dinoprost tromethamine or cloprostenol at standard intramuscular sites or at the lumbosacral acupuncture points in mares. Am J Vet Rev 2001; 62:1285-1289.
6. Bristol F: Studies on estrous synchronization in mares. Proceedings of the Annual Meeting of the Society of Theriogenology, p 258, 1981.
7. Asbury AC: The use of prostaglandins in broodmare practice. Proceedings of the 34th Annual Convention of the American Association of Equine Practitioners, pp 191-196, 1988.

8. Holtan DW, Douglas RH, Ginther OJ: Estrus, ovulation and conception following synchronization with progesterone, prostaglandin F$_2$a and human chorionic gonadotropin in pony mares. J Anim Sci 1977; 44:431.

9. Voss JL, Wallace RA, Squires EL et al: Effects of synchronization and frequency of insemination on fertility. J Reprod Fertil Suppl 1979; 27:256.

10. Irvine CHG: Endocrinology of the estrous cycle of the mare: applications to the embryo transfer. Theriogenology 1981; 15:895.

11. Meyers PJ: Control and synchronization of the estrous cycle and ovulation. In Youngvist RS (ed): Current Therapy in Large Animal Theriogenology, pp 97-102, Philadelphia, WB Saunders, 1997.

12. Lofstedt RM, Patel JH: Evaluation of the ability of altrenogest to control the equine estrous cycle. J Am Vet Med Assoc 1989; 194:361.

13. Blanchard TL, Varner DD, Schumacher J: Manual of Equine Reproduction, pp 22-23, St Louis, Mosby, 1998.

14. Farquhar VJ, McCue PM, Nett TM et al: Effect of deslorelin acetate on gonadotropin secretion and ovarian follicle development in cycling mares. J Am Vet Med Assoc 2001; 218:749-752.

15. Farquhar VJ, McCue PM, Carnevale EM et al: Deslorelin acetate (Ovuplant™) therapy in cycling mares: effect of implant removal on FSH secretion and ovarian function. Equine Vet J 2002; 34:417-420.

16. McCue PM, Farquhar VJ, Carnevale EM et al: Removal of deslorelin (Ovuplant™) implant 48 hours after administration results in normal interovulatory intervals in mares. Theriogenology 2002; 58:865-870.

17. Stich KL, Wendt KM, Blanchard TL et al: Effects of a new injectable short-term release deslorelin in foal-heat mares. Theriogenology 2004; 62:831-836.

18. McKinnon AO, Perriam WJ, Lescun TB et al: Effect of a GnRH analogue (Ovuplant), hCG and dexamethasone on time to ovulation in cycling mares. World Equine Vet Rev 1997; 2:16-18.

19. Lübbecke M, Klug E, Hoppen HO et al: Attempts to synchronize estrus and ovulation in mares using progesterone (CIDR-B) and GnRH-analog deslorelin. Reprod Domest Anim 1994; 29:305-314.

20. Arbeiter K, Barth U, Jöchle W: Observations on the use of progesterone intravaginally and of deslorelin Sti in acyclic mares for induction of ovulation. J Equine Vet Sci 1994; 14:21-25.

21. Klug E, Jöchle W: Advances in synchronizing estrus and ovulations in the mare: a mini review. J Equine Vet Sci 2001; 21:474-479.

22. Grimmett JB, Hanlon DW, Duirs GF et al: A new intravaginal progesterone-releasing device (Cue-Mare) for controlling the estrous cycle in mares. Theriogenology 2002; 58:585-587.

23. Varner DD, Blanchard TL, Brinsko SP: Estrogen, oxytocin and ergot alkaloids: uses in reproductive management of mares. Proceedings of the 34th Annual Conference of the American Association of Equine Practitioners, 1998, pp 219-241.

24. Loy RG, Pemstein R, O'Canna D et al: Control of ovulation in cycling mares with ovarian steroids and prostaglandin. Theriogenology 1981; 15:191-197.

25. Bergfelt DR, Adams GP: Ovulation synchrony after follicle ablation in mares. J Reprod Fertil Suppl 2000; 56:257-269.

CHAPTER 4
Estrous Suppression

GARY J. NIE

Horses are a seasonally polyestrous species. Known as long-day breeders, mares will experience cyclic reproductive activity during the spring and summer months. During multiple estrous cycles experienced by a mare each season, gonadal steroids, estrogen and progesterone, alternate dominance. Each estrous cycle is roughly 21 to 22 days in length. In general, behavioral signs of estrus are typical of a period (usually 5 to 7 days) during a cycle when estrogen dominates and progesterone is at basal levels, whereas the opposite is true during diestrus. Owners, trainers, managers, and veterinarians may all from time to time feel it necessary to suppress behavioral signs of estrus in their mares. Behavioral signs of estrus are suppressed in mares by suspending cyclicity. The primary indications for suspending cyclicity include the following:

- Synchrony for breeding management
- Pain/colic during estrus
- Cycle-related behavior/performance problems

Some indications are specific and well defined with treatments that are efficacious and have measurable outcomes. In contrast, other indications are nonspecific and poorly defined with treatments that can be questionable with immeasurable outcomes.

INDICATIONS FOR SUPPRESSING ESTRUS

Estrous Synchronization for Breeding Management

Estrous synchronization is discussed in depth in the preceding section; therefore specific protocols for synchrony will not be covered here. Synchronizing estrus in mares is necessary or at least highly advantageous in a variety of breeding management circumstances, including shipped cool or frozen semen breedings, scheduling around stallion availability, delaying the first postpartum ovulation, and embryo or gamete transfers, to name a few. Protocols typically involve suspending cyclicity in a mare by administering a progestin (with or without estrogen) for a defined/finite period. Treatment suppresses hypothalamic-pituitary-gonadal activity with resultant suspension of cyclic activity and suppression of behavioral signs of estrus. When treatment is removed, the hormonal axis again becomes active and the cycle resumes as the mare enters estrus. In this case the indication is specific, the treatment highly efficacious, and the outcome measurable.

Pain/Colic During Estrus

Some mares experience pain related to the preovulatory follicle or postovulatory luteinizing structure. This condition appears variable and rarely occurs during every estrous cycle in an afflicted mare. Evaluating the reproductive tract when discomfort is observed allows a veterinarian to document an association with ovarian structures. Some mares may benefit from use of ovulatory agents to reduce the interval that a large preovulatory follicle is present on the ovary. The outcome in these mares is measurable in that upon ovulation the discomfort rapidly dissipates. However, a response in others experiencing discomfort associated with a postovulatory structure is less dramatic. In some cases, nonsteroidal antiinflammatory agents may alleviate some of the discomfort. Suspending cyclic activity may benefit the rare mare in which discomfort is irregularly associated with multiple estrous periods each season.

Alternating hormonal dominance during the estrous cycle, between estrogen and progesterone, may also affect the physical condition of a mare.[1] Muscles relax during periods of estrogen dominance, providing less support than when progesterone dominates.[1] As a result, a minor lameness may become more uncomfortable for a mare during estrus and therefore more conspicuous to the owner.[1] Tolerance of discomfort may also vary with hormone levels.[1] This condition is nonspecific and difficult to accurately define. A response to treatment may also be difficult to objectively measure. Nevertheless, mares afflicted with discomfort associated with the cyclic changes in gonadal steroids may benefit from suspension of cyclic activity.

Cycle-Related Behavior/Performance Problems

When mares behave or perform in ways contrary to owner desire or expectation in the absence of obvious pathologic conditions, the reason is often felt to be estrous cycle–related. Common names used for this behavior are "Painful," "Moody," "Feisty," or "Pissy Mare Syndrome" or simply "Mare Madness." In fact, the behavior is most often not associated with estrus or the estrous cycle.[1] Many behaviors displayed by mares can be misinterpreted as estrous behaviors. An explanation for problematic behaviors that are not estrous behaviors include the following[1]:

- Submissive behavior
- Urogenital discomfort
- Stallion-like behavior

When evaluating an owner complaint of a cycle-related behavior/performance problem in a mare, a veterinarian should rule out these other conditions as part of a complete workup. In order to thoroughly evaluate the mare, additional expertise may be needed in the form of consults with or referrals to behavior and/or reproduction experts. A team approach to evaluating and solving the problem may be beneficial for everyone involved.

Once other potential causes of an undesirable behavior/performance problem have been ruled out, we should consider the estrous cycle. There are behavior problems that are truly estrous cycle–related.[1] Some mares simply display intense behavioral signs when in a normal estrus. This can create an unruly situation during training and performance. In other mares the condition may be much more subtle. Owners and trainers often report that the mare is less cooperative or attentive during estrus. Changes in estrogen and progesterone dominance during the estrous cycle may indeed affect physical condition.[1] Supportive muscles relax under estrogen influence and tone in response to progesterone. A minor lameness may become more pronounced during estrus. The ability to tolerate discomfort may also vary with hormonal dominance during the cycle.[1]

Unfortunately, today our understanding of the reasons for cycle-related behavior/performance problems is incomplete. Once the problem has been thoroughly evaluated and all other causes have been ruled out, we might consider treating the mare to suppress estrus. Depending on the nature of the behavior/performance problem, complete suspension of cyclicity may be necessary. However, some mares apparently respond to progestin treatment at levels that do not suppress ovarian activity.[2]

Using hormonal treatments that are not approved and have not been objectively evaluated for efficacy and safety is a concern to many veterinarians. But there is pressure from some horse owners for hormonal treatments. An informal survey was conducted of several veterinarians in preparing this work, representing every region in the United States and most segments of the horse industry. The demand for treatment varies widely among segments of the horse industry. Most commonly, owners and trainers seek treatment for mares that are actively engaged in some sort of training or performance. Some veterinarians routinely use unapproved hormones to treat cycle-related behavior/performance problems in mares, whereas others offer only approved products. A few veterinarians report that their owners have even "begged" them to implant their mares. Other veterinarians will reluctantly treat the mares but provide their clients with an extensive information sheet and have them sign a liability release form. Some owners go to the extent of purchasing hormones from international sources and treating the mares themselves.

There is very little published information on the use, response, and safety of many of the progestin products labeled for use in other species. Much of the information on treatment, response, side effects, and safety is from anecdotal information. Careful consideration is suggested before using any of the methods discussed below for suppressing estrus.

METHODS OF SUPPRESSING ESTRUS

There are a number of methods used to suppress behavioral signs of estrus. Some methods employ approved products with well-documented efficacy, whereas others are not approved and use is based entirely on anecdotal information. Every method, whether efficacious or not, has advantages and disadvantages. The primary methods that have been used include the following:

- Hormonal
- Surgical
- Immunologic
- Other methods

Hormonal Methods

Altrenogest
Altrenogest (Intervet, Millsboro, DE) is a synthetic progestin approved for use in horses for the purpose of suppressing estrus. Administered orally as an oil solution, the labeled dose of altrenogest is 0.044 mg/kg (1 ml per 110 lb of body weight). It is highly effective for suppressing estrus when administered daily in mares and has been demonstrated to be safe when administered long-term.[3-6] However, it has a labeled contraindication for use in mares with uterine inflammation.

Although it is effective for estrous suppression, there are a number of disadvantages to its use. As an oil solution, it can be messy to administer, and owners often complain about the expense and inconvenience of daily dosing. Human safety must also be considered for individuals handling the solution and when used in horses that may be intended for use as food.

It may take several days to effectively suspend cycling and fully suppress estrus. Therefore administration should be planned in accordance with the need for estrous suppression. In general, daily dosing is required to maintain adequate suppression of estrus. The duration of treatment is often tailored to individual management needs. Surveyed veterinarians indicated an overwhelming preference by practitioners for altrenogest when recommending a method of estrous suppression to their clients.

Progesterone
Progesterone in oil, administered intramuscularly, will effectively suppress signs of estrus in mares.[7] Daily doses of 100 mg or greater are sufficient to maintain circulating progesterone concentrations comparable to production from a functional corpus luteum.[8,9] Progesterone in oil is available from several sources, including compounding pharmacies. The duration of estrous suppression achieved with injectable progesterone appears variable in mares, because surveyed veterinarians report dosing once every 1 to 4 days. Though effective, a significant disadvantage of the form of progesterone is muscle soreness at the injection site. Side effects associated with short-term use have not been reported; however, as with altrenogest, progesterone administration is contraindicated in mares with uterine inflammation. The effects of long-term administration have not been evaluated.[10]

Pregnancy

Pregnancy is another means of suspending cyclicity by taking advantage of naturally produced progestins. This method has obvious disadvantages and is undesirable for many owners, particularly if the pregnancy is allowed to go to term. However, a pregnant mare can be aborted between days 50–60 of gestation. By then endometrial cups have developed and the mare will usually not return to estrus for another 60 days or more. This approach provides 120 days or more of elevated progestin concentrations and often is enough to get a performance mare through a critical period. Although—veterinarians should also consider—a small portion of pregnant mares will also readily display behavioral signs of estrus at various stages during gestation.

Medroxyprogesterone Acetate

Manufactured and marketed as a human contraceptive, medroxyprogesterone acetate (Depo-Provera, Pfizer, New York, NY) suppresses ovulation in women for 3 months. Routinely recommended by some veterinarians for suppression of estrus, it has not been evaluated for suspension of cyclicity in mares. Medroxyprogesterone acetate (MPA) was unable to maintain pregnancy in mares following induced luteolysis when administered at 1000 mg intramuscularly every 7 days.[11] After pregnancy loss the mares also returned to estrus and ovulated in spite of being treated with high doses of MPA.[11] Dose and frequency of administration, reported by surveyed veterinarians, for estrous suppression varied widely from 200 mg every 8 to 14 days to 1800 mg monthly for a 1000- to 1200-lb (450- to 550-kg) mare. Interpretation of therapeutic response is also widely varied. Some suggest no effect, whereas others say it works as well as altrenogest and suppresses estrus for 6 weeks to 3 months. Short- or long-term safety studies have not been conducted in horses, and there is concern among some practitioners that an occasional horse may be more prone to tying-up following administration of MPA.

Hydroxyprogesterone Caproate

Hydroxyprogesterone caproate (HPC) is a synthetic progestin available through human and veterinary pharmacies under a number of labels (one source is Wedgewood Pharmacy, Swedesboro, NJ). McKinnon et al[12] demonstrated an inability of HPC to maintain pregnancy in ovariectomized mares. The same synthetic molecule, repackaged as hydroxyprogesterone hexanoate (Gesteron-500, Illium Veterinary Products), though labeled for pregnancy maintenance was also unable to maintain pregnancy in mares following induced luteolysis.[11] Hydroxyprogesterone caproate was demonstrated to have a very low binding affinity for equine endometrial progesterone receptors.[13] This illustrates that basic physiologic differences in one species may negate the effective use of a hormonal product developed for another species. Nevertheless, HPC is being used for estrous suppression in mares. Doses recommended by surveyed veterinarians range from 500 to 1500 mg, administered intramuscularly at monthly intervals. Veterinarians using HPC report that estrous suppression lasts from 3 weeks to 2 months. However, HPC is reported to have a very poor ability to suppress estrus in mares.[11] As with MPA, short- and long-term safety studies have not been conducted in horses.

Melengestrol Acetate

Melengestrol acetate (MGA, Pfizer, New York, NY), a synthetic progestin, is labeled as a feed additive for estrous suppression in cattle. However, when fed to mares at 10 to 20 mg/day for up to 15 days or at 500 mg/day for up to 10 days, it failed to suppress estrus.[7,11] Neely[14] suggested higher doses (>100 mg/day) may be more effective. No information is available on the short- and long-term safety of MGA use in horses. Very little use of MGA for estrous suppression in mares is currently reported by surveyed veterinarians.

Implants

A variety of progestin-containing implants, labeled and marketed for use in other species, have been used in mares with an intent of suppressing estrus. The most widely used has been the Synovex S (Peptech, Macquarie Park, NSW, Australia) implants. Labeled for increasing feed efficiency in steers, each dose of 8 pellets contains 200 mg progesterone and 20 mg estradiol benzoate, which is slowly absorbed over months. McCue et al[15] were unable to suppress estrus or cyclicity in mares with 80 Synovex S pellets (10 times the labeled dose for steers). This is understandable considering Loy and Swan[7] reported 100 mg or greater of progesterone in oil was required on a daily basis to suppress estrus in mares. Absorption of progesterone from Synovex S implants over extended periods will provide far less than the equivalent of 100 mg/day. Nevertheless, surveyed veterinarians report recommending Synovex S at doses ranging from 8 to 80 pellets and implanted every 1 to 6 months. Veterinarians are widely split on the response to treatment that they report observing. Some report not observing any effect and no longer offer it as a service, whereas others report estrous suppression for up to 6 months. Veterinarians report implanting the pellets subcutaneously in a variety of locations, including the pectoral region, under the mane, and in the vulva. A major drawback to using the implants is the potential for inflammation and scar tissue at the site of administration. Short- and long-term safety of Synovex use in mares has not been evaluated.

An implantable norgestomet pellet and intramuscular injectable combination of norgestomet/estradiol valerate (Crestar, Intervet Australia, Bendigo East Victoria, Australia) is marketed for estrous suppression or preventing ovulation in mares, even when up to 5 norgestomet pellets were simultaneously implanted.[11,16-18] Nevertheless, some veterinarians recommend it at 1 pellet (6 mg) per 500 lb of body weight in mares. No reports on the response to treatment were provided. Safety has not been evaluated.

Levonorgestrel (Norplant, Wyeth, Collegeville, PA), an implantable progestin, is used as a contraceptive in women with an ultralong duration of action of up to 5 years. Interest in levonorgestrel for suppressing estrus was expressed by some surveyed veterinarians; however, no information was available regarding dose, frequency, response, or safety.

Zeranol (Ralgro, Schering-Plough, Kenilworth, NJ), an implantable anabolic agent, is marketed as a growth stimulant for beef cattle. Surveyed veterinarians reported minimal use of zeranol for suppression of estrus in mares. Doses ranged from 1 to 3 pellets (12 to 36 mg) per mare. All reports indicated it was ineffective for suppressing estrus.

Intrauterine Device

There is evidence to suggest placing a glass marble in the uterus will suspend cyclicity and suppress estrus in some mares. Cyclicity is suspended by endogenously produced progesterone as luteal function is extended following a normal diestrus. A Dutch veterinarian reported estrous suppression in approximately 75% of the mares in which a glass marble was placed.[19] However, only 40% of mares experienced extended luteal function and estrous suppression in work recently completed by this author.[20,21] Luteal function was maintained for approximately 90 days before the mare cycled again. Follow-up work showed that there was no detrimental effect to the uterus or fertility by the glass marble. The biggest disadvantage is that it does not appear to work in the majority of mares. In fact, the efficacy of a glass marble for extending luteal function appears only to be moderate. However, if it does work in a given mare, it offers several advantages. First, it takes advantage of natural progesterone production. Second, it is inexpensive. Finally and most importantly, the luteal function appears to last for approximately 3 months.

The protocol for using a glass marble to suppress estrus in mares is relatively simple. As with any long-term progestin protocol, the mare should be evaluated for uterine inflammation before treating. First, a glass marble (http://www.glassmarble.com), 35 mm in diameter, is sterilized by autoclaving. Avoid breakage by autoclaving at a temperature of 250°F (121°C) and pressure of 16 psi, without a prevacuum or dry-cycle and a slow cool-down phase. The mare is positioned in late estrus or within 24 hours after ovulation, while the cervix is relaxed. The perineum is prepared as for any clean procedure. A sterilized sleeve is donned, and a small amount of sterile lubricant applied to the back of the hand. The marble is manually carried through the vagina to the caudal os of the cervix and placed in the lumen. Using a finger, the marble is pushed forward to the caudal uterine body. After removing the hand from the vagina, locate the ball per rectum and push it forward to the horn-body junction if it has not already moved to that position. After the ball is placed, the uterus can be infused with antibiotics and the mare treated with oxytocin if there is concern about uterine contamination during the procedure.

In order to remove the glass marble from the uterus, position the mare in peak estrus. Occasionally a mare may require sedation during the removal procedure. Mares with pendulous horns present the most difficulty. Removal is accomplished by manipulating the glass marble, per rectum, caudally toward the cervix, through the cervix, and then to the vulva for retrieval. If the cervix is not fully dilated, a gloved hand is taken per vagina to the caudal cervical os and the glass marble retrieved from the lumen.

Glucocorticoids

There are conflicting reports about the ability of glucocorticoids to suppress estrus in mares.[22–24] Asa and Ginther[23] reported administering dexamethasone (30 mg/day) to mares starting on day 10 after ovulation. Estrus was suppressed in 7 of 8 mares compared with control mares. In contrast, McKinnon et al[24] were unable to prevent follicular development or suppress estrus when dexamethasone was administered late in estrus. Though there is some evidence of efficacy, undesirable side effects potentially associated with long-term use would suggest caution when using glucocorticoids to suppress estrus. None of the surveyed veterinarians reported using glucocorticoids as a method of suppressing estrus in mares.

Gonadotropin-Releasing Hormone (GnRH)

Deslorelin acetate (Ovuplant, Fort Dodge), a potent GnRH analogue, will induce ovulation in estrual mares with follicles greater than 35 mm in diameter.[12,25] Implanting a double dose (two 2.1 mg Ovuplant implants) of deslorelin acetate will suspend cyclicity in most mares, suppressing follicular development for 30 days or more.[26] Cyclicity was rapidly suspended in 50% and 80% of mares treated with 10 or 20 mg of deslorelin acetate on the longest day of the year, respectively.[27] Mares resumed normal cycling the following season. Fitzgerald et al[28] reported suppressing ovulation for 30 to 90 days in 15 of 20 mares that were treated with multiple doses of another GnRH analogue (goserelin acetate). Based on this information, treating mares with repeated doses of a potent GnRH analogue may be beneficial for suspending cyclicity and suppressing estrus in mares for extended periods.

Surgical

Ovariectomy is recommended in some circumstances for suppressing estrus in mares. The ovaries can be removed through a ventral abdominal or flank laparotomy, laparoscopy, or a colpotomy.[29-32] Cyclicity will certainly cease with removal of the ovaries; however, estrous behavior may not. Unlike other species that require elevated estrogen levels to stimulate estrous behavior, mares can display behavioral signs of estrus in the absence of progesterone and in spite of low estrogen levels.[1] This phenomenon should be considered when weighing the advantages and disadvantages of ovariectomy. This option offers an advantage of being a permanent solution to a cycle-related behavior/performance problem; however, there are significant disadvantages as well. The procedure is expensive, though when compared to repeated hormonal treatments may in fact be less costly. There are also risks associated with the surgical procedure, though newer laparoscopic procedures have significantly reduced them. The permanency of the procedure can also be a significant disadvantage because all possibility for future reproduction is eliminated. If the behavior/performance problem is truly related to estrus, removing the ovaries may not solve the problem if the mare continues to display behavioral signs of estrus. This option should be weighed carefully before proceeding.

Immunologic

Immunizing a mare against GnRH would eliminate the stimulus for gonadotropin release from the pituitary, resulting in suspension of cyclicity. Tshewang et al[33] reported successfully suspending ovarian activity and suppressing estrus for 25 to 30 weeks in mares after treating with a GnRH vaccine. All of the vaccinated mares recovered from the effect of immunization with normal cyclicity and estrous behavior. Over the next two seasons, each mare also conceived and produced a normal foal. It appears immunization against GnRH is effective, safe, and reversible. Several other groups around the world are also working on vaccines against GnRH as a means of suppressing estrus in mares. Currently there is a GnRH vaccine (Equity, Pfizer Australia, West Ryde NSW, Australia) available for use in Australia. Equity is marketed as "not for use in animals intended for breeding," presumably to avoid litigation with clients who have mares that fail to conceive (for other reasons) after using the vaccine.[27] A mare is vaccinated twice, 30 days apart, and the response is reported as excellent.[27]

Other Methods

A number of dietary supplements are promoted for the treatment of cycle-related behavior/performance problems in mares. Products currently on the market contain various herbs, spices, prebiotics/probiotics, and food stuffs. However, there is little or no scientific evidence supporting the marketing claims. The existence of these products is mentioned only for completeness.

Claims are also made for the use of physical therapy/massage and acupuncture. Again there is little or no documented evidence to support these claims. These types of treatments may be beneficial in cases where a very specific and clearly defined problem exists but are questionable at best for a general and nonspecific problem.

PLAN FOR DEALING WITH A SUSPECTED CYCLE-RELATED BEHAVIOR/ PERFORMANCE PROBLEM

First, the problem should be well defined by all parties involved working in concert to benefit the mare. All non–cycle-related problems including behavioral stereotypies should be identified and treated to avoid attempts to mask more serious sources of pain or irritation in a mare simply for human benefit. Once a behavior/ performance problem is confidently defined as cycle-related, methods of suppressing estrus can be evaluated for effect and advantage. Currently the two most plausible methods to suspend cyclicity are progestins or spaying.

As mentioned, spaying a mare has a number of significant disadvantages. In spite of the risks and disadvantages of spaying, if an owner wants to proceed, a veterinarian can determine whether the procedure will be effective or not. The inactive state of ovaries during the nonbreeding season (anestrus) is analogous to the absence of ovaries in a spayed mare. Therefore it is advisable to evaluate the behavior/performance problem in a mare during anestrus before proceeding with an ovariectomy. If the problem is not resolved or at least significantly improved during anestrus, it is unlikely ovariectomy with be of any advantage.

Cyclicity can be effectively suspended by administering progestins to mares. There is ample evidence that altrenogest is a very effective progestin for suspending cyclicity and suppressing behavioral signs of estrus. Therefore, if an owner decides progestins are the most acceptable way to suspend cyclicity in the mare, a veterinarian would be advised to try altrenogest first. If it is effective at suppressing behavioral signs of estrus and alleviating the behavior/performance problem, a decision can be made to continue or not. If the owner objects to routinely using altrenogest, other progestins that are more satisfactory to the owner can be evaluated. However, if the behavior/performance problem continues in spite of suppression of behavioral signs of estrus with altrenogest, it is highly unlikely that other progestins will be effective.

CONCLUSION

The major objections to approved and effective means of suppressing behavioral signs of estrus, such as altrenogest, are expense and inconvenience. However, veterinarians would be well advised to carefully evaluate the available evidence for efficacy and consider all safety issues before recommending unlabeled progestins to their clients for suppressing estrus in mares. In some cases, when extensive evaluation of a behavior/performance problem in a mare rules out other causes, progestin treatment may be beneficial. Perhaps progestins have some calming effect that is not easily detected. Regardless, hormonal treatments of cycle-related behavior/performance problems need to be investigated using blinded, controlled study designs. Treatments should be evaluated for dose, frequency, response, safety/side effects, and reversibility. Until such work is reported, responsible use of unlabeled hormonal products in our client mares dictates that we follow up with an objective evaluation of response to treatment. Veterinarians and owners should also consider that when hormones are used to suppress estrus in mares, especially in combination or for extended periods of time, it is highly likely an individually variable period will be required for normal estrous cycles to resume.

Perhaps in time, methods that are more satisfactory will be developed. Immunization against GnRH seems to hold such promise.

References

1. McDonnell S: Mare madness. The Horse Interactive 2000; April:1.
2. McDonnell S: Estrous cycle-related performance problems. J Equine Vet Sci 1997; 17:196.
3. Squires EL, Stevens WB, McGlothlin DE et al: Effect of an oral progestin on the estrous cycle and fertility of mares. J Anim Sci 1979; 49:729.
4. Webel SK: Estrus control in horses with a progestin. J Anim Sci 1975; 41:385.
5. Shidler RK, Voss JL, Aufderheide WM et al: The effect of altrenogest, an oral progestin, on hematologic and bio-

chemical parameters in mares. Vet Hum Toxicol 1983; 25:250.

6. Squires EL, Shidler RK, Voss JL et al: Clinical applications of progestin in mares. Comp Cont Educ Pract Vet 1983; 5:516.

7. Loy RG, Swan SM: Effects of exogenous progestogens on reproductive phenomena in mares. J Anim Sci 1966; 25:821.

8. Hawkins DL, Neely DP, Stabenfeldt GH: Plasma progesterone concentrations derived from the administration of exogenous progesterone to ovariectomized mares. J Reprod Fertil Suppl 1979; 27:211.

9. Ganjam VK, Kenney RM, Flickinger G: Effect of exogenous progesterone on its endogenous levels: biological half-life of progesterone and lack of progesterone binding in mares. J Reprod Fertil Suppl 1975; 23:183.

10. Squires EL: Use of progestins in open and pregnant mares. Anim Reprod Sci 1993; 33:183.

11. McKinnon AO, Lescun TB, Walker JH et al: The inability of some synthetic progestogens to maintain pregnancy in the mare. Equine Vet J 2000; 32:83.

12. McKinnon AO, Nobelius AM, Figuerosa STD et al: Predictable ovulation in mares treated with an implant of the GnRH analogue deslorelin. Equine Vet J 1993; 25:321.

13. Nobelius AM: Gestagens in the mare: an appraisal of the effects of gestagenic steroids on suppression of oestrus in mares. MSc Thesis, Melbourne, Australia, Monash University, 1992.

14. Neely DP: Progesterone/progestin therapy in the broodmare. Proceedings of the 34th Annual Convention of the American Association of Equine Practitioners, p 203, 1988.

15. McCue PM, Lemons SS, Squires EL et al: Efficacy of Synovex-S implants in suppression of estrus in the mare. J Equine Vet Sci 1997; 17:327.

16. Bristol F: Studies on estrous synchronization in mares. Proceedings of the Society for Theriogenology, p 258, 1981.

17. Scheffran NS, Wiseman BS, Vincent DL: Reproductive hormone secretions in pony mares subsequent to ovulation control during late winter. Theriogenology 1982; 17:571.

18. Wiepz GJ, Squires EL, Chapman PL: Effects of norgestomet, altrenogest and/or estradiol on follicular and hormonal characteristics of late transitional mares. Theriogenology 1988; 30:181.

19. de Greef RJ: Personal communication. March 19, 2000.

20. Nie GJ, Johnson KE, Wenzel JGW: Use of a glass ball to suppress behavioral estrus in mares. Proceedings of the 47th Annual Convention of the American Association of Equine Practitioners, p 246, 2001.

21. Nie GJ, Johnson KE, Braden TD et al: Use of an intra-uterine glass ball protocol to extend luteal function in mares. J Equine Vet Sci 2003; 23:266.

22. Cunningham GR, Goldzieher JW, de la Pena A et al: The mechanism of ovulation inhibition by triamcinolone acetonide. J Clin Endocrinol Metab 1978; 46:8.

23. Asa CS, Ginther OJ: Glucocorticoid suppression of oestrus, follicles, LH and ovulation in the mare. J Reprod Fertil Suppl 1982; 32:247.

24. McKinnon AO, Perriam WJ, Lescun TB et al: Effect of GnRH analogue (Ovuplant), hCG and dexamethasone on time to ovulation in cycling mares. World Equine Vet Rev 1997; 2:6.

25. Mumford EL, Squires EL, Jochle E et al: Use of deslorelin short-term implants to induce ovulation in cycling mare during three consecutive estrous cycles. Anim Reprod Sci 39:129, 1995.

26. McCue PM, Farquhar VJ, Squires EL: Effect of the GnRH agonist deslorelin acetate on pituitary function and follicular development in the mare. Proceedings of the 46th Annual Convention of the American Association of Equine Practitioners, p 355, 2000.

27. McKinnon AO: Personal communication. August 21, 2001.

28. Fitzgerald BP, Peterson KD, Silvia PJ: Effect of constant administration of a gonadotropin-releasing hormone agonist on reproductive activity in mares: preliminary evidence on suppression of ovulation during the breeding season. Am J Vet Res 1993; 54:1746.

29. Rodgerson DH, Belknap JK, Wilson DA: Laparoscopic ovariectomy using sequential electrocoagulation and sharp transaction of the equine mesovarium. Vet Surg 2001; 30:572.

30. Ross MW: Standing abdominal surgery. Vet Clin North Am Equine Pract 1991; 7:627.

31. Slone DE: Ovariectomy, ovariohysterectomy, and cesarean section in mares. Vet Clin North Am Equine Pract 1988; 4:451.

32. Hooper RN, Taylor TS, Varner DD et al: Effect of bilateral ovariectomy via colpotomy in mares: 23 cases (1984-1990). J Am Vet Med Assoc 1993; 203:1043.

33. Tshewang U, Dowsett KF, Knott LM et al: Preliminary study of ovarian activity in fillies treated with a GnRH vaccine. Aust Vet J 1997; 75:663.

CHAPTER 5

The Normal Uterus in Estrus

JUAN C. SAMPER
JONATHAN F. PYCOCK

Once the mare has entered the ovulatory season, the estrous cycle is on average 22 days long. The follicular phase, or estrus, typically lasts 5 to 7 days, and the luteal phase, or diestrus, lasts 14 to 16 days. Enormous variability, however, has been recognized in the number of days during which mares exhibit estrus, particularly early in the breeding season, when standing heat can be prolonged for weeks. The variation between mares is mostly due to differences in duration of estrous behavior, rather than in diestrus—depending on the mare and the time of the year, estrous behavior can last from 24 hours to several days.

Pregnancy rates are maximized when normal mares are bred within 72 hours before ovulation with a fertile stallion. For mares bred artificially, insemination should be performed within 12 to 24 hours before ovulation when chilled semen is used and within 8 hours when frozen semen is used. Accordingly, a very important aspect of the practitioner's job in working with broodmares is careful and well-timed examination to ensure that the animals are suitable to breed, to determine the stage of the estrous cycle, and to predict ovulation so that each mare is bred in a timely fashion. A wide range of parameters are used to estimate the time of ovulation and thus the optimal time for breeding.

Circulating concentrations of estrogen and progesterone have been well documented for the estrous cycle of the mare and reviewed by Ginther.[1] Most of the cyclic changes in the reproductive tract of the mare are under the control of the ovarian steroids. The changes during estrus and diestrus are due to the presence of the ovarian steroid that predominates during a given phase of the cycle—that is, estrogen and progesterone, respectively. In mares, estradiol is thought to be responsible for estrous behavior,[2] and estrogen concentrations during estrus correlate well with sexual behavior and grossly observable changes in the reproductive tract. During diestrus, when circulating levels of progesterone are greater than 2 ng/ml, estrus is inhibited, and the mare is aggressive toward the stallion. During estrus, progesterone concentrations in plasma are less than 1 ng/ml.[1] The effects of progesterone on behavior and morphologic characteristics of the uterus are reported to be dominant over the effects of estrogen.[3]

For the most part, estrus in mares that are at breeding farms is detected by exposing the mare to a stallion (teasing) and observing the typical squat and wink of estrus. The introduction of transrectal ultrasonography to visualize the reproductive tract in mares[4] has allowed study of cyclic changes in tissue morphology. Both the ovaries and the uterus need to be examined thoroughly at every examination of a mare. One of the most striking characteristics visualized at ultrasonography is the appearance of the endometrium during the estrous cycle. During diestrus in a normal mare, individual endometrial folds are not routinely detected, and the uterus has a homogeneous echotexture. The lumen of the body of the uterus often is visible as a white line formed by specular reflections at the closely apposed luminal surfaces, in marked contrast with the features typically seen during estrus, when individual endometrial folds can be visualized.[5] It is thought that endometrial folds become edematous during estrus as a result of increased concentrations of circulating estrogen.[6] These changes give a heterogeneous image, with the dense central portions of the folds appearing echogenic and the edematous portions of the folds represented by nonechogenic areas. When the uterine horn is imaged in cross section, the appearance suggests a sliced orange or wagon wheel (Figure 5-1).

Occasionally, free estrous fluid can be imaged. It also is possible to grade the degree of endometrial edema; this concept was introduced by Ginther and Pierson[5] and later developed by Squires et al.[7] The endometrial edema scores have been found to reflect changes in circulating estrogen and progesterone concentrations and to correlate with sexual behavior scores.[6] Endometrial folds first become visible at the end of diestrus, become more prominent as estrus progresses, and generally diminish from approximately 2 days from ovulation until the day of ovulation, when edema may have disappeared. This sequence is supported by three studies that used Thoroughbred and Standardbred or pony-type mares.[5,8,9] However, one recent study using Belgian Draft mares reported that peak edema was detected at 6.6 days before ovulation and abruptly regressed at 5.5 days before ovulation.[10] Breed differences may therefore be important for veterinarians to take into account.

The interpretation of endometrial morphologic characteristics on ultrasound examination constitutes an important part of establishing an accurate estimate of the stage of the estrus cycle. The appearance of edema precedes the onset of estrous behavior by 1, 2, or 3 days, although estrous behavior generally persists for 24 to 48 hours after edema has disappeared. In many instances, mares are presented for examination when they are in their first day of standing estrus. On ultrasonography the absence of a corpus luteum in the ovaries should be confirmed, and the presence of any follicle larger than 25 mm in diameter should be noted. Single follicles or a small number of nonadjacent follicles in an ovary usually retain their spherical shape until they are greater than 40 mm in size and within 48 hours of ovulation. Accurate measurement of the follicle is important to monitor its growth. When the follicle size is measured accurately, diameter correlates well with volume while the follicle remains spherical. Ovulation usually occurs when follicular size reaches 40 mm or greater and rarely occurs at a follicular size of less than 35 mm.

In our experience, none of these factors are consistently reliable for making practical estimates of the timing of ovulation. In some instances, changes in shape or echogenicity are not seen, even close to ovulation. Follicular size at ovulation also is variable: Some mares will ovulate off small (35-mm) follicles, whereas other mares do not ovulate until follicular size is 50 mm or more. It is important to use all of the parameters in combination to make the decision; serial examinations at 24- or 48-hour intervals are recommended.

The ability to predict ovulation can be improved by observing the pattern of endometrial edema.[9] It is possible to grade the degree of endometrial edema detected using a subjective scoring system of 0 to 5, presented in Box 5-1. Figures 5-2 to 5-5 show the various grades of uterine edema.

Endometrial edema first becomes visible at the end of diestrus, becomes more prominent as estrus progresses, and generally decreases from 48 to 24 hours before ovulation (Figures 5-6 and 5-7). Edema may be detectable on the day of ovulation but is always of lesser degree than at some point earlier during estrus; in any case, edema should not persist more than 36 hours after ovulation.[11] Mares will respond most predictably to ovulation-inducing agents when such agents are given at the time

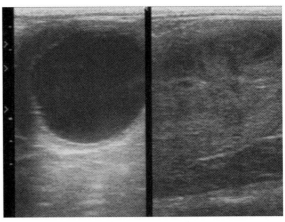

Figure 5-2 An ultrasound image of the uterine horn with edema grade 2, obtained using a 5-7.5 MHz transducer. Notice that the endometrial folds are clearly defined within the uterine horn, in contrast with grade 1.

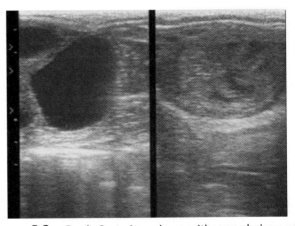

Figure 5-3 Grade 3 uterine edema with very obvious edematous uterine folds and the associated large follicle indicative of estrus. Distortion of follicular shape is due to pressure from smaller follicles on either side of the larger follicle.

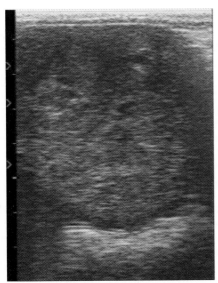

Figure 5-1 An ultrasound image of the uterine horn with edema grade 1, obtained using a 5 to 7.5 MHz transducer during estrus. Edema is barely detectable within the endometrium.

Box 5-1

Subjective Scoring System for Endometrial Edema

0 No edema, with a typical homogeneous echotexture characteristic of diestrus
1 Smallest amount of readily detectable uterine edema
2 Moderate amount of edema, heavier in the uterine body
3 Obvious edema throughout the entire uterus
4 Maximal amount of normal edema detected throughout the uterus; small amount of free fluid sometimes detected in the lumen; edema heavier in uterine body
5 Abnormal uterine edema characterized by irregular and disorganized uterine edema

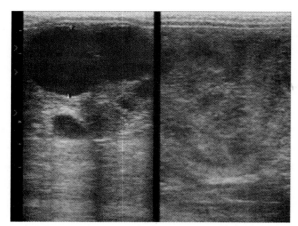

Figure 5-4   Grade 4 uterine edema, Notice the hyperechoic borders of the uterine folds and the hypoechoic body of the folds.

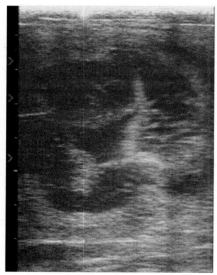

Figure 5-5   Abnormal uterine edema detected on the uterine horn. Notice the distorted pattern, the thickness of the folds, and a slight amount of free fluid within the uterine lumen.

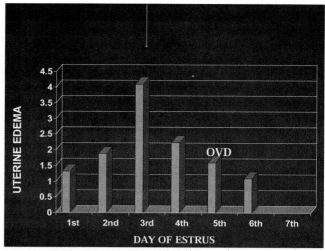

Figure 5-6   Normal pattern of uterine edema in mares during the estrous period. *Arrow* indicates time of treatment with an ovulation-inducing agent.

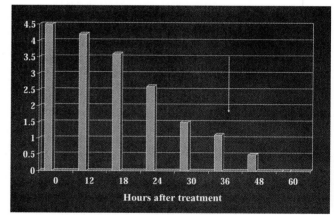

Figure 5-7   Decrease in the pattern of uterine edema in normal mares treated with an ovulation-inducing agent at time 0. *Arrow* indicates average time of ovulation.

maximal edema is recognized, together with an open cervix and follicular size greater than 35 mm. The appearance of edema preceded the beginning of estrous behavior by 1, 2, or 3 days, although estrous behavior generally persisted 1 day after edema disappeared.

Uterine edema is associated with basal (<1.0 ng/ml) progesterone values. It seems reasonable, therefore, to attribute edema to increasing circulating estrogen concentrations. Detection of endometrial edema is thus a reliable indicator of estrus in the mare. This finding is particularly useful in mares that cannot be teased with a stallion or that do not respond to teasing. Many mares may be kept at premises where no teasing facilities are available and the veterinarian needs to be able to diagnose a true follicular phase in the absence of any teasing infor-

mation. Nonhormonal influences such as endometrial swabbing, uterine infusions, breeding, or the presence of air or urine also can stimulate uterine edema, however. In addition, mares at the first estrus post partum ("foal heat") have a more intense endometrial edema pattern, which may not decline as much as at subsequent estrous periods as ovulation approaches (Figure 5-8).

The usefulness of assessment of endometrial edema in the breeding management of mares can be summarized as follows. Frequently a mare is presented for breeding when she is in standing heat. Veterinarians often are puzzled about when to breed these mares, particularly when they should be bred to a heavily booked stallion. The degree of uterine edema combined with follicular size is an important marker to determine when these mares should be bred. Low score of uterine edema (1 to 2) in the presence of a large follicle, often greater than 40 mm diameter, is a good indication of imminent ovulation. On

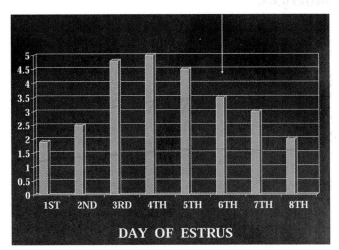

Figure 5-8 Abnormal pattern of uterine edema during estrus in mares. Notice that mares with abnormal patterns already have marked edema on the first day of estrus, and that ovulation (*arrow*) occurs without the normal edema reduction observed in normal mares.

the other hand, low SEE with follicular size less than 38 mm is suggestive of early estrus. Furthermore, the presence of uterine edema is the most reliable indicator of heat in the normal mare, even when she does not respond to teasing or a teaser is not available. Mares presented to a breeding farm often are in diestrus. It is not uncommon, however, for these mares to have large-size follicles on one or both ovaries. The absence of uterine edema together with a tight cervix generally constitutes an indication that the mare is in diestrus. Such mares often are given prostaglandin to induce their heat. The appearance of endometrial edema in these mares will depend on the size of the follicle at the time of treatment. Mares with follicular size greater than 30 mm will display uterine edema sooner than those mares with smaller follicles.

Mares that are susceptible to persistent postbreeding endometritis may ovulate with endometrial edema scores higher than normal. Susceptibility to postbreeding endometritis is known to involve fluid accumulation and possible lymphatic stasis, so it is not surprising that edema scores are not as reliable in this category of mares.

In conclusion, the timing of ovulation in the mare is a key skill for the practitioner working with mares to acquire. Detection of the pattern of endometrial edema, along with accurate assessment of follicle size, shape, and texture, constitutes the most helpful approach to deter-mine the appropriate time to breed or inseminate the mare. Ideally, these examinations should be performed on a regular basis.

References

1. Ginther OJ: Endocrinology of the ovulatory season. In Reproductive Biology of the Mare, ed 2, Wisconsin, Equiservices, pp 233-290, 1993a.
2. Nett TM: Oestrogens. In McKinnon AO, Voss JL (eds): Equine Reproduction, Philadelphia, Lea & Febiger, pp 65-68, 1993.
3. Daels PF, Hughes JP: The normal oestrous cycle. In McKinnon AO, Voss JL (eds): Equine Reproduction, Philadelphia, Lea & Febiger, pp 121-133, 1993.
4. Palmer E, Driancourt M: Use of ultrasonic echography in equine gynaecology. Theriogenology 1980; 13:203-216.
5. Ginther OJ, Pierson RA: Ultrasonic anatomy and pathology of the equine uterus. Theriogenology 1994; 2:505-516.
6. Hayes KEN, Pierson RA, Scraba ST, Ginther OJ: Effects of oestrous cycle and season on ultrasonic uterine anatomy in mares. Theriogenology 1985; 24:465-477.
7. Squires, E.L., McKinnon, A.O. and Shideler, R.K. (1988) Use of ultrasonography in reproductive management of mares. Theriogenology 1988; 29:55-70.
8. McKinnon AO, Squires EL, Carnevale EM et al: Diagnostic ultrasonography of uterine pathology in the mare. Proceedings of the 33rd Annual Convention of the American Association of Equine Practitioners, pp 605-622, 1988.
9. Samper JC: Ultrasonographic appearance and the pattern of uterine edema to time ovulation in mares. Proceedings of the 43rd Annual Convention of the American Association of Equine Practitioners, pp 189-191, 1997.
10. Plata-Madrid H, Youngquist RS, Murphy CN et al: Ultrasonographic characteristics of the follicular and uterine dynamics in Belgian mares. J Eq Vet Sci 1994; 14:421-423.
11. Pycock JF, Dieleman S, Drifjhout P et al: Correlation of plasma concentrations of progesterone and estradiol with ultrasound characteristics of the uterus and duration of estrous behavior in the cycling mare. Reprod Dom Animals 1995; 30:224.

Suggested Reading

Ginther OJ: Characteristics of the ovulatory season. In Reproductive Biology of the Mare, ed 2nd, Wisconsin, Equiservices, pp 173-233, 1993b.
Munro CD, Renton JP, Butcher R: The control of oestrous behaviour in the mare. J Reprod Fertil Suppl 1979; 27:217-227.
Nelson EM, Kiefer BL, Roser JF, Evans JW: Serum oestradiol-17 concentrations during spontaneous silent oestrus and after prostaglandin treatment in the mare. Theriogenology 1985; 23:241-262.

CHAPTER 6

Intrauterine Diagnostic Procedures

PATRICIA L. SERTICH

The character of the uterus is influenced by the reproductive status of the mare and the stage of the estrous cycle. Many of these changes are influenced by the presence of hormones. Dramatic changes occur during pregnancy and uterine involution. Thorough evaluation of the uterus is necessary to assess the status and predict the function of the uterus.

ANATOMY

The uterus has a single, relatively large uterine body and two uterine horns separated by a short septum at the bifurcation of the horns. The uterus is suspended in the broad ligament that is composed of smooth muscle and contains arteries, veins, lymphatic vessels, and nerves. The arteries supplying blood to the uterus are the uterine branch of the vaginal artery (caudal uterine artery), the uterine artery (middle uterine artery), and the uterine branch of the ovarian artery (cranial uterine artery). These three arteries form prominent anastomoses and contribute to arterial arches near the mesometrial attachment.[1] The uterine veins follow a similar course relative to the uterine arteries. The uterine artery (middle uterine artery) is the largest uterine artery and the main supplier of blood to the uterus, whereas the main venous drainage of the uterus is via the uterine branch of the ovarian artery (cranial uterine vein). Interstitial fluid drains from the uterus through the lymphatic vessels and lymph glands to the thoracic duct that empties into the venous system near the heart. The uterus does not have sensory fibers and therefore does not require anesthesia locally for surgical biopsy. Pelvic nerves have parasympathetic fibers coming from the sacral area. Hypogastric nerves and the pelvic plexus supply sympathetic innervations from the caudal mesenteric ganglion that is located near the origin of the caudal mesenteric artery. These nerves join branches of the sacral nerves.[2] The broad ligament is divided into indistinct regions defined by the part of the genital tract that it supports; the mesovarian supports the ovary, the mesosalpinx supports the oviduct, and the mesometrium supports the uterus. The uterus has several layers that from lumen to serosal surface include the luminal epithelium, endometrium composed of the stratum compactum and the stratum spongiosum, longitudinal muscle layer, circular muscle layer, and the perimetrium or serosal surface. Five to seven folds of endometrium are present in the collapsed uterus. These endometrial folds are arranged longitudinally and extend through the uterine body and cervix.

MARE RESTRAINT

The restraint necessary for most of the uterine diagnostic procedures that will be discussed in this chapter can be accomplished in most broodmares with simple standing restraint using a halter and lead shank. The horse handler should stand on the same side as the examiner, such that a left-handed examiner would stand to the right of the mare's hindquarters and the handler at the mare's head would also stand to the right or off side of the mare. Alternately, a right-handed examiner would stand to the left of the mare's hindquarters and the handler at the mare's head would stand to the left or near side of the mare. Positioning a mare in a stall doorway such that the body of the mare is against the wall of the stall and the hindquarters of the mare are just outside the door threshold may help keep a restless mare in position for the examination. The examiner can then stand behind the outside wall of the neighboring stall and reach over to the mare's hindquarters. Fractious mares may be distracted with the use of a nose twitch. Palpation stocks can be used to contain mares and appear to offer some protection from kicks, but the examiner must remain alert because severe injury may be sustained should a mare suddenly squat or kick out with both hind legs. Fractious or anxious mares may require sedation if there is significant risk that the mare or examiner will be injured. A combination of acepromazine (0.02 mg/kg) and xylazine (0.6 mg/kg) administered intravenously often provides sufficient relaxation for an adequate length of time to ease examination. Lengthy procedures may require a longer-acting sedative such as detomidine intravenously (0.01 to 0.02 mg/kg).[3] An attempt to assess the perineal conformation of the mare should be made before sedation, because the tranquilizers will dramatically relax the perineum, causing it to appear incompetent.

Tail hairs should be contained in a tail wrap or plastic bag that is secured to the tail by taping the bag to the base of the tail, being sure to enclose all the stray hairs. The tail can be tied using a quick-release knot or held to the side.

Palpation Per Rectum

Most mares are large enough to allow examination of the internal genital tract by palpation per rectum. The examiner should don a plastic shoulder-length examination sleeve and generously lubricate the forearm that will be used for the examination. Most commonly a nonsterile methylcellulose water-based lubricant is used. All feces must be removed from the rectum at the time of the internal examination. The uterine body is difficult to access adequately because it is bounded by the broad ligament. The entire length of each uterine horn should be systematically allowed to slip between the examiner's opposing thumb and forefingers and a conscious note be made of the palpable presence of the endometrial folds. The endometrial folds should be palpable in the nonpregnant mare. The character of the pregnant mare's uterine wall changes remarkably as early as 14 to 16 days after ovulation so that the endometrial folds are no longer palpable in the pregnant mare. A nonpregnant status must be confirmed before conducting any intrauterine procedures, because most intrauterine procedures would be detrimental to the maintenance of that pregnancy. The position of the uterus may be within the pelvic canal or cranial and/or ventral to the pelvic brim. The diameter of the horns should be estimated manually and the presence of any cysts, uterine fluid, or uterine masses noted. The tone of the anestrous uterus tends to be flaccid because steroid ovarian hormones are not present at this time. Progesterone present during diestrus will cause an increase in the tone of the uterus, resulting in a round, firm, tubular character of the uterine horns. During estrus the uterus tends to become edematous and have a plump but less turgid character. The cervix and ovarian structures should be assessed at the time of uterine palpation, and the character of these structures should be consistent with the character of the uterus and the stage of the mare's estrous cycle.

Ultrasonography Per Rectum

A linear 5-mHz probe that allowed adequate depth of penetration (8 cm) has traditionally been used for transrectal ultrasonography of the genital tract. Superior probes are now available with greater resolution (5 MHz and 10 MHz) and still have at least 8 cm of penetration. Ultrasound equipment should be properly adjusted and maintained to produce optimal images. Stable positioning of the ultrasound machine at shoulder height in a dimly lit area will enhance the examiner's ability to view the image. The use of palpation stocks positioned near a grounded electrical outlet and a strong broad shelf or cart to support the ultrasound machine will allow comfortable and safe operation of the ultrasound equipment. Farms with a number of suckling mares may consider the construction of a stock with a small enclosure positioned at the front of the stock to allow mares to be close to their foals during the examination, which may decrease the anxiety associated with separation during the examination.

The density of the tissue will determine the echogenicity of the image produced. Clear fluid such as follicular fluid appears black or anechoic (without echo), because it does not produce an echo. Tissue is more echogenic or hyperechoic and appears lighter or gray. Denser structures appear hyperechoic and more white. The terms *hypere-*

choic and *hypoechoic* are used to describe structures that are lighter or darker gray, respectively, than the comparative tissue.

Ultrasonography per rectum can be best used after complete and thorough palpation per rectum.[4] All fecal material must be removed from the rectum during the examination. The footprint of the probe can be lubricated with nonsterile rectal lubricant. Upon entering the rectum with the ultrasound probe, one should locate the bladder and its neck because the urethra marks the caudal limit of the vagina. The presence of any material in the vagina (located dorsal to the bladder) should be noted. The cervix is not particularly distinct ultrasonographically. Each uterine horn should be systematically and consecutively examined in its entirety so that no portion of the uterus is overlooked. The diameter of each uterine horn can be measured ultrasonographically at its base. During estrus, edema of the endometrial folds appears hypoechoic and allows the folds to be seen more distinctly. A cross section of an estrous uterine horn has a spoked-wheel appearance because each fold projects towards the center or lumen of the horn. Although a very slight amount of anechoic uterine fluid may be seen in the uterine lumen during estrus normally, most accumulations of fluid not associated with pregnancy are considered abnormal and may be a clinical sign of endometritis. The character of uterine fluid may range from anechoic to quite hyperechoic. Unfortunately, there is not a direct correlation between echogenicity of the fluid and severity of the abnormality. Air mixed with uterine fluid, as seen in pneumometra, causes bright white lines or hyperechoic flecks in hypoechoic fluid. Equine urine is quite hyperechoic due to the urine crystals and mucus typically present. Therefore urine present in the uterus would appear hyperechoic. The uterine fluid associated with a hydrometra due to segmental aplasia of the tubular genital tract or a nonpatent hymen may appear anechoic. The fetal fluids seen in the pregnant uterus are black or anechoic during early gestation and are confined within the membranes of the conceptus.

Uterine cysts can be seen using ultrasonography per rectum as round to irregularly shaped anechoic structures within the uterus. The clinical significance of uterine cysts is not known, but it is thought that cysts that protrude into the uterine lumen as pedunculated or broad-based luminal cysts may interfere with the early migration of the less than 16-day equine embryo and probably should be removed. Although cysts located deep within the endometrium are likely to interfere with the surrounding endometrial gland function, their removal is likely to damage the surrounding endometrium and result in scar tissue because the equine endometrium is not known to be regenerative. The location of cysts can be determined by endoscopy or infusing the uterus with sterile saline and subsequently reexamining the uterus using ultrasonography per rectum. Luminal cysts will be obviously and clearly outlined by the infused fluid. Deep cysts will be surrounded by uterine tissue. Care should be taken to evacuate the exogenous fluid following the procedure by siphon or administration of a low dose (10 to 20 IU) of oxytocin.

Endometrial Microbiology—Aerobic Culture of an Endometrial Swab

An endometrial swab can be cultured aerobically to identify the causative agents associated with a uterine infection. The independent results of a culture of an endometrial swab rarely are sufficient to make an accurate diagnosis of endometritis. To make a diagnosis of clinically significant endometritis one must consider the reproductive history of the mare, the stage of the reproductive cycle (anestrus versus breeding season), stage of estrous cycle (estrus versus diestrus), previous uterine therapy or uterine manipulations (including breeding) and time interval since the uterine procedures, character of the uterus, and ultimately histologic evaluation of an endometrial biopsy sample. After considering all of these factors, a clinician must be confident with his or her swabbing technique, sample handling, and the competence of the microbiology laboratory because the decision to treat endometritis usually results in a significant financial investment, and inappropriate therapy is not without potential ill effects.

It has been shown that the normal caudal genital tract has a considerable number of different microorganisms present, including microorganisms known to be significant uterine pathogens such as β-hemolytic *Streptococcus zooepidemicus* and *Escherichia coli*.[5] Care must be taken to avoid harvesting microorganisms from the caudal genital tract (cervix, vagina, vestibule, clitoris) when procuring an endometrial swab. If examination or environmental conditions are not ideal, one may wish to perform the uterine swabbing while the mare is in estrus when uterine defenses (open cervix, increased cellular immunity) are optimal for dealing with iatrogenic contamination. Procurement of the swab during diestrus will allow detection of microorganisms that the mare was not able to eliminate on her own during estrus. Examination during diestrus also allows the examiner ideal conditions to thoroughly evaluate the mare's cervix for presence of a competent canal or cervical laceration while the cervix is closed and under the influence of progesterone. The mare should be restrained so that procedures will be safe for the mare and the examiner as described in the section on palpation per rectum. In addition, swabs should be obtained in as clean an environment as possible. This can be challenging in a farm situation. Avoid dusty areas near hay storage and drafts.

The mare's tail hairs should be secured in a tail wrap and the tail held to the side. The rectum should be emptied to reduce the chance of fecal elimination during the procedure. Regardless of history provided, it is the examiner's responsibility to determine that the mare is not pregnant. Intrauterine manipulations in a pregnant mare are likely to cause an abortion or ascending placentitis. The perineum should be washed thoroughly with povidone-iodine scrub solution, rinsed, and then patted dry with clean paper toweling. The examiner should wear a sterile examination sleeve or clean sleeve covered by a sterile surgical glove. A water-soluble lubricant that is free of bacteriostatic chemicals is placed on the dorsum of the hand and lower arm. A double-guarded, occluded uterine swab should be used to prevent contamination of the swab in the caudal genital tract.[6]

The double-guarded occluded swab is carefully carried through the caudal genital tract; the examiner's forefinger should be placed into the cervix and the culture instrument slid alongside the finger. Once the end of the outer guard is in the uterine body, the examiner's finger should be withdrawn into the vagina. The inner guard is pushed through the occlusion and outer guard, and then the swab tip is passed into the uterine body. Care should be taken to avoid excessive manipulation of the swap tip because some instruments are quite brittle and may snap from the tip. The swab should be left in the uterine lumen for 30 to 60 seconds to absorb uterine contents and then be retracted into the inner guard, the inner guard then retracted into the outer guard and only then removed from the genital tract. One should note the competency of the vulvar musculature, vestibulovaginal ring, and the cervix at this time. After withdrawal, the swab tip should be transferred into the transport medium for transport to the laboratory to maintain viability of any microorganisms. This can be smoothly done by placing the inner guard directly in the opening of the transport system and then sliding the swab directly into the medium without exposing the tip to the external environment. A transport medium such as modified Stuart's bacterial transport medium should preserve the microorganisms for 72 hours if maintained between 15° and 30° C. Laboratories usually streak the swabs on 5% sheep blood agar for general growth and MacConkey agar that selects for growth of gram-negative organisms and incubate the plates aerobically at 37° C. Incubation on Sabouraud agar should be requested to isolate fungal organisms if one suspects fungal endometritis. A sensitivity test should be performed on microorganisms that are isolated to determine which antibiotics might be effective against a uterine infection. The following microorganisms have been isolated from mares that have clinical evidence of endometritis:

β-hemolytic *Streptococcus* sp.—most commonly
Streptococcus zooepidemicus
Escherichia coli
Klebsiella pneumoniae
Pseudomonas aeruginosa
Pasturella sp.
Citrobacter sp.
Candida albicans
Candida parapsilosis

Other microorganisms isolated in moderate or heavy pure growth may be associated with an endometritis, but one would also expect to see other positive signs of infection such as uterine edema during diestrus, uterine fluid, uterine discharge, or chronic failure to establish pregnancy. In the absence of positive clinical signs of endometritis, the isolation of other microorganisms, particularly a mixed growth of a number of different bacteria, usually indicates that contamination of the uterine swab occurred.

Endometrial Cytology—Cytologic Evaluation of an Endometrial Swab

Cytologic evaluation of an endometrial swab is not a diagnostic substitute for the histologic evaluation of an endometrial biopsy sample, but it can be helpful when making a prompt decision regarding a mare's suitability for immediate breeding.[7] An endometrial swab is obtained using a double-guarded swab in a similar fashion, as one would obtain a swab for aerobic culture. A more cellular sample may be obtained if the endometrium is scraped gently with the swab tip. Care should be taken to avoid contaminating the sample with sterile lubricant, which can cause confusion with the interpretation of the smear. The swab tip is then rolled gently onto a clean glass micro slide. The specimen is fixed onto the slide immediately with methanol or other suitable cytology fixative or spray. Once fixed, the specimen is stable and can remain unstained for 24 to 48 hours. A simple cytology stain such as Diff-Quik produces good results (Protocol, Kalamazoo, MI). This stain set consists of just three reagents, the first of which is a cell fixative. Simply dip the fixed slide slowly into each reagent 7 times, being sure to blot the end of the slide between fluids onto absorbent paper. After the last reagent, gently rinse the back of the slide with distilled water to remove excess stain. The slide can be air-dried and viewed with a bright light microscope. Cell types can be identified with high, dry magnification (400×), but detection of bacteria may require oil immersion at 1000× magnification. Swabs of a normal endometrium will include predominantly columnar epithelial cells and occasional red blood cells. A few white blood cells, bacteria, yeasts, or urine crystals may be seen in a normal mare but should be considered potentially abnormal.

Inflammatory exudate consisting predominantly of neutrophils is seen in mares having an acute endometritis (Figure 6-1). Although the method of sample and slide preparation does not allow for accurate quantification of cell numbers, it is generally accepted that more than one neutrophil per five high-power fields (400×) is considered abnormal. There will be large numbers of neutrophils in endometrial swabs from mares with pyometra or acute suppurative endometritis. Bacteria and fungi may be seen inside or surrounding the neutrophils. A Gram's stain of a sample smear will allow differentiation of the gram-positive organisms from the gram-negative organisms. As only a few microorganisms are typically associated with equine endometritis, the character of the cell as seen when stained with Gram's stain can provide useful clinical information. The presence of chains of gram-positive cocci would be most consistent with a β-hemolytic *Streptococcus* sp., which is almost always sensitive to ampicillin or penicillin. Gram-negative microorganisms typically isolated from mares with endometritis include *E. coli, P. aeruginosa,* and *K. pneumoniae.* An accurate identification of the gram-negative organisms can be made on the basis of their colony morphology on aerobic culture and biochemical reactions. Antibiotic selection for the therapeutic plan must be based on the sensitivity of the cultured organisms to different antibiotics. Macrophages, lymphocytes, and neutrophils may be seen in mares with chronic endometritis. Mares with chronic fibrotic endometritis may have little changes evident on cytologic examination.

The presence of urinary crystals would suggest that urovagina and subsequent urometra is present. Definitive diagnosis of these conditions would require detection of urine in the vagina and uterus by laboratory methods or by vaginoscopy along with other clinical evidence such as inappropriate voiding patterns, perineal soiling, and chronic vaginal and uterine irritation.

Endometrial Histology—Histologic Evaluation of an Endometrial Biopsy Sample

An endometrial biopsy sample can provide histologic evidence of uterine inflammation and provide information regarding the chronicity, severity, and distribution of the endometritis. This information is useful in developing a therapeutic plan for managing the endometritis. Histologic evaluation of an endometrial biopsy sample can also reveal the presence of periglandular fibrosis, cystic glandular distension, and lymphatic lacunae. In the mare there is a correlation between the character of the endometrial glands and the ability of the endometrium to carry a foal to term.[8] The secretions of the endometrial glands may be more important in maintaining the equine conceptus because functional placentation occurs rather late in the mare as compared to the cow and ewe. It is thought that periglandular fibrosis may interfere with gland function and be detrimental to the survival of the embryo. Therefore the histologic evaluation of an endometrial biopsy sample has prognostic value in predicting a mare's ability to carry a foal to term.

An endometrial biopsy sample may be obtained at any time of the reproductive cycle of a nonpregnant mare. Samples can even be taken during estrus after breeding without interfering with pregnancy. Diestrous mares with a mature corpus luteum may experience luteolysis subsequent to the biopsy procedure. The mare should be restrained, its tail wrapped, rectum emptied, and the perineum cleansed. The pregnancy status of the mare must be ascertained because the biopsy procedure is contraindicated during pregnancy. The clinician should wear a clean or sterile shoulder-length examination sleeve

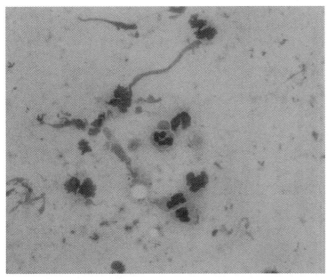

Figure 6-1 Neutrophils seen on a slide prepared from an endometrial swab of a mare with acute inflammation. (Diff-Quik.)

covered by a sterile surgical glove. Sterile water-soluble lubricant is placed on the dorsum of the operator's positioning hand and lower arm. The endometrial biopsy instrument has an overall length of 70 cm with an alligator forceps type of sample basket of 20 × 43 mm. The closed sampling end of the sterile biopsy instrument is carried through the caudal genital tract and, using the forefinger of the gloved hand as a guide, is passed through the cervix and into the uterine body. While holding the closed biopsy instrument stable and inside the uterus with the outside opposite hand, the gloved hand is withdrawn from the genital tract and placed into the rectum. By manipulations per rectum, the sample basket is positioned on the ventral aspect at the base of one of the uterine horns. The forceps are opened and an endometrial fold is pushed into the sides of the basket jaws per rectum. While the forceps are held closed, the instrument is withdrawn from the genital tract. Typically one can feel the biopsy instrument pull away from the uterine wall when the sample is incised. This procedure does not require anesthesia or tranquilization of the mare, because the equine uterus does not have sensory innervation. When sectioned and processed, the procured tissue sample should be large enough to provide endometrial sections with greater than 2 cm of linear lumen epithelium present for histologic evaluation. The biopsy sample should be placed into Bouin's fixative and submitted for tissue processing. If tissue processing will be delayed for more than a few days, Bouin's fixative should be replaced with fresh 10% formalin or 70% ethanol. Fixed tissue samples are embedded in paraffin, and a microscope slide is prepared and stained with hematoxylin and eosin. Tissue samples can also be fixed in 10% formalin, but this results in shrinkage of the tissue and a different cytologic detail. If specific areas of the uterus seem abnormal when examined by palpation or ultrasonography per rectum, additional endometrial biopsy samples can be obtained from those affected areas.

It is essential that the reproductive history of the mare, the stage of the estrous cycle, and character of the genital organs at the time of biopsy be supplied with the sample submission to the pathologist. Knowledge of this information and especially any recent breedings or uterine therapy is needed by the pathologist to develop an accurate epicrisis.

Interpretation of the histologic changes in the endometrial sample will discuss the patterns of distribution (widespread versus scattered) of lesions with regard to the frequency of changes (infrequent, moderately frequent, or frequent). The description of the anatomic pattern of lesion location may include the stratum compactum, stratum spongiosum, perivascular, or periglandular. Inflammatory cells in the sample may include neutrophils, lymphocytes, plasma cells, hemosiderophages, or eosinophils, and the character of the distribution of these cells may be focal, multifocal, diffuse, perivascular, or periglandular. Inflammatory lesions are classified as small (<120 μm), moderate (120 to 300 μm), or large (>300 μm). The severity of periglandular fibrosis is described by the number of layers of fibrosis present, slight (1 to 3 layers), moderate (4 to 10 layers), or severe (>10 layers).

A summary evaluation of the changes present in an endometrial sample was initially made by assigning the endometrium a classification in one of three endometrial categories (I, II, III).[8] Studies were performed to determine the foaling rate of mares with endometrium in the different categories. Since 1986, classifications have been divided into four categories with an attempt to allow prognostication of the ability of the endometrium to carry a foal to term.[9]

Category I.   The endometrium has little or no pathologic changes and is neither hypoplastic nor atrophic. The changes in this endometrium should not interfere with the ability of this endometrium to carry a foal to term. No abnormalities are present, and this endometrium would be expected to carry a foal to term at a rate of 80% to 90%.

Category IIA.   The inflammatory changes are slight to moderate, diffuse infiltrations of the stratum compactum or scattered but frequent foci in the stratum compactum and stratum spongiosum (Figure 6-2). Fibrotic changes may be infrequent to frequent, scattered, and involve individual gland branches with less than three layers of fibrosis or fibrotic nests averaging less than two per 5.5-mm linear field in an average of four or more fields. Extensive lymphatic lacunae that cause changes in the uterus that can be detected by palpation per rectum would relegate the endometrium to category IIA. These changes are mild, and this endometrium would be expected to carry a foal to term at a rate of 50% to 80%.

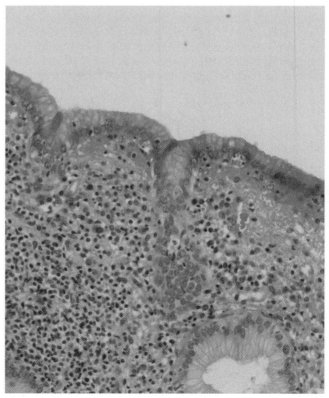

Figure 6-2 Histologic appearance of a category II endometria with widespread, diffuse, moderate infiltration of lymphocytes. (Hematoxylin and eosin; 400×.)

Category IIB. The endometrium from any mare that has been barren for 2 or more years and has the changes consistent with a category IIA endometrium would be assigned to category IIB. Inflammation that is widespread, diffuse, moderately severe, and focal would be included. Fibrotic changes are more extensive, with up to four or more layers of fibrosis surrounding individual gland branches and two to four fibrotic nests per 5.5-mm linear field in an average of four or more fields. These changes are moderate, and this endometrium would be expected to carry to term at a rate of 10% to 50% (Figure 6-3).

Category III. Inflammatory changes are widespread, diffuse, and severe. This category also includes other changes that not only interfere with the ability of the endometrium to carry a foal to term but also cannot be improved by uterine therapy. Uniformly widespread periglandular fibrosis or greater than an average of five fibrotic gland nests per 5.5-mm linear field in an average of four or more fields will automatically relegate the endometrium to category III. These changes are severe, and this endometrium would be expected to carry to term at a rate of only 10%.

Histologic evaluation of an endometrial biopsy sample is routinely performed in barren mares after the end of the breeding season to determine the cause of their infertility so therapy can be instituted to correct any abnormalities. Regarding financial decision making, one may consider performing an endometrial biopsy before booking a mare to the stallion or deciding to perform expensive surgical corrective procedures. Mares with category III endometria are less likely to produce a foal, and the costs associated with getting them in foal may out-weigh the probability of having only a 10% chance of carrying a foal to term. Knowledge of the histologic character of the endometrium during the breeding season can help when making decisions whether to breed or perform therapy at any particular time during the season.

Culture of an Endometrial Biopsy Sample

Occasionally an etiologic microorganism cannot be isolated from the genital tract of a mare displaying obvious clinical evidence of endometritis using traditional endometrial swabbing and aerobic culture of the swab. In these cases there may be value in aerobic culture of an endometrial biopsy sample. Prepare the mare as one would for a routine endometrial biopsy sample. The tissue sample must be collected aseptically. This can be accomplished using a sterile occluded outer guard over the sterile biopsy instrument. The biopsy instrument should not be exposed from the guard until it is positioned inside the uterine lumen. The biopsy instrument should be pulled back into the guard while being withdrawn from the genital tract. A sterile needle can be used to remove the biopsy sample from the forceps jaws. The sample can be sent to the laboratory in a sterile vial covered with sterile water and cooled to 4° C if transport time is less than 4 to 6 hours. If transport time for sample submission is longer than 4 to 6 hours, the tissue sample should be laid upon the surface of the media in a culture transport vial (Port-A-Cul, Becton Dickinson & Co, Sparks, MD) and maintained at ambient temperature. Culture results should be interpreted in a fashion similar to endometrial swab culture results.

Transmural Palpation

Integrity of the uterine wall can be evaluated by transmural palpation. The mare must not be under the influence of progesterone (anestrus, immediately postpartum, or estrus) so that the cervix is relaxed in order to accommodate one of the examiner's hands. The mare must be restrained well because the examiner will be in a precarious position when fully engaged in the procedure. The mare is prepared routinely for a vaginal procedure, including thorough palpation per rectum and perineal cleansing. One of the examiner's arms is covered with a clean or sterile shoulder-length sleeve and sterile surgical glove, lubricated with a sterile water-soluble lubricant, and placed in the vagina, through the cervix and into the uterine lumen. The other arm is covered with a clean shoulder-length sleeve, lubricated with water-soluble lubricant, and placed into the mare's rectum. The uterine wall can then be examined, systematically feeling the entire uterus between one's hands. This procedure is particularly useful in detecting uterine lacerations postpartum when the distal portions of the uterine horns may need to be pulled caudally over the vaginally located arm to permit contact with the tips of the uterine horns.

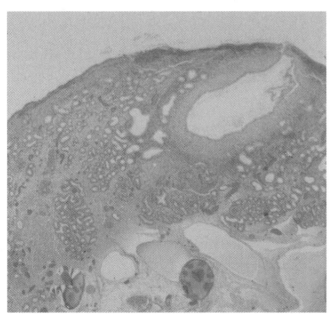

Figure 6-3 Histologic appearance of category IIB endometria with evidence of periglandular fibrosis and cystic glandular distension and a huge glandular cyst. Note the moderate lymphatic lacunae located to the glands. (Hematoxylin and eosin; 400×.)

Luminal Palpation

Direct manual palpation of the uterine lumen may reveal the character and position of luminal uterine cysts and transluminal adhesions. Using sterile sleeve and gloved hand, the uterine lumen can be directly examined if the cervix is relaxed. This should be possible during anestrus or estrus when the cervix is not under the influence of progesterone. Care should be taken to be sure to examine both uterine horns and the uterine body.

Hysteroscopy

Endoscopy of the uterus may reveal pathologic conditions of the uterus, including endometrial cysts, luminal adhesions, foreign bodies, uterine neoplasia, and exudate.[10] Other diagnostic techniques may detect these abnormalities, but endoscopy may allow more thorough evaluation of them.

Ideally the mare should be in diestrus at the time of the examination, because a closed cervix will help to maintain the fluid or air insufflated to cause uterine distension. The mare is restrained in stocks to maintain proximity to the endoscopic equipment. A flexible fiberoptic video endoscope 1 m in length and 8.8 mm or greater in diameter is most typically used to view the endometrium. The endoscope must be cleaned and sterilized for hysteroscopy. The portion of the scope that will be placed inside the mare can be soaked in Cidex OPA (Advanced Sterilization Products, Johnson & Johnson, Irvine, Calif.) for 10 minutes. Avoid leaving the equipment in the antiseptic solution too long because the scope may be damaged. The outer surface and inner channels must be thoroughly rinsed with sterile water before use.

The mare will require tranquilization and some pain control during the procedure. Although the uterus does not have sensory pain receptors, the mares seem to become quite uncomfortable due to the pressure of the distended uterus. Administration of 1.1 mg/kg intravenous (IV) xylazine and 0.01 to 0.02 mg/kg butorphanol IV may produce adequate relaxation and analgesia for the hysteroscopy. Longer procedures may require administration of 0.02 mg/kg detomidine IV. The mare is prepared for vaginal procedure as described in the endometrial microbiology section. One examiner should wear one clean or sterile shoulder-length examination sleeve covered by a sterile surgical glove and a sterile surgical glove on the other hand. Sterile water-soluble lubricant is placed on the back of the hand and lower arm. A second examiner manipulates the controls for fine movements within the genital tract, insufflation, and rinsing of the lens. A video monitor enhances the ability of both examiners to negotiate and evaluate the genital tract. The endoscope is manually carried into the vagina, and one finger is passed into the cervix. The endoscope is guided alongside the finger and is slowly advanced into the uterus. Once the endoscope is inside the uterine lumen, the uterus must be distended to allow visualization of the uterus. The uterus may be distended with room air or sterile water. The water may provide a clearer view and require less distension, but if exudate is present within the lumen, it will mix with the water and obstruct the view. The instrument should be advanced slowly and care be taken to maintain the viewer's orientation within the tract. The uterine bifurcation is a major landmark, and one must be certain that both horns are evaluated.

The visualization of the oviduct papilla confirms that the entire length of the uterine horn has been examined. If images seen are not clear, one should slightly retreat the endoscope, distend the uterus a bit more, and rinse the lens of the endoscope. A gentle, patient technique may be necessary to completely view the entire uterus. Air should be aspirated as the endoscope is being withdrawn. Oxytocin (10 to 20 IU) may be administered at the completion of the procedure to help evacuate the uterus.

Lesions that may be viewed include the following:

- Uterine fluid may be due to urine accumulations, exudates that are a result of chronic irritation of the endometrium, or blood from hemorrhage associated with neoplasia.
- Uterine cysts that are on the surface of the endometrium or pedunculated and positioned in the lumen may be seen as fluid-filled, thin-walled structures. It may be difficult to see broad-based cysts that are located on the surface of the endometrium if the examination is performed during estrus because the estrous endometrium is easily irritated and becomes quite edematous with little manipulation.
- Adhesions may be fine synechiae or wide bands of pale or white fibrous tissue that are transluminal or completely occlude the uterine lumen. Obstruction of the uterine lumen may also be due to segmental aplasia, which might be detected by hysteroscopy but usually is better evaluated using ultrasonography.
- Foreign bodies that include remnants of previous pregnancies or diagnostic equipment may be in the lumen. Mares that experience fetal loss between 40 and 120 days may have endometrial cups present at the base of the previously gravid uterine horn. Endometrial swab tips can break from the culture instrument and become lodged in the uterine lumen.

SUMMARY

Mares are usually tolerant of most uterine procedures and rarely require aggressive restraint or chemical sedation. Ultrasonography helps to confirm findings obtained by palpation per rectum, but skilled palpation per rectum is essential to thoroughly scan the uterus ultrasonographically. Nonpregnant status must be confirmed before uterine manipulation per vaginam because manipulation will result in abortion. A clinical diagnosis of endometritis must be based on reproductive history, clinical signs, and culture results with histologic evaluation of an endometrial biopsy sample confirming its presence. Evaluation of an endometrial biopsy sample for the presence of abnormalities, including endometritis, periglandular fibrosis, and cystic glandular distension, provides prognostic information regarding the ability of a mare's endometrium to carry a foal to term. Transmural palpation and hysteroscopy are not routinely performed but can provide additional diagnostic information in difficult cases.

References

1. Ginther OJ: Reproductive Biology of the Mare, ed 2, Madison, Wis, Equiservices, 1992.
2. Nickel R, Schummer A, Seiferle E et al: The Viscera of the Domestic Mammals, Berlin, Verlag Paul Parey, 1973.
3. Plumb DC: Veterinary Drug Handbook, White Bear Lake, MN, PharmaVet Publishing, 1991.
4. Ginther OJ: Ultrasonic Imaging and Animal Reproduction: Horses Book 2, Cross Plains, Wis, Equiservices, 1995.
5. Hinrichs K, Cummings MR, Sertich PL et al: Clinical significance of aerobic bacterial flora of the uterus, vagina, vestibule and clitoral fossa of clinically normal mares. JAMA 1988; 193:72-75.
6. Blanchard TL, Garcia MC, Hurtgen JP et al: Comparison of two techniques for obtaining endometrial bacteriologic cultures in the mare. Theriogenology 1981; 16:85-93.
7. Couto MA, Hughes JP: Technique and interpretation of cervical and endometrial cytology in the mare. J Equine Vet Sci 1984; 4(6):265-273.
8. Kenney RM: Cyclic and pathologic changes of the mare endometrium as detected by biopsy, with a note on early embryonic death. JAMA 1978; 172:241-262.
9. Kenney RM, Doig PA: Equine endometrial biopsy. In Morrow DA: Current Therapy in Theriogenology, vol 2, Philadelphia, WB Saunders, 1986.
10. Mather EC, Refsal KR, Gustafsson BK et al: The use of fibreoptic techniques in clinical diagnosis and visual assessment of experimental intrauterine therapy in mares. J Reprod Fertil Suppl 1979; 27:293-297.

CHAPTER 7

Uterine Contractility

TERTTU KATILA

The best known task of uterine contractions is the expulsion of the fetus at the term of pregnancy, but the contractile ability of the nonpregnant uterus is also important. Uterine contractions are necessary for sperm transport and, on the other hand, in the elimination of excessive semen, bacteria, and inflammatory by-products after breeding. Probably the susceptibility of some mares to uterine infections is determined by their ability to evacuate uterine contents, which depends on uterine contractions and on the degree of cervical opening. The contractility of the myometrium is controlled by steroid and ecbolic hormones. Also, some clinically used drugs affect uterine contractions. This overview focuses on the nonpregnant uterus only.

PHYSIOLOGICAL BASIS OF MYOMETRIAL CONTRACTILITY

The myometrium consists of two layers of smooth muscle with a vascular zone in between. The muscle fibers of the outer longitudinal layer are arranged parallel and those of the inner circular layers concentrically around the long axis of the uterus. The spindle-shaped, membrane-bound muscle cells are arranged into bundles of 10 to 50 cells. Neighboring cells come in close apposition in certain specialized regions of their plasma membranes forming cell-to-cell contacts, which are termed gap junctions. They are modifications of the apposing plasma membranes of the adjacent cells and couple them electrically and metabolically. The gap is a narrow space of about 2 to 3 nm, and it is composed of a few thousand channels.[1]

The contractile activity in the uterus is a direct consequence of the electrical activity in the smooth muscle cells. This activity is characterized by cyclic depolarization and repolarization of the plasma membrane and termed action potentials. Depolarization is mainly due to an increased permeability to Ca^{2+} and, to a lesser extent, to Na^+. Both ions have higher concentrations in the extracellular space and hence easily move into the intracellular space, making the membrane potential more positive. The membrane repolarizes by increasing the permeability to K^+ (high concentration in intracellular fluid), which results in outward movement of K^+.[1]

Some muscle cells are specialized for pacesetting uterine contractions. Pacemaker regions are 2 to 4 mm in size and contain one or more specialized pacemaker cells. Any myometrial cell is capable of assuming the role of a pacemaker. Therefore pacemaker regions can shift from one site to another. The individual muscle cell is the unit for excitation of the myometrium, but a bundle of muscle cells is the unit of propagation of the electrical stimulus.

Gap junctions are the sites of intercellular propagation of action potentials. The gap junction channels exhibit rapid transformations between open and closed states.[1]

The number of gap junctions and their permeability determines the efficiency of electrical and metabolic coupling of cells in the myometrium and the speed of conduction of action potentials.

The magnitude of uterine contractions is dependent on the total number of simultaneously and synchronously active smooth muscle cells. A single action potential can generate a twitch contraction. A synchronized contraction of many uterine smooth muscle cells (estimated to be billions) decreases the diameter of uterine lumen. At an action potential discharge rate around 1 cycle per second, a tetanic type of contraction is produced.[1]

MEASURING UTERINE CONTRACTILE ACTIVITY IN MARES

Electromyography

Electromyography (EMG) measures electrical changes in the membrane potential of the myometrium,[2,3] but neither the direction of contractions nor movement of intraluminal fluids can be studied using this technique. The method is sensitive to environmental stimuli (e.g., entry to the mare's stall, feeding, and human voices induced temporary changes in electrical activity).[4] Four pairs of electrodes are surgically implanted in the myometrium (tip, middle, and base of a horn and uterine body) under general anesthesia, which makes the technique unsuitable for routine use. Troedsson and his co-workers[2,3] have used the following system for quantification of the data for statistical analysis. A burst is defined as activity consisting of at least 10 peaks per minute and separated from other bursts by at least 1 minute. Frequency is the number of activity bursts per hour. Intensity is the number of spikes per minute. Amplitude is the highest recorded amplitude of spikes in a burst for each minute. All registered electrical activity is classified as total uterine activity. The presence of synchronous activity is expressed as the number of implantation sites that are active simultaneously.

Intrauterine Pressure Transducers

Intrauterine pressure (IUP) transducers record intraluminal pressure changes by responding to increases and decreases in the diameter of uterine lumen. Nowadays the transducers are electronic catheter–tipped and have one or two ultraminiature pressure sensors at the distal end coupled by a cable to a computer.[5,6] Also, IUPs are sensitive to various environmental stimuli. Respiration, resting a hind leg, stretching, urination, snorting, and whinnying induced transient variations in uterine pressure.[5] Jones et al[7] compared EMG and IUP in mares and found very little correlation between the two methods. They questioned the validity of IUP recordings, because intestinal motility and intraabdominal pressure changes can influence IUP responses.

Ultrasonography

The noninvasive technique of transrectal ultrasonography allows visualization of uterine contractions both in nonpregnant and pregnant animals. Active bowel movements near the uterus can confound uterine examination, and therefore it has been recommended that the uterus is examined only when the ventral limits of the uterus can be delineated above a full urinary bladder.[8] However, this would mean visualizing mostly the uterine body, and the body displays much less uterine contractile activity (UCA) than the horns.[9] Another concern has been the effect of rectal palpation itself, because it has been known to increase briefly the electrical activity of the myometrium.[4] It was shown that mean oxytocin (OT) and prostaglandin F_2 metabolite (PGFM) levels and mean UCA scores did not change significantly at any time throughout a 10-minute scanning procedure. It was concluded that transrectal ultrasonography is a useful tool for monitoring and evaluating UCA and does not appear to stimulate ecbolic hormone release.[10] B-mode (brightness mode) ultrasonography has been used most commonly, but Campbell and England[9] applied M-mode (motion mode) ultrasonography in the imaging of contractions in the equine uterus. This technique produces a graph of motion, contractions being positive deviations from the horizontal axis. The amplitude, duration, and frequency of contractions are recorded.

Scintigraphy

Scintigraphy is a technique where radioactive material is imaged in the body of an animal or a human being using a gamma-camera. Static scintigrams have been used to study uterine clearance in mares.[11] Dynamic scintigrams (one to two pictures per second) allow the visualization of uterine contractions, their direction, and the movement of intraluminal fluid.[12] The radioactive material infused into the uterus, as well as the possible use of sedatives, may cause uterine contractions. It is obvious that none of the techniques presented above is fully reliable in distinguishing natural uterine contractions from the ones induced by the use of the method itself or by environmental stimuli.[13] In practice conditions, the only method available is ultrasonography, preferably equipped with the M-mode technique.

HORMONAL CONTROL OF UTERINE CONTRACTILITY

Steroid hormones regulate uterine contractility. High progesterone levels maintain the quiescence of the uterus, whereas a decrease in progesterone and an increase in estrogens stimulate contractility. Progesterone suppresses the formation of gap junctions, thereby decreasing the coupling between the cells. Estrogens induce the formation of gap junctions, depolarize the muscle plasma membrane, increase prostaglandin (PG) production, and enhance the expression of OT receptors (OT-Rs) in the smooth muscle. OT stimulates uterine contractions and release of arachidonic acid and thus formation of PGs. Prostaglandins enhance uterine contractions by causing membrane depolarization and by increasing the number of gap junctions.[1]

Cyclicity and Stage of the Estrous Cycle

Anestrous mares showed significantly less uterine contractions than steroid-treated mares[14] when examined by ultrasonography. EMG recordings of anestrous mares were variable, but transitional mares resembled estrous mares.[7]

In transrectal M-mode ultrasonography, the number of contractions was lowest on the day of ovulation, but no significant differences were found between the other days of the cycle.[9] Transrectal B-mode ultrasonography of cyclic mares demonstrated a postovulatory decrease in UCA followed by a progressive increase between days 2 and 4. Another increase was detected on days 11 and 12, reaching the maximum on days 13 to 14, at the onset of luteolysis, and was followed again by a decrease on days 14 to 16.[15] In EMG, frequent phases of high-amplitude, low-density spikes alternated with short periods of inactivity during spontaneous luteolysis.[4] Estrus was characterized in EMG by well-defined but short phases of activity, closely grouped high-amplitude spikes, or high-intensity bursts separated by periods of relative inactivity.[2,4] During diestrus, more diffuse phases of activity with low-amplitude spikes were separated by variable periods of relative inactivity.[2,4] Because of the prolonged duration of activity bursts, the total time of electrical activity was higher during diestrus than during estrus.[2] This correlates well with the increased tone and tubularity that is characteristic of the equine uterus at diestrus upon rectal palpation.[2,16] Synchronization of electrical activity at different sites of the uterus was more marked during estrus than in diestrus.[2] A wave of synchronized activity is a prerequisite for a contraction to occur. It can be concluded that lowest UCA occurs on the day of ovulation and in the postovulatory period and highest during the time of luteolysis and that the type of activity during estrus is most likely to result in effective contractions.

Effects of Ecbolic Hormones

Oxytocin Receptors

The action of OT is mediated via oxytocin receptors (OT-Rs), which are located on the plasma membrane of smooth muscle cells. The number of binding sites was threefold greater in the myometrium than in the endometrial layer.[17] Lowest concentrations of OT-Rs were found during estrus and on days 1 to 13 of diestrus, whereas highest concentrations were detected on day 14[18] or on days 14 to 17 of the cycle.[17] Increasing amounts of estradiol induce estrogen and OT binding sites.

It is assumed that the release of PGF$_{2\alpha}$ is induced by OT and mediated by occupied OT-Rs. Therefore the increase in OT-Rs during days 14 to 17 may enhance PGF$_{2\alpha}$-production.[17,18]

Endogenous Oxytocin and Prostaglandin Release

Because OT and PGF$_{2\alpha}$ are known to induce uterine contractions, it is of interest to know the pattern of endogenous OT release and the stimulants of release. OT has been shown to be secreted in a pulsatile manner throughout the estrous cycle of the mare, but no differences in pulse frequencies were observed during the cycle.[19] Mean plasma OT concentrations were greater on day 15 after ovulation compared with days 0, 3, and 7.[19]

The release of PGF$_{2\alpha}$ in response to OT injection has been shown to change throughout the estrous cycle, being maximal at the time of luteolysis.[20] When only two periovulatory days were compared, PGFM response after OT administration was higher on the day of ovulation than 2 days after ovulation.[21] Taking of an endometrial biopsy transcervically elicited prompt OT release in all mares, followed by a PGFM increase after 15 minutes, and highest OT and PG releases were detected on days 12 and 14 of the cycle, respectively.[18]

Sexual stimulation, stallion's call, teasing, and artificial insemination (AI), induce pituitary OT secretion in estrous mares, and therefore it has been suggested that it could increase reproductive tract motility.[22] Madill et al[23] measured OT in pituitary venous fluid after the mares were exposed to sexual stimulation (stallion call, visual contact with a stallion, active teasing, or AI). All treatments increased significantly electrical activity of the myometrium and OT release, but the onset of OT secretion was simultaneous with uterine contractility, rather than preceding it.

Another study investigated the effects of teasing, mating, and manual manipulation of the genital tract and intrauterine infusion of fluid on venous OT and PGFM concentrations. Mating and genital tract manipulation caused a significant increase in OT in all mares. Teasing provoked a significant OT response in 6 of 10 estrous mares and in 3 of 5 diestrous mares. Three mares of 5 responded to intrauterine infusion with OT release. No significant effects were detected on PGFM concentrations, with the exception of two mares, which showed significant PG responses after manual manipulation of clitoris, vagina, and cervix or intrauterine infusion.[24] Vaginal distension appeared to be a potent stimulant for OT release associated with mating. Mating constantly induced an OT release, but PGFM was not detected.

Oxytocin Treatments

It has been demonstrated that OT injections increase UCA in mares[3,6,7,25] and uterine clearance in mares.[26] Anovulatory mares are an exception. Although they were primed with progesterone for 16 days, OT did not significantly alter contractility but did increase uterine tone.[27] A better effect of OT on contractility has been demonstrated during estrus than in diestrus.[3,7] Gutjahr et al[28] compared three periovulatory days and found best

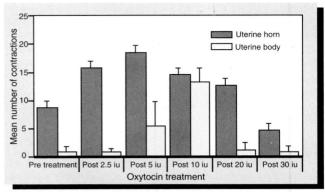

Figure 7-1 Total number of uterine contractions (± standard error of mean) in four mares during 4-minute recording periods before and after treatment with various doses of IV oxytocin. (From Campbell MLH, England GCW: A comparison of the ecbolic efficacy of intravenous and intrauterine oxytocin treatments. Theriogenology 2002; 58:473.)

uterine contractile response to exogenous OT 2 days before ovulation, followed by day of ovulation, and with the lowest response on day 2 after ovulation.

The effect of OT is probably mediated through PG-release. Intravenous OT injection increased PGFM concentration within 5 to 6 minutes[21,29] and peak values were observed within 10 minutes. The half-life of exogenous OT is 6.8 minutes.[21] The duration of effect is dose-dependent: 10 to 18 minutes after 2 IU,[25,30] 17 to 41 minutes after 5 IU,[30,31] 24 to 50 minutes after 10 IU,[30,31] 60 to 90 minutes after 20 IU,[3,31] and 99 minutes after 40 IU.[31] The route of administration differed in these studies: Madill et al[31] used intramuscular injections, and the others intravenous (IV) injections.[3,25,30] The contractile effect is also dose-dependent, usually increasing with higher doses.[30,31] However, when a high dose is given IV, it may result in uterine spasm instead of contractions.[10,32] In the study of Campbell et al[32] using M-mode ultrasonography, 2.5, 5, 10, and 20 IU of OT IV increased uterine contractions numerically, but only 5 IU resulted in significantly higher UCA (Figure 7-1). The dose of 30 IU decreased contractions, because it caused a sustained contraction. Likewise, an IV administration of 1 IU/20 kg body weight of OT (20 to 30 IU per mare) caused a significant reduction in UCA scores in both resistant and susceptible mares.[10]

Prostaglandin Treatments

The ability of prostaglandins, PGF$_{2\alpha}$,[3,14,25,27] cloprostenol,[7,25] and fluprostenol,[4] to induce uterine contractions has been demonstrated in mares. More pronounced effects have been reported during estrus than in diestrus,[3,7] but PGs increase uterine contractions also during diestrus.[27] However, seasonally anestrous mares failed to respond to PGF$_{2\alpha}$, whereas anovulatory mares treated with steroids showed a positive response. This indicates that the mare's uterus may require prior exposure to estrogen, progesterone, or both.[14] The action of PG starts within 8 to 10 minutes after an intramuscular (IM) injection.[7,25,27,33] The duration of the effect has been reported to vary from 40 minutes[25] to 5 hours,[3] but the doses have also been different: from 2.5 mg[25] to 10 mg[3] of PGF$_{2\alpha}$. Cloprostenol appears to be the drug of choice in augmenting uterine clearance; it is more consistent and effective than PGF$_{2\alpha}$ or fenprostalene.[34]

EFFECTS OF SEDATIVES AND UTERINE RELAXANTS

α$_2$-Agonists and Antagonists

It is well known that α$_2$-adrenergic receptor agonists increase UCA in nonpregnant mares,[35,36] but in pregnant mares detomidine seems to decrease myometrial activity.[37] Schatzmann et al[35] did not see any difference between detomidine, xylazine, and romifidine in the degree or duration of increased intraluminal pressure. In contrast, Gibbs and Troedsson[36] demonstrated significant differences between detomidine and xylazine in the increase of EMG activity of the myometrium and its duration: detomidine, 60 minutes; xylazine, 30 minutes. The latter study was carried out in diestrous mares. Schatzmann et al[35] used both estrous and diestrous mares, but the stage of the estrous cycle did not affect uterine contractility. An α$_2$-adrenergic receptor antagonist, acepromazine, suppressed myometrial contractions for 90 minutes.[36] The different results on α$_2$-agonists may be related to the different examination methods (IUP versus EMG).

Clenbuterol

Clenbuterol is a ß$_2$-agonist, which is considered to act as an antagonist to OT and PGF$_{2\alpha}$. It is a broncholytic and tocolytic drug, and it is commonly used in pregnant mares to suppress premature uterine contractions.[38] Jones et al[7] reported inconsistent effects on UCA (EMG) of three mares after an IV dose of 3 mg clenbuterol. Contrary to this study, clenbuterol (0.8 μg/kg or 600 μg/mare IV) depressed uterine contractility and tone in anovulatory, progesterone-primed mares and in pregnant mares as examined by ultrasonography.[27] Uterine motility, as assessed by ultrasonography, decreased also in estrous mares after the administration of clenbuterol (1 μg/kg IV), and the effect lasted for 6 to 8 hours.[39] In conclusion, uterine activity is not totally abolished by the clenbuterol treatment, but it is significantly reduced.

THE ROLE OF UTERINE CONTRACTIONS IN SPERM TRANSPORT

In insemination trials it is sometimes difficult to separate the effects of genital tract manipulations from the effect of the inseminate. AI without any manipulations is not possible. Usually it is preceded by rectal palpation, which may increase UCA.[4,7] Insertion of a hand into the vagina is a similar procedure as insertion of a speculum into the vagina, which has been shown to increase EMG activity.[4] In a study by Campbell and England,[40] mechanical stimulation of the vagina and cervix increased the number of uterine contractions but did not affect the amplitude or duration. However, transcervical insertion of a catheter reduced the number of uterine horn contractions.

During AI, EMG activity of the myometrium has been shown to be similar to that observed during rectal palpation, but after AI the activity increased markedly, persisting for 2 to 7 hours.[4] In another study, breeding caused a short-lived increase in EMG activity.[7] Madill et al[23] showed AI to increase myometrial contractility, and the effect was significantly stronger than the ones elicited by different kinds of contacts with the stallion. Intrauterine infusion of 10 and 80 ml of saline increased uterine contractions after 4 minutes in M-mode ultrasonography, whereas 150 ml decreased contractions in the uterine horns.[40] In another study where B-mode ultrasonography was used, a large volume inseminate (150 ml) induced more uterine contractions than a small volume (2 ml) 4 hours after AI.[41]

After AI with 5 ml of skim milk extended radiolabeled sperm (technetium 99m), strong and frequent uterine contractions were seen in dynamic scintigrams, but there was a lot of variation between mares in the number of contractions (from 5 to 65 within the first 30 minutes). Radioactivity was seen in the tips of the horns for the first time between 8 and 20 minutes after AI. The contractions pushed sperm continuously back and forth between the body and tips of the horns during the first half hour. Sometimes there were four to seven circular movements of sperm in the most ventral parts of the horns, which was followed by a rapid influx into the tip of the horn and subsequent return to the body. Localized horn contractions seemed occasionally to almost close the uterine horn for very short periods of time. Probably the uterine dynamics served to spread sperm effectively in the uterus and at the same time eliminate sperm. Obviously, some of the sperm that were returned caudally never made their way back to the horn but were discharged through the cervix.[12] Figure 7-2 shows how quickly radioactive sperm had been eliminated from the uterus. Only 20% of

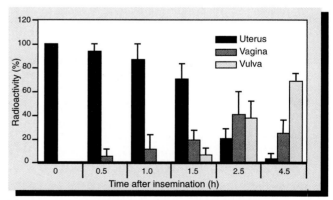

Figure 7-2 Distribution of radioactivity (mean ± SEM; n = 3) in the uterus (*solid black bar*), vagina (*dark gray bar*), and vulva (*light gray bar;* vulva includes radioactivity observed around the vulva and removed from the reproductive tract) of three mares during the 4.5 hours after insemination with radiolabeled spermatozoa. (From Katila T, Sankari S, Mäkelä O: Transport of spermatozoa in the reproductive tracts of mares. J Reprod Fertil Suppl 2000; 56:571.)

the activity was left in the uterus $2^1/_2$ hours after AI, and almost all sperm had left the uterus $4^1/_2$ hours after AI. These findings suggest that the selected sperm that manage to enter the oviduct make their journey very quickly. Elimination of sperm by mechanical drainage via the cervix and through phagocytosis by neutrophils also takes place very rapidly.[42]

Sperm motility is necessary for the access to the uterotubal junction and into the oviducts, but its role in the transport through the uterus is probably not very important. Uterine contractions are responsible for the rapid sperm transport. Without the aid of uterine contractions, even highly motile sperm could not make their long journey through the large uterus in such a short time.[43]

What causes uterine contractions after AI or breeding? Ecbolic hormones in the semen could be one explanation, because semen has been shown to contain oxytocin[44] and prostaglandins.[45] OT and $PGF_{2\alpha}$ are present in high concentrations in stallion semen, so it could contribute to uterine contractions. However, the highest concentrations were found in gel,[44] which is removed for AI. Therefore it is unlikely that semen could have induced myometrial contractions in the studies of Taverne et al[4] and Madill et al,[23] who used AI. Mechanical stretching of the uterus caused by the volume of the inseminate has also been suggested, as well as the inflammatory influence of semen.[4] However, the inflammatory response starts the first $^1/_2$ hour after AI,[42] so it cannot contribute at the time of AI, but it can continue to stimulate contractions because uterine fluid during inflammation is rich in prostaglandins.[46] In the study of Madill et al,[23] AI was associated with rapid onset of myometrial contractions. However, no association was observed between uterine contraction and pituitary OT release. The onset of OT secretion was simultaneous with the increase in uterine contractions, not preceding it.[23] The authors concluded that the commencement of the contractile response may be mediated neurogenically but with the concurrent OT release augmenting the myometrial contractions. Activation of the autonomic nervous system by mating or insemination stimuli could be mediated by α-adrenergic receptors.[24]

THE ROLE OF MYOMETRIAL CONTRACTIONS IN UTERINE EVACUATION

As early as 1986, Evans et al[47] demonstrated the importance of uterine clearance and the effect of steroids on the physical clearance. In the progesterone-dominated uterus the physical clearance of the inoculated material was impaired. This was very likely due to reduced uterine contractions or cervical patency or both. Later, Troedsson et al[48] showed that mares susceptible to uterine infections differed in uterine contractility from resistant mares. Although an increase in myometrial electrical activity was seen in all mares following intrauterine bacterial infusion, susceptible mares demonstrated weaker contractility between 10 and 20 hours after the inoculation. The important role of uterine contractility in uterine clearance was demonstrated also by Nikolakopoulos and Watson.[39] They reduced uterine contractions by treat-

ment with clenbuterol and then infused bacteria into the uteri of resistant estrous mares. Although most mares were able to eliminate bacteria, they all accumulated intrauterine fluid, which they did not do during the control cycle.

Insemination has been shown to cause the same kind of significant OT release in susceptible and resistant mares, but $PGF_{2\alpha}$ release was significantly higher in the resistant group than in the group of susceptible mares for the first 30 minutes after AI (Figure 7-3). Similarly, exogenous OT induced significantly higher $PGF_{2\alpha}$ release in resistant mares compared with susceptible mares (Figure 7-4). The authors thought this indicated a possible defect in $PGF_{2\alpha}$ release at the OT-R or postreceptor level.[49] Opposing results were obtained in another study.[50] An IV injection of 20 IU of OT 120 minutes after intrauterine radiocolloid infusion did not increase PGFM concentrations in normal mares, whereas in mares with delayed uterine clearance (DUC) it did. The difference between the mares was not related to the presence of intrauterine fluid, but it could have been associated with the uterine inflammation.[50] The authors suggested that the rapid clearance of radiocolloid induced by OT could be either

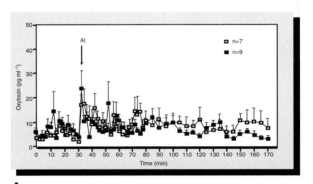

A

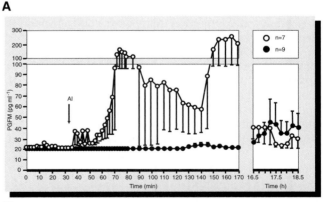

B

Figure 7-3 Mean ± SEM (**A**) oxytocin and (**B**) 13,14-dihydro-15-keto $PGF_{2\alpha}$ (PGFM) concentrations around the time of artificial insemination (AI) in mares resistant (*white square or white circle;* n = 7) and susceptible (*black square or black circle;* n = 9) to persistent mating-induced endometritis. (From Nikolakopoulos E, Kindahl H, Watson ED: Oxytocin and $PGF_{2\alpha}$ release in mares resistant and susceptible to persistent mating-induced endometritis. J Reprod Fertil Suppl 2000; 56:363.)

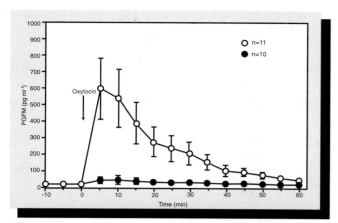

Figure 7-4 Mean ± SEM 13,14-dihydro-15-keto PGF$_{2\alpha}$ (PGFM) concentrations after IV oxytocin administration (1 IU per 20 kg body weight; Oxytocin-S; Intervet, Cambridge, UK) to estrous mares resistant (*white circle;* n = 11) and susceptible (*black circle;* n = 10) to persistent mating-induced endometritis. (From Nikolakopoulos E, Kindahl H, Watson ED: Oxytocin and PGF$_{2\alpha}$ release in mares resistant and susceptible to persistent mating-induced endometritis. J Reprod Fertil Suppl 2000; 56:363.)

independent of or synergistic with uterine prostaglandin secretion. The authors speculated that the PG release could have been induced by the introduction of a pipette through the cervix. However, transcervical insertion of a catheter or dilation of the catheter with a balloon induced OT release but did not increase PGFM levels.[51]

OT, xylazine (predominantly α_2-agonist but also with some α_1-agonist effect), and detomidine (α_2-agonist), increase uterine contractions, whereas acepromazine (an α_1-antagonist) decreases uterine contractions. However, the duration of increased intrauterine pressure was longer in mares with DUC than in normal mares when the mares had been sedated with xylazine before OT administration. In addition, acepromazine administration had no effect on the OT-induced contraction pattern in normal mares, but it decreased contractions in mares with DUC. It was proposed that this might be due to denervation supersensitivity. This condition results from chronic stretching of the myometrium in late gestation, leading to the increase of myometrial cells and to degeneration and reduction in the number of adrenergic nerve endings within the muscle. This is followed by functional denervation and supersensitivity of the myometrium to catecholamines. This supersensitivity, combined with an increase in the number of postsynaptic α-adrenoreceptor sites as a result of increased estrogen concentrations, renders the myometrium very sensitive to the adrenergic amines.[52]

But a combination of detomidine and OT gave totally different results. Normal mares experienced more uterine contractions than mares with delayed clearance. The authors explained the controversy between these two studies by the differences of the two drugs in the specificity for α-adrenoreceptors.[53] In the same study, differences were noted also in the pattern of propagation of uterine contractions. In normal mares, the contraction

originated in the horn and propagated towards the cervix. In mares with DUC, the contractions often started from the body or they were seen simultaneously in the body and horn. Transcervical insertion of a catheter or dilation of the catheter with a balloon induced OT release on days 5 and 7 of diestrus but did not increase PGFM levels. However, PG release after OT stimulation differs during the cycle.

The hypothesis about intrinsic weakness in myometrial contractility in susceptible mares was confirmed in an in vitro study using longitudinal and circular uterine muscle strips. For all contractile agonists that the authors tested (KCl, OT, and PGF$_{2\alpha}$), myometrium from mares with DUC failed to generate as much tension as myometrium from older normal mares. Rigby et al[54] concluded that an intrinsic contractile defect of the myometrium may contribute to reduced uterine contractility following breeding.

CONCLUSIONS

Susceptibility to uterine infections is a multifactorial condition, and myometrial contractility is one of these factors. A large percentage of susceptible mares probably have intrinsic contractile defects in myometrial contractility. This results in the accumulation of intrauterine fluid after breeding, predisposing the mares to persistent postbreeding endometritis.

Uterine contractions are vital in the transport of sperm through the uterus to the oviductal junction. This function of myometrium may also be impaired in problem mares because of deficient PG release in association with breeding. Intrauterine fluid accumulations have been successfully treated in the practice by OT injections, but this treatment may not be equally effective in mares susceptible to uterine infections. It has been shown that susceptible mares do not release PG in the same way as normal mares after exogenous OT administration. Small intravenous OT doses or intramuscular doses are probably more effective than high OT doses, which may cause a tetanic contraction. OT and PG treatments are not effective in anestrous mares, which appear to need steroid priming for an effect to occur. Best contractile responses have been reported after treatments given during estrus.

Clenbuterol reduces uterine contractility, which is a desired effect in pregnant mares. Many mares are treated with clenbuterol because of respiratory problems. In these mares the effect on uterine contractions has to be borne in mind when these mares are bred and managed for maximum reproductive efficacy. If mares need sedation in connection with breeding or uterine treatments, detomidine and xylazine are better alternatives than acepromazine. Acepromazine reduces uterine contractions, whereas detomidine and xylazine increase them.

References

1. Jain TL, Saade GR, Garfield RE: Uterine contraction. In Knobil E, Neill JD (eds): Encyclopedia of Reproduction, vol 4, Academic Press, p 932-942, 1999.

2. Troedsson MHT, Wiström AOG, Liu IKM et al: Registration of myometrial activity using multiple site electromyography in cyclic mares. J Reprod Fertil 1993; 99:299.

3. Troedsson MHT, Liu IKM, Ing M et al: Smooth muscle electrical activity in the oviduct, and the effect of oxytocin, prostaglandin F$_{2\alpha}$, and prostaglandin E2 on the myometrium and the oviduct of the cycling mare. Biol Reprod Mono 1995; 1:475.

4. Taverne MAM, van der Weyden GC, Fontijne P et al: In-vivo myometrial electrical activity in the cyclic mare. J Reprod Fertil 1979; 56:521.

5. Goddard PJ, Allen WE, Gerring EL: Genital tract pressures in mares. I. Normal pressures and the effect of physiological events. Theriogenology 1985; 23:815.

6. Ko JCH, Lock TF, Davis JL et al: Spontaneous and oxytocin-induced uterine motility in cyclic and postpartum mares. Theriogenology 1989; 32:643.

7. Jones DM, Fielden ED, Carr DH: Some physiological and pharmacological factors affecting uterine motility as measured by electromyography in the mare. J Reprod Fertil Suppl 1991; 44:357.

8. Griffin PG, Ginther OJ: Uterine contractile activity in mares during the estrous cycle and early pregnancy. Theriogenology 1990; 34:47.

9. Campbell MLH, England GCW: M-mode ultrasound imaging of the contractions of the equine uterus. Vet Rec 2002; 150:575.

10. Nikolakopoulos E, Watson ED: Can uterine contractile activity be evaluated by transrectal ultrasound? Theriogenology 2002; 58:483.

11. Neuwirth L, LeBlanc M, Mauragis F et al: Scintigraphic measurement of uterine clearance in mares. Vet Radiol Ultrasound 1995; 36:64.

12. Katila T, Sankari S, Mäkelä O: Transport of spermatozoa in the reproductive tracts of mares. J Reprod Fertil Suppl 2000; 56:571.

13. Katila T: Uterine contractility in non-pregnant mares. Pferdeheilkunde 1999; 15:574.

14. Cross DT, Ginther OJ: The effect of estrogen, progesterone and prostaglandin F$_{2\alpha}$ on uterine contractions in seasonally anovulatory mares. Domest Anim Endocrinol 1987; 4:271.

15. Griffin PG, Ginther OJ: Effects of day of estrous cycle, time of day, luteolysis, and embryo on uterine contractility in mares. Theriogenology 1993; 39:997.

16. Bonafos LD, Carnevale EM, Smith CA et al: Development of uterine tone in nonbred and pregnant mares. Theriogenology 1994; 42:1247.

17. Stull CL, Evans JW: Oxytocin binding in the uterus of the cycling mare. Equine Vet Sci 1986; 6:114.

18. Sharp DC, Thatcher M-J, Salute ME et al: Relationship between endometrial oxytocin receptors and oxytocin-induced prostaglandin F$_{2\alpha}$ release during the oestrous cycle and early pregnancy in pony mares. J Reprod Fertil 1997; 109:137.

19. Tetzke TA, Ismail S, Mikuckis G et al: Patterns of oxytocin secretion during the oestrous cycle of the mare. J Reprod Fertil Suppl 1987; 35:245.

20. Goff AK, Pontbriand D, Sirois J: Oxytocin stimulation of plasma 15-keto-13,14-dihydro prostaglandin F$_{2\alpha}$ during the oestrous cycle and early pregnancy in the mare. J Reprod Fertil Suppl 1987; 35:253.

21. Paccamonti DL, Pycock JF, Taverne MAM et al: PGFM response to exogenous oxytocin and determination of the half-life of oxytocin in nonpregnant mares. Equine Vet J 1999; 31:285.

22. Alexander SL, Irvine CHG, Shand N et al: Is luteinizing hormone secretion modulated by endogenous oxytocin in the mare? Studies on the role of oxytocin and factors affecting its secretion in estrous mares. Biol Reprod Mono 1995; 1:361.

23. Madill S, Troedsson MHT, Alexander SL et al: Simultaneous recording of pituitary oxytocin secretion and myometrial activity in oestrous mares exposed to various breeding stimuli. J Reprod Fertil Suppl 2000; 56:351.

24. Nikolakopoulos E, Kindahl H, Gilbert CL et al: Release of oxytocin and prostaglandin F$_{2\alpha}$ around teasing, natural service and associated events in the mare. Anim Reprod Sci 2000; 63:89.

25. Goddard PJ, Allen WE: Genital tract pressures in mares. II. Changes induced by oxytocin and prostaglandin F$_{2\alpha}$. Theriogenology 1985; 24:35.

26. LeBlanc MM, Neuwirth L, Mauragis D et al: Oxytocin enhances clearance of radiocolloid from the uterine lumen of reproductively normal and infertile mares. Equine Vet J 1994; 26:279.

27. Gastal MO, Gastal EL, Torres CAA et al: Effect of oxytocin, prostaglandin F$_{2\alpha}$, and clenbuterol on uterine dynamics in mares. Theriogenology 1998; 50:521.

28. Gutjahr S, Paccamonti DL, Pycock JF et al: Effect of dose and day of treatment on uterine response to oxytocin in mares. Theriogenology 2000; 54:447.

29. Cadario ME, Thatcher M-JD, LeBlanc MM: Relationship between prostaglandin and uterine clearance of radiocolloid in the mare. Biol Reprod Mono 1995; 1:495.

30. Cadario ME, Merritt AM, Archbald LF et al: Changes in intrauterine pressure after oxytocin administration in reproductively normal mares and in those with a delay in uterine clearance. Theriogenology 1999; 51:1017.

31. Madill S, Troedsson MHT, Santschi EM et al: Dose-response effect of intramuscular oxytocin treatment on myometrial contraction of reproductively normal mares during estrus. Theriogenology 2002; 58:479.

32. Campbell MLH, England GCW: A comparison of the ecbolic efficacy of intravenous and intrauterine oxytocin treatments. Theriogenology 2002; 58:473.

33. Cross DT, Threlfall WR, Rogers RC et al: Uterine electromyographic activity in horse mares as measured by radiotelemetry. Theriogenology 1991; 35:591.

34. Combs GB, LeBlanc MM, Neuwirth L et al: Effects of prostaglandin F$_{2\alpha}$, cloprostenal and fenprostalene on uterine clearance of radiocolloid in the mare. Theriogenology 1996; 45:1449.

35. Schatzmann U, Josseck H, Stauffer J-L et al: Effects of α$_2$-agonists on intrauterine pressure and sedation in horses: comparison between detomidine, romifidine and xylazine. J Vet Med Assoc 1994; 41:523.

36. Gibbs III HM, Troedsson MHT: Effect of acepromazine, detomidine, and xylazine on myometrial activity in the mare. Biol Reprod Mono 1995; 1:489.

37. Jedruch J, Gajewski Z, Kuussaari J: The effect of detomidine hydrochloride on the electrical activity of uterus in pregnant mares. Acta Vet Scand 1989; 30:307.

38. Santschi M: The management of equine high-risk pregnancy. Equine Pract 1995; 17:22-25.

39. Nikolakopoulos E, Watson ED: Uterine contractility is necessary for the clearance of intrauterine fluid but not bacteria after bacterial infusion in the mare. Theriogenology 1999; 52:413.

40. Campbell MLH, England GCW: Effect of teasing, mechanical stimulation and the intrauterine infusion of saline on uterine contractions in mares. Vet Rec 2004; 155:103.

41. Sinnemaa L, Järvimaa T, Lehmonen N et al: Effect of insemination volume on uterine contractions and inflammatory response and on elimination of semen in the mare uterus—

scintigraphic and ultrasonographic studies. J Vet Med A 2005; 52:466.

42. Katila T: Onset and duration of uterine inflammatory response of mares after insemination with fresh semen. Biol Reprod Mono 1995; 1:515.

43. Katila T: Sperm-uterine interactions: a review. Anim Reprod Sci 2001; 68:267.

44. Watson ED, Nikolakopoulos E, Gilbert C et al: Oxytocin in the semen and gonads of the stallion. Theriogenology 1999; 51:855.

45. Claus R, Dimmick MA, Gimenez T et al: Estrogens and prostaglandin $F_{2\alpha}$ in the semen and blood plasma of stallions. Theriogenology 1992; 38:687.

46. Watson ED, Stokes CR, David JSE et al: Concentrations of uterine luminal prostaglandins in mares with acute and persistent endometritis. Equine Vet J 1987; 19:31.

47. Evans MJ, Hamer JM, Gason LM et al: Clearance of bacteria and non-antigenic markers following intra-uterine inoculation into maiden mares: effect of steroid hormone environment. Theriogenology 1986; 26:37.

48. Troedsson MHT, Liu IKM, Ing M et al: Multiple site electromyography recordings of uterine activity following an intrauterine bacterial challenge in mares susceptible and resistant to chronic uterine infection. J Reprod Fertil 1993; 99:307.

49. Nikolakopoulos E, Kindahl H, Watson ED: Oxytocin and $PGF_{2\alpha}$ release in mares resistant and susceptible to persistent mating-induced endometritis. J Reprod Fertil Suppl 2000; 56:363.

50. Cadario ME, Thatcher WW, Klapstein E et al: Dynamics of prostaglandin secretion, intrauterine fluid and uterine clearance in reproductively normal mares and mares with delayed uterine clearance. Theriogenology 1999; 52:1181.

51. Handler J, Königshofer M, Kindahl H et al: Secretion patterns of oxytocin and PGF2α-metabolite in response to cervical dilatation in cyclic mares. Theriogenology 2003; 59:1381.

52. De Lille AJAE, Silvers ML, Cadario ME et al: Interactions of xylazine and acepromazine with oxytocin and the effects of these interactions on intrauterine pressure in normal mares and mares with delayed uterine clearance. J Reprod Fertil Suppl 2000; 56:373.

53. von Reitzenstein M, Callahan MA, Hansen PJ et al: Aberrations in uterine contractile patterns in mares with delayed uterine clearance after administration of detomidine and oxytocin. Theriogenology 2002; 58:887.

54. Rigby SL, Barhoumi R, Burghardt RC et al: Mares with delayed uterine clearance have an intrinsic defect in myometrial function. Biol Reprod 2001; 65:740.

SECTION II

Female Reproductive Problems: Diagnosis and Management

CHAPTER **8**

Fertility Expectations and Management for Optimal Fertility

SIDNEY RICKETTS

MATS H.T. TROEDSSON

The aim of commercial horse breeders is to achieve a live foal every year from their brood mares. Although small family bands of feral horses and native ponies may sometimes achieve this, most populations of commercial brood mares have conception and pregnancy failures that result in some mares entering the next breeding season not pregnant, i.e., "barren." Assuming normal stallion fertility and adequate management, in most cases this is a matter of sporadic mare subfertility, most commonly associated with obstetric injuries, age-related genital tract disease, or managerial problems. True infertility and epidemic subfertility (e.g., epidemic venereal infections or viral pregnancy failures) are uncommon in mares.

It is the responsibility of the equine theriogenologist to do the following:

1. Maximize the reproductive health and efficiency of all mares under his or her care, in general terms, so that conception and pregnancy failures are kept to a minimum
2. Specifically aid individual mares with reproductive problems to overcome or compensate for their problems in order that they may undergo a normal pregnancy and produce a healthy live foal at normal term

FERTILITY EXPECTATIONS

Historically, it has been suggested that the equine species inherently achieves relatively low fertility figures and that domestication makes matters worse. With good management, this is not the case. Mare fertility results vary between populations. The 2003 Weatherbys' Statistical Review[1] records that 23,136 Thoroughbred mares were mated by 783 registered Thoroughbred stallions at stud in the United Kingdom (UK) and Ireland. After excluding those mares for which no returns were made, those that were exported or that died, the pregnancy rate (number of mares pregnant/number of mares bred) was 89.30%, the live foal rate was 82.04%, the gestational failure rate was 7.42%, and the barren mare rate was 10.70%. In well-managed populations of Thoroughbred horses, pregnancy rates in excess of 90% and live foal rates in excess of 80% can be achieved.[2] Occasionally, young fashionable stallions, covering between 60 and 80 mares, achieve 100% pregnancy rates during a breeding season. Although similar statistics are not published for North America, there is no reason to suspect that results are substantially different. These are now the targets for both equine stud farm clinicians and stud managers. Because the only accurate measure of fertility is pregnancy rate per cycle, any figures such as those above are also related to breeding opportunity (i.e., number of cycles the mare is available to be bred). This is governed by not only gestation length but economic considerations of when a late foal may not be financially viable. If people are prepared to keep breeding outside what would be termed a normal breeding season, then even better figures can be expected.

Population statistics help little when considering aspirations for individual mares. Weatherbys' data demonstrates a linear decline in the fertility potential of mares with age[3] (Figure 8-1). During the years researched, the live foal rate of 4-year-old mares was approximately 75%, whereas that of 20-year-old mares was approximately 50%. It is vital that clinicians, stud managers, and owners

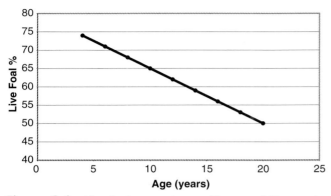

Figure 8-1 Live foal percentage with age of Thorough-bred mares. (Original data from Weatherbys' Returns for Mares 1973-77.)

understand that age has a major and irrevocable limiting effect on a mare's fertility potential.

By definition, an infertile mare is incapable of conceiving when mated by a fertile stallion and is thus, by true definition, a sterile mare. The latter is uncommon and is often associated with congenital defects of the reproductive tract or gonadal dysgenesis, often manifesting in demonstrable karyotype abnormality. In contrast, temporary breeding failures are relatively common, and these mares are more correctly termed subfertile. A barren mare is one who is not pregnant at the end of the breeding season, for whatever reason.

Preparing Barren Mares for Next Season

In order to achieve maximal breeding efficiency, all barren mares should receive a thorough examination after the end of the breeding season[4-8] and before they go into winter anestrus (e.g., in September [Northern Hemisphere]), with the following aims:

1. Making a diagnosis of genital abnormality, if one is present
2. Making a provisional breeding prognosis based on the abnormalities diagnosed
3. Formulating and carrying out a logical treatment program, if indicated
4. Assessing the response to treatment after a period of rest
5. Making a more accurate breeding prognosis based on the abnormalities diagnosed and their response to treatment
6. Repeating or substituting alternative treatment if their response to treatment is unsatisfactory, until improvement occurs or retirement is recommended
7. Allowing an extended period of rest before the next breeding season

Without this preparation, mares may enter the next breeding season with persistent genital abnormalities that then require diagnosis, treatment, reassessment and recovery, delaying mating and wasting valuable time.

The Autumn Barren Mare Examinations and Treatments

An accurate diagnosis is, as always in veterinary medicine, a prerequisite to prognosis, treatment, and successful management. This requires a detailed, logical investigatory approach, which, after taking a detailed reproductive history, may include a variety of tests to examine the mare's ovaries, uterus, cervix, vagina, vulva, and perineum and evaluation of the hypothalamic-pituitary-ovarian hormonal axis. Diagnoses are then made, and specific treatments are performed.

Reproductive History
The mare's age and breeding history are vital pieces of information with which to start the diagnostic process and are essential data that allow meaningful interpretations of gynecologic abnormalities to be made. A young barren maiden mare (not pregnant after her first season at stud with no history of conception) may be immature or even have gonadal dysgenesis (e.g., X0 or XY sex reversal, manifesting with very small and persistently inactive ovaries), whereas an 18-year-old mare that has produced 10 foals, suffered an early fetal death, an abortion, and two barren years will not have gonadal dysgenesis but is most likely to have perineal and/or uterine problems. A mare that has failed to conceive or maintain a pregnancy after dystocia should be examined carefully for cervical injury and/or incompetence.

Examination of the Vulva and Perineum
The conformation of the mare's perineum and the integrity, shape, and angle of slope of her vulva in relation to her anus is first evaluated to determine if she is likely to have pneumovagina (i.e., she requires Caslick's vulvoplasty surgery to be performed)[9-11] (Figure 8-2). Sometimes, small fistulas (Figure 8-3) are found in the vulval scar after surgery, and these need to be repaired. If the mare's perineal shape is very poor to the extent that Caslick's operation is insufficient to prevent pneumovagina, Pouret's perineal reconstruction operation (Figure 8-4) may be recommended.[10-12] The vulval lips are examined for signs of accidental injury leading to incompetent closure. For broodmares, all vulval injuries need careful repair and successful reconstruction to avoid incompetent closure leading to pneumovagina. The vulval lips should be manually separated while the examiner pays attention to aspiration of air into the vagina. In mares with a dysfunctional or weak vestibulovaginal fold, separation of the vulval lips creates a characteristic sound when air is aspirated into the vagina. These mares should be considered to be prone to pneumovagina.

In the UK, Ireland, France, Germany, and Italy, samples are routinely collected from the urethral opening, clitoral fossa, and sinuses (Figure 8-5) for annual screening for the potential equine venereal disease organisms *Taylorella equigenitalis*, *Klebsiella pneumoniae* (capsule types 1, 2, and 5), and *Pseudomonas aeruginosa*, as recommended by the Horserace Betting Levy Board's Code of Practice for the Control of Equine Venereal Diseases. These pathogens may exist in all of these sites and, if found, constitute carrier status.[13,14] Carrier mares are

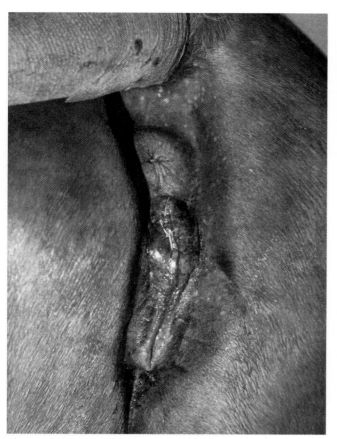

Figure 8-2　Caslick's vulvoplasty surgery, at completion.

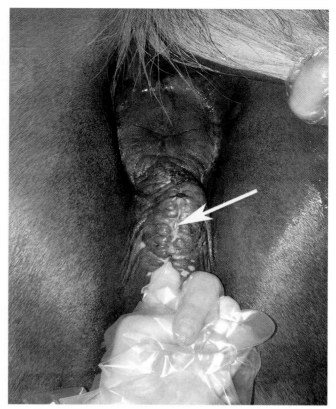

Figure 8-3　Small fistula *(arrow)* in healed Caslick's vulvoplasty scar.

excluded from mating until they have been successfully treated and have been proven so by repeated follow-up culturing. *T. equigenitalis* is sensitive to environmental conditions, and samples should be placed into Amies charcoal transport medium immediately after collection to preserve the organism during transportation to the diagnostic laboratory. The samples should not be subjected to high or low temperatures during transportation.

Vaginoscopic (Speculum) Examination

The cervix and vagina are examined, via a sterile vaginoscope (speculum), for their appearance in relation to cyclic state (moist, pink, and relaxed in estrus; dry, pale, and tight in diestrus) and for signs of injury, incompetence, discharge, and/or vaginal urine pooling.[15] Cervical lacerations that impair normal function, particularly closure, always carry a poor prognosis for future breeding. Some require attempts at surgical repair,[16-18] but such mares often remain "high risk" for ascending placentitis, which often results in abortion or the birth of an impoverished foal.[19] Other cases heal sufficiently to allow functional closure without surgical interference. In such cases some clinicians recommend that the mare is supplemented with oral progestagens (altrenogest), to aid tight cervical closure, on empirical grounds.

If the mare is in estrus, samples are collected from the endometrium, through the open cervix, and also directly via a sterile speculum (Figure 8-6) for cytologic screening

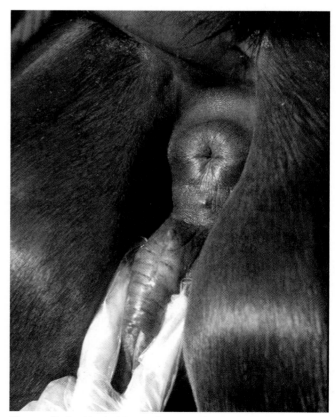

Figure 8-4　Healed Pouret's perineal reconstruction surgery.

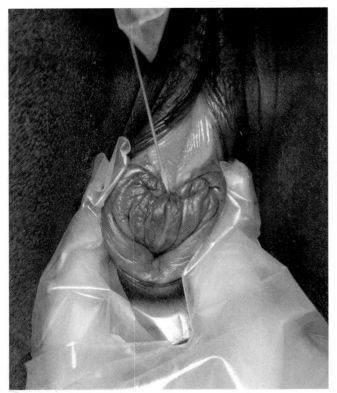

Figure 8-5 Narrow-tipped culturette being used to obtain specimens from the central clitoral sinus.

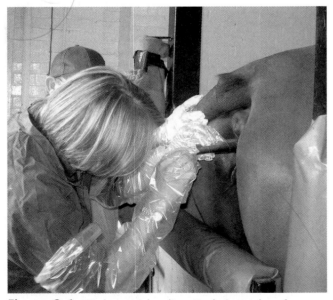

Figure 8-6 Endometrial culturette being taken from an estrous mare via a sterile disposable vaginal speculum.

for inflammation (the presence of polymorphonuclear leukocytes (PMNs) [i.e., PMNs in a smear test]), for the equine venereal disease organisms *T. equigenitalis, K. pneumoniae* (capsule types 1, 2, and 5), and *P. aeruginosa,* and for any of the multitude of opportunist pathogens (most

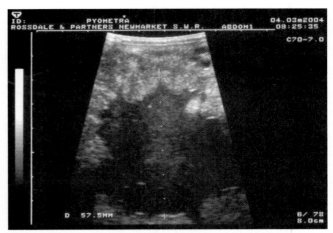

Figure 8-7 Transrectal ultrasonic appearance of pyometritis.

commonly β-hemolytic streptococci [i.e., *Streptococcus zooepidemicus*], *Escherichia coli,* and *Staphylococcus aureus,* and the anaerobe *Bacteroides fragilis*).[13,20] These opportunist organisms are only considered to be of significance (i.e., causing endometritis) if there is cytologic evidence of inflammation in the smear sample.[21-23]

If the mare is not in estrus, samples for bacterial culture are taken from the endometrial biopsy sample after it has been collected (see later).

Rectal Palpation and Ultrasonographic Examination
During estrus, the uterus has minimal palpable tone and, especially in early estrus, endometrial edema[4,5] delineates the endometrial folds on ultrasonographic examination.[24-26] During diestrus, the normal uterus should have uniformly palpable tone and no palpable enlargements. Ventral dilations (areas of fold atrophy and myometrial stretching) may contain luminal fluid accumulations that may be either hypoechoic or hyperechoic on scan, the former indicating clear fluid and the latter indicating hemorrhage or, more commonly, inflammatory fluids. In pyometra, which is less commonly seen in mares than some other species, the uterus is uniformly enlarged, palpably distended or "doughy," and contains particulate fluid, giving a "scintillating" hyperechoic ultrasonographic appearance (Figure 8-7).

Equine ovaries are highly variable in size and activity depending on cyclic state.[24] During estrus they may be large and contain follicles in varying stages of development, in addition to old, nonfunctional corpora lutea.[27] During diestrus there will be at least one functional corpus luteum in addition to follicles in varying stages of development. During anestrus they will be small and inactive, containing neither active follicles nor corpora lutea.

The most commonly diagnosed ovarian abnormality is the granulosa cell tumor (GCT).[28,29] This benign tumor causes one ovary to enlarge, sometimes enormously, and appear full of cysts on ultrasonographic examination (Figure 8-8), while the other ovary is characteristically inhibited and becomes small, hard, and inactive. Granulosa cell tumors are hormonally active, and a clinical diag-

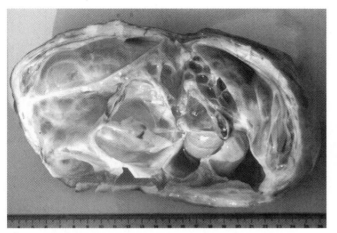

Figure 8-8 Sectioned gross appearance of granulosa cell tumor after surgical removal.

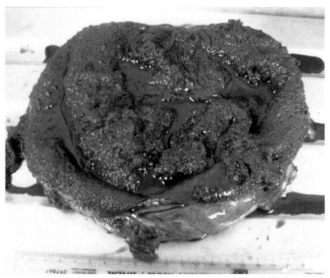

Figure 8-9 Gross appearance of sectioned ovarian hematoma after surgical removal.

nosis can be supported by measuring the mare's blood hormone profile. Diagnostic assays to detect granulosa cell tumors include inhibin, testosterone, and progesterone.[30] In a single blood sample of a mare with a granulosa cell tumor, α-inhibin is elevated in approximately 90% of cases, serum testosterone in approximately 50% of cases, and progesterone concentrations should be below 1 ng/ml because these mares are mostly not cycling.[30,31] There have certainly been enough reports of cyclicity with early cases of GCT to have caution about acyclicity.[32]

The cancerous ovary is removed surgically, allowing the inhibited ovary to regain normal function within 2 to 12 months. Other, much less common ovarian tumors are cystadenomas, dysgerminomas, teratomas, and malignant adenocarcinomas.

True cystic ovarian disease is rarely confirmed in mares. Occasionally mares hemorrhage excessively into an ovary after ovulation, causing enlargement and pain. A typical homogeneous hyperechoic ultrasonographic appearance of the blood clot allows the diagnosis to be confirmed (Figure 8-9). Most cases resolve with time, but occasionally pain cannot be controlled without removing the affected ovary surgically. Rarely, large ovarian hematomas are at risk of rupture, with fatal peritoneal exsanguinations, so persistent or uncontrollably painful ovarian hematomas should be treated by unilateral ovariectomy. Ovulation failure is a normal physiologic event for the mare during the spring and fall transition periods, but it may also occur occasionally in the cycling mare. Persistent anovulatory follicles (PAFs) are large (5 to 15 cm in diameter) and may result in prolonged interovulatory intervals. The cause of ovulation failure is not fully understood but has been suggested to be endocrine in nature. PAF has been reported to occur in approximately 8.2% of estrous cycles, and the incidence was found to increase with age.[33] PAFs may contain blood, which can be detected ultrasonically as scattered free-floating echogenic spots within the follicular fluid (Figure 8-10). Eventually the hemorrhage will organize into echoic fibrous bands traversing the follicular lumen. The majority of PAFs develop into luteal tissue, which can be confirmed by elevated plasma progesterone

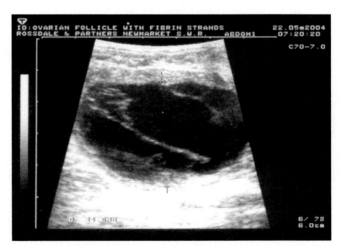

Figure 8-10 Transrectal ultrasonic appearance of persistent anovulatory ovarian follicle (PAF).

concentrations. Luteinized PAF can be treated with prostaglandins, and nonluteinized PAF will regress spontaneously in 1 to 4 weeks. Pregnancy obviously will not occur if the follicle becomes hemorrhagic or luteinized without ovulating (see Chapters 12 and 13).

Endometrial Biopsy

Special long (55 cm) basket-jawed forceps are essential to provide interpretable endometrial biopsy specimens[34-37] (Figure 8-11). Unfortunately, specimens obtained via endoscopic biopsy instruments are inadequate for histopathologic appraisal. Nonpregnancy must be confirmed before biopsy. One biopsy taken from a midhorn region is diagnostically representative unless there are palpable uterine abnormalities, when more than one sample should be taken.[37-38] A mid-diestrual biopsy is recommended as a routine. The sample is retrieved

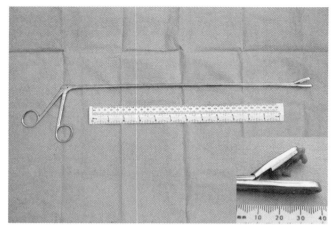

Figure 8-11   Mare endometrial biopsy forceps with basket jaw (inset).

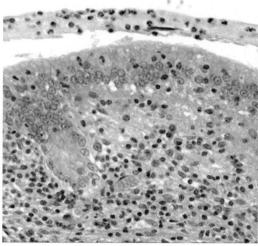

Figure 8-12 Photomicrograph of endometrial biopsy sample with signs of acute endometritis (polymorphonuclear leukocyte infiltration in uterine lumen and tissues).

carefully from the instrument with fine forceps or a needle to avoid artifactual damage and then placed into fixative without delay. If the mare is not in estrus and a specimen for bacteriologic examination was not collected via the cervix, then the inside of the biopsy forceps should be cultured immediately after removal of the tissue specimen. On some occasions, additional tissue (usually an adjacent endometrial fold) is retrieved, not required for fixation for histopathologic examination, and this can be used for bacteriologic examinations. Bouin's fluid is preferred as histopathologic fixative for reproductive tissues in general and endometrial samples in particular because their high water content leads to excessive artifactual shrinkage in more conventional fixatives (i.e., formol saline). The fixed tissues should be processed for microscopic examination and interpreted at a laboratory that has specific experience with equine endometrial biopsy samples and with equine gynecology.

Cyclic histology.   The microscopic architecture of the endometrium reflects the hormonal status of the mare, so changes that occur during estrus, diestrus, and anestrus can be classified accordingly.[37]

Histopathology. Microscopic pathologic abnormalities are usually mixed, so specific changes are classified and their significance is assessed in terms of the mare's age and gynecologic history.[37] They can be conveniently classified as inflammatory (acute and chronic endometritis) and noninflammatory conditions, including endometrial hypoplasia, hyperplasia, and chronic degenerative conditions.

Persistent superficial (acute) endometritis. Persistent superficial (acute) endometritis is diagnosed by the presence of PMNs (Figure 8-12) and, in severe cases, luminal epithelial degenerative changes, in endometrial biopsy samples taken at any stage of the nonpregnant mare's cycle.[34-37] It is recognized that as mares age and suffer the gynecologic and obstetric effects of a busy breeding career, their natural uterine defense mechanisms become less competent and they become more susceptible to recurrent/persistent acute endometritis.[39,40] These defense mechanisms involve local endometrial factors and myometrial function.[41-44]

Ultrasonography may help to demonstrate the severity of inflammation by the degree of endometrial edema and the volume and scan appearance of retained luminal fluid. Persistent endometritis indicates an inflammatory response to semen and/or a contaminating microorganism or microorganisms. Spermatozoa induce a physiologic inflammatory reaction in the uterus, which is an important part of normal sperm elimination. However, the inflammation should be resolved within 24 to 36 hours in normal mares, and a failure to resolve within this time results in persistent endometritis. If the endometritis is of bacterial origin, the associated organism(s) can be determined by bacteriologic examinations.

Persistent breeding-induced endometritis may resolve spontaneously with sexual rest. Waiting for this to happen is often not practical during a short breeding season, and treatment options include the intravenous administration of 10 to 25 IU oxytocin and/or uterine lavage with a large volume (1 to 2 L) of a buffered saline solution at 6 to 12 hours after breeding. The mare should be considered susceptible to recurrent endometritis each time she is mated, and appropriate prophylactic measures should be taken. Infectious endometritis is treated with local infusions of appropriate nonirritant, water-soluble antibiotics (e.g., ceftiofur sodium is recommended as a useful "first choice," although choice of antibiotics varies among clinicians, on grounds of availability, experience, and cost).[45] Where there are signs of uterine fluid accumulation or pyometritis/pyometra, large-volume (3 L) sterile saline irrigation (sometimes including 3% hydrogen peroxide) is recommended to remove uterine luminal inflammatory fluids and debris before starting antibiotic treatment. Irrigation is best performed via a uterine flushing catheter. Uterine fluid clearance can be stimulated by transrectal massage of the uterus or by the intravenous administration of 10 to 25 IU oxytocin. Large-volume uterine flushing, antibiotic therapy, and oxytocin treatment may be repeated daily or, if indicated, twice daily until ultrasonographic examina-

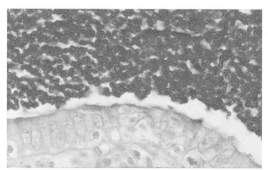

Figure 8-13 Photomicrograph of endometrial biopsy sample with signs of acute fungal (packed *Candida* spp. spores in the uterine lumen) endometritis (polymorphonuclear leukocyte infiltration) (PAS × 400).

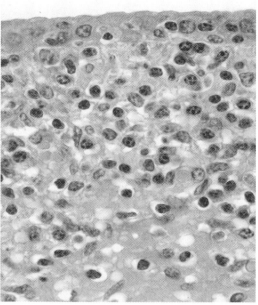

Figure 8-14 Photomicrograph of endometrial biopsy sample with signs of chronic infiltrative endometritis (mononuclear cell infiltration).

tions suggest resolution. In addition to local treatment with antibiotics, systemic treatment may, on occasion, be indicated. In the experience of the authors, systemic antibiotic treatment alone is of little value in the treatment of equine uterine infections. In most cases the infecting organism is in the uterine lumen and the most superficial part of the endometrium rather than in the deeper parts of the endometrial tissues. Thus local uterine luminal treatments are likely to be the most successful. The suitability of the preparation used for intrauterine irrigation is very important (irritant and incompletely dissolvable materials should be avoided), and 1 g ceftiofur sodium in 20 ml sterile water for injection has been found to be an excellent "first choice" pending identification of the pathogen(s) and specific antibiotic sensitivity test results.[23,45]

Fungal infections of the uterus (Figure 8-13) may produce clinical signs that vary from none, in which the infection is luminal and there is no tissue invasion, to severe purulent endometritis, demonstrable by ultrasonography.[46] If persistent, these infections lead to conception failure or, if infection occurs during pregnancy, to ascending placentitis and abortion. Treatment of mares with fungal infections is generally more challenging than for bacterial infections. Common treatment strategies include initial large-volume (3 L daily or twice daily) uterine irrigations with sterile saline solution (sometimes with added 3% hydrogen peroxide solution). Irrigation with dilute (0.5%) povidone-iodine solutions has been used, but care must be taken to avoid severe genital inflammation in individual mares. Culture and sensitivity will determine the choice of antifungal drugs. Daily intrauterine infusions for 7 to 10 days may be required to effectively resolve the infection. A single dose of a benzoylphenyl urea (Lufenuron) has been suggested to be effective in treating mares with fungal endometritis.[47] Initial data from four mares was encouraging but needs to be confirmed by controlled studies using larger groups of mares. Additional systemic (oral) treatment with ketoconazole may help resolution in some cases.

The success or failure of treatment for acute endometritis is monitored by "follow-up" endometrial smear/bacterial culture, ultrasonography, and/or biopsy examinations, taken 3 to 4 weeks after the end of the course of treatment.

Chronic infiltrative endometritis. Chronic infiltrative endometritis is diagnosed by the presence of mononuclear cells (histiocytes/lymphocytes and plasma cells) (Figure 8-14) in biopsy specimens.[34-37] The presence of these cells indicates a local immune response and therefore previous or ongoing challenge by semen or infectious agents. If uncomplicated by other abnormalities, this natural immune response is considered normal and no specific treatment is indicated. Occasionally, the immune response appears excessive, occasionally to granulomatous proportions, when treatment with a prolonged course of appropriate intrauterine antibiotics may be indicated to help remove deep-seated foci of infection.

Chronic degenerative endometrial disease (endometriosis). Chronic degenerative endometrial disease (endometriosis) is diagnosed by the presence of glandular degenerative changes in biopsy specimens in the form of "nests" (Figure 8-15), surrounded by lamellae of fibrous tissue or, less commonly, "cysts" (Figure 8-16), lined by glandular epithelial cells.[34-37] Periglandular, perivascular, or, less commonly, diffuse stromal fibrosis and angiopathy[48] are seen. These degenerate glands are malfunctional. Diffuse stromal fibrosis is considered to be a poor prognostic sign for the maintenance of future pregnancies.[34] Pools of tissue fluid (lymphatic "lacunae") (Figure 8-17) may be seen scattered in the stroma. As these develop, they become larger and migrate into the uterine lumen, attached to the endometrium by a "stalk" of lymphatic duct[37] (Figure 8-18). These uterine cysts (strictly speaking they are not endometrial cysts),[49] when large enough, can be seen by ultrasonography (Figure 8-19). It is unusual to sample a lymphatic cyst using conventional biopsy techniques.

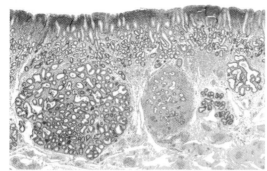

Figure 8-15 Photomicrograph of endometrial biopsy sample gland "nests" associated with chronic endometrial degenerative disease (degenerative glands with periglandular fibrosis).

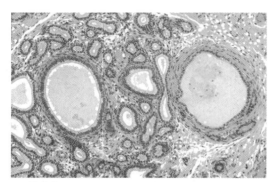

Figure 8-16 Photomicrograph of endometrial biopsy sample with gland cysts associated with chronic endometrial degenerative disease (cystic glands with periglandular fibrosis).

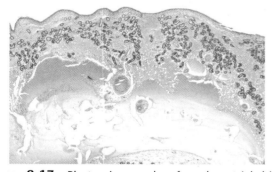

Figure 8-17 Photomicrograph of endometrial biopsy sample with lymphatic lacunae associated with chronic endometrial degenerative disease (degenerative glands with periglandular fibrosis).

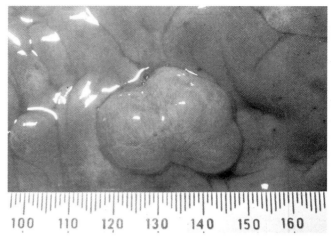

Figure 8-18 Endometrial lymphatic cyst.

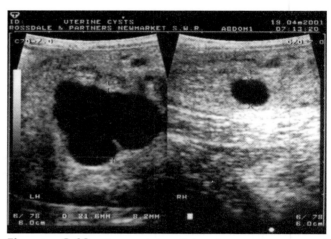

Figure 8-19 Transrectal ultrasonic appearance of endometrial lymphatic cyst.

Chronic endometrial degenerative changes are progressive and are associated most importantly with the normal aging process and cyclic hormonal effects[50] (Figure 8-20). The repeated stimulatory challenges of semen, microorganisms, external genital and environmental debris, and the physical challenges of obstetric difficulties may accelerate the progression of these changes, and it is possible that they may, to a large extent, account for the linear decline in fertility seen in the Thoroughbred mare population (see Figure 8-1). These degenerative changes are frequently seen in mares that suffer repeated pregnancy failure or prolonged gestation with fetal dysmaturity. Degenerative changes are inevitable to a degree, and thus each biopsy specimen must be assessed in terms of the mare's age and parity. The severity of these changes has been shown to be correlated with age to an extent that suggests that, in general terms, mares up to 9 years of age should have no signs, mares up to 13 years of age should have no more than mild signs, mares up to 15 years of age should have no more than moderate signs, and mares of 17 years and older are likely to have advanced signs (see Figure 8-20). Paradoxically, successful normal reproductive activity also appears to slow the development of these changes,[50] suggesting that repeated successive normal pregnancy, without obstetric difficulty, helps maintain a healthy endometrium. It is well recognized that older maiden mares (e.g., performance mares that retire later in life than Thoroughbred mares) frequently have degenerative changes in their biopsy speci-

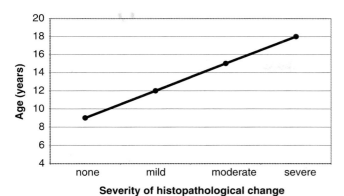

Figure 8-20 The progression of equine chronic degenerative endometrial disease (endometriosis) with age. (Data from Ricketts SW, Alonso S: The effect of age and parity on the development of equine chronic endometrial disease. Equine Vet J 1991; 23:189-192.)

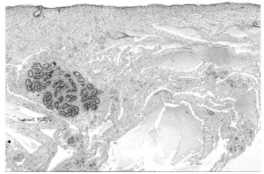

Figure 8-21 Photomicrograph of endometrial biopsy sample with signs of endometrial atrophy (loss of endometrial glands).

mens to degrees that are markedly in excess of what would be considered acceptable for their age. These mares often find difficulty in achieving a successful first pregnancy. Conversely, old Thoroughbred mares that have produced foals year after year since 4 years of age, without failures and while managing to avoid obstetric difficulties, have chronic endometrial degenerative changes that suggest a much younger age. The "moral" of the story is therefore good gynecologic and obstetric management and avoiding years of reproductive rest.

Where the degree of degenerative change is considered excessive for age, treatment with mechanical endometrial curettage may be attempted.[51] Improvements in histopathologic appearance and fertility can be expected in some mares, more reliably in those who are less than 17 years old. If this technique is of value, it must be by mild stimulation of endometrial blood supply. Attempts at chemical curettage are best avoided because the severity and complications of its effects in individual mares are unpredictable and uncontrollable. If transluminal adhesions or cervical damage occur, these may end the mare's reproductive career.

Endometrial atrophy. Endometrial atrophy is diagnosed by the loss of normal glands from the endometrium.[34-37] Temporary diffuse glandular atrophy is seen after prolonged ovarian inactivity and is therefore a normal feature during winter anestrus. This is seen in some mares with ovarian functional depression associated with ovarian granulosa cell tumors. True endometrial atrophy, with luminal and glandular atrophy, may be seen in aged mares, usually in association with senile ovarian malfunction, and is an "end-stage" process (Figure 8-21). Rarely, true endometrial atrophy has been seen in younger mares after severe recurrent acute endometritis with *P. aeruginosa* infection. No treatment is successful for true endometrial atrophy, and retirement is the most practical option.

Endometrial hypoplasia. Endometrial hypoplasia is diagnosed by signs of diffuse glandular underdevelopment and has been seen in young barren maiden mares, sometimes in association with ovarian cyclic irregulari-

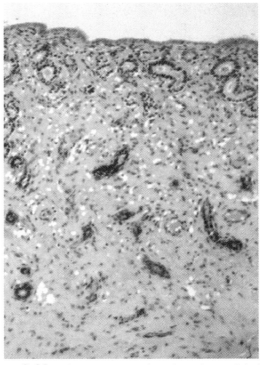

Figure 8-22 Photomicrograph of endometrial biopsy sample with signs of endometrial hypoplasia (failure of development of endometrial glands).

ties[34-37] (Figure 8-22). It appears to be a feature of relative genital immaturity and usually resolves, without treatment, in time. In a young maiden mare, where the degree of hypoplasia is marked and ovarian size is minimal, or where the condition persists, the possibility that fundamental ovarian abnormality (gonadal dysgenesis) is involved should be considered and chromosome analysis (karyotype) should be performed.[52]

Endometrial hyperplasia. Endometrial hyperplasia is diagnosed by signs of endometrial glandular overactivity.[34-37] Glandular hyperplasia with hypersecretion is a normal feature of the postpartum or postpregnancy

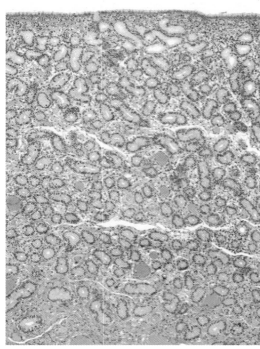

Figure 8-23 Photomicrograph of endometrial biopsy sample with signs of endometrial hyperplasia (persistent glandular hyperplasia).

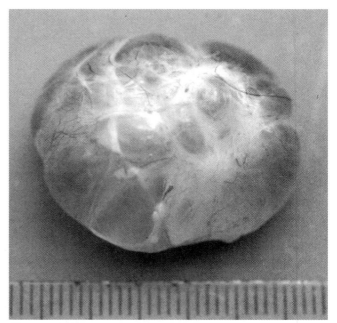

Figure 8-24 Endometrial lymphatic cysts removed by hysterendoscopic loop wire thermocautery.

failure period, and normal glandular architecture and secretory activity is usually achieved by 10 to 12 days but occasionally may persist for weeks if not months, when it is considered pathologic[37] (Figure 8-23). In such cases, acute endometritis is often a complicating feature. Treatment with the intravenous administration of 10 to 25 IU oxytocin has been used by the authors with good results. It is believed that oxytocin may reduce endometrial hyperplasia via its endometrial vasoconstrictive effect, as reported in other species.[53] Acute endometritis, where involved, should be treated as discussed above.

In some cases, recurrent acute endometritis appears to produce diffuse glandular hyperplasia, probably associated with short cycling and hyperestrogenism.[37] Successful treatment of the acute endometritis will reduce the signs of diffuse glandular hyperplasia, and treatment with oxytocin appears to aid resolution.

Other Uterine Abnormalities

Endometrial lymphatic cysts. The development of endometrial lymphatic cysts has been discussed above. They are observed in multiparous mares over 14 years old[37] (see Figure 8-19) and are commonly detected with ultrasonography. They can be seen during ultrasonographic examination because the lymphatic fluid that they contain is anechoic. The cysts may be unilocular or multilocular. They are frequently inconvenient in that they may confuse pregnancy examinations. Otherwise, unless they are very large, where they may prevent the normal intrauterine mobility of the pre-fixed embryo,

essential for early recognition of pregnancy, and/or they are widespread throughout the uterus, they appear to have no specific effect on fertility.[54] They can, if considered necessary, be visualized and removed with laser ablation or loop-wire thermocautery via a videoendoscope (Figure 8-24).

Transluminal fibrous adhesions. Transluminal fibrous adhesions may follow obstetric injuries or the injudicious intrauterine use of irritant chemicals. If widespread and diffuse, these are untreatable and the mare is most sensibly retired. If focal and discrete, they may be removed with laser ablation, thermocautery, or by biopsy attachment, via a videoendoscope.

Intrauterine foreign bodies. Use of the videoendoscope in mares with recurrent nonresponsive endometritis has revealed, in some cases, luminal foreign bodies consisting of placental remnants, cotton wool (presumably culturette tip fragments), and amorphous debris with a central core of multiplying bacteria or unidentifiable degenerate debris (Figure 8-25). Once removed with a biopsy attachment, via a videoendoscope, these cases responded to treatment for acute endometritis.

Endometrial neoplasia. Leiomyomas and fibroleiomyomas are uncommon but are the most frequently diagnosed equine endometrial tumors (Figure 8-26). They are usually small and benign and have no primary effect on fertility. They may be obstructive and may bleed. Treatment by laser surgery, via a videoendoscope, or surgical removal via hysterotomy, via laparotomy or laparoscopy, is only indicated where the tumor is large, when it may be pedunculated, and may cause persistent endometrial hemorrhage and secondary endometritis. Malignant endometrial adenocarcinoma has been only rarely recorded. One such case had respiratory signs, and necropsy examination confirmed pulmonary metastases.

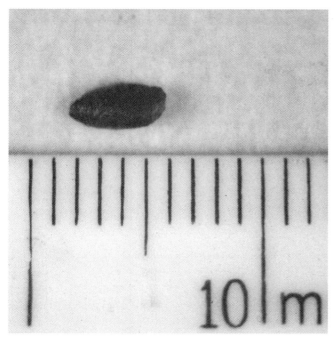

Figure 8-25 Uterine luminal foreign body removed by hysterendoscopic biopsy instrument retrieval.

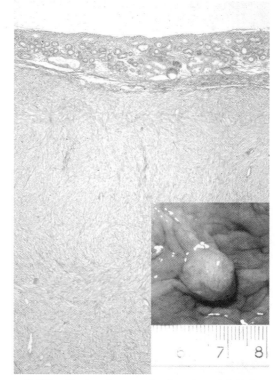

Figure 8-26 Photomicrograph of endometrial leiomyoma with gross appearance (inset).

Hysteroscopy

Examinations are best made with the videoendoscope, which gives better visualization than is possible with conventional fiber technology endoscopes. Endometrial lymphatic cysts (see Figure 8-24), fluid accumulations, fibrous adhesions, foreign bodies (see Figure 8-25), and endometrial tumors may be visualized and sometimes removed, using laser or thermocautery instruments. Biopsy specimens obtained with instruments supplied for passage through the endoscope are too small to be diagnostically useful. Conventional basket-jawed endometrial biopsy forceps can be passed alongside the endoscope, and visually directed samples can be obtained.

Laparoscopy

This technique has been used to study ovulation in mares and to treat fallopian tubes with external applications of prostaglandins for research purposes. Fallopian tube blockage is a rare condition in mares. Expertise and experience with this technique has improved markedly during recent years, and neoplastic ovaries and intractable ovarian hematomas (Figure 8-27) are now most commonly removed with the laparoscope, with the mare standing under sedation and local anesthetic. The technique may be used for intrapelvic exploration of the genitalia in specific cases.

Laparotomy

Rarely, midline or flank laparotomy (i.e., surgically opening the abdomen with the mare under general anesthesia) may be indicated for the investigation and/or treatment of uterine abnormality.

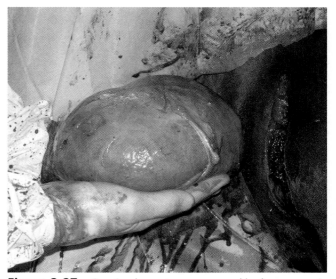

Figure 8-27 Ovarian hematoma removed by laparoscopic surgery.

Extrauterine Abnormalities

Organizing broad ligament hematomas or pelvic adhesions may be detected by their palpably hard consistency and their homogeneous appearance on ultrasonographic examination. Periuterine abscesses sometimes follow obstetric injuries, and these require intensive medical treatment with systemic antibiotic therapy.

Box **8-1**

Prognosis 1: After the First Examination, Before Treatment

Category 1	Mares that have no significant demonstrable gynecologic abnormalities	Good prognosis
Category 2	Mares that have gynecologic abnormalities that are expected to respond to treatment and/or that are unlikely to significantly affect their reproductive performance	Satisfactory prognosis
Category 3	Mares that have gynecologic abnormalities that are expected not to respond to treatment and/or are likely to significantly affect their reproductive performance	Poor prognosis

Box **8-2**

Prognosis 2: After Treatment and the Second Examination

Category 1	Mares that have no significant gynecologic abnormalities or whose abnormalities have recovered, apparently completely, following treatment	Good prognosis
Category 2	Mares that have gynecologic abnormalities that are unlikely to significantly affect their reproductive performance or whose abnormalities have recovered, following treatment, to a degree that should allow adequate compensation	Satisfactory prognosis
Category 3	Mares that have gynecologic abnormalities that are likely to significantly affect their reproductive performance or whose abnormalities have not recovered, or have become worse, following treatment, to a degree that will preclude adequate compensation	Poor prognosis

PROGNOSIS FOR FUTURE BREEDING

Some mare owners request a prognosis for the chances for successful future breeding to help with mating plans or to help with the decision to retire the mare. Although this is an understandable request, prognoses[34,55] should be made with great caution. Prognoses are most usefully and more accurately made in two stages,[8] on the following basis (Box 8-1).

Aged mares with true (not seasonally induced) endometrial atrophy (i.e., in effect, senility) and young maiden mares with fundamental chromosome abnormalities (gonadal dysgenesis) are appropriately retired at this stage.[8] Troedsson et al[42] demonstrated a significant association between biopsy grade and susceptibility to chronic uterine infection in mares with severe endometrial pathologic conditions (Box 8-2).

Failure to improve or deterioration after specific uterine treatments and, where necessary, further examinations and further specific treatments having been performed are considered very poor prognostic signs.[8]

SUBSEQUENT MANAGEMENT

After a satisfactory follow-up examination, a management plan is formulated to help the individual mare compensate for her residual abnormalities. The aim is to limit uterine exposure to semen and bacteria and to assist the uterus to physically clear contaminants and inflammatory products after breeding. This can be achieved, in populations of horses where registration authorities allow, by the use of artificial insemination (AI) with antibiotic-extended semen:

1. Satisfactory endometrial culturette and smear test results are obtained at the current estrous period.
2. An apparently normal, developing, mature ovarian follicle is palpable.
3. Mating is arranged as close as possible to the estimated time of likely ovulation. This can be aided by the administration of human chorionic gonadotropin (hCG) or a gonadotropin-releasing hormone (GnRH) analogue.
4. AI using a semen extender that contains antibiotics is performed.
5. Physical clearance after breeding can be assisted by the use of uterotonic drugs and/or uterine lavage.
   A. Oxytocin or $PGF_{2\alpha}$ treatment at 4 to 8 hours after breeding will effectively aid in uterine clearance, resulting in improved pregnancy rates in susceptible mares.[56,57] Data suggest that a lower dose of oxytocin (5 to 10 IU) may be more effective than higher doses in promoting uterine clearance.[58,59] Care must be taken with regard to the timing of $PGF_{2\alpha}$ treatment. Recent reports have demonstrated that

PGF$_{2\alpha}$ can cause a delay in the formation of a functional corpus luteum when administered within 2 days after ovulation. This was associated with pregnancy failure in two of the reports.[60,61]

B. Large-volume uterine lavage at 6 to 12 hours after breeding will also effectively assist in clearing the uterus from fluid and inflammatory products.[62] Because sperm transport to the oviduct is completed within 4 hours after breeding, uterine lavage between 6 and 12 hours after breeding will have no adverse effect on fertility.[63,64]

C. Manual dilation of the cervix in mares with poor cervical dilation may help these mares to more effectively clear their uteri of fluid.

6. AI should be limited to once per estrous period because each exposure to semen induces an inflammatory response.

Where AI is not applicable (i.e., in Thoroughbred horses), "minimal contamination breeding techniques" may be used.[65] These consist of the following:

1. Satisfactory endometrial culture and smear test results are obtained at the current estrous period.
2. An apparently normal, mature, developing ovarian follicle is palpable.
3. Mating is arranged as close as possible to the estimated time of likely ovulation.
4. Prebreeding semen extender, containing antibiotics, may be instilled into the mare's uterus as soon as possible before mating, if considered appropriate.
5. Luteinizing hormone in the form of hCG or a GnRH analogue is used to hasten ovulation.
6. The uterus is flushed with 1 to 3 L sterile saline (depending on size of mare/uterus) and then treated with a water-soluble, nonirritant, broad-spectrum antibiotic solution to which the common equine uterine aerobic and anaerobic pathogens are sensitive (e.g., 1 g ceftiofur sodium in 20 ml sterile water for injection), 12 to 24 hours after mating, followed by 10 to 25 IU oxytocin administered intravenously to aid uterine clearance. This may be repeated 24 hours and occasionally 48 hours later, depending on the circumstances of the individual case.
7. A second mating during that estrous period is not recommended.

Management for "High Risk" During Achieved Pregnancies

Pregnancies achieved from such mares should be identified as "high risk" and should be monitored by watching the mare's udder and in appropriate cases by serial ultrasonographic examinations. Unnecessary maternal stress should be avoided throughout pregnancy. Prolonged gestation sometimes occurs in mares with advanced chronic endometrial degenerative disease, and this identifies the fetus as "high risk" and neonatal critical care facilities should be prepared for use, when required.

Ultrasonographic examinations of the placenta in mares that are considered to be at risk for abortion during late gestation can be performed by transabdominal and transrectal approaches.

Transabdominal Ultrasonography

Using a 3.5- or 5-MHz sector scanner, four quadrants of the placenta (right cranial, right caudal, left cranial, and left caudal) should be examined by the transabdominal approach. Mares with normal pregnancies should have a minimal combined thickness of the uterus and the placenta (CTUP) of 7.1 ± 1.6 mm and a maximal CTUP of 11.5 ± 2.4 mm. Pregnancies with an increased CTUP have been associated with the delivery of abnormal foals.[66] The caudal portion of the allantochorion cannot be imaged by this approach, preventing the clinician from diagnosing ascending placentitis in its early stages. However, placental thickening and partial separation of the allantochorion from the endometrium may be observed in mares with placentitis originating from a hematogenous infection.

Transrectal Ultrasonography

Imaging the caudal allantochorion in late gestational mares provides an excellent image of the placenta close to the cervical star (Figure 8-28).[67] A 5-MHz linear transducer should be positioned 1 to 2 inches cranial of the

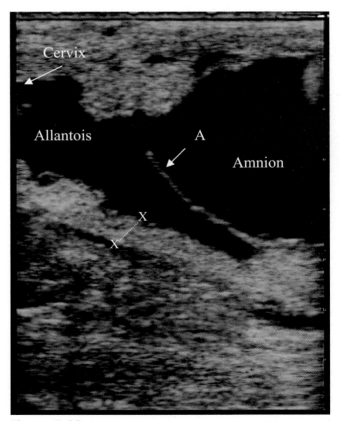

Figure 8-28 Transrectal ultrasonographic examination of the caudal part of the placenta in a late gestational mare. *A,* Amniotic membrane; *x–x,* CTUP.

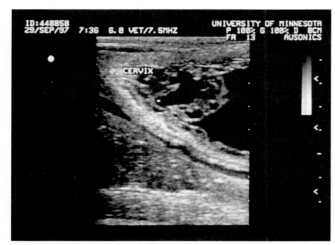

Figure 8-29   Transrectal ultrasonographic examination of the caudal part of the placenta in a late gestational mare with ascending placentitis. Note the thickness of the CTUP and the separation of the allantochorion from the endometrium in an area adjacent to the cervical star.

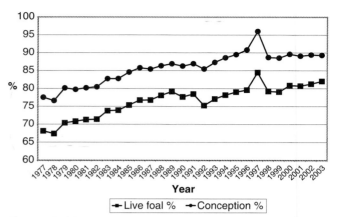

Figure 8-30   Weatherbys' annual returns for UK and Irish Thoroughbred mares, 1977-2003, conception and live foal rates.

cervical-placental junction and then moved laterally until the middle branch of the uterine artery is visible at the ventral aspect of the uterine body. The CTUP should then be measured between the middle branch of the uterine artery and the allantoic fluid. The clinician must make sure that the amnion is not adjacent to the allantochorion, because this may result in a false increased CTUP. It is important to obtain all CTUP measurements from the ventral aspect of the uterine body, because edema of the dorsal aspect of the allantochorion has been noted in normal pregnant mares during the last month of gestation. Increases in CTUP greater than 8 mm between day 271 and 300, greater than 10 mm between day 301 and 330, and greater than 12 mm after day 330 have been associated with placental failure and impending abortion.[68] In advanced stages of placentitis, hyperechoic fluid may be imaged in the space between the uterus and the placenta (Figure 8-29).

The equine placenta is part of an endocrine fetoplacental interaction, which synthesizes and metabolizes progestagens. Mares with advanced stages of placentitis or placental separation may have increased plasma concentrations of progestagens as a result of stress to the fetoplacental unit. Because fetoplacental progesterone is rapidly metabolized to 5α-pregnanes, its metabolites may not be recognized by all commercial progesterone assays. Therefore maternal serum progesterone concentrations in late pregnant mares do not always reflect the conditions in the uterus. Using an experimental model to induce placentitis, it was found that mares that develop a chronic form of placentitis responded with increased plasma progesterone concentrations, whereas mares that developed acute placentitis and abortion soon after infection experienced a drop in plasma progesterone concentrations.[69,70] These authors suggested that measurement of repeated samples of plasma progestin concentrations in mares with placentitis might be a useful method to identify mares that may abort or deliver prematurely.

Treatment of mares with placentitis should be aimed toward elimination of the infectious agents, reduction of the inflammatory response, and reduction of the increased myometrial contractility in response to the ongoing inflammation. Poor perineal confirmation, urine pooling, and cervical lesions should be corrected before breeding to prevent an ascending route of infection during pregnancy. Mares with clinical signs of placentitis or abnormal placental findings upon ultrasonographic evaluation should be treated with broad-spectrum antibiotics (e.g., trimethoprim sulfa), antiinflammatory medication (flunixin meglumine, 1.1 mg/kg q12h or phenylbutazone, 4 mg/kg q12h), and tocolytics (altrenogest, 0.088 mg/kg q24h or clenbuterol, 0.8 μg/kg q12h). Pentoxifylline (7.5 mg/kg PO q12h) has been suggested to increase oxygenation of the placenta.[71,72] Bacterial and fungal cultures should be obtained in mares with vaginal discharge for isolation of a causative agent and sensitivity to antibiotics. After foaling or abortion, the entire placenta (and foal in case of abortion) should be submitted for necropsy examinations. The endometrium should be cultured, and the mare should be treated for endometritis if the placental cultures suggest infection.

HAS PROGRESS BEEN MADE?

Weatherbys' annual returns made by owners of Thoroughbred mares in the United Kingdom and Ireland report that during the 26 years from 1977 to 2003 the number of mares registered as "mated by registered Thoroughbred stallions" increased from 14,556 to 23,136 and the number of live foals from 8,099 to 15,333. When these data are presented in terms of percentage of mares mated (minus "no returns" and "mares dead and exported," for whom accurate data is not available), encouraging trends emerge. Overall pregnancy rate (number of mares bred/numbers of mares pregnant) (%) has increased from 77.5% to 89.3% (Figure 8-30). Similarly, live foal rate (%) has increased from 68.1% to 82.0% (see Figure 8-30). Barren mare rate (%) has decreased from 22.5% to 10.7% (Figure 8-31). Gestational failure rate (%)

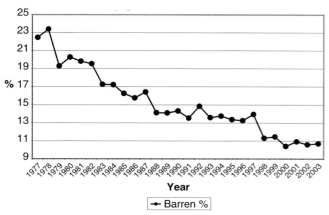

Figure 8-31 Weatherbys' annual returns for UK and Irish Thoroughbred mares, 1977-2003, barren mare rate.

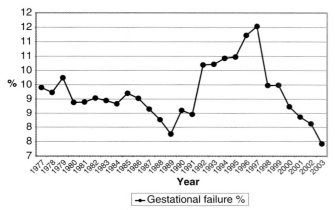

Figure 8-32 Weatherbys' annual returns for UK and Irish Thoroughbred mares, 1977-2003, gestational failure rate.

has reduced from 9.4% to 7.4% (Figure 8-32). Closer examination of the latter data shows a downward trend from 1977 to 1989, followed by a rise that is believed to be associated with the widespread use of ultrasonographic examinations, making possible the diagnosis of early gestational failure, which has since been reflected in mare owners' returns. Since then it appears that some progress has been made to decrease pregnancy losses.

The progressive fall in the barren mare rate by more than 50% over the last 23 years is particularly encouraging. Although it is only possible to speculate on the probable multifactorial causes of this improvement, one must hope that progress in management and equine gynecology has at least played a useful part.

CONCLUSION

Few mares are truly infertile, and with an accurate diagnosis, rational treatment, and careful management, most can be encouraged to breed successfully. Preparing the barren mare for the new breeding season early is essential to maximize chances for an early successful pregnancy and to help prolong the mare's long-term breeding

career. Management "teamwork" is a vital factor, and sufficient commitment is required from the owner, in terms of interest and finance, from the stud farm manager, in terms of interest and staff time and facilities, and from the veterinarian, in terms of interest, time, knowledge, expertise, experience, and provision of the necessary equipment.

References

1. Weatherbys, 2003
2. Morris LHA, Allen WR: Reproductive efficiency of intensively managed Thoroughbred mares in Newmarket. Equine Vet J 2002; 34:51-60.
3. Jeffcott LB, Rossdale PD, Freestone J et al: An assessment of wastage in Thoroughbred racing from conception to 4 years of age. Equine Vet J 1982; 14:185-198.
4. Greenhof GR, Kenney RM: Evaluation of the reproductive status of nonpregnant mares. J Am Vet Med Assoc 1975; 167:449.
5. Baker CB, Kenney RM: Systematic approach to the diagnosis of the infertile or subfertile mare. In Morrow DA (ed): Current Therapy in Theriogenology, Philadelphia, WB Saunders, 1980.
6. Ricketts SW: The barren mare: diagnosis, prognosis, prophylaxis and treatment for genital abnormality, part 1. Practice 1989; 11:119-125.
7. Ricketts SW: The barren mare: diagnosis, prognosis, prophylaxis and treatment for genital abnormality, part 2. Practice 1989; 11:156-164.
8. Ricketts SW, Alonso S: Assessment of the breeding prognosis of mares using paired endometrial biopsy techniques. Equine Vet J 1991; 23:185-188.
9. Caslick EA: The vulva and vulvo-vaginal orifice and its relation to genital health of the Thoroughbred mare. Cornell Vet 1937; 27:178.
10. Ricketts SW: Perineal conformation abnormalities. In Robinson NE (ed): Current Therapy in Equine Medicine, 2nd edition, pp 518-520, Philadelphia, WB Saunders, 1987.
11. Trotter GW: Surgery of the perineum of the mare. In McKinnon AO, Voss JL (eds): Equine Reproduction, pp 417-427, Philadelphia, Lea & Febiger, 1993.
12. Pouret EJM: Surgical technique for the correction of pneumo- and urovagina. Equine Vet J 1982; 14:249.
13. Ricketts SW, Young A, Medici EB: Uterine and clitoral cultures. In McKinnon AO, Voss JL (eds): Equine Reproduction, pp 234-245, Philadelphia, Lea & Febiger, 1993.
14. Ricketts SW: Contagious endometritis (CEM). Equine Vet Educ 1996; 8:166-170.
15. LeBlanc MM: Vaginal examination. In McKinnon AO, Voss JL (eds): Equine Reproduction, pp 221-224, Baltimore, Williams & Wilkins, 1992.
16. Evans LH, Tate LP, Cooper WL et al: Surgical repair of cervical lacerations and the incompetent cervix. Proceedings of the 21st Annual Convention of the American Association of Equine Practitioners, pp 483-486, 1975.
17. Brown JS, Varner DD, Hinrichs K et al: Surgical repair of the lacerated cervix in the mare. Theriogenology 1984; 22:351.
18. Aanes WA: Cervical laceration(s). In McKinnon AO, Voss JL (eds): Equine Reproduction, pp 444-449, Lea & Febiger, 1993.
19. Whitwell KE: Investigations into fetal and neonatal losses in the horse. Vet Clin North Am Large Anim Pract 1980; 2:313-331.
20. Ricketts SW: Bacteriological examinations of the mare's cervix: techniques and interpretation of results. Vet Rec 1981; 108:46.

21. Wingfield Digby NJ: The technique and clinical interpretation of endometrial cytology in mares. Equine Vet J 1978; 10:167-170.

22. Wingfield Digby NJ, Ricketts SW: Results of concurrent bacteriological and cytological examinations of the endometrium of mares in routine studfarm practice 1978-1981. J Reprod Fertil Suppl 1982; 32:181-185.

23. Ricketts SW, Mackintosh ME: The role of anaerobic bacteria in equine endometritis. J Reprod Fertil Suppl 1987; 35:343-351.

24. Ginther OJ: Ultrasonic Imaging and Reproductive Events in the Mare, Cross Plains, Wis, Equiservices, 1986.

25. Ricketts SW: Uterine abnormalities. In Robinson NE (ed): Current Therapy in Equine Medicine, 2nd edition, pp 503-507, Philadelphia, WB Saunders, 1987.

26. McKinnon AO, Carnevale EM: Ultrasonography. In McKinnon AO, Voss JL (eds): Equine Reproduction, pp 211-220, Baltimore, Williams & Wilkins, 1992.

27. Ginther OJ: Ultrasonic imaging of equine ovarian follicles and corpora lutea. Vet Clin North Am Equine Pract 1988; 10:197-213.

28. Kenney RM, Ganjam VK: Selected pathological changes of the mare uterus and ovary. J Reprod Fertil Suppl 1975; 23:335-339.

29. Liu IRW: Ovarian abnormalities. In Robinson NE (ed): Current Therapy in Equine Medicine, 2nd edition, pp 500-502, Philadelphia, WB Saunders, 1987.

30. McCue PM: Equine granulosa cell tumors. Proceedings of the 38th Annual Convention of the American Association of Equine Practitioners, pp 587-593, 1992.

31. Bailey MT, Wheaton JE, Troedsson MHT: Inhibin concentrations in mares with granulosa cell tumors. Theriogenology 2002; 57:1885-1895.

32. Hinrichs K, Watson ED, Kenney RM: Granulosa cell tumor in a mare with a functional contralateral ovary. J Am Vet Med Assoc 1990; 197:1037-1038.

33. McCue PM, Squires EL: Persistent anovulatory follicles in the mare. Theriogenology 2002; 58:541-543.

34. Kenney RM: Cyclic and pathologic changes in the mare endometrium as detected by biopsy with a note on early embryonic death. J Am Vet Med Assoc 1987; 172:241.

35. Ricketts SW: The technique and clinical application of endometrial biopsy in mares. Equine Vet J 1975; 7:102-109.

36. Ricketts SW: Endometrial biopsy as a guide to diagnosis of endometrial pathology in the mare. J Reprod Fertil Suppl 1975; 23:341-345.

37. Ricketts SW: Histological and histopathological studies on the endometrium of the mare. Fellowship Thesis, London, Royal College of Veterinary Surgeons, 1978.

38. Bergman RV, Kenney RM: Representativeness of a uterine biopsy in the mare. Proceedings of the 21st Annual Convention of the American Association of Equine Practitioners, pp 355-362, 1975.

39. Hughes JP, Loy RG: Investigations on the effect of intrauterine inoculations of *Streptococcus zooepidemicus* in the mare. Proceedings of the 15th Annual Convention of the American Association of Equine Practitioners, pp 289-292, 1969.

40. Peterson FB, McFeely RA, David JSE: Studies on the pathogenesis of endometritis in the mare. Proceedings of the 15th Annual Convention of the American Association of Equine Practitioners, pp 279-288, 1969.

41. Watson ED: Uterine defence mechanisms in mares resistant and susceptible to persistent endometritis: a review. Equine Vet J 1988; 20:397-400.

42. Troedsson MH, deMoraes MJ, Liu IK: Correlations between histologic endometrial lesions in mares and clinical response to intrauterine exposure with *Streptococcus zooepidemicus*. Am J Vet Res 1993; 54:570-572.

43. Troedsson MH: Uterine clearance and resistance to persistent endometritis in the mare. Theriogenology 1999; 52:461-471.

44. Watson ED: Post-breeding endometritis in the mare. Anim Reprod Sci 2000; 60-61, 221-232.

45. Ricketts SW: Treatment of equine endometritis with intrauterine irrigations of ceftiofur sodium: a comparison with mares treated in a similar manner with a mixture of sodium benzylpenicillin, neomycin sulphate, polymyxin B sulphate and furaltadone hydrochloride. Pferdeheilkunde 1997; 5:486-489.

46. Blue MG: Fungal endometritis. In Robinson NE (ed): Current Therapy in Equine Medicine, 2nd edition, pp 511-512, Philadelphia, WB Saunders, 1987.

47. Hess MB, Parker NA, Purswell BJ, et al: Use of lufenuron as a treatment for fungal endometritis in four mares. J Am Vet Med Assoc 2002; 221:266-267.

48. Gruninger B, Schoon H-A, Schoon D et al: Incidence and morphology of endometrial angiopathies in mares in relationship to age and parity. J Comp Pathol 1998; 119:293-309.

49. McKinnon AO, Squires EL, Carnevale EM et al: Diagnostic ultrasonography of uterine pathology in the mare. Proceedings of the 33rd Annual Convention of the American Association of Equine Practitioners, pp 605-622, 1987.

50. Ricketts SW, Alonso S: The effect of age and parity on the development of equine chronic endometrial disease. Equine Vet J 1991; 23:189-192.

51. Ricketts SW: Endometrial curettage in the mare. Equine Vet J 1985; 17:324-328.

52. Chandley A, Fletcher J, Rossdale PD et al: Chromosome abnormalities as a cause of infertility in mares. J Reprod Fertil Suppl 1975; 23:377-383.

53. Porter DG: Personal communication.

54. Eilts BE, Svholl DT, Paccamonti DL et al: Prevalence of endometrial cysts and their effect on fertility. Biol Reprod Mono 1995; 1:527-532.

55. Doig PA, McNight JD, Miller RB: The use of endometrial biopsy in the infertile mare. Can Vet J 1981; 22:72-76.

56. Pycock JF: Assessment of oxytocin and intrauterine antibiotics on intrauterine fluid and pregnancy rates in the mare. Proceedings of the 40th Annual Convention of the American Association of Equine Practitioners, pp 19-20, 1994.

57. Rasch K, Schoon H-A, Sieme H et al: Histomorphological endometrial status and influence of oxytocin on the uterine drainage and pregnancy rates in mares. Equine Vet J 1996; 28:455-460.

58. Madill S, Troedsson MHT, Santschi EM: Individual registration of longitudinal and circular muscle in the equine endometrium using electromyography and strain gauges: preliminary data [abstr]. In Havermeyer Foundation International Workshop on Uterine Defense Mechanisms in the Mare: Aspects of Physical Clearance, p 10, 1997.

59. Campbell MLH, England GCW: A comparison of the ecbolic efficacy of intravenous and intrauterine oxytocin treatments. Theriogenology 2002; 58:473-478.

60. Troedsson MHT, Ohlgren AF, Ababneh M et al: Effect of periovulatory prostaglandin $F_{2\alpha}$ on pregnancy rates and luteal function. Theriogenology 2001; 55:1891-1899.

61. Brendemuehl JP: Effect of oxytocin and cloprostenol on luteal formation, function and pregnancy rates in mares. Theriogenology 2002; 58:623-626.

62. Troedsson MHT, Scott MA, Liu IKM: Comparative treatments of mares susceptible to chronic uterine infection. Am J Vet Res 1995; 56:468-472.

63. Brinsko SP, Varner DD, Blanchard TL et al: The effect of postbreeding uterine lavage on pregnancy rate in mares. Theriogenology 1990; 33:465-476.

64. Brinsko SP, Varner DD, Blanchard TL: The effect of uterine lavage performed four hours post insemination on pregnancy rate in mares. Theriogenology 1991; 35:1111-1120.

65. Kenney RM, Bergman RV, Cooper WL et al: Minimal contamination techniques for breeding mares: technique and preliminary findings. Proceedings of the 21st Annual Convention of the American Association of Equine Practitioners, p 327, 1975.

66. Reef VB, Vaala WE, Worth LT et al: Ultrasonographic assessment of fetal well being during late gestation: development of an equine biophysical profile. Equine Vet J 1996; 28:200-208.

67. Renaudin C, Troedsson MHT, Gillis C et al: Ultrasonographic evaluation of the equine placenta by transrectal and transabdominal approach in pregnant mares. Theriogenology 1997; 47:559-573.

68. Troedsson MHT, Renaudin CD, Zent WW et al: Transrectal ultrasonography of the placenta in normal mares and in mares with pending abortion: a field study. Proceedings of the 43rd Annual Convention of the American Association of Equine Practitioners, pp 256-258, 1997.

69. Stawicki RJ, Ruebel H, Hansen PJ et al: Endocrinological findings in an experimental model of ascending placentitis. Theriogenology 2002; 58:849-852.

70. Sheerin PC, Morris S, Kelleman A et al: Diagnostic efficiency of transrectal ultrasonography and plasma progestin profiles in identifying mares at risk of premature delivery. Proceedings of the 1st Annual Focus Meeting of the American Association of Equine Practitioners, pp 22-23, 2003.

71. Kucheriavenko AN: Effect of Trental on placental transport function and fetal development in hypotrophy. Akush Ginekol (Moscow) 1985; 4:67-69.

72. Geor RJ, Weiss DJ, Burris SM et al: Effects of furosemide and pentoxifylline on blood flow properties in horses. Am J Vet Res 1992; 53:2043-2049.

CHAPTER 9

Endocrine Tests

ROBERT H. DOUGLAS

To provide some insight into the growth rate of routine endocrine diagnostics in equine practice the following time line may be of interest. In 1984 BET Labs of Lexington, Kentucky, was launched to provide a commercial endocrine diagnostic service for veterinarians. In that first year approximately 6,000 hormone assays were performed, mostly for progesterone and predominantly for veterinarians in the Lexington area. Twenty years later this laboratory performs approximately 60,000 assays annually, with progestins still most commonly assayed, for veterinarians throughout North America. When accompanied by a United States Department of Agriculture (USDA) import permit, it is possible for our laboratory to receive serum for assay from almost any part of the world. Application of endocrine diagnostic testing in other countries has been greatly limited due to lack of knowledge and economics. For example, BET Labs do Brasil has been in existence for over 5 years in Rio de Janeiro, Brazil, and performs less than 1,000 assays per year in equine patients, even though the number of horses in Brazil is about equal to the number in the United States. The Brazilian dog owner is much more willing to pay for endocrine diagnostics than the horse owner.

As mentioned previously, diagnostic endocrinology in equine practice has been used for over 20 years. By far the most common assay is for progesterone. It is important to distinguish between progesterone, progestins, and progestagens because the difference is not recognized by most veterinary practitioners. It should be noted that the metabolites of pregnenolone (P5) and progesterone (P4) are usually referred to as progestagens. The term *progestins* will be used here to refer to progesterone and its metabolites. It is recognized that the assay used in our laboratory may also measure some fraction of pregnenolone and therefore a more correct term might have been *progestagens*.

The radioimmunoassay kit used to generate the data for this chapter is for progesterone. It should be noted that the antibody used in this progesterone kit cross-reacts with progesterone metabolites and thus the kit can be used to measure progestins as well as progesterone.

PROGESTINS

In the pregnant broodmare progesterone is present only through 150 days of pregnancy, and thereafter the predominant progestins are 5α-pregnanes and 17α-hydroxy progesterone. The ovaries are no longer needed after 100 days of pregnancy to support pregnancy; thus only progestin concentrations during the first 100 days of pregnancy will be addressed in this chapter. In 1975 Holtan et al[1] reported that progesterone became very low, dropping to levels below 2 ng/ml by 180 days of pregnancy, and remained low until 30 days before parturition, at which time levels rose dramatically until the mare foaled. By 1990 Holtan et al[2] found that by using more specific assay techniques, including gas chromatography and mass spectrometry, progesterone was not detectable during the last half of pregnancy; however, progestins were detectable during this time and consisted predominantly of 5α-pregnanes. These progestins were actually what was rising before parturition. Recently it was suggested that 5α-pregnane-3, 20-dione (5αDHP) may be more biologically important than progesterone in late gestation in the mare.[3] This importance is related to its greater binding by uterine P4 receptors than P4 or other progestagens and that its concentration rises during the last 20 to 30 days of gestation, falling rapidly during the last few days before birth.[4] It is also a major precursor for other progestagens. Interestingly, 5αDHP concentrations were elevated by exogenous Regumate (altrenogest) but not by P4 in oil in late gestation in mares.[5] Species crosses, such as in jennies pregnant with a hinny fetus, have significantly higher serum progestins than horse mares carrying a horse fetus. Mares pregnant with a mule fetus appear to have progestin concentrations similar to mares pregnant with a horse fetus.[6] Progestin data in this chapter are from mares carrying horse fetuses.

Assaying serum or plasma levels has generated all data in the literature regarding progestins in mares. However, currently in human monitoring programs, especially in postmenopausal women, the focus is on salivary levels of progesterone and other steroids. The hypothesis is that a salivary level may represent the delivery of the hormone to tissue membranes, whereas serum concentrations measure the quantity of hormone not yet delivered to the tissue.[7] Apparently, salivary progestins have not been measured in mares and compared to serum concentrations.

EXPECTED CONCENTRATIONS OF PROGESTINS

Progestins are the most important endocrine diagnostic end point to assess ovarian function. Progestin assays are routinely used to assess ovulatory status of the mare. For example, a mare not exhibiting estrous behavior and having a serum progestin concentration of less than 1.0 ng/ml would be considered anovulatory. If the same mare had a progestin concentration of more than 1.0 ng/ml, she would be considered ovulatory. An excep-

Table 9-1

Mean Progestin Concentrations During the First 30 Days of Pregnancy

Days of Pregnancy	No. of Mares	Mean	SEM
3	2	7.35	0.45
4	4	4.42	1.62
5	39	6.94	0.45
6	30	7.01	0.62
7	46	6.48	0.45
8	5	8.40	1.40
9	2	5.75	1.50
10	21	5.23	0.54
11	25	6.28	0.59
12	36	5.40	0.44
13	28	5.37	0.41
14	123	5.45	0.25
15	238	6.60	0.19
16	116	5.23	0.30
17	73	4.82	0.34
18	85	5.20	0.36
19	36	6.61	0.82
20	42	4.91	0.43
21	33	4.99	0.51
22	16	3.94	0.67
23	30	6.17	0.59
24	19	4.45	0.76
25	22	6.54	1.70
26	11	5.28	1.33
27	6	4.48	0.83
28	27	4.59	0.61
29	10	3.89	0.82
30	67	4.95	0.46

Table 9-2

Relationship Between Serum Progestin (P4) Concentrations on Day 12 Post Ovulation and Pregnancy Rates

Serum P4 Concentration	No. of Mares	Pregnancy Rate (%)
>2.5 ng/ml	50	71*
<2.5 ng/ml	25	37†

Means with different superscripts are different.

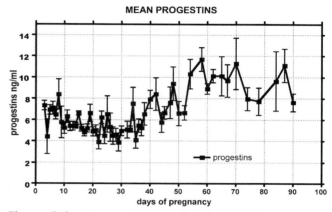

Figure 9-1 Mean and standard deviation (SD) serum concentrations of progestins during the first 90 days of pregnancy (n = 1695 mares).

tion to this rule would be the mare in race training that chronically exhibits estrous behavior but consistently has a progestin concentration between 1.0 and 4.0 ng/ml. Apparently these patients have a partially luteinized follicle that is persistent, similar to ovarian cysts in cows. When a luteolytic dose of prostaglandin $F_{2\alpha}$ ($PGF_{2\alpha}$) is given twice a day to these females until serum progestins drop below 1.0 ng/ml, the estrous behavior stops. This is due presumably to the lysis of the luteinized tissue present in the persistent follicle.

Data for mean progestin concentrations during the first 30 days of pregnancy in mares are shown in Table 9-1. There is no significant difference in progestin concentrations between pregnant and nonpregnant mares during the first 15 days post ovulation, and progestin concentrations during estrus will be less than 1.0 ng/ml. Most samples for progestin determinations are taken around the time of the first ultrasound examination, between days 14 and 18 post ovulation.

Placentitis is the single greatest cause of pregnancy loss, stillbirth, and premature foals in the United States.[8,9] Endometritis may be the greatest cause of low progestin

concentrations during the first 30 days of pregnancy. Data in Table 9-2 compare pregnancy rates in mares with low versus normal progestin levels on day 12 post ovulation. Pregnancy rates were almost double when progestins were above 2.5 ng/ml. Approximately 85% of mares were positive for pathogenic bacteria in uterine lavage effluents[10] when day 12 progestins were low (<2.5 ng/ml).

Figure 9-1 illustrates serum progestin concentrations throughout days 5 to 90 of pregnancy. As would be expected, progestins rise after formation of accessory corpora lutea around day 45 of pregnancy. The range of progestins throughout pregnancy as denoted by the two bold lines in the figure averaged between 4 and 10 ng/ml. It therefore can be assumed that values outside this range are abnormal for clinical diagnostic purposes.

ESTROGENS

During the estrous cycle the predominant estrogen secreted by the ovary is estradiol-17β. Little clinical information can be obtained by performing assays for estradiol during either estrus or diestrus. Values throughout the luteal phase are below 50 pg/ml. During estrus, serum concentrations rise from the first day of estrus and peak at approximately 150 to 300 pg/ml 24 hours before ovulation. Estrogens are elevated in mares with some types of ovarian tumors. Serum concentrations of mostly conjugated estrogens rise before formation of accessory corpora lutea around days 40 to 80 of pregnancy.

SUMMARY

Serum testing for progestins provides the clinician with data relative to the following: the presence of a corpus luteum, persistent luteinized follicle, possible endometritis, and if exogenous progestagen therapy may be indicated.

References

1. Holtan DW, Nett TM, Estergreen VL: Plasma progestins in pregnant, postpartum and cycling mares. J Anim Sci 1975; 40:251.
2. Holtan DW, Houghton E, Silver M et al: Plasma progestagens in the mare, fetus and newborn foal. J Reprod Fertil Suppl 1991; 44:517-528.
3. Fowden AL, Taylor PM, White KL, Forhead AJ: Ontogenic and nutritionally induced changes in fetal metabolism in the horse. J Physiol Lond 2000; 528:209-219.
4. Hamon M, Clarke SW, Houghton E et al: Production of 5α-pregnane-3, 20-dione during late pregnancy in the mare. J Reprod Fertil Suppl 1991; 44:529.
5. Ousey JC, Rossdale PD, Palmer L et al: Effects of progesterone to mares during late gestation. Theriogenology 2002; 58:793.
6. Ginther OJ: Reproductive Biology of the Mare, Cross Plains, Wis, Equiservices, 1992.
7. Gilson GR, Zava DT: A perspective on HRT for women. Int J Pharm Compounding 2003; 7:330.
8. Giles RC, Donahue JM, Hong CG et al: Causes of abortion, stillbirth and perinatal death in horses: 3527 cases (1986-1991). J Am Vet Med Assoc 1993; 1170.
9. Hong CB, Donahue JM, Giles RC et al: Etiology and pathology of equine placentitis. J Vet Diagn Invest 1993; 5:56.
10. Douglas, Unpublished data, 1990.

CHAPTER 10

Cytogenetic Evaluation

TERI L. LEAR

Many factors can lead to reproductive failure in horses; however, one factor commonly overlooked is a chromosome or karyotypic abnormality. Normal horses have 64 chromosomes including two sex chromosomes, XX in females and XY in males. When horse chromosomes are analyzed for abnormalities, the chromosomes are paired according to their size, morphology, and banding patterns into a standardized karyotype (ISCN 1990). The horse karyotype is composed of 13 pairs of metacentric or submetacentric and 18 pairs of acrocentric autosomes, plus a submetacentric X and an acrocentric Y chromosome.

Mares that are infertile or exhibit reduced fertility may have an abnormal chromosome complement, particularly with regard to the sex chromosomes (Table 10-1). The most common abnormalities affecting mares are X monosomy, often referred to as XO syndrome or equine Turner's syndrome; sex chromosome mosaicism; and sex reversal syndrome. Sex chromosome abnormalities sometimes cause the failure of reproductive organs to function normally, or they can result in unviable gametes lacking a normal sex chromosome complement. Other chromosome abnormalities affecting mare fertility, such as partial X chromosome deletions and autosomal duplications and translocations, are rare but have been identified. These abnormalities result in failure to produce gametes with complete sets of chromosomes, or they produce developmental abnormalities in the embryo.

Most samples submitted for karyotyping are from horses with poor reproductive performance. The incidence of chromosome abnormalities in the general horse population is unknown, since no systematic survey has been done. However, Power (1990) summarized the number of chromosome abnormalities observed in samples submitted for clinical analyses from 47 publications, and in 29% of the cases a chromosome abnormality was observed. Among the chromosome abnormalities observed, 36% were X monosomy, 28% were sex reversal syndrome, 5% were autosomal abnormalities, and the remaining 31% were mosaic for sex chromosomes. Equine heterosexual twins with XX/XY blood chimerism have been observed occasionally; however, this chimerism does not appear to affect sexual development or fertility in the female co-twin such as that seen in the freemartin condition described in cattle and sheep (Power, 1990).

CLINICAL SIGNS

Sex Chromosome Abnormalities

Mares exhibiting chronic primary infertility, failure to cycle regularly or at all, small ovaries, or lack of follicular activity, may have a numerical chromosome abnormality known as XO monosomy. These individuals have a karyotype of 63,XO instead of the normal 64,XX. Some XO mares may also exhibit small body size, angular limb deformities, and poor conformation. This is the most common chromosome abnormality described in horses and is thought to be the equine equivalent of human Turner's syndrome.

A few cases of X chromosome duplication, or trisomy, have been described in the horse. These mares have a karyotype of 65,XXX and appear phenotypically normal but are infertile.

Another variation of numerical sex chromosome abnormalities is X chromosome mosaicism, which may be the third most common sex chromosome abnormality described in the horse. Mares with mosaicism may exhibit one or more of the symptoms described above and have a variety of cells, each with different numbers of sex chromosomes, such as 63,X;64,XX or 63,X;64,XX;65,XXX.

Some infertile mares may have a more common but complicated abnormality called XY sex-reversal syndrome. XY sex-reversed individuals have a female phenotype and a male karyotype of 64,XY and can exhibit a wide range of phenotypes. Some mares may be quite feminine with normal external genitalia, underdeveloped uterus, and slightly infantile ovaries with follicles present, whereas others exhibit classic gonadal dysgenesis, ovotestes, testicular feminization, and sometimes, masculine behavior. This condition has been attributed to a deletion of the sex-determining region (*SRY* gene) on the Y chromosome. Although a Y chromosome is present, SRY deletion causes these genotypic males to develop into phenotypic females with gonadal dysgenesis (Pailhoux et al, 1995).

Autosomal Chromosome Abnormalities (Non–Sex Chromosomes)

Deletions, duplications, or rearrangements of autosomal chromosomes are rare because they lead to severe abnor-

Table **10-1**

Common Chromosome Abnormalities in Mares

Chromosome Number	Common Name	Phenotype
63,X	XO syndrome	Normal external genitalia; irregular or absent estrous cycles; gonadal dysgenesis; no follicular development; poor conformation; small stature
63,X/64,XX	XO mosaicism	Normal appearance but with gonadal dysgenesis; rare follicular activity/estrous cycles
64,XY	Sex reversal syndrome	Normal external genitalia; no estrous cycles; gonadal dysgenesis; intraabdominal testes/ovotestes; may exhibit stallion-like behavior and secondary sex characteristics

Box **10-1**

Laboratories Providing Diagnostic Service for Chromosome Abnormalities

Molecular Cytogenetics Laboratory
Dr. Teri L. Lear
Maxwell H. Gluck Equine Research Center
Department of Veterinary Science
University of Kentucky
Lexington, KY 40546
Phone: (859) 257-4757 ext 8-1108
Fax: (859) 257-8542
E-Mail: equigene@uky.edu

Molecular Cytogenetics Laboratory
Dr. Terje Raudsepp
Dr. Bhanu Chowdhary
Room 318B Bldg. 1197
Department of Veterinary Anatomy and Public Health
Texas A&M University
College Station, TX 77843
Phone: (979) 458-0519 ext 20
Fax: (979) 845-9972
E-Mail: bchowdhary@cvm.tamu.edu

malities in gametic or embryonic development. In fact, only 15 or so cases have been reported in the literature. This may be due to the low number of horses that have been karyotyped in comparison to humans. Mares with balanced chromosome rearrangements or chromosome duplications may appear phenotypically normal but exhibit irregular estrous cycles with or without ovulation, or they may conceive but experience early embryonic loss. While these mares have reduced fertility, they may produce viable foals that have a normal chromosome complement or foals that are carriers of the same chromosome abnormality. The reproductive status of a few of these mares has been followed, and a few normal foals from these mares have been produced: to a mare with an extra copy of chromosome 30 (65,XX,+30) (Bowling and Millon, 1990) and to two mares with reciprocal translocations [64,XX,t(1;3)] (Power, 1991) and [64,XX, t(1;16)] (Lear and Layton, 2002).

DIAGNOSIS

A blood sample is collected into tubes containing sodium heparin. Sodium heparin is critical to prevent red blood cell clotting. The tubes should be packed well in an insulating material to prevent breakage and shipped by overnight express service to the clinical cytogenetics laboratory (Box 10-1). It is important that the blood sample be fresh and of good quality in order to obtain good results. The sample should not be exposed to extremes of temperature, because living cells, lymphocytes, are needed for cell cultures. The lymphocytes are placed in a culture medium containing mitotic agents such as pokeweed mitogen or phytohemagglutinin to stimulate cell division. After approximately 72 hours, the cells are treated with colcemid to arrest them at metaphase when the chromosomes are most condensed in preparation for cell division. The cells are then separated from the culture medium by centrifugation and treated with a hypotonic solution causing them to swell. Following hypotonic treatment the cells are fixed in several changes of methanol/acetic acid and dropped onto slides. During this step the nuclear membranes rupture, allowing the chromosomes from each cell nucleus to spread out onto the slide into a "metaphase spread."

In order to count the number of chromosomes in each cell, the slides are stained routinely with Giemsa stain. Each metaphase spread is analyzed for chromosome number under a microscope, an image of a single metaphase spread is captured, and the chromosomes are arranged in a karyotype based on their morphology and

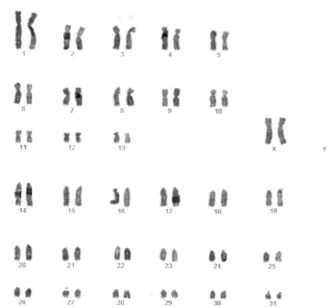

Figure 10-1 Giemsa-stained karyotype from a normal mare, 64,XX.

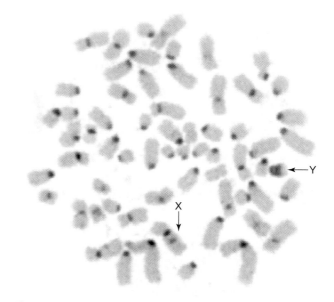

Figure 10-2 C-banded metaphase spread from a normal stallion, 64,XY, demonstrating the distinctive banding patterns of the X and Y chromosomes *(arrows)*.

size (Figure 10-1). Using this method, only the total chromosome number per cell and general morphology can be determined. The individual chromosomes, including the sex chromosomes, cannot be identified by Giemsa stain alone.

Sex chromosome identification is generally done by two methods, C-banding or G-banding. C-banding is specific for heterochromatic regions on chromosomes, specifically at the centromeres and along the arms of some chromosomes. The horse submetacentric X chromosome has a heterochromatic band along the long arm that stains distinctively using this method. The Y chromosome is composed mainly of heterochromatin and is easily distinguishable from the other small, acrocentric chromosomes. C-bands are created by treating the slides in a dilute solution of hydrochloric acid, followed by brief immersion in barium hydroxide solution, incubation in a sodium citrate-sodium chloride solution, and staining with Giemsa. Figure 10-2 shows a C-banded metaphase from a normal stallion demonstrating the distinctive banding pattern of the X and Y sex chromosomes.

If further analysis is warranted, G-banding enables identification of each chromosome specifically. G-bands are prepared by treating the chromosomes briefly in a trypsin solution then staining the chromosomes with Giemsa. The resulting banding pattern is specific for each chromosome pair. Each pair is arranged according to size, morphology, and banding pattern in a karyotype based on an accepted G-banded karyotype standard. Using this method the chromosomes can be analyzed for potential translocations, duplications, or deletions. Figure 10-3 shows a G-banded karyotype from a normal stallion. G-banding may be necessary when other less sensitive methods do not demonstrate an obvious chromosome abnormality.

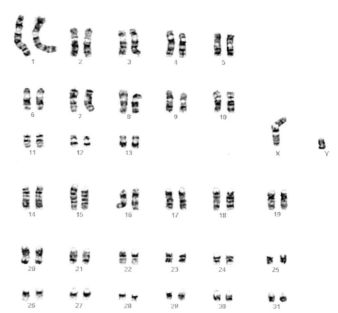

Figure 10-3 G-banded karyotype from a normal stallion, 64,XY. The chromosomes are paired by size, morphology, and banding patterns into a standardized karyotype for the domestic horse.

With the improvement in molecular technologies, another method that may be used to identify chromosome abnormalities is fluorescent in situ hybridization (FISH). FISH is generally used to confirm a chromosome abnormality identified using standard banding methods. It requires tagging horse chromosome-specific DNA with a fluorescent molecule. This tagged DNA or "probe" is

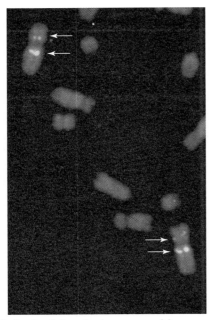

Figure 10-4   Partial metaphase spread from a mare with a normal karyotype demonstrating fluorescence in situ hybridization with two markers that map to both arms of the horse X chromosome *(arrows),* confirming that both arms of the X chromosome are present.

then applied to horse metaphase chromosomes on slides and allowed to bind to the chromosome. This method takes advantage of the double-stranded nature of DNA because the DNA of the probe will find its complementary DNA sequence on the chromosomes and form a hybrid molecule, thus the term *hybridization.* After a series of washes to remove unbound probe, the chromosomes are stained with a fluorescent stain and then analyzed using a fluorescent microscope. Both the probe and the chromosomes can be viewed simultaneously, permitting identification of the chromosome on which the probe is located. In cases of X chromosome monosomy, DNA from the horse X chromosome is hybridized to the chromosomes of the patient. Fluorescence will only be seen from the one X chromosome in mares with a 63,X karyotype instead of two X chromosomes of a normal mare (Figure 10-4). In cases of translocations, duplications, or deletions, DNA probes from the chromosomes thought to be involved in the abnormality can be used for further confirmation. Progress on the horse gene map has developed rapidly, and there are now hundreds of chromosome-specific horse genes available that can be used as probes. Testing for deletion of the *SRY* gene in these XY mares is done by extracting DNA from the affected individual, either from blood cells or hair root bulbs, and amplifying the *SRY* gene in a polymerase chain reaction (PCR). DNA fragments specific to the gene are amplified and observed on an agarose gel. Although these mares have the Y chromosome, no *SRY* gene fragment will be observed (Figure 10-5).

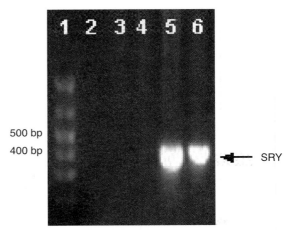

Figure 10-5   SRY PCR Test. Lanes: *1,* DNA ladder for sizing PCR products; *2,* water control; *3* and *4,* 64,XY, SRY-negative sex reversal mare; *5* and *6,* normal SRY-positive stallion.

PROGNOSIS

Mares diagnosed with X monosomy are always infertile unless only a small portion of the X chromosome is deleted, such as the short arm; then the mare may produce a live foal. Mares diagnosed with X chromosome mosaicism have been reported to conceive, although long-term studies have not been done to determine if these mares have ever produced a live foal. There are rare reports of 64,XY sex-reversed mares that have produced normal male and female offspring and XY sex-reversed female offspring. Mares with chromosome translocations may exhibit reduced fertility due to an imbalance of genetic material during chromosome segregation at gametogenesis. Although these mares may produce a live foal, the risk of transmitting the chromosome abnormality to the offspring should be considered.

The causes of infertility in many mares remains unknown. If the causes are due to genetic factors such as small genome deletions, duplications, or mutations it may be possible to identify them in the near future due to advances in genome technologies. The horse genome may be sequenced by the National Human Genome Research Institute (March 2006). As the sequence information becomes available, researchers will mine the horse genome sequence in search of genetic variations such as single nucleotide polymorphisms (SNPs). New technologies, such as SNP microarrays currently under development, permit high resolution identification of human chromosomal abnormalities (called "molecular karyotyping") that are not identifiable by current cytogenetic methods (Slater et al, 2005; Rauch et al, 2006). These technologies will pave the way for applications in equine clinical cytogenetics and enable us to identify even the most subtle changes in the horse karyotype that may cause infertility or other congenital abnormalities.

Supplemental Readings

Bowling AT: Horse Genetics, Wallingford, 1996, CAB International.

Bowling AT, Millon LV: Two autosomal trisomies in the horse: 64,XX,−26,+t(26q26q) and 65,XX,+30. Genome 1990; 33:679-682.

Chowdhary BP, Bailey E: Equine genomics: galloping to new frontiers. Cytogenet Genome Res 2003; 102:184-188.

Chowdhary BP, Raudsepp T: Cytogenetics and Physical Gene Maps. In Bowling AT, Ruvinsky A, editors: The Genetics of the Horse, New York, 2000 CABI Publishing.

ISCNH 1997: International system for cytogenetic nomenclature of the domestic horse (ISCNH). Bowling AT, Breen M, Chowdhary BP, Hirota K, Lear TL, Millon LV, Ponce de Leon FA, Raudsepp T, Stranzinger G (Committee). Chromosome Res 1997; 5:443-453.

Lear TL, Layton G: Use of Zoo-FISH to characterize a reciprocal translocation in a Thoroughbred mare: t(1:16)(q16;q21.3). Equine Vet J 2002; 34:207-209.

Pailhoux E, Cribiu EP, Parma P, Cotinot C: Molecular analysis of an XY mare with gonadal dysgenesis. Hereditas 1995; 122:109-112.

Power MM: Chromosomes of the Horse. In McFeely RA, ed: Advances in Veterinary Science and Comparative Medicine, vol 34, San Diego, 1990, Academic Press, Inc.

Power MM: The first description of a balanced reciprocal translocation [t(1q;3q)] and its clinical effects in a mare. Equine Vet J 1991; 23:146-149.

Rauch A, Rüschendorf F, Huang J et al: Molecular karyotyping using an SNP array for genomewide genotyping. J Med Genet 2004; 41:916-922.

Slater HR, Bailey DK, Hua R et al: High-resolution identification of chromosomal abnormalities using oligonucleotide arrays containing 116,204 SNPs. Am J Hum Genet 2005; 77:709-726.

CHAPTER 11

Diagnosis of Oviductal Disorders and Diagnostic Techniques

SCOTT D. BENNETT

Diagnosis of disorders involving the oviduct, along with associated fimbrial and ovarian disorders, should be one of the last procedures employed to diagnose infertility in the mare. However, these isolated reproductive disorders may deserve attention in a select group of barren mares that defy routine explanation for infertility.

Evaluation of the reproductive tract of the mare should involve a thorough evaluation of reproductive history, transrectal palpation, ultrasonography, endometrial culture, endometrial biopsy, cytologic examination, hormonal evaluation, and hysteroscopy before considering oviductal infertility. Diagnosis of infertility due to oviductal disorders should be considered when all avenues of evaluation have failed to provide a definitive diagnosis in cases of barren mares that have had sophisticated veterinary management. In these cases, early detection of pregnancy via ultrasonography or embryo flushing has failed to demonstrate evidence of conception. Oviduct disorders are more prevalent in older mares.[1,2,3] A mean age of 18 years has been reported, with a range of 9 to 26 years of age.[3]

Hysteroscopic evaluation of the uterus and evaluation of the uterotubal junction (UTJ) is of primary importance. The normal UTJ will project slightly into the insufflated uterine horn, giving a papilla type of appearance (i.e., pimplelike). The area around the UTJ should be examined for cysts, adhesions, fibrosis, or any other uterine abnormality that may cause obstruction of the UTJ. Many of these issues can be addressed endoscopically with the use of the Nd:YAG laser[4] (Surgical Laser Technologies Inc., Oaks, Pa.) or treated via uterotomy during an exploratory reproductive surgery. Flattening and/or scarring of the UTJ papillae is also considered an abnormal finding warranting further oviduct evaluation (Figures 11-1 and 11-2). The inability to visualize the papillae hysteroscopically is also an abnormal finding.

Catheterization of the equine oviduct through the UTJ papillae from the uterine lumen is technically an extremely difficult procedure, unlike other mammalian species. This is because the equine oviduct is anatomically distinct from other mammalian species. The distal one third of the equine oviduct has a well-developed muscularis, which acts as a sphincter apparatus, making mechanical entry from the uterus exceedingly difficult.[5]

The distal one third of the oviduct is also extremely convoluted, which further complicates catheterization from the uterine approach. Maintaining catheter placement from the uterine approach is also tenuous, because the muscularis-induced back-pressure that occurs during oviduct irrigation invariably ejects the catheter from the oviduct. Balloon catheterization of the oviduct from the uterine approach is not possible with current technology. Again, because of the well-developed distal oviduct muscularis, balloon insufflation is prevented within the distal one third of the oviduct (Figure 11-3).

Salpingitis in the equine species does not result in visible, physical enlargement of the oviduct as is seen in other species. The previously discussed muscularis prevents visible distension of the oviducts. Thus the diagnosis of salpingitis in the equine is difficult and has different criteria from the distension of the oviduct seen in other species.

Oviductal masses and occlusions of the lumen of the oviduct with a collagen type of material has been described[1,6,7] and has a prevalence in older mares.[1,2] The mare frequently retains oocytes in various stages of degeneration within the oviductal lumen.[1,2,5, 6, 8-10] It is not known at this time if these oviductal collagen type of masses and degenerated oocytes are interrelated or separate entities, and more research is needed. Due to the oviductal muscular sphincter apparatus, transport of collagen type of masses to the UTJ is thought to be difficult, thus occluding the oviductal lumen or interfering with proper oviductal function.[1,7,8] Any change within the oviductal environment can affect sperm transport, sperm nutrients, oocyte viability, fertilization, and embryo transport. Because of these oviductal disorders, the evaluation of patency and treatment of blockage may be of value in mares that are barren due to otherwise undetermined cause.[3] Disease of the oviduct is not easily evaluated or treated, thus pathologic conditions of these structures may be more common than reported in the literature.

Evaluation and treatment of the fimbria is similarly difficult. Unlike other species, the horse has few fimbria permanently attached to the ovary.[11] Parafimbrial cysts and adhesions may distort the ability of the fimbria to receive the oocyte for further transport into the oviduct and fertilization. Fimbrial cysts and adhesions may pull the fimbria off the ovary in such a manner that the mare

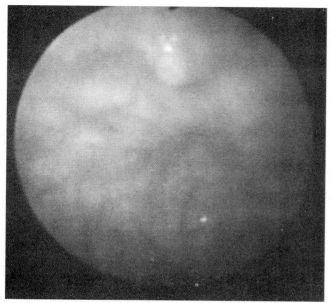

Figure 11-1 Normal oviduct papillae (tubal uterine junction).

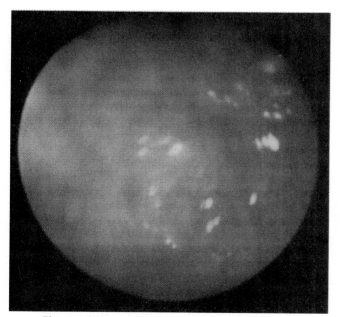

Figure 11-2 Diseased tubal uterine junction.

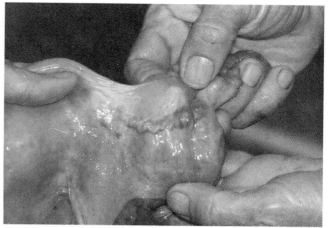

Figure 11-3 Oviduct showing distal one third of muscularis.

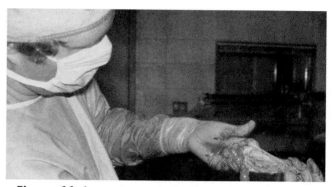

Figure 11-4 Fimbrial cyst pulling fimbria from ovary.

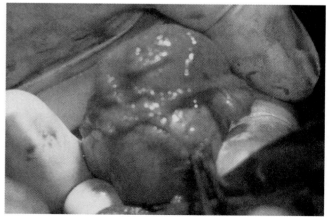

Figure 11-5 Fimbrial cystic disease with fimbrial adhesions.

would ovulate into the abdomen, thus making conception unlikely (Figures 11-4 and 11-5). The fimbria-ovarian interaction may also be disrupted by ovarian disease such as tumors, hematomas, adhesions, fibrosis, and ovaritis. Small, early granulosa cell tumors and ovarian fossa leiomyomas can affect the function of the ovary and its fimbrial interaction. Ultrasonographic evaluation of early ovarian dysfunction, fimbrial disorders, and oviductal disorders can be subjective and difficult to definitively diagnose. Deposition of fluorescent microspheres[12] and starch granules[13] on the ovary and fimbria has been described to diagnose oviduct obstruction. This can be accomplished using laparoscopic technique or ultrasound-guided transvaginal deposition. These procedures are cumbersome and do not treat the disorder once diagnosed.

Laparoscopic evaluation in the standing horse of the ovaries and oviducts is possible with a bilateral flank approach. Laparoscopy of the ovaries and oviducts can also be used through a ventral abdominal approach under general anesthesia. Ovariectomy can be accomplished laparoscopically when the ovaries are not greatly enlarged. Laparoscopic normograde catheterization of the oviduct, although possible, results in the same difficulty as the uterine-side catheterization and irrigation. Because of the sphincterlike muscularis of the distal oviduct, passage of a balloon catheter and oviduct irrigation will result in ejection of the catheter. Thus, laparoscopic evaluation of the cranial reproductive tract allows visualization but limited diagnostic and treatment capabilities for oviductal reproductive disorders.

Currently the best technique available for diagnosis and treatment of oviductal reproductive disorders is exploratory surgery.

REPRODUCTIVE EXPLORATORY SURGERY

Mares undergoing an oviductal exploratory surgery are fasted for 24 hours preoperatively and given 4 L of mineral oil via nasogastric tube 18 to 24 hours before surgery. Preoperative antibiotics and anti-inflammatories (penicillin G procaine, 30,000 IU/kg IM b.i.d.; gentamicin, 6.6 mg/kg IV s.i.d.; and flunixin meglumine, 1.1 mg/kg IV s.i.d.) are administered and continued for 3 days.

The mare is placed in dorsal recumbency under general anesthesia. A pelvic tilt apparatus is used to flex the mare at the lumbosacral junction, allowing for better access to the reproductive tract (Figure 11-6). A 10-cm ventral midline incision is made just cranial to the udder. An ovary and ipsilateral uterine horn are isolated and exteriorized through the incision. The ovary, fimbria, oviduct, and uterine horns are examined for any obvious abnormalities. Occasionally, either the large or small bowel can be adhered to the ovary and/or uterus, particularly if there is a history of previous abdominal surgery or uterine trauma (i.e., dystocia).

A Doyen intestinal forceps is placed across the uterine horn approximately 5 cm from the tip of the horn to occlude this portion of the horn (Figure 11-7). The oviduct is catheterized in a normograde fashion with a flexible balloon-tipped catheter (Cook V-PFC 8-30, 8.0 French Foley 30-cm 5-ml balloon catheter, Cook Veterinary Products Inc., Bloomington, Ind.). After the catheter

has been advanced into the ampulla, the balloon catheter is inflated with 1 to 1.5 ml of air to occlude the ampulla. Strong digital pressure is applied just cranial to the balloon to avoid catheter ejection from the back-pressure developed while flushing the oviduct. Careful attention to placement of the tip of the catheter is necessary to avoid pushing against the wall of the ampulla. This will help prevent iatrogenic damage to the oviduct.

A 20-ml solution of sterile 5% new methylene blue dye in normal saline is slowly injected through the catheter into the oviduct (Figure 11-8). The oviduct will distend under pressure down to the muscular distal third, which should fatigue, allowing the solution to pass into the tip

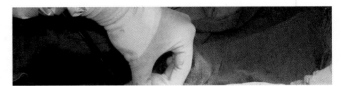

Figure 11-7   Doyen intestinal forceps placed across the uterine horn.

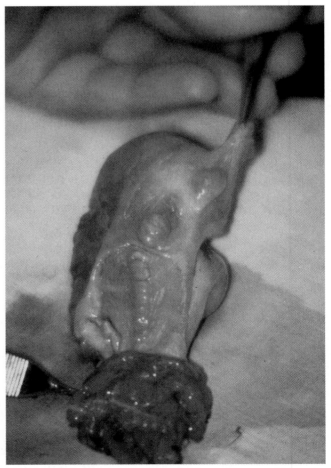

Figure 11-8   Dye flow through the oviduct and into the uterine horn. Note poor dye visualization through the distal one third of oviduct due to muscularis.

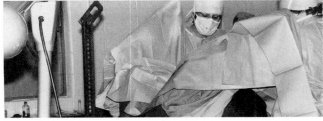

Figure 11-6   Pelvic tilt apparatus bending patient at the lumbosacral junction.

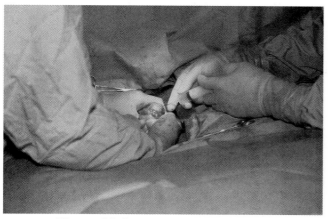

Figure 11-9 Oviduct catheterization.

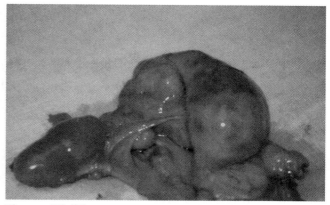

Figure 11-11 Dye rupture of oviduct into mesosalpinx due to complete blockage of the oviduct.

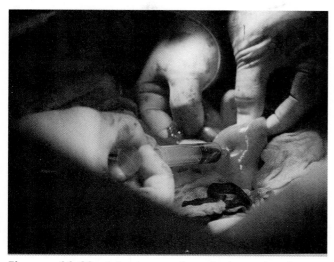

Figure 11-10 Injection and aspiration of saline in occluded horn to confirm dye.

of the uterine horn. If there is difficulty with fluid passage, then the oviduct should be saturated with 2% lidocaine hydrochloride, which may aid in establishing patency (Figure 11-9). Following passage of the dye solution, 20 ml of air is injected into the oviduct, giving a characteristic gurgling sound as air passes into and distends the occluded uterine horn. Injection and aspiration of 10 to 20 ml normal saline into the distended uterine horn should confirm the presence of dye in the aspirate (Figure 11-10). The contralateral ovary and uterine horn are then exteriorized before the Doyen forceps is released from its original position and replaced as previously described. The oviduct catheterization and lavage procedure is then repeated.

Complete occlusion will result in the inability of the dye solution or air to pass into the uterine horn (Figure 11-11). Intense pressure against a completely occluded oviduct may cause rupture of the oviduct, at which time dye will be visualized in the mesosalpinx. Unilateral irreversible occlusion of the oviduct may be treated with uni-lateral ovariectomy, and bilateral blockage of the oviduct deletes the mare from conventional breeding methods.

Fimbrial adhesions are removed, and fimbrial cysts are reduced if present. The Nd:YAG laser has proved to be beneficial with prevention of postoperative adhesions of the fimbria. The fimbria is highly vascular, and hemorrhage occurs easily with harsh manipulation. Fimbrial disease results in a guarded prognosis for fertility.[3]

A routine abdominal closure is performed following the procedure. Postoperative care involves stall rest for 4 weeks, followed by turnout in a small paddock for an additional 4 weeks. Breeding can be resumed as early as 3 weeks postoperatively.

References

1. Liu IKM, Lantz KC, Schalafke S et al: Clinical observations of oviductal masses in the mare. Proceedings of the 48th Annual Convention of the American Association of Equine Practitioners, pp 41-45, 1991.
2. Oguri N, Tsutsumi Y: Studies on lodging of equine unfertilized ova in fallopian tubes. Res Bull Livestock Farm Hokkaido U 1972; 6:32-43.
3. Bennett S, Griffin R, Rhoads W: Surgical evaluation of oviduct disease and patency in the mare. Proceedings of the 48th Annual Convention of the American Association of Equine Practitioners, pp 347-349, 2002.
4. Griffin R, Bennett S: Nd:YAG laser photoablation of endometrial cysts: a review of 55 cases (2001-2002). Proceedings of the 48th Annual Convention of the American Association of Equine Practitioners, pp 58-60, 2002.
5. Kainer RA: Reproductive organs of the mare. In McKinnon AO, Voss JL (eds): Equine Reproduction, Philadelphia, Lea & Febiger, 1993.
6. Saltiel A, Paramo R, Murcia C et al: Pathologic findings in the oviducts of mares. Am J Vet Res 1986; 47:594-597.
7. Tsutsami Y, Suzuki IT, Takeda T et al: Evidence of the origin of gelatinous masses in the oviducts of mares. J Reprod Fertil 1979; 57:287-290.
8. Onuma IT, Ohnami Y: Retention of tubal eggs in mares. J Reprod Fertil (Suppl) 1975; 23:507-511.
9. Steffenhagen WP, Pineda MH, Ginther OJ: Retention of unfertilized ova in the uterine tubes of mares. Am J Vet Res 1972; 33:2391-2398.

10. VanNickerk CH, Gerneke WH: Persistence and pathogenic cleavage of tubal ova in the mare. Onderstepoort J Vet Res 1966; 23:195-232.

11. Kenney RM: A review of pathology of the equine oviduct. In Antazcak A, Oriole B (eds): Equine Embryo Transfer III. Equine Vet J Suppl 15; Oct 1993.

12. Ley WB, Bowen JM, Purswell BJ et al: Modified technique to evaluate uterine tubal patency in the mare. Proceedings of the 44th Annual Convention of the American Association of Equine Practitioners, pp 56-59, 1998.

13. Allen WE, Kessy BM, Noakes DE: Evaluation of uterine tube function in pony mares. Vet Rec 1979; 105:364-366.

CHAPTER 12

Ovulation Failure

PATRICK M. MCCUE

Failure of ovulation of large follicles can be part of a normal physiologic process, a pathologic event, or may constitute lack of response to an ovulation-inducing agent. Clinically, ovulation failure should be distinguished from failure of follicular development, which is discussed in the chapter on ovarian abnormalities. Development of anovulatory follicles is common during the spring and fall transition periods and in some postpartum mares. Failure of mares to ovulate during the normal breeding season is less common but represents a significant cause of reproductive inefficiency in the mare and may be responsible for significant economic loss. The incidence of ovulation failure during the physiologic breeding season has been reported to range from 3.1% to 8.2%.[1,2]

PHYSIOLOGIC OVULATION FAILURE

The spring and fall transition periods are characterized by waves of follicular development and regression without ovulation.[3] The spring transition or resurgence phase may last 2 to 3 months. Dominant follicles of a follicular wave may reach preovulatory size (i.e., >35 mm in diameter) late in the spring transition period and yet still regress without ovulating. Ovulation of a dominant follicle marks the end of the spring transition period. A majority of mares subsequently ovulate at approximately 21-day intervals. In the fall, mares may exhibit waves of follicular growth and regression for several weeks after the last ovulation of the year. Follicular activity gradually decreases in association with the diminishing photoperiodic stimulation, and the ovaries of most mares become inactive during the winter months. Large anovulatory follicles may form during the fall transition period and have historically been referred to as "autumn follicles."[4,5] Autumn follicles are classically described as being hemorrhagic, with a liquid to gelatinous consistency.[3]

Postpartum mares may also exhibit physiologic ovulation failure. A majority of mares develop follicles and ovulate within the first 2 weeks postpartum and continue to cycle thereafter. Alternatively, a foal heat ovulation may be followed by a variable period of anestrus or anovulation until the mare resumes normal cyclic activity. Finally, some mares may have no significant follicular development or may exhibit moderate to substantial follicular development without ovulation during the immediate postpartum period. Mares in the latter groups may remain anestrous or anovulatory for weeks or months before cyclic ovarian activity is initiated.

A majority of mares that do not cycle after giving birth are mares that foal early in the year. Consequently, it may be difficult to distinguish between postpartum anestrus due to a short ambient photoperiod versus anestrus due to the effects of lactation. In general, failure to ovulate postpartum is more likely to be attributed to seasonal effects than lactation effects.[6,7] However, some mares that do not exhibit significant follicular development in the first 40 to 60 days after foaling or become anestrous following a foal heat ovulation will have rapid follicular development and associated estrus soon after the foal is weaned.[3,8] The incidence of lactation-associated anestrus in mares has been reported to be 21% to 74%.[7] In contrast, other investigators have reported that suckling had no effect on postpartum ovarian activity.[9]

Poor body condition in late gestation and the early postpartum period may also contribute to poor reproductive performance. The effects of inadequate nutrition and poor body condition may be manifested in delayed return to reproductive cyclicity postpartum, reduced pregnancy rates, and increased embryo loss rates.[10] The phenomenon of "lactational anestrus" may, in fact, represent the combined effects of season, body condition, and lactation.[3] Maintenance of late-term pregnant mares due to foal between January and March (Northern Hemisphere) under a stimulatory artificial photoperiod for the last 2 to 3 months of pregnancy may be beneficial. Pregnant mares housed under lights have been reported to foal approximately 10 days earlier than mares not maintained under lights,[11] are more likely to have a foal heat ovulation and continued estrous cycles,[7] and ovulate earlier in the postpartum period.[12]

PATHOLOGIC OVULATION FAILURE

Ovulation failure occasionally occurs during the physiologic breeding season. Anovulatory follicles may be large (5 to 15 cm in diameter), persist for up to 2 months, and result in a prolonged period of behavioral anestrus and a long interovulatory interval.[13] Specific causes of ovulation failure in the mare are not known but have been suggested to be insufficient pituitary gonadotropin stimulation to induce ovulation,[14] insufficient estrogen production from the follicle itself,[15] or hemorrhage into the lumen of the preovulatory follicle.[3] Mares may develop anovulatory follicles without prior exposure to exogenous hormones.[2]

Anovulatory follicles were reported in a recent study to occur in approximately 8.2% of equine estrous cycles.[2] The incidence of anovulatory follicles increases with age. Mares 16 to 20 years old were noted to form anovulatory

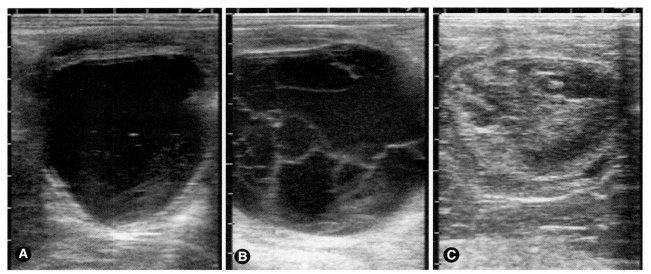

Figure 12-1 Ultrasonographic images of anovulatory follicles with (**A**) multiple echogenic spots, (**B**) echogenic strands traversing the follicular lumen, and (**C**) a completely echogenic follicular lumen.

follicles during 13.1% of estrous cycles during the physiologic breeding season. A high percentage (43.5%) of mares that developed anovulatory follicles experienced subsequent estrous cycles with anovulatory follicle formation during the same breeding season. The interval between actual ovulations for mares that developed anovulatory follicles was noted to be 38.5 days.

It is often difficult to determine in advance if a dominant follicle in an estrual mare will fail to ovulate. Formation of an anovulatory follicle is usually preceded by development of normal endometrial folds or edema. Initial growth patterns of follicles destined to become anovulatory are usually within normal limits, and the first indication of a problem is typically detection of echogenic particles within the follicular fluid during ultrasonographic examination (Figure 12-1, *A*).

Anovulatory follicles may contain blood and have consequently also been called hemorrhagic anovulatory follicles. Scattered, free-floating echogenic spots within the follicular fluid detected during ultrasound examination of a dominant follicle may be a result of hemorrhage or the shedding of granulose cells from the follicular wall. Hemorrhagic follicular fluid may form a gelatinous mass within the follicular lumen. Ultrasonographically, hemorrhagic follicles may contain echogenic fibrous bands or strands traversing the follicular lumen (Figure 12-1, *B*). A progression from echogenic particles and strands to complete infiltration of the follicular lumen with echogenic material (Figure 12-1, *C*) is commonly observed. In other instances, the only ultrasonographic sign observed during development of an anovulatory follicle is a thickening of the follicular wall.

A majority of anovulatory follicles eventually become luteinized (85.7%), although some remain as follicular (nonluteal) structures (14.3%). Progesterone levels may be used to determine the luteal status of anovulatory follicles.[2] Mares with anovulatory follicles containing a highly echogenic lumen invariably have elevated progesterone

levels. Administration of prostaglandins will result in the destruction of the luteal cells in mares with luteinized anovulatory follicles, a rapid decline in serum progesterone levels, and a return to estrus. Prostaglandin therapy is most consistently effective when administered 7 to 10 days after the onset of formation of a luteinized anovulatory follicle is recognized. Prostaglandin treatment has no apparent effect on nonluteinized anovulatory follicles. Fortunately, a majority of nonluteinized anovulatory follicles will spontaneously regress in 1 to 4 weeks. Administration of human chorionic gonadotropin (hCG) or the gonadotropin-releasing hormone (GnRH) agonist deslorelin is generally not effective in inducing ovulation or luteinization of a follicular type of anovulatory follicle.

Pregnancy obviously will not occur if the follicle becomes hemorrhagic or luteinized without ovulating. In many instances mares are bred before it is recognized that a dominant follicle is destined to become anovulatory. In addition, it may be difficult to discern between a partially luteinized anovulatory follicle and a corpus hemorrhagicum or early corpus luteum in mares that are not examined frequently (i.e., daily) by ultrasonography.

Anovulatory follicles in mares have some characteristics that are similar to the cystic ovarian syndrome in cattle.[16] Nonechogenic (nonluteal) equine anovulatory follicles appear to be analogous to follicular cysts in cattle and echogenic (luteal) equine anovulatory follicles are similar to luteal cysts in cattle.

TREATMENT-ASSOCIATED OVULATION FAILURE

hCG is a large dimeric glycoprotein hormone produced by cytotrophoblasts of the human placenta. hCG has luteinizing hormone (LH) biological activity when administered to horses and many other species. Administration of hCG to mares in behavioral estrus, with mild to moderate uterine edema and a follicle greater than or equal to 35 mm in diameter will usually induce ovulation in approximately 36 ± 4 hours.[17,18] Dosages of hCG commonly used to induce ovulation range from 1,000 to 3,300 IU.

hCG is very effective in inducing ovulation in young mares that have not received the hormone previously and in middle-age to older mares receiving the hormone for the first time in the breeding season. It may be less predictable in inducing a timed ovulation in older mares. Conflicting evidence and opinions exist as to whether the efficacy of hCG in inducing a predictable, timed ovulation is reduced when the drug is used on an individual mare repeatedly during a single breeding season.

hCG is a foreign protein to the mare, and administration of hCG will lead to development of anti-hCG antibodies. It has been speculated over the years that a potential cause of reduced efficacy after repeated use is formation of anti-hCG antibodies.[18] Roser et al[19] and Wilson et al[20] noted that repeated administration of hCG led to development of anti-hCG antibodies. However, presence of antibodies against hCG was not associated with a decrease in efficacy of the drug at inducing ovulation. In addition, it was determined that antibodies against hCG did not bind to equine LH (eLH) or equine chorionic gonadotropin (eCG) in vitro and did not interfere with the ability of endogenous eLH to induce ovulation in vivo. Blanchard et al[21] did not note any decrease in efficacy of hCG when administered to mares for up to four estrous cycles within the same breeding season or up to seven different estrous cycles over two consecutive breeding seasons.

In contrast, other studies have reported that use of hCG multiple times during a breeding season or intentional immunization of mares against hCG does result in decreased efficacy of subsequent hCG administration in inducing a timed ovulation.[18,22] Sullivan et al[18] reported a complete failure of the expected induced ovulation when hCG was administered for the third consecutive cycle. Additional potential reasons for a failure of hCG to induce ovulation are use of an inappropriate dose, use of outdated drugs, administration when the follicle is not sufficiently mature, when attempting to induce ovulation of an atretic, regressing follicle, or a persistent anovulatory follicle. Also, response to hCG is less predictable when administered in the transition period[23] and when administered to mares greater than 16 years of age.[24]

Clinicians should be aware of the potential for a decrease in efficacy following repeated use of hCG. It has been recommended that mares not be administered more than two doses of hCG within the same breeding season.[25] Consequently, in situations in which a mare is being bred during multiple estrous cycles during a breeding season (i.e., embryo transfer or problem breeding mares), periodic use of an alternative agent for induction of ovulation, such as the GnRH agonist deslorelin, should be considered.

Deslorelin is a small (nine amino acid) peptide hormone that stimulates a prolonged release of LH from the anterior pituitary of the mare. Follicular maturation and ovulation is induced by the endogenous LH. The mechanism of action of deslorelin is thus different than that of hCG, which has inherent LH activity. Mares that fail to ovulate in response to hCG may be induced to ovulate with deslorelin. Repeated use during a breeding season does not result in antibody formation or a decrease in efficacy.[26] However, removal of the implant after ovulation is detected is recommended to prevent the possibility of subsequent pituitary down-regulation and a delay in return to estrus.[27,28] A compounded injectable formulation containing deslorelin has also been reported to be effective in inducing ovulation in estrual mares.

References

1. Hughes JP, Stabenfeldt GH, Evans JW: Clinical and endocrine aspects of the estrous cycle of the mare. Proceedings of the 18th Annual Conference of the American Association of Equine Practitioners, p 119, 1972.
2. McCue PM, Squires EL: Persistent anovulatory follicles in the mare. Theriogenology 2002; 58:541.
3. Ginther OJ: Reproductive Biology of the Mare, ed 2, Cross Plains, Wis, Equiservices, 1992.
4. Burkhardt J: Some clinical problems of horse breeding. Vet Rec 1948; 60:243.
5. Stangroom JE, de Weevers RG: Anticoagulant activity of equine follicular fluid. J Reprod Fertil 1962; 3:269.
6. Loy RG: Characteristics of postpartum reproduction in mares. Vet Clin North Am Large Anim Pract 1980; 2:345.
7. Palmer E, Driancourt MA: Some interactions of season of foaling, photoperiod and ovarian activity in the equine. Livest Prod Sci 1983; 10:197.
8. Nagy P, Huszenicza G, Juhasz J et al: Factors influencing ovarian activity and sexual behavior of postpartum mares under farm conditions. Theriogenology 1998; 50:1109.
9. Ginther OJ, Whitmore HL, Squires EL: Characteristics of estrus, diestrus, and ovulation in mares and effects of season and nursing. Am J Vet Res 1972; 33:1935.
10. Henneke DR, Potter GD, Kreider JL: Body condition during pregnancy and lactation and reproductive efficiency of mares. Theriogenology 1984; 21:897.
11. Hodge SL, Kreider JL, Potter GD et al: Influence of photoperiod on the pregnant and postpartum mare. Am J Vet Res 1982; 43:1752.
12. Koskinen E, Kurki E, Katila T: Onset of luteal activity in foaling and seasonally anoestrous mares treated with artificial light. Acta Vet Scand 1991; 32:307.
13. Meyers PJ: Ovary and oviduct. In Kobluk CN, Ames TR, Geor RJ (eds): The Horse, Philadelphia, WB Saunders, 1995.
14. McKinnon AO: Ovarian abnormalities. In Rantanen NW, McKinnon AO (eds): Equine Diagnostic Ultrasonography, Baltimore, Williams & Wilkins, 1997.
15. Pierson RA: Folliculogenesis and ovulation. In McKinnon AO, Voss JL (eds): Equine Reproduction, Philadelphia, Lea & Febiger, 1993.
16. Kesler DJ, Garverick HA: Ovarian cysts in dairy cattle: a review. J Anim Sci 1982; 55:1147.
17. McCue PM: Induction of ovulation. In Robinson NE (ed): Current Therapy in Equine Medicine, ed 5, Philadelphia, WB Saunders, 2003.
18. Sullivan JJ, Parker WG, Larson LL: Duration of estrus and ovulation time in nonlactating mares given human chorionic gonadotropin during three successive estrous periods. J Am Vet Med Assoc 1973; 162:895.
19. Roser JF, Kiefer BL, Evans JW et al: The development of antibodies to human chorionic gonadotrophin following its repeated injection in the cyclic mare. J Reprod Fertil Suppl 1979; 27:173.

20. Wilson CG, Downie CR, Hughes JP et al: Effects of repeated hCG injections on reproductive efficiency in mares. J Equine Vet Sci 1990; 10:301.

21. Blanchard TL, Varner DD, Schumacher J et al: Manual of Equine Reproduction, ed 2, St. Louis, Mosby, 2003.

22. Duchamp G, Bour B, Combarnous Y et al: Alternative solutions to hCG induction of ovulation in the mare. J Reprod Fertil Suppl 1987; 35:221.

23. Webel SK, Franklin V, Harland B et al: Fertility, ovulation and maturation of eggs in mares injected with HCG. J Reprod Fertil 1977; 51:337.

24. Barbacini S, Zavaglia G, Gulden P et al: Retrospective study on the efficacy of hCG in an equine artificial insemination programme using frozen semen. Equine Vet Educ 2000;12: 404, 2000.

25. Palmer E: Induction of ovulation. In McKinnon AO, Voss JL (eds): Equine Reproduction, Baltimore, Williams & Wilkins, 1993.

26. Mumford EL, Squires EL, Jochle W et al: Use of deslorelin short-term implants to induce ovulation in cycling mares during three consecutive estrous cycles. Anim Reprod Sci 1995; 39:129.

27. Farquhar VJ, McCue PM, Nett TM et al: Effect of deslorelin acetate on gonadotropin secretion and subsequent follicular development in cycling mares. J Am Vet Med Assoc 2001; 218:749.

28. Farquhar VJ, McCue PM, Carnevale EM et al: Deslorelin acetate (Ovuplant) therapy in cycling mares: effect of implant removal on FSH secretion and ovarian function. Equine Vet J 2002; 34:417.

CHAPTER 13

Ovarian Abnormalities

PATRICK M. McCUE

Abnormalities of ovarian function are not uncommon in the mare. Ovarian problems may be due to a permanent developmental condition (i.e., chromosomal abnormality), transient physiologic condition (i.e., anovulatory follicle), or an acquired pathologic condition (i.e., ovarian tumor). Clinical techniques that may be used in the diagnosis and differentiation of ovarian abnormalities include behavioral observations, general physical examination of the mare, palpation of the ovary per rectum, ultrasonography of the ovary per rectum, hormone analysis, laparoscopy/laparotomy, ovarian biopsy, and karyotyping.

It is often helpful to develop a differential diagnosis list when presented with a mare that may have an ovarian problem. In most instances the list of potential diagnoses can be narrowed to one or two based on clinical observations and ultrasonographic examination. Measurement of ovarian hormone levels, chromosomal evaluation, and other more expensive and/or invasive diagnostic tests are only occasionally required to provide a diagnosis or confirm a presumptive diagnosis. A list of diagnoses for small/inactive ovaries and enlarged ovaries are presented in Box 13-1.

CHROMOSOMAL AND DEVELOPMENTAL ABNORMALITIES

Chromosomal abnormalities, especially of the sex chromosomes, have been associated with infertility in the horse (see Chapter 10). The prevalence of sex chromosome abnormalities in the mare has been reported to be less than 3%. A chromosomal abnormality may be suspected in a mare of breeding age with primary infertility and gonadal hypoplasia, especially if the mare is presented during the physiologic breeding season and has not been administered exogenous hormones.

The normal chromosome number of the domestic horse is 64, which consists of 62 autosomes and 2 sex chromosomes.[1] The karyotype of the normal mare and stallion are 64,XX and 64,XY, respectively. Horses of all domestic breeds have the same number, size, and shape of chromosomes. The most commonly reported chromosomal abnormality of the horse is 63,X gonadal dysgenesis, in which only a single sex chromosome is present.[2] The condition may occur when the sex chromosome pair fails to separate during meiosis, producing one gamete without a sex chromosome and another with two sex chromosomes. The equine condition is analogous to Turner's syndrome in humans. The 63,X (or XO) condition has been detected in most domestic horse breeds, including draft and miniature breeds.

Horses with gonadal dysgenesis develop as phenotypic females because of the absence of a Y sex chromosome, or more specifically absence of the sex-determining region (Sry) normally present on the Y chromosome. Affected horses may be normal or small in size for their age and breed and have small ovaries with limited or no follicular development. The uterus and cervix are generally small and flaccid, and the endometrial glands are hypoplastic. The external genitalia are female, but the vulva may be smaller than normal and there is no clitoral hypertrophy. XO mares may exhibit anestrus or irregular estrous behavior and occasionally stand to be mated. True XO mares are considered to be sterile. However, mares with a mosaic or chimeric karyotype (i.e., 63,XO/64,XX) are not always small in stature, and some have been reported to produce a foal. Mosaic mares account for approximately 15% to 30% of all cases of gonadal dysgenesis. Numerous other chromosomal abnormalities have been reported in the mare in addition to XO gonadal dysgenesis.[3]

Occasionally a horse that has a developmental abnormality of the reproductive tract may present for evaluation. Although true equine hermaphrodites have been reported,[4] the most common developmental abnormality of the reproductive tract is male pseudohermaphroditism (XY sex reversal syndrome).[5] Affected horses are phenotypic mares or masculinized intersex horses with a male karyotype (64, XY) and cryptorchid testes. Sex phenotype and behavioral traits (i.e., expression of aggressive or stallion-like behavior) are correlated with blood testosterone levels.[6] The point to be made is that not every mare exhibiting male behavior has a granulosa-theca cell ovarian tumor. Other possibilities should be on a differential diagnosis list, including pregnancy, exposure to anabolic steroids, and intersex conditions.

Diagnosis of a chromosomal or developmental abnormality may be based, in part, on chromosome analysis or karyotyping. Karyotyping can be performed on any tissue with actively dividing cells. A fresh blood sample collected into acid citrate dextrose or heparin may be sent by overnight courier to a laboratory specializing in animal karyotyping. Measurement of blood testosterone levels may be beneficial in the detection of cryptorchid testes in some phenotypic mares with XY sex reversal. Transrectal ultrasonography and/or laparoscopic evaluation of the abdominal cavity may also be used to locate and evaluate gonads and internal genitalia. Histologic evaluation of biopsied or excised gonadal tissue may be necessary to confirm a diagnosis of true hermaphroditism.

Due to the etiology of the conditions, no treatments are possible to correct chromosomal or developmental

Box   **13-1**

Differential Diagnosis for Small/Inactive Ovaries and Enlarged Ovaries in the Mare

Small/Inactive Ovaries

1. Season (i.e., winter anestrus)
2. Age (i.e., prepubertal or advanced age)
3. Chromosomal abnormality
4. Exogenous hormone administration
5. Equine Cushing's disease

Enlarged Ovaries

1. Ovarian tumor (unilateral)
2. Anovulatory or hemorrhagic follicle (unilateral)
3. Pregnancy (bilateral)
4. Cystic ?? ovaries
5. Ovarian hematomas??

abnormalities of the reproductive tract. Castration is recommended for male pseudohermaphrodite horses.

AGE-RELATED OVARIAN DYSFUNCTION

Geriatric mares may have reduced reproductive performance due to age-related changes in ovarian function, uterine health, perineal conformation, and other factors.[7] Older mares may experience a delay in their initial ovulation of the year by an average of 2 weeks. Geriatric mares may have a longer interovulatory interval than younger mares because of a longer follicular phase.[8,9] A lengthening of the follicular phase in association with elevated gonadotropin concentrations may indicate impending reproductive senescence in older mares.[10] Aged mares may also have decreased oocyte viability and a higher incidence of early embryonic loss and abortion. Complete ovulation failure or ovarian senescence has been observed in aged mares and may be due to an insufficient number of primordial follicles. The incidence of pituitary adenoma (pituitary pars intermedia dysfunction, also known as Cushing's disease) is also increased in older mares and may contribute to poor reproductive performance.

No effective treatments are currently available in the mare for promoting follicular growth in senescent ovaries.

EXOGENOUS HORMONE TREATMENT

Anabolic steroid administration may affect estrous behavior and ovarian function. Treatment of mares with low doses of anabolic steroids may cause aggressive or stallion-like behavior, whereas high doses may inhibit ovarian activity and result in failure of follicular development and ovulation.[11] Anabolic steroids may also suppress pituitary gonadotropin secretion.[12] Administration of anabolic steroids to prepubertal fillies may result in cli-

toral hypertrophy. The use of anabolic steroids should be avoided in fillies and mares intended to be used for breeding.

Progestins are commonly given to cycling mares for the suppression of estrus or synchronization of ovulation.[13] Mares may continue to ovulate during progestin administration, especially if treatment is started late in the luteal phase. A high incidence of persistent corpus luteum formation has been noted for mares ovulating during progestin treatment.[14]

Deslorelin acetate is a potent gonadotropin-releasing hormone (GnRH) agonist used to induce a timed ovulation in mares. The commercial product (Ovuplant) is a biocompatible implant designed for subcutaneous administration. The GnRH agonist stimulates release of luteinizing hormone (LH) from the anterior pituitary, which induces follicular maturation and ovulation. After the implant was used extensively in the United States in 1999 and 2000, reports suggested that some individual mares treated to induce ovulation that did not become pregnant may have experienced a delayed return to estrus and a prolonged interovulatory interval.[15] Subsequent studies determined that use of the implant may be associated with prolonged suppression (down-regulation) of follicle-stimulating hormone (FSH) secretion from the pituitary, a decrease in follicular development in the diestrous period following the induced ovulation, and a lengthened interovulatory interval.[16,17] Administration of prostaglandins 7 to 8 days after ovulation to induce luteolysis, as routinely provided after an embryo collection attempt, increases the risk of delayed follicular development. Removal of the deslorelin implant 48 hours after administration has been reported to prevent the adverse effects on pituitary function and does not alter ovulation rates.[18] For ease of removal, the implant may be inserted subcutaneously by using the implant device provided by the manufacturer in a region of the vulva that has been infused with a small amount of local anesthetic.[19] After ovulation, the implant may be removed through the original tract created by the implant device by using gentle topical pressure.

EQUINE CUSHING'S DISEASE

Mares with hypertrophy, hyperplasia, or adenoma formation in the pars intermedia of the pituitary (equine Cushing's disease [ECD]) have been reported to have a variety of medical and reproductive problems. Reproductive abnormalities reported in mares with ECD have included abnormal estrous activity,[20] estrous suppression,[21] and reduced fertility.[22] Potential cause(s) of the reproductive abnormalities in mares with ECD may be destruction of the gonadotrophs of the anterior pituitary due to compression by the enlarged pars intermedia[23] or suppression of gonadotropin secretion due to elevated levels of glucocorticoids or androgens produced by the adrenal cortex.[23,24] In support of the glucocorticoid hypothesis, administration of dexamethasone to intact mares has been reported to cause reduced estrous behavior, LH concentrations, follicular growth, and incidence of ovulation.[25] In addition, administration of dexamethasone to ovariectomized mares results in suppression of pituitary LH and FSH secretion,[26,27] and treatment of pony mares with dexamethasone during the winter eliminates estrous behavior.[28]

A majority of horses diagnosed with ECD are older, with the average age being approximately 20 years. Consequently, the decrease in reproductive efficiency in mares with ECD may be partly due to advanced age.

Clinical signs of ECD include hirsutism and abnormal hair-coat shedding patterns, polyuria, polydipsia, and hyperhidrosis.[29,30] Diagnostic tests for ECD include measurements of serum glucose, insulin, adrenocorticotropic hormone (ACTH) and cortisol levels and dexamethasone suppression, ACTH stimulation, and thyrotropin-releasing hormone response tests.

The medical management of ECD includes the administration of pergolide mesylate, a dopamine receptor agonist, at a dosage of 0.5 to 2 mg q24h per adult horse. Cyproheptadine, a serotonin antagonist, has also been used, but it may not be as efficacious as pergolide. The dose of cyproheptadine is 0.25 mg/kg q24h, given once in the morning.

ANOVULATORY FOLLICLES (CYSTIC FOLLICLES)

This topic is discussed in Chapter 12.

OVARIAN HEMATOMAS

In the older literature, ovarian hematomas were reported to be one of the most common causes of unilateral ovarian enlargement.[31,32] Hematomas were noted to be a result of excessive hemorrhage into the follicular lumen following ovulation, or essentially greatly enlarged corpora hemorrhagica. The contralateral ovary was reported to be normal in size and function, and mares with this condition continued to cycle normally. No specific behavioral abnormalities were noted, and endocrine patterns of the mare were normal.

With the common use of ultrasonography to closely monitor ovarian function, the occurrence of the ovarian hematoma as a postovulatory structure should be reconsidered. It is likely that most structures previously reported to be ovarian hematomas are anovulatory (hemorrhagic) follicles. Dramatic enlargement of a corpus hemorrhagicum following detection of a true ovulation probably does not occur. In contrast, formation of a blood-filled follicular lumen in an anovulatory follicle is relatively common.

PERSISTENT CORPUS LUTEUM

The corpus luteum that forms after ovulation is usually functional for 14 to 15 days in the nonpregnant mare. Corpora lutea that fail to regress at the normal time postovulation are considered to be pathologically persistent.[33] Luteolysis, or destruction of the corpus luteum, occurs as a result of prostaglandin release from the endometrium. Occasionally, a mare may fail to regress her corpus luteum spontaneously at the normal time. The most common causes of a persistent corpus luteum are (1) ovulations late

in diestrus, resulting in corpora lutea that are immature (<5 days old) at the time of prostaglandin release; (2) embryonic loss after the time of maternal recognition of pregnancy; and (3) chronic uterine infections, resulting in destruction of the endometrium and therefore diminished prostaglandin release.[34] Spontaneous persistence of the corpus luteum due to inadequate prostaglandin release has been suggested but inadequately documented. A prolonged period of luteal activity may also follow formation of a luteinized anovulatory follicle.

The corpus luteum may persist for 2 to 3 months, during which time the mare will not express behavioral estrus. A differential diagnosis for failure to express estrus during a physiologic breeding cycle-period would include persistent corpus luteum, silent heat (especially in maiden and postfoaling mares), pregnancy, and reduced ovarian activity.

Diagnosis of a persistent corpus luteum may be made by behavioral observations, palpation, ultrasonography, analysis of plasma progesterone concentrations, or clinical response to prostaglandin administration. Progesterone concentrations greater than 1.0 ng/ml are indicative of the presence of luteal activity. Mares with a persistent corpus luteum will have good tone in the cervix and uterus on palpation, and the cervix will appear tight and dry on vaginal speculum examination because of the influence of progesterone. The retained corpus luteum is almost always visible with ultrasonography. A persistent corpus luteum will usually be eliminated by the administration of a single intramuscular dose of prostaglandins (PGF$_{2\alpha}$, 10 mg; or cloprostenol, 250 mg).

SHORTENED LUTEAL PHASE (PREMATURE LUTEOLYSIS)

Diestrus in the normal mare lasts approximately 15 days. Premature destruction of the corpus luteum (luteolysis) may be associated with an early onset of estrus and a decrease in the interovulatory interval. The most common cause of premature luteolysis in the mare is endometritis. Inflammation of the endometrium can result in sufficient synthesis and release of prostaglandins to cause luteal regression.[35] Consequently, a mare that exhibits a shortened diestrus should be examined for endometritis. A cytologic examination, culture, and/or biopsy of the uterus would be indicated.

LUTEAL INSUFFICIENCY

Primary luteal insufficiency implies a deficiency in ovarian progesterone production. Luteal insufficiency has been suggested to be a cause of subfertility in mares,[36] although data are limited. Experimental data confirm that premature luteolysis caused by endotoxin-induced prostaglandin release will result in pregnancy loss before formation of secondary corpora lutea.[37] Simultaneous administration of exogenous progestogen prevents endotoxemia-induced abortion.[38] Maintenance of pregnancy in some habitually aborting mares following administration of exogenous progestogens offers circumstantial evidence that progesterone insufficiency may be responsible for some cases of pregnancy loss.

Documentation of progesterone insufficiency as a cause of pregnancy loss would necessitate (1) an accurate initial pregnancy diagnosis, (2) ruling out other potential causes of pregnancy loss, and (3) measurement of low progesterone concentrations in a series of daily blood samples. Minimum concentration of progesterone required to maintain pregnancy in the mare has been suggested to be 4.0 ng/ml. The most common treatment for luteal insufficiency is supplementation with the synthetic progestogen altrenogest (Regumate) at a dose of 0.044 mg/kg orally once daily. Options for duration of altrenogest supplementation include (1) treatment until day 60 of pregnancy or greater *and* measurement of endogenous progesterone level of greater than 4.0 ng/ml, (2) treatment until day 120 of pregnancy, or (3) treatment until the end of pregnancy. Administration of other synthetic progestins resulted in pregnancy failure in the absence of endogenous progesterone support.[39] An excellent review of the topic of luteal deficiency in the mare has recently been published.[40]

OVARIAN TUMORS

The most common ovarian tumor in the mare is the granulosa cell tumor (GCT).[41] Granulosa cell tumors are almost always unilateral, slow growing, and benign. An examination of the affected ovary by using transrectal ultrasonography often reveals a multicystic or honeycombed structure, but the tumor may also present as a solid mass or as a single large cyst.[42] The contralateral ovary is usually small and inactive, although mares with a GCT on one ovary and a functional contralateral ovary have been reported.[43] Behavioral abnormalities such as prolonged anestrus, aggressive or stallion-like behavior, and persistent estrus or nymphomania may be expressed in affected mares.

Granulosa cell tumors are hormonally active, and clinical diagnostic assays for the detection of a GCT include the measurement of inhibin, testosterone, and progesterone.[44,45] Inhibin is elevated in approximately 90% of the mares with a GCT.[44] Serum concentrations of monomeric (free) inhibin alpha-subunit are inversely correlated with tumor size.[46] It is hypothesized that inhibin produced by the GCT is responsible for the inactivity of the contralateral ovary through the suppression of pituitary follicle-stimulating hormone release. Serum testosterone levels may be elevated if a significant theca cell component is present in the tumor (i.e., a granulosa-theca cell tumor [GTCT]). Testosterone is elevated in approximately 50% to 60% of affected mares and is usually associated with stallion-like behavior.[44] Progesterone concentrations in mares with a GCT are almost always below 1 ng/ml, because normal follicular development, ovulation, and corpus luteum formation do not occur often.

Therefore measurements of inhibin levels greater than 0.7 ng/ml, testosterone levels greater than 50 to 100 pg/ml, and progesterone levels of less than 1 ng/ml are suggestive of a granulosa cell tumor in a nonpregnant mare (Table 13-1).

Granulosa cell tumors are usually surgically removed if the tumor affects follicular development on the contralateral ovary, causes behavioral abnormalities, or is a

Table　**13-1**

Hormone Concentrations in the Normal Nonpregnant Mare

Hormone	Normal Range
Inhibin	0.1-0.7 ng/ml
Testosterone	20-45 pg/ml
Progesterone	
Estrus	<1 ng/ml
Diestrus	>1 ng/ml

source of colic. Surgical approaches for tumor removal include colpotomy, flank and ventral midline laparotomy, and laparoscopy.

Ovulation from the remaining ovary will occur approximately 6 to 8 months after tumor removal. Attempts at inducing follicular development and ovulation in the remaining ovary within 1 month after tumor removal by the administration of gonadotropin-releasing hormone (GnRH) have not been successful. Attempts at stimulation of follicular development in the contralateral ovary using purified equine follicle-stimulating hormone (eFSH) have not been reported.

The most common tumor of the surface epithelium of the equine ovary is the cystadenoma. Cystadenomas occur unilaterally, and the contralateral ovary is normal. The ultrasonographic appearance of the affected ovary may include one to many cystlike structures. In general, cystadenomas are rare and benign and are not considered to be hormonally active, although a case involving a mare with a cystadenoma and elevated plasma testosterone concentration has been reported.[47]

The treatment of choice for an ovarian cystadenoma is surgical removal. The decision to remove the affected ovary does not have to be made immediately, because the tumor is slow growing and has not been reported to metastasize. However, if the tumor does continue to enlarge, the mare may exhibit episodes of abdominal pain.

Teratomas and dysgerminomas are rare ovarian tumors of germ cell origin.[48,49] Teratomas are considered to be benign, whereas dysgerminomas are potentially malignant. Both are unilateral, hormonally inactive, and associated with normal contralateral ovaries. Germ cell tumors may contain hair, bone, muscle, and other tissues. They do not alter the behavior of the mare and do not interrupt the estrous cycle. The treatment of choice for germ cell tumors is surgical removal. This is especially true for the dysgerminoma, because of its potential for metastasis.

SUMMARY

A majority of ovarian abnormalities can be diagnosed with a minimum of equipment and diagnostic tests. However, some abnormalities require a more extensive evaluation, which may include blood samples for hormone analysis or karyotyping or other procedures.

Disorders such as anovulatory follicles and persistent corpora lutea usually will resolve spontaneously over time if treatment is not administered. Surgical intervention is warranted for ovarian tumors that have potential effects on the contralateral ovary, cause recurrent abdominal pain, or have potential for metastasis.

A decision to remove one or both ovaries should be made only after careful deliberation. If a clear diagnosis cannot be determined on clinical signs, palpation, ultrasonography, hormone analysis, or other diagnostic tests, it may be prudent to postpone surgery until it is certain that the ovary will not return to normal function.

References

1. Bowling AT: Horse Genetics, Wallingford, Oxon, UK, CAB International, 1996.
2. Hughes P, Benirschke K, Kennedy PC et al: Gonadal dysgenesis in the mare. J Reprod Fertil Suppl 1975; 23:385.
3. Zhang TQ, Buoen LC, Weber AF et al: Variety of cytogenetic anomalies diagnosed in 240 infertile equine. Proceedings of the 12th International Congress on Animal Reproduction and Artificial Insemination, p 1939, 1992.
4. Meyers-Wallen VN, Hurtgen J, Schlafer D et al: Sry-negative XX true hermaphroditism in a Paso Fino horse. Equine Vet J 1997; 29:404.
5. Kent MG, Shoffner RN, Buoen L et al: XY sex-reversal syndrome in the domestic horse. Cytogenet Cell Genet 1986; 42:8.
6. Kent MG, Schneller HE, Hegsted RL et al: Concentration of serum testosterone in XY sex reversed horses. J Endocrinol Invest 1988; 11:609.
7. Madill S: Reproductive considerations: mare and stallion. Vet Clin North Am Equine Pract 2002; 18:591.
8. Carnevale EM, Bergfelt DR, Ginther OJ: Aging effects on follicular activity and concentrations of FSH, LH, and progesterone in mares. Anim Reprod Sci 1993; 31:287.
9. Vanderwall DK, Peyrot LM, Weber JA et al: Reproductive efficiency of the aged mare. Proceedings of the Annual Meeting of the Society for Theriogenology, p 153, 1989.
10. Carnevale EM, Bergfelt DR, Ginther OJ: Follicular activity and concentrations of FSH and LH associated with senescence in mares. Anim Reprod Sci 1994; 35:231.
11. Maher JM, Squires EL, Voss JL et al: Effect of anabolic steroids on reproductive function of young mares. J Am Vet Med Assoc 1983; 183:519.
12. Turner JE, Irvine CH: Effect of prolonged administration of anabolic and androgenic steroids on reproductive function in the mare. J Reprod Fertil Suppl 1982; 32:213.
13. McCue PM: Estrus suppression in performance horses. J Equine Vet Sci 2003; 23:1.
14. Daels PF, McCue PM, DeMoraes M et al: Persistence of the luteal phase following ovulation during altrenogest treatment in mares. Theriogenology 1996; 46:799.
15. Morehead JP, Blanchard TL: Clinical experience with deslorelin (Ovuplant®) in a Kentucky Thoroughbred broodmare practice. J Equine Vet Sci 2000; 20:358.
16. Farquhar VJ, McCue PM, Nett TM et al: Effect of deslorelin acetate on gonadotropin secretion and subsequent follicular development in cycling mares. J Am Vet Med Assoc 2001; 218:749.
17. Johnson CA, Thompson DL Jr, Kulinski KM et al: Prolonged interovulatory interval and hormonal changes in mares following use of Ovuplant™ to hasten ovulation. J Equine Vet Sci 2000; 20:331.
18. Farquhar VJ, McCue PM, Carnevale EM et al: Deslorelin acetate (Ovuplant) therapy in cycling mares: effect of implant removal on FSH secretion and ovarian function. Equine Vet J 2002; 34:417.
19. McCue PM, Niswender KD, Farquhar VJ: Induction of ovulation with deslorelin: options to facilitate implant removal. J Eq Vet Sci 2002; 22:54.
20. Love S: Equine Cushing's disease. Br Vet J 1993; 149:139.
21. Beech J: Tumor of the pituitary gland (pars intermedia). In Robinson NE (ed): Current Therapy in Equine Medicine, ed 2, Philadelphia, WB Saunders, 1987.
22. Dybdal NO, Hargreaves KH, Madigan JE et al: Diagnostic testing for pituitary pars intermedia dysfunction in horses. J Am Vet Med Assoc 1994; 204:627.
23. Daels PF, Hughes JP: The abnormal estrous cycle. In McKinnon AO, Voss JL (eds): Equine Reproduction, Baltimore, Williams & Wilkins, 1993.
24. Troedsson MHT, Barber JA: Diseases of the ovary. In Robinson NE (ed): Current Therapy in Equine Medicine, ed 4, Philadelphia, WB Saunders Co, 1997.
25. Asa CS, Ginther OJ: Glucocorticoid suppression of oestrus, follicles, LH and ovulation in the mare. J Reprod Fertil Suppl 1982; 32:247.
26. Thompson DL Jr, Garza F Jr, St George RL et al: Relationships among LH, FSH and prolactin secretion, storage and response to secretagogue and hypothalamic GnRH content in ovariectomized pony mares administered testosterone, dihydrotestosterone, estradiol, progesterone, dexamethasone or follicular fluid. Domest Anim Endocrinol 1991; 8:189.
27. McNeill-Wiest DR, Thompson DL, Wiest JJ: Gonadotropin secretion in ovariectomized pony mares treated with dexamethasone or progesterone and subsequently with dihydrotestosterone. Domest Anim Endocrinol 1988; 5:149.
28. Pope NS, Sargent GF, Kesler DJ: The dexamethasone induced suppression of androgen secretions suppressed estrous behavior in pony mares during the winter. J Equine Vet Sci 1995; 15:119.
29. Dybdal N: Pituitary pars intermedia dysfunction (equine Cushing's-like disease). In Robinson NE (ed): Current Therapy in Equine Medicine, ed 4, Philadelphia, WB Saunders, 1997.
30. McCue PM: Equine Cushing's disease. Vet Clin North Am Equine Pract 2002; 18:533.
31. Meyers PJ: Ovary and oviduct. In Kobluk CN, Ames TR, Geor RJ (eds): The Horse, Philadelphia, WB Saunders, 1995.
32. Bosu WTK, Van Camp SC, Miller RB et al: Ovarian disorders: clinical and morphological observations in 30 mares. Can Vet J 1982; 23:6.
33. Stabenfeldt GH, Hughes JP, Evans JW et al: Spontaneous prolongation of luteal activity in the mare. Equine Vet J 1974; 6:158.
34. Ginther OJ: Prolonged luteal activity in mares—a semantic quagmire. Equine Vet J 1990; 22:152.
35. Neely DP, Kindahl H, Stabenfeldt GH et al:. Prostaglandin release patterns in the mare: physiological, pathophysiological, and therapeutic responses. J Reprod Fertil Suppl 1979; 27:181.
36. Douglas RH, Burns PJ, Hershman L: Physiological and commercial parameters for producing progeny for subfertile mares by embryo transfer. Equine Vet J Suppl 1985; 3:111.
37. Daels P, Starr M, Kindahl H et al: Effect of *Salmonella typhimurium* endotoxin on PGF-2a release and fetal death in the mare. J Reprod Fertil Suppl 1987; 35:485.
38. Daels PF, Stabenfeldt GH, Kindahl H et al: Prostaglandin release and luteolysis associated with physiological and pathological conditions of the reproductive cycle of the mare: a review. Equine Vet J Suppl 1989; 8:29.

39. McKinnon AO, Lescun TB, Walker JH et al: The inability of some synthetic progestagens to maintain pregnancy in the mare. Equine Vet J 2000; 32:83.
40. Allen WR: Luteal deficiency and embryo mortality in the mare. Reprod Domest Anim 2001; 36:121.
41. Hughes JP, Kennedy PC, Stabenfeldt GH: Pathology of the ovary and ovarian disorders in the mare. Proceedings of the 9th International Congress on Animal Reproduction and Artificial Insemination, p 203, 1980.
42. Hinrichs K, Hunt PR: Ultrasound as an aid to diagnosis of granulosa cell tumour in the mare. Equine Vet J 1990; 22:99.
43. McCue PM, LeBlanc MM, Akita GY et al: Granulosa cell tumors in two cycling mares. J Equine Vet Sci 1991; 11:281.
44. McCue PM: Equine granulose cell tumors. Proceedings of the 38th Annual Convention of the American Association of Equine Practitioners, p 587, 1992.
45. Stabenfeldt GH, Hughes JP: Clinical aspects of reproductive endocrinology in the horse. Compend Contin Educ 1987; 9:678.
46. Bailey MT, Troedsson MH, Wheato JE: Inhibin concentrations in mares with granulosa cell tumors. Theriogenology 2002; 57:1885.
47. Hinrichs K, Frazer GS, deGannes RVG et al: Serous cystadenoma in a normally cyclic mare with high plasma testosterone values. J Am Vet Med Assoc 1989; 194:381.
48. McEntee K: Reproductive Pathology of Domestic Animals, New York, Academic, 1990.
49. Frazer GS, Threlfall WR: Differential diagnosis of enlarged ovary in the mare. Proceedings of the 32nd Annual Convention of the American Association of Equine Practitioners, p 21, 1986.

CHAPTER 14

Therapy for Mares with Uterine Fluid

JONATHAN F. PYCOCK

Reduced fertility associated with fluid accumulation has been recognized for many years in broodmares. This subfertility is due to an unsuitable environment within the uterus for the developing conceptus, and in some instances the ensuing endometritis persists and causes early regression of the corpus luteum. The term *endometritis* refers to the acute or chronic inflammatory process involving the endometrium. These changes frequently are the result of microbial infection, but they also can be due to noninfectious causes. The objective of the veterinary surgeon and the stud farm owner or manager should be to produce the maximum number of live, healthy foals from mares mated during the previous season. One of the main obstacles to this goal is susceptibility in individual mares to persistent acute endometritis, manifested as fluid accumulation in the uterus after mating.

Persistent mating-induced endometritis has come to be recognized as a major reason for failure of mares to conceive. Persistent sperm-induced inflammation may be a more important cause of infertility in susceptible mares than infectious endometritis.[1]

PATHOGENESIS

The Inflammatory Response to Semen

Semen is deposited directly into the uterus when mares are bred by either natural service or artificial insemination. This means that bacterial and seminal components, as well as debris, contaminate the uterus, which results in uterine inflammation. It was previously thought that the inflammatory response to breeding was due to bacterial contamination of the uterus at the time of insemination. It is now accepted that the spermatozoa themselves, rather than bacteria, are responsible for the acute inflammatory response in the equine uterus after insemination.[2] Spermatozoa are transported rapidly to the oviducts, but only a small number actually reach the site of fertilization. The greater part of the ejaculate remains in the uterus, where it induces an acute inflammatory reaction.

Kotailen et al[3] showed that the intensity of the reaction was dependent on the concentration and/or volume of the inseminate: Concentrated semen (frozen semen) induced a stronger inflammatory reaction in the uterus than that observed for fresh or extended semen. The inflammatory reaction of the uterus is not different for live or for dead spermatozoa.[4]

Work by Nikolakopoulos and Watson[5] found that the number of uterine neutrophils (polymorphonuclear leukocytes [PMNs]) was greater when smaller numbers of sperm were infused. Because the volumes used in this study were larger, however, it may be that a significant amount of inseminate was lost via cervical reflux. In addition, the mares were not sampled for PMNs until 48 hours after insemination. It is likely that the inflammatory reaction was well past its peak by then.[6,7]

That the intensity of the inflammatory response following insemination depends on the sperm themselves, rather than on any extender, was the conclusion of Parlevliet and her co-workers,[8] who measured the inflammatory response after insemination with raw semen, extended semen, and various extenders.

Seminal plasma is the fluid portion of the ejaculate and suspends the cells present in semen. Seminal plasma improves sperm transport either directly or by protecting the sperm from phagocytosis while in the uterus, thereby improving survival time. Seminal plasma is rich in oxytocin and prostaglandins, both of which cause uterine contractions. The precise role of seminal plasma in sperm transport in the horse is not known. Seminal plasma prolongs sperm life within the uterus because it suppresses PMN chemotaxis and phagocytosis of sperm. The mechanism is thought to involve more than simply complement inactivation.[9,10]

Evidently, then, seminal plasma modulates the inflammatory response to spermatozoa. A reduction in the inflammatory response after insemination can be expected to have both positive and negative effects. Any suppression of phagocytosis will reduce the elimination of sperm but also of bacteria. The amount of fluid produced after insemination may be reduced. Seminal plasma has a low buffering capacity, and in a freshly collected ejaculate, by-products rapidly accumulate in seminal plasma as a result of the high metabolic activity of the sperm cells. During freezing of sperm, seminal plasma is removed. This may be why the inflammatory response is greater with frozen/thawed semen. The increased response also may be due to the high sperm concentration.[3] Recently, it has been reported that seminal plasma decreases uterine contractility and increases the inflammatory response of the uterus to semen.[11] Thus, the evidence for the role seminal plasma plays in inflammation within the uterus of the mare is conflicting.

The first inflammatory cells to enter the uterus are PMNs, observed in the uterus within 30 minutes after insemination.[12] The equine uterus produces fluid that has chemoattractant properties for PMNs.[6] Complement is thought to be the crucial component that serves as a chemoattractant for PMNs, although other products may serve as chemoattractants.[6,7] It is now believed that spermatozoa initiate chemotaxis of PMNs through activation of complement,[13] suggesting that a transient uterine inflammation following insemination is physiologic and serves to clear the uterus of excess spermatozoa, seminal plasma, and contaminates associated with insemination. Damaged sperm may be more readily phagocytosed by PMNs. In normal mares, the inflammation peaks at approximately 10 to 12 hours and subsides appreciably within 24 hours after insemination.

In most mares, this transient endometritis resolves spontaneously within 24 to 72 hours, so that the environment of the uterine lumen is compatible with embryonic life. It is important not to regard this endometrosis as a pathologic condition. Rather, it is a physiologic reaction to clear excess sperm, seminal plasma, and inflammatory debris from the uterus before the embryo descends from the oviduct into the uterine lumen 5.5 days after fertilization.

If the endometritis persists beyond day 3 or 4 of the luteal phase, however, in addition to being incompatible with embryonic survival, the premature release of the prostaglandin $PGF_{2\alpha}$ results in luteolysis with a rapid decline in progesterone and an early return to estrus. Mares in which this occurs are referred to as **susceptible**, and they develop a persistent endometritis.[6] The concept of susceptibility to endometritis was first suggested by Farrely and Mullaney,[14] who stated that infective endometritis is essentially the failure of an individual mare to limit the uterine and cervical microflora to a non-resident type. At the same time, Knudsen[15] reported the discrete collection of fluid in permanent ventral dilatations at the base of one or (rarely) both horns of the uterus that could be palpated per rectum. Hughes and Loy[16] developed the concept of susceptibility to endometritis and confirmed that resistant mares could eliminate induced infection without treatment, whereas susceptible mares could not. In general, reduced resistance to endometritis is associated with advancing age and multiparity.

Susceptibility to endometritis is not an absolute state, because failure of uterine defense mechanisms need only slow the process of eliminating infection. In the practice situation, a wide range in degrees of susceptibility to endometritis is seen, and it must not be thought that mares can be neatly classified as either resistant or susceptible.[17] Studies on immunoglobulins, opsonins, and the functional ability of PMNs in the uterus of susceptible mares have not confirmed the presence of an impaired immune response (see the review by Allen and Pycock[18]). Evans et al[19] first suggested that reduced physical drainage may contribute to an increased susceptibility to uterine infection. The physical ability of the uterus to eliminate bacteria, inflammatory debris, and fluid is now known to be the critical factor in uterine defense. It is a logical conclusion that any impairment of this function—that is, defective myometrial contractility—renders a mare susceptible to persistent endometritis.[20-22] The reason for this defective contractility in susceptible mares is not known. It has been suggested that the regulation of muscle contraction by the nervous system may be impaired.[23]

The resulting fluid accumulation also could be due to failure to drain via the cervix or to decreased reabsorption by lymphatic vessels. Lymphatic drainage potentially may play an important role in the persistence of postbreeding inflammation, and it is interesting that lymphatic lacunae (lymph stasis) are a common finding in endometrial biopsy specimens taken from susceptible mares.[24,25]

Other factors can be involved in a delay in uterine clearance. In older mares that have had several foals, the uterus may have dropped ventrally within the abdomen. Such mares can have a delay in uterine clearance.[26]

An adequate cervical opening is vital to allow drainage, and any failure of the cervix to dilate can cause fluid accumulation (see Chapter 21). This failure of the cervix to open is particularly relevant in the case of the older mare in general and the older maiden mare in particular, leading to the term "old maiden mare syndrome." Recognition and appropriate management of the older maiden mare are particularly important because a susceptibility to postbreeding endometritis is common in such mares even though they have never been bred before. Mares that have had a showjumping or dressage career often may not be presented to be bred until they are in their teens, and such mares can be very difficult to get in foal.

Older maiden mares have some common characteristics that resemble a syndrome. Endometrial biopsy samples reveal glandular degenerative changes and stromal fibrosis (endometriosis) as an inevitable consequence of ageing even in mares that have not been bred.[27] Another common characteristic is presence of uterine fluid. The older maiden mare often has an abnormally tight cervix that fails to relax properly during estrus, so that fluid is unable to drain and then accumulates in the uterine lumen.[28] In many instances, this fluid tests negative for bacterial growth and presence of PMNs. Once the mare is bred, the fluid accumulation will be aggravated as a result of poor lymphatic drainage and impaired myometrial contraction compounded by the cervical tightness. The amount of intrauterine fluid will vary in individual mares, ranging from a few milliliters to greater than a liter in extreme cases. Recently, endometrial vascular degeneration also has been suggested as a contributing factor in delayed uterine clearance.[29] To maximize the fertility of these mares, it is vital that the veterinarian be aware of the possibility of this type of uterine and cervical pathology. All too often, owners assume that the fertility of these mares is comparable to that of younger maiden mares; one of the most important aspects of breeding the old maiden mare is to make the owner aware of the increased risk of problems. These mares must be regarded as highly susceptible and managed accordingly.

DIAGNOSIS

Identification of the Fluid-Producing Mare

Identifying the susceptible mare can be difficult because only subtle changes may be present in the uterine environment, not readily detected by current diagnostic procedures. Many mares show no signs of inflammation before mating but will fail to resolve the inevitable endometritis that follows mating. Response to bacterial challenge has been used in a research setting. Scintigraphic and other methods based on charcoal clearance have been used to make an accurate diagnosis of a clearance problem in a mare,[22] but such methods are difficult to apply in practice. History of repeat breeding and/or fluid accumulation at the time of breeding is perhaps the most useful indicator of susceptibility to mating-induced endometritis in an individual mare.

Detection of Intraluminal Uterine Fluid Using Transrectal Ultrasound Imaging

Ultrasonographic examination to detect uterine luminal fluid (Figure 14-1) has proved useful to identify mares with a clearance problem and is the most useful technique in practice. The presence of free intraluminal fluid before breeding strongly suggests susceptibility to persistent endometritis.[30] Excessive production of fluid due to glandular alterations, rather than a failure of lymphatic drainage, has been postulated to cause intrauterine fluid accumulation.[31] It is currently not known for certain, however, whether the fluid accumulates as a result of excess production, delay in physical clearance via the open cervix, or decreased reabsorption by lymphatic vessels; a combination of all three mechanisms may well be involved.

Since the first description of the identification of collections of small volumes of intrauterine fluid using ultrasound imaging, which could not be palpated per rectum,[32] general awareness of the frequency of this abnormality has increased. The detection of uterine fluid during both estrus and diestrus has been reported.[33,34] Endometrial secretions and the formation of small volumes of free fluid may be associated with the same mechanism responsible for normal estral edema formation. In many instances, the uterine luminal fluid that accumulates before mating is sterile and contains no neutrophils.[30] The importance of these sterile fluid accumulations is that although initially sterile, the fluid may act as a culture medium for bacteria that gain entry to the uterus at mating and also may be spermicidal.[35]

The amount of fluid that should be considered significant is not clear, and it may be that quantity is more important than nature, particularly for fluid appearing during estrus. Brinsko et al[36] concluded that the presence of more than a 2-cm depth of fluid during estrus was a predictor of susceptibility. The significance depends to some extent on when during estrus the fluid is observed: Fluid detected early in estrus may disappear subsequently when the mare is further advanced in estrus and the cervix relaxes more. Small volumes of intrauterine fluid during estrus do not affect pregnancy rates in mares, in contrast with larger (>2 cm in depth) collections of fluid.[30] Mares that are susceptible to endometritis demonstrate greater accumulation of fluid than that observed in resistant mares.

In general, if greater than a 1-cm-depth of fluid is present during estrus, some attempt should be made to remove this fluid before breeding using oxytocin. If the depth is greater than 2 cm, the fluid is drained and may need to be investigated for the presence of inflammatory cells and bacteria. The mare may then need to undergo large-volume uterine lavage. Visualization of intrauterine fluid on ultrasonography performed later than 18 hours after breeding is diagnostic of defective uterine clearance in the mare. Intrauterine fluid during diestrus is indicative of inflammation and is associated with subfertility related to early embryonic death and a shortened luteal phase.[37]

Intraluminal uterine fluid can be graded I to IV according to the degree of echogenicity (Figure 14-2). The more echoic the fluid, the more likely the fluid is contaminated with debris including white blood cells. Cellular fluid can appear relatively anechoic, however, so care is needed in interpretation. Inspissated pus can be so echoic that it is overlooked. It may be that the actual character of the fluid and the ultrasonographic appearance are not as closely linked as was once thought.

Ultrasonographic appearance may be proportional to the size and concentration of particulate matter within the fluid, rather than the viscosity of the fluid; for example, purulent exudates can appear nonechogenic. Air has hyperechoic foci (Figure 14-3), and fluid with air bubbles appears cellular. Urine in the bladder can appear echoic, despite being a watery liquid (Figure 14-4).

TREATMENT OPTIONS FOR MARES WITH FLUID ACCUMULATION

The aim of treatment for mares with fluid accumulation should be to assist the uterus to physically clear the normal inflammatory by-products of the response to breeding.[38-41] Because within 4 hours of mating, the spermatozoa necessary for fertilization are present within the oviduct, and because the embryo does not descend into the uterus for approximately 5.5 days, treatment may be

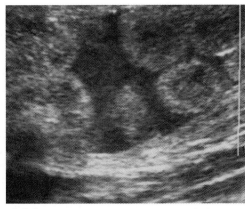

Figure 14-1 Ultrasonographic image of the uterus of a mare with fluid accumulation.

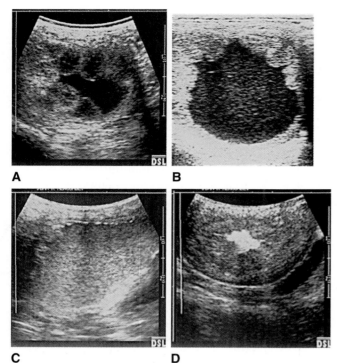

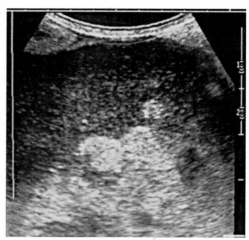

Figure 14-4 Ultrasonographic image of a full urinary bladder.

Figure 14-2   A, Ultrasonographic image of grade I uterine fluid: Anechogenic. **B,** Ultrasonographic image of grade II uterine fluid: Hypoechogenic with hyperechogenic particles. **C,** Ultrasonographic image of grade III uterine fluid: Moderately echogenic. **D,** Ultrasonographic image of grade IV uterine fluid: Hyperechogenic fluid in the uterus of an infected mare.

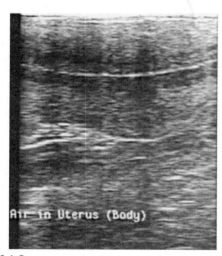

Figure 14-3 Hyperechogenic reflections appearing as a *line* at the opposed luminal surfaces of the uterine body. The reflections are caused by air in the uterine body.

safely given from 4 hours after mating until 2 days from ovulation, provided that isotonic solutions are used. Progesterone concentrations rise rapidly following ovulation in the mare, however, and it is preferable to avoid treatment involving uterine interference beyond 2 days after ovulation. Both coitus and artificial insemination can be

a source of uterine contamination; it is well known that spermatozoa themselves are responsible for initiating a marked inflammatory response leading to a persistent endometritis in susceptible mares.[12] Susceptible mares, therefore, may be bred only once per estrus, regardless of whether natural mating or artificial insemination is used. If repeated breedings are necessary, uterine lavage should be performed after each mating.

The successful management of susceptible mares will logically require some form of postmating therapy such as uterine lavage, intravenous administration of oxytocin, and intrauterine antibiotic infusion; these may be used alone or in combination. The emphasis should be on treatment in relation to timing of breeding, rather than ovulation. Too often in the past, veterinarians have waited until ovulation before providing appropriate treatment for these mares. By then, a large amount of fluid usually has accumulated and the bacteria are in a logarithmic phase of growth.

Uterine Lavage

Recognition of the importance of the mechanical evacuation of uterine contents accounted for the introduction of large-volume uterine lavage. The technique involves infusion of 2 to 3 liters of previously warmed (to 42° C) sterile physiologic (buffered) saline or lactated Ringer's solution into the uterus via a catheter that has been retained within the cervix via a cuff. The fluid is then siphoned out of the uterus by gravity flow. The most convenient device is a large-bore (30 French), 80-cm autoclavable equine embryo flushing catheter (EUF-80, Bivona, Ind) (Figure 14-5). The cuff is useful to effectively seal the internal cervical os. The catheter should be inserted only after thorough cleansing of the perineum (Figure 14-6). The rationale for such an approach includes the following considerations:

The removal of accumulated uterine fluid and inflammatory debris, which may interfere with neutrophil function and the efficacy of antibiotics

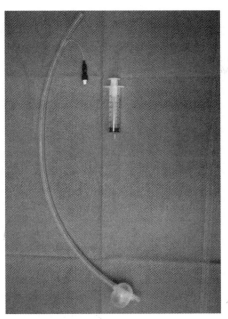

Figure 14-5 Large-bore (30 French) embryo flushing catheter, 80 cm in length. Note the inflated cuff.

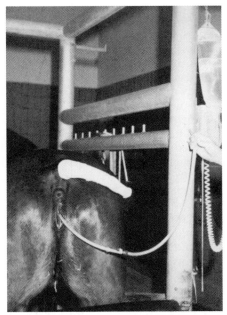

Figure 14-6 Performing large-volume lavage with a flushing catheter in position.

Stimulation of uterine contractility
Recruitment of fresh neutrophils through mechanical
   irritation of the endometrium

The saline is infused by gravity flow 1 L at a time, and the washings are inspected to provide immediate information concerning the nature of the uterine contents. The lavage should be repeated until the fluid that is recovered is clear (Figure 14-7). In most instances, the fluid evenly distributes in both horns, making transrectal

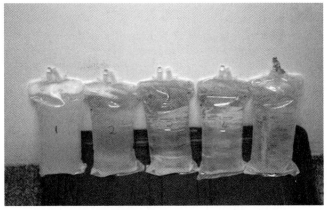

Figure 14-7 Sterile saline should be infused 1 L at a time until the recovered fluid is clear.

massage of the uterus unnecessary. If a rectal examination is performed while the catheter is in the uterus, it is essential to avoid contaminating the catheter. The fluid should be recovered in the same container in which it is infused, thereby preventing air from being aspirated into the uterus through the catheter. During lavage, oxytocin should be given intravenously. Measurement of the recovered fluid and ultrasonographic examination of the uterus should be performed after flushing to ensure that all the fluid has been recovered. This is necessary because the patient is a mare with an impaired ability to spontaneously drain the uterus. For this reason, the process usually is combined with oxytocin injection.

The optimal time to perform a large-volume uterine lavage in relation to insemination or mating represents a balance between risk and benefit. On the one hand, uterine contaminants should be removed as soon as possible after mating, whereas on the other, sperm cells may be detected in the oviduct between 2 and 4 hours after insemination.[42] Additionally, studies have found that uterine lavage performed 4 hours after insemination did not harm the sperm cells or influence pregnancy rate, whereas the pregnancy rate was reduced when the lavage was performed 0.5 or 2 hours after insemination.[38,43] The lavage usually is performed between 4 and 18 hours after breeding.

The optimal time of treatment in highly susceptible mares was found to be between 4 and 6 hours in a study by Knutti.[44] Eighteen barren mares with a mean age of 15 years were selected. They had been barren for more than 1 year, had been inseminated during greater than 6 estrous periods, had a history of fluid accumulation after breeding, and had failed to become pregnant with the standard protocol for management as described previously. In nine mares, the standard protocol was repeated (control). In the other nine mares, the standard protocol was performed, with the only change that the mare's uterus was flushed 4 to 6 hours after insemination. Twice as many mares with the early lavage were pregnant compared with the group of mares not lavaged until 18 to 20 hours after insemination.

The combination of both treatment options was effective in clearing even large amounts of intraluminal fluid.

The decision to perform uterine lavage only when more than 2 cm of intraluminal fluid was detected was based on the clinical experience that smaller amounts of fluid usually could be cleared from the uterus with oxytocin alone, which is a time- and cost-saving treatment. To be certain that oxytocin injection would not interfere with sperm transport in the uterus and oviduct, the drug was not administered immediately before or after insemination. The results of this study correlate with the findings of Brinsko et al[38] that a uterine lavage performed 4 hours after insemination does not adversely affect conception rate.

In my practice, known susceptible mares are routinely treated the day after breeding. In keeping with the principle that the longer a foreign particle stays in the uterine lumen, the more PMNs accumulate, an earlier treatment is given to reduce the inflammatory reaction and improve the chances for these susceptible mares to get pregnant. In mares believed to be highly susceptible to endometritis, as indicated by the history of fluid accumulation, the lavage should be performed within 4 to 6 hours.

Oxytocin

Oxytocin is the ideal method of treatment that is non-invasive and frequently provides early and complete elimination of any intrauterine fluid. The beneficial effect of oxytocin is widely accepted.[31,39] Oxytocin stimulates uterine contractions in the cyclical, pregnant, and postpartum mare and was first suggested to promote uterine drainage in mares with defective uterine clearance by Allen.[45] Until then, use of oxytocin was not considered to be an appropriate treatment for endometritis, probably because it was taught that oxytocin induced uterine contractions only in the first 48 hours after foaling. Alternatively, use of oxytocin was discouraged because of the concern that it would cause severe colic. After the pioneering study of Allen,[45] however, subsequent clinical experience[31,39,40,46,47] has allayed early fears that oxytocin would cause severe colic when given as an intravenous bolus. Various investigators have reported improved pregnancy rates in susceptible mares after oxytocin administration. Oxytocin is now well accepted as an effective agent for aiding mechanical clearance mechanisms and improving fertility.

Myometrial response to oxytocin depends partly on the time for which oxytocin remains in the circulation after administration and partly on the type of local cellular effects within the uterus, including prostaglandin $F_{2\alpha}$ ($PGF_{2\alpha}$) production.[48] Oxytocin is known to stimulate prostaglandin release,[22,49] although the precise mechanism that controls myometrial contraction remains unclear. The uterine response to oxytocin may be due in part to a direct effect of oxytocin on the myometrium and in part to the indirect effect of oxytocin causing $PGF_{2\alpha}\alpha$ release.[50,51] Support for this dual mode of action comes from the fact that oxytocin has been shown to override the inhibitory effect of phenylbutazone on uterine clearance.[52] Phenylbutazone inhibits prostaglandin synthesis and has been shown to slow uterine clearance in reproductively normal mares.[50] Phenylbutazone is a commonly used drug in broodmares for conditions such as lamini-

tis, and oxytocin would be preferable to $PGF_{2\alpha}$ analogues to improve uterine clearance in mares on phenylbutazone therapy. Even reproductively normal mares receiving phenylbutazone for lameness should be given oxytocin after breeding.

If oxytocin is to be advocated as a treatment for mares with mating-induced endometritis or uterine clearance problems, it would be best to first know how reproductively normal mares respond to the doses used clinically. In a recent study in reproductively normal mares, Paccamonti et al[49] reported that the half-life of oxytocin was 6.8 minutes. Mares were given intravenous oxytocin, 10 or 25 IU, on the day of ovulation or 2 days afterward. Neither dose of oxytocin nor day of treatment affected the half-life of the exogenous oxytocin.

No advantage is associated with use of oxytocin in doses greater than 25 IU, and it may even be that the same effect can be obtained by use of 10 IU, so long as treatment is given during the preovulatory period.[51] Although the initial change in intrauterine pressure appeared more pronounced with a larger dose (25 IU) of oxytocin at 5 and 10 minutes after treatment, the change in pressure at subsequent time intervals was similar between the two doses (25 IU and 10 IU). These authors also found an effect of day of administration of oxytocin on the uterine response, with a weaker response when oxytocin was administered after ovulation. Statistical significance was not present, however. A later study[49] has shown that prostaglandin metabolite (PGFM) release was more obvious with mares given 25 IU versus 10 IU of oxytocin. PGFM is the main metabolite of $PGF_{2\alpha}$ in plasma. Likewise, PGFM release was elevated when oxytocin was given on the day of ovulation compared with 2 days after ovulation. Again, these differences were not statistically significant. Further work is needed to establish the pattern of PGFM response in vivo to oxytocin administration in subfertile versus normal mares. It has been shown that in reproductively normal mares, the uterus itself may produce oxytocin.[53,54] This could mean that the uterus of susceptible mares may exhibit inadequate oxytocin synthesis, which may affect uterine clearance both directly and indirectly through reduced PGF release. It is therefore important that we now know the half-life of oxytocin, and further work needs to be done on patterns of PGF release after oxytocin administration. No untoward effects have been noted, apart from a very occasional mild and transient discomfort. Any possible adverse effect on gamete transport would seem to be outweighed by the ability to improve uterine fluid clearance. In most mares, the response is rapid, with fluid voided almost immediately.

Larger doses of oxytocin (25 IU) have been associated with a decreased pregnancy rate.[31] This dose frequently is used in clinical practice, however, and no other studies have reported this finding. The dose of oxytocin used in my practice in mares weighing approximately 500 kg is 20 IU given by either the intravenous or the intramuscular route. Smaller mares are given 15 IU of oxytocin. Campbell and England[55] confirmed a dose effect of oxytocin on uterine contractions: doses between 2.5 and 20 IU increased uterine contractions, and the number of contractions was reduced at a dose of 30 IU. This study also looked at intrauterine use of oxytocin and concluded that at equivalent 30 IU doses of oxytocin intrauterine treatment is more ecbolic than intravenous.

Recently a long-acting analogue of oxytocin, carbetocin (Reprocine, Vetoquinol), has become available and may have an indication in situations in which a more prolonged uterine contraction is desired. My own preliminary work has shown it to be safe and effective at inducing uterine clearance. Two intramuscular injections of 0.14 mg carbetocin are given 12 and 24 hours after breeding in mares with marked uterine edema or free fluid before breeding or in mares with uterine fluid greater than 2 cm deep at 12 hours after breeding.

Prostaglandin Analogues

Prostaglandins are known to be released very early in mares with endometritis.[7] A useful role for prostaglandins in increasing myometrial activity and assisting uterine clearance has been described in several studies.[13,50,56] The investigators showed that the prostaglandin analogue cloprostenol (Estrumate, Intervet), given intramuscularly in a dose of 500 µg, caused increased clearance of radiocolloid in susceptible mares, but significantly slower than that caused by oxytocin. The uterus did contract for a longer time, however—5 hours versus 45 minutes. Of the prostaglandins administered (PGF$_{2\alpha}$, cloprostenol, and fenprostalene), cloprostenol produced the most consistent response. Cloprostenol would seem to be indicated in mares that have lymphatic stasis as shown by excessive fluid within the endometrium or large lymphatic cysts.[52] The suggested dose of cloprostenol is 250 µg given at 12 and 24 hours after breeding.[29] Cloprostenol should not be given after ovulation in case of inducing premature luteal regression.[1]

Intrauterine Antibiotics

The intrauterine infusion of broad-spectrum antibiotics after breeding is controversial.[30,47,57] It has been shown in at least one scientific experiment in which an endometritis model was used that saline lavage and uterotonic drugs such as prostaglandin F$_{2\alpha}$ are as effective as antibiotics in eliminating bacteria from the uterus.[57] In this controlled experiment–type situation, however, a single bacterial species (usually streptococci) was infused into the uterus, and lavage treatment was performed at a fixed time (within 12 hours of mating).

Under normal clinical conditions, a mixed bacterial contamination is present, and lavage cannot always be performed within 12 hours. Accordingly, I prefer to continue to use intrauterine antibiotics as part of the therapeutic protocol. The treatments have different effects on the uterus: The uterine lavage provides mechanical evacuation of intraluminal fluid and inflammatory products, whereas the single infusion of broad-spectrum antibiotics should prevent any growth of bacteria introduced during insemination or uterine lavage. Furthermore, mares susceptible to postbreeding endometritis have, according to their history, a reduced capacity for uterine clearance and impaired defense mechanisms. Therefore, they cannot be compared with healthy mares used in experiments.

Routine administration of intrauterine antibiotics has no negative effect on pregnancy rates in treated mares.[30,47,58]

Intrauterine Plasma Infusions

On the basis of research findings of the 1970s and 1980s that emphasized the immunologic aspects of the uterine defense mechanisms, intrauterine plasma has been used in the susceptible mare. Studies following its use have indicated an improvement in fertility.[59,60] Two different groups of investigators suggested that the plasma had an enhancing effect on phagocytosis by uterine neutrophils. Adams and Ginther,[61] in a study that included control groups of mares, found that intrauterine plasma was not efficacious in treating endometritis because it was not associated with any improvement in pregnancy rates. In addition, transfer of infectious agents also is possible. Troedsson et al[62] suggested that plasma treatment may benefit only certain susceptible mares. This latter point was also alluded to recently by Pascoe,[60] who, while remaining enthusiastic about the use of plasma in the management of immunoincompetent mares, conceded that this may be beneficial only in mares without a mechanical clearance problem. Consequently, plasma is best used in mares that repeatedly fail to become pregnant but have no history of fluid accumulation. Because mares that are susceptible to endometritis do not possess a quantitative deficiency of immunoglobulins, it is questionable if such treatment is truly effective.

HOW TO BREED THE MARE THAT ACCUMULATES FLUID

Breeding or inseminating a mare induces an immediate inflammatory response in the uterus. This is a physiologic reaction against foreign material. In most mares, this inflammation clears within 1 or 2 days.

Mares susceptible to mating-induced endometritis are known to accumulate fluid in the uterus as a result of impaired clearance of inflammatory products. Reduced myometrial contractions, poor lymphatic drainage, a large, overstretched uterus, and cervical incompetence are predisposing factors for persistent mating-induced endometritis.

Reduction of myometrial activity and endometrial deterioration are correlated with age and parity. Therefore, older pluriparous mares suffer more often than younger mares from mating-induced endometritis. The often very tight, nonrelaxing cervix seen in older mares also can be associated with postbreeding endometritis, however. A mare that from past experience or history is known to produce a large amount of luminal fluid (to a depth of several centimeters) after mating should be managed using the following protocol that optimizes the condition of the mare before breeding:

Hygiene. Good hygiene at foaling is essential, and all mares should be thoroughly examined post partum for the presence of traumatic injury that might compromise the physical barriers to uterine contamination. Gynecologic examinations, particularly of the vagina, should be performed as aseptically as possible. Thorough digital examination of the cervix can identify fibrosis, lacerations, or adhesions that may need treatment before breeding. Because air in the vagina can cause irritation of the mucosa, it should be expelled by applying downward pressure with the hand through the rectal wall. Attention can be paid to hygiene at mating by using a tail bandage and washing the mare's vulva and perineal area with clean water (ideally from a spray nozzle, which avoids the need for buckets).

Correct timing of breeding.   Breeding should occur at the optimal time, and the number of breedings should be restricted to one. Thus, these mares will need very close monitoring of the estrous period by rectal palpation and ultrasonography. The use of ovulation induction agents is strongly recommended in such mares in an attempt to ensure they are bred only once. Prediction of ovulation is made easier by not breeding these mares too early in the year, before they have begun to cycle regularly. If feasible, the use of artificial insemination with fresh semen can be helpful to reduce (but not eliminate) the inevitable postbreeding endometritis.

Ultrasound evaluation of the uterus.   The uterus should be evaluated by ultrasound examination to detect intraluminal fluid, in addition to conventional endometrial cytologic and bacteriologic techniques, before mating. Even if cytologic and bacteriologic studies have yielded negative results before breeding, mares susceptible to postbreeding endometritis usually accumulate fluid in the uterine lumen for more than 12 hours after breeding.

Correction of any external conformational defects. The mare should be evaluated for any conformational defects, and such defects should be corrected.

Tailoring of the treatment regime to the individual mare.   No standard approach can be given. Susceptibility to endometritis is not an absolute state: failure of the defense mechanisms need be only of the degree necessary to slow the process of clearance past a critical point. The treatment adopted should be based on history and clinical findings, including those on ultrasonographic evaluation of the uterus before and after breeding.

Before Breeding

Recent work has shown that among mares with uterine fluid accumulation before mating, although the fluid initially is sterile and free of neutrophils, the pregnancy rate is reduced when no treatment is performed.[30,47] If greater than a 0.5-cm depth of fluid is detected, 20 IU oxytocin should be given as an intravenous bolus. The next ultrasound examination should confirm that the fluid has been cleared. If intraluminal fluid is still visible, the dose of oxytocin is repeated, possibly with digital dilation of the cervix. If more than 2 cm of fluid is present, the uterus is lavaged as described earlier. In general, instillation of antibiotics before breeding should be avoided owing to possible irritant and/or spermicidal action.

A single breeding must be arranged 1 or 2 (or even 3) days before the anticipated time of ovulation (if natural covering or fresh semen is to be used). It is my experience that most stallion spermatozoa are viable at least 48 to 72 hours after mating, as supported by the findings of Umphenour et al.[63] In any case, records based on previ-

ous early pregnancy examinations will soon indicate if the semen from a particular stallion is not viable after 48 hours. This early mating allows more time for drainage of fluid via an open estrous cervix and also utilizes the natural resistance of the tract to inflammation during estrus. It allows sufficient time to flush the uterus more than once before ovulation if necessary. Although uterine lavage is possible after ovulation, it is more complicated because the cervix starts closing. Moreover, the resistance of the tract is reduced and the uterotonic effect of oxytocin is reduced as a result of the increasing amount of circulating progesterone.[64]

Treatment for endometritis is ideally performed before ovulation. Progesterone concentrations rise rapidly in the mare, and any postovulation treatment carries an increased risk of uterine contamination. In addition, uterine fluid is less likely to drain if the cervix is beginning to close.

After Breeding

Doses of 20 IU of oxytocin are given by the intramuscular route every 4 to 6 hours after breeding by the stud farm personnel. Ultrasound examination of the uterus the day after mating is performed to assess the amount and echogenicity of any intrauterine fluid. If more than 2.0 cm of fluid is present in the uterine lumen, lavage of the uterus with warmed, buffered, sterile saline using a uterine flushing catheter is performed. During lavage, 20 IU of oxytocin is given by the intravenous route. In instances in which the cervix has failed to relax adequately, digital dilation of the cervix, with scrupulous attention to cleanliness, is indicated.

This is followed by infusion of a small volume (25 ml) of water-soluble, broad-spectrum antibiotics such as a combination of neomycin sulfate (1 g), polymyxin B (40,000 IU), furaltadone (600 mg) (Utrin Wash, Vetoquinol UK), and crystalline benzylpenicillin (5 MU) instilled through the cervix into the uterus via a sterile irrigation catheter. Instillation of a low volume of antibiotic solution (the minimum effective volume) seems logical because these mares have a drainage problem. Older, pluriparous mares may need larger volumes (up to 50 ml). It is my experience that with larger volumes (greater than 100 ml), some of the solution is lost via cervical reflux. It is vital that the antibiotic used not irritate the endometrium or predispose to overgrowth with fungal organisms. Neither of these problems has been observed using the antibiotic combination described here.

Further doses of 20 IU of oxytocin are given by the intramuscular route every 4 to 6 hours by the stud farm personnel. In mares with lymphatic stasis, the slower release of carbetocin (0.14 mg IM) or prostaglandin (cloprostenol 250 μg IM) may be useful in addition to oxytocin. The carbetocin or cloprostenol should be given some 6 to 8 hours after the first oxytocin injection.

The mare is re-examined the following day, and oxytocin treatment is repeated if fluid is still present. Only rarely will a second infusion of antibiotics or lavage procedure be performed, owing to the risk of uterine contamination. The day after mating is a crucial time to assess all mares, but too many clinicians fail to perform postbreeding evaluation of the uterus. Another important concept is to treat in relation to time of breeding and not wait for ovulation.

CONCLUSIONS

A problem mare, once inseminated or mated, should be checked not only for ovulation but also for fluid accumulation in the uterus, one of the most reliable clinical signs of susceptibility to postbreeding endometritis. If a mare is recognized as being susceptible to persistent mating-induced endometritis, intensive postbreeding monitoring and, eventually, treatment will be necessary to improve the chances of conception. The combination of early postbreeding lavage supported by oxytocin and the infusion of broad-spectrum antibiotics has proved to be an effective management strategy for mares susceptible to mating-induced endometritis.

Some questions remain unanswered: Hearn[65] voiced the concern that the early embryonic or fetal loss rate in susceptible mares with endometritis who receive aggressive postmating therapy will be much higher despite the temporary improvement in uterine environment. Undoubtedly the live foal rate in the mares that receive such therapy after breeding is less than in young, genitally healthy mares. Often, however, susceptible mares are old, and uterine biopsy results, when available, frequently confirm degenerative changes within the endometrium. Consequently, live foal rates can be expected to be lower in these mares in any case.

This consideration does not constitute a reason to avoid postmating treatment, however. Of course the practitioner should optimize the chances for conception by the foregoing methods, but the susceptible mare still requires treatment after mating.

In my daily routine, I assume that most multiparous mares are at risk for either clinical or subclinical endometritis after insemination, be it natural or artificial. Routine postmating treatment of mares believed to be at risk for the development of persistent acute endometritis is dependent on balancing cost and time against benefits to the breeder. This view also is held by Australian colleagues (e.g., DR Pascoe, personal communication, 2005) who claim increased pregnancy rates and subsequent foaling rates through adoption of a routine postmating treatment.[60] The results of published clinical studies[30,39,40,47,60] and field experience with large numbers of mares over many breeding seasons have demonstrated the effectiveness of a single postmating treatment to combat endometritis. This has certainly been the case in the mares with which I have been involved.

Against this demonstrable improvement in pregnancy rate, a point of concern is whether, apart from economic considerations, routine treatment of *all* mares after mating is indicated. Certainly, management standards must not fall. Postmating treatment should not be seen as a means of getting away with poor management practices.

No bacterial resistance problems or increase in fungal endometritis must be apparent with the intrauterine antibiotics used. At the first International Symposium on Equine Endometritis, Zent[58] reported that, of 4000 broodmares under the care of members of his Kentucky veterinary practice, all those except maiden mares were routinely given at least one postmating intrauterine antibiotic infusion. He believed that this treatment had improved pregnancy rates without the development of a resistance problem or an increased incidence of fungal endometritis.

At what point the susceptible mare should be bred and when she should be treated and either short-cycled or bred at the next natural estrus are difficult decisions to be dogmatic about. This must be a matter of clinical experience based on the history and findings on clinical and laboratory examinations.

PYOMETRA

Pyometra is the accumulation of large quantities of inflammatory exudate in the uterus, causing its distention.[66] It must be distinguished from the smaller, and intermittent, accumulations of fluid that can be detected by ultrasonography in acute endometritis. Pyometra occurs because of interference with natural drainage of fluid from the uterus, which may be due to the presence of cervical adhesions or an abnormally constricted, tortuous, or irregular cervical canal. In some cases, the fluid accumulates in the absence of cervical lesions, presumably because of an impaired ability to eliminate the exudate. Other predisposing factors include chronic infection with *P. aeruginosa* or fungi.

When the endometrium is severely damaged, the extensive loss of surface epithelium, severe endometrial fibrosis, and glandular atrophy result in a prolonged luteal phase, presumably secondary to interference with the synthesis or release of $PGF_{2\alpha}$. (In mild endometritis, by contrast, accumulation of small amounts of intraluminal uterine fluid is more likely to cause premature release of $PGF_{2\alpha}$ and luteolysis.)

Some clinicians restrict the term *pyometra* to describe cases in which, in addition to the accumulation of exudate within the uterine lumen, the corpus luteum persists beyond its normal lifespan. Some mares with pyometra have normal, regular cyclical ovarian activity. Persistence of the corpus luteum probably is due to the failure of synthesis and/or release of prostaglandins from the uterus. Mares that have prolonged luteal activity demonstrate the greatest endometrial damage.

The mare with pyometra seldom shows overt signs of systemic disease even when up to 60 L of exudate is present in the uterine lumen. Very occasional findings include weight loss, depression, and anorexia. Pyometra in mares has been classified as either open or closed.[67] In closed pyometra, the fluid accumulates because of a closed cervix. In open pyometra, the cervix remains open, but purulent material accumulates because of impaired uterine clearance. A vulval discharge often is observed in open pyometra, especially at estrus, which may vary in consistency, ranging from watery to cream-like. Although the culture of endometrial swabs sometimes can result in the growth of mixed organisms, or no bacterial growth at all, in most instances the organism isolated is *S. zooepidemicus*.

The diagnosis of pyometra is based on rectal palpation, ultrasonographic examination of an enlarged, fluid-filled uterus (Figure 14-8), and analysis of the uterine fluid.

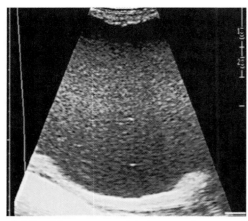

Figure 14-8 Ultrasonographic image of uterus of a mare with pyometra.

The possibility of pregnancy must be eliminated, together with rare conditions such as mucometra and pneumouterus.

Because of the absence of clinical signs of systemic illness, the pyometra often becomes a chronic condition before treatment is sought. In such cases, the prognosis is poor because of severe endometrial damage, so that the uterus is unlikely to be able to sustain a normal pregnancy.

The aim of treating pyometra is to expel the purulent material from the uterus. In the absence of systemic illness or an unsightly vulvar discharge, treatment of chronic pyometra may not be indicated, although some mares can show signs of discomfort during exercise.

In many cases, significant improvement can be obtained by repeated large-volume lavage with several liters of warm saline delivered through a wide-bore tube such as a nasogastric tube. Initially, $PGF_{2\alpha}$ can be used to induce luteolysis of the corpus luteum if present, which should allow the cervix to relax sufficiently for digital exploration for the presence of any adhesions. Estradiol or PGE_2 also may help relax the cervix. The broad-spectrum combination of antibiotics (Utrin Wash, Vetoquinol UK) should be infused after repeated large-volume lavage and oxytocin to achieve drainage of exudate, and an endometrial biopsy is useful in assessing the degree of endometrial damage. Monitoring the uterus by a combination of rectal palpation and ultrasound examination provides information on the response to treatment. Even if the pyometra is successfully treated, the mare must be considered susceptible to this condition if she is to be bred and must be managed accordingly.

In nonresponsive cases, hysterectomy can be performed after aspiration of the exudate from the uterus, although great care must taken to prevent contamination of the peritoneal cavity.

References

1. Troedsson MHT, Loset K, Alghamdi AM et al: Interaction between equine semen and the endometrium: the inflammatory response to semen. Anim Reprod Sci 2001; 68:273.
2. Katila T: Sperm-uterine interactions: a review. Anim Reprod Sci 2001; 68:267.
3. Kotilainen T, Huhtinen M, Katila T: Sperm-induced leukocytosis in the equine uterus. Theriogenology 1994; 41:629.
4. Katila T: Interactions of the uterus and semen. Pferdeheilkunde 1997; 13:508.
5. Nikolakopoulos E, Watson ED: Effect of infusion volume and sperm numbers on persistence of uterine inflammation in mares. Equine Vet J 2000; 32:164.
6. Pycock JF, Allen WE: Pre-chemotactic and chemotactic properties of uterine fluid from mares with experimentally induced bacterial endometritis. Vet Rec 1988; 123:193.
7. Pycock JF, Allen WE: Inflammatory components in uterine fluid from mares with experimentally induced bacterial endometritis. Equine Vet J 1990; 22:422.
8. Parlevliet JM, Tremoleda JM, Cheng FP et al: Influence of semen, extender and seminal plasma on the defence mechanism of the mare's uterus (abstract). Pferdeheilkunde 1997; 13:540.
9. Troedsson MHT, Franklin RK, Crabo BG: Suppression of PMN-chemotaxis by different molecular weight fractions of seminal plasma. Pferdeheilkunde 1999; 115:568.
10. Troedsson MHT, Lee CS, Franklin R, Crabo BG: Post-breeding uterine inflammation: the role of seminal plasma. J Reprod Fertil Suppl 2000; 56:341.
11. Portus BJ, Reilas T, Katila T: Effect of seminal plasma on uterine inflammation, contractility and pregnancy rates in mares. Equine Vet J 2005; 37:515.
12. Katila T: Onset and duration of uterine inflammatory response of mares after insemination with fresh semen. Biol Reprod Mono 1995; 1:515.
13. Troedsson MHT, Scott MA, Liu IKM: Comparative treatment of mares susceptible to chronic uterine infection. Am J Vet Res 1995; 56:468.
14. Farrelly BY, Mullaney PE: Cervical and uterine infections in thoroughbred mares. Irish Vet J 1964; 18:210.
15. Knudsen O: Partial dilatation of the uterus as a cause of sterility in the mare. Cornell Vet 1964; 54:423.
16. Hughes JP, Loy RG: Investigations on the effect of intrauterine inoculations of Streptococcus zooepidemicus in the mare. Proceedings of the 15th Annual Convention of the American Association of Equine Practitioners, p 289, 1969.
17. Pycock JF, Paccamonti D, Jonker H et al: Can mares be classified as resistant or susceptible to recurrent endometritis? Pferdeheilkunde 1997; 13:431.
18. Allen WE, Pycock JF: Current views on the pathogenesis of bacterial endometritis in mares with lowered resistance to endometritis. Vet Rec 1989; 125:298.
19. Evans MJ, Hamer JM, Gason LM et al: Clearance of bacteria and non antigenic markers following intrauterine inoculation into maiden mares: effect of steroid hormone environment. Theriogenology 1986; 26:37.
20. Troedsson MHT, Liu IKM: Uterine clearance of non-antigenic markers (51-Cr) in response to a bacterial challenge in mares potentially susceptible and resistant to chronic uterine infections. J Reprod Fertil Suppl 1991; 44:283.
21. Troedsson MHT, Liu IKM, Ing M: Multiple site electromyography recordings of uterine activity following an intrauterine bacterial challenge in mares susceptible and resistant to chronic uterine infection. J Reprod Fertil 1993; 99:307.
22. LeBlanc MM, Neuwirth L, Mauragis D et al: Oxytocin enhances clearance of radiocolloid from the uterine lumen of reproductively normal mares and mares susceptible to endometritis. Equine Vet J 1994; 26:279.
23. Liu IKM, Rakestraw P, Coit C et al: An in vitro investigation of the mechanism of neuromuscular regulation in myometrial contractility (abstract). Pferdeheilkunde 1997; 13:557.

24. Kenney RM: Cyclic and pathologic changes of the mare endometrium as detected by biopsy, with a note on early embryonic death. J Am Vet Med Assoc 1978; 172:24.

25. LeBlanc MM, Johnson RD, Calderwood Mays MB et al: Lymphatic clearance of india ink in reproductively normal mares and mares susceptible to endometritis. Biol Reprod Mono 1995; 1:501.

26. LeBlanc MM, Neuwirth L, Jones L et al: Differences in uterine position of reproductively normal mares and those with delayed uterine clearance detected by scintigraphy. Theriogenology 1998; 50:49.

27. Ricketts SW, Alonso S: The effect of age and parity on the development of equine chronic endometrial disease. Equine Vet J 1991; 23:189.

28. Pycock JF: Cervical function and uterine fluid accumulation in mares. Proceedings of JP Hughes International Workshop on Equine Endometritis, summarised by W.R. Allen. Equine Vet J 1993; 25:191.

29. LeBlanc MM: Persistent mating induced endometritis in the mare: pathogenesis, diagnosis and treatment. In Ball BA (ed): Recent Advances in Equine Reproduction. Ithaca, NY, International Veterinary Information Service, 2003.

30. Pycock JF, Newcombe JR: The relationship between intraluminal uterine fluid, endometritis and pregnancy rate in the mare. Equine Pract 1996a; 18:19.

31. Rasch K, Schoon HA, Sieme K et al: Histomorphological endometrial status and influence of oxytocin on the uterine drainage and pregnancy rate in mares. Equine Vet J 1996; 28:455.

32. Ginther OJ, Pierson RA: Ultrasonic anatomy and pathology of the equine uterus. Theriogenology 1984; 21:505.

33. Adams GP, Kastelic JP, Bergfelt DR et al: Effect of uterine inflammation and ultrasonically detected uterine pathology on fertility in the mare. J Reprod Fertil Suppl 1987; 35:445.

34. Allen WE, Pycock JF: Cyclical accumulation of uterine fluid in mares with lowered resistance to endometritis. Vet Rec 1988; 122 :489.

35. McKinnon AO, Voss JL, Squires EL et al: Diagnostic ultrasonography. In McKinnon AO, Voss JL (eds): Equine Reproduction. Philadelphia, Lea & Febiger, pp 266-302, 1993.

36. Brinsko SP, Rigby SL, Varner DD, Blanchard TL: A practical method for recognizing mares susceptible to post-breeding endometritis. Proceedings of the 49th Annual Convention of the American Association of Equine Practitioners, pp 363-365, 2003.

37. Newcombe JR: The effect of the incidence and depth of intrauterine fluid in early dioestrus on pregnancy rates in mares (abstract). Pferdeheilkunde 1997; 13:545.

38. Brinsko SP, Varner DD, Blanchard TL: The effect of uterine lavage performed four hours postinsemination on pregnancy rates in mares. Theriogenology 1991; 35:1111.

39. Pycock JF: A new approach to treatment of endometritis. Equine Vet Educ 1994a; 6:36.

40. Pycock JF: Assessment of oxytocin and intrauterine antibiotics on intrauterine fluid and pregnancy rates in the mare. Proceedings of the 40th Annual Convention of the American Association of Equine Practitioners, pp 19-20, 1994b.

41. Troedsson MHT: Therapeutic considerations for mating-induced endometritis. Pferdeheilkunde 1997; 13:516.

42. Bader H: An investigation of sperm migration into the oviducts of the mare. J Reprod Fertil Suppl 1982; 32:59.

43. Brinsko SP, Varner DD, Blanchard TL, Meyers SA: The effect of postbreeding uterine lavage on pregnancy rates in mares. Theriogenology 1990; 33:465.

44. Knutti B, Pycock JF, van der Weijden GC, Kupfer U: The influence of early postbreeding uterine lavage on pregnancy rates in mares with intrauterine fluid accumulations after breeding. Equine Vet Educ 2000; 12:267.

45. Allen WE: Investigations into the use of oxytocin for promoting uterine drainage in mares susceptible to endometritis. Vet Rec 1991; 128:593.

46. LeBlanc MM: Oxytocin—the new wonder drug for treatment of endometritis? Equine Vet Educ 194; 6:39.

47. Pycock JF, Newcombe JR: Assessment of the effect of three treatments to remove intrauterine fluid on pregnancy rate in the mare. Vet Rec 1996b; 138:320.

48. Watson ED: Release of immunoreactive arachidonate metabolites by equine endometrium in vitro. Am J Vet Res 1989; 50:1207.

49. Paccamonti DL, Pycock JF, Taverne MAM et al: PGFM response to exogenous oxytocin and determination of the half-life of oxytocin in nonpregnant mares. Equine Vet J 1999; 31:285.

50. Cadario ME, Thatcher MJD, LeBlanc MM: Relationship between prostaglandin and uterine clearance of radiocolloid in the mare. Biol Reprod Mono 1995; 1:495.

51. Paccamonti DL, Gutjahr S, Pycock JF et al: Does the effect of oxytocin on intrauterine pressure vary with dose or day of treatment (abstract). Pferedeheilkunde 1997; 13:553.

52. LeBlanc MM: Effects of oxytocin, prostaglandin and phenylbutazone on uterine clearance of radiocolloid. Pferdeheilkunde 1997; 13:483.

53. Behrendt CY, Adams MH, Daniel KS, McDowell KJ: Oxytocin expression by equine endometrium. Biol Reprod 1997; 56(Suppl 1):206.

54. Watson ED, Bjorksten TS, Buckingham J, Nikolakopoulos E: Immunolocalisation of oxytocin in the uterus of the mare. J Reprod Fertil Abstract Series 1997; 20:31.

55. Campbell MLH, England GCW: A comparison of the ecbolic efficacy of intravenous and intrauterine oxytocin treatments (abstract). Theriogenology 2002; 58:473.

56. Combs GB, LeBlanc MM, Neuwirth L et al: Effects of prostaglandin $F_{2\alpha}$, cloprostenol and fenprostalene on uterine clearance of radiocolloid in the mare. Theriogenology 1996; 45:1449.

57. Troedsson MHT: Uterine response to semen deposition in the mare. Proc Soc Theriogenol 1995; 130:130-135.

58. Zent W: Post-ovulation intrauterine antibiotics. Proc. of J.P. Hughes International Workshop on Equine Endometritis, summarised by W.R. Allen. Equine Vet J 1993; 25:192.

59. Asbury AC: Uterine defence mechanisms in the mare: the use of intrauterine plasma in the management of endometritis. Theriogenology 1984; 21:387.

60. Pascoe DR: Effect of adding autologous plasma to an intrauterine antibiotic therapy after breeding on pregnancy rates in mares. Biol Reprod Mono 1995; 1:137.

61. Adams GP, Ginther OJ: Efficacy of intrauterine infusion of plasma for treatment of infertility and endometritis in mares. J Am Vet Med Assoc 1989; 194:372.

62. Troedsson MHT, Scott MA, Liu IKM: Pathogenesis and treatment of chronic uterine infection. Proceedings of the XXth Annual Convention of the American Association of Equine Practitioners, p 595, 1992.

63. Umphenour NW, Sprinkle TA, Murphy HQ: Natural service. In McKinnon AO, Voss JL (eds): Equine Reproduction, Philadelphia, Lea & Febiger, pp 798-808, 1993.

64. Gutjahr S, Paccamonti D, Pycock JF et al: Intrauterine pressure changes in response to oxytocin application in mares. Reprod Domest Anim Suppl 1998; 5:118.

65. Hearn P: The relationship of uterine inflammation to fertility. Proc Soc Theriogenol 1993; 139-147.

66. Hughes JP, Stabenfeldt GH, Kindahl H et al. Pyometra in the mare. J Reprod Fertil Suppl 1979; 27:321-329.

67. Hughes JP, Loy RG, Asbury AC et al: The occurrence of *Pseudomonas* in the reproductive tract of mares and its effect on fertility. Cornell Vet 1966; 56:595.

Suggested Reading

Hinrichs K: The role of endometrial swabs in the diagnosis (and pathogenesis?) of endometritis. Cornell Vet 1991; 81:233.

Kenney RM:The aetiology, diagnosis and classification of chronic degenerative endometritis (CDE) (endometriosis). Proceedings of J.P. Hughes International Workshop on Equine Endometritis summarised by W.R. Allen (abstract). Equine Vet J 1993; 25:186.

Knutti B, Pycock JF, Paccamonti D et al: The influence of early post-breeding uterine lavage on uterine fluid accumulation in the mare highly susceptible to acute endometritis (abstract). Pferdeheilkunde 1997; 13;545.

Ricketts SW: Histological and histopathological studies on the endometrium of the mare. Fellowship Thesis, Royal College of Veterinary Surgeons, London, 1978.

Ricketts SW, Mackintosh ME: Role of anaerobic bacteria in equine endometritis. J. Reprod Fertil Suppl 1987; 35:343.

CHAPTER 15

Uterine Therapy for Mares with Bacterial Infections

ROBERT C. CAUSEY

Infertility caused by bacterial uterine infections inflicts major losses on the equine industry. The expense of breeding, palpation, ultrasonography, board, mare transport, semen shipment, stallion collection fees, and many booking fees can never be recovered if a mare fails to conceive. In addition, the client does not have an item for sale in the future. Consequently, successful prevention and management of uterine infections in the broodmare is an essential part of equine reproductive practice.

The term *uterine infections* can apply to many conditions, but this chapter will focus on bacterial uterine infections causing infertility in the cycling mare. The culprit in these infections is probably persistent endometrial inflammation that prevents survival of the early conceptus.[1] The inflammation is most commonly caused by a mixture of semen, bacteria, extender, and debris introduced at breeding. In healthy mares such inflammation is a normal postbreeding phenomenon and often subsides within hours post breeding.[2] However, in some mares the inflammation is prolonged by the persistence of bacteria, and the mare may remain persistently infected on subsequent cycles. The embryo is unable to survive when it enters the uterus at day 6 (144 hours) post ovulation. These barren mares, so called "susceptible" mares, are believed to have defects in their defense against reproductive infections.[3,4] The aim of diagnosis and therapy for uterine infections is to identify and if necessary treat mares with compromised defenses before breeding and to aggressively manage endometrial inflammation post breeding.

PATHOGENESIS

Organisms

There is no "normal flora" in the uterus of the cycling mare. If culture technique is good, any organism isolated from the uterus is a potential cause of inflammation and infertility. Organisms most often isolated from mares with uterine infection include *Streptococcus zooepidemicus, Escherichia coli, Klebsiella pneumoniae, Pseudomonas aeruginosa,*[5] and very rarely the microaerophilic venereal pathogen *Taylorella equigenitalis.*[6] Anaerobic bacteria such as *Bacteroides fragilis* also appear to be significant causes of endometritis, especially in postpartum and foal heat mares.[7] Causative organisms are usually found in the caudal genital tract of the healthy mare, with numbers decreasing as one proceeds past the vaginovestibular sphincter into the vagina and uterus.[8] The clitoral sinus

is an important reservoir for these bacteria and for introducing them into the uterus during breeding or vaginal procedures.[8] This is especially true of *T. equigenitalis* and anaerobic bacteria.[7,9] Outbreaks of *T. equigenitalis* and early recognition of infection are of great concern to the equine industry and animal health regulators.[9-11] *T. equigenitalis* is a reportable disease in the Northern Hemisphere and a notifiable disease in the United Kingdom (UK) and most other countries.

Types of Infection

Bacterial uterine infections usually appear as either venereal, chronic, or postbreeding infections.[12] Venereal infections are caused by a stallion spreading a reproductive pathogen between mares. The classic example of such a pathogen is *T. equigenitalis,*[6] the causative agent of contagious equine metritis (CEM). *Klebsiella*[13] and *Pseudomonas*[14] are also capable of inducing venereal infections. Chronic infections are probably caused by a combination of potentially virulent bacteria and weakened reproductive defenses, especially in mares predisposed to self-contamination.[12] These may appear as persistent infections with gram-negative bacteria in older mares with poor perineal conformation and are frequently difficult to treat. Postbreeding infections occur following deposition of semen in the uterus, following either natural mating or artificial insemination. Isolated organisms are commensals of the mare, differentiating the condition from a venereal infection. Postbreeding infections are usually transient, with rapid expulsion of semen and bacterial contaminants within hours of breeding,[2,15] but in susceptible mares they can become persistent due to failure of the uterus to expel fluid.[16] Persistent postbreeding infections are a major cause of infertility, with *S. zooepidemicus* being a commonly isolated organism.[17]

Uterine Defense in Health and Disease

When discussing therapy and prevention of bacterial uterine infections it is valuable to understand how reproductive defenses against infection function in health and disease. Reproductive defenses include physical barriers to contamination and uterine defenses.

The physical barriers of the reproductive tract are the first line of defense against infection. These barriers include the vulva, vaginovestibular sphincter, and cervix. They prevent feces, air, and environmental bacteria from entering the reproductive tract. Feces tends to enter because of the proximity of the anus; air tends to enter as a result of negative pressure in the cranial vagina. In young mares the vulva lies mostly below the level of the pelvic brim. This orientation allows fecal material to fall past without adhering and requires upward movement to penetrate the vestibule, providing an effective barrier to feces and air. In older mares the perineal conformation may shift, pulling the vulva onto the pelvic floor.[18] Feces falls directly onto the vulva, predisposing the mare to fecal contamination and facilitating the entry of air.

The vaginovestibular sphincter forms a second physical barrier. Parting of the vulval lips should not elicit a "sucking sound," because the vaginovestibular sphincter prevents entry of air into the cranial vagina. Caslick's procedure allows one to increase the effectiveness of the vulval seal or to compensate for an ineffective vaginovestibular sphincter.[19]

The cervix is the final physical barrier to infection of the uterus. It is a dynamic seal, opening in estrus and closing in diestrus and pregnancy. When open it allows semen into and fluid out of the uterus; when closed it forms a seal against the inward passage of microorganisms or the outward passage of the embryo.[20] The more tenacious cervical mucus of diestrus and pregnancy, in comparison with estrus, probably improves the cervical seal. Mares can remain fertile with anatomic imperfections in either the vulva or vaginovestibular sphincter, but less so the cervix. Damage to the cervix, such as from dystocia, can impair the ability of a mare to conceive or carry a foal, especially in cases of complete cervical lacerations. However, some mares with incomplete cervical lacerations may successfully carry foals to term. If the cervical seal is broken, the mare becomes vulnerable to inflammation by ascending organisms or air. If the cervical lumen is blocked by an adhesion or failure to dilate, pyometra may result from the inability to drain fluid. Surgical repair is an option in mares with cervical lacerations.[21]

An array of uterine defenses protects the uterus when the physical barriers to infection are breached. Physical barriers are always breached during breeding, when either the stallion ejaculates forcefully into the uterus or the artificial inseminator deliberately penetrates the cervix to deposit semen in the uterine body or even the uterine horns. Other intrauterine procedures, including culture, cytology, biopsy, endoscopy, lavage, infusion, embryo transfer, etc., are breaches of the physical barriers and may induce inflammation and even infection.[8] Researchers have experimentally breached the physical barriers of mares with infusions of bacteria, irritants, or semen to determine how uterine defenses fight infection.

From these studies it is clear that the young, healthy mare is highly resistant to infection and quickly eliminates irritants from the uterus; the uterus of a healthy estrous mare can eliminate experimental infection with good subsequent fertility.[3,4] The sequence of events appears to be as follows: immediately following introduction of bacteria there is an acute uterine response, peaking at about 6 hours, in which plasma proteins and neutrophils move into the uterine lumen. Uterine contractions propel any inflammatory fluid retrograde through the cervix, and after about 12 to 24 hours uterine cultures are usually negative.[15] During the acute response, especially within the first 6 hours following inoculation,

serum complement and antibody facilitate the phagocytosis of bacteria by neutrophils.[22] Meanwhile, uterine contractions facilitate removal of fluid through the cervix, helping to clear the uterus of debris.[16] The postbreeding response of mares to spermatozoa is identical.[2,23] In both situations the rapid, aggressive response observed would be necessary to eliminate exponentially growing bacteria. However, in some mares, although bacterial numbers decline during the acute uterine response, they rebound 12 to 24 hours later, and a more persistent inflammation develops.[15] Thus a failure to eliminate all remaining bacteria allows infection to persist.

Failure to eliminate uterine fluid by uterine contraction appears to be related to persistent uterine infections.[24,25] It appears that a defect in the myometrium of susceptible mares is responsible for this failure to expel fluid,[16,26] although hypersecretion may contribute to fluid accumulation.[27] If fluid accumulates in the uterus, hypothesized uterine defenses may be disrupted.[28] Inflammatory fluid that is retained in the uterus appears to lose its ability to support phagocytosis.[29] Furthermore, it has been known since the 1920s that in free fluid, neutrophils and bacteria will stratify to different levels of suspension, allowing bacteria an opportunity to escape.[30] Lymphatic drainage has been proposed to play an important role in uterine clearance[31] but is disrupted when fluid accumulates in the uterine lumen. Similarly, the cleansing of the uterine surface by a mucus blanket propelled by cilia[32] would be rendered ineffective in the presence of a large volume of free fluid. Any accumulations of uterine fluid cause major disruptions to proposed uterine defenses, whether the uterine defense be phagocytosis, lymphatic drainage, or mucociliary clearance.

The stage of the reproductive cycle greatly influences uterine defenses. During estrus the ability to clear infection is greater than in diestrus.[33] This is probably due to the open cervix,[20] expulsive myometrial contractions,[34,35] more active phagocytosis,[36-38] and by more frequent posturing to urinate. During diestrus the ability to clear infection is significantly reduced. Mares maintained on high progesterone often establish infection.[39] Uterine contamination during diestrus is usually less than in estrus due to the tight cervix, thick cervical mucus, sexual refusal, and less iatrogenic introduction. Because mares may develop large follicles during diestrus, artificial insemination of mares with large follicles, but no other signs of heat, should be avoided.

Microbial Pathogenesis

Although many uterine infections arise from defects in the mare's uterine defenses, bacteria themselves play significant roles in causing disease. The pathogenesis of bacteria during uterine infections in horses have not been well studied. In the 1920s, workers in Kentucky first noted that exudates in streptococcal mare uterine infections are watery, whereas those in *Klebsiella* infections are tenacious,[13,40] providing an interesting insight into potential differences in pathogenesis of different bacteria. More recent studies in other species and in horses have provided more detail. Some bacteria tenaciously adhere to epithelial surfaces, preventing their physical removal. This is well known in colonization of the genitourinary tract in humans[41] and probably true in many persistent equine uterine infections. It appears that *S. zooepidemicus* has adhesive ability,[42-44] probably mediated in part by fibronectin binding[45] and the hyaluronic capsule.[46] Similarly, both pili and capsule on *K. pneumoniae* appear to mediate attachment to epithelial cells.[47] Furthermore, biochemically complex biofilms secreted by several genera of bacteria, especially *P. aeruginosa,* provide an adhesive matrix contributing to persistent, opportunistic infections with tenacious microcolonies.[48,49] Biofilms also provide inherent resistance to antibiotics and both cellular and humoral immune defenses.[50,51] The persistence of *T. equigenitalis* in the equine genital tract may also be due in part to secretion of extracellular material.[52,53]

Streptococci may disrupt uterine defense by promoting the inflow of uterine fluid. Superantigens,[54,55] streptokinases,[56-58] and other toxins released by streptococci may cause hyperirritation of the endometrium, contributing to hyperemia and the in-rush of fluid. Superantigens probably play a significant role in the pathogenesis of strangles, though their role in uterine infections is less clear.[59] If fluid can be eliminated, for example by saline lavage, then streptococci appear to become vulnerable to uterine defenses.[60]

Resistance to phagocytosis is an important property of many uterine pathogens, including *S. zooepidemicus*[46,61] and *K. pneumoniae.*[62] This is probably mediated with *S. zooepidemicus* by a combination of antigenic variation,[63] antiphagocytic M-like proteins,[64] the hyaluronic capsule,[46] and Fc receptors.[65,66] Furthermore, because Fc receptors on the streptococcal cell wall disrupt the complement cascade, they may provide opportunities for gram-negative bacteria to colonize the uterus in mixed infections.[67] Resistance of *K. pneumoniae* to phagocytosis is mediated in part by the polysaccharide capsule.[62]

DIAGNOSIS

The goal of diagnosis of uterine infections in mares is to accurately identify uterine infections when they occur and to identify susceptible mares requiring management. An accurate diagnosis of a uterine infection includes evidence of uterine inflammation and isolation of typical bacteria. A history of infertility and a tendency to accumulate uterine fluid, especially post breeding, is especially useful in identifying susceptible mares.

History

The classic history of a susceptible mare is one who has foaled successfully for several consecutive breeding seasons but now is consistently failing to conceive or carry a foal. These mares are usually in their teens when the condition becomes apparent. A common presenting complaint is that she has failed to conceive despite repeated breedings on multiple cycles to a fertile stallion.[17] A history of repeated bouts of uterine infections is an excellent predictor of susceptibility to infection.[68] To construct a useful reproductive history can be challenging because infertile mares tend to change hands frequently. Where possible, it is helpful to obtain from the owner a brief year-by-year account of the mare's production (i.e., In what years did she foal? Who was she bred to? In those years that she did not foal, had she been bred

and failed to carry the pregnancy or had the owners chosen to leave her open?) Did the mare have any previously diagnosed uterine infections? Identifying past years when the mare had dystocia or abortion is particularly important because it can indicate trauma to the cervix. This information can usually be obtained quickly over the phone or immediately before examining the mare.

Having obtained an overall picture of the mare's reproductive life, more detailed questions concerning the most recent season can be asked. On how many cycles has the mare been bred and roughly how many breedings per cycle? What is the quality of the stallion's semen, and what is the breeding method (i.e., live cover or artificial insemination with fresh, chilled, or frozen semen)? When was the first breeding of the year, and how was it determined that the mare was cycling? Commonly mares are bred during spring transition; the contamination of the uterus that results from wasted breedings associated with lack of ovulation may significantly retard the mare's fertility during subsequent cycles. Were cycles of normal length, or did she have short or long interestrous intervals, or was the mare short cycling? The inflammation of an infected/inflamed uterus can induce the release of prostaglandin, causing luteolysis and thus shortening the estrous cycle.[69] It is also useful to review management of the mare to determine how closely the mare was monitored. Was fluid detected in the uterus before or after breeding, and, if so, how was it managed? Was ovulation date determined? What were the results of uterine cultures, cytologic examinations, or other diagnostic work if they were performed? What previous treatment has the mare received, and what was the result? From these types of questions it will be possible to determine the nature, severity, and duration of the infertility, uncover management problems, and help identify uterine infection as a possible cause of infertility.

Physical Examination

Physical examination of the mare may provide clues to potential causes of infertility. A forward-tilted pelvis, poor perineal conformation, tendency to suck air into the vagina, and overall health of the mare can quickly be determined. A forward tilt to the pelvis may indicate impaired drainage of the reproductive tract or a tendency to pool urine in the cranial vagina. Although urine pooling is not usually associated with uterine infections, the sterile inflammation is sufficient to compromise fertility. Mares in poor condition may be more predisposed to infection overall and may tend to have poorer perineal conformation. Mares who have failed to shed their hair coat are probably not cycling,[70] and this may indicate contamination due to wasted breedings if presented for current infertility.

Palpation, Ultrasonography, and Scintigraphy

Transrectal palpation and ultrasonography of the reproductive tract and ovaries are powerful aids in diagnosing uterine infections and identifying susceptible mares, especially in the first 12 hours post breeding. Through ultrasonography one can quickly determine whether the mare is cycling or not, determine the stage of cycle, whether there is fluid in the uterus, the nature of the fluid, the number and size of endometrial cysts, confirm that the mare is not pregnant, and detect uterine inflammation.[71] Accumulation of fluid in the uterus is one of the cardinal signs of a mare susceptible to infection and may indicate an ongoing infection. In a field setting, mares predisposed to uterine infection tend to have ultrasonographically more fluid in the uterus than normal mares over the course of an estrous cycle.[24] Whereas normal mares will have little or no fluid in the uterus (a trace of fluid is common during estrus), susceptible mares may accumulate significant volumes of fluid in the uterus during estrus that distend the lumen. In the postbreeding period, susceptible mares will retain fluid in the uterus, whereas normal mares should have little or no uterine fluid 6 to 12 hours after breeding. Accumulations of uterine fluid during the ovulatory period are consistently associated with decreased pregnancy rates.[72,73]

Ultrasonographic examination of the uterus 24 hours post breeding is a valuable diagnostic procedure to diagnose and treat mares susceptible to uterine infections. Examination at 6 to 12 hours is even better[74] but may not always be possible. It is at this early postmating stage that the differences between healthy and susceptible mares are most apparent, and there is still time to institute effective therapy to evacuate the uterus.

Measurement of clearance of radiocolloid by scintigraphy is a powerful technique for diagnosing mares with a delay in uterine clearance, especially in a research setting,[25] but it is a technique currently unavailable to many practitioners. The technique involves intrauterine infusion of 10 mCi of technetium 99m-albumin colloid and monitoring rate of clearance using a large field-of-view gamma camera. Reproductively normal mares clear >50% of radiocolloid within 2 hours of infusion.

Through ultrasonography one can gain valuable insight into the nature of the uterine fluid during a uterine infection.[71] If it is homogeneous and appears dark or black on the ultrasound screen, this usually indicates that the fluid is probably a mucoid transudate, suggesting that oxytocin alone may be appropriate for its evacuation. If it appears heterogeneous and flocculent, gray with white specks floating in it, this indicates cellular debris of an active infection; uterine lavage with saline may be necessary for most effective cleansing. Ultrasonography is particularly useful for detecting the presence of air in the uterus. The air-fluid interface is highly echogenic and appears as white sparkles within the uterus or vagina. Although a normal finding after intrauterine procedures, presence of air indicates that the mare's external barriers to contamination may be failing.

Determining the exact day of ovulation by ultrasonography is also important in management of uterine infections. The embryo enters the uterus on day 6 (~144 hours) post ovulation, allowing a short window of opportunity to cleanse the uterus. Monitoring day of ovulation allows one to institute intrauterine therapy with confidence before ovulation and up to about day 2 or at the most 3 post ovulation.[75] As the cervix tightens after ovulation, intrauterine therapy becomes less effective and more hazardous because evacuation of fluid by oxytocin is more difficult through the tighter cervix; the risk of introducing infection by intrauterine procedures increases as progesterone rises; the transient inflammation that intrauterine procedures induce may not subside before the embryo enters the uterus.

Vaginal Speculum Examination

Vaginal speculum examination is a useful way to detect mucoid or purulent exudates, urine accumulation, or inflammation of the reproductive tract.[76] The cervix of mares with uterine infections frequently appears "fire engine" red due to hyperemia. The anterior vagina may also be red and congested. Discharges from the uterus may pool on the floor of the anterior vagina and occasionally be seen dripping from the vaginal lips. Mucoid exudates resembling watery skim milk can sometimes be difficult to see on the floor of the vagina if the light is dim. More tenacious exudates may be seen clinging to the folds of the cervix. Urine pooling in the anterior vagina may sometimes appear as a thick yellow mucoid fluid, which can be mistaken for a suppurative exudate. Distinction between urine and suppurative exudate can be made by microscopic examination or by a reagent strip used to estimate blood urea nitrogen (Azostix).[77] Similarly, serum transudates may flow out of the uterus and pool on the vaginal floor, with a straw color very similar to urine. Distinction between serum and urine can also be made by using Azostix. Fluids may be obtained from the anterior vagina by tipping the speculum so fluid flows back into a specimen cup, or using an infusion pipette through the speculum attached to a syringe. Odor may also be helpful in determining the identity of the different fluids found in the mare's vagina but is subjective.

Uterine Culture and Cytologic Examination

Uterine culture can provide much useful information in the diagnosis of uterine infections if used in conjunction with uterine cytologic examination. Uterine culture will provide misleading results if uterine cytologic examination is neglected.[78] Uterine cytologic examination provides direct evidence of uterine inflammation, usually in the form of large numbers of neutrophils relative to endometrial cells, adding significance to the culture results. If the examination is negative for neutrophils, then isolation of a few organisms on culture indicates a contaminated swab and should be regarded as a negative culture. Typical contaminants may include alpha-hemolytic streptococci, *Enterobacter* spp, and *Staphylococcus epidermidis*.[75] If cytologic examination results are positive, isolation of bacteria is probably significant, especially if in high numbers and in pure culture. Organisms such as *S. zooepidemicus, E. coli, Klebsiella* sp, and *Pseudomonas* sp are typical pathogens of uterine infections. *Corynebacterium* spp, *Proteus* spp, and *Staphylococcus* spp should be considered pathogens only if inflammation is present, or if they are strongly implicated by history.[75] If uterine culture and cytologic examination results are negative, then it is unlikely the mare has a uterine infection. If negative culture is accompanied by positive cytologic examination results, then inflammation has been detected, but the cause remains undetermined; if one strongly suspects a bacterial cause, one may reculture the uterus. Occasionally, inflammation is associated with other irritants such as air or urine.

Where possible, antibiotic sensitivities should be obtained. Sensitivity to specific antibiotics is a useful way of labeling isolates and tracking them on subsequent cultures. Most uterine infections in horses can be treated using oxytocin alone, or in conjunction with saline lavage, and usually do not require intrauterine antibiotics. However, some infections will not respond to oxytocin or saline. If the same organism is recovered on successive estrous cycles, despite oxytocin or saline therapy, antibiotics are probably indicated. Antibiotic sensitivities would be helpful both to confirm reisolation of the same organism and to select an appropriate antibiotic. Typical antibiotics used to treat uterine infections and to request in sensitivities include penicillin, ampicillin, amoxicillin, ticarcillin, neomycin, gentamicin, amikacin, kanamycin, polymyxin, ceftiofur, etc. Unfortunately, in vitro sensitivity may not always lead to in vivo treatment success,[75] perhaps a result of biofilm production preventing antibiotic penetration of bacterial micro-colonies.[50]

We know too little about the role of anaerobes in uterine infections. *B. fragilis* is the most common anaerobe isolated from the mare. It is resistant to most penicillins or aminoglycosides but sensitive to nitrofurantoin or metronidazole.[7] In situations of persistent inflammation that yield no aerobic pathogens, or in postpartum, foal heat, or traumatized uteri, anaerobic culture is probably a valuable adjunct to diagnosis. In the midst of heavy growth of facultative anaerobes, metronidazole disks on culture plates may help to identify obligate anaerobes such as *B. fragilis* by growth inhibition.[7]

Where venereal transmission of pathogens is of concern, negative cultures of *K. pneumoniae, P. aeruginosa,* and *T. equigenitalis* should be obtained from both endometrium and clitoris of mares before natural service. Isolation of a few colonies of other bacteria should not prevent breeding, provided cytologic examination results are normal.[79]

A variety of methods of culture and cell collection are available. For routine endometrial cytologic examination and culture a guarded swab should be used to minimize contamination.[80] A more accurate flush technique is probably appropriate when searching for specific pathogens in persistent infections of barren mares and in cases where suspected false negatives have been obtained with guarded swabs.[81] Culture of the clitoral fossa may be accomplished with a standard nonguarded swab, although a narrow-tipped pediatric swab should be used for the clitoral median sinus.[9,79] For isolation of *T. equigenitalis* swabs should be placed in Amies charcoal transport medium and within 48 hours reach a laboratory approved for culture of the CEM organism.[9]

Uterine Biopsy

The author prefers to avoid uterine biopsy during uterine infection because the damaged epithelium at the biopsy site might provide a site for bacterial attachment or cause systemic exposure to bacterial pathogens. Nevertheless, it provides valuable information in the barren mare that may help rule in or out susceptibility to uterine infection.[82] Due to a persistently inflamed state of their uteri,

susceptible mares have more pronounced infiltration of the endometrium by mononuclear infiltration.[83,84] Such findings on a uterine biopsy specimen can alert one to suspect some defect in uterine defenses, either a barrier defect such as pneumovagina or a uterine defect such as a delay in uterine clearance. However, history of repeated bouts of infection is a better predictor of susceptibility.[68] Mares with fibrotic changes will also be detected by uterine biopsy.[83]

Endoscopy

Like biopsy, endoscopy should be avoided in the infected uterus because of the irritation it causes.[85] It may be a helpful adjunct to diagnosis of the susceptible mare when she is not infected, but it should be reserved for unusual or diagnostically challenging cases. (The author has employed endoscopy to perform endometrial biopsy in a miniature horse.) The endometrium of healthy mares is normally thrown into heavy longitudinal folds, which can be seen clearly on endoscopy. In subfertile mares the folding of the endometrium is greatly reduced. In addition, susceptible mares may have received potentially harmful intrauterine treatments that cause necrosis and scarring of the endometrium.[86] The aftereffects of these treatments, such as transluminal adhesions, may be detected on endoscopic examination.[87]

THERAPY

Management of uterine infections, referenced in detail in subsequent paragraphs, begins with maintaining hygiene of the breeding shed and the mare's genital tract. Mares should be free of uterine inflammation prior to breeding, and post-breeding inflammation should be aggressively controlled in susceptible mares. Most bacterial infections in the uterus respond during estrus to removal of fluid by oxytocin, often used in conjunction with saline lavage. If, despite this therapy, the uterus remains infected with the same organism at a subsequent estrus, antibiotics may be considered. Because of the effectiveness of oxytocin and saline lavage, the intrauterine infusion of potentially irritating antiseptics is now generally avoided. Plasma, once commonly used to treat uterine infections, is now rarely employed, though it has performed well in clinical trials. Therapy for uterine infections should be employed during estrus when uterine defenses are strongest, in some cases as early as 4 hours post breeding. If the mare is in diestrus when an infection is detected then she should be brought into estrus using a luteolytic dose of prostaglandin. Recently a mannose preparation has been proposed to prevent adhesion of bacteria to the uterus, but has yet to be tested in clinical trials.[44]

Hygiene

Minimizing contamination to the genital tract during breeding and vaginal and intrauterine procedures is an essential component of managing uterine infections in mares. Defects in the mare's perineal conformation should be corrected. Minimal contamination techniques for breeding have been described for artifical insemination and natural sevice.[88] Maintaining cleanliness of breeding equipment and the use of antibiotic-containing semen extender all help to reduce bacterial insult to the uterus during breeding. The stallion's penis should be washed and dried before semen collection or breeding; the mare's tail should be wrapped and pulled to the side, and the vulva should be washed clean and dried before insemination. Fecal soiling of the vestibule should be identified and removed. For invasive procedures, alternating washes of the vagina with povidone-iodine scrub applied with wet cotton with clean water rinses may be repeated until the labia are clean. The labia and clitoris are then blotted dry. Whenever possible, sterile lubrication, sterile sleeves, and sterile instruments should be used when entering the vagina or uterus. Adherence to cleanliness will both prevent introduction of bacteria and help win the client's confidence.

Oxytocin

First reported by Allen in 1991,[89] oxytocin has now become the mainstay for treating uterine infections in horses. It is safe, inexpensive, noninvasive, nonirritating, effective, and a powerful adjunct to host defenses.[73] In estrus, oxytocin induces uterine contractions, which expel fluid through the cervix.[90] The indication for oxytocin is the detection of free uterine fluid before or after breeding. Oxytocin may be given as early as 4 hours post insemination and dosed repeatedly over the next 24 to 48 hours to eliminate fluid from the uterus.[74,91] The average 1000-lb mare responds to a dose of 10 IU administered intravenously (IV) or 20 IU given intramuscularly (IM). The dose may be doubled if necessary, but further increases in dose may decrease uterine contractions.[92,93] Because of its 8-minute half-life, oxytocin can be given repeatedly, such as every 6 hours or as frequently as every hour.[91] There does not appear to be any evidence that oxytocin interferes with ovulation or corpus luteum function in the horse, though the same is not true of cloprostenol.[91,94] Oxytocin is most effective when given during estrus when the cervix is open. It is valuable to monitor response to oxytocin by ultrasonography and to adjust dosages and frequency of administration accordingly.[12]

Analogues of Prostaglandin

Prostaglandin $F_{2\alpha}$ ($PGF_{2\alpha}$) causes weaker uterine contractions than oxytocin and is less effective at evacuating the uterus.[95] However, if a uterine infection is discovered in diestrus, $PGF_{2\alpha}$ should be used (5 to10 mg IM in a 1000-lb mare) to bring the mare into estrus.

Cloprostenol, a prostaglandin analogue, produces weaker but more prolonged contractions than oxytocin.[96] It is particularly useful in mares with excessive uterine edema that are refractory to oxytocin. Although 250 mcg IM has been administered as frequently as once every 24 hours through the second day post ovulation without depressing fertility, circulating progesterone levels were transiently depressed; higher or more frequent doses should therefore probably be avoided.[91,94]

Uterine Lavage

Uterine lavage with sterile, isotonic saline is a powerful method to remove uterine contaminants, debris, old semen, and inflammatory exudate and to improve the phagocytic environment.[17,60] A large-bore catheter (30 French, 80 cm) with a 100-ml inflatable cuff (Bivona Inc, Gary, Ind.) is introduced into the uterus, and the large cuff is inflated with air or liquid to form a seal against the internal cervical os. A liter of saline is introduced into the uterus, agitated, and then uterine contents are siphoned off into a collection vessel. Samples from the first flush may be submitted for cytologic examination and culture. The procedure is repeated until the recovered fluid is almost clear, usually after three or four flushes. The mare is given 10 IU of oxytocin IV after the final flush to assist in removing all remaining fluid. Immediately turning the mare into a paddock and encouraging her to exercise also helps uterine drainage after lavage.[97]

In some mares postbreeding inflammatory reaction may be severe, especially following frozen semen inseminations. Aggressive removal of debris and inflammatory exudates early is often helpful in these mares to allow uterine inflammation to subside before arrival of the embryo. At 4 hours post breeding, uterine lavage may be performed safely in normal mares, without fear of preventing fertilization or disrupting sperm transport.[98] This may be repeated at 24 hours post breeding if fluid is still retained in the uterus. If the clinician suspects defective sperm transport, lavage at 4 hours may be premature. Because it is labor intensive, uterine lavage should be performed in conjunction with ultrasonography to monitor effectiveness and need for continued therapy.

Exercise

As previously mentioned, exercise is helpful in draining the uterus. Increased intraabdominal pressure associated with movement will help evacuate uterine contents. Allowing broodmares to stand idle in stalls, especially post breeding, should probably be avoided. Walking mares to a teasing stallion may also help uterine drainage through oxytocin release in response to the stallion's call[99] and through frequent posturing to urinate.

Intrauterine Antibiotics

Intrauterine antibiotics have been used extensively for the treatment and prevention of uterine infections.[97] However, with a better understanding of pathogenesis, the proven effectiveness of oxytocin and saline lavage, social concerns about overuse of antibiotics, and the risk of inducing fungal infections, antibiotic use is becoming less frequent in individually managed mares. However, they may be used extensively on farms where clinicians are required to breed large numbers of mares as efficiently as possible. As a first line or routine treatment for susceptible mares, the author prefers postbreeding oxytocin or saline lavage combined with oxytocin.[74] Intrauterine antibiotics are held in reserve for persistent venereal or chronic infections with specific pathogens that do not respond to oxytocin or saline. Recovery of the same isolate at estrus of different cycles, despite oxytocin or saline lavage, would confirm such an infection, and antibiotic choice can be based on sensitivity results to the reisolated organism. Intrauterine antibiotics would be included in a first-line treatment for venereal infection with *K. pneumoniae* capsule types 1, 2, and 5 or *T. equigenitalis*.[9] If cultures from different cycles yield different isolates, then antibiotics probably should be avoided; such cases of various organisms being isolated is common in susceptible mares but can lead to persistent fungal infections if antibiotics are used.[100]

The author's preference notwithstanding, reports of large clinical studies clearly demonstrate a therapeutic benefit from routine use of broad-spectrum intrauterine antibiotics to large numbers of mares.[73,101] Conception rates are equivalent in mares treated with single doses of oxytocin or broad-spectrum antibiotics but are highest in mares who receive both.[73] Some cases of fungal endometritis may be encountered with repeated (e.g., four or more) administration of antibiotics.[101] The purpose of such studies is not to recommend widespread use of antimicrobials to all mares, regardless of susceptibility to infection. Rather, it is to make clear that oxytocin and antibiotics have entirely different modes of action, often resulting in an additive benefit. Oxytocin alone will not successfully treat all cases of uterine infections; inclusion of antibiotics, with due concern to the added cost and risks, can sometimes succeed when oxytocin alone would fail.[73]

Practical recommendations for intrauterine antibiotic use are as follows: to treat active infections, intrauterine antibiotics should be administered daily for 3 days through estrus, and response to therapy ideally should be determined by uterine culture and sensitivity. Uterine cytology can provide a more rapid indication that treatment has been successful. Mares may be bred as soon as signs of inflammation have resolved. Ultrasonographic absence of fluid accumulation is also a useful indication of treatment success. If necessary, treated mares can be returned early to the next estrus for reculture and breeding by administration of 5 to 10 mg $PGF_{2\alpha}$ IM (in a 1000-lb mare) at day 5 or greater post ovulation. Some recommend infusing a volume of approximately 30 to 60 ml to prevent expulsion of the drug.[12] Others prefer to infuse a larger volume (e.g., 200 ml) to ensure thorough coverage of the entire endometrium.[75,97] A 250-ml volume was shown to maintain higher endometrial drug concentration than 60 ml in the case of ticarcillin.[102] If the lower volume is used, rectal massage is recommended to distribute the drug throughout the uterus.[103] Preparations must be soluble and nonirritating. Sterile aqueous diluents should be used such as water, saline, or lactated ringer's solution. The acidic aminoglycosides should be buffered with equal volume of 7.5% sodium bicarbonate to minimize irritation. Tetracyclines should be avoided due to irritation.[104] Table 15-1 is a compilation of recommendations for common intrauterine antibiotics.[12,75,97,101,103]

Systemic Antibiotics

Systemic antibiotics are rarely used to treat uterine infections in horses because minimum inhibitory concentration is more easily and cheaply achieved by intrauterine administration.[102,105,106] Nevertheless, systemic administration may be advantageous in certain circumstances.[97] For example, systemic administration can achieve minimum inhibitory concentrations in the endometrium without inducing contamination of the uterus and with less fluctuation of antibiotic levels. If one wished to maintain antibiotic levels through diestrus, then systemic administration would be preferable to intrauterine administration. Situations can arise where intrauterine delivery is not possible, and the systemic route the only alternative (such as temperament, recent urogenital surgery, trauma to the caudal genital tract, etc.). Systemically administered antibiotics include procaine penicillin G, gentamicin, amikacin, ampicillin, and trimethoprim sulpha, at usual systemic doses.[97] Systemic ciprofloxacin (2.5 g/day) and probenecid (1 g/day) have been reported to be effective against *Pseudomonas* infections.[12]

Intrauterine Antiseptics and Other Intrauterine Solutions

A variety of preparations have been infused into the uterus of mares in attempts to treat uterine infection.[104] The discomfort, inflammation, necrosis, and reproductive sterility that injudicious use of intrauterine antiseptics can induce should be a warning to all practitioners.

Table 15-1

Antibiotics for Treatment of Bacterial Uterine Infections in the Mare

Drug	Dose	Comments
Amikacin sulfate	2 g	Buffer with equal volume of 7.5% sodium bicarbonate.
Ampicillin	3 g	Use soluble preparation.
Carbenicillin	6 g	Some *Pseudomonas* are sensitive.
Ceftiofur	1 g	Broad spectrum, probably including the anaerobe *B. fragilis*.
Gentamicin sulfate	1-2 g	Gram-negative spectrum; buffer with equal volume of 7.5% sodium bicarbonate.
Kanamycin sulfate	1-2 g	Most *E. coli* are sensitive.
Neomycin	4 g	*E. coli* and some *Klebsiella* are sensitive.
Penicillin G	5 million units	Use sodium or potassium salts (soluble). Preferred for streptococci.
Polymyxin B	1 million units	Despite in vitro sensitivity of *Pseudomonas* and *Klebsiella* lack of clinical response is often seen.
Ticarcillin	6 g	Broad spectrum.
Ticarcillin/clavulanic acid	6 g/200 mg	Broad spectrum.

Mares can be highly variable in their responses to such products.

A 50-ml infusion of a 0.2% iodine solution induced acute hemorrhage, edema, necrosis, and chronic fibrosis in endometrial biopsy specimens in mares.[86] Chlorhexidine-gluconate (Hibiclens-ICI) caused vulval blistering, vaginal straining at concentrations as low as 0.5%, and at 0.25% caused acute endometrial inflammation and degenerative changes on uterine biopsy.[107] Mares have been reportedly rendered sterile by administration of dilute solutions of chlorhexidine-diacetate (Nolvasan, Fort Dodge Animal Health, Kansas City, Kan.), and its use as a uterine lavage is contraindicated.[75,97] However, vigorous scrubbing of the clitoris with a 4% chlorhexidine solution followed by packing with nitrofurazone ointment is currently recommended for treatment of *T. equigenitalis,* in conjunction with intrauterine administration of antibiotics (e.g., 5 to 10 million units of potassium penicillin for 5 to 7 days).[9,108]

In careful hands, some antiseptics may be administered safely. Dilute povidone-iodine solution (0.05% to 5 ml of 10% povidone-iodine in 1 L of saline) 4 hours post breeding had no adverse effects on pregnancy rates in reproductively sound mares when compared with saline and did not cause inflammation on endometrial biopsy. Because antimicrobial activity is maintained to concentrations as low as 0.01%, this lavage at 0.05% may have a role in management of some bacterial uterine infections.[98,103]

Because of its in vitro activity against *P. aeruginosa,* including alteration of antibiotic sensitivities, ethylenediaminetetraacetic acid (EDTA)-tris (250 ml at 38° C of 3.5mM EDTA, 0.05 M tris, pH 8) has been evaluated for safety as a uterine infusion in mares.[109] The inflammation induced was no greater than saline, suggesting that this solution may be a safe adjunct to uterine therapy, especially against antimicrobial-resistant pseudomonads. However, the author is not aware of any clinical studies documenting in vivo efficacy against *Pseudomonas.*

Plasma

Intrauterine administration of plasma has been used to strengthen host defenses of susceptible mares, but its use has diminished because of questions about its efficacy. The ability of uterine fluid to support the phagocytosis of *S. zooepidemicus* is greatly enhanced by the addition of serum or plasma. This is probably due to both complement and antibody acting via the classical pathway of complement activation to promote opsonization of streptococci.[110,111] This is consistent with the findings of others that streptococci require both a source of specific antibody and complement to be effectively phagocytized.[112] Clinical experiences with intrauterine infusions of plasma showed considerable early promise, with several barren mares being successfully bred.[113] Subsequent attempts to document efficacy by others were unsuccessful, but none replicated the original protocol.[60,114,115] Because there are several strains of streptococci, one cannot be sure that mares have specific antibodies to a given strain, a fact that may have influenced the results of some of these studies.[61] One study showed that intrauterine infusions of serum

hyperimmunized against a given strain of *S. zooepidemicus* were more effective than nonimmune serum in promoting intrauterine phagocytosis, confirming the importance of specific antistreptococcal antibody.[116]

A large clinical study found a significant therapeutic benefit to intrauterine plasma administration.[117] Significantly higher pregnancy rates were seen in mares treated with plasma and antibiotics than with antibiotics alone. In this study, plasma was collected into sterile blood collection bottles using citric acid/sodium citrate as anticoagulant, refrigerated for 12 hours at 6° C to allow settling of red cells, then poured off into 90-ml aliquots and stored at −20° C. Heparin is also an acceptable anticoagulant, although calcium binders should be avoided because of their disruption of the complement cascade.[111]

Whether or not to use intrauterine plasma is a decision for the individual practitioner. Because of improved conception rates, plasma appears to have some efficacy.[117] Whether this efficacy outweighs the effort required to collect, store, and administer plasma must be decided. In a given case there may be a role for intrauterine administration of plasma, especially if a hyperimmune source is available and applicable. A detailed account of how to collect and store equine plasma for intrauterine infusion is available.[97]

Other Treatments

A variety of other treatments have been proposed for uterine infections, but some await results of clinical efficacy. Because of its ability to disrupt bacterial adhesion, mannose and other sugars have been proposed as adjuncts to uterine therapy.[44] The approach is a logical one given the potential importance of adhesion in bacterial pathogenesis. A cell-free streptococcal filtrate has shown considerable promise in resolving uterine inflammation.[118] Cell wall preparations of *Mycobacterium phlei* may help to modulate postbreeding inflammation.[119] The protective effect of seminal plasma on spermatozoa in an inflamed uterus may become an important consideration in breeding with frozen semen.[120]

From the foregoing it is clear that new therapies for bacterial uterine infections in mares are continuing to be developed. Selecting the best treatments will keep researchers and practitioners occupied for many years to come.

References

1. Adams GP, Kastelic JP, Bergfelt DR et al: Effect of uterine inflammation and ultrasonically-detected uterine pathology on fertility in the mare. J Reprod Fertil Suppl 1987; 35:445-454.
2. Katila T: Onset and duration of uterine inflammatory response of mares after insemination with fresh semen. Biol Reprod Mono 1995; 1:515-517.
3. Peterson FB, McFeely RA, David JSE: Studies on the pathogenesis of endometritis in the mare. Proceedings of the 15th Annual Convention of the American Association of Equine Practitioners, pp 279-287, 1969.
4. Hughes JP, Loy RG: Investigations on the effect of intrauterine inoculations of *Streptococcus zooepidemicus* in the mare. Proceedings of the 15th Annual Convention of the

American Association of Equine Practitioners, pp 289-292, 1969.

5. Shin SJ, Lein DH, Aronson AL et al: The bacteriological culture of equine uterine contents, in-vitro sensitivity of organisms isolated and interpretation. J Reprod Fertil Suppl 1979; 27:307-315.
6. Timoney PJ: Contagious equine metritis. Comp Immunol Microbiol Infect Dis 1996; 19:199-204.
7. Ricketts SW, Mackintosh ME: Role of anaerobic bacteria in equine endometritis. J Reprod Fertil Suppl 1987; 35:343-351.
8. Hinrichs K, Cummings MR, Sertich PL et al: Bacteria recovered from the reproductive tract of normal mares. Proceedings of the 35th Annual Convention of the American Association of Equine Practitioners, pp 11-16, 1989.
9. Watson ED: Swabbing protocols in screening for contagious equine metritis. Vet Rec 1997; 140:268-271.
10. Swerczek TW: The first occurrence of contagious equine metritis in the United States. J Am Vet Med Assoc 1978; 173:405-407.
11. Pierson RE, Sahu SP, Dardiri AH et al: Contagious equine metritis: clinical description of experimentally induced infection. J Am Vet Med Assoc 1978; 173:402-404.
12. Troedsson MHT: Treatment strategies in mares with endometritis. Paper presented at Mare Reproduction Symposium, Kansas City, Mo, Society for Theriogenology, pp 40-50, 1996.
13. Dimock WW, Edwards PR: Genital infection in mares by an organism of the encapsulatus group. J Am Vet Med Assoc 1927; 70:469-480.
14. Hughes JP, Loy RG, Asbury AC et al: The occurrence of *Pseudomonas* in the reproductive tract of mares and its effect on fertility. Cornell Vet 1966; 56:595-610.
15. Williamson P, Munyua S, Martin R et al: Dynamics of the acute uterine response to infection, endotoxin infusion and physical manipulation of the reproductive tract in the mare. J Reprod Fertil Suppl 1987; 35:317-325.
16. Troedsson MHT, Liu IKM, Ing M et al: Multiple site electromyography recordings of uterine activity following an intrauterine bacterial challenge in mares susceptible and resistant to chronic uterine infection. J Reprod Fertil 1993; 99:307-313.
17. Asbury AC: Post-breeding treatment of mares utilizing techniques that improve uterine defenses against bacteria. Proceedings of the 30th Annual Convention of the American Association of Equine Practitioners, pp 349-356, 1984.
18. Easley J: External perineal conformation. In McKinnon AO, Voss JL (eds): Equine Reproduction, Philadelphia, Lea & Febiger, pp 20-24, 1993.
19. Caslick EA: The vulva and the vulvo-vaginal orifice and its relation to genital health of the thoroughbred mare. Cornell Vet 1937; 27:178-187.
20. Ginther OJ: Reproductive anatomy. In Reproductive Biology of the Mare, Cross Plains, Equiservices, pp 1-40, 1992.
21. Aanes WA: Cervical laceration(s). In McKinnon AO, Voss JL (eds): Equine Reproduction, Philadelphia, Lea & Febiger, pp 444-449, 1993.
22. Pycock JF, Allen WE: Inflammatory components in uterine fluid from mares with experimentally induced bacterial endometritis. Equine Vet J 1990; 22:422-425.
23. Kotilainen T, Huhtinen M, Katila T: Sperm-induced leukocytosis in the equine uterus. Theriogenology 1994; 41:629-636.
24. Allen WE, Pycock JF: Cyclical accumulation of uterine fluid in mares with lowered resistance to endometritis. Vet Rec 1988; 122:489-490.
25. LeBlanc MM, Neuwirth L, Asbury AC et al: Scintigraphic measurement of uterine clearance in normal mares and mares with recurrent endometritis. Equine Vet J 1994; 26:109-113.
26. Troedsson MHT, Liu IKM: Uterine clearance of non-antigenic markers (51Cr) in response to a bacterial challenge in mares potentially susceptible and resistant to chronic uterine infections. J Reprod Fertil Suppl 1991; 44:283-288.
27. Ozgen S, Rasch K, Kropp G et al: Aetiopathogenesis and therapy of equine hydromucometra: preliminary data. Pferdeheilkunde 1997; 13:533-536.
28. Allen WE, Pycock JF: Current views on the pathogenesis of bacterial endometritis in mares. Vet Rec 1989; 125:298-301.
29. Troedsson MHT, Liu IKM, Thurmond M: Function of uterine and blood-derived polymorphonuclear neutrophils in mares susceptible and resistant to chronic uterine infection: phagocytosis and chemotaxis. Biol Reprod 1993; 49:507-514.
30. Todd EW: A method of measuring the increase or decrease of the population of haemolytic streptococci in blood. Br J Exp Pathol 1927; 8:1-5.
31. Leblanc MM, Johnson RD, Mays MBC et al: Lymphatic clearance of India ink in reproductively normal mares and mares susceptible to endometritis. Biol Reprod Mono 1995; 1:501-506.
32. Causey RC, Ginn PS, Katz BP et al: Mucus production by endometrium of reproductively healthy mares and mares with delayed uterine clearance. J Reprod Fertil Suppl 2000; 56:333-339.
33. Ganjam VK, McLeod C, Klesius PH et al: The effect of ovarian hormones on the pathophysiologic mechanisms involved in resistance versus susceptibility to uterine infections in the mare. Proceedings of the 26th Annual Convention of the American Association of Equine Practitioners, pp 141-153, 1980.
34. Evans MJ, Hamer JM, Gason LM et al: Clearance of bacteria and non-antigenic markers following intra-uterine inoculation into maiden mares: effect of steroid hormone environment. Theriogenology 1986; 26:37-50.
35. Troedsson MHT, Wistrom AOG, Liu IKM et al: Registration of myometrial activity using multiple site electromyography in cyclic mares. J Reprod Fertil 1993; 99:299-306.
36. Washburn SM, Klesius PH, Ganjam VK et al: Effect of estrogen and progesterone on the phagocytic response of ovariectomized mares infected in utero with B-hemolytic streptococci. Am J Vet Res 1982; 43:1367-1370.
37. Asbury AC, Hansen PJ: Effects of susceptibility of mares to endometritis and stage of cycle on phagocytic activity of uterine-derived neutrophils. J Reprod Fertil Suppl 1987; 35:311-316.
38. Watson ED, Stokes CR, David JSE et al: Effect of ovarian hormones on promotion of bactericidal activity by uterine secretions of ovariectomized mares. J Reprod Fertil 1987; 79:531-537.
39. Colbern GT, Voss JL, Squires EL et al: Development of a model to study endometritis in mares. J Equine Vet Sci 1987; 7:73-76.
40. Dimock WW, Edwards PR: Pathology and bacteriology of the reproductive organs of mares in relation to sterility. Ky Agr Exp Sta Res Bull 1928; 286:157-237.
41. Beachey EH: Bacterial-adherence: adhesin-receptor interactions mediating the attachment of bacteria to mucosal surfaces. J Infect Dis 1981; 143:325-345.
42. Watson ED, Stokes CR, Bourne FJ: Influence of ovarian steroids on adherence (in vitro) of *Streptococcus zooepidemicus* to endometrial epithelial cells. Equine Vet J 1988; 20:371-372.
43. Ferreira-Dias G, Nequin LG, King SS: Influence of estrous cycle stage on adhesion of *Streptococcus zooepidemicus* to equine endometrium. Am J Vet Res 1994; 55:1028-1031.

44. King SS, Young DA, Nequin LG et al: Use of specific sugars to inhibit bacterial adherence to equine endometrium in vitro. Am J Vet Res 2000; 61:446-449.

45. Lindmark H, Jacobsson K, Frykberg L et al: Fibronectin-binding protein of *Streptococcus equi* subsp. *zooepidemicus*. Infect Immun 1996; 64:3993-3999.

46. Wibawan IWT, Pasaribu FH, Utama IH et al: The role of hyaluronic acid capsular material of *Streptococcus equi* subsp. *zooepidemicus* in mediating adherence to HeLa cells and in resisting phagocytosis. Res Vet Sci 1999; 67:131.

47. Favre-Bonte S, Joly B, Forestier C: Consequences of reduction of *K. pneumoniae* capsule expression on interactions of this bacterium with epithelial cells. Infect Immun 1999; 67:554-561.

48. Costerton JW, Lewandowski Z, Caldwell DE et al: Microbial biofilms. Annu Rev Microbiol 1995; 49:711-745.

49. Parkins MD, Ceri H, Storey DG: *Pseudomonas aeruginosa* GacA, a factor in multihost virulence, is also essential for biofilm formation. Mol Microbiol 2001; 40:1215-1226.

50. Costerton JW, Stewart PS, Greenberg EP: Bacterial biofilms: a common cause of persistent infections. Science 1999; 284:1318-1322.

51. Olson ME, Ceri H, Morck DW et al: Biofilm bacteria: formation and comparative susceptibility to antibiotics. Can J Vet Res 2002; 66:86-92.

52. Strzemienski PJ, Benson CE, Acland HM et al: Comparison of uterine protein content and distribution of bacteria in the reproductive tract of mares after intrauterine inoculation of *Haemophilus equigenitalis* or *Pseudomonas aeruginosa*. Am J Vet Res 1984; 45:1109-1113.

53. Hitchcock PJ, Brown TM, Corwin D et al: Morphology of three strains of contagious equine metritis organism. Infect Immun 1985; 48:94-108.

54. Muller-Alouf H, Alouf JE, Gerlach D et al: Cytokine production by murine cells activated by erythrogenic toxin type A superantigen of *Streptococcus pyogenes*. Immunobiology 1992; 186:435-448.

55. Rikiishi H, Okamoto S, Sugawara S et al: Superantigenicity of helper T-cell mitogen (SPM-2) isolated from culture supernatants of *Streptococcus pyogenes*. Immunology 1997; 91:406-413.

56. McCoy HE, Broder CC, Lottenberg R: Streptokinases produced by pathogenic group C streptococci demonstrate species-specific plasminogen activation. J Infect Dis 1991; 164:515-521.

57. Schroeder B, Boyle MDP, Sheerin BR et al: Species specificity of plasminogen activation and acquisition of surface-associated proteolytic activity by group C streptococci grown in plasma. Infect Immun 1999; 67:6487-6495.

58. Caballero AR, Lottenberg R, Johnston KH: Cloning, expression, sequence analysis, and characterization of streptokinases secreted by porcine and equine isolates of *Streptococcus equisimilis*. Infect Immun 1999; 67:6478-6486.

59. Anzai T, Sheoran AS, Kuwamoto Y et al: *Streptococcus equi* but not *Streptococcus zooepidemicus* produces potent mitogenic responses from equine peripheral blood mononuclear cells. Vet Immunol Immunopathol 1999; 67:235-246.

60. Troedsson MHT, Scott MA, Liu IKM: Comparative treatment of mares susceptible to chronic uterine infection. Am J Vet Res 1995; 56:468-472.

61. Causey RC, Paccamonti DL, Todd WJ: Antiphagocytic properties of uterine isolates of Streptococcus zooepidemicus and mechanisms of killing in freshly obtained blood of horses. Am J Vet Res 1995; 56:321-328.

62. Domenico P, Salo RJ, Cross AS et al: Polysaccharide capsule-mediated resistance to opsonophagocytosis in *Klebsiella pneumoniae*. Infect Immun 1994; 62:4495-4499.

63. Walker JA, Timoney JF: Molecular basis of variation in protective SzP proteins of *Streptococcus zooepidemicus*. Am J Vet Res 1998; 9:1129-1133.

64. Timoney JF, Mukhtar MM: The protective M proteins of the equine group C streptococci. Vet Microbiol 1993; 37:389-395.

65. Myhre EB, Kronvall G: Demonstration of a new type of immunoglobulin G receptor in *Streptococcus zooepidemicus* strains. Infect Immun 1980; 27:808-816.

66. Jonsson H, Lindmark H, Guss B: A protein G-related cell surface protein in *Streptococcus zooepidemicus*. Infect Immun 1995; 63:2968-2975.

67. Lyle SK, Asbury AC, Boyle MDP et al: Pathogenesis of equine endometritis: proposed interaction between streptococcal immunoglobulin-binding proteins and other uterine pathogens (abstract). J Reprod Fertil Suppl 1991; 44:741.

68. Williamson P, Munyua SJM, Penhale J: Endometritis in the mare: a comparison between reproductive history and uterine biopsy as techniques for predicting susceptibility of mares to uterine infection. Theriogenology 1989; 32:351-357.

69. Neely DP, Kindahl H, Stabenfeldt GH et al: Prostaglandin release patterns in the mare: physiological, pathophysiological, and therapeutic responses. J Reprod Fertil Suppl 1979; 27:181-189.

70. Sharp DC, Davis SD: Vernal Transition. In McKinnon AO, Voss JL (eds): Equine Reproduction, Malvern, Lea & Febiger, pp 133-143, 1993.

71. McKinnon AO, Voss JL, Squires EL et al: Diagnostic ultrasonography. In McKinnon AO, Voss JL (eds): Equine Reproduction, Malvern, Lea & Febiger, pp 266-302, 1993.

72. McKinnon AO, Squires EL, Harrison LA et al: Ultrasonographic studies on the reproductive tract of mares after parturition: effect of involution and uterine fluid on pregnancy rates in mares with normal and delayed first postpartum ovulatory cycles. J Am Vet Med Assoc 1988; 192:350-353.

73. Pycock JF, Newcombe JR: Assessment of the effect of three treatments to remove intrauterine fluid on pregnancy rate in the mare. Vet Rec 1996; 138:320-323.

74. Troedsson MHT: Therapeutic considerations for mating-induced endometritis. Pferdeheilkunde 1997; 13:516-520.

75. Asbury AC: Endometritis in the mare. In Morrow DA (ed): Current Therapy in Theriogenology. Philadelphia, WB Saunders, pp 718-722, 1986.

76. LeBlanc MM: Vaginal examination. In McKinnon AO, Voss JL (eds): Equine Reproduction, Malvern, Lea & Febiger, pp 221-224, 1993.

77. Althouse GC, Seager SWJ, Varner DD et al: Diagnostic aids for the detection of urine in the equine ejaculate. Theriogenology 1989; 31:1141-1148

78. Wingfield-Digby NJ, Ricketts SW: Results of concurrent bacteriological and cytological examinations of the endometrium of mares in routine stud farm practice 1978-1981. J Reprod Fertil Suppl 1982; 32:181-185.

79. Ricketts SW, Young A, Medici EB: Uterine and clitoral cultures. In McKinnon AO, Voss JL (eds): Equine Reproduction, Malvern, Lea & Febiger, pp 234-245, 1993.

80. Blanchard TL, Garcia MC, Hurtgen JP et al: Comparison of two techniques for obtaining endometrial bacteriologic cultures in the mare. Theriogenology 1981; 16:85-93.

81. Ball BA, Shin SJ, Patten VH et al: Use of a low-volume uterine flush for microbiologic and cytologic examination of the mare's endometrium. Theriogenology 1988; 29:1269-1283.

82. Troedsson MHT, deMoraes MJ, Liu IKM: Correlations between histologic endometrial lesions in mares and clinical response to intrauterine exposure with *Streptococcus zooepidemicus*. Am J Vet Res 1993; 54:570-572.

83. Kenney RM: Cyclic and pathologic changes of the mare endometrium as detected by biopsy, with a note on early embryonic death. J Am Vet Med Assoc 1978; 172:241-262.

84. Waelchli RO, Winder NC: Mononuclear cell infiltration of the equine endometrium: immunohistochemical studies. Equine Vet J 1991; 23:470-474.

85. LeBlanc MM: Endoscopy. In McKinnon AO, Voss JL (eds): Equine Reproduction, Malvern, Lea & Febiger, pp 255-257, 1993.

86. Van-Dyk E, Lange LA: [The detrimental effect of the use of iodine as an intra-uterine instillation in mares], J S Afr Vet Assoc 1986; 57:205-210.

87. Bracher V, Mathias S, Allen WR: Videoendoscopic evaluation of the mare's uterus. II. Findings in subfertile mares. Equine Vet J 1992; 24:279-284.

88. Kenney RM, Bergman RV, Cooper WL et al: Broodmare problems and management panel: minimal contamination techniques for breeding mares: technique and preliminary findings. Proceedings of the 21st Annual Convention of the American Association of Equine Practitioners, pp 327-336, 1975.

89. Allen WE: Investigations into the use of exogenous oxytocin for promoting uterine drainage in mares susceptible to endometritis. Vet Rec 1991; 128:593-594.

90. LeBlanc M, Neuwirth L, Mauragis D et al: Oxytocin enhances clearance of radiocolloid from the uterine lumen of reproductively normal mares and mares susceptible to endometritis. Equine Vet J 1994; 26:279-282.

91. Nie GJ, Johnson KE, Wenzel JGW et al: Effect of periovulatory ecbolics on luteal function and fertility. Theriogenology 2002; 58:461-463.

92. Campbell MLH, England GCW: A comparison of the ecbolic efficacy of intravenous and intrauterine oxytocin treatments. Theriogenology 2002; 58:473-477.

93. Madill S, Troedsson MHT, Santschi EM et al: Dose-response effect of intramuscular oxytocin treatment on myometrial contraction of reproductively normal mares during estrus. Theriogenology 2002; 58:479-481.

94. Brendemuehl JP: Influence of cloprostenol, PGF2a and oxytocin administered in the immediate post ovulatory period on corpora luteal formation and function in the mare. In Society for Theriogenology Annual Conference, San Antonio, Tex, p 267, 2000 (abstract).

95. Cadario ME, Thatcher MD, LeBlanc MM: Relationship between prostaglandin and uterine clearance of radiocolloid in the mare. Biol Reprod Mono 1995; 1:495-500.

96. LeBlanc MM: Effects of oxytocin, prostaglandin and phenylbutazone on uterine clearance of radiocolloid. Pferdeheilkunde 1997; 13:483-485.

97. Asbury AC, Lyle SK: Infectious causes of infertility. In McKinnon AO, Voss JL (eds): Equine Reproduction, Malvern, Lea & Febiger, pp 381-391, 1993.

98. Brinsko SP, Varner DD, Blanchard TL: The effect of uterine lavage performed four hours post insemination on pregnancy rate in mares. Theriogenology 1991; 35:1111-1119.

99. Alexander SL, Irvine CHG, Shand N et al: Is luteinizing hormone secretion modulated by endogenous oxytocin in the mare? Studies on the role of oxytocin and factors affecting its secretion in estrous mares. Biol Reprod Mono 1995; 1:361-371.

100. Davis LE, Abbitt B: Clinical pharmacology of antibacterial drugs in the uterus of the mare. J Am Vet Med Assoc 1977; 170:204-207.

101. Ricketts SW: Treatment of equine endometritis with intrauterine irrigations of ceftiofur sodium: a comparison with mares treated in a similar manner with a mixture of sodium benzylpenicillin, neomycin sulphate, polymyxin B sulphate and furaltadone hydrochloride. Pferdeheilkunde 1997; 13:486-489.

102. Spensley MS, Baggot JD, Wilson WD et al: Pharmacokinetics and endometrial tissue concentrations of ticarcillin given to the horse by intravenous and intrauterine routes. Am J Vet Res 1986; 47:2587-2590.

103. Brinsko SP: Treatment of infectious infertility. In Mare Reproduction Symposium, Kansas City, Mo, Society for Theriogenology, pp 150-155, 1996.

104. Bennett DG, Poland HJ, Kaneps AJ et al: Histologic effect of infusion solutions on the equine endometrium. Equine Pract 1981; 3:37-44.

105. Brown MP, Embertson RM, Gronwall RR et al: Amikacin sulfate in mares: pharmacokinetics and body fluid and endometrial concentrations after repeated intramuscular administration. Am J Vet Res 1984; 45:1610-1613.

106. Pedersoli WM, Fazeli MH, Haddad NS et al: Endometrial and serum gentamicin concentrations in pony mares given repeated intrauterine infusions. Am J Vet Res 1985; 46:1025-1028.

107. Jackson PS, Allen WR, Ricketts SW et al: The irritancy of chlorhexidine gluconate in the genital tract of the mare. Vet Rec 1979; 105:122-124.

108. Couto MA, Hughes JP: Sexually transmitted (venereal) diseases of horses. In McKinnon AO, Voss JL (eds): Equine Reproduction, Malvern, Lea & Febiger, pp 845-854, 1993.

109. Youngquist RS, Blanchard TL, Lapin D et al: The effects of EDTA-Tris infusion on the equine endometrium. Theriogenology 1984; 22:593-599.

110. Asbury AC, Schultz KT, Klesius PH et al: Factors affecting phagocytosis of bacteria by neutrophils in the mare's uterus. J Reprod Fertil Suppl 1982; 32:151-159.

111. Asbury AC, Gorman NT, Foster GW: Uterine defense mechanisms in the mare: serum opsonins affecting phagocytosis of Streptococcus zooepidemicus by equine neutrophils. Theriogenology 1984; 21:375-385.

112. Jacks-Weiss J, Kim Y, Cleary PP: Restricted deposition of C3 on M+ group A streptococci: correlation with resistance to phagocytosis. J Immunol 1982; 128:1897-1902.

113. Asbury AC: Uterine defense mechanisms in the mare: the use of intrauterine plasma in the management of endometritis. Theriogenology 1984; 21:387-393.

114. Colbern GT, Voss JL, Squires EL et al: Intrauterine equine plasma as an endometritis therapy: use of an endometritis model to evaluate efficacy. J Equine Vet Sci 1987; 7:66-68.

115. Adams GP, Ginther OJ: Efficacy of intrauterine infusion of plasma for treatment of infertility and endometritis in mares. J Am Vet Med Assoc 1989; 194:372-378.

116. Watson ED, Stokes CR: Use of hyperimmune serum in treatment of endometritis in mares. Theriogenology 1988; 30:893-899.

117. Pascoe DR: Effect of adding autologous plasma to an intrauterine antibiotic therapy after breeding on pregnancy rates in mares. Biol Reprod Mono 1995; 1:539-543.

118. Couto MA, Hughes JP: Intrauterine inoculation of a bacteria-free filtrate of Streptococcus zooepidemicus in clinically normal and infected mares. J Equine Vet Sci 1985; 5:81-86.

119. Fumuso E, Giguere S, Dorna IV et al: Use of immunomodulation in persistent post-breeding endometritis: effect on proinflammatory cytokines IL1B, IL6, and TNFa mRNA transcription studied by real time PCR. In Annual Conference of the Society for Theriogenology, Colorado Springs, Colo, p 41, 2002.

120. Troedsson MHT, Alghamdi AS, Mattisen J: Equine seminal plasma protects the fertility of spermatozoa in an inflamed uterine environment. Theriogenology 2002; 58:453-456.

CHAPTER 16

Treatment of Fungal Endometritis

JOHN J. DASCANIO

Treating equine fungal endometritis can be a frustrating endeavor to undertake. Oftentimes mares become reinfected or remain infected with fungi, are culture positive with a bacterial endometritis the next cycle, or are classified as susceptible to infection/uterine fluid accumulation. Generally, mares affected are 10+-years-old with a history of infertility. Most treatments for fungal endometritis have been extrapolated from other species or from other disease processes. Specific controlled intrauterine fungal treatment studies are lacking in the horse. The information presented in this chapter is based on what is available in the literature, the author's experience, and information from colleagues. This chapter will be broken down into a description of fungi, fungal endometritis, and the diagnosis and treatment of fungal endometritis. By following a systematic approach with a longer duration of therapy, infection can be eliminated in many mares, allowing for subsequent breeding.

Fungi are classified either as single-celled organisms, called yeast, or multi-cellular filamentous organisms, called molds. The filamentous cells within molds are called hyphae. Hyphae may also form tangled masses called mycelia. Cytological specimens may demonstrate yeast or hyphae (Figures 16-1 and 16-2), whereas mycelia are usually identified in fluid from a uterine lavage (Figure 16-3). Yeasts are typically more suited to growth in liquids, whereas hyphae are better adapted for penetrating solid substrates. Thus, when hyphae are identified on cytology or biopsy, thought should be directed toward treatment of a more deep seated infection within the endometrium. Yeasts are 3 to 5 μm round-to-oval single-cell organisms and often have a capsule surrounding them that excludes dyes (Figure 16-2). By comparison, neutrophils are typically 10 μm in diameter.

Most fungi have a plasma membrane surrounded by a cell wall made of chitin. Rarely, some fungi may have cell walls composed of cellulose. Chitin is a polysaccharide made from acetylglucosamine. It is closely related to cellulose, where 1 hydroxyl group of cellulose is replaced by an acetylamino group in chitin. The cell wall has a structural support function and also serves to protect the fungus from osmotic stress. In addition, the cell wall may protect the fungus from the entry of molecules that may be toxic. Fungi that form hyphae may or may not have cell walls separating their nuclei. The cell membrane of fungi is different from the cell membrane of bacteria, with fungi having ergosterol and bacteria having cholesterol in their membranes. Many antifungal antibiotics are directed at ergosterol, causing defects in fungal cellular membranes but leaving bacterial membranes intact. There are also other drugs directed at fungal cell wall function/formation, such as chitin inhibitors. Depending on the treatment, the effects may be on current cell wall/membrane function or future cell wall/cell membrane formation. All these factors are important when deciding on treatment modalities and dealing with treatment failures.

A number of different fungi have been isolated from the mare's reproductive tract, with *Candida* spp and *Aspergillus* spp identified most commonly. Table 16-1 lists the fungi that have been isolated from the mare's reproductive tract. Certain fungi, such as *Candida* spp, may normally be present as commensal organisms in the gastrointestinal tract, vagina, or oral mucosa. *Candida* may be present as both yeast cells and hyphal elements on cytology. *Candida albicans* is able to adhere to vaginal epithelium better than other *Candida* spp; thus it is isolated from the majority of *Candida* infections. Estrogen enhances the ability of *Candida* to adhere to vaginal tissue; consequently, drug therapy with estrogens may increase the risk for this fungal infection. Nystatin, clotrimazole, ketoconazole and amphotericin B have been reported as effective against *Candida* spp. Some of the newer azole drugs, such as fluconazole, may also be effective. In contrast to *Candida*, *Aspergillus* spp are in hyphal form and may exhibit conidiophores. *Aspergillus* has been reported to invade tissues, making topical therapy less effective. Macrophages are particularly effective against *Aspergillis*, and when macrophage function is decreased, tissue invasion is more likely. Hyphal forms are too large for phagocytosis by polymorphonuclear cells; consequently, they must be damaged by substances released by polymorphonuclear leukocytes and mononuclear phagocytes. Amphotericin B is often employed in the treatment of *Aspergillis* infections, although the azole compounds should also be effective, as described later.

Predisposing factors to fungal infections include immunosuppression, malnutrition, tissue trauma, endocrine dysfunctions such as equine pituitary disorders, physiologic changes associated with pregnancy or growth, and changes induced by antimicrobial and immunosuppressive drug therapy. Specifically, antibiotic, corticosteroid, and chemotherapeutic agents have been implicated in the altering of immune function leading to opportunistic fungal infections. Antibiotics are believed

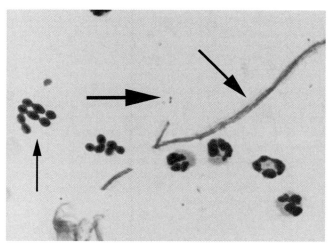

Figure 16-1 Magnification 1000× oil immersion view of endometrial cytology from a mare stained with Diff-Quik. Four neutrophils are present in the lower right quadrant of the picture. *Large arrow* is pointed at bacteria, *medium arrow* is pointed at hyphae, and *small arrow* is pointed at budding yeast. Neutrophils are approximately 10 microns in diameter.

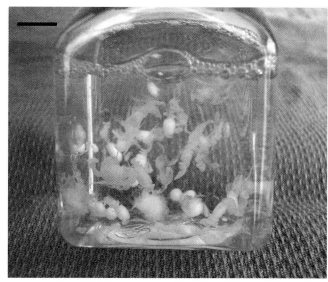

Figure 16-3 Mycelia obtained from a mare with fungal endometritis during uterine lavage. *Black bar* in upper left corner is ~1 cm.

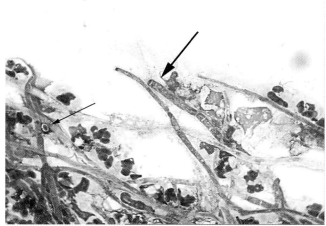

Figure 16-2 Magnification 1000× oil immersion view of endometrial cytology from a mare stained with Diff-Quik. The *large arrow* is pointed at fungal hyphae and the *small arrow* is pointed at a yeast organism with a capsule. There are multiple neutrophils scattered throughout the picture. Neutrophils are approximately 10 microns in diameter.

to predispose to fungal infections by eliminating competing bacteria within the vagina, allowing opportunistic fungi to colonize. Pneumovagina has been identified as a predisposing condition to fungal endometritis, probably leading to fecal contamination of the cranial reproductive tract. The use of progesterone therapy may increase the risk of endometritis as cervical tone may increase, uterine muscular activity is altered, and neutrophil function may be decreased. Exposure to a moist environment, large numbers of fungi, and necrotic tissue will also increase the risk of infection.

Both humeral and cell mediated immunity (CMI) are important in combating fungal infections, with CMI cited as being more effective. *Candida* infections have been identified with T cell disturbances and with disruptions of mucosal surfaces. Complement-dependent and complement-independent phagocytosis by macrophages may be interfered with in immunodeficient states. A common predisposing factor in *Candida* infections is neutropenia, thus, polymorphonuclear leukocyte mediated phagocytosis is decreased. Some types of fungal infections may be contagious, such as *Candida* infections, which can pass from one individual to the next through skin-to-skin contact. This is important in situations where natural service is employed as the primary means for breeding. Enzymes may also be associated with some types of fungi such as *Apergillus* spp, including endotoxins, mycotoxins, and elastases. This may lead to increased endometrial damage, as evident on uterine biopsies subsequent to resolution of infection. With *Cryptococcus* infections, the presence of a capsule around the fungi makes it resistant to phagocytosis and opsonization. *Coccidiodes immitis* infections in humans are not highly virulent and nearly all are self-healing in nonimmunocompromised patients.

Fungal endometritis is a condition usually affecting older multiparous mares that have been treated for bacterial endometritis in the past. Fungal uterine infections have also been documented in mares without previous history or treatment for endometritis. Approximately 2% to 3% of all positive uterine cultures will be positive for fungi. The perineal conformation of many of these older mares is not optimum with greater than two-thirds of their vulvar opening above the pelvic floor, an incompetent vulvar seal from multiple Caslick's procedures or trauma, and/or a tilted conformation to their vulva. These decreased physical barriers potentially lead to fecal contamination of the cranial reproductive tract, predisposing these mares to bacterial and fungal infections.

Table **16-1**

Fungi that have Been Reported in Isolates from the Mare's Reproductive Tract with Associated Form

Fungal organism	Yeast, pseudohyphae, filamentous hyphae, hyphae
Actinomyces spp	Filamentous hyphae
Aspergillus fumigatus	Hyphae
Aspergillus spp	Hyphae
Candida albicans	Yeast, pseudohyphae
Candida guillermondii	Yeast, pseudohyphae
Candida krusei	Yeast, pseudohyphae
Candida lusitaniae	Yeast, pseudohyphae
Candida parapsilosis	Yeast, pseudohyphae
Candida rugosa	Yeast, pseudohyphae
Candida tropicalis	Yeast, pseudohyphae
Candida stellatoides	Yeast, pseudohyphae
Candida zeylanoides	Yeast, pseudohyphae
Coccidiodes immitis	Hyphae
Cryptococcus neoformans	Yeast
Fusarium spp	Hyphae
Hansenula anomala	Yeast, pseudohyphae
Hansenula polymorpha	Yeast, pseudohyphae
Monosporium apiospermum	Hyphae
Monosporium spp	Hyphae
Mucor spp	Hyphae
Nocardia spp	Filamentous hyphae
Paecilomyces spp	Hyphae
Rhodotorula glutinis	Yeast, pseudohyphae
Rhodotorula minuta	Yeast, pseudohyphae
Rhodotorula rubra	Yeast, pseudohyphae
Rhodotorula spp	Yeast, pseudohyphae
Scedosporium apiospermum	Hyphae
Saccharomyces cerevisiae	Yeast, pseudohyphae
Torulopsis candida	Yeast
Trichosporon beigelii	Hyphae, pseudohyphae
Trichosporon cutaneum	Hyphae, pseudohyphae
Trichosporon spp	Hyphae, pseudohyphae

The diagnosis of fungal endometritis may be made from a cytological uterine specimen, uterine culture, or uterine biopsy. In the author's experience, the identification of fungi on cytology is a relatively straightforward procedure. Most commonly, fungi are seen on cytology first and confirmed with culture second. Cells obtained from a uterine swab are placed on a microscope slide, air dried, and stained with a modified Wright's stain, such as Diff-Quik (Becton Dickinson and Company, Cockeysville, Md.). It is important to perform the isolation and identification of the fungi for further classification to allow for antifungal drug sensitivities to be performed. Mares with fungal endometritis may have uterine fluid accumulation, as detected on ultrasonographic uterine examination, a grayish vulvar discharge, or no apparent clinical signs.

A confounder in diagnosis is that culture results may only demonstrate fungi even though bacteria are present, especially if bacteria are in low numbers. Consequently, when a fungal infection is resolved by antifungal antibiotics, the bacteria may then have a less competing environment in which to grow and subsequent uterine cultures then demonstrate a bacterial infection. The possibility also exists that treatments used to combat fungal infections may decrease the normal microflora of the vagina, allowing overgrowth of pathogenic bacteria. When fungi are identified on uterine cytology, care should be taken during examination to inspect for the presence of bacteria.

The treatment of fungal endometritis should be a carefully orchestrated plan. **Step one:** Assess the integrity of the physical barriers to uterine infection: the vulva, the vestibulovaginal fold, and the cervix. Defects in any of these barriers will predispose the uterus to contamination from fecal sources. Feces have been implicated as one origin of fungi that infect the reproductive tract. Vulvoplasty (Caslick's procedure), involving suturing of the vulvar lips, should be considered even with minor anatomical deficits, in order to prevent fecal contamination and spread of opportunistic intestinal fungi to the reproductive tract. Surgical staples without a mucosal incision may be used as a temporary vulvoplasty procedure to allow for easy removal of the vulvoplasty and access to the reproductive tract. **Step two:** Consider treatment of all possible major reproductive tissues that may harbor fungi. These include the clitoris, clitoral fossa, vagina, cervix, and uterus. Remember with multiple mare infections to examine the stallion as a potential source. Fresh semen, extended semen, and urethral cultures from stallions have yielded positive fungal cultures, although there are no reports of fungal endometritis caused from natural cover or artificial insemination. **Step three:** Obtain a uterine cytological sample, culture, and possible biopsy. Additional culture specimens may also be acquired from other tissue sources, such as vagina and clitoral fossa. Fungi will grow on blood agar and can be subcultured on Sabaroud's agar but may take more time to grow than bacteria. To examine mares for invasive forms of fungi, a uterine biopsy stained with a silver stain such as Gomori's methanamine silver stain can provide useful information. Isolated fungi should be examined for antifungal antibiotic sensitivity patterns to determine effective drugs. **Step four:** Identify if yeasts, hyphae, or both are present in cytological samples. Yeasts alone are associated more with superficial infections, whereas hyphae are associated with more tissue invasive fungal forms. Deep seated infections may be more difficult to resolve and require longer duration of therapy. **Step five:** Perform large volume uterine lavage to remove any potential uterine fluid, decrease fungal/bacterial numbers, and expose organisms to antifungal solutions, such as 2% (v/v) acetic acid (white vinegar—20 ml of white vinegar in 1 liter of 0.9% saline), 0.1% (v/v) povidone-iodine solution, or 20% DMSO. Acidic and alkaline environments are not conducive to fungal growth. Uterine lavage will also cause an influx of neutrophils, which enhance fungal destruction. Oxytocin (5-20 IU intramuscularly or intravenously) or prostaglandins (cloprostenol, 125-250 µg or dinoprost tromethomine, 5-10 mg intramuscularly) may be used to augment uterine contractility to remove residual uterine fluid. **Step six:** Infuse specific antifungal agents into the uterine lumen. Ideally agents are selected from antifungal sensitivity patterns run on uterine culture results. Antifungal antibiotics should also be placed in the vagina and clitoral fossa to remove potential reservoirs of fungi to prevent reinfection of the uterus. Longer-term treatments may be necessary to suppress fungi. In humans prone to reinfection, a 10- to 14-day treatment period may be recommended. In horses, our treatment periods are usually limited to the duration of estrus (5-7 days). By starting treatment during diestrus, on the day of prostaglandin administration to cause return to estrus, a longer treatment period may be achieved. **Step seven:** Address any immunodeficient conditions affecting the reproductive tract. This may include removal of steroid use for other systemic issues such as dermatologic conditions or recurrent airway obstruction (RAO) or treatment of pituitary disorders such as anterior pituitary dysfunction (equine Cushing's disease). More controversial is the use of immunomodulators to enhance immune function. A *Mycobacterium phlei* cell-wall extract (MCWE) preparation has been shown to decrease production of Interleukin-1β, decreasing the inflammatory response to artificial insemination. This product may have benefit in modulating inflammation associated with other inflammatory insults such as uterine infection, but work in this area has not been conducted. Use of prostaglandin therapy to induce estrus will allow an affected mare to return to a stage of her reproductive cycle where there is an enhanced immunologic response to infection.

Reestablishing normal bacterial flora within the vaginal canal is important in preventing recurrence. Use of Lactobacillus acidophilus and garlic (antibacterial and antifungal) orally has been suggested in humans. Antioxidants including vitamins A, C, E, and B complex may also be useful.

The polyene and imidazole antifungal antibiotics work by affecting ergosterol in the cell membrane of fungi. This results in an increase in permeability of the cell and eventual cell lysis. Amphotericin B, nystatin, and natamycin are examples of polyene antibiotics. Clotrimazole, miconazole, ketoconazole, fluconazole, and itraconazole are examples of azole derivatives. It is believed that antifungal drugs are more effective with a slightly acid environment to aid in their absorption; consequently, prior lavage with a 2% acetic acid solution may be beneficial. The typical administration of antifungal antibiotics is through direct contact with affected tissues because oral absorption from the gastrointestinal tract is poor for most of these drugs. An exception to this is fluconazole, which has excellent absorption, but is costly to use via the oral route in horses. Systemic administration may be beneficial with tissue invasive fungi. Drug dosages are not well defined for antifungal drugs in the horse. Suggested dosages are presented in Table 16-2 for those drugs that have been reported in the literature. Minimum inhibitory concentrations for these drugs in the mare's uterus have not been established.

Chitin inhibitors have been investigated recently for their use in treatment of fungal infections. These sub-

Table 16-2

Intrauterine Antifungal Antibiotic Dosages That Have Been Reported in the Literature

Antifungal Antibiotic	Dosage
Clotrimazole	500 to 700 mg
Nystatin	0.5 to 2.5 million units
Amphotericin B	100 to 200 mg
Fluconazole	100 mg

stances work by affecting new chitin formation and usually have no effect on fungal cell walls that have already formed. Their role in treatment might include deposition during or at the end of a treatment period to prevent new fungal growth and thus reinfection. Lufenuron is an example of a chitin inhibitor that has been suggested as a treatment for equine fungal endometritis. However, recent studies have suggested that lufenuron does not appear to have good antifungal properties. Nikkomycin Z is another chitin inhibitor that has shown promise either alone or in combination with itraconazole. Further investigation into intrauterine chitin inhibitors is warranted before they can be recommended for use.

A suggested treatment regime for a mare with fungal endometritis is morning lavage with 2% acetic acid with afternoon placement of an antifungal antibiotic. This is repeated daily for a minimum of 7 to 10 days. Uterine cytology and culture are obtained on the first day of the next naturally occurring estrus. If clean, the mare is bred once in coordination with follicular development. The veterinarian should limit the number of times the reproductive tract is entered for insemination to prevent accidental seeding with bacteria/fungi from reservoir sources. A double-guarded insemination pipette should be used to limit vaginal contamination of the uterus.

The prognosis for mares with fungal endometritis is guarded to poor for future fertility. This is based on past reports of treatment failures, subsequent bacterial infections, and the low fertility of an aged population of affected mares. In addition, some of the fungal infections may cause significant endometrial damage if they have been present for longer than a few estrous cycles. Once the fungal infection is cleared, it may be prudent to obtain a uterine biopsy to detail endometrial grade. Diligence in diagnosis and treatment gives the best opportunity for resolution.

Suggested Reading

Abou-Gabal M, Hogle RM, West JK: Pyometra in a mare caused by *Candida rugosa*. J Am Vet Med Assoc 1977; 170:177-178.
Arora DK, Ajello L, Mukerji KG: Handbook of applied mycology: Humans, animals and insects, ed 2, New York, Marcel Dekker, Inc, 1991.
Asbury AC, Lyle SK: Infectious causes of infertility. In McKinnon AO, Voss JL (eds): Equine reproduction, Philadelphia, Lea & Febiger, pp 381-391, 1993.

Blue MG: Mycotic invasion of the mare's uterus. Vet Rec 1983; 113:131-132.

Chengappa MM, Maddux RL, Greer SC et al: Isolation and identification of yeasts and yeast-like organisms from clinical veterinary sources. J Clin Microbiol 1984; 19:427-428.

Collins SM: Study of the incidence of cervical uterine infections in Thoroughbred mares in Ireland. Vet Rec 1964; 76:673-676.

Doyle AW: Genital tract infection with *Candida albicans* (Monilia) in a Thoroughbred mare. Irish Vet J 1969; 23:90-91.

Eschenbach DA: Lower genital tract infections. In Galask RP, Larsen B (eds): Infectious diseases in the female patient, New York, Springer-Verlag, pp 163-186, 1986.

Farelly BT, Mullaney MA: Cervical and uterine infection in Thoroughbred Mares. Irish Vet J 1964; 18:201-212.

Freeman KP, Roszel JF, Slusher SH et al: Mycotic infections of the equine uterus. Eq Pract 1986; 8:34-42.

Fumuso E, Giguère S, Wade J et al: Endometrial IL-1, IL-6 and TNF-, mRNA expression in mares resistant or susceptible to post-breeding endometritis. Vet Immuno and Immunopath 2003; 96:31-41.

Garcia-Tamayo J, Castillo C, Martinez AJ: Human genital candidiasis. Acta Cytol 1982; 26:7-14.

Granger SE: The aetiology and pathogenesis of vaginal candidosis: an update. Brit J Clin Pract 1992; 46:258-259.

Grant SM, Clissold SP: Fluconazole: A review of its pharmacodynamic and pharmacokinetic properties, and therapeutic potential in superficial and systemic mycoses. Drugs 1990; 39:877-916.

Hector RF, Davidson AP, Johnson SM: Comparison of susceptibility of fungal isolates to lufenuron and nikkomycin Z alone or in combination with itraconazole. Am J Vet Res 2005; 66:1090-1093.

Hess MB, Parker NA, Purswell BJ et al: Use of lufenuron as a treatment for fungal endometritis in four mares. J Am Vet Med Assoc 2002; 221:266-267.

Hinrichs K, Cummings MR, Sertich PL et al: Bacteria recovered from the reproductive tracts of normal mares. Proc Am Assoc Eq Pract 1989; 35:11-16.

Horowitz BJ, Edelstein SW, Lippman L: Sexual transmission of *Candida*. Obstet Gynecol 1987; 69:883-886.

Hurtgen JP, Cummings MR: Diagnosis and treatment of fungal endometritis in mares. Proc Annu Meet Soc Theriogenol 1982; 18-22.

Katila T: Uterine defense mechanisms in the mare. Anim Repro Sci 1996; 42:197-204.

Kenny RM: Minimum contamination techniques for breeding mares: techniques and preliminary findings. Proc Am Assoc Eq Pract 1975; 21:327.

Larone DH: Medically important fungi: a guide to identification, ed 3, Washington, DC, ASM Press, 1995.

Ley WB: Current thoughts on the diagnosis and treatment of acute endometritis in mares. Vet Med 1994; 89:648-660.

Malmgren L, Olsson Engvall E, Engvall A et al: Aerobic bacterial flora of semen and stallion reproductive tract and its relation to fertility under field conditions. Acta Vet Scand 1998; 39: 173-182.

Petrites-Murphy MB, Robbins LA, Donahue JM et al: Equine cryptococcal endometritis and placentitis with neonatal cryptococcal pneumonia. J Vet Diagn Invest 1996; 8:383-386.

Pottz GE, Rampey JH, Benjamin F: The effect of dimethyl sulfoxide (DMSO) on antibiotic sensitivity of a group of medically important microorganisms: preliminary report. Ann NY Acad Sci 1967; 141:261-272.

Pugh DG, Bowen JM, Kloppe LH, et al: Fungal endometritis in mares. Compend Contin Educ Pract Vet 1986; 8:S173-S181.

Ross RA, Mei-Ling TL, Onderdonk AB: Effect of *Candida albicans* infection and clotrimazole treatment on vaginal microflora in vitro. Obstet Gynecol 1995; 86:925-930.

Schafer-Korting M: Pharmacokinetic optimization of oral antifungal therapy. Clin Pharmacokinet 1993; 25:329-341.

Tortora GJ, Funke BR, Case CL: Functional anatomy of procaryotic and eucaryotic cells. In Microbiology, an Introduction, Menlo Park, Addison Wesley Longman, Inc, pp 76-111, 1998.

Tortora GJ, Funke BR, Case CL: Fungi, algae, protozoa, and multicellular parasites. In Microbiology, an Introduction, Menlo Park, Addison Wesley Longman, Inc, pp 320-358, 1998.

Troedsson MHT: Diseases of the uterus. In Troedsson MHT (ed): Current Therapy in Equine Medicine, ed 4, Philadelphia, Saunders Company, pp 517-524, 1997.

Volk WA: Bacterial morphology. In Basic Microbiology, New York, HarperCollins Publishers, Inc, pp 38-56, 1992.

Witkin SS: Immunology of recurrent vaginitis. Am J Reprod Immunol Microbiol 1987; 15:34-37.

Zafracas AM: *Candida* infection of the genital tract in Thoroughbred Mares. J Reprod Fert 1975; 23(Suppl):349-351.

CHAPTER 17

Management Regimens for Uterine Cysts

G. REED HOLYOAK
WILLIAM B. LEY

Uterine cysts are diagnosed clinically either during routine examination per rectum of the internal genital tract if of sufficient size by palpation, or by ultrasonography if smaller. There is controversy over the effect of uterine cysts on fertility, and there are a number of different recommended treatments indicating the inability of any one treatment to be consistently successful. Almost invariably, uterine cysts are associated with some degree of chronic degenerative change within the endometrium referred to as endometrosis.

ENDOMETROSIS

Endometrosis refers to the described wide range of degenerative histopathologic characteristics of the endometrium in mares.[1] The condition is degenerative and lacks the typical features of active inflammation. Historically the term *endometritis* was and often still is indiscriminately used for this condition. However, the use of the modifying suffix "-itis" in association with this pathologic condition is felt to be misleading and inaccurate. Infiltrates of lymphocytes, plasmacytes, and macrophages are the predominant cell types observed in the submucosal periglandular endometrial tissues of such mares. Endometrosis is a feature of uterine "wear and tear" that develops during a mare's advancing reproductive lifetime. Its development is age related, but the age of onset varies between individual mares. The major histopathologic changes that characterize endometrosis are considered to be fibrosis, lymphatic stasis, uterine sacculation, transluminal adhesions, and glandular or lymphatic cysts.[2,3] Cystic glandular changes are often observed in endometrial biopsy specimens from older mares.[4] These are thin walled and contain fluid with large numbers of lymphocytes, suggesting that they may be due to stromal fibrosis causing obstruction of uterine glands. Glandular duct obstruction is postulated to arise by one of several mechanisms: (a) a strangling effect produced by periglandular fibrosis; (b) decreased myometrial tone and peristaltic activity associated with either prolonged anestrous or age-related changes; and/or (c) epithelial hypertrophy, one of the first responses to periglandular fibrosis observed in the equine endometrium.

Reliable and specific treatments have not been described that can permanently alter or reverse the course of endometrosis. Treatments that have been described attempt to induce superficial endometrial inflammation, necrosis, and tissue loss in the hope that the tissue that regenerates is in a better state to support any subsequent pregnancy.[5-7] A few of the treatments studied in critically controlled settings have shown to be of some benefit in improving endometrial histomorphologic architecture in the posttreatment evaluation period. These therapies also have the potential for inducing irreversible damage to the urogenital tract of mares treated if treated too vigorously or if used inappropriately. They must therefore be used in a cautious and controlled manner. Overly aggressive application of mechanical modalities, such as endometrial curettage,[8] or too caustic a chemical irritant may induce superficial mucosal, and possibly submucosal, necrosis and potentially lead to the development of intrauterine, cervical, and/or vaginal adhesions. The long-term effects of such therapies have received little study. Whether or not there is increased endometrial fibrosis in mares years after receiving such treatments is unknown. With all such therapies, it is cautioned that they are to be reserved for use in mares that have otherwise failed to respond to more traditional intrauterine treatments. It is of the utmost importance in each case to mate treated mares using a breeding management technique to minimize uterine contamination and optimize her chances for conception.[9]

UTERINE CYSTS

There are two distinct types of uterine cysts recognized. Endometrial glandular cysts are smaller (5 to 10 mm) and usually are the result of periglandular fibrosis. Lymphatic lacunar cysts are areas of lymphangiectasia. They can be from one to several centimeters in diameter and tend to be more problematic for the mare's future breeding serviceability. Uterine cysts are diagnosed clinically either during palpation per rectum examination of the uterus (e.g., when they are either large or numerous), during ultrasonography (e.g., when they are smaller or fewer in number) (Figure 17-1), or during hysteroscopy (Figure 17-2). The prevalence of uterine cysts recorded by investigators in one study found at least one cyst in 27% of 295 mares examined by ultrasonography during one breeding season.[10] They determined that mares greater

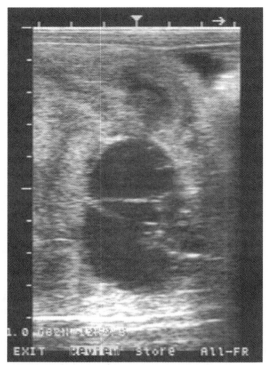

Figure 17-1 Ultrasonographic image of a nest of uterine cysts. Markers on the left and top of image equal 1 cm.

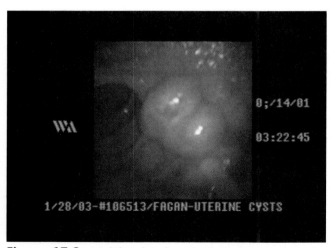

Figure 17-2 Multiloculated nest of uterine cysts at the base of the right uterine horn. Nd:YAG fiber can be seen in the lower right corner.

than 11 years of age were 4.2 times more likely to have endometrial cysts than mares less than 11. Logistic regression models failed to show a significant impact on the presence of endometrial cysts and successfully establishing and maintaining pregnancy. Adams et al[11] reported that single small cysts or even groups of small cysts do not adversely affect fertility. However, mares with greater than five cysts or cysts larger than 1 cm in diameter have lower 40-day pregnancy rates when compared with mares with fewer or smaller cysts. Uterine cysts were associated with a greater embryonic loss rate between means of 22

and 44 days (embryo loss of 24% in mares with cysts versus 6% in mares without cysts), but no effect of fetal loss (44 to 310 days) was found.[12] Another report involving 259 mares[13] found a slightly lower overall incidence of cysts (22%). However, a significantly lower (P < 0.01) overall day 40 pregnancy rate was found among mares with cysts (71.4%) when compared with mares without cysts (88%). A report from Germany[14] documenting endometrial cysts in 11 (13.4%) of 82 mares stated that they found no evidence of cysts in mares less than 10 years of age. Also, mares with endometrial cysts had a 10% higher history of disturbed fertility than mares without endometrial cysts. However, seven of nine mares with cystic structures in the uterus became pregnant.[14] Assigning clinical significance to the presence of uterine cysts is therefore a problem in broodmare practice.

It is held that the presence of numerous or large cysts can prevent or obstruct embryonic mobility during prefixation stages and thus jeopardize maternal recognition of pregnancy. Later in pregnancy, nutrient absorption between the yolk sac, or allantois, and endometrial glands may be limited due to intervening contact with large cyst wall(s), thus jeopardizing embryonic or fetal survival. Newcombe[15] suggested that when the conceptus begins development adjacent to normal endometrium it is likely to have normal development; however, if it begins development directly adjacent to a cyst, nutrient deprivation may cause pregnancy loss. The observation that larger uterine cysts frequently develop at the junction of the uterine body and horn[16] may on occasion lead to problems associated with misdiagnosis of singleton and/or twin pregnancies.

There is a positive correlation between the presence of uterine cysts and degree of endometrial fibrosis observed in histopathologic samples,[1-4] as well as with age of the mare.[10,13-16] One report, involving the use of videoendoscopic examination of the uterus of subfertile mares, documented that all mares with more than one cyst were classified as category II (Kenney system[2]), or worse, on their corresponding endometrial biopsies.[17] However, the absence of cysts did not exclude the presence of significant histopathologic changes. In the same study, only 4 of the 48 mares that were observed to have had uterine cysts were younger than 10 years of age.

THERAPIES

Multiple treatment modalities have been described for uterine cysts. These have included mechanical curettage,[8] rupture of large, discrete cysts either by manual rupture per vaginam or by endometrial biopsy forceps,[18] hysteroscopy and rupture by biopsy forceps or fine-needle aspiration,[19] electrocoagulative removal of cysts,[20,21] repeated uterine lavage with warmed (40° to 45°C) hypertonic saline or with warmed (40° to 45°C) magnesium sulfate solution,[22,23] and endoscopically guided photoablation using laser technology.[24-26]

Six mares selected for treatment by hysteroscopically directed electrocoagulative removal of endometrial cysts were reported by Brook and Frankel.[19] Of these, three mares subsequently conceived and presumably carried to term. All mares had previously exhibited poor breeding performance, and endometrial cysts were described as their only detectable abnormality.

Photoablation of uterine cysts in the mare is an extension of earlier work done in human medicine. Photoablation of endometriosis tissue using a CO_2 laser in human gynecologic surgery was first reported by Bruhat et al in 1977.[26] The first successful use of an operative hysteroscope with neodymium:yttrium-aluminum-garnet (Nd:YAG) laser to destroy endometrium was reported in 1981.[27] Nd:YAG has surfaced as the predominant laser in the field of gynecologic surgery because of its coagulative properties. It is not well absorbed by blood, so the energy is able to penetrate through the vessel wall, causing contraction of surrounding tissues and therefore contributing to the control of bleeding. When compared with other laser modalities, vessels of much greater diameter can be coagulated up to 3 to 5 mm with Nd:YAG. It also has a wide power range from 15 to 100 watts and can be used in water or saline solutions without altering its thermal effect, therefore making it one of the most versatile of medical lasers. Because it can be conducted safely down optical fibers, it is the laser of choice for uterine surgery.[28] Endometrium has amazing regenerative capabilities, and women can become pregnant following Nd:YAG laser ablation of the endometrium for menorrhagia.[29-31] With this information Nd:YAG has been used for uterine cyst photoablation in the mare.

Laser ablation of uterine cysts using Nd:YAG has been described in the mare.[24-26] The laser is directed hysteroscopically through a flexible endoscope using the biopsy channel port (Figures 17-2 and 17-3) for introduction of the laser fiber.[25] Six mares received this treatment by Blikslager,[23] and three subsequently produced live foals. Griffin and Bennett[26] reported on 55 barren mares treated with laser photoablation to remove uterine cysts; 26 of the 39 (66.7%) mares that were available for follow-up survey were reported to have conceived.

The authors in collaboration with multiple clinicians have been actively involved in clinical research in this area over the past 7 years. In our program mares with cysts greater than 20 mm in diameter or those that may be less

than 20 mm but are cylindrical and cover more surface area are considered candidates for laser ablation. These large lymphatic cysts are often pedunculated, and vaporization of these cysts at their base allows quick drainage and tissue excision. This method appears to be the most desirable approach for complete elimination of the structure. Cysts with large bases may require multiple passes for complete ablation. Cysts embedded deeper in the endometrium are usually small and possibly cystic dilations of degenerated endometrial glands. These can be lysed by linear vaporization, thus allowing evacuation of the contents and apparent dissolution following necrosis of the margins. It is necessary to destroy the endometrial gland dilations within the stratum compactum or cause coagulation of the lymphatic lacuna to prevent regrowth of endometrial cysts and lymphatic cysts, respectively.

The Nd:YAG laser produces tissue coagulation necrosis for about 2 to 4 mm in all directions around the zone of vaporization. This causes a point destruction of the endometrium to the superficial myometrium without threatening the integrity of the deeper myometrium. Immediately post laser ablation of large lymphatic cysts or detectable endometrial cysts, the remaining structure is reduced to a small area of carbonized or blanched tissue with a concomitant radius of erythematous tissue.

Although it has been stated that frequently the endometrium associated with uterine cysts and dilations is atrophied with a resultant decrease in the number of glands and an increase in collagen[19] and therefore may not regenerate after their removal,[32] we have found the endometrium capable of restoration at the site of photoablation. Within 14 days post vaporization, often the only marker remaining is a small (<2 mm) foci of carbon and hemosiderin, and by 28 days post vaporization nothing more can be found than a focal area of white scar tissue, usually 1 to 2 mm in diameter if found at all. When comparing endometrial histopathology of biopsies taken before laser treatment, 14 days and 28 days post treatment, preliminary results indicate no concomitant increase in endometrial fibrosis or glandular degeneration in the area of cyst ablation over that found in the uterus before laser surgery. There is also no significant indication of cyst redevelopment in the site of the previous cyst. However, some mares develop both lymphatic and endometrial cysts in other areas of the uterus. The exact mechanism(s) behind this has not been elucidated. One critical point is that photoablation of uterine cysts does not improve the general health of the endometrium. Although there appears to be no significant increase in diffuse or periglandular fibrosis at ablation sites, the mare with a grade IIb endometrium due to fibrosis remains at a grade IIb following treatment.

Because laser therapy involves invading the uterine lumen, the evacuation of cyst contents into the lumen, and the destruction of endometrial and lymphatic tissue, an acute inflammatory response ensues, peaking within 24 to 48 hours. Immediately following laser surgery, the uterus is lavaged with 2 to 3 L of sterile lactated Ringer's solution. The subsequent inflammatory response may help clear necrotic debris, depositing it as a mucopurulent accumulation within the uterine lumen for 2 to 3 days post treatment. To clear this material the uterus is volume

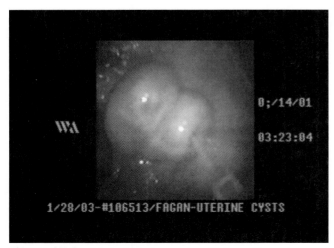

Figure 17-3 Nest of uterine cysts with laser fiber advanced and in contact just before photoablation.

lavaged during this period and beyond, if indicated. Ultrasonography is performed concomitant to the lavage therapy to reevaluate the need for further clearance treatment. To assist in uterine emptying, adjunct therapy may include oxytocin or prostaglandin $F_{2\alpha}$ to increase myometrial activity and tone. Volume lavage continues until no further fluid accumulates within the uterine lumen. Usually two to three flushes are all that are needed.

Although we have ample anecdotal evidence of improved fertility, until our current study is completed we cannot say that pregnancy rates are significantly increased after laser cyst ablation. However, we have had mares come into our program with a history of being barren that have successfully become pregnant and carried foals to term following laser ablation of cystic structures in the uterine lumen. Combining the reports of Blikslager[23] and Griffin and Bennett[25] with our preliminary findings, there is a growing body of evidence suggesting an improvement in fertility post photoablation of large uterine cysts. It appears that larger cysts, greater than 20 to 25 mm in diameter, present a challenge to the conceptus for complete prefixation migration. Location of these larger cysts may also play a role. Those located at the angle of the uterine horn near the bifurcation, which is the site of normal fixation, may also affect proper fixation and orientation. Further study in this area is warranted.

Although the availability of photoablative technology is an important advance in the field of equine theriogenology, its access to the practitioner remains limited to university clinics and larger equine referral clinics.

The number of different treatments attempted for this problem suggests the inability of any one treatment to be consistently successful. When looking toward the horizon, reports from human gynecologic studies suggest future therapies that may find their way into veterinary medicine and the treatment of uterine cystic structures. Magnetic resonance imaging (MRI) has been reported in delimiting and contributing to the diagnosis of adenomyotic cysts and other neoplastic lesions in the uterus,[33,34] and percutaneous MRI-guided laser ablation has been reported as a minimally invasive treatment of symptomatic fibroids.[35] A combination of ultrasonographically guided aspiration followed by an injection of the antimetabolite methotrexate has been reported to effectively treat endometriotic cysts[36] and may hold potential for treatment of intrauterine neoplastic lesions. Also, color flow Doppler combined with gray scale ultrasound used in detecting uterine vascular flow dynamics may lead to a greater understanding of the development of uterine cysts and their impact on early gestational events.[37,38] With the adaptation and implementation of these or similar therapy and diagnostic modalities, a greater understanding of the impact and treatment of uterine cystic structures may emerge.

References

1. Kenney RM: Chronic degenerative endometritis (CDE). Endometrosis. Equine endometritis: The John P. Hughes International Workshop. Equine Vet J 1993; 25:184-193.

2. Kenney RM: Cyclic and pathological changes of the mare endometrium as detected by biopsy with a note on early embryonic death. J Am Vet Med Assoc 1978; 172:241-262.

3. Ricketts SW: Endometrial biopsy as a guide to diagnosis of endometrial pathology in the mare. J Reprod Fertil Suppl 1975; 23:341-345.

4. Kenney RM, Ganjam VR: Selected pathological changes of the mare's uterus and ovaries. J Reprod Fertil Suppl 1975; 23:335-339.

5. Ley WB: Treating endometrosis in mares. Vet Med 1994; 89(8):778-788.

6. Ley WB, Bowen JM, Sponenberg DP et al: Dimethyl sulfoxide intrauterine therapy in the mare: effects upon endometrial histomorphological features and biopsy classification. Theriogenology 1989; 32(2):263-275.

7. Bracher V, Neuschaefer A, Allen WR: The effect of intrauterine infusion of kerosene on the endometrium of mares. J Reprod Fertil Suppl 1991; 44:706-707.

8. Ricketts SW: Endometrial curettage in the mare. Equine Vet J 1985; 17(4):324-328.

9. Pycock JF: Breeding management of the problem mare. In Samper JC (ed): Equine Breeding Management and Artificial Insemination, pp 223-224, Philadelphia, WB Saunders, 2000.

10. Eilts BE, Scholl DT, Paccamonti DL et al: Prevalence of endometrial cysts and their effect on fertility. Biol Reprod Mono 1995; 1:527-532.

11. Adams GP, Kastelic JP, Bergfelt DR et al: Effect of uterine inflammation and ultrasonically-detected uterine pathology on fertility of mares. J Reprod Fertil Suppl 1987; 35:445-454.

12. Chevalier-Clement F: Pregnancy loss in the mare. Anim Reprod Sci 1989; 20:231-244.

13. Tannus RJ, Thun R: Influence of endometrial cysts on conception rate of mares. J Vet Med 1995; 42:275-283.

14. Leidl W, Kaspar B, Kahn W: Endometrial cysts in the mare. II. Clinical studies: occurrence and significance. Tierartzl Prax 1987; 15:281-289.

15. Newcombe JR: Embryonic loss and abnormalities of early pregnancy. Equine Vet Educ 2000; April, pp 115-131.

16. Kaspar B, Kahn W, Laging C et al: Endometrial cysts in the mare. I. Post-mortem examinations: occurrence and morphology. Tierartzl Prax 1987; 15:161-166.

17. Bracher V, Mathias S, Allen WR: Videoendoscopic evaluation of the mare's uterus. II. Findings in subfertile mares. Equine Vet J 1992; 24(4):279-284.

18. Neeley DP: Evaluation and therapy of genital disease in the mare. In Hughes JP (ed): Equine Reproduction, pp 40-56, New Jersey, Nutley, Hoffman-LaRouche, Inc, 1983.

19. Brook D, Frankel K: Electrocoagulative removal of endometrial cysts in the mare. J Equine Vet Sci 1987; 7(2):77-81.

20. Van Ittersum AR: Electrosurgical treatment of endometrial cysts. Tijdschr Diergeneeskd 1999; 124:630-633.

21. Bowman RT: New distinctions advance knowledge of infertility. Mod Horse Breed 1993; 10:7-13.

22. Dascanio JJ, Parker NA, Ley WB et al: Effect of magnesium sulfate on the equine endometrium. Proceedings of the 42nd Annual Convention of the American Association of Equine Practitioners, pp 148-149, 1996.

23. Blikslager AT, Tate LP, Weinstock D: Effects of neodymium:yttrium aluminum garnet (Nd:YAG) laser irradiation on endometrium and on endometrial cysts in six mares. Vet Surg 1993; 22(5):351-356.

24. Ley WB, Higbee RG, Holyoak GR: Laser ablation of endometrial and lymphatic cysts. Clin Tech Eq Pract 2002; 1(1):28-31.

25. Griffin RL, Bennett SD: Nd:YAG photoablation of endometrial cysts: a review of 55 cases (2000-2001). Proceedings of the 48th Annual Convention of the American Association of Equine Practitioners, pp 58-60, 2002.

26. Bruhat MA, Mage G, Manhes H: Use of CO_2 laser by laparoscopy. In Kaplan I (ed): Laser Surgery III: Proceedings of the Third International Congress on Laser Surgery, Tel Aviv, Jerusalem, 1977.

27. Goldrath MH, Fuller TA, Segal S: Laser photovaporization of the endometrium for treatment of menorrhagia. Am J Obstet Gynecol 1981; 140:14-19.

28. Davis J: The principles and use of the neodymium-YAG laser in gynaecological surgery. In Baillier's Clinical Obstetrics and Gynaecology, vol 1, pp 331-352.

29. Garry R, Erian J, Grochmal SA: A multi-centre collaborative study into the treatment of menorrhagia by Nd-YAG laser ablation of the endometrium. Br J Obstet Gynaecol 1991; 98:357-362.

30. Pugh CP, Crane JM, Hogan TG: Successful intrauterine pregnancy after endometrial ablation. J Am Assoc Gynecol Laparosc 2000; 7:391-394.

31. Pinette M, Katz W, Drouin M et al: Successful planned pregnancy following endometrial ablation with the YAG laser. Am J Obstet Gynecol 2001; 185:242-243.

32. Van Camp SD: Uterine abnormalities. In McKinnon AO, Voss JL (eds): Equine Reproduction, pp 392-396, Media, Pa, Williams & Wilkins, 1993.

33. Kataoka ML, Togashi K, Konishi I et al: MRI of adenomyotic cyst of the uterus. J Comput Assist Tomogr 1998; 22:555-559.

34. Robert Y, Launay S, Mestdagh P et al: MRI in gynecology. J Gynecol Obstet Biol Reprod 2002; 31:417-439.

35. Hindley JT, Law PA, Hickey M et al: Clinical outcomes following percutaneous magnetic resonance image guided laser ablation of symptomatic uterine fibroids. Human Reprod 2002; 17:2737-2741.

36. Mesogitis S, Anatsaklis A, Daskalakis G et al: Combined ultrasonographically guided drainage and methotrexate administration of endometriotic cysts. Lancet 2000; 355: 1160.

37. Carter JR, Lau M, Saltzman AK et al: Gray scale and color flow Doppler characterization of uterine tumors. J Ultrasound Med 1994; 13:835-840.

38. Jauniaux E, Greenwold N, Hempstock J et al: Comparison of ultrasonographic and Doppler mapping of the intervillous circulation in normal and abnormal early pregnancies. Fertil Steril 2003; 79:100-106.

CHAPTER 18

Some Unusual Conditions of the Uterus

JOHN P. HURTGEN

A wide variety of conditions may affect the uterus of the mare but occur at a low frequency. Many of these conditions are frequently overlooked, in part because the uterine size and consistency may not be altered and/or the mare's cyclicity may not be affected. A few of these unusual conditions will be presented, but this list is not exhaustive.

ASYNCHRONY OF ESTROUS BEHAVIOR AND OVARIAN ACTIVITY, WITH ENDOMETRIAL HISTOLOGY

During the transitional phase at the beginning of the breeding season, it is common for mares to exhibit erratic estrous cycles, ovulatory patterns, and estrous behavior not necessarily in synchrony with ovarian activity. This transitional pattern normally becomes quite predictable after one or two estrous cycles. However, each year in private veterinary practice a number of mares appear to be normal in all respects but fail to become pregnant for three or more estrous cycles.

Asynchrony of estrous and ovarian activity with uterine histology, however, has been observed during the natural breeding season (May, June, July, and August). Affected mares have normal estrous cycles and develop normal ovulatory follicles during estrus yet fail to conceive following breeding. The uterine consistency seems normal on rectal evaluation, but the pattern of uterine edema during estrus is less pronounced compared with subsequent cycles. In order to determine the cause of infertility, an endometrial biopsy specimen has been obtained from some of these mares. In general the histologic appearance of the endometrium is suggestive of the anestrous or the early transitional phase of the mare's reproductive cycle. The luminal epithelium is frequently cuboidal or low columnar, the density of the endometrial glands is reduced, and the endometrial glands are straight, have a small diameter, and appear inactive. Frequently, one or two estrous cycles later, these mares become pregnant or have an endometrial biopsy specimen representative of the breeding season. The uterine consistency seems normal on rectal evaluation, but the pattern of uterine edema during estrus is less pronounced compared with subsequent cycles.

The cause of the asynchrony of the endometrial architecture with ovarian activity is unknown. Hormonal profiles of these mares have not been recorded. Possible explanations may include inappropriate lighting schemes before the breeding season, such as inadequate lighting or constant 24-hours-per-day lighting. Mares that exhibit this syndrome are not likely to repeat this pattern in subsequent breeding seasons. In most cases these mares are identified after three or four cycles have passed, so specific therapy is not initiated. If these mares can be identified before breeding, supplemental estrogen and progesterone may stimulate the endometrium to develop the architecture expected for cyclic mares during the natural breeding season.

FOREIGN BODIES IN THE UTERUS

A wide variety of foreign bodies are occasionally found in the uterus. The majority of the foreign bodies or substances do not interfere with the mare's estrous cycle pattern. The most commonly recognized foreign body in the uterine lumen is the mummified fetus. In most cases of fetal mummification the mare will have normal estrous cycles during the breeding season. The mummified fetus may not be evacuated from the uterus during estrus due to the configuration of the fetus, size of the fetus, and lack of uterine fluids. Presence of a mummified fetus has been identified many days after a mare has delivered a live foal. In some cases the mummified fetus may become trapped in the cervical canal. Fetal mummification usually occurs during the second trimester but has been observed as early as 40 to 50 days of gestation. The presence of a mummified fetus can usually be identified by rectal palpation and ultrasonographic evaluation of the uterus. In the case of very early mummification of the fetus, the foreign body may not be recognized without the aid of endoscopy.

Treatment of fetal mummification involves regression of the corpus luteum, if present, to induce estrous and cervical dilation. The degree of cervical dilation should be evaluated, per vaginam, 3 to 4 days following prostaglandin. If the cervix is not adequately dilated, it may be useful to repeat the use of prostaglandin or administer estradiol (or PGE) to aid dilation. In many cases the cervix may need to be manually dilated to retrieve the mummified fetus. Infusion of the uterus with approximately 1 L of fluid may aid lubrication of the uterus and cervix. With slow deliberate manual dilation of the cervix, the fetus can usually be grasped and removed. The uterine environment is usually bacteriologically sterile. However, following manual manipulation and removal of the mummified fetus, the mare should be monitored for an induced endometritis.

On rare occasions the tip of an endometrial culture swab may break off within the uterus. In most cases the swab tip can be retrieved by passing two fingers through the cervix. The swab tip can also be visualized and recovered from the uterus with an endoscope that is equipped with a small biopsy forceps. If an endoscope is not available, the swab can be located using ultrasonography per rectum while a grasping instrument (forceps or biopsy punch) is passed through the cervix in a sterile fashion to grasp the swab.

Certain medications may precipitate or crystallize in the uterine lumen, leaving a residue on the endometrial surface. Although ampicillin and gentamicin are the antibiotics most frequently implicated, the formulation and pH of these medications are important factors. If this material is allowed to remain in the uterus, the mare may become infertile. Therapy involves the removal of the residual material by copious uterine lavage and induction of estrus using prostaglandin. The lavage should be repeated until the flush fluid is void of residual medication. Following removal of the foreign material, fertility should be normal.

TRANSLUMINAL ADHESIONS

Transluminal adhesions are occasionally encountered following endometritis associated with dystocia, tissue damage to the endometrium, or following the use of harsh medications or fluids in the uterus. The most commonly implicated caustic medications involved in transluminal adhesion formation include chlorhexidine, iodine, and unbuffered gentamicin. These products have been used safely in the uterus of mares, but the appropriate frequency of use, stage of cycle, and concentration of medication have not been determined in controlled studies of normal endometria and seriously inflamed uteri. In the majority of cases when these caustic treatments are used, other medications are available with much reduced endometrial irritation and possible subsequent transluminal adhesions.

Transluminal adhesions are usually diagnosed with the use of endoscopic evaluation of the uterine lumen. The adhesions appear as scar tissue and bands of tissue traversing the uterine lumen and occasionally completely occlude an entire uterine horn or portion of it. Dilation of the uterus with fluid or air may result in a nonuniform filling of the uterine lumen. Affected mares usually have markedly reduced fertility because of intraluminal adhesions, underlying periglandular or endometrial fibrosis, and altered early embryo mobility.

The transluminal adhesions may be broken down manually by passing a gloved hand through the dilated cervix. The adhesions may also be freed using laser surgery. Although the uterine condition of the treated mares may appear clinically improved, fertility usually remains poor because of the underlying scar tissue formation and periglandular fibrosis.

PELVIC AND VISCERAL ADHESIONS INVOLVING THE UTERUS

Adhesions of the uterus or cervix to other structures in the pelvic cavity or abdomen can interfere with fertility and maintenance of pregnancy. These adhesions may develop in association with uterine surgery such as cesarean section, uterine or ovarian artery rupture, postpartum metritis, peritonitis, uterine laceration associated with fetal movement, forced fetal extraction or fetotomy, and uterine trauma associated with ovariectomy. The uterine adhesions may involve the pelvic cavity, bladder, ovary, or viscera. If the adhesions are not extensive, mares may still become pregnant and carry a foal to term with the adhesions resolving or breaking down during the course of uterine descent during pregnancy. The periuterine adhesions may alter uterine position or uterine motility, resulting in increased risk of uterine fluid accumulation and susceptibility to endometritis.

Periuterine adhesions are usually not treated because of the inaccessibility of the uterus for surgery. The advent of laser treatment of adhesions may allow some of the more accessible structures to be freed by laser surgery using a paralumbar or midline approach. Before this type of abdominal surgery is performed, the health of the uterus should be evaluated by manual examination of the uterus, vagina, and cervix, bacteriologic culture of the uterus, and endometrial biopsy.

CHAPTER 19

Congenital Abnormalities Involving the Cervix and Uterus

JOHN P. HURTGEN

Congenital abnormalities involving the uterus or cervix are rare in the horse. However, these abnormalities are frequently associated with infertility, even sterility. Many mares with congenital abnormalities of the cervix or uterus are bred on repeated cycles and for years before a thorough examination identifies the abnormality. Congenital abnormalities of the cervix or uterus may be associated with normal or abnormal estrous behavior patterns and ovarian function.

CHROMOSOMAL ABNORMALITIES

Mares with chromosomal abnormalities, such as 63XO, 64XY, 65XXY, and others, usually have gonadal dysgenesis. In addition to very small ovaries or even testicular tissue, the mares usually have very underdeveloped uteri and an infantile, open cervix. A cytogenetic evaluation (see Chapter 10) should be performed on blood or tissue samples from mares with developmental abnormalities of the cervix, uterus, oviducts, or ovaries.[1] On rare occasions, mares with congenital absence of the cervix or uterus may have normal ovaries. The reproductive tract of mares with gonadal dysgenesis may still be responsive to progesterone and estrogen. Pregnancy has been established in XO mares in an embryo transfer program when the mares were treated with estrogen and progesterone.[2]

CERVICAL ABNORMALITIES

Rare cases of double cervix have been reported in the mare. Each cervical canal may not communicate with the uterine body but end as a blind-ended canal, or the two canals may converge to enter the uterus. These mares are usually fertile and deliver foals uneventfully. However, artificial insemination procedures could be frustrating if the selected canal ends blindly.

An occasional mare has been identified with a double cervix connected to separate uterine horns. The uterine horns do not communicate. These mares are likely to be sterile due to lack of embryo migration and lack of uterine space for pregnancy development. Luteal regression is likely to occur due to the systemic prostaglandin release, which is normally prevented with embryo migration throughout the uterus.[3] However, the author has had a Clydesdale mare with separate cervical canals associated with independent uterine horns deliver a small viable foal at term. However, due to the mare's breeding history of prior pregnancy loss, the mare was maintained on oral altrenogest during the entire successful gestation. In an embryo transfer program, this mare produced numerous embryos and foals. Interestingly, this mare also had a total aplasia of one ovary and had normal endometrial edema in both horns during estrus. Another case of uterus bicollis has also been reported in a Clydesdale.[4]

Although congenital abnormalities of the müllerian and paramesonephric ducts can occur in any breed, there seems to be an increased incidence of these abnormalities in Clydesdale and Shire horses. The author has had two unrelated Shire mares with segmental aplasia of a uterine horn (uterus unicornis). Both mares were bred repeatedly by live cover or artificial insemination (AI) without success. The mares had been diagnosed pregnant a number of times due to the localized accumulation of fluid in the uterine horn not connected to the cervix. Ultrasonographic evaluation should identify these mares before breeding and determine pregnancy status with certainty in those that have been bred. Embryo transfer should be successful in obtaining embryos from uterine segmental aplasia mares if ovulation occurs from the ovary associated with the patent cervix and uterine horn.

Extreme tortuosity of the cervix is occasionally encountered in the mare. The cervical canal does not appear to relax during estrus as expected. These mares also tend to accumulate varying amounts of fluid in the uterine body during estrus. These mares are capable of becoming pregnant if fluid accumulation is prevented and semen is deposited in the uterine body. Fertility of affected mares is likely to be improved when artificial insemination is employed. A breed predisposition has not been noted. Although not documented, there is some suggestion that mares with Cushing's disease may be prone to cervical tortuosity.

A single case of cervical hyperplasia has been reported in a 5-year-old maiden mare.[5] The mare was presented for evaluation due to chronic vulvar prolapsing of cervical tissue.

Hypoplasia of the cervix is extremely rare in the mare with normal ovarian function and a normal karyotype.[6]

Although congenital abnormalities of the cervix and uterus are rare in the mare, a thorough evaluation of these organs by manual evaluation, rectal palpation, and ultrasonography should identify the majority of these individuals before mating. In the majority of the above cases, therapy is unrewarding.

References

1. Bowling AT, Millon L, Hughes JP: An update of chromosomal abnormalities in mares. J Reprod Fertil Suppl 1987; 35:149-155.
2. Hinrichs K, Riera FL, Klunder LR: Establishment of pregnancy after embryo transfer in mares with gonadal dysgenesis. J In Vitro Fert Embryo Transf 1989; 6:305-309.
3. Ginther OJ, Garcia MC, Squires EL et al: Anatomy of vasculature of uterus and ovaries in the mare. Am J Vet Res 1972; 33:1561-1568.
4. Volkmann DH, Gilbert RO: Uterus bicollis in a Clydesdale mare. Equine Vet J 1989; 21:71.
5. Riera FL, Hinrichs K, Hunt PR et al: Cervical hyperplasia with prolapse in a mare. J Am Vet Med Assoc 1989; 195:1393-1394.
6. Blanchard TL, Evan LH, Kenney RM et al: Congenitally incompetent cervix in a mare. J Am Vet Med Assoc 1982; 181:266.

CHAPTER 20

Cervical Tears

ROLF M. EMBERTSON
CORTNEY E. HENDERSON

Cervical lacerations or tears, which often form defects when healed, have long been recognized as a cause of mare infertility. The cervix can function as a physical barrier, separating the uterus from the vagina. During pregnancy and diestrus, when under the influence of progesterone, this muscular tube is tightly closed. This barrier protects the uterus from infectious agents and debris that may have gained access to the cranial vagina. Depending on size, a defect in the cervix may adversely affect cervical function and thus the ability of the mare to conceive and carry a foal to term. It is important for fertility that cervical defects be promptly recognized and managed appropriately.

ANATOMIC FEATURES OF THE EQUINE CERVIX

The cervix of a nongravid mare in diestrus typically is a strong and resilient tubular smooth muscle sphincter measuring 2.5 to 5.0 cm in diameter and 5.0 to 7.5 cm in length.[1] The muscular cervix is an extension of the uterine body, with the distal portion protruding caudally into the anterior vagina and containing the external cervical os. The endometrial folds of the uterine body continue longitudinally along the length of the cervical canal and create the folded mucosal surface of the cervical lumen. The cervical epithelium is made up of ciliated epithelial and mucus-producing cells.[2] The vascular and nerve supply to the cervix comes primarily from the vaginal artery, vein, and nerve. The vaginal artery arises from the internal pudendal artery, branching from the internal iliac artery, which is a terminal branch of the abdominal aorta.[3]

ETIOLOGY OF CERVICAL LACERATIONS

An important characteristic of the equine cervix is the inherent elasticity of the cervical tissue. This elasticity allows the cervical walls to expand greatly for passage of the fetus during parturition. Cervical lacerations occur most commonly from excessive and/or abrupt cervical stretching during foaling. This is especially true if the cervix has not relaxed sufficiently. Cervical tears are more likely to occur during dystocia than during normal parturition. Nevertheless, a cervical tear can occur during unassisted, normal foaling. In fact, one study showed that 86% of the mares presented for cervical defect repair sustained the injury after an apparently normal foaling.[4] Manipulations performed to deliver a fetus vaginally from a mare in dystocia, are sometimes done with swollen tissues and inadequate lubrication.[5,6] This places the cervix at increased risk for injury. A fetotomy also increases the risk for cervical trauma.

Other causes of cervical defects are rare. Cervical laceration in an Arabian mare as a result of cervical penetration by the stallion's penis during breeding has been reported.[7] Cervical incompetency due to congenital failure of cervical closure has been reported in a 2-year-old filly.[8]

No site around the circumference of the cervix has been reported to be predisposed to tearing.[9] This finding is supported by our clinical experience. Presentation for cervical defect repair in the thoroughbred is most commonly done in the middle-aged, multiparous mare.[4]

DIAGNOSTICS

The most common problems associated with cervical defects are endometritis and infertility. Failure to conceive and early term abortion are problems more commonly seen with large cervical defects. Late-gestation abortion is more commonly seen with medium size defects.

Careful examination of the cervix is an important part of the reproductive examination of the mare. A vaginal speculum is routinely used in evaluation of the cervix. Cervical defects can be overlooked, however, on the basis of visual inspection alone. This is especially true during the estrous period, when visualization of the defect may be obstructed because of the presence of tissue edema. Edematous cervical folds may overlap and obscure the laceration site from view.[7] The cervix ideally is examined with the mare in diestrus. The cervix exhibits minimal edema and is contracted and tight, allowing accurate evaluation of the competency of the cervical wall. Digital palpation is necessary for full appreciation of a cervical defect.

Recording or describing the site of a cervical abnormality is simplified by considering the external margin of the cervix as analogous to the face of a circular clock (Fig. 20-1). The most dorsal aspect of the cervix corresponds to the 12 o'clock position, whereas the ventral-most aspect corresponds to the 6 o'clock position. Palpation of the cervix is done using a sterile glove or sleeve and an ample amount of sterile lubricant. The cervical wall is evaluated between the operator's thumb and index finger, with either the thumb or finger inserted into

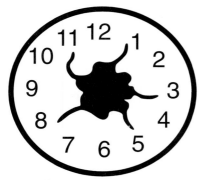

Figure 20-1 The clock face analogy used to identify location on the cervix (normal).

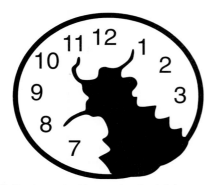

Figure 20-2 A cervical laceration is visible extending from the 4 o'clock to the 6 o'clock position.

the lumen. The circumference of the cervix is carefully palpated to identify any defect in the cervical wall. The clock face analogy is used to characterize the location of the defect (Fig. 20-2).

The severity and extent of the cervical laceration should be determined. Most lacerations affect the vaginal part of the cervix, but some extend cranially into the uterine cervix. Findings on palpation of the cervix soon after foaling can be difficult to interpret, but this examination may be warranted after known birthing trauma. Examination findings are more accurate after resolution of the edema and contraction of the cervical muscle. Rarely, palpation of a recently torn cervix reveals penetration into the abdomen, which requires immediate attention.

INDICATIONS FOR SURGICAL REPAIR

If the cervix proves to be competent under the influence of progesterone and the defect involves less than 50% of the length of the cervix, surgical repair may not be needed.[9] Repair is indicated for defects greater than 50% of the cervical length and for smaller defects if the mare is infertile with few other obvious reproductive abnormalities. As the width of the defect increases, the degree of surgical difficulty also increases, and the prognosis decreases. Although less than ideal, defects involving up

to 50% of the circumference of the cervix can be successfully repaired. It is not unusual for a cervical defect to have mucosa bridging a gap in the cervical muscle. These defects should follow the same guidelines as above regarding cervical repair.

SURGICAL REPAIR OF THE DEFECT

Surgical Considerations

Surgical repair of a cervical laceration should ideally be delayed for at least 60 days after injury, to allow for healing and contraction of the tissues. Some pressure to rebreed the mare as soon as possible is a frequent consideration, however. Surgical repair of a cervical defect 3 to 4 weeks after injury can be consistently and successfully done. The surgery is routinely accomplished as a standing procedure and on an outpatient basis. We prefer the mare to be in diestrus, with the cervix as tight as possible. These conditions afford the best opportunity for accurate apposition of tissue layers during the repair. If two defects are present in the cervix, it is preferred to repair them at least 3 to 4 weeks apart.

Anesthetic Considerations

Surgical repair of a cervical laceration is facilitated by having the mare standing, restrained in stocks, and under the influence of sedation and epidural anesthesia. The procedure can be performed with the mare under general anesthesia and positioned in dorsal or sternal recumbency, if needed. Different medications and methods of administration can be used to provide adequate sedation and analgesia to yield a cooperative patient for a standing procedure. We have used the following protocol for several years to provide generally consistent results in a 500-kg mare. The mare initially is sedated with 18 mg of detomidine given intramuscularly. As the sedation takes effect, she is placed in stocks, her tail wrapped, and the site prepared for epidural anesthesia. Just before placement of the epidural needle, 150 mg of xylazine is administered intravenously. The epidural anesthetic solution is prepared in a 10-ml syringe by combining 85 mg of xylazine and 20 mg or 1 ml of 2% lidocaine HCl. This mixture is diluted to a volume of 6 ml with sterile saline solution (0.9% NaCl). A 20-gauge, 3.5-inch (9-cm) spinal needle is directed into the aperture between the first two coccygeal vertebral arches (usually at the first movable joint in the tail). The needle is inserted over the dorsal spinous process of the second vertebra and then directed at a 30-degree angle to the skin surface toward this aperture. Generally the entire length of the needle is used to penetrate the epidural space. The hub of the needle is then filled with anesthetic solution. If the needle is accurately placed, the negative pressure within the epidural space will draw this fluid in from the hub. The remaining solution is then administered and the needle withdrawn. The effect of the epidural should become apparent within 15 minutes and persist for 2 to 3 hours. It is not unusual, with use of this technique, to find that cutaneous perineal and vulvar sensation is still present.

Patient Preparation

In preparation for surgery, the mare is administered pre-operative medication. The drug selection typically consists of intravenous potassium penicillin G at a dosage of 10,000 IU/kg, intravenous gentamicin at a dosage of 6.6 mg/kg, intravenous flunixin meglumine at a dosage of 1.1 mg/kg, and an intramuscular dose of tetanus toxoid of 1 ml. The mare's tail is wrapped and tied securely to the upper crossbar of the stocks with a knot that can be released in the event of an emergency. Tying the tail overhead serves to provide stabilization for the mare if significant ataxia occurs or if she loses footing on the often wet floor of the operating room. It also serves the purpose of mechanically removing the tail from the surgery site and helps to secure the retractors in place. Feces should be evacuated from the rectum. The perineal area is prepared for surgery using pieces of roll cotton, mild dish soap, and warm water. The perineum is cleansed from the vulva outward to the tailhead and including approximately 6 inches of the skin over the gluteal region on each side of the perineum. If the dorsal vulva has been sutured closed, the tissue should be blocked with local anesthetic solution and incised to the very dorsal extent of the vulva. This maneuver allows placement of large modified Finochietto retractors (Sontec Instruments, Englewood, Colo.) and provides access to the cervix.

Surgical Equipment

Equipment needed to repair a cervical laceration in the mare is not extensive but is specific for surgery within the vagina. Adequate lighting of the surgical field is a necessity and can be provided by a standing or hand-held lamp. A surgeon's head lamp, however, is far superior for illumination of the surgical site. The lamp should be positioned between and just below the level of the operator's eyes. A lamp positioned on the forehead creates problematic shadows. Long-handled instruments are essential for cervical surgery, because even with caudal traction of the cervix, the surgery is performed in the depths of the vagina. The instruments we use for this procedure are a long Bard-Parker No. 3 scalpel handle and No. 10 scalpel blade, a 12- to 16-inch tissue forceps, a 12- to 18-inch Mayo-Hegar needle holder, two 10-inch Allis tissue forceps, three Kelly forceps and a 12- to 16-inch Metzenbaum scissor. A modified Finochietto retractor with long detachable blades is invaluable for cervical surgery because the long blades extend cranial to the vaginovestibular junction, enabling visualization and manipulation of the cervix.

Surgical Procedure

The surgical repair of a cervical laceration begins by positioning of the modified Finochietto retractor within the caudal vaginal vault and retracting the vulva and caudal vagina to the maximal extent safely possible. The cervix is retracted caudally within the vaginal vault to gain access for surgical manipulation. This can be done with Knowles cervical forceps or stay sutures. We prefer stay sutures because they can be placed and held in a manner that does not interfere with the surgical repair. Two sutures (No. 2 or 3 braided suture on a large curved needle) are placed manually through the wall of the cervix, one on either side of the defect. A Kelly forceps is clamped onto the distal ends of each stay suture. The cervix is then retracted caudally, and another stay suture is placed through the wall of the cervix opposite from the defect. Use of a needle holder facilitates placement of this latter suture, because now the cervix is more easily reached. An assistant(s) applies caudal traction to the stay sutures. Alternatively, they may be secured to the modified Finochietto retractor to accomplish continuous caudal traction on the cervix. Allis tissue forceps are used to grasp and apply tension to the mucosa at the caudal edge of both sides of the defect. Next, an incision is made with a No.10 scalpel blade through the outer cervical mucosa along the edge of the defect. Long-handled scissors are then used to resect a strip of tissue along the margins of the defect. This maneuver exposes three distinct tissue layers and creates a V-shaped piece of tissue, which is then excised from the surgery site.

The three tissue layers are apposed individually, using No. 1 braided absorbable suture, to provide a secure closure of the defect. The suture is started at the cranial-most extent of the defect and continued caudally to the external os for each layer. The inner cervical mucosa is sutured first, in a continuous horizontal mattress pattern, inverting mucosa into the cervical lumen. During closure of this layer, the cervical lumen should be periodically evaluated for patency by digital exploration. This precaution will prevent creation of a partial obstruction caused by inadvertent catching of cervical mucosa by a misguided suture across the lumen from the defect. The cervical muscle is then sutured using a simple continuous pattern. The outer cervical (vaginal) mucosa is then closed in a simple continuous pattern, catching cervical muscle with each bite.

A two-layer repair technique also has been used successfully.[5,7] Using this technique, after débridement of the laceration, absorbable suture material on a cutting needle placed in a continuous pattern was used to close the cervical mucosal layer, with incorporation of the fibromuscular layer of the cervix into the suture line. The second continuous suture layer is placed in the vaginal mucosal layer and also incorporates the fibromuscular layer.

A post-breeding single-layer repair has been tried with some success.[10] This approach has been used in mares at the end of breeding season, when adequate time for tissue healing after traditional repair techniques was not available. This technique is performed 2 to 3 days after ovulation, with breeding by artificial insemination. The closure is accomplished using No. 0 monofilament absorbable suture in a simple continuous pattern. The suture line extends through the vaginal mucosal surface and bisects the fibromuscular layer, with consecutive sutures placed less than 1 cm apart. Four out of five mares were reported to have conceived as a result of the breeding preceding a single-layer repair.

Aftercare

Immediately after surgery, the uterus is infused with 3 g of ticarcillin disodium. Flunixin meglumine is continued for 3 to 5 days after surgery. The mare should have routine turnout exercise on return to the farm. Recently, we have recommended uterine lavage through a soft silicone tube for 3 to 5 days for postoperative management if the uterus became contaminated during the repair. The cervix should be re-evaluated 3 to 4 weeks after the repair. Healing of the cervical tissues should be adequate by 4 weeks for breeding to resume.

Complications

Complications related directly to the surgical repair of a cervical defect are uncommon. Although the procedure involves working in a surgical field that must be considered contaminated, problems with infection at the surgical site in the cervix are very unusual. As mentioned earlier, however, it is not usual for the uterus to become contaminated during this procedure, necessitating appropriate treatment.

Adhesions across the lumen of the cervix infrequently occur. These usually can be broken down using the fingers. Adhesions between the cervix and the vaginal wall are rare after this surgical procedure. In the latter instance, adhesions generally are the result of foaling trauma.

PROGNOSIS AND IMPLICATIONS FOR MARE FERTILITY

The prognosis for conception and carrying a foal to term generally is favorable after repair of a cervical defect. Several factors, however, play a role in postoperative fertility. Factors involving the cervix include the size of the defect, the presence of more than one defect, the amount of functional cervical muscle actually present, cervical adhesions and/or adjacent scar tissue, and the experience of the surgeon. Many other causes of infertility affecting the reproductive tract may be present, in addition to the cervical defect. The experience of the attending veterinarian and the expertise of the farm personnel also play a large role in foaling rates. Thus, it is difficult to accurately interpret foaling rates in mares that have undergone cervical defect repair. A 1984 study of 13 mares yielded a conception rate of 62.5% after cervical surgery.[9] A 1996 study of 53 thoroughbred mares indicated a pregnancy rate of 75.3% after surgical repair of a cervical defect.[4]

Mares that have had cervical surgery are at risk for reinjury occurring at a subsequent foaling. The 1996 study revealed that 26.4% of the mares had more than one surgical repair of their cervix. In a majority of mares, the cervix was reinjured at the same site of the previous defect. This susceptibility to reinjury probably is due to the decreased elasticity of scar tissue at the repair site, in comparison with that of normal cervical muscle, so that the risk of tearing is higher with stretching of the cervix during foaling. The cervix should be closely examined after foaling in mares that have had previous cervical surgery.

References

1. Walker DF, Vaughan JT: Bovine and Equine Urogenital Surgery. Philadelphia, Lea & Febiger, 1980.
2. Ley WB: Anatomy and physiology of the female reproductive system. In Wolf DF, Moll HD (eds): Large Animal Urogenital Surgery, Baltimore, Williams & Wilkins, 1999.
3. Dyce KM, Sack WO, Wensing CJ: Textbook of Veterinary Anatomy, 2nd ed, Philadelphia: WB Saunders, 1996.
4. Miller CD, Embertson RM, Smith S: Surgical repair of cervical lacerations in thoroughbred mares: 53 cases (1986-1995). Proceedings of the 42nd Annual Convention of the American Association of Equine Practitioners, pp 154-155, 1996.
5. Moll HD, May KA: Cervical lacerations. In Wolf DF, Moll HD (eds): Large Animal Urogenital Surgery, Baltimore, Williams & Wilkins, 1999.
6. Evans LH, Tate LP, Copper WL, et al: Surgical repair of cervical lacerations and the incompetent cervix. Proceedings of the 18th Annual Convention of the American Association of Equine Practitioners, pp 483-486, 1979.
7. Aanes WA: Surgical management of foaling injuries. Vet Clin North Am Equine Pract 1988; 4:417.
8. Blanchard TL, Evans LH, Kinney RM, et al: Congenitally incompetent cervix in a mare. J Am Vet Med Assoc 1982; 181:266.
9. Brown JS, Varner DD, Hinrichs K, et al: Surgical repair of the lacerated cervix in the mare. Theriogenology 1984; 22:351.
10. Foss RR, Wirth NR, Kutz RR: Post-breeding repair of cervical lacerations. Proceedings of the 40th Annual Convention of the American Association of Equine Practitioners, pp 11-12, 1994.

CHAPTER 21

Cervical Failure to Dilate

ANDRÉS J. ESTRADA

JUAN C. SAMPER

The uterine cervix, with the vulva and the vestibular fold, forms the natural barrier that separates the uterus from the external environment, thus protecting it from contamination. Some authors consider the cervix to include the most caudal part of the uterus, but because it is the main topic of this chapter we will refer to it as a single structure. The uterine cervix is a complex organ that works under neural, hormonal, and myogenic influences and is amazingly able to dilate during parturition. A brief review of the anatomy is necessary before we explore the different scenarios that the clinician may experience when the cervix fails to dilate. Some reported anomalies that interfere with the ability of the cervix to relax and dilate will also be discussed.

ANATOMY

The cervix averages 5 to 7 cm in length and 3 to 4 cm in width.[1,2] The cervix communicates cranially with the body of the uterus and caudally with the vagina, into which the caudal cervical portion projects. The cervix has a thick layer of smooth muscle and is rich in elastic fibers. Its degree of tone depends on the presence of progesterone, and its relaxation is determined by circulating estrogens during estrus. A distinctive feature of the mare's cervix is the complete absence of cervical rings, such as those found in cows. The cervix of the mare is arranged in longitudinal mucosal folds that are continuous with the endometrial folds of the uterine body and horns.[3] Each dorsal and ventral fold may continue onto the floor of the vagina as a prominent frenulum.[4] Among its different functions are the production of a large amount of mucus that may act as a lubricant for breeding purposes (especially natural breeding) or as a sealant during pregnancy, and the occlusion of the uterine lumen so that it is impermeable to foreign material and bacteria. The other important function is the dilation and expansion to its maximal diameter to allow the passage of the foal during parturition.

CONDITIONS IN WHICH THE CERVIX FAILS TO DILATE

The cervix does not normally dilate during two physiologic conditions in the mare. The first occurs when the mare is in the diestrus period of the estrous cycle, which falls between day 1 (day 0 = ovulation) and day 14 or 15, before the development of the follicular wave that will result in the next estrus period. The second physiologic condition in which the mare does not relax the cervix occurs during pregnancy. From the moment the mare recognizes her pregnancy status (maternal recognition between day 14 and 16), until hours before parturition when cervical dilation occurs due to hormonal changes to permit the delivery of the foal, the cervix is very tight. The hormonal changes that cause cervical relaxation include a decrease in progesterone and an increase in estrogens promoted by the cortisol released by the fetal adrenal glands.[5] It is worth noting that this closing of the cervix is due to the progesterone produced by the primary corpora lutea during diestrus and the progesterone/progestagens that are produced by the secondary corpora lutea and placenta when pregnant.

Adhesions

Cervical adhesions are the most common noninfectious abnormalities of the cervix. Adhesions are internal scars made up of strandlike fibrous tissue that forms an abnormal bond between two parts of the cervix after trauma, through complex processes involving the cervical area. Depending on the extension and the location, adhesion formation can compromise the ability of the cervix to dilate during estrous or parturition.

Adhesions usually occur in response to trauma or injury of various kinds. Any cervical injury can result in fibrous adhesion formation.[6]

Adhesion formation can be viewed as a variant of the normal physiologic healing process. Usually adhesions start with a fibrin matrix that occurs during coagulation. Over a period of a few days (in the rat model) a variety of cellular elements become encased in the fibrin matrix, which is gradually replaced by vascular granulation tissue containing macrophages, fibroblasts, and giant cells. By 4 days postinjury, most of the fibrin is gone and more fibroblasts and collagen are present. During days 5 through 10, fibroblasts align within the adhesion. At 2 weeks, the relatively few cells present are predominantly fibroblasts. At 1 to 2 months, the collagen fibrils organize into discrete bundles. Eventually, the adhesion matures into a fibrous band, often holding small calcifications. Extensive adhesions often contain blood vessels.[7]

Adhesions of the cervix can be caused by trauma at parturition or mating. They can be broken manually, but this must be done daily to prevent recurrence and some Vaseline should be placed over the site at least twice a day to avoid reattachment or scar formation due to bleeding.

The application of a steroid-antibacterial cream to the cervical lumen on a daily basis has also been recommended.[8]

Fibrosis

Fibrosis of the cervix is a condition that occurs in older mares, especially older maiden mares. Impaired cervical drainage of uterine fluid can predispose the mare to chronic endometritis. This inability of the cervix to dilate results in delayed uterine clearance in which mares (usually pluriparous mares older than 14 years) are not capable of expelling fluids that accumulate in the uterus after breeding.[9] LeBlanc et al[9] reported that the condition is not common in nulliparous mares, and when present, there is usually a history of poor cervical relaxation during estrus. In a study by Santschi et al,[10] six mares underwent ovariohysterectomy (OVH) because of a fibrotic and/or stenotic cervix. The mares were suffering from recurrent endometritis with cervical narrowing or inability of the cervix to drain because of the tightness of the cervix. No particular breed disposition to this condition was identified in this study, because each of the mares was a different breed. A cervix that does not dilate completely may reduce the stallion to vaginal ejaculation, as opposed to an intrauterine ejaculation, and may make delivery of the foal difficult.[11] In a retrospective study by Watkins et al,[12] eight mares underwent cesarean sections, and of those eight, one was submitted because of previously diagnosed cervical adhesions. Artificial insemination and embryo transfer have been used successfully in mares with abnormally narrow cervixes.

The administration of prostaglandin E_2 gel within the cervix of women has been shown to promote dilation without manifestation of collateral effects.[13,14] The prostaglandin E_2 gel works by increasing soluble collagen structures, which cause softening and relaxation of the cervix.[15] Rigby et al[15] demonstrated that the same protocol could be extrapolated to mares that were induced to foal. In this study, prostaglandin E_2 was suspended in 0.5 ml of saline solution and then applied within the cervical lumen to promote softening of the area. The results showed that this ripening of the cervix before induction with oxytocin reduced the labor length and facilitated the passage of the fetus; alternatively, mares that delivered with a tight cervix were more prone to have prolonged labor, premature separation of the placenta, birth hypoxia, and reduced foal vigor.[16] Prostaglandin E can be combined with estrogens (Estradiol cypionate 6 mg given 24 hours before induction) to dilate the cervix in case of foaling induction followed by oxytocin. Although the use of Prostaglandin E has been mentioned as an aid to ripe the cervix of old mares, some studies in humans report poor results may be due to an increase in the amount of fibrotic tissue and a decrease in the elastic tissue.

Although not reported very often in mares, congenital or anatomic abnormalities of the cervix and disorders of the opening/dilating function have been described by many authors. Volkmann and Gilbert[17] described the presence of a double uterus in a Clydesdale mare. Although the mare foaled normally one time, she aborted the next two foals. According to the authors, there is no evidence to suggest that the anatomic abnormality was the cause of either of the abortions, but it would be impossible to deny that possibility. It may therefore be possible to describe this condition as a breed-related abnormality.

Another interesting case was reported by Foster et al[18] in which the presence of varices with thrombosis in the cervical area of a Peruvian Paso Fino mare was found. Although an uncommon finding in mares, it has been reported in the dorsal wall of the vagina; however, this was the first time this abnormality was found in the cervix. Weakness of venous valves, weakness in the valve of the vein, multiple arteriovenous communications, reduced venous outflow and increased venous pressure, and greater arterial flow have been proposed as possibilities, but none has been confirmed.

Uterocervical leiomyomas have been reported in two Appaloosa fillies by Romagnoli et al.[19] The two half-sibling fillies were referred due to masses that protruded through the vulvar opening. After histologic evaluation, the masses were classified as multicentric leiomyoma and multicentric fibroleiomyoma. According to the authors, the tumors were attached to the dorsal aspect of the external os of the cervix and by a pedicle originating from the cervical tissue. Amazingly, a third filly (a paternal half-sibling) had been previously euthanized for the same reason. The stallion was reported to be the sire of two normal colts. This led the authors to believe that this condition may be controlled by a sex-limited or sex-linked form of inheritance.

Riera et al[20] reported on postmortem examination the presence of a mass that arose from the right lateral wall of the cervix of a mare. The mass weighed 745 g, and upon histologic evaluation scattered, infrequent cystic distension of the basal areas of the cervical crypts, with inspissated, eosinophilic hyaline secretion were found. The presence of small numbers of superficial endometrial glands indicated that the sample came from the cervical-endometrial junction.

References

1. Kainer RA: Reproductive organs in the mare. In McKinnon AO, Voss JL (eds): Equine Reproduction, Philadelphia, Lea & Febiger, 1993.
2. Timothy JE, Constantinescu GM, Ventatataseshu KG: Clinical reproductive anatomy and physiology of the mare. In Youngquist RS, (ed): Current Therapy in Large Animal Theriogenology, p 51, Philadelphia, WB Saunders, 1997.
3. Bergfelt DR: Anatomy and physiology of the mare. In Samper JC, (ed): Equine Breeding Management and Artificial Insemination, p 146, Philadelphia, WB Saunders, 2000.
4. Ginther OJ: Reproductive Biology of the Mare: Basic and Applied Aspects, 2nd edition, p 29, Cross Plains, WI, Equiservices, 1992.
5. Vivrette S: The endocrinology of parturition in the mare. Vet Clin North Am Equine Pract 1994; 10(1):1-17.
6. Causes and consequences of adhesions. [http://www.adhesions.org.uk/adhesions.html]. September 23, 2003 (accessed).
7. Contemporary adhesion prevention. [http://www.centerforendo.com/news/adhesions/adhesions.htm]. September 23, 2003 (accessed).

8. Trotter GW: The vulva, vestibule, vagina and cervix. In Auer J, Stick J, (eds): Equine Surgery, 2nd edition, pp 558-575, Philadelphia, WB Saunders, 1999.

9. LeBlanc MM, Neuwirth L, Jones L et al: Differences in uterine position of reproductively normal mares and those with delayed uterine clearance detected by scintigraphy. Theriogenology 1998; 50:49-54.

10. Santschi EM, Adams SV, Robertson JT et al: Ovariohysterectomy in six mares. Vet Surg 1995; 24:165-171.

11. Van Camp SD: Breeding soundness evaluation of the mare and common abnormalities encountered. In Morrow DA, (ed): Current Therapy in Theriogenology, 2nd edition, pp 654-661, Philadelphia, WB Saunders, 1986.

12. Watkins JP, Talor TS, Day WC et al: Elective cesarean section in mares: eight cases (1980-1989). J Am Vet Med Assoc 1990; 197(12): 1639-1645.

13. Ekman G, Forman A, Marsal K et al: Intravaginal versus intracervical application of prostaglandin E_2 in viscous gel for cervical priming and induction of labor at term in patients with unfavorable cervical stage. Am J Obstet Gynecol 1983; 147:657-661.

14. Laube DW, Zlatnik FJ, Pitkin RM: Preinduction cervical ripening with prostaglandin E_2 intracervical gel. Obstet Gynecol 1986; 68:54-57.

15. Rigby S, Love C, Carpenter K et al: Use of prostaglandin E_2 to ripen the cervix of the mare prior the induction of parturition. Theriogenology 1998; 50:897-904.

16. Macpherson ML, Chaffin MK, Carroll GL et al: Three methods of oxytocin induced parturition and their effects on foals. J Am Vet Med Assoc 1997; 210:799-803.

17. Volkmann DH, Gilbert RO: Uterus bicollis in a Clydesdale mare. Equine Vet J 1989; 21(1):71.

18. Foster RA, Gartley CJ, Newman S: Varices with thrombosis in the cervix and uterus of a mare. Can Vet J 1997; 38:375-376.

19. Romagnoli SE, Momont HW, Hilbert BJ et al: Multiple recurring uterocervical leiomyomas in two half-sibling Appaloosa fillies. J Am Vet Med Assoc 1987; 191(11):1449-1450.

20. Riera FL, Hinrichs K, Hunt PR et al: Cervical hyperplasia with prolapse in a mare. J Am Vet Med Assoc 1989; 195(10):1393-1394.

CHAPTER 22

Cervical Adhesions

PATRICIA L. SERTICH

The clinical problems caused by a cervical adhesion will depend on the location of the adhesion on the cervix. Translumenal cervical adhesions can prevent a cervix from opening properly and pericervical adhesions involving the portio vaginalis may prevent a cervix from closing adequately. Adhesions of the portio vaginalis are often present with a cervical laceration and clinically will be associated with infertility because of cervical incompetency. Complete resolution of a cervical adhesion is rarely achieved, but some procedures may enhance the cervical function that remains.

ANATOMY

The cervix develops from a fusion of the paramesonephric duct system. It is supported by the caudal aspect of the broad ligament, and its serosal surface is confluent with the broad ligament. The lumen of the cervix consists of longitudinal cervical folds that extend from the longitudinal folds of the uterus. The dorsal and the ventral cervical fold may extend caudally to form a sagittal dorsal and/or ventral frenulum to the vaginal wall. A circular layer of smooth muscle contracts and relaxes to close and open the cervix, respectively. The caudal portion of the cervix (portio vaginalis) extends into vaginal fornix.[1] During diestrus, when the genital tract is under progesterone influence, the cervical muscle contracts to close the cervix and the portio vaginalis is erect and protrudes into the cranial vagina. During estrus, estrogen concentrations are elevated and progesterone is absent. Consequently, the cervix dilates, and the portio vaginalis is edematous, flaccid, and lies on the floor of the cranial vagina. During anestrus, ovarian steroids are baseline and the cervix has little shape and does not close. Although in some anestrous mares the cervix may be closed, any manipulation will easily open it and it will remain dilated until ovulation occurs at the onset of the breeding season.

ETIOLOGY

Cervical lacerations or damage and associated adhesions can occur in a spontaneous and otherwise uneventful parturition. Stage II of parturition can be described as explosive in the mare with most normal foals passing through the birth canal in less than 20 minutes. If cervical softening is inadequate due to maiden status or anxiety, the cervix may not have sufficient time to fully relax before fetal expulsion. Cervical adhesions are frequently present with cervical lacerations and seem to develop as the laceration heals. Abraded or lacerated cervical mucosa tends to heal rapidly and adheres to any mucosal surface that it contacts. Adhesions present with cervical lacerations most often form from flaps of portio vaginalis tissue that adhere to the vaginal fornix. These adhesions are clinically significant because they prevent the caudal aspect of the cervix from closing and forming a competent canal of sufficient length. More extensive and severe cervical adhesions may develop after a dystocia. The mare's pelvic canal seems to be prone to pressure necrosis caused by the fetus being wedged in the cervix and pelvic canal. This results in tissue ischemia and subsequent sloughing of cervical and vaginal mucosa. The raw tissue that is exposed is at risk for developing transluminal adhesions. Mares undergoing fetotomy have the potential for even more extensive pressure necrosis and additional lacerations inflicted by the obstetric wire and equipment. Subsequent metritis exacerbates the mucosal inflammation and prolongs the healing time, often resulting in an irregular, firm, and inelastic cervix.

Although administration of some uterine therapy using caustic irritants is thought to stimulate and improve the endometrium, the cervix and vagina seem to be less tolerant of irritants. The cervix and vagina are more likely to become severely inflamed and form extensive transluminal adhesions between mucosal surfaces in the lumen of the cervix. The serosal surface of the cervix may adhere to the vaginal fornix, resulting in pericervical adhesions. Forced manual delivery of a greater-than-60-day conceptus during elective pregnancy termination that was initiated by repeated prostaglandin administration frequently results in circumferential tight rings of fibrotic tissue that constrict the cervical lumen.[2]

CLINICAL SIGNIFICANCE

The clinical significance of cervical adhesions is not simply based on the sheer amount of fibrotic tissue that develops. A completely nonpatent cervix will prevent both natural and artificial insemination, resulting in obvious infertility. An equally serious condition exists when much smaller strands of fibrotic tissue hinder dilation and prevent complete drainage of natural endometrial secretions or postbreeding debris.

Mares with an incompetent cervix caused by a laceration of the portio vaginalis with portions of the cervical mucosa adhered to the vaginal fornix may conceive readily and easily resolve any postbreeding endometritis. The author has seen mares with these changes become pregnant but fail to carry the foal to term, with pregnancy loss occurring at different stages of gestation.

CERVICAL EXAMINATION

Mare Preparation

Thorough evaluation of the cervix must be performed when the cervix is under the influence of progesterone. One must determine what proportion of the cervix is intact and can form a competent canal. The significance of the adhesions can be better estimated when the cervix is fully closed. Diestrus is the stage of choice, but anestrous mares can be examined satisfactorily if progesterone in oil (300 mg intramuscularly [IM]) is administered for 3 to 4 days before the cervical examination.

Most broodmares will tolerate cervical examination with simple standing restraint using a halter and lead shank. The horse handler should stand on the same side as the examiner. Positioning a mare in a stall doorway may help keep a restless mare in position for the examination. Fractious mares may be distracted with the use of a nose twitch. Palpation stocks can be used to contain mares and appear to offer some protection from kicks. The examiner must remain alert because severe injury may be sustained should a mare suddenly squat or kick out with both hind legs. One should avoid the administration of sedatives that may artificially alter the tone of the genital tract, preventing accurate assessment of the cervical competency. If there is significant risk that the mare or examiner will be injured, a combination of acepromazine (0.02 mg/kg) and xylazine (0.6 mg/kg) administered intravenously should provide sufficient tolerance for a brief examination.

Tail hairs should be contained in a tail wrap, and the tail should be secured to the side. The rectum should be emptied to reduce the chance of fecal elimination during the procedure. Regardless of history provided, it is the examiner's responsibility to determine that the mare is not pregnant. Cervical manipulations in a pregnant mare may cause abortion or ascending placentitis. The perineum should be washed thoroughly with povidone-iodine scrub solution, rinsed, and then patted dry with clean paper toweling. The examiner dons a sterile examination sleeve or clean sleeve covered by a sterile surgical glove. A sterile water-soluble lubricant is placed on the dorsum of the hand and lower arm.

Palpation per Vaginam

The examiner's forefinger should be placed inside the lumen of the cervix. All three layers (serosal mucosa, luminal mucosa, and muscularis) of the complete circumference of the portio vaginalis must be palpated between the thumb and forefinger. Any portion of the portio vaginalis that is adhered to the vaginal fornix should be noted. The entire length of the cervical canal should the assessed for degree of closure and presence of adhesions. Adhesions may be thick or strandlike and transluminal or pericervical.

CLINICAL MANAGEMENT

Some mares that have a cervical laceration and minor adhesions can maintain a pregnancy to term. The success seems to depend on the absence of chronic uterine fluid accumulations, competency of the mare's perineum and vestibulovaginal ring, body condition, length of residual competent canal, and cervical patency. It may be a reasonable decision to defer surgical correction if greater that 70% to 75% of the length of the canal is competent and patent. However, if the mare also has a history of otherwise unexplained pregnancy loss, then surgical correction of any lacerations and adhesions is recommended. Pericervical adhesions may need to be dissected to free sufficient cervical tissue for suturing. Long retention sutures are often placed near the incision edges and are manipulated several times a day for several days in an attempt to decrease the formation of adhesions postsurgically.

Thick ventral adhesions and transluminal adhesions can usually be disrupted but are difficult to prevent from reforming. Daily application of antibiotic and steroid ointments are effective at keeping the tissue free, but adhesions tend to reform soon after the daily manipulations and ointment applications cease.[3] Efforts to keep the cervix open by installing retention drainage tubes or inert devices are usually futile.

Mares with adhesions that prevent adequate drainage of uterine debris are at risk for chronic pyometra. In cases in which the uterine exudate can be controlled temporarily with uterine lavage and ecbolics, embryo transfer may be the most efficient method to obtain offspring. In mares that have continuous severe uterine exudate accumulations regardless of therapy, oocyte harvesting and transfer may offer the only hope of producing a foal. Fortunately, chronic pyometra caused by cervical adhesions is usually not life-threatening in mares. Hysterectomy may be considered in performance mares that are aesthetically unacceptable due to the persistent uterine discharge.

SUMMARY

Cervical adhesions may occur concurrently with cervical lacerations following spontaneous uneventful parturitions, dystocia, and fetotomies. Adhesions may also be a sequela to caustic intrauterine manipulations. Cervical adhesions may interfere with normal uterine clearance and predispose a mare to developing chronic pyometra. Mares with cervical lacerations and adhesions may benefit from cervical surgery. Transluminal and pericervical adhesions are difficult to resolve completely even with persistent, aggressive treatment. Assisted reproductive techniques may allow production of offspring from mares having chronic pyometra due to significant cervical adhesions.

References

1. Ginther OJ: Reproductive Biology of the Mare: Basic and Applied Aspects, 2nd edition, Cross Plains, Wis, Equiservices, 1992.
2. Sertich PL: Cervical problems in the mare. In McKinnon AO, Voss JL (eds): Equine Reproduction, Philadelphia, Lea & Febiger, pp 404-407, 1993.
3. Haibel GK: Disorders of the cervix. In Robinson NE (ed): Current Therapy in Equine Medicine, Philadelphia, WB Saunders, pp 409-410, 1983.

CHAPTER 23

Vulvar Conformation

REGINALD R. PASCOE

In 1937 Caslick[1] made the first reference to the importance of the conformation of the mare's vulva in relation to infections of the genital tract and subsequent infertility of the mare. He discussed the principal factors related to this infertility as being changes in conformation and persistent relaxation of the vulva. He considered a vulval angle of 80 degrees to the horizontal to be desirable, whereas angles below 50 degrees lead to windsucking (pneumovagina) becoming a clinical problem. He described a simple surgical procedure to close the upper vulvar lips, now universally known as Caslick's operation, which was found to markedly improve the fertility in the mares so treated.

This operation has also been successfully used to prevent pneumovagina in yearlings, 2-year-olds,[2] and racing maiden fillies.[3] Other surgeons have described various techniques that must be carefully followed to ensure maximum benefits from this simple operation.[2,4]

Scientific evidence was presented by Pascoe[5] in 1979 that described a simple measuring device to determine the slope (angle of declination) of the vulva and the length of the vulvar lips (Figure 23-1).

In a study on 9020 mares made on Thoroughbred, Standardbred, and Arabian mares, measurements of these two parameters were recorded; a simple mathematical formula produced a Caslick Index, which allowed a scientific determination of the necessity for Caslick's operation to be performed in mares not exhibiting classical signs of pneumovagina.

ANATOMIC CONSIDERATIONS

The perineum of the horse is the area that includes the anus, vulva, and the adjacent skin (usually hairless) under the tail. The normal conformation of the perineum prevents the entrance of air and bacteria into the genital tract. This is a very important area because of its protective role for the internal genital tract and its implications in creating some forms of infertility in particular. It is commonly a site for injury at parturition. The anatomic arrangement of the perineum, including its length relative to the pelvic bones and its angle relative to the vertical plane, is an important feature for the fertility of the mare; for example, mares that experience bouts of infertility frequently have a flat-topped croup with a tail setting that is level with the sacral iliac joint and a sunken anus (Figure 23-2). Alterations of angle and length have been used to determine a Caslick Index, which is used to provide an index of the need to perform Caslick's operation.

CASLICK INDEX

Calculation and measurements (Figure 23-3):

$$\text{Caslick Index} = (\text{length of vulva in cm}) \times (\text{angle of declination in degrees})$$

Interpretation

- Values of less than 100 are associated with a normal anatomic arrangement and better fertility than a score approaching 150 or higher.
- The Caslick Index increases with age and can vary with nutritional status.
- Continuous evaluation is essential, especially if loss of body condition occurs.

As a rule, a Caslick's operation must be performed when the dorsal vulvar commissure is located more than 4 cm ($1^1/_2$ inches) dorsal to the pelvic floor.

- Conformational characteristics that correlate with high fertility include a long sloping hip, a sacral iliac joint located dorsal to the tail setting, and a vulva that is no more than 10 degrees from the vertical. Various degrees of vulvar length and angulation and their relationship to fertility are illustrated in Figure 23-4.
- The normal/ideal anatomic arrangement is that the vulva should be vertical (or at least less than 10 degrees from the vertical) and that more than 80% of its length (from dorsal commissure to ventral commissure) should lie below the level of the ischial tuberosities (Figure 23-5). Variations in either the relative length below the ischium or an increase in the angle of declination (or both) result in a tendency for the vulva to be drawn forwards into the perineum below the anus (Figure 23-6). This combination results in an increased chance of aspiration of air into the vagina and a higher Caslick Index.
- Endometritis secondary to pneumovagina may resolve spontaneously after the operation.
- Natural defense mechanisms can become effective again after eliminating the continued irritation from aspirated contaminants.
- Once pneumovagina is corrected, it is essential that the mare remains Caslicked for the remainder of her reproductive life.

Breeding soundness examinations are performed to determine a mare's suitability as a broodmare and for

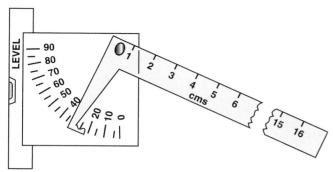

Figure 23-1 A stainless steel measuring device (vulvometer) for determination of effective length and angle of declination (Caslick Index).

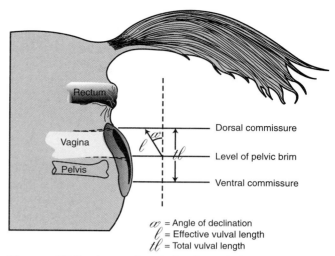

a° = Angle of declination
l = Effective vulval length
tl = Total vulval length

Figure 23-3 Anatomic relationship of the vulva of the mare showing measurement site. *a,* angle of declination; *l,* effective length of vulva; *tl,* total length of vulva.

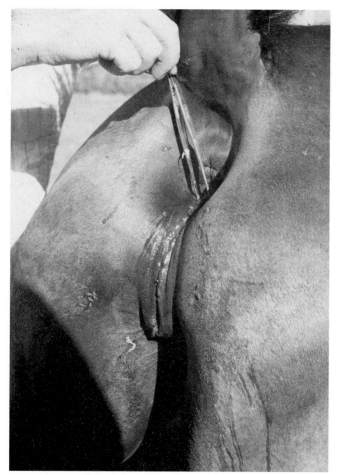

Figure 23-2 Clinical case showing sunken anus and high angle of declination—indication for Caslick's repair.

identifying causes of infertility. Portions of the examination are performed routinely on normal mares during the breeding season to determine when they should be bred. Common uses of new technologies, such as artificial insemination (AI) of mares with shipped, cooled or frozen semen and embryo transfer, require that the veterinarian excel in reproductive examination skills. A com-

plete breeding soundness examination is most commonly performed to identify a cause of infertility.

EXTERNAL EXAMINATION (RELATED TO VULVAR CONFORMATION)

- Examination of the external genitalia should include the entire perineal area, as well as the tail and buttocks, to detect changes in conformation, presence of signs of equine herpesvirus type 3 (EHV-3), signs of vulvar discharge, and the presence of tumors (e.g., melanoma or squamous cell carcinoma).
- Perineal and pelvic conformation needs to be examined thoroughly because the anatomic alignment of the mare's perineum is important for reproductive soundness. The perineal body may be defective in older, pluriparous mares. The defect most likely occurs from repeated foalings and poor reproductive conformation and results in a sunken anus and lack of tissue between the rectum and the vagina.
- The pelvic conformation should be viewed laterally and caudally.
- Mares that experience bouts of infertility frequently have a flat-topped croup with a tail setting that is level with the sacral iliac joint and a sunken anus. These conformational defects lead to pneumovagina, urovagina, and accumulation of intrauterine fluid.
- The vulva is best evaluated during estrus, when relaxation and elongation of the vulvar lips are greatest. The integrity of the vulvar lips, the angulation of the vulva, and the location of the dorsal commissure of the vulva in relation to the pelvis need to be evaluated. The vulvar lips should meet evenly and appear full and firm. They function as a seal against external contamination of the uterus.

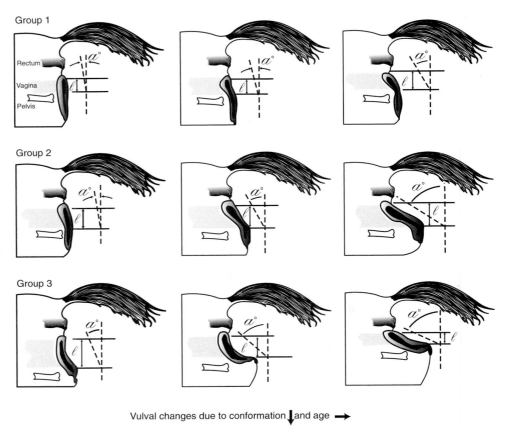

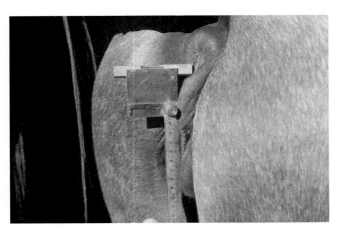

Figure 23-4 Vulvar changes in three conformation groups as effected by increasing angle of declination *(α)* and length of vulva *(l)*.

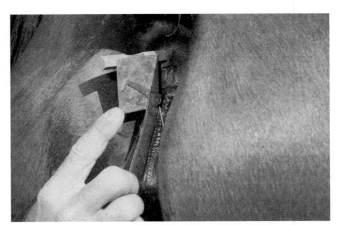

Vulval changes due to conformation ↓ and age ➡

$a°$ = Angle of declination
l = Effective vulval length

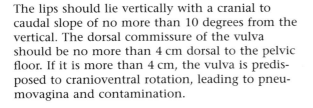

Figure 23-5 Application of vulvometer with angle of 5 degrees and l of 8 cm; Caslick Index = 40. Caslick's operation would not be required.

Figure 23-6 Application of vulvometer with angle of 30 degrees and l of 8 cm; Caslick Index = 240. Caslick's operation is necessary.

The lips should lie vertically with a cranial to caudal slope of no more than 10 degrees from the vertical. The dorsal commissure of the vulva should be no more than 4 cm dorsal to the pelvic floor. If it is more than 4 cm, the vulva is predisposed to cranioventral rotation, leading to pneumovagina and contamination.

- The lips of the vulva should be parted to determine the integrity of the vestibulovaginal sphincter. An intact sphincter is present in a mare when the labia can be spread slightly without air entering the cranial vagina. By parting the labia, the color and moisture of the vestibular walls can be assessed. Estrus produces a glistening pink to red mucosa. Anestrus generally is reflected by a pale, dry mucosa; a dark-red or muddy color suggests inflammation. A white, tacky mucosa indicates progesterone dominance.

- The integrity of the perineal body can be assessed by placing one finger into the rectum (usually the second finger) and the thumb into the vestibule. There should be at least 3 cm of muscular tissue between the two fingers. Surgical correction of the defect can be possible in some cases.

Three seals protect the genital tract:

- The vulvar seal (created by close contact between the vulvar lips or labia and the skin and muscles of the perineum)
- The vestibulovaginal seal (formed by the posterior vagina, the pillars of the hymen, and the floor of the pelvic girdle)
- The cervix, which acts as a final barrier for the uterus

Any deficiency in one or more of these "seals" has implications for the reproductive efficiency of the mare. During a normal reproductive examination these seals are broken and air is allowed into the vagina. Inevitably this air carries bacteria, and the presence of the air itself is responsible for a typical inflammatory response with blood vessel engorgement. When any of the three seals is disrupted (either through trauma, acquired faults or congenitally poor perineal conformation, or poor body condition), air may be aspirated into the vagina and the resulting contamination and infection can be a serious cause of infertility. The vulvar and vestibulovaginal seals to the vulvar lips and immediate vestibule usually restrict the ingress of clinically significant bacteria. The vagina and uterus should be free of significant infection, although some incidental bacteria are commonly found.

Simply gently parting the lips of the vulva and listening for aspiration of air into the vagina can test the integrity of the vaginal seal.

- Normally the vestibulovaginal seal will maintain an airtight seal when the lips of the vulva are parted in this way. In-rushing air suggests poor vestibulovaginal seal efficiency.

Vulva and Vestibule

The vulva comprises the two vulvar lips (labia and clitoris) and is the region of the reproductive tract that is in common with the urinary system. The two vulvar lips meet dorsally at the tightly angled dorsal commissure and ventrally at the more rounded ventral commissure. Just inside the vulvar lips lies the junction between the highly glandular skin and the nonglandular mucous membrane of the vestibule (the area of the reproductive tract that lies outside the level of the vestibulovaginal seal/hymen). The mucocutaneous junction is continuous with the clitoral prepuce or fold. The vulvar constrictor muscle continues into the external anal sphincter dorsally. The clitoral retractor muscle lies over the vulvar constrictor muscle ventrally. These muscles are variously responsible for the protective function of the vulva and the winking of the clitoris that occurs at the end of urination and

during estrus, and the arrangement allows considerable expansion during delivery of the foal.

The vestibule is the tubular portion of the tract between the lips of the vulva and the vestibulovaginal seal. The lateral and ventral walls contain the strong vestibular constrictor muscles. The vestibular wall and the muscles of the anus create the roof.

The vulvar lips should be vertically orientated and approximately two thirds of the vulvar cleft should lie below the level of the ischial arch.

- The anus should not be located anterior to the dorsal commissure of the vulva.
- There should be no aspiration of air into the vagina (vaginal wind-sucking) during normal walking or trotting. If this occurs, it suggests a poor vulvar seal and an inefficient vestibulovaginal seal.

Clitoris

The erectile clitoris of the mare is held in a protective pouch (the clitoral prepuce) just inside the ventral commissure of the vulva. It can readily be everted by gentle manual pressure applied across the ventral commissure of the vulva. This process reveals the clitoral glans itself, which has a wrinkled appearance in most mares. The clitoris lies in the clitoral fossa created by the clitoral prepuce, and it is common to encounter an accumulation of moist smegma in this area. On the crown of the clitoris are three depressions (the clitoral sinuses) with a deep central sinus and two smaller, shallower lateral sinuses. All of these commonly harbor a variable amount of smegma derived from the clitoral sebaceous glands.

Caslick's Operation

Caslick's operation is probably the most important procedure in the treatment of pneumovagina and infertility caused by infection of the genital tract. With numerous foals, loss of condition, and aging, the shape of the perineal area of the mare changes. There is usually an insidious loss of fertility, but continuous contamination of the breeding tract with air and fecal material lowers the mare's uterine tone and resistance to infection and, as the mare ages, creates a lowered plane of fertility.

Careful adherence to the measurements and calculation required to define the Caslick Index removes much of the doubt as to whether a mare will or will not benefit from the surgery.

Mares requiring Caslick's operation should always have the vulvar dorsal commissure carefully closed and kept closed. Failure to be meticulous about this reduces fertility.

Incision and resuturing for breeding and foaling are necessary management tools, and any delay in resuturing after foaling or service for as little as a few days may allow reinfection.

Technique

1. The mare is restrained in stocks/chute/crush (or behind a doorway), twitched or in a small

number of cases may need to be tranquilized (an α_2-adrenoreceptor agonist, such as romifidine or detomidine, with butorphanol is effective and safe).This usually applies to maiden and racing mares.

2. The tail may be wrapped in a disposable plastic sleeve or a clean bandage, or have the upper tail hairs clipped at the commencement of the breeding season. The tail is then elevated or held to one side (either by an assistant or by tying it to the stocks).

3. The rectum can be manually evacuated to reduce the risks of defecation during the procedure; however, on most breeding farms with experienced operators this is regarded as unnecessary.

4. The vulva and perineum are carefully cleaned with soap and water or a dilute surgical scrub. Strong, irritating antiseptics and surgical spirits should be avoided.

5. The labial margins are infiltrated with local anesthetic (2% lignocaine hydrochloride or mepivacaine) using a 21-gauge (or smaller) needle.

6. The tissues should be distended sufficiently to stretch the skin along the labial margins.

7. A 6- to 8-mm strip of mucosa is then removed along the mucocutaneous junction with sharp scissors.

8. Care should be taken not to remove skin with mucosa because a shortage of skin will occur in the course of many repairs, leading to difficulties in the repair process.

9. Because the vulva will need to be opened at foaling time (and possibly at breeding time), it is important that no more than a 6- to 8-mm strip of mucosa is removed from the stretched labial margin during the initial procedure.

10. Removal of a narrower strip less than 6 mm may lead to gaps between the adherent labia, especially at the dorsal commissure.

11. Careful removal of mucosa should occur to ensure that an uninterrupted raw surface is obtained from the dorsal commissure to approximately 1 cm ventral to the pelvic floor.

12. The raw edges of the labia are sutured together, starting at the dorsal vulvar commissure.

13. The preferred suture material is a nonabsorbable monofilament (nylon or polypropylene).

14. Many suture patterns, including simple-continuous, interrupted, vertical mattress, and continuous interlocking, have been used successfully. All are effective if sutures are placed carefully no more than 8 mm apart.

15. Continuous repetition of the procedure can lead to excessive scarring and loss of plasticity of the vulvar tissues. It is therefore important to perform the surgery with the utmost care.

Alternatively, the "breeding stitch" is sometimes used:

- A single suture of umbilical tape is placed sufficiently dorsal to allow intromission and protect the ventral aspects of the closed labia from tearing during service.

- In many mares it cannot protect the vulva effectively and still allow intromission by the stallion.
- This type of stay suture carries the danger of trauma to the stallion's penis at the time of mating.
- Its usefulness is limited.

MANAGEMENT

- At the time of foaling (and in some mares at the time of breeding), the vulvar repair must be opened and resutured immediately after foaling or service to prevent laceration of the vulva and aspiration of contamination (or infection).
- Reopening of the vulva should be left as close to foaling as possible to prevent contamination of the vagina and cervix and ascending infection from occurring. Reopening too soon can occasionally lead to infection of the placenta and even premature foaling and/or abortion.
- The procedure is simply performed following the infiltration of local anesthetic as above. The "healed scar" is cut directly upward with sharp scissors or scalpel blade.
- Quite frequently the Caslick's repair is opened 20 to 30 days before foaling, but it is better to reduce this to 7 to 10 days if good supervision is available before foaling.
- Mares should have Caslick's repairs carried out as soon as possible after foaling.
- Delay may be necessary if the fetal membranes have not been passed.

Vestibulovaginal Sphincter Insufficiency

If labial vestibular sphincter function is not reestablished by a routine Caslick's procedure, surgical reconstruction of the perineal body is indicated. Incompetency of the vulvar and vestibular sphincters can result from repeated stretching during further foalings or from second- or third-degree perineal lacerations. Perineal body reconstruction restores the reliability of the vestibular sphincter by reducing the diameter of the vestibule and surgically enlarging and suturing the perineal body dorsoventrally and craniocaudally.

Perineal Reconstruction (Vestibuloplasty)

Technique

1. The mare is restrained in stocks/chute/crush (or with a suitable protective kickboard or door) and sedated (with an α_2-adrenoreceptor agonist such as romifidine or detomidine and butorphanol).

2. Epidural anesthesia is preferred (see technique in standard surgical and anesthesia texts); local infiltration can be used but may be less effective and can slow healing.

3. The tail is wrapped in a sterile bandage or a plastic sleeve so that all hair is covered and is then held or fastened to one side.

4. The rectum is carefully evacuated manually, and gauze sponges or a portion of rolled cotton lint

or wool is placed in the rectum to prevent passage of feces into the surgical field during the procedure.

5. The animal's perineum and vulva are scrubbed thoroughly.
6. The mare's tail and buttocks and the stocks are then draped.
7. Stay sutures of umbilical tape or long-jaw Balfour retractors are placed either side and are used to provide retraction of the vulvar lips.
8. An incision is made along the mucocutaneous junction of the dorsal labia and the dorsal commissure, and a triangular section of mucosa is then dissected submucosally from the dorsum and dorsolateral aspects of the vestibule.
9. The apex of the mucosal triangle is located at or near the dorsal vestibulovaginal junction and the base of the triangle at the mucocutaneous junction of the labia.
10. This triangular section of mucosa is then removed, usually with curved scissors. During the submucosal dissection care must be used not to enter the rectum. Should the rectum be entered, the defect should be repaired immediately with sutures that invert the rectal mucosa into the rectum, and then the dissection is continued and completed.
11. The two incised edges of the mucosa of the vestibule are then sutured together with a simple, continuous pattern of 3.5 polypropylene.
12. The raw surfaces dorsal to this suture line are apposed with simple, interrupted through and through "quilting" sutures of polypropylene.
13. Suturing must proceed from deep layers to superficial layers, alternating first the continuous line in the mucosa, then the "quilting" sutures above.
14. The skin of the perineum and vulva are closed as for the Caslick's operation.
15. Complete healing of deep tissues takes 4 to 8 weeks; complete sexual rest must be observed until healing is completed.

Perineal Body Transection (Pouret's Operation)

An alternative surgery was described by Pouret[6] in 1982 to totally free the attachments between the ventral terminal rectal wall and the dorsal vaginal wall, allowing the vulva to assume a more normal vertical positioning and at the same time allowing the pull of the sunken anus on the dorsal vagina to be reduced. This surgery does not reduce the size of the vaginal opening.

Technique
- Tranquillize and surgically prepare perineum.
- Administer 2% Xylocaine epidural, and drape perineum.
- Make a 4- to 6-cm transverse incision in perineal skin midway between ventral anus and dorsal vulvar commissure; blunt dissect from skin incision anteriorly.
- Dissect shelf through perineal muscles anteriorly for 8 to 14 cm until all muscles connecting the caudal rectum and anus are sectioned and vulva is vertically orientated.
- Skin closure is recommended; another option is to leave wound open to heal by secondary intention because frequently the sutured wound dehisces.
- Mares may be bred with AI almost immediately; natural service should be delayed until the wound is fully healed.
- This procedure is of more value to correct pneumovagina than urinary pooling.

Vulvar laceration and vulvar insufficiency:

- Vulvar lacerations are most commonly an aftermath of foaling.
- With extensive pressure on the labia during foaling, circulation of the vulva may be disrupted, resulting in vulvar necrosis.
- Small tears in a previously sutured dorsal vulvar commissure may occur at the time of breeding.
- These are usually of no consequence to the mare's health or fertility at that mating.
- Depending on perineal conformation, repair by Caslick's operation may be necessary.
- If the laceration is severe, the inflammation must be resolved before repair is attempted.
- Immediate care should include cleansing of the laceration and administration of systemic antimicrobials and tetanus toxoid.
- The damage may reduce the amount of vulvar tissue and require a deeper closure than the simple Caslick's operation.
- In the worst cases, more healing time is allowed and repair should be delayed until after the mare is mated.
- After repair of a cranial full-thickness vaginal tear, a Caslick's operation reduces the possibility of air aspiration into the peritoneal cavity.

References

1. Caslick EA: The vulva and the vulvo-vaginal orifice and its relation to genital health of the thoroughbred mare. Cornell Vet 1937; 27:178.
2. Sager FC: Care of the reproductive tract of the mare. J Am Vet Med Assoc 1966; 149:1541.
3. Roberts SJ: Veterinary Obstetrics and Genital Diseases (Theriogenology), 3rd edition, Noodstock, VT, p 11, 1971.
4. Trotter GW: The vulva, vestibule, vagina, and cervix. In Auer J, Stick J (eds): Equine Surgery, 2nd edition, Philadelphia, WB Saunders, pp 558-575, 1999.
5. Pascoe RR: Observations on the length and angle of declination of the vulva and its relation to fertility in the mare. J Reprod Fertil Suppl 1979; 27:299.
6. Pouret EJM: Surgical technique for the correction of pneumo- and urovagina. Equine Vet J 1982; 14:249.

CHAPTER 24

Selected Reproductive Surgery of the Broodmare

ANGUS O. MCKINNON
JAMES R. VASEY

The notes herein are a compilation of some of the techniques that are used at the Goulburn Valley Equine Hospital and are not intended as an exhaustive, heavily referenced treatise of all available techniques. No attempt has been made to discuss all reproductive techniques or conditions requiring intervention. The procedures herein work very well for us. However, readers should be aware that different methods are employed successfully by others. We would be grateful to those who have different ideas and experiences if they would communicate them by e-mailing Dr. McKinnon at aom@iinet.net.au. Many of the techniques presented are modifications of existing techniques, newer techniques, and/or areas we feel warrant special attention. We have assumed that readers are at least familiar with both relevant anatomy and standard documented surgical correction of reproductive-related problems.

Topics discussed have been dictated by our experience and preference for an individual or alternate technique when many techniques exist. A busy equine practitioner can expect to encounter most of these problems in any individual breeding season. Most of the techniques relate to restoring or improving fertility, and most are elective and require experience to make the correct diagnosis and therapeutic approach.

PATIENT SELECTION

In consideration of the client, patient, and general perception of our professional abilities as well as the merit of our interference, care should be exercised to select only those patients that are likely to respond favorably to surgery (Box 24-1). For example, it is pointless to perform a sophisticated, expensive surgery for vesico vaginal reflux if the mare has sustained chronic uterine damage and fibrosis that will render her infertile despite an excellent surgical outcome. Full reproductive evaluation is necessary before surgery in any candidate subjected to physical insults such as recto-vaginal lacerations and fistulas for longer than 1 year.

SEDATION AND ANESTHESIA

Most procedures are performed with the mare standing, using local infiltration or epidural anesthesia. Apart from minor procedures (Caslick's vulvoplasty), we prefer to have mares tranquilized and restrained in appropriate stocks such as facilities for cross tying and/or tail elevation. Tranquilization and analgesia are provided most commonly with intravenous (IV) detomidine (mg) and butorphanol (mg). Longer surgeries may require the repeated IV use of low doses of xylazine (100 mg). Cost and length of tranquilization/analgesia are important considerations. Some have other physiological effects, such as increased urinary output with xylazine. Detomidine provides excellent tranquilization and analgesia; however, effects are often still apparent hours after administration. Epidural anesthesia may be extremely effective; however, variation in response and individual susceptibility and time before appropriate anesthesia is obtained occasionally make it less rewarding than tranquilization and local infiltration for some of the procedures discussed here. Techniques for epidural anesthesia have been discussed elsewhere.[1] One word of warning: epidural administration of more than 7 to 9 ml of 2% local anesthetic to a 500 kg mare can be associated with loss of motor control to the hind limbs and recumbency. These mares are difficult to manage and may require support for 2 to 4 hours.

Epidural injection of xylazine for perineal analgesia has been reported to be very efficacious. A dose of 0.17 mg/kg (around 75-100 mg in an average horse) was as effective as local anesthetic agents for analgesia and had nil or minimal effects on depression of motor nerves in the lumbosacral intumescence. Another advantage was demarcation of the area of analgesia with an area of sweating (dermatome) that was consistent both temporally and topographically.[2] In our experience the perineal dermatome is not always obvious. In addition it takes around 35 to 40 minutes for good analgesia to be recognized associated with xylazine epidural anesthesia. Currently we prefer to use a combination of xylazine (70 mg) and lidocaine (60 mg [3 ml]), q.s. saline to 10 ml for most horses. With this regime, loss of tail tone has occurred associated with a successful "block" within 5 to 10 minutes and surgery generally has begun by approximately 30 to 45 minutes post administration. Our most common method of epidural anesthesia is to begin with the infusion of 1 ml of local anesthetic through a 25 gauge needle subcutaneously above the first moveable coccygeal/sacral joint (usually C1 and C2). Next, a 38-mm, 18-gauge needle (bevel forward and introduced at 45 degrees) that has a small amount of fluid left to create a meniscus on the needle hub is introduced through the

Box 24-1

Considerations for Favorable Response to Surgery

The probability of a successful outcome (i.e., pregnancy, live foal, etc.) must be evaluated with regard to the following:

- Severity and nature of the problem
- Breeding history of the mare
- Value of the mare and/or offspring (commercial or sentimental)
- Cost of the procedure
- Mare age
- Fertility of the stallion
- Availability and suitability of sophisticated breeding techniques such as AI, ET, etc.
- Long-term value of interference (i.e., temporary or permanent improvement)
- General health of the candidate
- Perpetuation of heritable conditions
- Insurance and informed client consent
- Ethical considerations
- Experience of the veterinarian
- Quality of on-farm management

local bleb. Recognition of the fluid being aspirated into the needle infers correct placement, and the appropriate amount of solution is injected slowly into the epidural space whilst continually evaluating the ease of administration to ensure that the needle tip is still in place.

Occasionally epidural anesthesia is difficult to achieve (infusion outside the spinal cord before proper epidural placement, hemorrhage through the needle and tissues, anatomic abnormalities and fat horses). Provided local anesthesia can be obtained by infiltration without adverse affects on wound healing, we prefer to perform surgery without the epidural and provide incremental IV administration of xylazine (i.e., 50-100 mg to already tranquilized patients when or if minor surgical discomfort is recognized).

In some instances we have been able to identify correct epidural placement by injecting the anesthetic slowly while moving the needle until there is an obvious change in the amount of pressure needed to advance the solution. These situations are usually associated with a mare with abnormal anatomy (i.e., after a traumatic foaling) and lack of movement of fluid in the needle hub.

VESTIBULE AND VULVAL LIPS

Pneumovagina

There are 3 barriers to aspiration of air and contaminants into the cranial reproductive tract.

1. The vulval/vaginal lips
2. The vestibular sphincter
3. The cervix

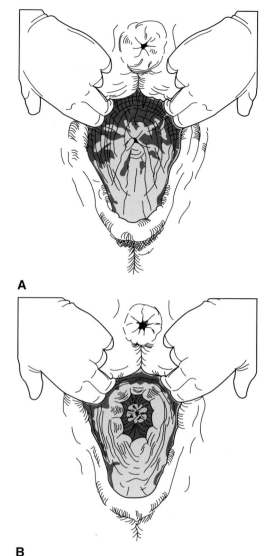

A

B

Figure 24-1 **A,** Retraction of vulval lips reveals an intact vestibular sphincter. **B,** Retraction of vulval lips reveals an open vestibular sphincter that is likely associated with pneumovagina.

It would appear that the vestibular barrier is more important than previously recognized; however, when any of these protective barriers are rendered incompetent, contamination and concomitant vaginitis, cervicitis, and metritis may result. Pneumovagina can result from faulty perineal conformation, previous injury to perineal tissues, or effects of poor body condition. Pneumovagina can also be iatrogenic (i.e., reproductive examination or breeding).

Recognition of potential candidates for pneumovagina are made from anatomical observations[3] (i.e., predisposition is associated with a low pelvis, tilted vaginal lips, and a sunken anus) (Figure 24-1). If possible, mares should be examined during estrus when the reproductive tract is relaxed. Parting the vulval lips results in loss of integrity of the vestibular sphincter and an audible ingress of air to the cranial vagina. Recognition of foamy exudates from the vaginal lips may often be noted during rectal examination. In addition, ultrasonography has been used to visualize air in the uterus.[4] If in doubt after clinical evaluation regarding a mare's potential to aspirate air into the vagina, we recommend treating by surgery all mares that have been barren one or more breeding seasons, unless other causes of reduced fertility are obvious (i.e., stallion, farm management).

Caslick's Vulvoplasty

Caslick's vulvoplasty was first described by Dr. E. A. Caslick in 1937 and involves apposition of the vulval lips.[5] Local anesthesia of vulval lips, removal of a thin portion of mucosa from the mucocutaneous junction, and apposition of the cut edges is simple, quick, and effective. Length of apposition is determined by height of pelvis relative to vulval lips. In general the join should continue to a point at least 3 to 4 cm below level of the pelvis, and approximately 3 cm should be left unopposed to allow for urination. If this is not possible, other surgical techniques (see below) may be necessary.

Points for consideration

- For suture material we use 0 catgut (Metric 4) on a continuous spool. The benefit of gut is that it is gone or degraded by either pregnancy testing (~15 days) or the next breeding cycle (if the mare is empty). Other materials that are nonabsorbable or delayed-absorbable may damage the stallion if the mare is rebred.
- For suture pattern, a simple continuous pattern is quicker and just as effective as a simple pattern interrupted. However, failure to appose the deepest layers of the exposed tissues may result in fistula forma-

tion. Failure to exit/enter in the middle of the cut tissue caused by taking bites too deep will result in wound breakdown.

- Method of mucosa removal:
  - Tissue should be removed from the mucosal surface of the vestibule, not the skin of the vulva lip.
  - Removing too much will result in fibrosis and difficulty for the next veterinarian (Figure 24-2, *A*).
  - If multiple procedures are performed in 1 season, freshening with a scalpel blade is sufficient, provided a careful suture pattern is placed (Figure 24-2, *B*).
  - Incision with a scalpel blade rather than mucosal removal is recommended for maidens (i.e., race mares) (Figure 24-2, *C*). This results in a thinner join that is easily opened at the breeding farm.

Postoperative treatment

- Frequent rectal palpation within 2 weeks will result in fistula formation.
- Remove (open) 2 to 3 weeks before anticipated foaling.

Variations. Placement of a breeding stitch (usually doubled heavy gauge suture material or umbilical tape) will save unnecessary replacement and facilitate breeding and some manual vaginal manipulations for treatment (Figure 24-2, *D*). Care is needed with natural service to prevent penile trauma. We routinely treat or bred (AI) mares by passage of an infusion pipette into the vagina (past the vestibular sphincter) and use rectal manipulation of the pipette through the cervix similar to, but with a little more difficulty than cattle.

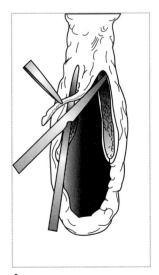 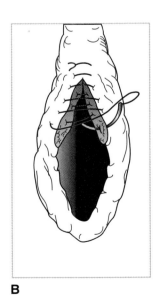 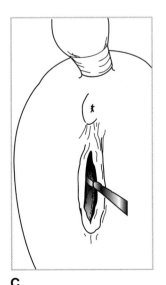 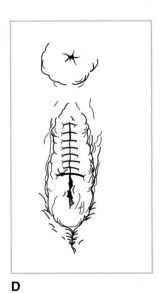

A **B** **C** **D**

Figure 24-2   **A,** Careful trimming of the mucocutaneous junction without removing skin from the vulval lips facilitates many more identical surgeries. **B,** Simple continuous suture is all that is necessary, but suture placement will help avoid fistulas. **C,** A scalpel blade is recommended for the first Caslick a mare has, especially maidens in work. **D,** A breeding stitch may be useful in preventing the Caslick from opening with vaginal examination or natural service.

Episioplasty

This procedure is used in cases with more severe anatomic abnormalities where the Caslick vulvoplasty is ineffective and in mares with extensive or repeated second-degree perineal lacerations. Technically the previous surgery is an episioplasty as well; however, we use the term to describe the more extensive procedure previously referred to as (1) a deep Caslick, (2) the Gadd technique, or (3) a perineal body reconstruction.[6] The procedure is designed to restore some degree of function to the perineal body. (Figure 24-3)

The surgery is performed on the standing mare with local anesthesia. Visualization is improved by good retrac-

tion and light sources. We prefer to perform all perineal surgeries using a centrally mounted beam as the light source.

A triangular portion of the dorsal caudal vestibule is removed from both sides. Apposition of the ventral borders of the incision and obliteration of the potential space above result in an increase in the size of the perineal body and a decreased propensity of the vestibule to create negative pressures.

The ventral borders are apposed with a continuous absorbable suture (2/0 vicryl) and dead space with single interrupted sutures. The mucocutaneous junction is closed similar to the Caslick procedure.

Points for consideration
- The procedure appears most beneficial when combined with a perineal body transection (see below).
- Failure to "open" the dorsal vestibule and vulval lips before foaling (2-3 weeks) may result in severe perineal laceration.
- The surgery usually takes longer (30-40 minutes) than expected (10-15 minutes) and is sometimes associated with significant and annoying obscuring hemorrhage.

Urovagina

Pooling of urine in the vagina is a problem for a variety of reasons. In 1985 Jay Belden, then of Fossil Creek Farms, showed me his technique for urovagina. Before this time, both of us had tried other described techniques and were not particularly happy with the outcome. After approximately 34 surgeries between us using Jay's technique, we decided the technique was efficacious and should be presented. The resultant publication is summarized below.[4]

The midline caudal border of the transverse vaginal fold is grasped with Allis tissue forceps and retracted caudally toward the surgeon 2 to 4 cm cranial from the caudal border of the transverse fold. A horizontal transverse incision to the submucosa is made with a No. 12 Bard Parker blade (Figure 24-4). The incision is continued laterad and then slightly dorsad to the vaginal wall. The vaginal retractors are then repositioned, and a No. 20 Bard Parker blade is used to extend the incision from the lateral border of the transverse folds caudad. This incision is made approximately one half to two thirds of the distance between the vaginal floor and roof and is extended to the vulvar labia. The caudal cut edge from the transverse fold incision and the ventral cut edge of the vaginal wall incision are dissected so that the free tissue flaps are reflected caudad and mediad, respectively. This causes vaginal mucous membranes of the free tissue flaps to be reflected ventrally and the underlying cut surface to be exposed dorsally. Next, the retractors are repositioned and an identical incision is made on the opposite vaginal wall, extending from the lateral extremity of the transverse fold caudally toward the surgeon.

Dissection of the tissue flap from the transverse fold is continued until the caudal cut edge can be reflected approximately 3 to 6 cm toward the surgeon. The dissection of both vaginal wall flaps is continued ventrally until the cut edges can be reflected without tension past the midline (Figure 24-4, *C*). The suture pattern used to appose the submucosal tissue layer is a continuous

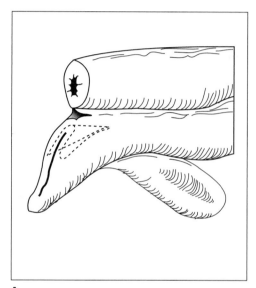

A

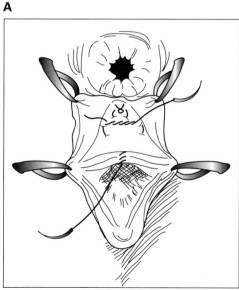

B

Figure 24-3 **A,** The *dotted lines* outline the area to be apposed with the formation of a new perineal body. **B,** The ventral layer of the perineal body consists of the vaginal mucosa. The perineal body is created from apposition of the vaginal mucosa where the tissue has been denuded.

modified Connell's, using 2-0 gut (Figure 24-4, *D*). The final configuration is in the shape of a Y, with the apex pointing caudally. The first suture line begins cranially and laterally at the junction of the transverse fold and vaginal wall incisions and is ended at the midpoint of the transverse fold reflection. Cut edges of the transverse fold and vaginal wall are inverted so that denuded tissues are in apposition. The second suture line begins on the opposite side, at the junction of the transverse fold and vaginal wall incisions, and is continued to the end point of the first suture pattern and then on the midline, toward the surgeon, to the caudal end of the vaginal wall reflections. The result is an extended tunnel from the urethral orifice (under the transverse fold) to the caudal vaginal vault. It is important to have minimal tension associated with the suture line and have all apposed edges inverted so that dissected or denuded tissues are in apposition (Figure 24-4, *E* and *F*)

The denuded tissues created dorsally by the dissection of the transverse and vaginal folds are allowed to heal by second intention. If necessary, an episioplasty is performed after surgery.

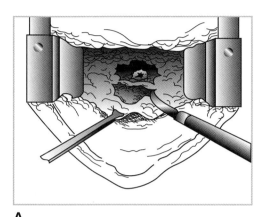

A

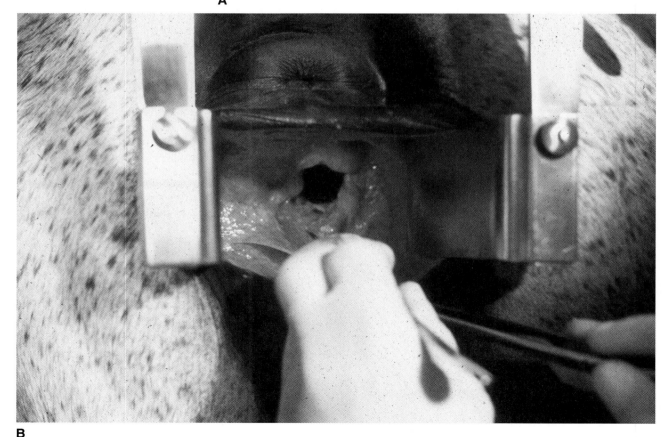

B

Figure 24-4 **A,** The first incision is along the transverse fold of the vestibular sphincter. **B,** A No. 12 blade (hook blade) facilitates the undermining of the transverse fold.

Continued

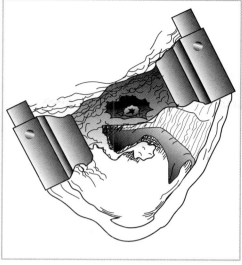

C

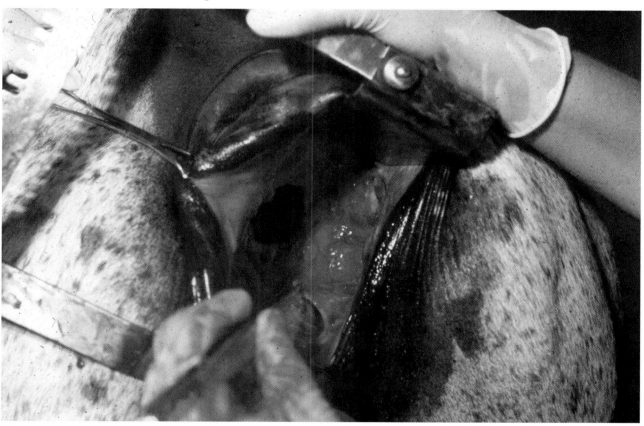

D

Figure 24-4, cont'd   **C**, The lateral vaginal wall is dissected after the retractors are repositioned. **D**, The vaginal wall is dissected from between one half to two thirds of the wall until the free mucosal flap can be passed across midline without undue tension.

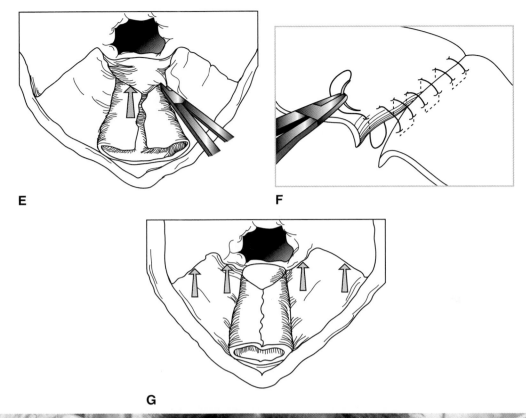

E

F

G

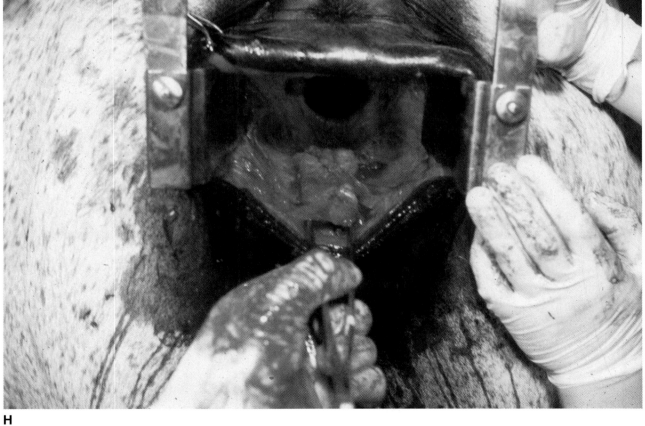

H

Figure 24-4, cont'd   E, The reflected two vaginal walls and the reflected undermined transverse fold are all brought together and inverted, leaving the denuded surface in the vestibule. **F,** The suture pattern is a modified Connell. **G,** The finished urethral tunnel. **H,** There is not much tension on the newly created urethra.

Additional points

- The technique described is our technique of choice for treatment of all mares with urovagina. Other treatments such as perineal body transection or caudal relocation of the transverse fold are often only temporarily effective.
- Episioplasty performed at the same time may result in excessive ablation of vestibule.
- In some mares, urine will pool in the caudal relocation of the urethral tunnel and it will be voided during exercise, commonly resulting in urine staining of the perineum. While this does not affect fertility, it is unsightly and may be treated by incision into the new urethral tunnel to a point 2 to 4 cm cranial to the vulval lips but not far enough to allow urovagina to recur.

Perineal Body

Surgeries of the perineal body are necessary to correct severe anatomic defects (perineal body transection [PBT]) or injuries due to foaling (perineal lacerations and fistulae).

Perineal Body Transection

Perineal body transection has been described to be beneficial for both pneumovagina and urovagina.[7] Our experiences suggest definitely the former but only occasionally the latter.

The primary indication for PBT is mares with such external reproductive conformation that we are not able to prevent pneumovagina after either Caslick's vulvoplasty or episioplastly (i.e., mares with a severely sunken anus and most or all of the vulval lips positioned above the brim of the pelvis (Figure 24-5, A and B).

The procedure is performed with local anesthesia with or without tranquilization. Local anesthesia (40-70 ml) is liberally infused into the perineal body and laterally to include the vaginal walls to a depth of 8 to 14 cm.

Towel clamps positioned just ventral to the anal sphincter and dorsal to the dorsal commissure of the vulva are used to provide retraction and tension while a 4- to 6-cm horizontal incision is made midway between the anus and dorsal vulva. The incision is continued for a short distance (2-5 cm) along either side of the vulva. Sharp and blunt dissection are used to completely transect the muscular and ligamentous supporting tissues between the rectum and vestibule (Figure 24-5, C, D, and E). Depending on the individual mare, the dissection proceeds cranially for 8 to 14 cm and finishes before entering the peritoneal cavity. The aim of the surgery is to allow the vulval lips to assume a more horizontal position by freeing them from attachments to the rectum. Generally the surgery is finished when the desired external conformation is achieved after allowing for wound contraction.

Closure of the skin incision was originally recommended[7]; however, we commonly leave the incision open. Closing the skin occasionally results in dehiscence and also seems to influence the result after wound contracture occurs. The wound heals by second intention, which is surprisingly rapid (2 to 3 weeks).

Points for consideration

- Placing a hand in the vestibule enables accurate dissection. Penetration of the vagina or rectum should be avoided.
- The wound is unsightly while healing, and we recommend careful client communication and/or hospitalization for 1 to 2 weeks.
- The benefits from corrective surgery are immediate, and mares can be bred at the first opportunity, provided that qualified personnel are available. Natural service is generally delayed 2 to 3 weeks to allow strengthening of the dorsal vestibule and vagina.
- Despite the surgery causing moderate hemorrhage, we have not had to take any special precautions or protective measures.

Perineal Lacerations

Most perineal injuries occur at the time of foaling and are associated with a mal-presented or oversized fetus, extensive, vigorous, inappropriate or sometimes unavoidable manual manipulation during parturition and/or violent expulsive efforts of the mare. Maiden mares are by far the most commonly injured with third degree perineal lacerations.

The injuries are commonly referred to as first, second, or third degree perineal lacerations (PL). First degree PL involve only the mucosa of vestibule and skin of the dorsal commissure of the vulva. Minor first degree PL may require no treatment. Extensive lacerations may require episioplasty or perineal body reconstruction. If tissue damage results in significant edema, inflammation, and infection, then surgical correction is often delayed for 2 to 3 weeks.

Second degree PL involve both the mucosa and submucosa of the dorsal vulva, and some of the musculature of the perineal body, in particular the constrictor vulvae muscle. There is no damage to rectal mucosa.

Third degree PL result in tearing of the vestibular and sometimes vaginal wall and disruption of the perineal body, anal sphincter, and rectal wall. This results in a common opening between the rectum and the vestibule.[8] The constant presence of feces in the vestibule and occasional unpleasant sound from air movement make repair imperative for breeding and recommended for future riding horses.

Immediate care for the mare at foaling involves antibiotics, anti-inflammatories, and protection against tetanus. The surgical correction is delayed at least 4 weeks to allow initial second intention wound healing to occur. Heroic repair at the time of foaling is almost never successful.[8] The longer the injury is left untreated, the more opportunities for continual contamination of the reproductive tract; however, this is related to functional capabilities of the vestibular sphincter, and many people will wait until weaning if a live foal was delivered. The cervix must be examined before surgical correction of PL, and if a prolonged time between foaling and repair has occurred, a full reproductive evaluation including biopsy is warranted.

Surgical technique. There are many methods described. Most importantly, the procedures are modifications of either a single- or two-stage repair. A modification of the single-stage repair is the technique we prefer.[9]

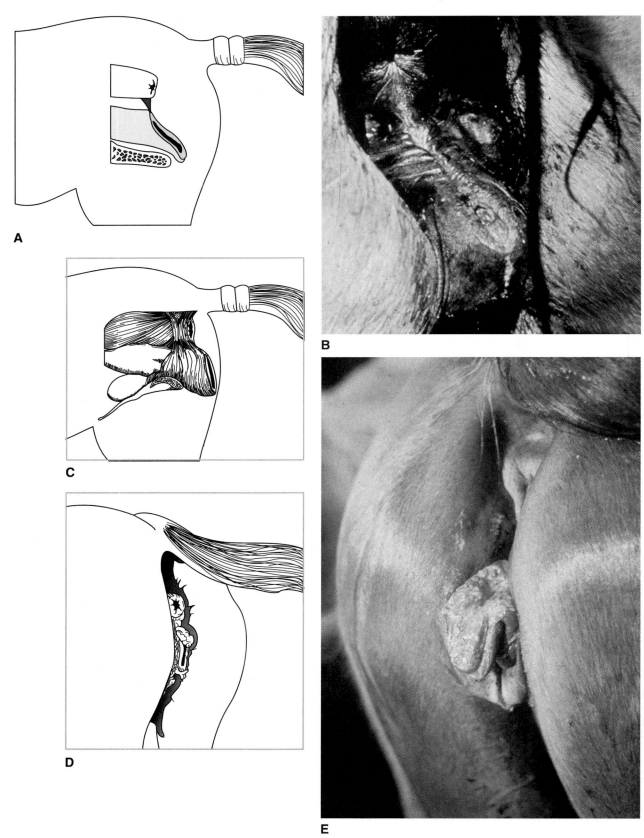

Figure 24-5 **A,** The ageing process of the mare and her conformation has allowed the vestibule and vagina to be positioned mostly above the pelvic brim. **B,** This conformation results in pneumovagina and occasional urine pooling. **C,** The musculature associated with the rectum and vestibule/vagina must be transected to allow the vulval lips to relax caudal. **D,** The surgery often results in the tip of the vulva relaxing to create a shelf if the incision is left not sutured. **E,** The final result, about 48 hours after surgery.

Before surgery vigorous efforts are made to modify the consistency of the feces. Mares are held off feed for at least 24 hours and given a mineral oil drench (2-3 liters) before beginning surgery. After surgery mares are placed on pasture if available, and mineral oil is administered by stomach tube daily for 3 days as necessary to maintain a soft fecal consistency.

Mares are restrained standing, tranquilized, and epidural anesthesia is employed.

Fecal material from the rectum is removed as far cranial as possible. Large wads of cotton are inserted into the cranial rectum to absorb fecal fluid and prevent fecal contamination of the surgical site. Tissues are cleansed and prepared for aseptic surgery. Towel clamps are inserted into the ventral anal sphincter in a configuration that when apposed represent the ideal surgical apposition point. In addition, towel clamps are placed on the dorsal vulval commissure and then retracted to provide visualization for surgical access or, alternatively, stay sutures are used to retract the vulva. An incision is made along the scar tissue line marking the junction between the vestibule/vagina and rectum. Tissues ventral to the incision are dissected to create mobilized vestibular mucosa and submucosa that when apposed from side to side will form the ventral border of the perineal body. Tissues dorsal of the incision are debrided, and rectal submucosa is undermined to allow sufficient mobilization to invert by side-to-side apposition the ventral border of the terminal rectum. All tissues are then sutured concurrently and incrementally from cranial to caudal. The rectal and vaginal reflections are apposed by a continuous modified inverting Connell suture. Suture material preferred is a No. 1 delayed absorbable (i.e., PDS) for the fibrous layer, 0 PDS for the vagina, and 2/0 for the rectal mucosa. When the suture pattern of the rectal submucosa has proceeded 2 to 3 cm, the suture material is retracted and then the vaginal or vestibular submucosa is similarly apposed. The resulting dead space in between, the *recreated perineal body*, is obliterated by multiple interrupted or continuous apposition sutures. The three areas of apposition are then alternatively progressed caudally, 2 to 4 cm each time, diverging at the perineal body, until the ventral vestibular submucosa stitch can be tied and vulval lips closed by a Caslick. The apposing suture of the rectal submucosa is terminated at the dorsal perineal body at the level of the defect in the anal sphincter. The anal sphincter may or may not be apposed at all. Adequate dissection of vestibular and rectal submucosa is necessary to prevent undue tension on the continuous suture patterns.

Postoperatively, apart from antibiotics, anti-inflammatories, and protection against tetanus, the management of fecal consistency is most important (Figure 24-6).

Two-stage repair. In the first stage the aim is to recreate the rectovestibular shelf (i.e., close the vestibular cavity and recreate a portion of the ventral perineal body). Because the rectal mucosa is not apposed and anal sphincter not repaired, there is less tension on the sutures, minimal straining, and potentially less dehiscence.

The surgical technique is described elsewhere; however, it is very similar to the single-stage repair except the rectal mucosa and dorsal perineal body are not apposed until 3 to 4 weeks later (second stage).[8,10]

Points for consideration

- Techniques are largely dictated by experience. We believe inexperienced surgeons will have less difficulty with the two-stage repair.
- The better the surgeon's anatomical and functional understanding of the perineal body, the more likely a favorable outcome will follow.
- If a two-stage repair is attempted, economic consideration for the client appears warranted as single-stage repair is just as successful with experienced surgeons.
- Fertility is good after successful repair. A slightly higher incidence of perineal trauma is expected with these mares.

Rectovestibular Fistula (RVF)

RVF most commonly results from foaling injuries, although it can occur from breeding, sadism, or other accidents. Some will heal without surgical intervention, so surgical correction is attempted at least one month or more after the injury. In the last five years we have been breeding the mares on an induced (prostaglandin) second postpartum estrous period and then immediately (within 2 days) performing the fistulae repair. The fertility of mares undergoing this technique has been excellent (~75% per cycle). For this to be successful, as much fecal material as possible is removed immediately before breeding (either natural or AI). After breeding the uterus is lavaged at least daily until repair is performed.

Most surgeons treat RVFs by converting them to third degree PL and repairing as previously described, either standing or under general anesthesia.[11] For deep (cranial) RVFs, a perineal body transection has been utilized.[9]

During the last 15 years we have repaired RVF with a transrectal approach, which we first described in 1991.[12] A similar technique was described in the 1996 AAEP proceedings by Dr. Stephen Adams.[13] In our hospital, modified Finochetto retractors (Scanlan Instruments, Englewood, Colorado) are inserted into the rectum through the anal sphincter.[9] These retractors make the surgery quite simple. The fistula is debrided and closed in three layers, with continuous suture patterns and without conversion into a third degree PL. The vestibular portion may be closed through the vagina or rectum and is inverted into the vestibule. The middle layer (perineal body) is closed from the rectum, and the rectal portion inverted into the rectum. When we previously described the surgical correction, it was recommended to alternate the orientation of the closure.[12] Now we recommend that all three layers are closed transversely, not longitudinally. The fistula middle layer is closed with 0 or 1 PDS, the vagina with 0 PDS, and the rectum with 0 or 2/0 PDS (Figure 24-7).

Restraint and postoperative care is similar to mares with perineal lacerations; however, not as much attention is given to fecal softening.

Points for consideration

- The caudal border of the fistula may be difficult to debride and is most commonly rotated toward the surgeon by grasping it with forceps (from the rectum) and everting it caudally. On occasion it may be helpful to have the surgeon's hand in the vagina while working on this part of the fistula. The use of a No. 12 blade greatly facilitates dissection of the fistula ring.

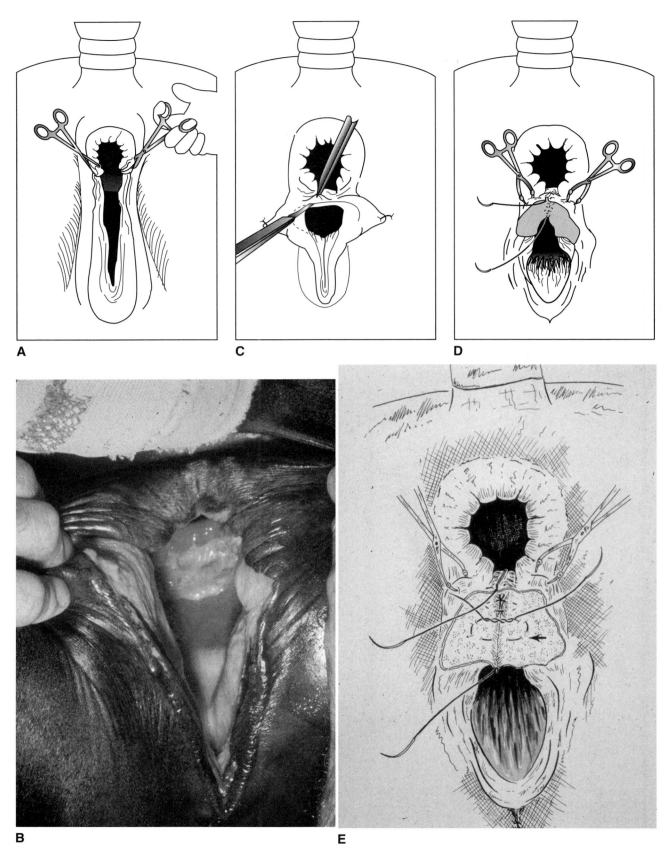

Figure 24-6 **A,** Towel forceps are used to identify the ideal position of the rectum at the end of the surgery. **B,** Typical appearance of a mare before surgery. **C,** The incision before beginning dissection. **D,** After dissection of the scar tissue, the tissues are sutured according to their origin (rectal mucosa, perineal body, and vaginal wall). **E,** The three suture patterns are incrementaly increased to ablate dead space in the perineal body and provide integrity of the rectal and vaginal layers.

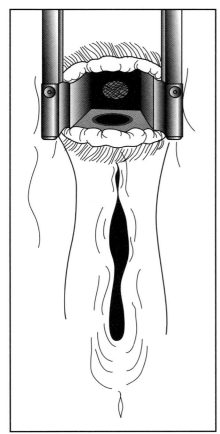

Figure 24-7 The fistula is easily approached per rectum if good retractors are available

Cervix

Cervical Lacerations
Injuries to the cervix most commonly occur at foaling. Many are not associated with a recognized dystocia. Assessing degree of compromise to the cervix as a barrier to intrauterine infection may be difficult. In general, examination immediately after foaling will reveal only the most major defects. Most cervical lacerations are identified later and are best evaluated in diestrus because increased tone facilitates assessment of degree of apposition of cervical folds and damage to the muscular layer. Manual palpation is essential for accurate diagnosis. Many mares with major cervical defects are still able to conceive and carry a foal to term.

In general only those mares with a cervical defect that progresses cranially to involve the junction of the external Os with the vagina are candidates for surgery at our practice. In addition, only mares with obvious subfertility are usually considered (i.e., uterine infection, barren one or more years, etc.)

Surgical technique. Mares are restrained standing and tranquilized. Local anesthesia is preferred with 40 to 60 ml of 2% lidocaine infused dorsally and laterally deep in the vaginal tissues around the cervix.

The most difficult aspect of cervix surgery in the mare is adequate exposure. Modified Finochietto retractors are

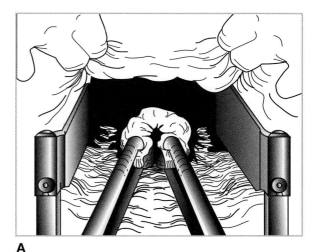

A

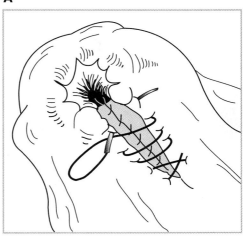

B

Figure 24-8 **A,** Knowles forceps applied to either side of the laceration facilitate the retraction and identification of the best place to debride and suture. **B,** Suture pattern recommended for cervix surgery.

preferred, and the cervix is drawn caudally by Knowles forceps.[9]

The forceps used must have large teeth that facilitate retraction with vigorous caudal pressure without tearing out of the cervix. With this technique it is generally not necessary to use specially extended cervical instruments (Figure 24-8).

The forceps are placed about 1 to 2 cm on either side of the defect or laceration. Slight rotational movement provides excellent access to the fibrous scar of the defect. The scar is debrided to the level of the cervical musculature, and the external vaginal mucosa of the cervix is slightly undermined. The internal cervical mucosa is undermined and trimmed. Original reports of cervical closure describe a three-layer closure.[9] We prefer two. The internal layer is closed with a 1 PDS with a cutting needle by a continuous pattern through the muscular layer. The external layer is closed with a simple continuous layer using 2/0 or 0 PDS. Occasionally it is necessary to trim excessive cervical folds that prolapse into the suture pattern and result in fistula formation; however, care in not removing too much is recommended to avoid creating a cervix with major orientation deviations. In addition, it is easy to inadvertently include cervical mucosa on the wrong side of the lumen if the cervical forceps are not positioned well. Patency of the cervical Os is continually confirmed during placement of sutures.

Postoperative treatments for the mare are antibiotics and protection against tetanus. After 21 days, patency of the lumen is assessed by careful manual examination. Frequently, mild adhesions attempt to form. Their occurrence is of no major concern, and gentle manipulation and daily application of a corticosteriod, antibiotic, and oil-based cream, after the surgical site has healed, result in return to normal function.

Points for consideration

- The most craniad portions of the external cervical Os appear to be the most important barriers to infection. Overzealous surgical apposition of the caudad cervix results in a very small external Os that broadens cranially and does not create a good enough seal in diestrus or relax enough during estrus to allow adequate drainage of uterine contents.
- Previously repaired cervix problems often are injured again at breeding and/or foaling. AI is recommended, or a breeding roll at the very least, if natural service is necessary.

Ovaries

Ovariectomy

Some indications for ovariectomy include: mares displaying continual annoying nymphomania; ovarian neoplasia; use of ovariectomized steroid treated mares as recipients for embryo transfer; or mares to be used as tease/jump mares (with or without exogenous hormone administration).

Most techniques describe ovariectomy by a ventral midline approach with ovarian pedicle ligature before excision. However, this is expensive and in our experience occasionally unnecessary. Ovariectomy by colpotomy (vaginal approach) with hemostasis and excision performed with an ecraseur ("crusher") is an approach not often utilized, despite having been described centuries before the advent of powerful restraining pharmaceuticals. Of course there are many occasions when flank or ventral midline approaches will be necessary, particularly for mares with ovarian neoplasia.

Colpotomy

Mares are not fed for 24 hours before surgery. Mares are restrained standing and tranquilized. The tail is secured dorsally. The external perineum is cleansed, and the vaginal cavity is lavaged with sterile saline (1 liter). No epidural anesthesia is necessary. Blunt/Blunt scissors (Metzenbaum) are used to puncture the cranial vaginal wall in a position between 4 and 5 o'clock relative to the external Os of the cervix and near the border of the pelvic canal. The scissors are advanced 4 to 6 cm, then opened and withdrawn through the vaginal wall in the opened position. The resultant hole enables a single finger to bluntly enlarge the opening to admit a hand. The peritoneum is punctured with a single digit, and ovaries and uterus identified and palpated. Swabs that have been previously sewn together and then sterilized are soaked with 50 ml of local anesthetic and applied circumferentially to each ovarian pedicle for at least 1 minute each. A "Hauptner" ecraseur is used to remove each ovary individually. Frequently the ovarian attachments to the ovary have to be manually stretched to allow ovarian removal. The vaginal incision is not closed; however, we recommend a Caslick be performed.

Mares are treated with anti-inflammatory medication (i.e., phenylbutazone, 2 g IV) approximately 10 to 20 minutes before beginning surgery. Delaying phenylbutazone administration or use of oral preparations may result in moderate abdominal discomfort manifested by sternal recumbency. Other prophylactic administrations are antibiotics and protection against tetanus. Mares are not cross tied but usually are boxed overnight and then turned out onto pasture the next day.

We have used this technique in many mares, including mares with small granulosa theca cell tumors up to approximately 10 cm, without complication.

Reported complications are evisceration, hemorrhage, removal or penetration of bowel, fatal peritonitis, and local infection. The incidence of these problems is likely related to the experience of the surgeon and speed of the surgery.

Clearly the technique has potential drawbacks (i.e., size of ovary or structure is limited to less than approximately 10 cm). However, the procedure is safe and efficacious in many instances and able to be performed expediently by personnel experienced with examination of female reproductive tract.

Points for consideration

- Occasionally some mares strain during the procedure. Allowing more time for improved analgesia or additional analgesia appears effective.
- Many of the complications such as evisceration and infection appear to be minimized by presurgical administration of IV phenylbutazone to prevent postsurgical recumbency; a Caslick; and prophylactic antibiotics.
- The procedure is safe, expedient, and efficacious, and the complication rate is similar to or less than male castration.
- Mares with uterine infection or urovagina are not considered for this technique.

Uterus

Uterine Torsion

Uterine torsion is an infrequent but serious complication of the late gestation mare. Most occur in the last two months of gestation and are recognized by mild to moderate colic that responds temporarily to analgesics. Unlike cattle, most uterine torsions of the mare are preterm and not associated with parturition. Definitive diagnosis is based on careful rectal examination. Identification of the ovarian pedicle and uterine ligaments should suggest whether the rotation is clockwise (to the right and downwards when viewed from behind) or counterclockwise. The uterine ligament on the side to which the rotation has occurred is pulled directly downward and under the uterine body. The other uterine ligament is displaced medially and runs over the uterine body toward the side of rotation and then downward. The greatest tension is on the ligament that the rotation is turned toward. Occasionally diagnosis of direction of torsion is difficult per rectum.

Technique for correction depends on stage of gestation and value of the animal. At term, manual rotation of the fetus through the cervix is often possible. Before imminent parturition, nonsurgical repositioning (rolling) is possible but may occasionally result in uterine rupture.

The mare is positioned in lateral recumbency on the side to which the uterus has rotated (i.e., clockwise torsions result in the mare being placed in right lateral recumbency). The mare is quickly flipped over to her other side and hopefully uterine weight allows the mare's body to pivot about the fetus and reposition the problem. Degree of success can be ascertained by repeated rectal palpation. Another approach is to place a board with weight (i.e., a person) on the upper flank and turn the mare slowly. In this case the board keeps the foal in position during rotation.

Alternative techniques for correction include standing flank laparotomy and ventral midline approach. Standing flank laparotomy has been our preferred method for correction if the mare and/or foal are valuable and there is no evidence of uterine rupture. This technique has a lower probability of creating uterine rupture and avoids the stress of anesthesia.

Standing Flank Laparotomy

For standing flank laparotomy, the mare is moderately sedated, and the paralumbar fossa on the side toward which the rotation is directed is clipped and prepared for aseptic surgery. Local anesthetic (40-80 ml) infused in a vertical line is administered at or slightly cranial to the anticipated incision in the middle of the paralumbar fossa. The skin and paniculus (cutaneous) muscle are incised vertically, and external and internal abdominal oblique muscles are separated along their direction of orientation (grid approach). The transverse adominus is bluntly dissected and the peritoneum punctured with a single finger. The direction of the torsion is confirmed, and a prominent part of the foal under the uterus is grasped and used to gently rock and lift the uterus toward the surgeon. Resolution of the torsion is usually immediately obvious; however, on occasion, lengthening the incision to allow two hands to enter the abdomen or a bilateral flank incision with two surgeons is sometimes necessary. The external and internal abdominal oblique muscles and subcutaneous tissues are apposed by a simple continuous suture pattern with a No. 1 or 2 absorbable material. The skin is closed with a continuous simple or interlocking pattern of nonabsorbable material.

Points for consideration

- Abdominal ultrasonography should be used to verify that the fetus is still alive and, if possible, assess uterine integrity.
- Survival of the mare and/or foal may be influenced by degree of uterine torsion, ease of correction, elapsed time before correction, and stage of pregnancy.
- Regardless of the stage of gestation, if the cervix is open at the time of recognition of uterine torsion, delivery after standing intravaginal/intrauterine manipulation or ventral midline access for reposition and caesarian section is preferable to standing flank laparotomy or rolling of the mare.
- Occasionally a standing flank laparotomy will not have a successful surgical outcome due to the degree of rotation. If a more severe rotation (>360 degrees) is suspected or an excessively elevated heart rate (>70 beats/min) is identified, it may be better to perform a ventral midline laparotomy to better assess uterine health and gain the best physical advantage for uterine positioning. In addition, the fetus can be removed.

References

1. Turner AS, McIlwraith CW: Techniques in large animal surgery, ed 2, Philadelphia, Lippincott Williams & Wilkins, 1989.
2. LeBlanc PH, Canon JP, Patterson JS et al: Epidural injection of xylazine for perineal analgesia in horses. J Am Vet Med Assoc 1988; 193:1405.
3. Pascoe RR: Observations on the length and angle of declination of the vulva and its relation to fertility in the mare. J Reprod Fert 1979; 27(Suppl):299.
4. McKinnon AO, Belden JO: A urethral extension technique to correct urine pooling (vesicovaginal reflux) in mares. J Am Vet Med Assoc 1988; 192:647-650.
5. Caslick EA: The vulva and the vulvo-vaginal orifice and its relation to genital health of the thoroughbred mare. Cornell Vet 1937; 27:178.
6. Trotter GW, McKinnon AO: Surgery for abnormal vulvar and perineal conformation in the mare. Vet Clin N Am 1988; 4:389.
7. Pouret EJM: Surgical technique for the correction of pneumo and urovagina. Eq Vet J 1982; 14:249.
8. Aanes WA: Surgical management of foaling injuries. Vet Clin N Am 1988; 4:417.
9. Stickle RL, Fessler JF, Adams SB: A single-stage technique for repair of rectovestibular lacerations in the mare. Vet Surg 1979; 8:25.
10. Colbern GT, Aanes WA, Stashak TS: Surgical management of perineal lacerations and rectovestibular fistulae in the mare: a retrospective study of 47 cases. J Am Vet Med Assoc 1985; 186:265.
11. Hilbert BJ: Surgical repair of recto-vaginal fistuas. Aust Vet J 1981; 57:85.
12. McKinnon AO, Arnold KS, Vasey JR: Selected reproductive surgery of the broodmare. In Equine reproduction: A seminar for veterinarians. Sydney, Post Graduate Committee in Veterinary Science 1991; 174:109-25.
13. Adams SB, Benker F, Brandenburg T: Direct rectovaginal fistula repair in five mares. Proc AAEP 1996; 42:156-9.

Additional Reading

Auer JA, Stick JA: Equine surgery, Philadelphia, W.B. Saunders, 1999.
Colahan PT, Mayhew IG, Merritt AM et al: Equine medicine and surgery, 4th ed, Goleta, American Veterinary Publicaitons Inc., 1991.

Jennings PB: The practice of large animal surgery, Philadelphia, W.B. Saunders, 1984.

McIlwraith CW, Turner AS: Equine surgery advanced techniques, Philadelphia, Lea and Febiger, 1987.

McKinnon AO, Squies EL, Carnevale EM et al: Urogenital surgery. Vet Clin N Am Vol 4 Equine Pract 1988.

Walker DF, Vaughan JT: Bovine and equine urogenital surgery. Philadelphia, Lea and Febiger, 1980.

White NA, Moore JN: Current practice of equine surgery. Philadelphia, J.B. Lippincott Company, 1990.

CHAPTER 25

Infectious and Neoplastic Conditions of the Vulva and Perineum

COREY D. MILLER

CONTAGIOUS EQUINE METRITIS

Etiology

In 1977 an outbreak of a transmissible venereal disease of horses, subsequently named contagious equine metritis (CEM), occurred in the Newmarket area of England and in Ireland. An outbreak affecting several Kentucky breeding farms occurred the following year, after the importation of two Thoroughbred carrier stallions from France in the fall of 1977. Since 1978 the disease has been reported only once in the United States, in one Thoroughbred stallion and two mares in 1982. The etiologic agent was identified to be a gram-negative microaerophilic coccobacillus and was initially identified as *Haemophilus equigenitalis* and later renamed *Taylorella equigenitalis*.[1]

More than 20 distinct genotypes among over 200 strains of *T. equigenitalis* have been identified through pulsed-field gel electrophoresis.[2] A recent study using polymerase chain reaction (PCR) assay indicates that *Taylorella* is endemic to the horse population by the presence of *Taylorella* DNA in the genital tract of 7 out of 24 horses in the isolated Icelandic horse population.[3]

In 1997, bacterial isolates of an atypical *T. equigenitalis* strain were obtained from donkey jacks in Kentucky and California. Although the isolates were phenotypically indistinguishable from *T. equigenitalis* in culture, comparisons of the DNA sequence revealed that the new isolates were different. Pulsed-field gel electrophoresis showed that the Kentucky and California isolates were also different.[4] This strain of *Taylorella* has been named *Taylorella asinigenitalis* sp. nov.[5] One study attempted to infect mares with both the California and Kentucky isolates of *T. asinigenitalis* sp. nov., along with *T. equigenitalis*. This study found that the two mares inoculated with the California isolate did not become infected, whereas the mares inoculated with the Kentucky isolate of *T. asinigenitalis* sp. nov. and with *T. equigenitalis* did develop infections. The Kentucky isolate produced a CEM-like infection that developed several days later and with less intensity than the *T. equigenitalis* infection, but otherwise showed clinical, serologic, and pathologic changes that closely resemble classic CEM.[6] Clearly, different isolates of *T. equigenitalis* are found among U.S.-origin Equidae, and one isolate has been shown to produce CEM-like symptoms in mares. A veterinarian must consider atypical *Taylorella* sp. infections as a differential diagnosis of equine infertility when examining U.S.-origin mares.[6] Any veterinarian who suspects that a horse in his care may be affected with *T. equigenitalis* is required under law to report such suspicions to his or her state veterinarian.

Diagnostics

Clinical Signs

Mares infected for the first time usually exhibit a copious grayish vulvar discharge 8 to 10 days after infection that persists for 13 to 17 days. The discharge typically disappears without treatment. Another clinical sign is a shortened interestrous interval due to acute endometritis. Most mares recover spontaneously; however, some mares become chronic carriers of the bacteria[7] and subsequently may transmit the bacteria to stallions. On the other hand, a mare may become infected by a stallion, show no clinical signs, and become an asymptomatic carrier. These mares can become pregnant and carry the pregnancy to term. The organism has been recovered from the placenta of positive mares[8] and from the genitalia of colts and fillies,[9] indicating that it can be transferred in utero and/or at parturition. There have been two reported cases of abortion in mares caused by a *T. equigenitalis* infection. In these cases the bacterium was cultured from several sites in the aborted fetuses.[10] However, the transmission of CEM primarily occurs during coitus or by fomites used in handling and treating infected mares and stallions.

Bacteriologic Cultures

Bacteriologic testing is the most reliable means of diagnosing CEM,[11] but a major disadvantage of this method is the extended culture time, resulting in delays in diagnosis.[12]

In one study a group of mares was experimentally infected by intrauterine inoculation with *T. equigenitalis* and subsequently necropsied at various intervals post inoculation.[13] During the first 2 weeks after infection the organism was isolated from the uterine and cervical

Box   25-1

States Approved to Accept Mares and Stallions for Contagious Equine Metritis Treatment and Testing

Alabama	New York
California	North Carolina
Colorado	Ohio
Florida	Oklahoma
Georgia	Oregon
Kentucky	Rhode Island
Louisiana	South Carolina
Maryland	Tennessee
Montana	Texas
New Hampshire	Virginia
New Jersey	Wisconsin

lumen, most commonly, and less frequently from the vaginal vestibule, clitoral fossa, clitoral sinuses, and oviducts. Between 3 and 4 months after infection, *T. equigenitalis* was only occasionally recovered from the ovarian surface, oviducts, uterus, cervix, and vagina, but more frequently from the clitoral sinuses and fossa.[13] As a result of this study, the culture sites for screening mares for CEM for import/export regulations are the mucosal surfaces of the clitoral sinuses and clitoral fossa.

All cultures for CEM must be performed at a licensed state facility (Box 25-1), under current U.S. Department of Agriculture (USDA) guidelines. Sets of specimens for culture must be collected from the mucosal surfaces of the clitoral sinuses and fossa on three separate occasions over a 7-day period (including days 1 and 7 of quarantine). The openings to the clitoral sinuses, located on the dorsal aspect of the clitoris, require a small swab. Culture specimen swabs submitted for culture must be placed in Amies transport media with charcoal and maintained at approximately 4° to 6°C for transit. Specimens must be received within 48 hours of collection by the National Veterinary Services Laboratories (NVSL) in Ames, Iowa, or by a diagnostic laboratory that is approved to conduct CEM cultures and tests.[14] *T. equigenitalis* requires chocolate agar plus 10% horse blood as its culture media. The plates are incubated at 37°C, in an atmosphere of 5% to 10% carbon dioxide. Growth is enhanced in an atmosphere of 90% hydrogen gas and 10% carbon dioxide.[12] All culture set plates must be negative and readable by an approved state or federal animal disease diagnostic laboratory. The organism is oxidase, catalase, and phosphatase positive but is otherwise biochemically nonreactive.

Serologic Testing

No serologic test described to date will, by itself, reliably detect infection. However, serologic tests can be used as an adjunct to culture for *T. equigenitalis* in screening mares but must not be used as a substitute for culture.

All methods of serologic testing are based upon detection of *T. equigenitalis* antibodies. The complement fixation (CF) test is the serologic test used by USDA regulatory officials but is only accurate 10 or more days after infection. CF testing is not reliable for identifying mares that are carriers of the *T. equigenitalis* bacteria.[12] An enzyme-linked immunosorbent assay (ELISA) has also been developed to test for *T. equigenitalis* and *T. asinigenitalis*. The ELISA test had comparable results to the traditional CF test, but results are ready in less than 3 hours, as opposed to the overnight incubation of the CF test.[15] A rapid microtitration serum agglutination test for the detection of CEM antibodies has also been described. This test was developed as a backup to the CF test and is useful as a serologic test early in the disease.[16]

Prognosis

Infertility associated with the infection is usually temporary, and no long-term effects on fertility have been reported.[17]

Therapy

The acute stage of CEM should be treated using similar protocols to routine endometritis cases: uterine lavage with large volumes of sterile physiologic fluids, oxytocin injections, and uterine infusions with antibiotics based on culture and sensitivity.

For carrier infections with *T. equigenitalis* and to meet U.S. import requirements, standard USDA protocol should be followed: after the three sets of specimens have been collected for culture, all organic debris and smegma should be manually removed from the clitoral sinuses and fossa of the mare and the areas should be flushed with 2% chlorhexidine solution, followed with saline solution. This must be done for 5 consecutive days. After each cleaning has been completed, the clitoral fossa and sinuses are to be filled with an antibiotic ointment that is effective against *T. equigenitalis*. Most antibacterial ointments and creams, except streptomycin, such as nitrofurazone ointment and Silvadene cream are effective against *T. equigenitalis*. If any of the culture sets test positive for *T. equigenitalis*, the mare must be treated as above and then recultured again on three separate occasions over a 7-day period (including days 1 and 7), starting no less than 21 days after the last day of treatment.[14] If the mare remains culture positive, the mare can be retreated or the owners may elect to have a clitoral sinusectomy performed.[18]

Managerial Considerations

After a mare has been treated and tested as negative for *T. equigenitalis*, it is important to remember that reinfection can occur. Prior exposure to the bacteria may attenuate future clinical signs, but will not prevent reinfection. Attempts have been made to produce a vaccine, including uterine inoculation with killed *T. equigenitalis*, but were unsuccessful, as the killed bacteria inoculating vaccine did not prevent an infection by *T. equigenitalis* after a subsequent uterine challenge.[19] Attention to detailed hygienic, gynecologic practice is essential to prevent the inadvertent spread of infection through dis-

Box   25-2

Countries Affected With Contagious Equine Metritis

Member States of the European Union (Austria, Belgium, Denmark, Finland, France, Germany, Greece, Ireland, Italy, Luxembourg, The Netherlands, Norway, Portugal, Spain, Sweden, and the United Kingdom [England, Northern Ireland, Scotland, Wales, and the Isle of Man])
   Countries of the Former Yugoslavia (Bosnia, Croatia, Herzegovina, Macedonia, Montenegro, and Serbia)

Czech Republic
Guinea Bissau
Japan
Slovakia
Slovenia
Switzerland

posable gloves, speculums, infusion pipettes, and other equipment. Also, transfer of *T. equigenitalis* by artificial insemination with semen from an infected stallion can be controlled by adding 1-2 mg/ml of gentamycin sulfate to the semen extender.[20]

It is important to note that all horses over 2 years of age that are imported into the United States from countries affected with CEM (Box 25-2) must fulfill the USDA import quarantine and testing requirements. The mare must be consigned to a state that has been approved by the administrator of the Animal and Plant Health Inspection Service (APHIS) to receive mares (see Box 25-1) from CEM-affected countries in order to undergo the prescribed CEM treatment and testing requirements. The treatment and collection of culture specimens for CEM has to be performed by an accredited veterinarian and monitored by a state or federal veterinarian. The area veterinarian in charge (AVIC) is responsible for reviewing all treatment activities with state animal health officials to ensure that proper procedures are being administered. For specific guidelines regarding importation of horses from areas affected by CEM, consult your current federal and state guidelines.

EQUINE COITAL EXANTHEMA

Etiology

Equine coital exanthema is caused by an infection with equine herpesvirus type 3 (EHV-3). There is some evidence that a combination of small- and large-plaque variant viruses are involved in the development of coital exanthema.[21] Due to the occurrence of neutralizing antibodies to EHV-3 in horses of breeding age, it is thought that spread of EHV-3 is primarily through genital contact.[22]

Diagnostics

Coital exanthema is typically diagnosed by characteristic clinical signs, which include multiple circular nodules up to 2 mm in diameter on the vulvar mucosa and perineal skin for 7 days after sexual contact.[7] These lesions progress to vesicles and pustules that eventually rupture, leaving naked, ulcerated areas approximately 3 to 10 mm in diameter. These shallow erosions have sharply defined borders, scab over, and heal within a few weeks, leaving behind small, depigmented spots on the vulvar and perineal skin.[23] Occasionally the virus can cause systemic signs of infection, including dullness, anorexia, fever, and regional edema of the vulvar, perineum, and inner thighs.[22] Extragenital lesions are uncommon but on occasion may be found on the lips and nasal mucosa.[7]

Additional diagnostics during the acute vesicular stage include viral isolation of swabs or scrapings taken from the edge of erosions using electron microscopy and histologic identification of typical herpesvirus inclusions in affected tissue.[24] In addition, serologic testing for EHV-3 antibodies may be performed by complement fixation and serum neutralization. Complement-fixing antibodies decline rapidly after exposure and are not detectable after 60 days post introduction, whereas serum-neutralizing antibodies remain high for at least 1 year post exposure.[25,26] Therefore comparison of complement fixation and serum neutralization antibodies may be useful in determining the time of exposure.

Prognosis

Coital exanthema is thought to be a benign infection in mares, although some investigators suggest that mares bred to stallions infected with EHV-3 may have reduced pregnancy rates for that mating.[24] However, investigation of two outbreaks of coital exanthema did not reveal any evidence supporting subfertility in mares bred by stallions infected with EHV-3, such that normal pregnancy rates occurred in the mares bred to actively infected stallions.[27] Lesions may appear repeatedly in some mares, usually during the later stages of pregnancy or after foaling, without reexposure to the virus.[24] Infertility, if it occurs at all, is associated with either pain that prevents copulation or ejaculation or a transient decrease in motility that accompanies severe swelling in some cases. Both problems are short lived.

Therapy

Primary therapy with topical antiviral preparations is not warranted due to the benign, self-limiting nature of this condition and because there is no evidence that such treatments speed recovery. Treatment with demulsifying antibiotic-containing ointment may be useful to prevent secondary bacterial infections.

Managerial Considerations

Sexual rest should be instituted to help prevent further spread of the disease by natural mating. Artificial insemination can be performed, as long as disposable equipment is used and personnel are aware of the risk of perpetuating the disease.

The disease is not contagious once the ulcerative lesions have healed (apart from recrudescence). Immunity to this virus is relatively short. However, some immunity to the virus is acquired after infection, because reinfection without recurrence of clinically apparent disease is common. Previously infected horses are subject to reinfection by this virus later in the same breeding season or in subsequent years.[24] It is likely that the virus remains in the genitalia in a latent form.[28]

NEOPLASTIC CONDITIONS OF THE VULVA AND PERINEUM

The most common tumors of the external genitalia of the mare are squamous cell carcinoma (SCC) and melanoma.[29]

Squamous Cell Carcinoma

Etiology

Squamous cell carcinoma of the perianal, vulva, and clitoral regions of mares accounts for 12% of all equine SCC cases. The average age of mares affected by SCC is 11.9 years. Draft breeds, Appaloosas, Paints, Pintos, and individual horses with little or no pigmentation around the mucocutaneous junctions are most likely to be affected.[30] The causes of SCC in mares have been suggested to include papilloma virus, trauma, chronic irritation, melanin deficiency, and sunlight.[31] SCC lesions may be erosive or productive and are usually locally aggressive tumors that invade surrounding tissue and metastasize to the local lymph nodes and the lungs in later stages of the disease.[32] Pseudohyperparathyroidism has been reported as a peri-neoplastic syndrome in a mare that had a large primary SCC of the vulva.[33]

Diagnostics

A definitive diagnosis of SCC is made by cytologic or histologic examination of the tissue.[31]

Prognosis

The prognosis is quite variable and is dependent upon the aggressiveness of the individual tumor, the size of the tumor, the location of the tumor, the degree of local invasion at the time of diagnosis/treatment, and the presence or absence of metastases. In addition, tumors of the perineal region can interfere with urination, defecation, or coitus.[34]

Therapy

Treatment options for SCC of the external genitalia of mares include surgical removal, cryotherapy,[35] topical 5-fluorouracil administration,[36] and intratumoral cisplatin administration.[37] Typically, a combination of surgical and chemical intervention is the most efficacious means of treating the tumor.

Melanoma

Etiology

Melanomas are common in the perineal, perianal, and tail areas of older gray horses. It has been estimated that approximately 80% of gray horses over 15 years of age are afflicted with melanomas.[38] Melanomas vary greatly in size and are typically firm, black masses. Melanomas may be solitary or multiple, and benign or malignant. Melanomas may be locally invasive and may metastasize to regional lymph nodes or distant tissues via the lymphatics or blood vessels.[39]

Diagnostics

Diagnosis is by clinical appearance and is confirmed by histologic evaluation of the tissue. Histologic characteristics of melanomas are not predictive of malignancy in the majority of cases.[40]

Prognosis

The prognosis is quite variable and is dependent upon the aggressiveness of the individual tumor, the size of the tumor, the location of the tumor, the degree of local invasion at the time of diagnosis/treatment, and the presence of metastases. In addition, tumors of the perineal region can interfere with urination, defecation, or coitus.[34]

Therapy

Treatment options for melanomas of the external genitalia of mares may include surgical removal, cryotherapy, immunotherapy, radiotherapy, and cimetidine therapy.[34,38]

References

1. Sugimoto C, Isayama Y, Sakazaki R et al: Transfer of *Haemophilus equigenitalis* to the genus *Taylorella* gen. nov. as *Taylorella equigenitalis* comb. nov. Curr Microbiol 1983; 9:155-162.
2. Kagawa S, Moore JE, Murayama O et al: Comparison of the value of pulsed-field gel electrophoresis, random amplified polymorphic DNA and amplified rDA restriction analysis for subtyping *Taylorella equigenitalis*. Vet Res Commun 2001; 25:261-269.
3. Parlevliet JM, Bleumink-Pluym NMC, Houwers DJ et al: Epidemiologic aspects of *Taylorella equigenitalis*. Theriogenology 1997; 47:1169-1177.
4. Arata AB, Cooke CL, Spencer SJ et al: Multiplex polymerase chain reaction for distinguishing *Taylorella equigenitalis* from *Taylorella equigenitalis*-like organisms. J Vet Diagn Invest 2001; 13:263-264.
5. Jang SS, Donahue JM, Arata AB et al: *Taylorella asinigenitalis* sp. nov., a bacterium isolated from the genital tract of male donkeys (*Equus asinus*). Int J Syst Evol Microbiol 2001; 51:917-976.
6. Katz JB, Evans LE, Hutto DL et al: Clinical, bacteriologic, serologic, and pathologic features of infections with atypical *Taylorella equigenitalis* in mares. J Am Vet Med Assoc 2000; 216(12):1945-1948.
7. Couto MA, Hughes JP: Sexually transmitted (venereal) disease of horses. In McKinnon A, Voss JL (eds): Equine Reproduction, pp 845-854, London, Lea & Febiger, 1993.
8. Powell DG, Whitwell K: The epidemiology of contagious equine metritis (CEM) in England 1977-1978. J Reprod Fertil Suppl 1979; 27:331-335.
9. Timoney PJ, Powell DG: Isolation of the contagious equine metritis organism from colts and fillies in the United Kingdom and Ireland. Vet Rec 1982; 111:478-482.
10. Fontijne P, Terlack EA, Hartman EG: *Taylorella equigenitalis* isolated from an aborted foal. Vet Rec 1989; 125:485.

11. Brown BS, Timoney PJ: Contagious equine metritis and fluorescence. Vet Rec 1988; 123:38 (letter).
12. Timoney JF: The genus *Taylorella*. In Timoney JF, Gillespie JH, Scott FW et al (eds): Hagan and Bruner's Microbiology and Infectious Diseases of Domestic Animals, 8th edition, pp 100-103, Ithaca, NY, Comstock Publishing Associates, 1988.
13. Strezmienski PJ, Benson CE, Acland HM et al: Comparison of uterine protein content and distribution of bacteria in the reproductive tract of mares after intrauterine inoculation of *Haemophilus equigenitalis* or *Pseudomonas aeruginosa*. Am J Vet Res 1984; 45(6):1109-1113.
14. Veterinary Services Memorandum No. 558.4. Veterinary Services, Animal and Plant Health and Inspection Service, U.S. Department of Agriculture, 1997.
15. Katz J, Geer P: An enzyme-linked immunosorbent assay for the convenient serodiagnosis of contagious equine metritis in mares. J Vet Diagn Invest 2001; 13:87-88.
16. Gummow B, Herr S, Brett OL: A rapid microtitration serum agglutination test for the detection of contagious equine metritis antibodies. Onderstepoort J Vet Res 1987; 54:97-98.
17. Platt H, Taylor CED: Contagious equine metritis. In Easmon CSF, Jeljaszewicz J (eds): Medical Microbiology, p 49, New York, Academic, 1983.
18. Swerczek TW: Elimination of CEM organisms from mares by excision of clitoral sinuses. Vet Rec 1979; 105:131-132.
19. Widders PR, Stokes CR, David JS et al: Specific antibody in the equine genital tract following local immunization and challenge infection with contagious equine metritis organism *(Taylorella equigenitalis)*. Res Vet Sci 1986; 40:54-58.
20. Timoney PJ, O'Reilly PJ, Harrington AM et al: Survival of *Haemophilus equigenitalis* in different antibiotic-containing semen extenders. J Reprod Fertil Suppl 1979; 27:377-381.
21. Jacob RJ et al: Molecular pathogenesis of equine coital exanthema: identification of a new equine herpesvirus isolated from lesions reminiscent of coital exanthema in a donkey. In Powell DG (ed): Equine Infectious Diseases V: Proceedings of the Fifth International Conference of Equine Infectious Diseases, pp 140-146, Lexington, University Press of Kentucky, 1988.
22. Gibbs EPJ, Roberts MC, Morris JM: Equine coital exanthema in the United Kingdom. Equine Vet J 1970; 4:74.
23. Bryans JT: Herpesviral diseases affecting reproduction in the horse. Vet Clin North Am Large Anim Pract 1980; 2:303.
24. Blanchard T, Kenney R, Timoney P: Venereal disease. Vet Clin North Am Equine Pract 1992; 8:191.
25. Pascoe RR, Bagust TJ, Spradbrow PB: Studies on equine herpesviruses. IV. Infection of horses with a herpesvirus recovered from equine coital exanthema. Aust Vet J 1972; 48:99.
26. Pascoe RR, Bagust JL: Coital exanthema in stallions. J Reprod Fertil Suppl 1975; 23:147.
27. Pascoe RR: The effect of equine coital exanthema on the fertility of mares covered by stallions exhibiting the clinical disease. Aust Vet J 1981; 57:111.
28. Ladds PW: The male genital system. In Jubb KVF, Kennedy PC (eds): Pathology of Domestic Animals, 3rd edition, p 409, New York, Academic, 1985.
29. Sundberg JP, Burnstein T, Page EH: Neoplasms of Equidae. J Am Vet Med Assoc 1977; 170:150.
30. Burney DP, Theisen SK, Schmitz DG: Identifying and treating squamous cell carcinoma of horses. Vet Med 1992; 6:588.
31. MacFadden KE, Pace LW: Clinical manifestations of squamous cell carcinoma in horses. Compend Contin Educ Pract Vet 1991; 13:669.
32. Mullowney PC: Dermatologic diseases of horses. IV. Environmental, congenital, and neoplastic diseases. Compend Contin Educ Pract Vet 1985; 7:22.
33. Karcher LF, Le Net J, Turner BF et al: Pseudohyperparathyroidism in a mare associated with squamous cell carcinoma of the vulva. Cornell Vet 1990; 80:153.
34. Goetz TE, Ogilvie GK, Keegan KG et al: Cimetidine for treatment of melanomas in three horses. J Am Vet Med Assoc 1990; 196:449.
35. Hanson RR: Cryotherapy for equine skin conditions. In Robinson NE (ed): Current Therapy in Equine Medicine, p 370, Philadelphia, WB Saunders, 1997.
36. Fortier LA, Mac Harg MA: Topical use of 5 fluorouracil for treatment of squamous cell carcinoma of the external genitalia of horses: 11 cases (1988-1992). J Am Vet Med Assoc 1994; 205:1183.
37. Theon AP: Cisplatin treatment for cutaneous tumors. In Robinson NE (ed): Current Therapy in Equine Medicine, p 372, Philadelphia, WB Saunders, 1997.
38. Jeglum KA: Melanomas. In Robinson NE (ed): Current Therapy in Equine Medicine, p 399, Philadelphia, WB Saunders, 1997.
39. McCue PM: Neoplasia of the female reproductive tract. Vet Clin North Am Equine Pract 1998; 14(3):505-515.
40. MacGillivray KC, Sweeney RW, Del Piero F: Metastatic melanoma in horses. J Vet Int Med 2002; 16(4):452-456.

SECTION III

The Normal Male Reproductive System

CHAPTER 26

Anatomy and Examination of the Normal Testicle

TRACEY S. CHENIER

THE SCROTUM

The testes of the normal stallion are contained within the slightly pendulous scrotum located between the stallion's hindlimbs. In a normal stallion, the scrotum and contents should appear generally symmetric. The scrotum is formed from an outpouching of skin, with two distinct pouches separated by a median raphe. The scrotum contains the two testes, epididymides, spermatic cords, and cremaster muscles. The wall of the scrotum consists of four layers: (1) skin, (2) tunica dartos, (3) scrotal fascia, and (4) tunica vaginalis. The scrotal skin is essentially hairless and contains large numbers of sebaceous and sweat glands, which assist with thermoregulation of the testicles.[1-3] A longitudinal scrotal raphe marks the center line of the scrotum and continues cranially onto the prepuce and dorsocaudally onto the perineum. The tunica dartos layer consists of both muscular and fibroelastic tissue and is adhered to the inner surface of scrotal skin, lining both scrotal pouches and reflecting along the raphe to form the median septum. The degree of relaxation or contraction of this layer results in alterations in shape and positioning of the scrotum in relation to the body wall, assisting with testis thermoregulation.[3] The scrotal fascia is a loose connective tissue layer between the tunica dartos and tunica vaginalis and allows the testis to move freely within the scrotal pouch.[3] The tunica vaginalis is the innermost layer of the scrotum and is formed by evagination of the peritoneum during testicular descent. This layer is closely apposed to the tunica albuginea of the testis, but separated by a potential space termed the vaginal cavity. A thin layer of fluid lines the vaginal cavity to permit the testis to slide smoothly within the scrotum. On palpation the scrotal skin should be thin, consistent throughout without wrinkling, slide loosely over the testicles and be free of any lesions. The tunics should palpate as smooth layers without wrinkling.

THE TESTIS

The testis is encapsulated by the tunica albuginea, a layer of collagenous tissue and smooth muscle (Figure 26-1). Trabeculae of the tunica albuginea extend into the testicular parenchyma to provide a supporting framework and divide the testis into lobules.[3] The mediastinum testis of the stallion is located at the cranial pole of the testis where the excurrent ducts cross the tunica albuginea and enter the head of the epididymis. This results in a mediastinum testis that is less obvious ultrasonographically compared with other species such as the bull, where the mediastinum testis is oriented axially within the testis. On manual palpation the testes of a normal stallion lie horizontally within the scrotum with the tail of the epididymis directed caudad. Palpation of the tail of the epididymis and the ligament of the tail of the epididymis assist the examiner in determining normal orientation of the testicle. The ligament is palpable as a fibrous nodule attaching the tail of the epididymis to the caudal pole of the testis. The tone of the testicles on palpation should be firm to rigid and resilient. Excessive softness or firmness may be indicative of disease conditions.

TESTIS SIZE AND VOLUME

Testicular size varies among stallions depending upon breed, size, age, season, and reproductive status. Each testis of a normal postpubertal light horse breed stallion weighs between 150 and 300 g.[4] Testis size and parenchymal weight correlate highly with daily sperm production and is a useful predictor of a stallion's breeding potential. Because parenchymal weight cannot be measured in the live stallion, testicular measurements are used. Individual testis measurements have been shown to correlate well with parenchymal weight ($r^2 = 0.57$ to 0.82) and daily sperm output ($r^2 = 0.52$ to 0.76).[5-8] Testicular measure-

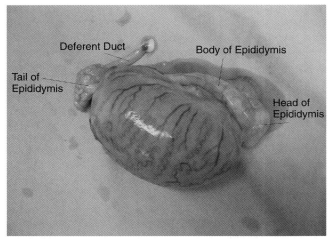

Figure 26-1 Lateral view of the right testis of a stallion showing relationship of the head, body, and tail of epididymis to the testis.

Table 26-1

Minimum Recommended Measurements for Total Scrotal Width for Light Horse Stallions

	2-3 Years	4-6 Years	7 Years and Up
Minimum	81 mm	85 mm	95 mm
Range	81-111 mm	85-115 mm	95-124 mm

Modified from Thompson DL, Pickett BW, Squires EL et al: Testicular measurements and reproductive characteristics in stallions. J Reprod Fertil Suppl 1979; 27:13-17.

ments therefore become a critical component of a breeding soundness evaluation in the stallion. The testes are measured individually using calipers for length, width, and height. Alternatively, ultrasonographic measurements can be taken to determine cross-sectional area (through the widest portion of the testicle) and length. In addition, the total scrotal width is measured using calipers. The testicles should be pushed downwards into the scrotum with one hand while the other hand operates the calipers. The average of three measurements should be used to reduce operator error. Recommended minimum guidelines for light horse stallions[9] for total scrotal width and individual testicular measures are given in Tables 26-1 and 26-2, respectively. The reproductive characteristics, including testicular measurements, of miniature stallions have also been determined.[10] Tables 26-3 and 26-4 give the mean total scrotal width and individual testis measurements for 216 miniature stallions in the study.

Because the shape of a testis is approximately that of an ellipsoid, the following formula has been suggested to convert measurements into testicular volume[11]:

$$\text{Testis Volume} = 0.5333 \times \text{Height} \times \text{Length} \times \text{Width}$$

Table 26-2

Mean (SD) Individual Testis Measurements of 46 Light Horse Stallions

Testis Measurement	Recommended Minimum in mm (±SD)
Left width	57.8 (5.2)
Left length	103.1 (8.2)
Right width	55.8 (5.8)
Right length	107.5 (8.0)

Modified from Thompson DL, Pickett BW, Squires EL et al: Testicular measurements and reproductive characteristics in stallions. J Reprod Fertil Suppl 1979; 27:13-17.

Table 26-3

Calculated Total Scrotal Width Measurements for Miniature Stallions (n = 216) by Stallion Size

Miniature Horse Size (Height Range in cm)	Total Scrotal Width Mean (mm)
Small/Medium (72-96)	72.5
Large (97-104)	79.5

TSW was calculated using the equation TSW = 1.74 + 0.696 (LW + RW).
Modified from Paccamonti DL, Buiten AV, Parlevliet JM et al: Reproductive parameters of miniature stallions. Theriogenology 1999; 51:1343-1349.

Table 26-4

Testicular Measurements for Miniature Stallions (n = 216) by Stallion Size

Testis Measurement	Recommended Minimum in mm (±SD) Small/Medium (72-96 cm)	Recommended Minimum in mm (±SD) Large (97-104 cm)
Left width	39.0 (0.05)	4.34 (0.07)
Left length	63.74 (0.08)	7.03 (0.10)
Right width	38.3 (0.05)	4.30 (0.07)
Right length	62.64 (0.08)	6.92 (0.10)

Minimum recommended values were taken as means minus 2 SD.
Modified from Paccamonti DL, Buiten AV, Parlevliet JM et al: Reproductive parameters of miniature stallions. Theriogenology 1999; 51:1343-1349.

The following formula is then used to predict daily sperm output (DSO) in the stallion:

$$\text{Predicted DSO} = [0.024 \times (\text{vol L} + \text{vol R})] - 0.76$$

For the stallion whose observed DSO is below that predicted on the basis of testicular measurements, additional evaluations for disease conditions of the testes, epididymides, and accessory glands may provide useful information.

THE SPERMATIC CORD

Examination of the stallion's scrotal contents must also include examination of the spermatic cord. A corresponding deferent duct, testicular artery, testicular veins, lymphatic vessels, nerves and cremaster muscle are contained within each spermatic cord and enveloped by the vaginal tunic.[1,2,3] The testicular artery, vein, lymph vessels and nerves are gathered together in the anterior aspect of the cord, whereas the deferent duct is found in the caudal aspect of the cord. The spermatic cord functions in testis thermoregulation through blood cooling via the pampiniform plexus and contraction/relaxation of the cremaster muscles to raise or lower the testis as required according to external temperature. On palpation it may be difficult to determine the individual components of the cord; however, any swellings, lumps, thickening, or pain should be considered abnormal.

ULTRASOUND EXAMINATION OF THE NORMAL STALLION TESTIS

Ultrasound examination of the testis is easily performed and can provide useful information for the clinician. The stallion should be suitably restrained either in stocks or against a wall. Most stallions are more tractable following semen collection and tolerate the procedure well. Some stallions may require the application of a twitch to divert their attention during the examination. A 5.0- or 7.5-mHz linear or sector transducer will provide quality imaging. The examiner stands on the left side of the stallion and uses the right hand under the bar of the stocks to place the probe on the scrotum. Contact lubricant applied liberally will maximize skin-probe contact and improve image quality. The left hand is used to push the opposite testis upwards into the scrotum and out of the way. The ultrasound probe is placed in vertical orientation across the testis at the cranial pole and slowly moved caudad until the entire testis and epididymis is visualized. The ultrasound probe can be used to take length, width, and height measurements of each testis for calculation of testis volume. This method is likely to be more accurate than caliper measurements, provided the operator takes care to avoid inadvertent oblique orientation of the ultrasound probe across the testis.

In the normal testis the scrotum appears as a thin uniformly echogenic layer, and a very small amount of fluid may be visible between the skin and testis. The testicular parenchyma should appear homogenous and uniformly echogenic (Figure 26-2). The central vein is visible as a

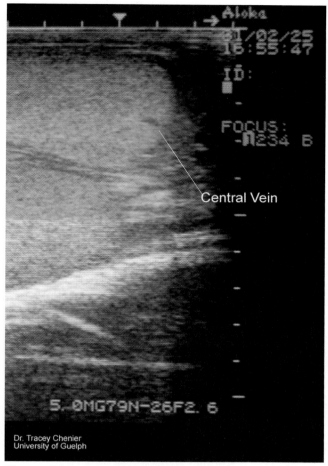

Figure 26-2 Ultrasound image of the left testis showing the homogenous nature of the normal testicular parenchyma. The central vein is visible as a small homogeneous structure in the cranial third of the testis.

small anechoic structure within the cranial third of the testis. The tail of the epididymis is visualized as a distinct heterogeneous structure at the caudal pole of the testis (Figure 26-3). The spermatic cord has a characteristic heterogenous, Swiss cheese–like appearance because of the many vessels of the pampiniform plexus (Figure 26-4). Recently, color Doppler ultrasound evaluation of the blood flow of the spermatic cord and testis of stallions has been described.[12] This technique shows promise in evaluation of some disorders of the testis, such as varicocele or tumor, where normal vascular supply to the testis may be disrupted.

The testis of the normal stallion is easily examined by inspection, palpation, and ultrasonography. All of these procedures should be routinely performed during the thorough physical examination of any breeding stallion. Additional procedures such as semen collection and evaluation, hormonal analysis, and testicular biopsy will also provide valuable information to the clinician regarding the health of the testis and are covered elsewhere in this text.

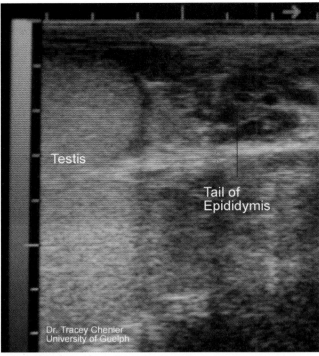

Figure 26-3 Ultrasound image of the left testis showing the heterogeneous nature of the tail of the epididymis, located at the caudal pole of the testis.

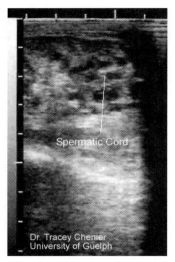

Figure 26-4 Ultrasound image of the spermatic cord. The many vessels of the pampiniform plexus are visualized as hypoechoic structures within the cord.

References

1. Dyce KM, Sack WO, Wensing CJG: Textbook of Veterinary Anatomy, Philadelphia, WB Saunders, 1987.
2. Sack WO: Isolated male reproductive organs. In Sack WO (ed): Rooney's Guide to the Dissection of the Horse, ed 6, Ithaca, NY, Veterinary Textbooks, 1991.
3. Sisson S: Equine urogenital system. In Getty R (ed): Sisson and Grossman's Anatomy of the Domestic Animals, 5th edition, Philadelphia, WB Saunders, 1975.
4. Nickel R: Male genital organs. In Nickel R, Schummer A, Seiferle E et al: The Viscera of Domestic Animals, New York, Springer-Verlag, 1973.
5. Thompson DL, Pickett BW, Squires EL et al: Testicular measurements and reproductive characteristics in stallions. J Reprod Fertil 1979; 27:13.
6. Burns PJ: Effects of season, age and increased photoperiod on reproductive hormone concentrations and testicular diameters in Thoroughbred stallions. Equine Vet Sci 1984; 4(5):202-208.
7. Love CC, Garcia MC, Riera FR et al: Use of testicular volume to predict daily sperm output in the stallion. Proceedings of the 36th Annual Convention of the American Association of Equine Practitioners, pp 15-21, 1990.
8. Gebauer MR, Pickett BW, Faulkner LC et al: Reproductive physiology of the stallion: daily sperm output and testicular measurements. J Am Vet Med Assoc 1974; 165(8):711-714.
9. Thompson DL, Pickett BW, Squires EL et al: Testicular measurements and reproductive characteristics in stallions. J Reprod Fertil Suppl 1979; 27:13-17.
10. Paccamonti DL, Buiten AV, Parlevliet JM et al: Reproductive parameters of miniature stallions. Theriogenology 1999; 51:1343-1349.
11. Love CC, Garcia MC, Riera FR et al: Evaluation of measures taken by ultrasonography and caliper to estimate testicular volume and predict daily sperm output in the stallion. J Reprod Fertil Suppl 1991; 44:99-105.
12. Pozor MA, McDonnel SM: Color Doppler ultrasound evaluation of testicular blood flow in stallions. Theriogenology 2004; 61:799-810.

CHAPTER 27

The Epididymis

THERESA BURNS

GROSS ANATOMY

The epididymis is a single tubule that connects the efferent ductules to the vas deferens and plays important roles in sperm transit, maturation, and storage. The structure identifiable grossly as the epididymis contains the efferent ductules, the highly convoluted epididymal tubule, and the surrounding connective tissue. The epididymis is conventionally divided into three contiguous regions based on gross appearance: the caput, the corpus, and the cauda epididymis. The caput epididymis extends over and is firmly attached to the cranial pole of the testicle. The corpus epididymis lies horizontally, dorsal to the testicle and lateral to the spermatic cord. The cauda epididymis is firmly attached to the caudal pole of the testicle by the proper ligament of the testis and to the parietal vaginal tunic by the ligament of the tail of the epididymis, both of which are remnants of the fetal gubernaculum (Figure 27-1).

ULTRASTRUCTURAL ANATOMY

Ultrastructurally, the proximal caput actually contains 13 to 15 coiled efferent ductules. The efferent ductule epithelium comprises ciliated and nonciliated pseudostratified columnar cells.[1,2] The efferent ductules fuse to form the epididymal tubule in the midcaput region. The transition from efferent ductule to epididymis is marked by the disappearance of ciliated cells and a dramatic increase in the epithelial cell height. The proximal epididymis has a thick epithelial lining and a narrow star-shaped lumen. Distally the epididymal epithelium becomes gradually lower, and the lumen widens and contains densely packed spermatozoa. In the cauda epididymis the mucosal layer forms folds that protrude into the lumen. A thin layer of longitudinally oriented smooth muscle cells surrounds the caput, corpus, and proximal cauda. A thick smooth muscle layer surrounds the distal cauda.

The most abundant cell type in the epididymal epithelium is the principal cell, which exhibits prominent vacuoles and apical microvilli typical of secretory and absorptive cells.[2,3] Less common basal cells and intraepithelial leukocytes are also present. Throughout the epididymis, epithelial cells are connected by tight junctions, which form a blood epididymal barrier.[4]

FUNCTIONS

The functions of the epididymis include spermatozoal transit, concentration, maturation, protection, and storage. In stallions, sperm cell transit through the epididymis lasts on average 7.5 to 11 days.[5] Spermatozoa are concentrated as testicular fluid is resorbed in the efferent ductules and proximal cauda epididymis.[1,6] Spermatozoa are immature after testicular development but become capable of progressive motion and fertilization by the time they reach the terminal epididymis. Changes occurring during maturation include enhanced chromatin cross-linking, redistribution of membrane proteins, and alterations in the activity of ion pumps. After maturation, spermatozoa are maintained in a protected, quiescent state by the luminal environment and cool temperature in the cauda epididymis. Approximately 87% of the extratesticular spermatozoa are in the epididymis, 66% in the cauda, and 20% in the caput and corpus; 13% are in the vas and ampulla.[5] In the stallion, the cauda holds approximately 66% of all extragonadal spermatozoa. The number of spermatozoa available is correlated with testicular weight and daily sperm output. During ejaculation, smooth muscle contracts under sympathetic control and propels sperm into the vas deferens. The epididymis may also function in removal of abnormal spermatozoa and seasonal changes in sperm output in the stallion. Spermatophagy occurs in the efferent ductules and possibly the epididymis.[1]

In the stallion the activities of the epididymal epithelium and their effects on spermatozoa are areas of active research. One hundred seventeen proteins are secreted over the length of stallion epididymis, with maximal protein secretion occurring in the distal caput epididymis.[6] Some proteins are present in equal concentration along the length of the tubule, whereas others are present only in discrete regions, creating multiple microenvironments in the epididymal lumen.

Secreted proteins appear to be active in many areas of sperm maturation and protection. Proteins such as clusterin may become adsorbed to the surface of sperm cells and participate in sperm-oocyte interactions.[7] Enzymes secreted in the epididymis may alter proteins and glycoproteins of testicular origin such as PH-20, resulting in their redistribution to specific regions of the sperm cell membrane.[8] Other epididymal proteins, such as lactoferrin and glutathione peroxidase, may act to prevent oxidative damage to sperm cells, helping to preserve their life span. The secreted epididymal protein ubiquitin adsorbs to abnormal spermatozoa in high levels and may be associated with their destruction.[9]

CLINICAL EXAMINATION

In the normal stallion the epididymis can be palpated along the dorsal rim of the testicle (Figure 27-2). It is of

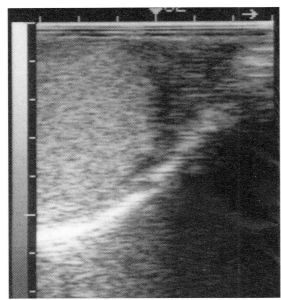

Figure 27-1   Ultrasound image of the caudal pole of the left testicle and the cauda epididymis from a normal stallion.

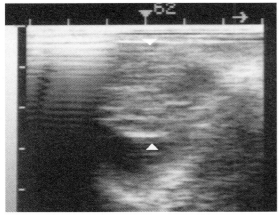

Figure 27-2   Ultrasound image of the cauda epididymis (*white arrowheads*) from a normal stallion.

consistent texture throughout and is less firm than the testicle. Normal ultrasonographic appearance is hypoechogenic compared to the testicle and is uniformly microcystic.

Evaluation of a stallion with suspected epididymal disease includes physical examination with transrectal palpation of the accessory sex glands and scrotal palpation. Complete blood count, semen collection, and complete semen evaluation and culture are performed. Staining of semen smears with a modified Wright's Giemsa stain will aid in observation of white blood cells. Scrotal ultrasonographic and videoendoscopic examination of the urethra and colliculus seminalis are also indicated. Fine needle aspirates and cytologic examination and culture may be useful in evaluating epididymal masses.

CONGENITAL ANOMALIES

Congenital abnormalities of the epididymis are rare in stallions. Bilateral congenital hypoplasia of the distal corpus epididymis has been reported and resulted in azoospermia despite normal libido and ejaculatory behavior.[10] A low alkaline phosphatase activity in the ejaculate indicates absence of the testicular fluid fraction.

Congenital failure of the gubernaculum to regress to form the proper ligament of the testis or the ligament of the tail of the epididymis results in cryptorchidism. In complete abdominal cryptorchidism both the testicle and epididymis are located intraabdominally and the ligament of the tail of the epididymis is not regressed. In incomplete cryptorchidism the ligament of the tail of the epididymis is regressed and the cauda epididymis is in a normal scrotal position; however, the proper ligament of the testicle is not regressed, and the testicle, caput, and corpus epididymis are located in the abdomen.

ACQUIRED DISEASE

Acquired epididymal disease in the stallion is rare and carries a poor prognosis for fertility. Reported conditions include bacterial epididymitis, sperm granuloma, and epididymal lymphosarcoma.

Bacterial epididymitis in the stallion is uncommon and may be unilateral or bilateral. Epididymitis is accompanied by orchitis or testicular degeneration (Figure 27-3). Stallions may present with abdominal or hindlimb pain, scrotal swelling, weight loss, and fever. Stallions may also present with reproductive problems such as poor fertility, failure to ejaculate, poor semen quality, or white blood cells in the semen. Physical examination findings include swollen and painful scrotal contents. Ultrasonographic appearance of the epididymis

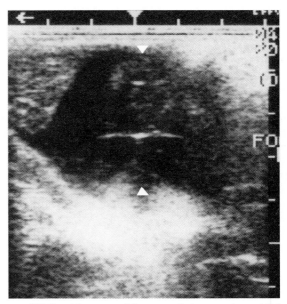

Figure 27-3   Ultrasound image of the cauda epididymis (*white arrowheads*) from a stallion with orchitis and cystic epididymal degeneration. (Courtesy Tracy Chenier.)

is less homogenous than normal with hypoechoic and hyperechoic regions.[11] *Streptococcus zooepidemicus* and *Proteus mirabilis* have been cultured from semen and epididymal fine needle aspirates in stallions with bacterial epididymitis.[12,13]

Medical treatment of epididymitis in the stallion has had poor success because disease is often chronic before diagnosis. Poor drug penetration into the equine excurrent ducts and immune-mediated attack on the reproductive organs also decrease prognosis. Attempts at medical treatment in valuable animals may be beneficial if white cells are detected in the semen and prompt evaluation reveals acute epididymitis. The antibiotic selected must have high efficacy against the cultured pathogen, high lipid solubility, and good activity in purulent tissue. Antiinflammatory medications, scrotal elevation, and physical cooling may limit edema, inflammation, and fibrosis of the epididymis and testicle. Unilateral or bilateral castration with perioperative antibiotic administration has been a successful treatment.

Sperm granuloma due to occlusion of tubules and extravasation of spermatozoa into connective tissue may be due to congenital abnormality of the efferent tubules, previous trauma, or parasite migration.[14-16] Findings include enlarged, painful epididymis; abnormal ultrasonographic appearance; and negative semen and fine-needle aspirate cultures. Histologically the tubule epithelium is disrupted, and there is leukocyte infiltration and severe peritubular fibrosis. Unilateral castration may preserve fertility if the contralateral testis and epididymis are normal.

Lymphosarcoma with invasion of the caput epididymis is a reported cause of testicular swelling.[17] Clinical findings include hard, nonpainful swelling of the epididymal heads with a variable ultrasonographic echotexture showing both hyperechoic and anechoic regions. Fine-needle aspiration of epididymal masses can be attempted, but castration and histopathologic examination may be required for definitive diagnosis. A diagnosis of epididymal lymphosarcoma necessitates evaluation for systemic disease.

References

1. Arrighi S, Romanello MG, Domeneghini C: Ultrastructure of the epithelium that lines the ductuli efferentes in domestic Equidae, with particular reference to spermatophagy. Acta Anat 1994; 149:174-184.
2. Johnson L, Amann RP, Pickett BW: Scanning electron microscopy of the epithelium and spermatozoa in the equine excurrent duct system. Am J Vet Res 1978; 39(9):1428-1434.
3. Lopez ML, Grez P, Gribbel I et al: Cytochemical and ultrastructural characteristics of the stallion epididymis (*Equus caballus*). J Submicrosc Cytol Pathol 1989; 21(1):103-120.
4. Lopez ML, Fuentes P, Retamal C, De Souza W: Regional differentiation of the blood-epididymis barrier in stallion (*Equus caballus*). J Submicrosc Cytol Pathol 1997; 29(3):353-363.
5. Gebauer MR, Pickett BW, Swiestra EE: Reproductive physiology of the stallion. Part 3. Extragonadal transit time and sperm reserves. J Anim Sci 1974; 39(4):737-742.
6. Fouchecourt S, Metayer S et al: Stallion epididymal fluid proteome: qualitative and quantitative characterization, secretion and dynamic changes of major proteins. Biol Reprod 2000; 62(6):1790-1803.
7. Cuasnicu PS et al: Changes in specific sperm proteins during epididymal maturation. In Robaire B, Hinton BT (eds): The Epididymis: From Molecules to Clinical Practice, pp 203-389, Sacaucus, NJ, Kluwer Academic/Plenum Publishers, 2002.
8. Rutlant J, Meyers SA: Posttranslational processing of PH-20 during epididymal sperm maturation in the horse. Biol Reprod 2001; 65:1324-1331.
9. Sutovsky P, Turner RM, Hameed A, Sutovsky M: Differential ubiquination of stallion sperm proteins: possible implications for infertility and reproductive seasonality. Biol Repod 2003; 68:688-698.
10. Blanchard TL, Woods JA, Brinsko SP: Theriogenology question of the month. J Am Vet Med Assoc 2000; 217(6):825-826.
11. Traub-Dargatz JL, Trooter GW, Kaser-Hotz B et al: Ultrasonographic detection of chronic epididymitis in a stallion. J Am Vet Med Assoc 1991; 198(8):1417-1420.
12. Held JP, Prater P, Toal RL et al: Bacterial epididymitis in two stallions. J Am Vet Med Assoc 1990; 197(5):602-604.
13. Brinsko SP, Varner DD, Blanchard TL et al: Bacterial infectious epididymitis in a stallion. Equine Vet J 1992; 24(4):325-328.
14. Braun WF: Physical examination and genital diseases of the stallion. In Morrow DA (ed): Current Therapy in Theriogenology 2, pp 646-651, Philadelphia, WB Saunders, 1986.
15. Blue MG, McEntee K: Epididymal sperm granuloma in a stallion. Equine Vet J 1985; 17(3): 248-251.
16. Held JP, Adair S, McGavin MD et al: Sperm granuloma in a stallion. J Am Vet Med Assoc 1989; 194(2):267-268.
17. Held JP, McCracken MD, Toal R, Latimer F: Epididymal swelling attributable to generalized lymphosarcoma in a stallion. J Am Vet Med Assoc 1992; 201(12):1913-1915.

CHAPTER 28

Stallion Reproductive Behavior

AHMED TIBARY

Evaluation of reproductive behavior is an integral part of the examination for breeding potential or problems in the stallion. An understanding of the sequence of behaviors displayed by the stallion in preparation for, during, and after mating is important for the diagnosis of disorders such as poor libido, erection, or ejaculation failure. Modern breeding practices do not allow display of the full array of stallion reproductive behavior. Therefore, knowledge of behavioral clues will be very useful in training the novice stallion for mating and implementing behavioral correction techniques.

NORMAL REPRODUCTIVE BEHAVIOR IN THE STALLION

Reproductive Behavior in Free-Ranging Stallions

Reproductive behavior of the stallion in feral or semiferal situation has been thoroughly described by several authors.[1-7] In these conditions, breeding occurs in what is described as a harem social organization. A harem is composed of a mature stallion and a few mares and their offspring. In some situations, the main (primary) stallion in the harem may be "assisted" by a second stallion. The second stallion helps with defense of the group and will breed only on rare occasions (usually with young mares).[5,7-12]

The stallion tends his mares all year round. Reproductive status of the mares is continually monitored by elimination marking behavior (olfactory investigation of the mare or her urine or feces).[13] Monitoring of the herd is increased during the peak of the foaling and breeding season. Stallions tend to spend more time closer to mature harem mares in estrus. The mare plays a primary role in initiation of reproductive behavior by soliciting the stallion, displaying strong estrous behavior signs, and allowing mounting.[1-4,6,7]

Precopulatory Behavior
Stallion display a characteristic precopulatory sequence beginning with nose-to-nose contact associated with a characteristic soft nicker vocalization. Oronasal investigation (sniffing, nibbling, nuzzling, and licking) follows, starting at the shoulder and elbows and proceeding to the ventral abdomen and udder and then to the hind legs and perineum.[14] Flehmen response generally is displayed when the stallion comes into contact with urine or vaginal fluid.[15,16] During this precopulatory behavior the stallion may nip the mare at the flank or hock. Rubbing or resting the chin on the rump may be displayed, as well as mounting without erection.

Copulatory Behavior
Copulatory behavior (mounting, insertion, thrusting, and ejaculation) may follow the precopulatory behavior immediately or may occur after several precopulatory sessions. The mare generally facilitates mounting and insertion, but the stallion needs a high degree of coordination and physical ability to complete this behavior.[5] Insertion and organized thrusting occur over a period of 20 to 25 seconds before ejaculation is observed. Mares may move forward during copulation to accommodate the stallion, which also may serve to prevent injuries. Dismount occurs approximately 20 to 30 seconds after ejaculation.[1]

Although mares remain in heat for a few days, the copulatory behavior generally is observed only during peak receptivity, which spans 1 to 2 days and during which the mare may be bred several times.

Erection and Ejaculation
Erection and ejaculation are controlled by nerves originating in the spinal cord. Erection occurs as a result of relaxation of smooth muscles of the corpus cavernosum and corpus spongiosum in combination with an increase in arterial blood flow to the penis.[17] Penile rigidity is improved by contraction of the perineal striated muscles after engorgement and erection of the penis.[18] The activity of the striated muscle is increased during copulation as a result of stimuli from the autonomic nerves to the corpus cavernosum and corpus spongiosum and from the somatic nerves to the ischiocavernosus and bulbospongiosus.[19,20] Continuous stimulation by the vagina and pelvic thrusting further enhances this activity and promotes emission and ejaculation.

Emission occurs as a reflex to proper stimulation after 7 to 9 pelvic thrusts.[21] During emission, the rhythmic contractions of the smooth muscle layer of the cauda epididymis, ductus deferens, and accessory sex glands serve to release spermatozoa and fluid into the urethra. Emission and bladder neck closure reflexes are primarily under α-adrenergic control involving preganglionic sympathetic fibers from the lumbosacral segment of the spinal cord and connecting with the caudal mesenteric plexus. Ejaculation occurs in 5 to 10 successive forceful jets produced by the rhythmic contractions of the ischiocavernosus, bulbospongiosus, and urethralis muscles, as well as sphincter muscles. Each ejaculatory jet is evident externally by a characteristic downward movement of the tail known as *tail flagging*. Ejaculation is controlled by the pudendal nerve and the sacral segment of the spinal cord.[21-24]

Postcopulatory Behavior

The stallion and the mare usually remain in proximity of each other for a few minutes after copulation. During this time, the stallion may engage in investigation of the spilled vaginal fluid and displays flehmen reaction. In some instances, stallions also may engage in rolling and dusting activity.

Masturbation

Spontaneous erection with penile movement and rubbing against the belly is described as masturbation in the male equine.[25] Several studies and clinical observations have shown this to be a normal behavior.[25] Masturbation occurs in all equids at regular intervals (every 90 minutes) and does not seem to be related to age, libido, fertility, or sociosexual conditions (e.g., type of housing, mare proximity).[26-29] Masturbation behavior does not occur during standing or recumbent sleep but rather is seen during periods of quiet rest and may be elicited within a few minutes of return to calm after startle.[25,30] Ejaculation during these periods of masturbation is extremely rare (less than 1 in 100 episodes); therefore, the common belief that semen "wastage" results from this behavior is not substantiated.[25]

Several devices—stallion rings, the brush, the basket, electrical collars—have been designed to inhibit or eliminate this behavior in show and performance horses. Clinical experience shows that these "anti-masturbation" devices are not effective and may even compromise stallion breeding ability.[25] Recent reports show that aversive conditioning to eliminate masturbatory behavior by means of electrical shock suppresses sexual arousal and adversely affects breeding efficiency and semen quality.[25] Stallions subjected to aversive conditioning showed an increase in erection latency, mount readiness latency, ejaculation latency, and mounts to ejaculation and a decrease in number of vocalizations, erection rigidity score, and ejaculatory pulses. Decreased ejaculation efficiency resulted in decreased sperm number in the ejaculate.[25]

Observation and documentation of spontaneous penile erection and movement may be helpful in the examination of stallions with erectile dysfunction.

Reproductive Behavior in Modern Breeding

Most species-specific sociosexual interactions are eliminated in domestic horse breeding. The precopulatory and copulatory behaviors are similar to those displayed in a free system but are much more restrained. In modern horse breeding and husbandry, strict limitations are imposed on horses, particularly colts and stallions, in sexual behavior development. Colts rarely have a chance to develop key behavioral clues, because they are separated from other animals, particularly in small operations with limited number of horses. In the performance horse, sexual behavior is considered undesirable and is discouraged or repressed. In addition, breeding stallions may be housed together in high-male-density situations (specialized stud farms). All of these factors may affect stallion reproductive behavior. Also, it is well known that stallion behavior is sensitive to aversive experiences and can be effectively suppressed, which may cause a problem later on when the colt or young stallion is introduced to the breeding shed. Domestic breeding management of stallions involves generally one of three types of systems: pasture or paddock mating, in-hand mating, and semen collection.

Paddock or Pasture Mating

The pasture or paddock mating system involves one or more mares housed in the same enclosure for the entire breeding season or until the mare is confirmed to be pregnant. This situation is similar in several ways to natural harem conditions, but the structure of the herd may be continuously modified by addition of new mares and removal of pregnant mares.

Introduction of a stallion to a group of mares or moving an established herd to a new unfamiliar surrounding results in increased snaking activity.[31] This behavior, characterized by extension of the head and neck, holding the ears back, and lowering the head, usually subsides within a day or 2. New mares do not reinitiate snaking and herding behavior, but they may be kept at a distance by the stallion for up to 4 days.[31,32] Stallion seem to adjust relatively quickly when moved from one paddock to another with different groups of mares.[33] Although stallions in this system breed often (every 1 to 2 hours), pregnancy and foaling rates achieved in these systems generally are good if the stallion does not have any physical or genital problem.[32,34,35] Unfortunately, this system is notorious for the increased incidence of stallion breeding injuries.[36]

In-Hand Mating

Complete supervision and control of the interaction between the stallion and the mare during natural cover is referred to as *in-hand mating.* This is the most common form of natural cover practiced in the modern equine breeding industry, particularly when artificial breeding is not allowed. The amount of restraint (breeding hobble, nose/lip/ear twitch) of the mare and the stallion is variable from one geographic region or farm to another. The level of restraint affects the ability of the mare to display receptive postures and adjustment to mounting, intromission, and thrusting (e.g., forward stepping), which may create discomfort and even lead to injuries if a breeding roll is not used.

In general, the mare is teased by a different stallion and restrained in the breeding shed. The stallion is brought to the breeding shed using a halter or a breeding bridle. The contact time between the mare and the stallion is variable, depending on several factors. Typically, the stallion is directed to approach the mare from the hindquarters, skipping the major part of precopulatory sequence. Stallions in this system learn that their role is to walk into the breeding shed and perform breeding, so that the opportunity for precopulatory behavior is very limited. Most stallions will walk into the breeding shed already in erection and ready to mount, insert, and complete the mating with minimal sexual preparation. In some stud farms, it is not uncommon for the process of natural cover to involve more than six people, each of whom specializes in a small detail of mare and stallion preparation and handling. This is hardly a natural breeding environment, and interpretation of stallion reaction should be done very carefully.

Mount without erection is not as frequently seen in this situation as with free-ranging horses, probably as a result of "specialization" of the stallion or repression of the handler.[37] In one study of experienced stud farm stallions, mounts without erection were observed in only 6 of 85 attempts.[37] In my experience, mount without erection is observed more frequently in young novice males and during the second ejaculation. Mount without erection is rarely observed during the breeding season in stallions that are used with moderate frequency for breeding. Although mounting without erection is a normal behavior, some stallion handlers may reprimand stallions, thereby conditioning them not to mount until they have achieved full erection. It is not known whether mounting without erection (false mount) results in improved seminal characteristics in terms of sperm concentration and volume.

Another characteristic of in-hand mating is the rush to dismount after ejaculation promoted by some stallion handlers. This unnatural dismount may cause added strain on some aged stallions or stallions with musculoskeletal or neurologic conditions, thus creating an aversive experience.

The time from introduction to the breeding shed to erection (erection latency) ranges from 10 to 163 seconds.[14,37,38] Variations observed in this latency may be due to differences in management procedures and in stimulation provided. In one study, no significant correlation was found between age of the stallion and erection latency.[37]

Ejaculation latency varies depending on the individual stallion and the frequency of mating. In a study conducted on French stud farms, a majority of first mounts (75%) resulted in ejaculation.[37] In another report, ejaculation occurred after 1.8 mounts.[39] The number of mounts per ejaculation generally is higher out of season than during the breeding season.[37,39] Ejaculation latency increases between the first and the second mounts.[37]

Semen Collection

Semen collection for the purpose of reproductive evaluation or for use in artificial insemination is widely practiced in modern horse breeding. Although semen collection can be performed on jump mares, the standard accepted method is to train the stallion to mount a phantom, or dummy. Stallions can be readily trained to serve the artificial vagina. Stallions trained to perform in these conditions do not necessarily lose their ability to breed naturally. Semen collection using a phantom, however, is characterized by a complete absence of auditory, olfactory, and vaginal contact and contraction stimuli. It is well established that these stimuli reinforce erection and ejaculation in the stallion.[40] Some studies have reported that more mounts are necessary per ejaculation for semen collection than in natural cover.[39] In a recent study comparing behavior during natural cover and semen collection on a phantom in 42 stallions, however, no statistically significant difference was found

in erection latency (62 ± 22 seconds for natural service versus 100 ± 13 seconds for phantom collection) and ejaculation latency (84 ± 18 seconds versus 86 ± 28 seconds, respectively).[37] These findings suggest that appropriate training and adjustment of artificial vagina conditions (temperature, pressure, and position) are important and should be adjusted for each stallion to allow a repeatable technique for adequate semen collection.[41,42]

In my experience, training of a novice stallion to semen collection using an artificial vagina and an estrous mare is successful in more than 90% of instances after one or two attempts. Training for semen collection on a phantom may take a little longer. Steps for training stallions for semen collection on dummies have been thoroughly described. The key points in this technique are to use an estrous mare for stimulation of the stallion and to allow a few mounts on the mare, alongside the phantom, before attempting in a later session to divert the stallion's mounting efforts to the phantom.[43] Presence of an estrous mare is not necessary after initial training.[37] Semen collection on a phantom or on the ground (i.e., standing collection) does not affect natural cover, and vice versa.[37,44]

NORMAL REPRODUCTIVE BEHAVIOR IN JACKS

Male donkeys (*Equus asinus*) are described as territorial.[45-47] Each jack has a territory in which breeding of solitary females takes places.[46] Jacks defend their territory against any adult males, particularly in the presence of estrous jennies. The jack typically interacts with jennies in a series of brief episodes, interrupted by a retreat to his resting area. The precopulatory sequence includes vocalization within the resting area; approach to and teasing of an individual jenny, followed by a retreat; and then a sudden approach with brief teasing or mounting. This sequence may be repeated several times before the jack retreats again to the resting place, where erection is achieved before he immediately approaches a jenny and copulates quickly without precopulatory behavior.[47] Specific precopulatory behaviors include nasonasal contact; nibbling or sniffing of the head, neck, back of the knee, body, flank, perineum, and tail; olfactory investigation of voided urine or feces; and flehmen.[47,48] Achieving an erection at a distance from jennies is one important characteristic of breeding behavior in the jack. Spontaneous erection and masturbation occur at the same rate as in the horse, with an episode every 90 minutes on average.[28]

Insertion latency, number of thrusts, and total time mounted for free-ranging donkeys have been described as similar to those for horses.[35] However, in hand-mating situations and, in particular, in situations of mule production (jacks breeding mares), my experience has been that all jacks take an extremely long time to erection and mount, but that once mount is achieved, ejaculation generally is easily obtained.[49]

Hand Breeding in Donkeys

In-hand mating of male donkeys may be used in either (1) breeding a jenny or (2) breeding a mare for mule production.

Breeding Donkeys to Jennies

Space for and freedom of interaction between the jack and the jenny seem to be key factors in sexual stimulation. The time to first mount increases if the jenny is restrained.[47,50] It is recommended that enough space be provided during in-hand mating of a jenny for the jack's retreating behavior to take place. The slow/fast retreat from the female is a unique behavior in jacks.[48,51] The number of retreats generally is higher for the first ejaculation than for successive ejaculations.[50] Presence of other receptive jennies may enhance sexual stimulation, whereas presence of other jacks may distract or inhibit sexual activity, in keeping with the territorial nature of this species.[52] The time from introduction to a female to mounting and ejaculation varies, ranging from 6 to 32 minutes in various studies.[47,50,52,53]

During the precopulatory and copulatory phases, jacks exhibit a sequence of behaviors including nasonasal contact, flehmen responses, mounting without erection, partial and total exposure of the penis, sniffing and biting specific areas of the female body, lip clapping, and slow/quick retreats with vocalization.[51-53] These behaviors show significant individual variation.[50]

The frequency of flehmen response (5 to 8) is generally higher than in stallions[47,50,51] and does not seem to be affected by rank of ejaculation.[50] The initial reaction of the jack in the breeding shed is vocalization, which is followed by one or several mounts without erection. The first mount is performed without erection in 70% of the cases.[47,50,52,53] The number of mounts without erection varies from one study to another and probably is affected by training and handling differences.[47,48,50]

Frequent partial exposure of the penis during the precopulatory phase is common in jacks.[47,48,52] Total exposure of the penis generally is followed by erection.[50] The first erection does not always result in ejaculation. Jacks may show several erections and masturbation before mounting and ejaculation.[47,48] The mean time from first contact with the female until the first erection varies, ranging between 10 and 15 minutes.[50] Depending on the individual animal, from 4 to 8 pelvic copulatory movements occur before ejaculation.[47,48,50] A seasonal effect on libido has been reported by some authors, with decreased latency to first mount, first erection, and ejaculation during spring and summer (breeding season).[52] This seasonal effect may vary from one geographic region to another.[50]

Breeding Donkeys to Mares

In my experience, breeding jacks to mares is more challenging, with often increased latency to erection, mount, and ejaculation. In pasture breeding systems, lack of conditioning of jacks to breed mares may result in lower reproductive efficiency. It has been suggested that jacks destined for mule production should be raised with horse fillies after weaning and prevented from any contact with jennies until they are adult.[48,54]

In pasture, precopulatory, copulatory, and postcopulatory behavior for jacks breeding mares are similar to those for jacks breeding jennies.[51] The interaction between mares and jacks is reportedly shorter in duration but more frequent. Also, mares do not display behavioral estrus with the same intensity to jacks as they do toward horse stallions. In one study, the percentage of estrous mares exhibiting signs toward a jack ranged between 28% and 43%, whereas 93% exhibited sexual behavior toward stallions.[51,54] In a stud farm situation, I have observed latency to erection and ejaculation of up to 120 minutes when stallions are bred to hobbled estrous mares.[49] In addition to these behavioral differences that may affect fertility results, size discrepancy may be another constraint in jack-mare breeding.

ABNORMAL REPRODUCTIVE BEHAVIOR

Sexual behavior dysfunction has long been recognized as an important cause of equine reproduction failure.[55-59] A variety of behavioral problems have been identified, including low sexual arousal, preferences for certain mares, preference for handler or handling conditions, aggressiveness toward the mare or handler, self-mutilation, abnormal copulatory behavior, failure of erection or ejaculation, and unruly behavior during mating.[14,43,56,57,60-63]

Despite this inventory of behavioral problems occurring in stallions, very few detailed studies on the prevalence of specific problems in the stallion population have been performed. In addition, most relevant reports are restricted to clinical observations and therapeutic trials based on a limited number of cases.[14] Several disorders manifesting as behavioral problems are secondary to a specific physical difficulty or endocrine disturbance. Therefore, diagnosis of the cause of what is perceived as a breeding-related behavioral problem requires a multidisciplinary approach involving an orthopedic specialist, a theriogenologist, and a behavioral specialist. A thorough medical and breeding history should be taken, including previous injuries during breeding, handling routine, changes in handling, and time of onset of the problem.

All attempts to breed or collect semen from the stallion should be thoroughly documented and videotaped. Videotaping the stallion in his stall and in a paddock may provide some clues regarding his ability to achieve erection (masturbation), stereotypic behavior, and so on. The use of at least two video cameras during each breeding session is recommended: one focusing on the head of the stallion and interaction with the handler(s) and the other focusing on the approach, penile exteriorization, mounting, positioning, and pelvic thrusting. Videotaping also should include observations of the stallion during the preparation stage (washing and teasing).

Stallion sexual behavior can be rapidly modified by negative experience. In addressing behavioral problems it is important to consider the main factors involved: the stallion's "attitude," training, and conditioning; the handler; the method used (use of a phantom or a mare for teasing or breeding); and the environment of collection (distractions from other animals, noise, or visitors).

Poor Libido

Failure to show sexual interest is relatively common in equine breeding. This problem often is encountered in young or novice stallions. Experienced breeders may show a decrease in sexual response expressed as increased length of time to react when brought to the breeding shed or display of a particular preference for certain mares, locations, handlers, or procedures, or a combination of these. Clinical observations, as well as experimental evidence, suggest that injury or pain during mating, disciplinary actions to inhibit sexual behavior (e.g., use of stallion rings for suppression of erection or disciplining the stallion for overt vocalization using shanks) may lead to anxiety and response-contingent aversive conditioning.[56,57,64,65]

A systematic approach is essential in the evaluation of stallions demonstrating poor libido. The evaluation should begin with a thorough history of the stallion's breeding activity and pinpoint the time of onset of the problem and the progression, as well as management changes implemented during the time when the decrease in libido was first observed. The stallion should be bred and evaluated under as natural conditions as possible (with mare in heat and the usual environment, handler, or paddock). The importance of direct interaction between mares and stallions in the establishment of normal breeding behavior should not be overlooked. The performance of slow-starting or low-libido stallions may improve substantially if adequate access to mares is provided (e.g., housing near mares, access to a paddock adjacent to mare pasture).[25]

The role of the mare is evidenced by the fact that most successful copulations (88%) are initiated by the mare,[35] A stallion will show different behavior toward different mares, depending on their social rank. What appears to be a libido problem, then, may be a refusal of the stallion to breed a particular mare.[35] Allowing a longer precopulatory period such as slow-walking the mare to the stallion, increased teasing time in the normal precopulatory behavior sequence, and encouraging the mare to display normal sexual behavior and posture will greatly improve stallion stimulation,[35]

Stallions that are housed together tend to have bachelor herd behavior and physiology, characterized by a reduction in sexual interest and arousal. Harem stallions have been shown to have increased circulating androgen levels, sexual drive, accessory sex gland size and activity, as well as increased testicular size and semen quality, compared with stallions in bachelor bands.[66,67] Moving the stallion to the proximity of mares may increase libido, androgen levels, and sperm production.[35]

Novel environment or handling during breeding has been shown to negatively affect sexual behavior in stallions.[68] This probably is due to the unfamiliarity of the new environment, which may elicit a fear or anxiety response.

Antianxiety drugs (benzodiazepine derivatives) may be considered in stallions with poor sexual arousal if they do not respond to retraining and increased exposure to estrous mares or if they show an increased confusion and aggressiveness toward mares.[65] Diazepam (0.05 mg/kg) given by slow intravenous infusion 5 to 7 minutes before breeding has been shown to be effective in blocking suppressive effects of novel environment and aversive conditioning.[25,65,68]

The use of testosterone or other exogenous androgens to increase libido is strongly discouraged. These hormones may increase aggressiveness without improving normal sexual behavior and have known deleterious effects on spermatogenesis and fertility.[69-72]

Gonadotropin-releasing hormone (GnRH) administered subcutaneously at a rate of 25 µg every 3 hours, or in a dose of 50 µg given 2 hours and again 1 hour before breeding, improves sexual arousal, erection, and ejaculation in some stallions. This treatment is particularly helpful in slow-starting or novice stallions.

Aggressive Behavior

Overt sexual behavior or aggressive behavior in the stallion will result in an unsafe working environment for the mare, stallion, handlers, and veterinarian. Such behavior, characterized as *unruly*, may include rushing to the mare or phantom, striking at the mare or handler, kicking, sudden turns and rearing, biting when washed or during mating, or excessive pelvic thrusting.[73] Retraining both stallion and handler is required in these conditions.

Detailed descriptions of behavioral modification techniques of unruly study are available in the literature; multiple daily short sessions of 5 to 10 minutes typically are used.[73] The retraining process generally takes 1 week. The goal of these retraining sessions is to reduce or eliminate the specific undesirable responses while maintaining the normal stallion sexual behavior responses. This is accomplished by working on specific short-term goals using a combination of negative reinforcement (appropriate punishment using verbal reprimand, shank chain pressure, or occasional slaps on the shoulder and belly) when an undesirable behavior is displayed and positive reinforcement when the stallion is responding normally. During the training sessions, special attention should be paid to maintaining consistency in terms of handler, clues, and environment.[73]

Overt Sexual Behavior

Strong sexual drive or libido in performance horses is undesirable and often is controlled by either behavioral modification or pharmacologic means—in particular, the administration of the progestagen altrenogest.[74] Overt sexual excitement in breeding stallions may pose some problems during copulation. One characteristic manifestation of overt sexual anticipation is the premature dilation of the glans penis (belling), which prevents normal intromission and may predispose the stallion to penile injuries. Some of these behaviors can be controlled by proper diet and exercise. As discussed later in this chapter, it is important to note that altrenogest treatment in breeding stallions affects semen quality.

Erection Failure

Erection failure (inadequate erection or loss of erection on insertion) has been reported in approximately 4% of stallions with sexual behavior dysfunction in a study of 250 cases.[14] In most instances, erection failure in a stallion is secondary to underlying traumatic damage to the erectile tissue (e.g., breeding injuries, stallion ring injuries) or a long-standing drug- or trauma-induced paraphimosis. A peculiar case of folding entrapment of the engorged penis within the prepuce has been described.[43]

Manual stimulation can be used to collect semen from stallions that are unable to mount or achieve erection.[44,75-77]

Ejaculatory Disorders

Ejaculation disorders include absence of ejaculation (aspermia or anejaculation), incomplete ejaculation (oligospermia), premature ejaculation, retrograde ejaculation, and urospermia. Premature ejaculation has been described but is relatively rare.[21,62,78] Perceived anejaculation may be due to retrograde ejaculation, spermastasis in the ampullae, or epididymal aplasia.[79-81]

Ejaculation Failure
Ejaculatory disorders were estimated to account for approximately 25% of all behavioral problems in stallions presented in one clinic.[21] In nearly 60% of all cases, the problem was complete failure of ejaculation (anejaculation), and in 36%, it was urospermia. The most commonly encountered ejaculatory disorder that may have a behavioral component in the stallion is incomplete or failure of ejaculation. Ejaculation disorders are caused mainly by physical or neurologic conditions.

The emission and ejaculation processes rely primarily on coordinated sets of stimuli involving specific nerves and anatomic penile structures, as well as musculoskeletal function. Disturbances at any level due to acute or degenerative diseases may interfere with ejaculation. Painful conditions (back pain, hind limb deficiencies or lameness, bladder pain, painful conditions of the penis, accessory glands and testis) may result in hesitation during thrusting and poor stimulation. These conditions should be ruled out before any attempt to diagnose purely behavioral or psychogenic problems.[82] Stallions with chronic pain may be managed by providing adequate environment to reduce strain during copulation (weight loss, good footing, adjusting phantom mount height and angle, lateral support). Treatment with nonsteroidal antiinflammatory drugs may be helpful. Extra stimulation to the penis during copulation can be provided by applying hot towels at the base of the penis or increasing pressure and temperature of the artificial vagina. Collection on the ground (standing collection) may be the only viable option with some severely affected stallions.[83]

Primary psychogenic causes of ejaculation failure in stallions generally are a consequence of handling errors or unpleasant or painful experiences during breeding or semen collection. Overuse of the halter or bit as a method to control the stallion during mounting, or to force him to dismount immediately after ejaculation or to mount without erection, and slippery breeding ground may lead to these problems.

The practice of "tail nerving" for the purpose of some horse show events may have deleterious effects on ejaculation. I have seen a stallion with ejaculatory failure due to unnerving the tail. In this particular case, treatment with imipramine 100 mg 2 hours before semen collection

or breeding resulted in ejaculation (Sue McDonnell, PhD, personal communication). Semen was of low volume (7.5 to 10 ml) but with an appropriate total number of spermatozoa consistent with testicular size.[84]

Sperm Accumulation Syndrome
Sperm accumulation syndrome (spermastasis) is seen in some stallions with ampulla-emptying defect. The ejaculate obtained after a long period of rest shows a very high sperm concentration and sperm abnormalities. Diagnosis is based on ultrasonographic evaluation of the ampullae and serial semen collections. Improvement of the ejaculate is seen after several collection procedures and intravenous administration of oxytocin (10 to 20 IU).[81]

Retrograde Ejaculation
Retrograde ejaculation into the bladder has been described in stallions.[80] This disorder is due to a failure of bladder sphincter closure due to a traumatic or infectious lesion. Strong rhythmic pulsations of the urethra are felt during collection, but the ejaculate is either absent or of small volume despite normal appearance of the internal and external genitalia. Confirmation of retrograde ejaculation is easily accomplished by cytologic evaluation of urine collected by catheterization of the bladder immediately after mating or a semen collection attempt.[21,80] Administration of imipramine before breeding may enhance bladder sphincter closure and reduce the chances of retrograde ejaculation.[21]

Urospermia
Elimination of urine in variable quantity may occur at any moment during ejaculation and results in the presence of urine in sperm.[85-90] Collection of semen in separate fractions using an open-ended artificial vagina may help determine the timing of urination in relationship to ejaculation.[22,85,90] The causes of urospermia remain unclear; some cases probably are related to ejaculatory disorders with failure of urinary bladder sphincter closure, which may be secondary to neurologic disorders, equine herpesvirus type 1 (EHV-1) infection, intoxication, or urolithiasis.[84] Urospermia may be seen intermittently on some ejaculates when the stallion is used on a regular basis. One stallion with neurologic hindlimb deficits showed urospermia only if used twice consecutively within 3 hours (Tibary A, 2003, personal observations).

Management of stallions with urospermia may be frustrating. Breeding after micturition may help. Urination may be induced by introducing the stallion to a fresh box stall or by exposure to feces from another stallion, or by the use of diuretics (furosemide, 250 mg IV).[87] Catheterization of the bladder before breeding also has been suggested but may result in complications if used too often.[91]

The use of imipramine in the treatment of urospermia has been advocated because of its tonic effect on the bladder sphincter.[21,91] In a study of 3 cases of urospermia, however, no improvement was obtained with the use of bethanechol, imipramine, or furosemide.[92] This finding suggests that response may be dependent on the degree of compromise of bladder sphincter function. Fractionation of the ejaculate or direct collection into an extender followed by centrifugation is beneficial if artificial insemination is possible.

Other Sexual Behavioral Problems

Other sexual behavior abnormalities include sexual arousal in response to other species of farm animals or people, excessive pacing in the paddock, self-mutilation, self-directed intermale aggression, and other stable vices that appear to be more common in stallions.[93] At one large stud farm where 85 stallions were housed with limited exercise, 60% of all stallions exhibited stereotypies that increased in frequency during the breeding season (Tibary A, 1988 personal observation). Sexual arousal toward humans most typically is seen in miniature horses and donkeys and in general in stallions that have been hand-reared.

Self-mutilation behavior is a syndrome characterized by compulsive nipping or biting of the genital area and flank or excessive floor-stomping, wall-kicking, and ramming.[14,94] This behavior may be continuous or seasonal and may lead to severe injuries, thereby compromising the well-being and/or fertility of the stallion.[56,58,61,95] Self-mutilation behavior has been described in closely related stallions, which suggests some genetic component. This behavior also has been associated with genital lesions such as squamous cell carcinoma of the urethral processes[96] and habronemiasis.[36]

Self-mutilation behavior in stallions reportedly has been decreased by treatment with imipramine[93] or clomipramine[97] (500 to 1000 mg, bid, per os). Maximal effect was seen 8 days after treatment. The narcotic antagonist nalmefen (0.08 to 0.4 mg/kg) also has been reported to be effective in some stallions.[60]

PHARMACOLOGIC MANIPULATION OF REPRODUCTIVE BEHAVIOR

Pharmacologic Manipulation of Libido

Overt expression of stallion-like behavior is undesirable in many performance horses. It is therefore a major complaint in veterinary practice. Judicious training is thought to be the most effective technique to control stallion behavior. In some instances, however, the use of tranquilizers and endocrine treatment to suppress androgen production have been advised. This treatment should not replace behavioral manipulation training.

Progestogen
Administration of the synthetic progestogen altrenogest temporarily creates a more manageable animal.[74,98-101] In a recent survey, 29% of 63 training facilities reported using altrenogest to manipulate stallions' behavior. In young stallions (2 to 4 years of age), treatment with 0.088 mg/kg of body weight for 8 weeks caused a decrease in testicular size and libido. Treated colts showed a decrease in flehmen frequency and duration, decreased duration of penile exteriorization, and decreased frequency and duration of erection.[99] The treatment also resulted in a decrease in sperm production and quality (increased abnormalities), which lasted for 8 weeks after

the last treatment.[99] Treatment with altrenogest at 0.044 mg/kg in 2-year-old colts[98] and 0.088 mg/kg in 3-year-old stallions[101] caused a decrease in estrogen levels, scrotal size, and spermatogenesis activity. In a group of mature stallions (3 to 18 years of age), altrenogest was administered in a dose of 0.088 mg/kg for 150 days. In addition to decreased testicular size, sperm output, and testosterone, these stallions showed altered sexual behavior characterized by an increased number of semen collection attempts associated with failure of ejaculation and increased time to first erection and ejaculation. A carry-over effect on sexual behavior was observed after the end of treatment. Testicular size and seminal parameters improved by 90 days after the end of the treatment.[100]

GnRH
Administration of the GnRH analogue busereline to normal stallions has a positive effect on libido, sperm concentration, sperm motility, and sperm membrane integrity, and on ability of sperm to withstand freezing.[102] GnRH given subcutaneously at a rate of 25 μg every 3 hours or in a dose of 50 μg, 2 hours and again 1 hour before breeding, improves sexual arousal, erection, and ejaculation in some stallions.

Immunization against GnRH has been used to control reproduction in feral horses.[103-105] Immunized stallions show reduced or absent libido, decreased testicular size, and azoospermia.[104,105] Similar effect may be obtained by administration of the luteinizing hormone–releasing hormone antagonist antarelix (100 μg/kg).[106]

Growth Hormone
It has been shown that growth hormone may be involved in testicular function.[107] Administration of growth hormone to normal stallions does not improve spermatogenesis but does increase ejaculate volume and the volume of gel fraction.[108]

Pharmacologic Manipulation of Ejaculation

Pharmacologic facilitation or induction of ejaculation often is used to obtain semen from stallions with erectile or ejaculatory dysfunction or from those incapable of performing a mount as a result of physical or neurological problems.[109] A series of experiments realized primarily by McDonnell[114] showed that α-adrenergic agonists or β-adrenergic blockers enhance smooth muscle contraction and promote ejaculation during copulation and are able to induce ejaculation ex copula.

Treatment with the α-agonist L-norepinephrine (0.01 mg/kg IM), 15 minutes before breeding, followed 5 minutes later with the β-antagonist carazolol (0.015 mg/kg), was successful in producing ejaculation in 71% (n = 24) of stallions treated for failure of ejaculation.[24,110]

Xylazine
Xylazine has central and peripheral $α_1$ and $α_2$ adrenergic effects, with a predominance of $α_2$ events.[111-113] Response to xylazine induction of ejaculation depends on the level of arousal at the time of treatment. Best results are obtained when the stallion is in a quiet, undisturbed environment.[111] Ejaculation rates may be improved by

prolonged teasing before treatment. Response rate with xylazine alone is quite variable, however. The ejaculate obtained generally is similar to in-copula ejaculates in terms of volume, sperm concentration, pH, and total sperm number.[111]

Imipramine

Tricyclic antidepressants of the dibenzazepine family—imipramine and clomipramine—are known for their effect on erection and spontaneous ejaculation in men.[21,114] In stallions, these drugs produce erection and masturbatory behavior, accompanied on occasion by ejaculation. Ejaculation occurs usually within 10 to 45 minutes after intravenous administration of imipramine alone.[112,115] Hemolysis has been reported after intravenous administration of imipramine.[112] Oral treatment produces similar results without the hemolysis side effect. Besides prolonged yawing, no other side effect has been reported in mature breeding stallions even after prolonged utilization.

Imipramine is thought to act centrally on norepinephrine, dopamine, and serotonin systems, which are involved in sexual behavior. Imipramine also is believed to act on the autonomic nervous system, particularly by inhibiting norepinephrine reuptake and mild anticholinergic proprieties to produce erection and ejaculation.[116,117] An increase in circulating testosterone has been observed in stallions after oral or intravenous treatment with imipramine. The erection and masturbation behavior observed in geldings after imipramine treatment, however, does not support a role for testosterone in this response.[116]

Ejaculates obtained after treatment with imipramine have lower volume, higher sperm concentration, higher total sperm numbers, and lower pH than in-copula ejaculates. This difference suggests that imipramine improves sperm output by enhancing contractions or the ampullae and reduces seminal plasma volume by inhibiting accessory sex gland contraction.[112,115]

Imipramine given orally twice daily in a dose of 100 mg, or 500 to 1000 mg 2 hours before collection or breeding, has been used to enhance sexual arousal in stallions with sexual dysfunction. This treatment generally is accompanied by increased frequency of erection and masturbation in the stall. I have successfully treated failure of ejaculation in two stallions by administration of 100 mg of imipramine orally 2 hours before semen collection or natural breeding. With use of this protocol, one stallion has been performing for three seasons without any effect on libido or fertility.

Detomidine

Ex-copula ejaculation has also been reported after detomidine (0.01 to 0.02 mg/kg) treatment.[118,119] Similar to imipramine, detomidine appears to enhance contractions of the ampullae and reduce contractions of the accessory sex gland.

Prostaglandin F2-alpha

The effects of prostaglandin F2-alpha ($PGF_{2\alpha}$) on ejaculation or seminal characteristics are somewhat controversial. Administration of $PGF_{2\alpha}$ (2.5 mg) before semen collection has been shown to increase semen volume and total sperm number.[120] In one study, however, administration of a dose of 10 mg at 1 hour before collection resulted in increases in sperm concentration and gel-free seminal volume without improvement in total sperm number and quality.[121]

In another report, the investigators described spontaneous ejaculation within 10 to 50 minutes after injection of $PGF_{2\alpha}$ (0.01 mg/kg IM) in 50% of treated stallions.[21] According to these investigators, the treatment seems to enhance contraction of the accessory sex gland and production of high-volume ejaculate with a higher gel fraction and pH. Although erection was observed in all treated animals within 1 hour of treatment, all ejaculations occurred when the penis was flaccid.[21] Masturbation behavior also was reported in some stallions within 20 to 30 minutes after treatment with $PGF_{2\alpha}$.[121] Treatment with $PGF_{2\alpha}$ generally is not recommended because of the low efficacy and significant side effects (sweating, abdominal cramping, urine dripping).

Oxytocin

Use of oxytocin to enhance ejaculation has been evaluated in normal stallions and was not found to be beneficial. However, in stallions with sperm accumulation syndrome (sperm-occluded ampullae), oxytocin (10 to 20 IU IV) has been used to stimulate smooth muscle contraction and helps in the elimination of stored semen.

Imipramine/Xylazine

The most commonly used and reliable protocols for the ex-copula induction of ejaculation in stallions are based on the combination of the tricyclic antidepressant imipramine, followed by administration of xylazine. Initial studies used intravenous imipramine, but more recently, oral administration of imipramine has proved to be more advantageous (the drug can be administered by the owner, and side effects due to hemolysis are less common).[112,113] The standard treatment consists of administration of oral imipramine (2 to 3 mg/kg), followed 2 hours later by administration of intravenous xylazine (0.66 mg/kg). Ejaculation usually occurs at the onset of sedation, within 1 to 3 minutes of xylazine administration or when the sedation is wearing off (15 to 25 minutes after xylazine injection). Reported success rates (as determined by induction of ejaculation) vary, ranging between 30% and 75%.[111-113,115,122] The ejaculation rate may be improved by titrating the doses of imipramine and xylazine for a particular stallion. Titration studies done in up to 8 trials at 2- to 3-day intervals with 3 or 5 mg/kg imipramine, followed 2 hours later by intravenous xylazine at 0.50, 0.60, 0.65, or 0.70 mg/kg, found success rates of 80% to 100%.[114]

Ejaculates obtained ex copula with imipramine-plus-xylazine treatment generally are of lower volume, higher concentration, and total sperm number and lower pH than in-copula ejaculates. Fertility and cryopreservation performance are adequate.[113,122] The high sperm concentration and low volume of seminal plasma make ex-copula ejaculates ideal for cryopreservation without the need for centrifugation.

Some anecdotal reports have described the use of the same imipramine plus xylazine protocol for ex-copula induction of ejaculation in jacks. However, in an ongoing large study in 42 jacks treated with varying doses of imipramine and xylazine, the ejaculation rate was disappointingly low despite a high frequency of erection and masturbation (Sghiri and Tibary, unpublished data).

References

1. McDonnell S: Reproductive behavior of the stallion. Vet Clin North Am Equine Pract 1986; 2:535-555.
2. Keiper R, Houpt KA: Reproduction in feral horses. An eight-year study. Am J Vet Res 1984; 45:991.
3. McCort WD: Behavior of feral horses and ponies. J Anim Sci 1984; 58:493.
4. Asa CS: Male reproductive success in free-ranging feral horses. Behav Ecol Sociobiol 1999; 47:89-93.
5. McDonnell SM: Sexual behavior. In Mills DS, McDonnell SM (eds): The Domestic Horse: The Origins, Development and Management of Its Behaviour, London, Cambridge University Press, pp 110-125, 2005.
6. Bahloul K, Pereladova OB, Soldatova N et al: Social organization and dispersion of introduced kulans (*Equus hemionus kulan*) and Przewalski horses (*Equus przewalski*) in the Bukhara Reserve, Uzbekistan. J Arid Envir 2001; 47:309-323.
7. Linklater WL, Cameron EZ: Tests for cooperative behaviour between stallions. Anim Behav 2000; 60:731-743.
8. Bowling AT, Touchberry RW: Parentage of Great Basin feral horses. J Wildlife Manag 1990; 54:424-429.
9. Linklater WL, Cameron EZ, Minot EO, Stafford KJ: Stallion harassment and the mating system of horses. Anim Behav 1999; 58:295-306.
10. Eagle TC, Asa CS, Garrott RA et al: Efficacy of dominant male sterilisation to reduce reproduction in feral horses. Wildlife Soc Bull 1993; 21:116-121.
11. Feh C: Alliances and reproductive success in Camargue stallions. Anim Behav 1999; 57:705-713.
12. Franke Stevens E: Instability of harems of feral horses in relation to season and presence of subordinate stallions. Behaviour 1990; 112:149-161.
13. Turner JW, Perkins A, Kirkpatrick JF: Elimination marking behavior in feral horses. Can J Zool 1981; 59:1561.
14. McDonnell SM: Normal and abnormal sexual behavior. Vet Clin North Am Equine Pract 1992; 8:71-89.
15. Crowell-Davis S, Houpt KA: The ontogeny of flehmen in horses. Anim Behav 1985; 33:739.
16. Stahlbaum CC, Houpt KA: The role of the flehmen response in the behavioral repertoire of the stallion. Physiol Behav 1989; 45:1207-1214.
17. Andersson KE, Wagner G: Physiology of penile erection. Physiol Rev 1995; 75:191–236.
18. Schmidt MH, Schmidt HS: The ischiocavernosus and bulbospongiosus muscles in mammalian penile rigidity. Sleep 1993; 16:171–183.
19. Beckett SD, Hudson RS, Walker DF et al: Blood pressures and penile muscle activity in the stallion during coitus. Am J Physiol 1973; 225:1072–1075.
20. Beckett SD, Walker DF, Hudson RS et al: Corpus spongiosum penis pressure and penile muscle activity in the stallion during coitus. Am J Vet Res 1975; 36:431–433.
21. McDonnell SM: Ejaculation, physiology and dysfunction. Vet Clin North Am Equine Pract 1992; 5:57-69.
22. Tischner M, Kosiniak K, Bielanski W: Analysis of the pattern of ejaculation in stallions. J Reprod Fertil 1974; 41:329-335.
23. Kosiniak K: Characteristics of the successive jets of ejaculated semen of stallions. J Reprod Fertil 1975; 23 (Suppl):59.
24. Klug E, Deegan E, Lazarz B: Effect of adrenergic neurotransmitters upon the ejaculatory process in the stallion. J Reprod Fertil 1982; 32 (Suppl):31.
25. McDonnell SM, Hinze AL: Aversive conditioning of periodic spontaneous erection adversely affects sexual behavior and semen in stallions. Anim Reprod Sci 2005; 89:77-92.
26. McDonnell SM: Spontaneous erection and "masturbation" in equids. Proceedings of the Second International Workshop on Erection and Ejaculation in Horses and Men, Mount Joy, PA, pp 29-30, 1995.
27. McDonnell SM: Spontaneous erection and masturbation in equids. Proceedings of the 35th Annual Convention of the American Association of Equine Practitioners, Boston, pp 567–580, 1989.
28. McDonnell SM, Henry M, Bristol F: Spontaneous erection and masturbation in equids. J Reprod Fertil 1991; 44 (Suppl): 664-665.
29. Boyd LE: The behavior of Przewalski's horses and its importance to their management. Appl Anim Behav Sci 1991; 29:301-318.
30. Wilcox S, Dusza K, Houpt K: The relationship between recumbent rest and masturbation in stallions. Equine Vet Sci 1991; 11:23-26.
31. Ginther OJ, Lara A, Leoni M, Bergfelt DR: Herding and snaking by the harem stallion in domestic herds. Theriogenology 2002; 57:2139-2146.
32. Ginther OJ, Scraba ST, Nuti LC: Pregnancy rates and sexual behavior under pasture breeding conditions in mares. Theriogenology 1983; 20:333-345.
33. Steinbjornsson B, Kristjansson H: Sexual behaviour and fertility in Iceland horse herds. Pferdeheilkunde 1999; 15:481-490.
34. Bristol F: Breeding behaviour of a stallion at pasture with 20 mares in synchronized oestrus. Proceedings of the Third International Symposium on Equine Reproduction, University of Sydney, pp 71-77, 1982.
35. McDonnell SM: Reproductive behavior of stallions and mares: comparisons of free-running and domestic in-hand breeding. Anim Reprod Sci 2000; 50/61:211-219.
36. Tibary A: Pathologie genitale. In Tibary A, Bakkoury M (eds): Reproduction Equine, tome II: L'etalon, Actes ed, pp 185-316, 2005.
37. Noue P, Bernabe J, Rampin O et al: Sexual behavior of stallions during in-hand natural service and semen collection: an observation in French studs. Anim Reprod Sci 2001; 68:161-169.
38. Wallach SJR, Pickett BW, Nett TM: Sexual behavior and semen concentration of reproductive hormones in impotent stallions. Theriogenology 1983; 19:833–840.
39. Pickett BW, Faulkner LC, Seidel GE Jr et al: Reproductive physiology of the stallion. VI. Seminal and behavioral characters. J Anim Sci 1976; 43:617-625.
40. Anderson TM, Pickett BW, Heird JC, Squires EL: Effect of blocking vision and olfaction on sexual responses of haltered or loose stallions. J Equine Vet Sci 1996; 16:254-261.
41. Hillman RB, Olar TT, Squires EL, Pickett BW: Temperature of the artificial vagina and its effect on seminal quality and behavioral characteristics of stallions. J Am Vet Assoc 1980; 177:720-722.
42. Love CC: Semen collection techniques. Vet Clin North Am Equine Pract 1992; 8:111-128.
43. McDonnell SM: Stallion sexual behavior. In Samper JC (ed): Equine Breeding Management and Artificial Insemination, Philadelphia, Saunders, pp 53-61, 2000.

44. McDonnell SM, Love CC: Manual stimulation collection of semen from stallions: training time, sexual behavior and semen. Theriogenology 1990; 33:1201-1210.

45. Klingel H: Observations on social organization and behaviour of African and Asiatic wild asses *Equus africanus* and *E. hemionus*. Z Tierpsychol 1977; 44:323–331.

46. Woodward SL: The social system of feral asses *Equus asinus*. Z Tierpsychol 1979; 49:304–316.

47. Henry M, McDonnell SM, Lodi LD, Gastal EL: Pasture mating behaviour of donkeys *Equus asinus* at natural and induced estrus. J Reprod Fertil 1991; 44 (Suppl):77–86.

48. Henry M, Lodi LD, Gastal MMFO: Sexual behaviour of domesticated donkeys (*Equus asinus*) breeding under controlled or free range management systems. Appl Anim Behav Sci 1998; 60:263-276.

49. Tibary A, Bakkoury M, Anouassi A, Sghiri A: Examen et evaluation de l'aptitude à la reproduction. In Tibary A, Bakkoury M (eds): Reproduction Equine, tome II: L'etalon, Actes ed, pp 39-184, 2005.

50. Gastal MO, Henry M, Beker AR et al: Sexual behavior of donkey jacks: influence of ejaculatory frequency and season. Theriogenology 1996; 46:593-603.

51. Lodi LD, Henry M, Paranhos da Costa MJR: Behavior of donkeys (*Equus asinus*) breeding mares (*Equus caballus*) at pasture. Biol Reprod 1995; monogr 1:591-598.

52. Kreuchauf A: Reproductive physiology in the jackass. Anim Res Dev 1984; 20:51-78.

53. Ostrowski JEB, Cortesano JA: Production de mulares por inseminaccion artificial Manejo del asno doador de semen. Rev Med Vet 1987; 68:210-216.

54. Henry M: Some reproductive characteristics of donkeys. Prat Vet Equine 2001; 33:11-20.

55. Mill J: [Clinical experiences in the treatment of hypersexual behaviour in stallions with sex hormones and tranquillizers to improve racing performance.] Monatsh Veterinarmed 1974; 29:951-956.

56. Pickett BW, Voss JL: Abnormalities of mating behaviour in domestic stallions. J Reprod Fertil 1975; 23(Suppl):129-134.

57. Pickett BW, Voss JL, Squires EL: Impotence and abnormal sexual behavior in the stallion. Theriogenology 1977; 8:329-347.

58. Houpt KA, Lein D: Equine behavior. The sexual behavior of stallions. Vet Clin North Am Equine Pract 1980; 2:8-22.

59. Veserat GM, Cirelli AA Jr: Stallion behavior. Vet Clin North Am Equine Pract 1996; 18:29-32.

60. Dodman NH, Shuster L, Court MH, Patel J: Use of a narcotic antagonist (nalmefene) to suppress self-mutilative behavior in a stallion. J Am Vet Med Assoc 1988; 192:1585-1586.

61. Houpt KA: Self-directed aggression: a stallion behavior problem. Vet Clin North Am Equine Pract 1983; 5:6-8.

62. Klug E, Bartmann CP, Gehlen H: Diagnosis and therapy of copulatory disorders of the stallion. Pferdeheilkunde 1999; 15:494-502.

63. Veeckman J: Aberrant sexual behaviour of a covering stallion. Vlaams Diergeneeskd Tijdschr 1978; 47:267-273.

64. Rasbech N: Ejaculatory disorders of the stallion. J Reprod Fertil 1975; 23(Suppl):123-128.

65. McDonnell SM: Conditioned suppression of sexual behavior in stallions and reversal with diazepam. Physiol Behav 1985; 34:951-956.

66. McDonnell SM, Haviland JCS: Agonistic ethogram of the equid bachelor band. Appl Anim Behav Sci 1995; 43:147-148.

67. McDonnell SM, Murray SC: Bachelor and harem stallion behavior and endocrinology. Biol Reprod 1995; monogr 1: 577-590.

68. McDonnell SM, Kenney RM, Meckley PE, Garcia MC: Novel environment suppression of stallion sexual behavior and effects of diazepam. Physiol Behav 1986; 37:503-505.

69. Carson RL, Thompson FN: Effects of an anabolic steroid on the reproductive tract in the young stallion. J Equine Med Surg 1979; 3:221-224.

70. Nagata S, Kurosawa M, Mima K et al: Effects of anabolic steroid (19-nortestosterone) on the secretion of testicular hormones in the stallion. J Reprod Fertil 1999; 115:373-379.

71. Berndtson WE, Hoyer JH, Squires EL, Pickett BW: Influence of exogenous testosterone on sperm production, seminal quality and libido of stallions. J Reprod Fertil 1979; 27 (Suppl):19-23.

72. Squires EL, Todter GE, Pickett BW: The effect of androgenic compounds on reproductive performance of stallions. Proc AAEP 1980; 25:421-438.

73. McDonnell SM, Diehl NK, Oristaglio Turner RM: Modification of unruly breeding behavior in stallions. Compend Contin Educ 1995; 17:411-417, 428.

74. Goolsby HA, Brady HA, Prien SD: The off-label use of altrenogest in stallions: a survey. J Equine Vet Sci 2004; 24:72-75.

75. Crump J Jr, Crump J: Stallion ejaculation induced by manual stimulation of the penis. Theriogenology 1989; 31:341-346.

76. Love CC, McDonnell SM, Kenney RM: Manually assisted ejaculation in a stallion with erectile dysfunction subsequent to paraphimosis. J Am Vet Med Assoc 1992; 200:1357-1359.

77. McDonnell SM, Pozor MA, Beech J, Sweeney RW: Use of manual stimulation for collection of semen from an atactic stallion unable to mount. J Am Vet Med Assoc 1991; 199:753-754.

78. McDonnell SM: Libido, erection, and ejaculatory dysfunction in stallions. Compend Contin Educ Pract Vet 1999; 21:263-266.

79. Blanchard TL, Woods J, Brinsko SP: Theriogenology question of the month. J Am Vet Med Assoc 2000; 217:825-826.

80. Brinsko SP: Retrograde ejaculation in a stallion. J Am Vet Med Assoc 2001; 218:551-553.

81. Love CC, Riera FL, Oristaglio RM, Kenny RM: Sperm occluded (plugged) ampulae in the stallion. Proceedings of the Annual Conference of the Society for Theriogenology, San Antonio, TX, pp 117-125, 1992.

82. Martin BB, McDonnell SM, Love CC: Effects of musculoskeletal and neurologic diseases on breeding performances in stallions. Compendium Contin Educ 1998; 20:1159.

83. Forney BD, McDonnell SM: How to collect semen from stallions while they are standing on the ground. Proceedings of the 45th Annual Convention of the American Association of Equine Practitioners, Albuquerque, NM, pp 142-144, December 5-8, 1999.

84. Tibary A: Diagnostic et traitement de l'infertilité. In Tibary A, Bakkoury M (eds): Reproduction Equine, tome II: L'etalon, Actes ed, pp 317-357, 2005.

85. Althouse GC, Seager SWJ, Varner DD, Webb GW: Diagnostic aids for the detection of urine in the equine ejaculate. Theriogenology 1989; 31:1141-1148.

86. Danek J, Wisniewski E, Krumrych W: A case of urospermia in a stallion. Med Weteryn 1994; 50:129-131.

87. Lowe JN: Diagnosis and management of urospermia in a commercial Thoroughbred stallion. Equine Vet J 2001; 13:4-7.

88. Leendertse IP, Asbury AC, Boening KJ, Von Saldern FC: Successful management of persistent urination during ejaculation in a Thoroughbred stallion. Equine Vet Educ 1990; 2:62-64.

89. Mayhew IG: Neurological aspects of urospermia in the horse. Equine Vet Educ 1990; 2:68-69.

90. Nash JGJ, Voss JL, Squires EL: Urination during ejaculation in a stallion. J Am Vet Med Assoc 1980; 176:224-227.

91. Turner RMO, Love CC, McDonnell SM et al: Use of imipramine hydrochloride for treatment of urospermia in a stallion with a dysfunctional bladder. J Am Vet Med Assoc 1995; 207:1602-1606.

92. Hoyos Sepulveda ML, Quiroz Rocha GF, Brumbaugh GW et al: Lack of beneficial effects of bethanechol, imipramine or furosemide on seminal plasma of three stallions with urospermia. Reprod Domest Anim 1999; 34:489-493.

93. Houpt KA, McDonnell SD: Equine stereotypies. Comp Cont Educ Pract Vet 1993; 15:1265-1272.

94. Marsden D: A new perspective on stereotypic behaviour problems in horses. In Pract 2002; 11/12:558-569.

95. Dodman NH, Normile JA, Shuster L, Rand W: Equine self-mutilation syndrome (57 cases). J Am Vet Med Assoc 1994; 204:1219-1223.

96. Bedford SJ, McDonnell SM, Tulleners E et al: Squamous cell carcinoma of the urethral process in a horse with hemospermia and self-mutilation behavior. J Am Vet Med Assoc 2000; 216:551-553.

97. McClure SR, Chaffin MK, Beaver BB: Non-pharmacological management of stereotypic self mutilation in a stallion. J Am Vet Med Assoc 1992; 200:1975-1977.

98. Heninger NL, Brady HA, Herring AD et al: The effects of oral altrenogest on hormonal, seminal and behavioral profiles of two-year-old stallions. Prof Anim Sci 1999; 17:75-80.

99. Johnson NN, Brady HA, Whisnant CS, LaCasha PA: Effects of oral altrenogest on sexual and aggressive behaviors and seminal parameters in young stallions. J Equine Vet Sci 1998; 18:249-253.

100. Squires EL, Badzinski SL, Amann RP et al: Effects of altrenogest on total scrotal width, seminal characteristics, concentrations of LH and testosterone and sexual behavior of stallions. Theriogenology 1997; 48:313-328.

101. Vartorella HA, Brady HA, Herring AD, Prien SD: Case study: the effects of an intermittent regimen of altrenogest on behavioral, hormonal, and testicular parameters of three-year-old stallions. Prof Anim Sci 2001; 17:317-321.

102. Weinrich S: Influence of GnRH treatment on sexual behaviour and spermatological parameters in Warmblood stallions during the nonbreeding season. Hanover, Germany, Tierarztliche Hochschule Hannover, p 131, 2002.

103. Dowsett KF, Knott LM, Tshewang U et al: Suppression of testicular function using 2 dose-rates of a reversible water-soluble gonadotropin-releasing-hormone (GnRH) vaccine in colts. Aust Vet J 1996; 74:228-235.

104. Tshewang U, Dowsett KF, Knott L, Jackson A: Effect of GnRH immunization on testicular function in colts. Asian-Australas J Anim Sci 1999; 12:348-353.

105. Malmgren L, Andresen O, Dalin AM: Effect of GnRH immunisation on hormonal levels, sexual behaviour, semen quality and testicular morphology in mature stallions. Equine Vet J 2001; 33:75-83.

106. Hinojosa AM, Bloeser JR, Thomson SRM, Watson ED: The effect of a GnRH antagonist on endocrine and seminal parameters in stallions. Theriogenology 2001; 56:903-912.

107. Aurich C, Kranski S, Aurich J et al: Involvement of growth hormone in the regulation of testicular function in the pony stallion. Theriogenology 2002; 58:429-432.

108. Storer WA, Thompson DLJ, Cartmill JA, Evans MJ: Does growth hormone treatment of stallions during the non-breeding season increase testis sensitivity to luteinizing hormone or pituitary sensitivity to GnRH? Theriogenology 2002; 58:433-436.

109. Turner ORM, McDonnell SM, Hawkins JF: Use of pharmacologically induced ejaculation to obtain semen from a stallion with a fractured radius. J Am Vet Med Assoc 1995; 206:1906-1908.

110. Klug E. Ejaculatory failure. In Robinson NE (ed): Current Therapy in Equine Medicine 2, Philadelphia, WB Saunders, p 562, 1987.

111. McDonnell SM, Love CC: Xylazine-induced ex copula ejaculation in stallions. Theriogenology 1991;36:73-76.

112. McDonnell SM, Odian MJ: Imipramine and xylazine-induced ex copula ejaculation in stallions. Theriogenology 1994; 41:1005-1010.

113. Johnston PF, De Luca J: Chemical ejaculation of stallions after the administration of oral imipramine followed by intravenous xylazine. Proceedings of the 44th Annual Convention of the American Association of Equine Practitioners, Baltimore, Md, 1998; 44:12-16.

114. McDonnell SM: Oral imipramine and intravenous xylazine for pharmacologically-induced ex copula ejaculation in stallions. Anim Reprod Sci 2001; 68:153-159.

115. McDonnell SM, Oristaglio Turner RM: Post-thaw motility and longevity of motility of imipramine-induced ejaculates of pony stallions. Theriogenology 1994; 42:475-481.

116. McDonnell SM, Garcia MC, Kenney RM, Van Arsdalen KN: Imipramine-induced erection, masturbation, and ejaculation in male horses. Pharmacol Biochem Behav 1987; 27:187-191.

117. McDonnell SM, Garcia MC, Kenny RM: Pharmacological manipulation of sexual behaviour in stallions. J Reprod Fertil 1987; 35(Suppl):45-49.

118. Blanco M, Serres C, Del Rio A et al: Induction of ex copula ejaculation in stallions using pharmacological methods. Proceedings of Congresso Iberico Reproducao Animal 1997; 2:32-37.

119. Rowley DD, Lock TF, Shipley CF: Fertility of detomidine HCl–induced ex copula– ejaculated stallion semen after storage at 5°C. Proceedings of the 45th Annual Convention of the American Association of Equine Practitioners, Albuquerque, NM, 1999; 45:221-223.

120. Klug E, Martin JC, Graser A et al: Effect of PGF2 alpha on ejaculate fractions in the horse. Zuchthygiene 1978; 13:80.

121. Kreider JL, Ogg WL, Turner JW: Influence of prostaglandin F2 alpha on sperm production and seminal characteristics of the stallion. Prostaglandins 1981; 22:903-913.

122. Card CE, Manning ST: Pregnancies from imipramine and xylazine-induced ex copula ejaculation in a disabled horse. Can Vet J 1997; 38:171-174.

Male Reproductive Problems: Diagnosis and Management

CHAPTER 29

Testicular Descent and Cryptorchidism

MIMI ARIGHI

TESTICULAR DESCENT

In the normal equine male fetus, the testes descend into the scrotum between 30 days before and 10 days after birth.[1] Three anatomic structures are involved in normal descent: the vaginal process, the gubernaculums, and the inguinal canal.

The vaginal process is a flask-shaped evagination of the peritoneum in the inguinal region. This evagination penetrates the abdominal wall at the inguinal canal and passes into the scrotum. In stallions, it is a large, flask-shaped structure that is divided into 2 parts: (1) a long, narrow neck containing the spermatic cord, which consists of the blood vessels, nerves, and lymphatics of the testis, the epididymis, the vas deferens, and the internal cremaster muscle, and (2) a dilated body containing the testes, epididymis, and the proximal section of the vas deferens.[2,3] The opening of the vaginal process, through which the gubernaculum proprium passes, forms the vaginal cavity.[1-4] The vaginal ring is at the level of the internal inguinal ring.[2,5] The testes are encased in the tunica albuginea and lie within an out pocket of abdominal peritoneum known as the tunica vaginalis. The tunica vaginalis consists of visceral and parietal tunics. The visceral tunic is tightly adhered to the testis, ducts, and vessels, and the parietal tunic is continuous with the parietal peritoneum.

The fetal gubernaculum is divided into 3 parts: (1) a portion connecting the testis to the tail of the epididymis—the proper ligament of the testis, (2) a portion between the tail of the epididymis and vaginal process—the caudal ligament of the epididymis, and (3) a remaining portion extending from the vaginal process to the scrotal fold—the scrotal ligament.[2,3,6,7] The gubernacular ligament passes from the end of the vaginal process to the scrotum but does not form a firm anchor to the process. The gubernaculum helps to keep the passageway open by expanding in size and stretching the vaginal ring.[1-4,6,8-12]

The inguinal canal is a passageway between the internal inguinal ring and the external inguinal ring. The internal inguinal ring is formed from the internal abdominal oblique muscle, and the external inguinal ring is formed from both the internal and external abdominal oblique muscles.[2,3] The external cremaster muscle, which lies on the outside of the vaginal tunic, is derived from the internal abdominal oblique muscle and is continuous with the parietal layer of the tunica vaginalis, inserting at the caudal pole of the testis. It helps bring the testis closer to the external inguinal ring when it contracts.[3,13]

During embryonic development, the equine gonad becomes differentiated into testes at $5\frac{1}{2}$ weeks of gestation and lies ventral to the mesonephric kidney.[2-4,8,14-16] At 4 months, the cranial pole of the testis overlies the caudal pole of the mesonephric kidney, while its caudal pole is still some distance from the vaginal ring. The equine gonad begins to hypertrophy at 6 weeks of age through an increase in the number of interstitial cells, and by 5 months of gestation this hypertrophy results in the caudal pole of the testis lying close to the vaginal ring.[1,4,8,14,17-19] The high growth rate of the fetal testes corresponds to a period of high blood estrogen in the pregnant mare.[17,19] The equine fetal testis weigh about 20 grams at 5 months of gestation, 50 grams at 8 months, and 30 grams at 10 months.[1,8,9,14]

After about $7\frac{1}{2}$ months, the testes begin to decrease in size due to degeneration of the interstitial cells, and by 10 months there is a clear separation between the testes and the kidneys.[1,4,8,14,16,19] Between 5 months and 10 months the inguinal canal is too small for the passage of the testes. The developing gubernaculum and vaginal process hold the testes at the vaginal ring. Other abdominal viscera also aid in retaining the testes in the pelvic region. After 5 months of gestation, the enlarged distal end of the gubernaculum proprium becomes the main force preventing inversion of the vaginal process. Firm fibrous connections between the process and the inguinal canal also exist. After 8 months of gestation, the gubernaculum proprium begins to decrease in size and only the fibrous connections in the inguinal canal hold the vaginal process outside the vaginal ring.[1,2,4,8-10,14,16,17,19]

The vaginal process and gubernaculum continue to lengthen at about the same rate up to $8^1/_2$ months of gestation. During this time, the caudal gonadal ligament, between the testis and caudal epididymis, increases in length faster than the gubernaculum, resulting in the caudal epididymis becoming progressively displaced from the caudal pole of the testis. The caudal epididymis does in fact descend into the inguinal canal at about 5 months of gestation in advance of the testes.[1-4,11,14,15,17,18] After $8^1/_2$ months there is a gradual decrease in the length of the gubernaculum while the vaginal process remains static, so that the caudal pole of the regressing testis is drawn into the opening of the vaginal ring, which has been dilated by the increasing diameter of the caudal gonadal ligament and the body of the epididymis.[2,4,14] Owing to the length of the caudal gonadal ligament, hypertrophy of the fetal testis, the small diameter of the vaginal ring, and the lack of tension on the gubernaculum, descent of the testes through the inguinal canal occurs late in gestation.[18]

The actual passage of the testis through the vaginal ring is a rapid process, which occurs during the last month of pregnancy. The gubernacular length continues to decrease while there is a rapid increase in the length of the vaginal process, which increases tension of the gubernaculum on the small flaccid testis. The testis does not pass immediately into the scrotum because the gubernaculum mass remains below it. At birth, most testes lie in the inguinal canal while the gubernaculum lies in the scrotal region and can easily be mistaken for a testis. Further passage of testis into the scrotum after birth is affected by progressive reduction in length and mass of the gubernaculum, which finally becomes a small, dense, fibrous band.[1,2,4,6,17,19] During the first 2 weeks of neonatal life, the internal vaginal ring constricts to about 1 centimeter in diameter and is fibroses; thus the testis cannot be forced through in either direction after this time.[4,6,8,9,16,17]

At birth the weight of each testis ranges from 5 to 20 grams and testicular size does not change much throughout the first 10 months of life. There is slight growth between 11 and 16 months of age, and rapid development of the testes starting around 18 months of age.[1] Puberty in pony stallions was reported to occur between 11 and 15 months of age based on the appearance of sperm in the ejaculate.[20-22] Puberty in Quarter horse stallions was found to occur between 13 months and 23 months of age.[23] Although stallions produce spermatozoa throughout the year, their testes show seasonality where maximum production of sperm occurs from May to July. In one study, 17 stallions were looked at and their testes were found to weigh an average of 167 grams, with an average length of 8.5 cm and an average width of 5.0 cm.[24] In another study, 48 stallions were looked at and their average weight was 164 grams, with an average length of 10.4 cm and an average width of 5.6 cm.[25]

Normal testicular descent involves a process in which the essential physical components are a testis with sufficient freedom of attachment to allow it to be moved from its original dorsal abdominal location to its final scrotal position; patent inguinal rings leading to a properly developed tunica vaginalis; proper size relationship between the testis and the inguinal ring; and sufficient force to move the testis to the inguinal ring.

Surgical Approaches to Castration of Normal Stallions

Castration is probably the most common surgical procedure performed in male horses. It is performed to prevent or eliminate aggressive male behavior in animals not intended to become breeding stallions. Other indications for castration include prevention of testicular neoplasia, testicular trauma, spermatic cord torsion, orchitis, hydrocele, and most cases of inguinal or scrotal hernia. Castration may be safely performed at any age, without complications, even before weaning. Some owners prefer to delay castration until a later age than weaning to allow for development of a more masculine appearance.[13,26]

Castration can be performed safely and acceptably either with the horse standing, using chemical restraint and local anesthesia, or with the horse in recumbency, under general anesthesia. Factors for choosing one method or the other include the surgeon's preference, practice tradition, owner's desire, behavior of horse, descent of the testes, and location where the surgery will be performed.[13,18,26] One must always make sure that the horse has been immunized for tetanus within the last 6 months before any surgical procedure. If not, then the horse should be vaccinated right before or right after the surgical procedure. Postoperatively the horse should be confined for 12 to 24 hours so that he may be monitored for bleeding or herniation. After that, moderate exercise is important so that drainage occurs and healing proceeds normally.[13,18,26]

Standing Castration
Standing castrations have been done for years. However, to be able to use this approach, both testes must be descended into the scrotum. Some of the types of chemical restraint used are the sedative-hypnotics, tranquilizers, and opioids, and include acepromazine, xylazine hydrochloride, romifidine, detomidine hydrochloride, and butorphanol tartrate. Detomidine (0.011-0.022 mg/kg intravenously [IV]) in combination with butorphanol (0.011-0.022 mg/kg IV) has been shown to provide excellent sedation and analgesia for standing castrations. Xylazine (0.3-0.5 mg/kg IV) has been added to this combination for a longer lasting sedative effect.[13] Once sedation takes place, anesthesia of the testis and spermatic cord is accomplished by injecting 10 to 25 ml of local anesthetic into the parenchyma of each testis and also in a subcutaneous line block along each side of the scrotal raphe.[13,18,26]

Standing castration should be performed with both the surgeon and handler positioned on the same side of the horse, with a right-handed surgeon standing on the left side of the horse, facing toward its rear. Both spermatic cords are grasped with the left hand, and the testes are displaced ventrally to tense the skin of the scrotum. Two parallel incisions are made through the scrotal skin on either side of the median raphae. The left incision is deepened so that the cut goes through the tunica dartos, scrotal fascia, and vaginal tunic. This allows the left testis to prolapse through the incision. The mesorchium is then separated so that separate emasculation can be done of the vascular spermatic cord and the vaginal tunic. This procedure is then repeated on the right testis.[13,26]

Care must always be taken to ensure that the emasculator has been applied so that the crushing component is proximal to the cutting blade (nut to nut), which means that the crushing will occur on the part of the tissue that is to be left in the horse. This should prevent major bleeding from occurring. Once both testes have been removed, any tissue that is protruding from the incisions should be excised and the wounds left open to heal by secondary intention.[13,26]

Recumbent Castration

Many veterinarians prefer general anesthesia for castration because surgical exposure is improved and it carries less risk for both the surgeon and patient.[13] A requirement for recumbent castration is a clean, safe area for induction and recovery. Again, before induction, a physical exam is necessary to make sure both testes are palpable in the inguinal/scrotal area and that the horse is healthy and a good candidate for general anesthesia. Ideally the animal should be taken off feed for 12 to 24 hours before anesthesia is carried out.[13,26]

In most cases only a short-term, general anesthetic is necessary and there are many safe and effective choices. The most commonly used anesthetic regimen is still xylazine (1.1mg/kg IV) administered first, then, once the horse is fully sedated, Ketamine (2.2-3.0 mg/kg IV). This protocol provides recumbency in 1 to 2 minutes and 10 to 15 minutes of surgical anesthesia. The administration of butorphanol (0.022-0.044 mg/kg IV) or diazepam (0.05-0.1 mg/kg IV) simultaneously with or just after xylazine may provide additional anesthetic time. If more time is necessary, more xylazine or Ketamine can be given intravenously at $1/3$ to $1/2$ the dose. If additional time is necessary, it is wise to use a longer lasting anesthetic from the start, for example, continuous infusion of 5% guaifenesin containing 2 mg/ml Ketamine and 0.5 mg/ml xylazine.[13,26]

Once the animal is anesthetized, he is placed in either lateral or dorsal recumbency, depending on surgeon's preference and the status of the animal. Lateral recumbency is easier on the cardiovascular status of the animal; however, it is easier to reach both testes in dorsal recumbency.[13,18,26]

The surgeon should stand behind the horse's croup and reach over the operative field. The lower testis is removed first in case there is dripping of blood. Parallel skin incisions are made on either side of the median raphae, as in the standing castration. The incision on the down testis is made deeper so that the scrotal fascia is cut exposing the vaginal tunic. The scrotal fascia is then stripped from the vaginal tunic as far proximally as the surgeon can go. Once this is done, the surgeon must make a decision as to whether to carry out a closed castration or an open cas-

tration. Young horses or horses with small testicular cords may be safely emasculated across the entire spermatic cord within the vaginal tunic (closed castration). In mature horses, it is safer to open the tunic, separate the vascular spermatic cord and ductus deferens from the vaginal tunic, and emasculate and/or ligate separately (open castration). One will have less chance of heavy bleeding postoperatively if an open castration is done.[26]

Traditionally castration wounds are left open to heal by second intention. However, primary closure of these wounds at the time of surgery is becoming more popular. It allows the wound to heal more quickly with less chance of a secondary bacterial infection. Once castration has occurred, scrotal ablation and closure of deeper fascial layers may be performed to reduce dead space. Cox described a closed castration, but instead of emasculating the spermatic cord and tunic, a transfixation suture was first placed and then the cord and tunic were emasculated distal to the ligature. The scrotal skin incision was then closed with suture. No complications were seen with this procedure, postoperative appearance of the animals was more acceptable, and convalescence time was dramatically reduced.[27] Castration with primary closure is probably ideal, however, it ideally should be done in a hospital using Halothane or Isoflurane, not in the field, so as to limit postoperative infection.[26]

There can be many complications after castration. Most common are hemorrhage and infection, with intestinal evisceration, omental prolapse, penile damage, and hydrocele being less common. Also there can be accidents during physical restraint, general anesthesia, and recovery from general anesthesia.[18,26,28-30]

After castration, the concentration of serum testosterone and estradiol rapidly decreases and stabilizes within 6 to 12 hours, while the concentrations of follicle stimulating hormone (FSH) and luteinizing hormone (LH) increase dramatically. It appears that testicular hormones exert negative control over FSH and LH secretion.[22,31,32] The desire to mount (libido) and the ability to ejaculate are gradually lost; however, libido is retained for a longer period than is the ability to ejaculate. Attainment of an erection is generally the last aspect of normal sexual behavior to disappear after castration.[31] Postcastration geldings could have enough motile sperm in their ejaculate to impregnate a mare for up to 1 week. This is due to the presence of extragonadal sperm. Frequency of ejaculation does not seem to hasten the disappearance of spermatozoa from the ejaculates. It is therefore important to keep a newly castrated horse separate from mares for at least a week to prevent unwanted pregnancy. Longer separation may help to diminish stallion-like behavior.[26,33]

PATHOGENESIS OF CRYPTORCHIDISM

Cryptorchidism, or the failure of normal testicular descent, is most frequently found in humans, swine, and horses, though it does occur in many other mammalian species.[8,34] In horses, cryptorchidism, with one or both testes retained, is a common problem. The percentage of foals having cryptorchidism is about 5% to 8%, with most being unilateral cryptorchids. It is not known how many diagnosed retained testes would descend at a later date, nor how many would remain undescended.[19,35] The highest incidence of cryptorchidism has been reported in Quarter horses, followed by Percheron, American Saddle horses, and ponies.[6,35,36] When both testes are retained in the abdomen, the animal is sterile due to the detrimental effect of higher temperatures on spermatogenesis, and the testes have been shown to be more prone to development of secondary tumors.[5,19,37] Unilateral cryptorchids may be fertile if spermatogenesis occurs in the descended testis.[19]

Cryptorchid testes are usually smaller than normal, are soft and flaccid, and weigh between 25 and 131 grams, which is considerably less than normal.[11,38-40] Histologically, cryptorchid testes have arrested spermatogenesis, with changes seen mainly in the germ cell layers. Their Leydig cells appear normal.[11,19,38,41,42] Spermatogenesis does not seem to proceed beyond A- or B-spermatogonia in abdominal testes, or primary spermatocytes in the case of inguinal testes.[3,17,18,39] Mean tubular diameters and spermatogenic cell layers were significantly less in inguinal and abdominal testes when compared to normally descended scrotal testes.[39] In horses, development of seminiferous tubules in abdominal testes appeared to proceed to the extent normally found in foals of 3 to 4 months of age, whereas development in the inguinal testes roughly corresponded to that of a 9- to 12-month-old normal foal.[3,6,11,17,18]

The interstitial (Leydig) cells, which produce testosterone and other hormones, are not as heat sensitive as are the cells of the seminiferous epithelium. Thus, although bilateral abdominal cryptorchid horses may not produce viable sperm, they will often still exhibit normal secondary sex characteristics, including libido.[37] This is especially true in horses, since Leydig cells are very abundant and increase in numbers with age.[43]

A cryptorchid horse may have either one or both testes retained in an abdominal and/or inguinal location, and diagnosis can be complicated if a single normal descended testis has been removed.[1,2,6,8-10,15,28,44] The retained abdominal testis can be complete or incomplete. When all parts of the testis and epididymis are located in the abdominal cavity, the cryptorchidism is complete. If either the epididymis or part of the testis is located in the inguinal canal, the cryptorchidism is incomplete.[8,19,36]

In the horse, the epididymis descends first, thus horses with an abdominal retained testis may have the epididymis in the inguinal canal. If the change in the gubernaculum does not occur at the proper time (decrease in size), or if sufficient gonadal shrinkage does not take place, abdominal testes will never descend because after birth, gonadal size again begins to increase and the vaginal ring constricts.[1,6,8,17] If the gonad does not escape the abdomen about the time of parturition, the horse will remain an abdominal cryptorchid.[6,8,17]

Causes of maldescent remain unresolved and may be due to several factors. Researchers have proposed several explanations for maldescent in humans.

- Defective hypothalamic-pituitary axis and deficiency of LH.[8,15,18]
- Mechanical defects, such as gubernacular abnormality.[8,15,18]
- Genetic factor, based on familial and inherited tendencies.[15,18,19]

- Defects in the testis itself, resulting in deficiency of testicular production of androgens, which influence ductus deferens, epididymis, and gubernaculum during descent.[8,15,18,45-47]
- Testicular dysgenesis based on abnormal "testicular" chromosomes.[18,41,48,49]

In humans, and perhaps horses, a deficiency of gonadotropic hormonal stimulation appears to be an attractive theory to explain bilateral cryptorchidism. Based on experiments with rats, it is now known that premature descent can be induced by treatment with gonadotropin. In addition, because normal testicular descent occurs at a time when endogenous gonadotropin levels are rising, it is assumed that descent of the testes into the scrotum in rats is under regulation of the pituitary gonadotrophins. Testicular descent can also be inhibited by daily injections of estradiol, which can be reversed by simultaneous treatment with human chorionic gonadotropin (hCG). It is thought that estrogen inhibits testicular descent by suppressing pituitary gonadotrophin release, at least in the rat. Only dihydrotestosterone, not testosterone or any other androgen, can induce premature testicular descent in the rat.[15] Although the findings in rats may not be directly applicable to humans or horses, the finding of bilateral cryptorchidism supports at least the need for an intact hypothalamic-pituitary axis and adequate levels of LH for appropriate testicular descent to occur.

Unfortunately, however attractive the hormonal theory is, it is difficult to apply to unilateral cryptorchidism, which is far more common in both humans and horses (3-5 times) than bilateral cryptorchidism.[15] Other causes of, or complicating factors in, failure of testicular descent are thought to be undue stretching of the gubernacular cord; abdominal pressure inadequate for proper expansion of the vaginal process; inadequate growth of the gubernaculum and epididymis, resulting in failure of the testis to expand the inguinal ring; and/or displacement of the testis into the pelvic cavity where it is held by organ pressure, resulting in ineffective gubernacular tension.[1,3,8,9,14] In addition, some authors have suggested that cryptorchidism in the horse can be an inherited abnormality with dominant inheritance,[17,18,48,50] whereas others have concluded that transmission is a simple autosomal recessive trait.[19] At least 2 genetic factors have been reported to be involved, one of which is located on the sex chromosome.[19]

The descent of the right testis in equine fetuses is more advanced than the left in the majority of the fetuses between 9 months of gestation and birth.[1,8,16] The right testis is also found to be significantly smaller in size than the left. The difference in size seems to persist after birth. According to some authors, the smaller size of the right testis predisposes its passage from the abdomen to the inguinal area, and retention in the inguinal area.[4,16,40] Overall, inguinal retention is reportedly more common than abdominal.[36] Some authors have reported more left abdominally retained testes,[4,6,16,28,29,41,51-56] while others have reported equal incidence on both the sides.[36] Reports of location of inguinal testes are more variable, with some authors reporting a higher incidence of right testis involvement,[4,11,16,17,52,55,57] while others have found an equal incidence on both sides.[6,28,41,53] Bilateral cryptorchid horses are much less commonly seen (14% of cryptorchid horses), but when encountered, both testes may be in the abdomen, in the inguinal areas, or one in each site.[35] Some studies report predominance of both retained testes being inguinal,[11] while others have reported a greater incidence of both being abdominal.[6,17,28,52,53] Inguinal testes are more commonly found in yearlings and 2-year-old horses than in older horses, and the ratio of inguinal to abdominal cryptorchid diagnoses decreases with advancing age.[16,36,41] These findings could be explained by the fact that some of the inguinal testes may advance into the scrotal area as the animal becomes older.[16,36]

Cryptorchid horses have a variety of undesirable behavior characteristics. They can be irritable and nervous, have abnormal sexual excitement, or vicious behavior. Owners normally want these animals castrated as soon as possible because their behavior traits make them poor riding horses, and their retained testis/testes usually make them poor breeding prospects.[19]

Diagnostic Tests for Cryptorchidism

Monorchidism is reported to be rare in horses. It is defined as the complete absence of one testis, and may result from agenesis of the testis and mesonephric duct or follow a unilateral testicular vascular accident. The diagnostic approach to monorchid and cryptorchid horses should be similar. A definitive diagnosis of monorchidism is based on history, behavior, physical examination, hormonal testing, and probably surgical exploration.[38,49,58,59]

At 1 to 2 years of age a stallion should receive an examination of the inguinal and scrotal areas to determine that both testes have descended into the scrotal sac. If one or both testes are not present, inguinal and possibly rectal examinations should be performed to determine the position of the retained testis/testes. If one or both testes cannot be palpated in the rectal and/or inguinal areas, then other tests must be done to determine the location of the testis/testes so the best surgical approach can be chosen to locate and remove the testis/testes.

Rectal Examination

Some practitioners do rectal exams on stallions to determine testis location; however, the usefulness of rectal palpation to determine location of retained testis is controversial. Some authors have found this test reliable while others have not. In a study done by Stickle and Fessler, preoperative diagnosis by rectal palpation of the vaginal rings was found to be 87% accurate. Incorrect diagnoses occurred usually because the ductus deferens was felt to enter the vaginal ring; however, the testis was still in the abdomen (partial abdominal cryptorchid).[6] Rectal palpation can also be dangerous, especially in a young stallion, because a rectal tear could occur or the veterinarian could be injured by the stallion's kick.

During rectal palpation, a normal vaginal ring is about 1.2 cm in diameter with the ductus deferens located at the caudo-medial aspect of the ring if the testicular structures have passed normally into the scrotum. Rectal palpation findings may include either the absence or presence of the ductus deferens passing through the vaginal ring toward the scrotum, or the presence of the testis in the abdomen. If the ductus deferens leaving the abdomen through the vaginal ring is not felt, the testis is most likely in the abdomen. If it is felt, then it has traditionally indicated that either the testis is in the inguinal canal or the ductus deferens is in the inguinal canal with the testis still in the abdomen.[6,60]

Ultrasonography

Ultrasonography can be either inguinal, rectal, or both. Animals need sedation in most cases before ultrasonography can be safely done and xylazine and butorphanol have successfully been used. A 5-MHz transrectal transducer is necessary for a successful ultrasonographic examination of this area. The operator first palpates the inguinal area and then places the transducer longitudinally over the external inguinal ring on the side of the retained testis and scans the inguinal ring thoroughly. Rectal scans are started at the pelvic brim and moved forward in an axial to abaxial pattern over the side of the retained testis. Most abdominal testes are located over or within 6 cm of the deep inguinal ring. In 11 horses reported by Jann, only 2 of the 11 retained testes could be palpated rectally or inguinally, whereas 100% of the testes were found via ultrasonography. Also, testicular size determined presurgically via ultrasound in all cases closely approximated the actual size obtained by gross measurement of the excised testis.[60]

Basal Testosterone Levels

Hormone concentrations of animals in which no scrotal/inguinal testes are palpable have been used to determine whether testicular tissue is present. Basal hormonal concentrations can differentiate geldings from animals with testicular tissue. Although low testosterone concentrations in some stallions and high concentrations in some geldings may overlap,[61,62] we found that in all ages of horses, resting testosterone was the most reliable method for differentiating geldings from animals with testicular tissue. Geldings had a mean testosterone value of 0.12 ng/ml (range 0.03-0.15 ng/ml) while animals with testicular tissue had mean values ranging from 0.72 to 0.98 ng/ml (range 0.38-1.2 ng/ml).[38,42] Only 5% of the animals (5/101) were incorrectly diagnosed using this method. Eleven percent (11/101) would have needed further testing.[38,42] In this study it was concluded that resting testosterone concentrations of less than or equal to 0.24 ng/ml were diagnostic of absence of testicular tissue (gelding) whereas resting concentrations of greater than or equal to 0.44 ng/ml were indicative of the presence of testicular tissue.[38,42] Others have confirmed this finding.[49] Values between 0.24 and 0.44 ng/ml were shown not to be diagnostic, and in these cases another type of hormonal testing, such as hCG stimulation or basal levels of estrone sulfate, should be run concurrently.[38,42]

hCG Stimulation Test

hCG has also been utilized to identify the presence or absence of testicular tissue in a horse. The administration of hCG increases synthesis and secretion of testosterone by Leydig cells in the stallion.[18,63] Testosterone secretion in response to hCG is longer than secretion following a natural, episodic discharge of LH.[1,64,65] The injection of hCG is followed within 1 to 2 hours by an elevation of testosterone to a level much higher than the normal episodic changes.

The testing procedure compares a base plasma testosterone level with a second one taken at either 1 hour, 3 hours, 24 hours, or even 3 days after the injection of 6,000 to 12,000 international units (IU) of hCG.[7,9,38,55,61,65-68] In known geldings, basal testosterone concentrations averaged 0.015 ng/ml (0.011-0.02 ng/ml). Stallions had basal concentrations ranging from 0.065 ng/ml to 1.6 ng/ml, while cryptorchids had a mean testosterone concentration of 0.42 ng/ml.[61] In intact stallions, testosterone concentrations increased 4- to 30-fold between 0 and 120 minutes after IV injection of hCG. In geldings, the concentration only increased 0- to 2-fold (values <0.04 ng/ml), and in cryptorchids, a 3-fold increase was seen (values >0.1 ng/ml).[16,61,67,69] We reported that a plasma sample taken before stimulation compared with 2 more samples taken at 1 hour and 24 hours after stimulation with 10,000 IU hCG IV captured 2 testosterone peaks if testicular tissue was present.[38,42]

Location of the testis, age of the animal, and time of year affect the response of testis to hCG. Abdominal testes were much less responsive to gonadotrophin stimulation compared to scrotal testes.[38,42] The response is more pronounced in the summer than in the winter, possibly due to the seasonal variation in testosterone production. Colts less than 18 months of age did not, in many instances, produce enough testosterone in response to hCG to differentiate them from geldings.[68] This was also seen with bilateral abdominal cryptorchid stallions.[38] In addition, stimulation with hCG did not cause an increase in estrogens in horses.[1,38,64]

Basal Estrone Sulfate Levels

Stallion testes produce uniquely high amounts of estrogens.[63,70,71] The stallion's daily estrogen output in urine exceeds that of a nonpregnant mare by a factor of 100 to 200.[66,72] The urine or blood of geldings contains very little estrogen.[72] Urinary estrogen levels in immature stallions are only 0.2% to 0.5% of a mature stallion, and as sexual maturity approaches, a rise in urinary estrogen secretion occurs.[72] The highest level of estrogen production and secretion is attained at the age of 4 to 5 years.[1] Estrone sulfate is by far the most abundant plasma estrogen in the stallion.[73,74] Findings of large quantities of estrone sulfate and only trace amounts of estrogens as free compounds in stallion testes may partly answer the question of how males retain their masculinity in spite of enormous estrogen secretion.[74]

Different groups of researchers have found significantly higher total estrogen levels in the peripheral plasma of bilaterally cryptorchid horses and boars, which suggests that the cryptorchid testis synthesizes more estrogens than does the scrotal testis.[32,56] One of these groups, Ganjam and Kenney,[32] also saw a higher concentration of total estrogens in the cryptorchid testis than in the scrotal testis in unilaterally cryptorchid animals. The germinal epithelium, along with the Sertoli cells, are destroyed in cryptorchid testes, and since the Sertoli cells in the testis normally secrete an FSH-inhibiting substance (inhibin), a lack of FSH inhibition could explain the marked increase in estrogen levels observed in bilateral cryptorchids. Because the total estrogen levels in unilateral cryptorchids are only slightly higher than those of normal stallions, the scrotal testis in the unilateral cryptorchid may be producing sufficient inhibin (an FSH inhibitor) to control the overall production and secretion of estrogen by the cryptorchid tissues.[1,32] Results also suggest that the measurement of total estrogen in horses may be useful in determining whether testicular tissue is still present in a particular suspect animal.[32]

Because the concentration of estrone sulfate in the plasma of mature stallions (>3 years of age) is nearly 100-fold greater than that of testosterone, and geldings' plasma contain very little, the measurement of estrone sulfate in the plasma of a horse greater than 3 years of age has been shown to be a good way to determine whether testicular tissue is still present in that horse.[38,49,69,75] This has been shown to not be true, however, for donkeys,[49] which have an absence of conjugated estrogen. Thus this test would not be good for determining whether testicular tissue was still present in a supposedly castrated donkey. We showed that geldings had resting estrone sulfate concentrations of ≤0.12 ng/ml, whereas animals with testicular tissue had concentrations of ≥1.0 ng/ml. There was less likely to be false positives if the animal being tested was greater than 3 years of age.[38,42] If the hormone concentration falls in the area between these 2 values, the test should be rerun or an assay for basal level testosterone and hCG stimulation should be done simultaneously.[38,42,49,76]

Surgical and Non-surgical Approaches to Castration of Cryptorchid Horses

Vaccination

One alternative to surgical castration of cryptorchid stallions is the use of a vaccination against LH-releasing hormone (LHRH). This immunological approach to castration has been successfully applied to cattle and sheep. This method was carried out on one cryptorchid stallion in which an inguinal testis had been removed but hormonal analysis indicated testicular tissue present in the abdomen. Although this report showed that cryptorchid stallions could be effectively immunized against LHRH, repeated booster injections were needed. Additional studies are necessary to evaluate the LHRH immunocastration and ascertain the most effective immunogen and vaccination schedule.[77]

Another study done by Dowsett et al utilized 2 different doses of a reversible water soluble gonadotrophin releasing hormone (GnRH) vaccine in colts and then monitored their testicular function. The results found that both dose rates suppressed testicular function and that the vaccine effects were reversible. However, the degree of immunosuppression was variable, and it was determined that further work was necessary to achieve a less variable response.[78]

Hemicastration

Hemicastration used to be commonly carried out on cryptorchid horses. Hemicastration is defined as removal of the scrotal testis, leaving the retained testis in the animal. It was once believed that removal of the scrotal testis would promote the descent of the second testis.[79] That has been shown to only occur in a small percentage of cases in which the retained testis was already outside the abdomen and just dorsal to the scrotum.[11] In stallions that have been hemicastrated, the remaining abdominal testis appears to undergo compensatory hyperplasia of interstitial cells with subsequent increase in secretion of hormones.[39,40,61] The significance of this hyperplasia is not well understood. Hemicastration can no longer be justified because it does nothing to promote the welfare of the horse, it creates confusion in the minds of the owners, and it presents veterinary surgeons with an unnecessarily complicated second operation.[79]

Surgical Approaches

Surgical options to remove retained testes include inguinal, parainguinal, suprapubic, paramedian,[7,13,51-53,55,80,81] and flank approaches,[9,13,16,17,55,82,83] and, recently, laparoscopic (both standing and recumbent). There are 3 common approaches now used: inguinal, parainguinal, and laparoscopic.

Inguinal Approach

The inguinal approach has been one of the more common surgical approaches to remove a retained testis for many years. It is one of the few approaches in which the surgeon does not have to be sure before surgery of the exact location of the retained testis since both the inguinal and abdominal areas can be explored.[84] The horse is anesthetized and the inguinal area prepared for aseptic surgery. Then 1 of 2 incisions is used. Either a 10 cm incision is made through the scrotal skin where the testis should be and digital dissection is continued toward the superficial inguinal ring, or an 8 to 10 cm incision is made directly over the superficial inguinal ring. With either approach, during dissection down to the inguinal ring, the testis and/or epididymis are sought. If they cannot be found in the inguinal area, the surgeon has to choose between a noninvasive or invasive approach to seek the abdominal testis.[6,9,44,83-85]

A noninvasive abdominal cryptorchidectomy has been defined as retrieval of the testis via traction on the gubernaculum, epididymis, or ductus deferens after rupture of the vaginal process.[6,84,85] With the noninvasive method, the surgeon must search for the inguinal extension of the gubernaculum (scrotal ligament). The inguinal extension of the gubernaculum is a thin, flat, fibrous band that courses from the vaginal process to the scrotum and is usually located on the caudo-lateral aspect of the superficial inguinal ring.[13,44,84] Gentle traction on that ligament using forceps will evert the vaginal process, which can then be carefully opened. This gives the surgeon access to the abdominal cavity. Commonly, the tail of the epididymis is the first structure that is identified because it is attached to the vaginal process. Gentle traction on the epididymis will expose the ductus deferens and then the testis. The testis is removed and subcutaneous tissue and skin then closed.[6,13,44,83-85]

An invasive technique allows introduction of the surgeon's fingers or entire hand into the abdominal cavity via the vaginal ring to search for the missing testis. Once the testis is found, it is brought out of the abdomen and removed. Closure of this large opening into the abdominal cavity can be difficult. Suturing of the inguinal ring and/or vaginal ring has been tried, as has packing of the inguinal canal for a few days until soft tissue swelling has closed the

opening enough to preclude herniation.[13] The invasive technique can cause more postoperative problems of postoperative bleeding or postoperative intestinal herniation, so most surgeons will attempt a noninvasive method first.

Parainguinal Approach

If the inguinal extension of the gubernaculum and/or the vaginal process cannot be located, the surgeon has to try other surgical methods. One method is the invasive approach described above. The other option the surgeon has is to make a parainguinal incision a few centimeters medial and parallel to the inguinal ring that is large enough to allow the surgeon to put his or her hand into the abdomen to find the testis. Once the testis is removed, the surgeon can close that incision as any abdominal incision, using multiple layers. With this approach, the inguinal ring is left intact. Very few postoperative complications have been noted with this approach, and those seen were minor.[13,16,55,84,86]

Laparoscopic Approach

Over the last 10 to 12 years, surgeons have been using the laparoscope to not only confirm that the retained testis was in the abdomen,[87] but also to remove the testis from the abdomen. Laparoscopic cryptorchidectomy offers improved visualization of the testis, secure closure of the abdominal wall preventing herniation without invading the inguinal canal, visualization of hemorrhage occurring at the time of surgery, and a shortened postoperative patient confinement time.[88,89]

Laparoscopic cryptorchidectomy is done either with the horses sedated, but standing, using a flank approach for both the instrument and laparoscope portals, or with the horses in dorsal recumbency with instrument/laparoscope portals both in a ventral midline or paramedian location.[87-95] If the procedure is performed standing, the horse is typically sedated with a combination sedative/ analgesic like xylazine hydrochloride (0.5 mg/kg IV) and butorphanol tartrate (0.015-0.02 mg/kg IV), or with detomidine (10-15 ug/kg IV) alone. Some surgeons will also do a caudal epidural in addition to sedation using xylazine (0.18 mg/kg diluted to 10-15 ml with 0.9% sodium chloride), or a combination of 2% mepivacaine and xylazine (0.18 mg/kg).[93] Once sedation takes effect, either lidocaine hydrochloride or 2% mepivacaine is infiltrated subcutaneously and intramuscularly at the sites of insertion of the laparoscope and instruments. If it is decided to anesthetize the horse and do the surgery in dorsal recumbency, the horse is induced and maintained on a gas anesthetic and O_2 with intermittent positive-pressure ventilation.[91,94]

Laparoscopic instrumentation is expensive and the anatomy of the region and surgical orientation must be learned. CO_2 or NO_2 insufflation equipment must also be available.[91,94,95] Intestinal damage may occur if the laparoscope is inserted without care and the intestinal wall is mistakenly penetrated, or if electro-surgical instruments are used too close to the intestinal wall and instead of cutting the testicular pedicle the intestinal wall is sliced open.[90,95] If the procedure is done on a horse under general anesthesia, the surgeon must raise the pelvis to displace the viscera cranially. Positive-pressure ventilation must also be provided. In a standing horse, visualization of the vaginal ring is easier because the viscera falls away from the ring and the testis is suspended adjacent to the ring. Also, the dorsal caudal aspect of the abdomen can be well visualized and explored in the standing horse and it avoids the use of general anesthesia, dorsal positioning of the animal, the need for positive pressure ventilation, and the dangers of anesthetic recovery.[91] The disadvantages of doing the procedure in a standing horse are the need to locally anesthetize the testis and the general complications of working on a sedated horse. Also, if both testes are retained, the surgeon must normally repeat the procedure on the opposite side to remove the second testis[91,95]; however, some surgeons have been successful in removing both testes from the same flank approach.[93] If the horse is a unilateral cryptorchid and removal of both testes is to be performed simultaneously, it makes more sense to remove the testes with the horse in dorsal recumbency under general anesthesia, using the laparoscope for the retained testis and the emasculator for the normal scrotal testis.[87]

Once the testis is found in the abdomen, it can be ligated, stapled, or cauterized in the abdomen,[87-89,93] or it can be retrieved from the abdomen and then ligated or emasculated.[91,94,95] If the testis and all associated structures are in the abdomen, the vaginal ring will look small since no structures will be coursing through it. If the horse has incomplete abdominal retention, the tail of the epididymis will be in the inguinal canal, with the testis and remaining structures intraabdominal. However, if both the ductus deferens and mesorchium are seen to be entering the vaginal ring, an extraabdominal location of the testis is present. This may necessitate removal of that testis through an inguinal surgical approach.[94] Otherwise the surgeon will need to enlarge the vaginal ring laparoscopically and attempt to bring the testis back into the abdomen so it can be grasped and removed. This has been successfully done with both inguinally- and scrotally-placed testes in both ponies and juvenile stallions. The vaginal ring is then stapled laparoscopically after bringing the testis back into the abdomen to ligate. Once ligated, the testis is removed via one of the laparoscopic portals. The closure of the vaginal ring is done to prevent intestinal herniation.[87] A third option is the transection of the spermatic cord of that testis so that avascular necrosis will occur. This is a relatively new technique and revascularization of the testis along with subsequent production of testosterone has been reported.[87,96]

False Rigs

Castration is not always successful in completely preventing or eliminating unwanted stallion-like behavior. These horses are called false rigs.[97] A false rig is a horse that has had both testes removed but still exhibits some stallion-like behavior. The majority of false rigs attempt to mount mares if allowed to do so, and about 75% are successful in mounting and achieving an erection and intromission. If they are not successful, it is usually due to the mare not being in heat, or a difference in relative size of the 2 animals. A false rig may be very selective in which mares he tries to mount. Some false rigs also show aggression, but it is a rare trait. Difficulty in handling or riding these animals is the most common owner complaint and is usually seen when the gelding is in the presence of a mare. Many people have reported that they have

seen no difference in the characteristics between a cryptorchid and a false rig.[97,98]

The behavior of a false rig has been attributed to androgens produced either from a piece of epididymis or spermatic sac left behind during castration. These horses are said to be "cut proud."[98] However, Crowe et al and others have shown convincingly that horses with intact epididymides but no testes are endocrinologically and behaviorally indistinguishable from geldings.[61,62] Also, very few false rigs have been found to have an epididymis present.[17,98] It has been shown that the spermatic sac and the adrenal glands of false rigs are not capable of producing testosterone.[41,98] Thus there is no evidence to support the belief that false rigs act like stallions because they are "cut proud" and are still producing testosterone.

The cause of retention of stallion-like behavior remains unknown, but it has been suggested that this may, in part, be due to normal social interaction between horses.[26,98,99] It can occur in horses that are castrated at a young age or in stallions that are castrated late in life. It may occur long after castration has taken place. In a study of the effectiveness of castration on modifying stallion-like behavior, the probability of eliminating sexual behavior or aggression toward people was found to be 60% 70%, and toward other horses was only about 40%. No behavioral differences were found between male horses castrated as adults or as juveniles (<2 years of age).[100] Behavior modification is one of the current recommended treatments, if hormone testing does not suggest the presence of testicular tissue.[98,99]

Another option besides behavior modification that is presently being used is the off-label use of Altrenogest (Regu-Mate). Altrenogest has been used within the equine industry to treat overly aggressive stallions and so potentially could be tried in these animals with stallion-like behavior that have no identifiable testicular tissue. Altrenogest is an oral synthetic progestogen that is normally used to suppress estrus in performance mares and to synchronize estrous cycles for breeding. Several studies in males of various species, including mice, boars, rams, and humans, have demonstrated that exogenous progesterone can cause a reduction of serum testosterone concentrations.[101]

A study done on younger stallions ranging from 2 to 4 years of age showed that there were decreases in the scrotal circumferences, daily sperm production, and flehmen frequency and duration when these animals were given Altrenogest orally for 56 days at 0.088 mg/kg. However, several of these parameters did not return to normal by 8 weeks postcessation of treatment.[102] Another study was done on stallions ranging from 3 to 18 years of age. In this study, the animals were administered a 0.088 mg/kg body weight dose over 150 days or 240 days. The use of Altrenogest alone caused lowered libido, testicular measurements, testosterone, and LH, with only partially reversible effects.[103]

There is concern that the use of Altrenogest in stallions could be detrimental to animals that owners want to use for breeding, but in the situation where the animal has been supposedly castrated and the only concern is the remaining stallion-like behavior, this should not be an issue. Whether the use of Altrenogest will lessen or eliminate the stallion-like behavior in these animals is yet to be determined.

References

1. Amann RP: A review of anatomy and physiology of the stallion. J Eq Vet Sci 1981; 1:83.
2. Ashdown RR: Symposium: The inguinal canal and its relationship to health and disease: I. the anatomy of the inguinal canal in the domestic mammals. Vet Rec 1963; 75:1345.
3. Nickel R, Schummer A, Séiferle E et al: The viscera of the domestic mammal, first English ed, New York, Verlag Paul Parey, Springer-Verlag, 1973.
4. Smith JA: The development and descent of the testis in the horse. Vet Annual 1975; 15:156.
5. Stick JA: Teratoma and cyst formation of the equine cryptorchid testicle. J Am Vet Med Ass 1980; 176:211.
6. Stickle RL, Fessler JF: Retrospective study of 350 cases of equine cryptorchidism. J Am Vet Med Ass 1978; 172:343.
7. Trotter GW, Aanes WA: A complication of cryptorchid castration in three horses. J Am Vet Med Ass 1981; 178:246.
8. Bergin WC, Gier HT, Marion GB et al: A developmental concept of equine cryptorchidism. Biol Reprod 1970; 3:82.
9. Collier MA: Equine cryptorchidectomy: surgical considerations and approaches. Mod Vet Pract 1980; 61:511.
10. Sisson S: Male genitalia. In Sisson S, Grossman JD (eds): The anatomy of the domestic animal, ed 5, Toronto, WB Saunders Co, 1975.
11. Bishop MWH, David JSF, Messervy A: Some observations on cryptorchidism in the horses. Vet Rec 1964; 76:1041.
12. Frank ER: Veterinary surgery, ed 7, Minneapolis, Burgess Publishing, 1964.
13. Searle D, Dart AJ, Dart CM et al: Equine castration: review of anatomy, approaches, techniques, and complications in normal, cryptorchid and monorchid horses. Aust Vet J 1999; 77:428.
14. Gier HT, Marion GB: Development of the mammalian testes. In Johnson AD, Gomes WR, Vandemark NL (eds): The Testis, vol 1, New York, Academic Press, 1970.
15. Shapiro SR, Bodai BI: Current concepts of the undescended testis. Surgery Gynec Obstet 1978; 147:617.
16. Genetzky RM, Shira MJ, Schneider EJ et al: Equine cryptorchidism: pathogenesis, diagnosis and treatment. Comp Cont Educ 1984; 6:S577.
17. Arthur GH: The surgery of the equine cryptorchid. Vet Rec 1961; 73:385.
18. Vaughan JT: Surgery of the male equine reproductive system. In Jennings PB (ed): The practice of large animal surgery, Toronto, WB Saunders Co, 1984.
19. Leipold HW, DeBowes RM, Bennett S et al: Cryptorchidism in the horse: genetic implications, Proceedings of Am Assoc of Eq Pract, Toronto, 1985.
20. Skinner JD, Bowen J: Puberty in the welsh stallion. J Reprod Fert 1968; 16:133.
21. Wesson JA, Ginther OJ: Plasma gonadotrophin concentrations in intact female and intact and castrated male prepubertal ponies. Biol Reprod 1980; 22:541.
22. Wesson JA, Ginther OJ: Puberty in the male pony: plasma gonadotropin concentrations and the effects of castration. Anim Repro Sci 1981; 4:165.
23. Naden J, Amann RP, Squires EL: Testicular growth, hormone concentrations, seminal characteristics, and sexual behavior in stallions. J Reprod Fert 1990; 88:167-176.
24. Love CC, Garcia MC, Riera FR et al: Use of testicular volume to predict daily sperm output in the stallion. Proc Am Assoc Equine Pract 1991; 36:15-21.
25. Thompson DL, Pickett BW, Squires EL, et al: Testicular measurements and reproductive characteristics in stallions. J Reprod Fert 1979; 27(Suppl):13-17.
26. Pleasant RS: Castration of the normal horse. In Wolfe DF, Moll HD (eds): Large animal urogenital surgery, Baltimore, Williams and Wilkins, 1999.
27. Cox JE: Castration of horses and donkeys with first intention healing. Vet Rec 1984; 115:372.
28. Stanic MN: Castration of cryptorchids. Mod Vet Pract 1960; 41:30.
29. Wright JG: The pattern of equine surgery as seen at the field station of the Liverpool school. Br Vet J 1955; 111:43.
30. Hoadley RE: Complications of equine castration, and the questions they raise. Calif Vet 1980; 6:27.
31. Thompson DL, Pickett BW, Squires EL et al: Sexual behavior, seminal pH and accessory sex gland weights in geldings administered testosterone and/or estradiol-17β. J Anim Sci 1980; 51:1358.
32. Ganjam VK, Kenney RM: Androgens and estrogens in normal and cryptorchid stallions. J Reprod Fert 1975; 23(Suppl):67.
33. Shideler RK, Squires EL, Voss JL: Equine castration—disappearance of spermatozoa. Equine Pract 1981; 3:31.
34. Williams WL: Diseases of the genital organs of domestic animals, ed 3, Massachusetts, Ethel Williams Plimpton Publishing Co., 1943
35. Hayes HM: Epidemiological features of 5009 cases of equine cryptorchidism. Equine Vet J 1986; 18:467.
36. Cox JE, Edwards GB, Neal PA: An Analysis of 500 cases of equine cryptorchidism. Equine Vet J 1979; 11:113.
37. Eik-Nes KB: Secretion of testosterone by the eutopic and the cryptorchid testes in the same dog. Can J Physiol Pharmacol 1966; 44:629.
38. Arighi M, Bosu WTK: Comparison of hormonal methods for diagnosis of cryptorchidism in horses. Eq Vet Sci 1989; 9:29.
39. Arighi M, Singh A, Bosu WTK et al: Histology of the normal and retained equine testis. Acta Anat 1987; 129:127.
40. Cox JE: Factors affecting testis' weight in normal and cryptorchid horses. J Reprod Fert 1982; 32(Suppl):129.
41. Coryn M, DeMoor A, Bouters R et al: Clinical, morphological and endocrinological aspects of cryptorchidism in the horse. Theriogenology 1981; 16:489.
42. Arighi M, Bosu WTK, Raeside JI: Hormonal diagnosis if equine cryptorchidism and histology of the retained testes. Proc Am Assoc of Equine Pract 1985; 31:591.
43. Johnson L, Neaves WB: Age-related changes in the leydig cell population, seminiferous tubules and sperm production in stallions. Biol Reprod 1981; 24:703.
44. Valdez H, Taylor TS, McLaughlin SA et al: Abdominal cryptorchidectomy in the horse using inguinal extension of the gubernaculum testis. J Am Vet Med Ass 1979; 174:1110.
45. Nalbandov AV: Reproductive physiology, ed 2, San Francisco, Freeman Publishers, 1964.
46. Cour-Palais IJ: Spontaneous descent of testicle. Lancet 1966; I:1403.
47. Federman DD: Disorders of sexual development. New Eng J Med 1967; 277:351.
48. Roberts SJ: Infertility in male animals. In Roberts, SJ (ed): Veterinary obstetrics and genital diseases, ed 2, Ann Arbor, Edwards Brothers Inc, 1971.
49. Cox JE, Redhead PH, Dawson FE: Comparison of the measurement of plasma testosterone and plasma estrogens for the diagnosis of cryptorchidism in the horse. Equine Vet J 1986; 18:179.
50. Jones WE, Bogart R: Genetics of the horse, East Lansing, Caballus Publishers, 1971.
51. Wright JG: Laparo-orchidectomy in the horse with abdominal cryptorchidism. Vet Rec 1960; 72:57.
52. Wright JG: The surgery of the inguinal canal in animals. Vet Rec 1963; 75:1352.
53. Lowe JE, Higginbotham R: Castration of abdominal cryptorchid horses by a paramedian laparotomy approach. Cornell Vet 1969; 59:121.

54. O'Connor JP: Rectal examination of the cryptorchid horse. Ir Vet J 1971; 25:129.

55. Moore JN, Johnson JH, Tritschler LG et al: Equine cryptorchidism: presurgical considerations and surgical management. Vet Surg 1978; 7:43.

56. Ryan PL, Friendship RM, Raeside JI: Impaired estrogen production by Leydig cells of the naturally retained testis in unilaterally cryptorchid boars and stallions. J Androl 1986; 7:100.

57. Arthur GH: The surgery of the inguinal canal in animals. Vet Rec 1963; 75:1365.

58. Parks AH, Scott EA, Cox JE et al: Monorchidism in the horse. Eq Vet J 1989; 21:215.

59. Strong M, Dart AJ, Malikides N et al: Monorchidism in two horses. Aust Vet J 1997; 75:333.

60. Jann HW, Rains JR: Diagnostic ultrasonography for evaluation of cryptorchidism in horses. J Am Vet Med Assoc 1990; 196:297.

61. Cox JE, Williams JW, Rowe PH et al: Testosterone in normal, cryptorchid and castrated male horses. Equine Vet J 1973; 5:85.

62. Crowe CW, Gardner RE, Humbug JM et al: Plasma testosterone concentrations and behavior characteristics in geldings with intact epididymis. J Equine Med Surg 1977; 1:387.

63. Amann RP, Ganjam VK: Effects of hemicastration or hCG-treatment on steroids in testicular vein and jugular vein blood of stallions. J Androl 1981; 3:132.

64. Cox JE, Redhead PH: Prolonged effect of a single injection of human chorionic gonadotrophin on plasma testosterone and estrone sulphate concentrations in mature stallions. Eq Vet J 1990; 22:36.

65. Silberzahn P, Pouret EJM, Zwain I: Androgen and estrogen response to a single injection of hCG in cryptorchid horses. Eq Vet J 1989; 21:126.

66. Lindner HR: Androgens and related compounds in the spermatic vein blood of domestic animals. J Endocr 1961; 23:171.

67. Cox JE, Williams JH: Some aspects of the reproductive endocrinology of the stallion and cryptorchid. J Reprod Fert 1975; 23(Suppl):75.

68. Cox JE: Experiences with a diagnostic test for equine cryptorchidism. Equine Vet J 1975; 7:179.

69. Cox JE: Testosterone or estrone sulphate assay for the diagnosis of cryptorchidism. Equine reproduction III: Proceedings of the Third International Symposium on Equine Reproduction, Sydney. J Reprod Fert 1982; 32(Suppl):625.

70. Nyman MA, Geiger JA, Goldzieher JW: Biosynthesis of estrogen by the perfused stallion testis. J Biol Chem 1959; 234:16.

71. Bedrak E, Samuels LT: Steroid biosynthesis by the equine testis. Endocrinology 1969; 85:1186.

72. Pigon H, Lunaas T, Velle W: Urinary estrogens in the stallion. Acta Endocr 1961; 36:131.

73. Raeside JI: Seasonal changes in the concentration of estrogens and testosterone in the plasma of the stallion. Anim Reprod Sci 1978/79; 1:205.

74. Raeside JI: The isolation of estrone sulphate and estradiol-17Ǝ sulphate from stallion testis. Can J Biochem Physiol 1969; 47:811.

75. Cox JE: Blood test for equine cryptorchidism. Vet Rec 1982; 110:211.

76. Burba DJ: Theriogenology question of the month. J Am Vet Med Assoc 1996; 15:1705.

77. Schanbacher BD, Pratt BR: Response of a cryptorchid stallion to vaccination against luteinising hormone-releasing hormone. Vet Rec 1985; 116:74.

78. Dowsett KF, Knott LM, Tshewang U et al: Suppression of testicular function using two dose rates of a reversible water soluble gonadotrophin releasing hormone (GnRH) vaccine in colts. Aust Vet J 1996; 74:228.

79. Cox JE: The castration of horses: or castration of half a horse? Vet Rec 1973; 93:425-426.

80. DeMoor A, Verschooten F: Paramedian incision for the removal of abdominal testicles in the horse. Vet Med Small Anim Clin 1967; 62:1083.

81. Cox JE, Edwards GB, Neal PA: Suprapubic paramedian laparotomy for equine abdominal cryptorchidism. Vet Rec 1975; 97:428.

82. Swift PN: Castration of a stallion with bilateral abdominal cryptorchidism by flank laparotomy. Aust Vet J 1972; 48:472.

83. Adams OR: An improved method of diagnosis and castration of cryptorchid horses. J Am Vet Med Ass 1964; 145:439.

84. Arighi M, Horney JD, Bosu, WTK: Noninvasive inguinal approach for cryptorchidectomy in thirty-eight stallions. Can Vet J 1988; 29:346.

85. Merriam JG: An inguinal approach to equine cryptorchidectomy. Vet Med Small Anim Clin 1972; 67:187-191.

86. Wilson DG, Reinertson EL: A modified parainguinal approach for cryptorchidectomy in horses. An evaluation in 107 horses. Vet Surg 1987; 16:1.

87. Wilson DG, Hendrickson DA, Cooley AJ et al: Laparoscopic methods for castration of equids. J Am Vet Med Assoc 1996; 209:112.

88. Fischer AT, Vachon AM: Laparoscopic intra-abdominal ligation and removal of cryptorchid testes in horses. Eq Vet J 1998; 30:105.

89. Ragle CA, Southwood LL, Howlett MR: Ventral abdominal approach for laparoscopic cryptorchidectomy in horses. Vet Surg 1998; 27:138.

90. Hanrath M, Rodgerson DH: Laparoscopic cryptorchidectomy using electrosurgical instrumentation in standing horses. Vet Surg 2002; 31:117.

91. Davis EW: Laparoscopic cryptorchidectomy in standing horses. Vet Surg 1997; 26:326.

92. Fischer AT: Laparoscopic management of the cryptorchid horse. Eq Vet Ed 1997; 9:242.

93. Hendrickson DA, Wilson DG: Laparoscopic cryptorchid castration in standing horses. Vet Surg 1997; 26:335.

94. Fischer AT, Vachon AM: Laparoscopic cryptorchidectomy in horses. J Am Vet Med Assoc 1992; 201:1705.

95. Fischer AT: Standing laparoscopic surgery. Vet Clin North Am 1991; 7:641.

96. Bergeron JA, Hendrickson DA, McCue PM: Viability of an inguinal testis after laparoscopic cauterization and transection of its blood supply. J Am Vet Med Assoc 1998; 213:1303.

97. O'Connor JJ: Dollar's veterinary surgery, ed 3, Chicago, Alexander Eger Inc., 1950.

98. Cox JE: Some observations on the behavior of false rigs. Vet Rev 1979; 25:86.

99. Cox JE: Behavior of the false rig: causes and treatments. Vet Rec 1986; 118:353.

100. Line SW, Hart BL, Sanders L: Effect of prepubertal versus postpubertal castration on sexual and aggressive behavior in male horses. J Am Vet Med Ass 1985; 186:249.

101. Goolsby HA, Brady HA, Prien SD: The off-label use of altrenogest in stallions: a survey. J Equine Vet Sci 2004; 24:72.

102. Johnson NN, Brady HA, Whisnant CS, et al: Effects of oral altrenogest on sexual and aggressive behaviors and seminal parameters in young stallions. J Equine Vet Sci 1998; 18:250.

103. Squires EL, Badzinski SL, Amann RP et al: Effects of altrenogest on total scrotal width, seminal characteristics, concentrations of LH and testosterone and sexual behavior of stallions. Theriogenology 1997; 48:313.

CHAPTER 30

Testicular Abnormalities

REGINA M. O. TURNER

A wide variety of testicular abnormalities have been reported in horses. Some adversely affect fertility, whereas others are benign lesions that have no significant impact on spermatogenesis. An accurate diagnosis of the pathologic condition will greatly aid in treatment recommendations and in forming a prognosis for future fertility.

ANORCHIA, MONORCHIA, AND POLYORCHIA

Anorchia is defined as an absence of testicular tissue and monorchia as a condition in which only one testis is present. These conditions can be congenital or acquired (as with surgical removal of a testicle). Congenital anorchia and monorchia are rare.[1-3] When seen as congenital pathologic conditions, the epididymides are usually missing, as well as the testes. In most cases of congenital monorchia in horses, a vaginal process can be identified on the side without a testicle, leading to the suggestion that the condition arose during gestation secondary to severe degeneration of a previously existing testis. Only rarely was a vaginal process not present, thus suggesting that the problem was due to unilateral testicular agenesis.[4] Polyorchia (the presence of one or more supernumerary testis) has been reported but is exceedingly rare.[2,5,6]

CRYPTORCHIDISM

A cryptorchid horse is one in which one or both testicles have not descended into the scrotum. This condition can be unilateral or bilateral and is relatively common in the stallion.[7-9] The retained testicle may be present either in the inguinal canal or in the abdominal cavity. Abdominal testicles can be located anywhere from just caudal to the kidney to within the internal inguinal ring; however, most are located in or adjacent to the internal inguinal ring.[10] Normal spermatogenesis does not occur in cryptorchid testicles, but hormone production is relatively unaffected. Thus, although stallions with one cryptorchid testicle and one normal descended testicle are usually fertile, bilaterally cryptorchid stallions are sterile but will continue to exhibit stallion-like behavior.

Cryptorchidism should be suspected in any stallion presenting with only one identifiable scrotal testicle or in a supposed gelding with excessively stallion-like behavior. A careful history must be obtained to determine if the missing testicle(s) was (were) surgically removed for reasons unrelated to cryptorchidism. In cases in which no scrotal testes are present, blood hormone profiles can be used to determine whether or not a nonscrotal testis is present. A single, baseline blood testosterone assay may be diagnostic because most cryptorchid animals have elevated testosterone when compared to geldings. However, there is some variation in baseline testosterone concentrations in both normal and cryptorchid animals. Thus this test can result in false-negative results on occasion. Alternatively, a human chorionic gonadotropin (hCG) stimulation test can be performed. Documentation of a rise in blood testosterone in response to hCG stimulation is considered diagnostic of a retained testicle and is a more accurate test than a single baseline blood testosterone assay. Paired plasma samples are drawn before and 30 to 120 minutes after administration of 6000 to 12000 IU hCG intravenously. If functional testicular tissue is present, a significant rise in plasma testosterone concentrations will occur.[11] This technique is reportedly over 90% accurate in detecting the presence of testicular tissue.[12] However, it has been reported that the response to hCG stimulation depends somewhat on the location and number of retained testicles.[13] Unilateral cryptorchids have been reported to have the greatest rise in peripheral plasma testosterone in response to hCG, regardless of the location of the cryptorchid testicle. Horses with bilateral inguinal testicles produced a lower response to hCG than did unilateral cryptorchids, and animals with bilateral abdominal testicles produced a still lower response.

Because of the potential variation in response to hCG, and because the standard hCG stimulation test results in a false-negative response in approximately 8% of cryptorchid animals, in cases in which clinical signs suggest that testicular tissue is present but standard hormone analyses do not confirm this suspicion, extended sampling (up to 72 hours post hCG administration) may be indicated to identify a rise in serum testosterone.[14]

Measurement of plasma total conjugated estrogens also has been used to diagnose the presence of a retained testicle and can be very reliable in differentiating cryptorchid stallions from geldings.[12] Animals with testicular tissue have significantly higher plasma conjugated estrogens than do geldings. Alternatively, or in addition to blood hormone testing, ultrasonography can be used to identify the presence and location of a retained testicle. In one report, 11 of 11 retained testicles were accurately identified, located, and measured using a 5-MHz linear array transducer either transrectally (abdominal testicles) or by scanning externally over the external inguinal ring (inguinal testicles).[15] Ultrasonography is particularly useful in animals with one scrotal testis because hormonal assays cannot differentiate between animals with two testicles (one in the scrotum and the other cryptorchid) and animals with only a single, scrotal testicle.

Debate exists over the heritability of cryptorchidism in the horse. The condition has been reported to be more prevalent in Quarter Horses, Percherons, and American Saddle Horses, thus suggesting a genetic component.[12] Because of the suspicion that cryptorchidism is at least partially heritable, because many breed registries consider cryptorchid animals to be unsound, and because cryptorchid testicles may be at increased risk for neoplasia,[16] bilateral castration of affected animals is strongly recommended.[17] Until more information becomes available on the heritability of cryptorchidism, cryptorchid stallions, whether fertile or not, should be classified as unsatisfactory prospective breeders.[18]

In humans, several hormonal treatments have been reported to cause the descent of cryptorchid testicles with mixed results.[19,20] To the author's knowledge, these protocols have not been evaluated in horses in controlled studies and so are not recommended. Orchiopexy can be used to anchor an undescended testis into the scrotum. However, this technique does not result in the return of normal spermatogenesis.[10] Any attempt to either medically or surgically correct a cryptorchid testicle for the purpose of selling, showing, or marketing the animal as a normal stallion is unethical.

TESTICULAR TORSION

Testicular torsion is more appropriately termed spermatic cord torsion. Torsion of the spermatic cord may cause resultant testicular problems if it results in vascular compromise to the testis. Torsions of less than 180 degrees often do not result in any overt clinical signs, and so treatment classically has not been recommended. Interestingly, recent Doppler ultrasonographic studies have shown that, in some animals with asymptomatic cord torsions, blood flow to the testicle is altered slightly. This raises some concerns that the problem may have more of an impact on testicular function than was previously believed.[21] However, to date, there is no information to suggest that asymptomatic torsions adversely affect testicular function or fertility, and the standard of care for asymptomatic animals remains no treatment.

In some cases of torsions less than 180 degrees, and in many torsions of greater than 180 degrees, blood flow to the testicle can be severely impaired. In addition, lymphatic and venous stasis can result. In these cases, clinical signs are usually apparent. Affected stallions present with signs of colic associated with an enlarged, painful testicle; enlarged scrotum; increased scrotal fluid; and an enlarged spermatic cord (Figure 30-1). Diagnosis typically can be made based on observation and palpation of the affected area. Analgesics and tranquilizers usually are required to adequately examine the affected testicle and spermatic cord. Careful palpation will reveal a twisted and enlarged spermatic cord. In association with the torsion, the tail of the epididymis is rotated from its normal caudal position. The exact location of the epididymal tail depends on the degree of rotation of the

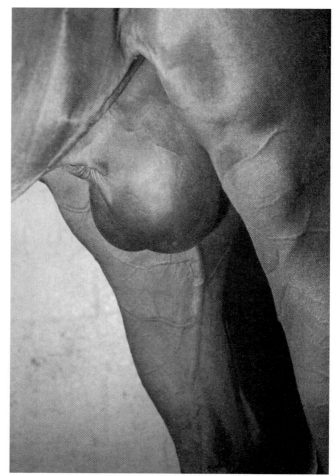

Figure 30-1 Clinical appearance of pathologic left spermatic cord torsion in the stallion. The scrotum is enlarged and painful. Although the torsion affects only the left cord, the scrotum is diffusely edematous and so in this case appears enlarged bilaterally.

cord. For example, 180-degree torsion would result in the tail of the epididymis pointing cranially. Ultrasonography can be used to confirm the diagnosis, if needed.[22] Ultrasonographically, the lumina of the vessels of the spermatic cord are distended. In addition, the ultrasonographic character of the testicular parenchyma is altered. In acute cases of spermatic cord torsion, echogenicity of the testicular parenchyma may be decreased due to static blood and lymph. In more chronic cases, echogenicity may be increased as a result of clotted blood and fibrin. Associated hydrocele often is present. Torsion of the spermatic cord has also been reported in cryptorchid testicles.[16]

The usual treatment for spermatic cord torsion with vascular compromise is castration of the affected testicle. However, if the affected testicle is viable, it can sometimes be salvaged surgically by correcting the torsion and performing an orchiopexy to prevent recurrence.[23] If the contralateral testicle was normal before the torsion, salvage of the affected testicle often is not necessary because sperm can still be obtained from the unaffected testis. If the torsion and associated inflammation and hydrocele cause an increase in scrotal temperature, a transient decline in semen quality from the contralateral testicle can be expected. Once thermoregulation is returned to normal, the contralateral testicle should return to normal function within one spermatogenic cycle and the stallion should again be fertile.

In some instances, spermatic cord torsion may be intermittent. If the stallion is asymptomatic and blood flow is not compromised, no treatment is required. If signs of discomfort are associated with the intermittent torsion, then unilateral orchiectomy or orchiopexy may be indicated. Prognosis for stallions with unilateral testicular torsion is very good, assuming prompt and appropriate treatment is provided.

NEOPLASIA

Testicular neoplasia is uncommon in the stallion.[24] Although one tends to associate neoplasia with an increase in size of the affected tissue, most testicular neoplasms in the stallion are relatively small and so are seen in association with either no change in testicular size or with a decrease in testicular size. Small testicular size in the presence of a testicular tumor most often is due to coincident testicular degeneration (TD). Because both testicular neoplasia and TD are seen most commonly in older stallions, it is not clear whether or not testicular neoplasia is a direct cause of TD. It seems likely that pressure necrosis of parenchyma surrounding a growing tumor will result in some localized degree of TD. However, in many cases, both testicles are uniformly degenerate, even though only one testicle is affected by a tumor. In these cases, is seems likely that the tumor and the degeneration are coincident, but not causative. Uncommonly, testicular tumors in the horse may result in an enlarged testicle.

Testicular neoplasms in the horse can arise from either germinal or nongerminal cells, and most are benign. Germinal neoplasms are the most common tumor type found in stallions. Teratomas, seminomas, teratocarcinomas, and embryonic carcinomas are all germinal neoplasms that have been described in the horse (Figure 30-2).[25] Nongerminal tumors arise from stromal cells and include Sertoli and Leydig cell tumors.[26] A mixed germ cell-sex cord-stromal neoplasia has also been reported.[27]

A tentative diagnosis of a testicular tumor can be made ultrasonographically. However, a definitive diagnosis requires histopathologic examination of the abnormal tissue. Ultrasonographically, testicular neoplasia results in a localized heterogeneous appearance to the normally very homogeneous testicular parenchyma. Most testicular tumors are well demarcated and are hyperechoic with respect to the surrounding testicular parenchyma (Figure 30-3).

Because most testicular tumors in the horse are benign, if a suspected tumor is small with respect to the surrounding testicular parenchyma, and if it does not appear to be aggressive, no treatment may be required other than periodic monitoring of the tumor's progression. If coincident TD is not present, it is likely that the unaffected testicular parenchyma will continue to function and con-

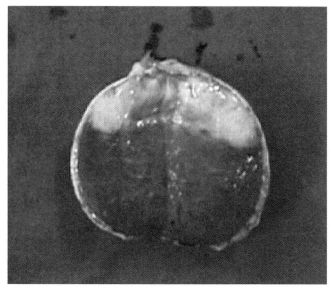

Figure 30-2 Gross appearance of a benign testicular seminoma in a stallion. In this example the tumor is relatively large, occupying approximately one third of the total mass of the testicle. In spite of the relatively large size of the mass, overall testicular size was small due to associated testicular degeneration.

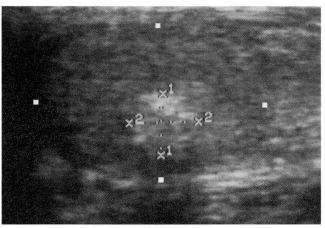

Figure 30-3 Ultrasonographic image of a testicular neoplasm in a stallion. The tumor is hyperechoic and heterogeneous (demarcated by the ultrasound calipers [*1* and *2*]) relative to the surrounding testicular parenchyma (*solid white squares*).

tribute sperm to the ejaculate. If a tumor is aggressive and is growing rapidly in size, orchiectomy can be considered. However, even locally invasive testicular tumors usually do not metastasize. So again, it may be possible to do nothing other than monitor the neoplasia. In theory, histologic evaluation of an ultrasonographically guided testicular biopsy sample can aid in the decision as to whether or not to remove the testicle. In practice, the additional information gained from a biopsy sample may not be worth the risk of damage to the testicle that may be incurred during procurement of the sample. In humans, testis-sparing surgery for removal of benign testicular tumors has been described.[28] Cryosurgery has been used in one horse in this author's clinic with a benign testicular tumor. The cryosurgery was intended to halt the growth of the tumor and prevent further pressure necrosis and degeneration of the surrounding testicular parenchyma. Unfortunately, regrowth of the tumor continued in spite of the procedure.

Keep in mind that malignant testicular tumors have been reported in equids.[29-32] In particular, seminomas in the stallion may have a greater tendency to metastasize than do seminomas in other species.[2] Should the decision be made to leave an affected testicle in place, this unlikely possibility should be discussed with the animal's owners.

ORCHITIS

Orchitis, or inflammation of the testis, is a rare cause of testicular enlargement in the stallion. Orchitis can arise secondarily to trauma, ascending or descending infection, parasites, or autoimmune disease.[33] The affected testicle is typically enlarged, hot, and painful. Systemic signs such as fever, leukocytosis, and hyperfibrinogenemia may also be present. If semen is collected and evaluated, large numbers of white blood cells are typically found and semen quality is often poor. Cultures of ejaculated semen may aid in identification of the causative organism in cases of infectious orchitis. In stallions the ultrasonographic appearance of an affected testicle appears to be similar to what has been described in humans.[34] The affected testis may be hypoechoic with respect to the unaffected testis. The decrease in echogenicity may involve the entire testicular parenchyma uniformly, or it may be seen isolated to focal areas within the parenchyma. Hydrocele, epididymitis, and thickening of the scrotal skin also may be present.[35]

Bilateral orchitis is associated with a guarded prognosis for future fertility[33] because, in severe cases, the resultant inflammation and increases in local temperature can result in fibrosis and degeneration of the testicular parenchyma. However, if one testicle is unaffected by the problem, the chances for return to normal fertility are greatly improved. If orchitis is suspected and the desire is to salvage the affected testis (testes), treatment should be initiated as soon as possible. Systemic antibiotics, ideally based on culture and sensitivity of the causative organism, should be included. In addition, antiinflammatory drugs and cold hydrotherapy should be included in the treatment plan. Alternatively, if the opposite testicle is normal, unilateral orchiectomy can be performed. After resolution of the inflammatory process, the unaffected testicle should return to its prior level of function and fertility may be restored.

TESTICULAR ABSCESS

Testicular abscesses can be the result of a penetrating wound through the scrotum and testicle, a testicular biopsy, a progression of orchitis, a descending infection from the bloodstream, or a descending infection from peritonitis (Figure 30-4). Stallions typically present as

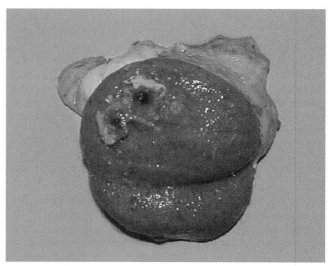

Figure 30-4 Gross appearance of a testicular abscess in a stallion. This abscess resulted from a penetrating wound. A small hematoma is present at the center of the lesion.

febrile with a unilaterally enlarged, warm, painful testicle. Evidence of a previous wound or trauma to the scrotum may be found. The abscess usually can be visualized ultrasonographically as a well-defined pocket of purulent debris within the surrounding parenchyma. Fibrin tags and adhesions may be visible around the testicle, and hydrocele may be present.

Because of the risk of possible rupture of the abscess with subsequent pyocele and possibly peritonitis, unilateral orchiectomy, together with systemic antibiotics and nonsteroidal antiinflammatory drugs, should be considered. Alternatively, if the testis is to be spared, aggressive medical treatment with careful monitoring can be started. Systemic antibiotics and nonsteroidal antiinflammatory drugs should be started. If available, culture of an ejaculate may help to identify the causative organism. An ultrasonographically guided aspiration of the abscess could be considered to obtain a sample for culture and sensitivity analysis; however, this procedure typically is not recommended because it may lead to spread of the infection and/or rupture of the abscess. The use of systemic therapy in the absence of orchiectomy may not be highly efficacious because, without establishing drainage of the abscess, pharmaceutical agents may have difficulty gaining access to the abscess cavity.

Any disease process that causes pyrexia or insulates the testicle can be expected to cause at least a temporary decrease in semen quality. However, if the contralateral testicle is normal, removal of the abscessed testicle or successful medical treatment of the abscess usually allows the contralateral testicle to return to normal function over time. If orchiectomy is not performed, the prognosis for future function of the abscessed testicle will depend on the size of the abscess and the extent of resulting fibrous tissue formation and pressure necrosis of the surrounding testicular parenchyma. Larger abscesses with extensive fibrous tissue will decrease the likelihood that the affected testis will return to normal function.

TESTICULAR HEMATOMA

Testicular trauma is the most common cause of testicular hematomas in the stallion. Small hematomas also may develop following testicular biopsy.[36] Hematomas can form within the testicular parenchyma or on the surface of the testicle. Although small intratesticular hematomas may not result in noticeable scrotal enlargement, usually in the acute stages of hematoma formation the affected testis does become enlarged, warm, and painful. A diagnosis of testicular hematoma often can be made ultrasonographically. Acutely, hematomas appear very similar to a fresh corpus hemorrhagicum in the mare ovary. As the hematoma organizes, its ultrasonographic appearance becomes more echogenic, eventually appearing hyperechoic relative to the surrounding testicle. Fibrin tags and adhesions may also form in the affected area.

Prognosis for future fertility of the affected testicle depends on the size of the hematoma and the degree of fibrous tissue formation. Small hematomas can be expected to cause only local changes in spermatogenesis, leaving the majority of the testicular parenchyma unaffected or only transiently affected by the temporary increase in temperature. Larger hematomas typically cause more severe effects on fertility. The degree of loss of testicular parenchyma will depend on the amount of pressure necrosis and fibrous tissue formation.

If the hematoma is contained, antiinflammatory drugs, cold hydrotherapy, and stall rest may be the only treatments required. Once the hematoma condenses and the testicular temperature returns to normal, any undamaged testicular parenchyma should once again be able to contribute sperm to the ejaculate. In cases of extremely large hematomas where bleeding is not contained, unilateral orchiectomy may be considered. However, this is rarely indicated.

TESTICULAR CYSTS

Testicular cysts in stallions are uncommon but have been reported as incidental findings noticed during testicular ultrasonography.[34] There have been no reports of testicular cysts having a negative impact on fertility.

TESTICULAR DEGENERATION

Background and Pathogenesis

TD is a common cause of acquired and often progressive infertility in stallions.[37,38] It is loosely defined by a common set of clinical findings, including decreasing fertility and testicular size and declining semen quality. TD can be subdivided in two ways: TD arising from a known cause and idiopathic TD (ITD).

Known causes of TD include, for example, trauma; exposure of the testis to heat, cold, radiation, specific toxins, or ischemia; certain nutritional deficiencies; administration of exogenous androgens; infection; autoimmune disease; sperm outflow obstructions; and neoplasia.[2,39-41] In these cases the length and the severity of the causative insult determine the extent of TD. If the testis is only mildly affected, some areas may recover once the insult is removed. Even if the testis is severely affected, TD generally does not progress once the inciting cause is removed.

On the other hand, and as its name implies, ITD has no known underlying cause.[42,43] ITD is most often seen in middle-aged or older stallions (senile or age-related TD) but also can affect much younger animals.[43] Regardless of the age of onset, ITD is typically progressive and results in a steady decline in fertility, sometimes ending in sterility. It is possible that the different forms of TD actually constitute a group of heterogeneous disorders that all lead to a common end point.[40,41,44]

TD, whether idiopathic or otherwise, can be focal or diffuse and can affect one or both testes (Figure 30-5).[38] Focal and/or unilateral TD often is associated with some sort of traumatic insult, whereas ITD more commonly uniformly affects both testes. Similarly, TD arising from increases in scrotal temperature, toxins, or nutritional deficiencies most often is bilateral. The pathogenesis of each of these conditions varies, and only the pathogenesis of ITD (the most common form of TD) will be discussed further in this chapter.

There is limited information available on the pathogenesis of ITD in the stallion. Several investigators have studied endocrine changes in aging, subfertile stallions,[45-48] many of which were probably affected by ITD. These and other studies all suggest that the testis, rather than the hypothalamus or pituitary, is the primary problem in cases of idiopathic stallion infertility.[49]

Endocrine values in subfertile stallions can vary widely. Because of this variability, hormone profiles by themselves often are of limited use in making a diagnosis of ITD. However, it has been suggested that low plasma estrogens in the presence of high plasma FSH is a reasonable indicator of low fertility and possibly TD.[46]

Researchers have begun to examine components of testicular steroidogenic signaling pathways in an attempt to determine the testicular defect that is responsible for ITD. In the stallion, the number of LH receptors (LH-R) on membrane preparations from subfertile stallion testicles is similar to the number found in normal, fertile controls.[50] The defect in the testis therefore may reside downstream of the LH-R, possibly in the steroidogenic pathway itself.[49] In addition, it has been shown that a decline in testicular inhibin concentrations is the first observed change in testicular steroid levels in subfertile stallions. This suggests that, in cases of idiopathic infertility, the primary defect resides in the Sertoli cell rather than in the Leydig cell.[48] Regardless of the primary cell type that is involved, these studies supply further evidence to support the hypothesis that the primary cause of ITD resides at the level of the testis, rather than in the hypothalamus or pituitary.

Some differences in testicular gene expression have been identified between normal, fertile stallions and stallions affected with severe ITD. However, the differentially expressed genes vary from individual to individual, thus adding further weight to the argument that what we currently call ITD comprises a heterogeneous group of problems.[51]

Blanchard and Johnson[52] reported increased germ cell degeneration rates in stallions producing low sperm

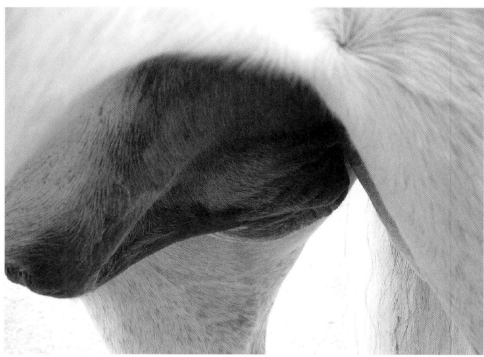

Figure 30-5 Clinical appearance of unilateral testicular degeneration in a stallion. The left testicle is remarkably small and palpably soft. In the past, both of this stallion's testicles had been of normal size. The cause of the degeneration in this case was unknown.

numbers. The germ cell loss was especially evident during early meiosis and spermiogenesis. In addition, a lower germ cell:Sertoli cell ratio was reported in these stallions. In general, earlier stage germ cells (e.g., spermatogonia) appear to be more resistant to degenerative changes. Thus, if the inciting cause of TD can be identified and removed, these remaining germ cells may have the ability to repopulate the testis with normal spermatogenesis. However, in cases of ITD in which no inciting cause can be identified, the disease is typically progressive.

History

An accurate history is critical to making a diagnosis of TD. Clinically and histologically, TD may be indistinguishable from testicular hypoplasia. Because TD is an acquired condition, whereas testicular hypoplasia is congenital, a firm diagnosis of TD can be made only if the stallion has a history of declining reproductive efficiency and/or declining testicular size. As such, information on the stallion's past book sizes, seasonal pregnancy rates, and average numbers of heat cycles per pregnancy is very important. Serial measurements of testicular size also are helpful. It should be kept in mind that many animals with testicular hypoplasia often are affected by degeneration as well.[38]

Information on a possible cause for TD also may be found in the history. For example, the history may include an incident of trauma to the testicle, a history of recent illness associated with fever, administration of anabolic steroids, or administration of other potentially damaging substances. In these cases the onset of infertility is generally sudden and closely associated with the cause. If an inciting cause can be identified and removed, the prognosis for future fertility is often better than for cases of true ITD.

If a stallion presents with a history of declining fertility over time, ITD should be suspected. This is particularly true in older animals. Although classic ITD is considered to be a slowly progressive problem, it is surprising how many stallions present for what is perceived to be an acute onset of infertility or subfertility.

Clinical Signs and Diagnosis

For cases in which TD results from a known, finite cause (such as an increase in scrotal temperature secondary to fever or trauma to the scrotum), a sudden decline in sperm numbers and semen quality and sometimes even azoospermia may be seen within the first 2 weeks after the insult. If the inciting factor is removed, semen quality should improve gradually over the next 2 months. In severe cases it may take up to 5 months for complete recovery and return to normal sperm production.[37]

Cases of ITD generally present with a range of clinical signs. Mild cases of ITD may not be associated with any noticeable change in testicular character. Studies on germ cell loss rates in stallions indicate that ITD can be present before any clinically significant decrease in testicular size can be appreciated.[52] As such, early signs of ITD may only be noticed if semen quality is being frequently and carefully monitored. A gradual decline in overall semen quality (including a decline in total sperm numbers and/or declines in the percentages of motile and morphologically normal sperm) may be the only clinical signs early in the disease. As the disease progresses, clinical signs become more apparent and include decreasing testicular size, palpable softening of the testicular parenchyma, decreasing sperm numbers, low daily sperm output (DSO) per milliliter of testis, the appearance of increasing numbers of immature round spermatogenic cells and/or multinucleate giant cells in the ejaculate, and an overall decline in semen quality.[2,38,42,53] In advanced cases, stallions may become azoospermic. Because the size of the epididymis usually does not change in cases of ITD, the epididymis may seem to be disproportionately large with respect to testicular size.[37] If a stallion's fertility is not regularly monitored, some cases of ITD may present for what is perceived to be an acute onset of subfertility or infertility. In fact, in many of these cases the problem was more likely progressive over time but went unnoticed until it had become a severe problem. In severe, end-stage ITD the testicles may become overly firm.[54]

In stallions that can be followed over time it is a good idea to measure total scrotal width, DSO, and testicular volume at least once annually. Any trends suggestive of ITD then can be identified early (e.g., decreasing testicular size/volume, declining semen quality, declining sperm numbers). ITD might be suspected if a stallion is producing low sperm numbers for his testicular volume.[55] In addition, DSO per milliliter of testis can be calculated by dividing the total number of sperm in the ejaculate at DSO by the total testicular volume.[53] Low DSO per milliliter of testis, together with a low percentage of morphologically normal sperm in the ejaculate, have been recommended as good indicators of the possible presence of TD.[53]

Another hallmark of TD (whether it results from a known cause or is idiopathic) is the appearance of immature spermatogenic cells (round cells) in the ejaculate. In an unstained semen sample, these cells can sometimes be confused with white blood cells. However, spermatogenic cells often vary in size because different stages of spermatogenic cells can appear in a single ejaculate. White blood cells are typically much more homogeneous. A simple Diff-Quik stain can quickly identify neutrophils and lymphocytes and so aid in the identification of spermatogenic cells. Multinucleated giant cells also may be present.[2,38] It should be kept in mind that low numbers of immature spermatogenic cells may be found in the ejaculates of normal stallions.[56] However, in normal stallions, other signs of abnormal spermatogenesis (small testicular size, poor semen quality, low sperm numbers, etc.) should not be found.

Because of the variation in plasma hormone levels seen in normal and subfertile stallions, circulating hormone levels may not be a good predictor of mild to moderate TD.[52] In severe cases, elevated follicle-stimulating hormone (FSH) and luteinizing hormone (LH), as well as low plasma estradiol, are consistent with a diagnosis of TD.

Histopathologic evaluation of affected testes reveals a common group of spermatogenic abnormalities, including cytoplasmic vacuolization and a loss of the normal architecture of the seminiferous epithelium.[2] The diameter of the seminiferous tubules may be decreased, and immature spermatogenic cells may be shed into the lumen of the seminiferous tubule. In more severe cases, these immature (or "round") spermatogenic cells may appear in the ejaculate in increasing numbers, as described above. As TD progresses, there is an increased loss of germ cells from the seminiferous tubule (Figure 30-6). In the most extreme cases, fibrous tissue may be present and tubules can become almost devoid of spermatogenic cells and may be left with only Sertoli cells and few spermatogonia. Fibrosis and calcification of the testicular parenchyma also may be seen.[57] It should be kept

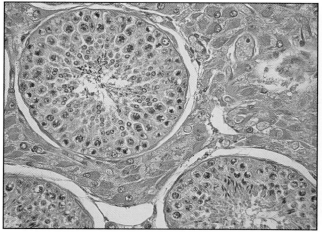 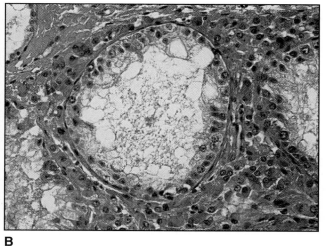

A   **B**

Figure 30-6 Histopathologic appearance of normal testicular parenchyma from a fertile stallion (**A**) and severe degeneration in a stallion affected with bilateral ITD (**B**). In the normal stallion, note that the tubules are full of germ cells in organized associations with one another and at varying stages of development. Meiotic and postmeiotic stages can be seen. Sperm are present in the lumen. In contrast, the seminiferous tubule of the stallion affected with severe ITD is relatively empty, and the normal architecture of the seminiferous epithelium is lost. The only apparent cells within the tubule are Sertoli cells and perhaps some remaining spermatogonia adjacent to the basement membrane. Many of the cells are vacuolated. The tubule is devoid of meiotic and postmeiotic germ cells.

in mind that even normal testes have some focal areas of abnormal spermatogenesis. Thus the percentage of the testicular parenchyma that is affected, as well as the severity of the histologic lesions, should be taken into account before a diagnosis of TD is made.

Because histopathologic findings can help to define TD (and testicular hypoplasia), evaluation of a testicular biopsy sample does provide definitive evidence of these conditions. However, in practice, testicular biopsy is rarely indicated. Once the clinician has obtained an adequate history and has performed a complete physical and reproductive examination, a diagnosis of TD can usually be made with some confidence and a biopsy sample is not necessary. In addition, there is some concern that a single biopsy sample may not be representative of the condition of the entire testis and thus may not be of significant prognostic value. If a biopsy sample is to be taken, the testes should be examined ultrasonographically before obtaining the biopsy.[34] The ultrasonographic appearance of the parenchyma can help the clinician to choose a representative site for sampling. Several reports have indicated that obtaining testicular biopsy samples in the stallion can be done safely and with minimal permanent damage to the remaining testicular parenchyma.[36,58] However, many of these studies were performed on normal stallions, and thus the risk to an already compromised testicle (e.g., a degenerating testicle) is more difficult to ascertain. Clinicians must carefully weigh the diagnostic benefits of obtaining a biopsy sample against the risk of damaging some portion of an already marginally functional testicular parenchyma.

Treatment

There is no known, proven successful treatment for TD. If the cause of the degeneration is known (e.g., fever, toxin), successful treatment of or removal of the inciting cause should at least prevent further progression of the disease. If the degeneration is not severe and if the inciting cause is removed, the testicle may at least partially, and sometimes fully, recover depending on the degree of damage sustained.

In cases of unilateral TD, some have recommended removal of the affected testis. The reasoning behind this recommendation is that the damaged testicular tissue could result in the production of antisperm antibodies[59] that might adversely affect sperm produced by the normal testis. In addition, removal of one testis often results in hypertrophy of the remaining testis and a resultant increase in sperm numbers. The practice of unilateral castration is debatable, however, because many stallions with unilateral TD in which the affected testicle is not removed have acceptable fertility.[37]

There are some reports of the successful use of gonadotropin-releasing hormone (GnRH) therapy as a treatment for infertility in stallions.[60,61] However, these successes have not been duplicated in controlled studies.[42,62,63] GnRH therapy has been highly successful in treating men with hypogonadotropic hypogonadism; however, this condition has not been clearly documented in stallions. As such, the use of GnRH implants or pulsatile administration of GnRH as a treatment for stallion infertility in general or ITD specifically is controversial. If this therapy is to be attempted, it has been suggested that treatment must start before the testis has reached a severe state of degeneration.[64]

Because there is no proven treatment for TD per se, the basis of dealing with this problem centers on stallion management. The veterinarian first should determine the number of progressively motile, morphologically normal sperm that the stallion is capable of producing on a regular basis. The stallion's mare book then should be adjusted accordingly to ensure that the stallion is not overused. If a stallion with low or marginal sperm numbers is required to breed daily, it is not uncommon for the animal's sperm numbers to drop below what would be required for a minimum insemination dose. Limiting the animal's book so that he has one or more days of sexual rest between each ejaculate often can help boost sperm numbers and improve pregnancy rates in mares. If possible, the semen quality of each ejaculate should be monitored to be certain that each mare is receiving a minimum insemination dose. Addition of an extender to the ejaculate may help improve longevity of sperm motility in some cases.

Semen from stallions with severe TD should be handled with particular care. Mares should be inseminated as quickly as possible after semen collection. Semen should be carefully evaluated as to its suitability for cooled transport. However, in many cases of moderate to severe TD, sperm longevity of motility is poorly maintained and pregnancy rates may be significantly reduced in mares bred with cooled semen. If this is the case, it may be prudent to discontinue the use of shipped semen and only breed mares on site with fresh, extended semen or by natural cover.

More intensive mare management also can be used to improve pregnancy rates. By breeding mares very close to the time of ovulation, the veterinarian can minimize the requirements for sperm longevity.

Summary

If a cause for TD can be identified, it should be treated or eliminated. In these cases, depending on the degree of testicular damage, testicular function should improve and possibly return to normal over a period of months.

If a cause for the TD is not known, then by definition the case should be classified as ITD. It should be kept in mind that this is a catch-all phrase and that it is possible and even likely that stallions diagnosed with ITD probably represent a very heterogeneous group. Changes in plasma hormone levels, particularly during the early stages of ITD, can be variable. In addition, no consistent differences in gene expression have been identified in normal versus ITD testes. As such, some of the most reliable signs of ITD can be identified as part of the routine breeding soundness examination. These include small, soft testes; poor semen quality; low numbers of sperm for testicular size; and the presence of immature germ cells in the ejaculate. Unfortunately, by the time changes in testicular size are noticed, the damage to the testes is already significant. Thus valuable animals should be monitored carefully with regular semen evaluations and testicular measurements to try to identify subtle changes in semen quality and sperm numbers over time. Currently there is no known successful treatment for ITD. If caught early, and if breed registries permit, semen can be frozen in anticipation of a gradual decline in the stallion's fertility over time. Stallions diagnosed with ITD should be managed intensely to maximize fertility in the face of progressively declining semen quality.

References

1. Johnson BD, Klingborg DJ, Heitman JM et al: A horse with one kidney, partially obstructed ureter, and contralateral urogenital anomalies. J Am Vet Med Assoc 1976; 169:217-219.
2. McEntee K: Reproductive Pathology of Domestic Mammals, San Diego, Academic Press, 1990.
3. Santschi EM, Juzwiak JS, Slone DE: Monorchidism in three colts. J Am Vet Med Assoc 1989; 194:265-266.
4. Parks AH, Scott EA, Cox JE et al: Monorchidism in the horse. Equine Vet J 1989; 21:215-217.
5. Foster AEC: Polyorchidism. Vet Rec 1952; 64:158.
6. Earnshaw RE: Polyorchidism. Can J Comp Med Vet Sci 1959; 23:66.
7. Wright JG: The inguinal canal and its relationship to health and disease. Part 2. The surgery of the inguinal canal in animals. Vet Rec 1963; 75:1352-1367.
8. Stickle RL, Fessler JF: Retrospective study of 350 cases of equine cryptorchidism. J Am Vet Med Assoc 1978; 172:343-346.
9. Cox JE, Edwards GB, Neal PA: An analysis of 500 cases of equine cryptorchidism. Equine Vet J 1979; 11:113-116.
10. Roberts SJ: Veterinary Obstetrics and Genital Diseases: Theriogenology, Woodstock, Vt, published by the author, 1986.
11. Vaughen JT: Surgery of the male equine reproductive system. In Morrow D (ed): Current Therapy in Theriogenology, pp 740-756, Philadelphia, WB Saunders, 1986.
12. Threlfall WR: Cryptorchidism in the horse. Annual Meeting of the Society for Theriogenology, pp 158-161, 1991.
13. Cox JE: Testosterone concentrations in normal and cryptorchid horses: response to human chorionic gonadotropin. Anim Reprod Sci 1989; 18:43-50.
14. Silberzahn P, Pouret EJ-M, Zwain I: Androgen and oestrogen response to a single injection of hCG in cryptorchid horses. Equine Vet J 1989; 21:126-129.
15. Jann HW, Rains JR: Diagnostic ultrasonography for evaluation of cryptorchidism in horses. J Am Vet Med Assoc 1990; 196:297-300.
16. Hunt RJ, Hay W, Collatos C et al: Testicular seminoma associated with torsion of the spermatic cord in two cryptorchid stallions. J Am Vet Med Assoc 1990; 197:1484-1486.
17. Braun WF: Physical examination and genital diseases of the stallion. In Morrow D (ed): Current Therapy in Theriogenology, pp 646-651, Philadelphia, WB Saunders, 1986.
18. Kenney RM: Clinical fertility evaluation of the stallion. Annual Meeting of the American Association of Equine Practitioners, p 336, 1975.
19. Palmer JM: The undescended testicle. Endocrinol Metab Clin North Am 1991; 20:231-240.
20. Rozanski TA, Bloom DA: The undescended testis: theory and management. Urol Clin North Am 1995; 22:107-118.
21. Pozor MA, McDonnell S: Color Doppler ultrasound evaluation of testicular blood flow in stallions. Theriogenology 2004; 61:799-810.
22. Turner RM: Ultrasonography of the genital tract of the stallion. In Reef VB (ed): Equine Diagnostic Ultrasound, pp 446-479, Philadelphia, WB Saunders, 1998.
23. Threlfall WR, Carleton CL, Robertson J et al: Recurrent torsion of the spermatic cord and scrotal testis in a stallion. J Am Vet Med Assoc 1990; 196:1641-1643.
24. Moulton JE: Tumors of the genital system. In Moulton JE (ed): Tumors in Domestic Animals, p 309, Berkeley, Calif, Davis Press, 1978.
25. Ladd PW: The male genital system. In Jubb KVF, Kennedy PC, Palmer N (eds): Pathology of the Domestic Animals, 3rd edition, pp 409-459, New York, Academic Press, 1985.
26. Caron JP, Barber SM, Bailey JV: Equine testicular neoplasia. Comp Contin Educ Pract Vet 1985; 7:53-59.
27. Cullen JM, Whiteside J, Umstead JA et al: A mixed germ cell-sex cord-stromal neoplasm of the testis in a stallion. Vet Pathol 1987; 24:575-577.
28. Rushton HG, Belman AB: Testis-sparing surgery for benign lesions of the prepubertal testis. Urol Clin North Am 1993; 20:27-37.
29. Becht JL, Thacker HL, Page EH: Malignant seminoma in a stallion. J Am Vet Med Assoc 1979; 175:292-293.
30. Trigo FJ, Miller RA, Torbeck RL: Metastatic equine seminoma: report of two cases. Vet Pathol 1984; 21:259-260.
31. Duncan RB: Malignant Sertoli cell tumour in a horse. Equine Vet J 1998; 30:355-357.
32. Pandolfi F, Roperto F: Seminoma with multiple metastases in a zebra (Equus zebra) X mare (Equus caballus). Equine Vet J 1983; 15:70-72.
33. DeVries PJ: Diseases of the testes, penis and related structures. In McKinnon AO, Voss JS (eds): Equine Reproduction, pp 878-884, Philadelphia, Lea & Febiger, 1993.
34. Turner RM: Ultrasonography of the reproductive tract of the stallion. In Reef VB (ed): Equine Diagnostic Ultrasound, Philadelphia, WB Saunders, 1998.
35. Arger PH: Scrotum. In Coleman BG (ed): Genitourinary Ultrasonography: A Text/Atlas. Tokyo, Igaku-Shoin, 1988.
36. DelVento VR, Amann RP, Trotter GW et al: Ultrasonographic and quantitative histologic assessment of sequelae to testicular biopsy in stallions. Am J Vet Res 1992; 53:2094-2101.
37. Blanchard T, Varner D: Testicular degeneration. In McKinnon AO, Voss JS (eds): Equine Reproduction, pp 855-860, Philadelphia, Lea & Febiger, 1993.
38. Watson ED, Clarke CJ, Else RW et al: Testicular degeneration in 3 stallions. Equine Vet J 1994; 26:507-510.
39. Freidman R, Scott M, Heath SE et al: The effects of increased testicular temperature on spermatogenesis in the stallion. J Reprod Fertil Suppl 1991; 44:127-134.
40. Blanchard T, Jorgensen JB, Varner DD et al: Clinical observations on changes in concentrations of hormones in plasma of two stallions with thermally-induced testicular degeneration. J Equine Vet Sci 1996; 16:195-201.
41. Blanchard T, Varner D, Johnson L: Testicular and hormonal changes occurring in stallions with thermally-induced testicular degeneration. J Reprod Fertil Suppl 2000; 56:51-59.
42. Blanchard T, Johnson L, Roser AJ: Increased germ cell loss rates and poor semen quality in stallions with idiopathic testicular degeneration. J Equine Vet Sci 2000; 20:263-265.
43. Gehlen H, Bartmann CP, Klug E et al: Azoospermia due to testicular degeneration in a breeding stallion. J Equine Vet Sci 2001; 21:137-139.
44. Garcia MC, Ganjam VK, Blanchard TL et al: The effects of stanozolol and boldenone undecylenate on plasma testosterone and gonadotropins and on testis histology in pony stallions. Theriogenology 1987; 28:109-119.
45. Burns PJ, Douglas RH: Reproductive hormone concentrations in stallions with breeding problems: case studies. J Equine Vet Sci 1985; 5:40-42.
46. Douglas RH, Umphenour N: Endocrine abnormalities and hormonal therapy. Vet Clin North Am Equine Pract 1992; 8:237-249.

47. Roser JF: Endocrine regulation of reproductive function in fertile, subfertile and infertile stallions. Reprod Domest Anim 1995; 30:245-250.
48. Stewart BL, Roser JF: Effects of age, season, and fertility status on plasma and intratesticular immunoreactive (IR) inhibin concentrations in stallions. Domest Anim Endocrinol 1998; 15:129-139.
49. Roser JF: Endocrine basis for testicular function in the stallion. Theriogenology 1997; 48:883-892.
50. Motton DD, Roser JF: HCG binding to the testicular LH receptor is similar in fertile, subfertile, and infertile stallions. J Androl 1997; 18:411-416.
51. Turner RM, Casas-Dolz R: Differential gene expression in stallions with testicular degeneration. Theriogenology 2002; 58:421-424.
52. Blanchard TL, Johnson L: Increased germ cell degeneration and reduced germ cell:Sertoli cell ratio in stallions with low sperm production. Theriogenology 1997; 47:655-677.
53. Blanchard TL, Johnson L, Varner D et al: Low daily sperm output per ml of testis as a diagnostic criteria for testicular degeneration in stallions. J Equine Vet Sci 2001; 21:11-35.
54. Varner D, Schumacher J, Blanchard T et al: Diseases and management of breeding stallions, Goleta, Calif, American Veterinary Publications, 1991.
55. Love CC, Garcia MC, Riera FR, et al: Evaluation of measures taken by ultrasonography and caliper to estimate testicular volume and predict daily sperm output in the stallion. J Reprod Fertil Suppl 1991; 44:99-105.
56. Swerczek TW: Immature germ cells in the semen of Thoroughbred stallions. J Reprod Fertil Suppl 1975; 23:135-137.
57. Humphrey JD, Ladds PW: A quantitative histological study of changes in the bovine testis and epididymis associated with age. Res Vet Sci 1975; 19:135-141.
58. Faber NF, Roser JF: Testicular biopsy in stallions: diagnostic potential and effects on prospective fertility. J Reprod Fertil Suppl 2000; 56:31-42.
59. Zhang J, Ricketts SW, Tanner SJ: Antisperm antibodies in the semen of a stallion following testicular trauma. Equine Vet J 1990; 22:138-141.
60. Evans JW, Finely M: GnRH therapy in a stallion of low fertility. J Equine Vet Sci 1990; 10:182.
61. Shiner KA, Pickett BW, Juergens TD: Clinical approaches to diagnosis and treatment of subfertile stallions. Proceedings of the 39th Annual Convention of the American Association of Equine Practitioners, p 149, 1993.
62. Blue BJ, Pickett BW, Squires EL et al: Effect of pulsatile or continuous administration of GnRH on reproductive function of stallions. J Reprod Fertil Suppl 1991; 44:145-154.
63. Roser JF, Hughes JP: Use of GnRH in stallions with poor fertility: a review. Proceedings of the 40th Annual Convention of the American Association of Equine Practitioners, pp 23-25, 1994.
64. Brinsko SP: GnRH therapy for subfertile stallions. Vet Clin North Am Equine Pract 1996; 12:149-160.

CHAPTER 31

Testicular Biopsy

JANET F. ROSER
NATHALIE F. FABER

HISTORICAL BACKGROUND

As its name implies, *testicular biopsy* consists of the operative removal of a piece of tissue from the testis, so small as to have no deleterious effect on the gland yet large enough to include a representative group of tubules.[1] Along with a carefully performed history, physical examination, semen analyses, and appropriate assessment of endocrinologic variables, testicular biopsy can afford the clinician the opportunity for more precise diagnosis and treatment of many male infertility disorders.[2] The technique was first applied to human beings and published by Charny in 1940.[1] This open surgical technique consisted of the removal of a minute piece of tissue from the periphery of the testis through a small incision in the scrotum. No undesirable side effects were reported. Rowley et al,[3] however, reported a transient decrease in sperm concentration in humans associated with testicular biopsy. The drop was observed in 39 of 100 men studied. The decrease occurred within 10 weeks of treatment; recovery began by 10 weeks of treatment and was complete at 18 weeks after bilateral testicular biopsy. With the development of gonadotropin radioimmunoassays (RIAs) in the 1970s and the demonstration of the relationship between serum follicle-stimulating hormone (FSH) concentrations and the histologic appearance of biopsy specimens in humans, a reappraisal of the value of testicular biopsy was made.[4] At present, testicular biopsy is recommended only for those cases in which serum FSH concentrations and clinical evaluation are inconclusive.[4] Fine needle aspiration (FNA) is the most recently described technique and currently is used clinically in human medicine.[5]

In recent years, methods have been developed for direct surgical sperm sampling from either the epididymis or the testis to be used for intracytoplasmic sperm injection (ICSI).[6] The main approach, proven to be effective for the retrieval of spermatozoa from the epididymis in patients with obstructive azoospermia, is microsurgical epididymal sperm aspiration, although recently the retrieval of spermatozoa by FNA was shown to be equally effective.[6] Recovery of spermatozoa also is now performed in patients with severely deficient spermatogenesis using open testicular biopsy as well as FNA.[6] Araki et al[7] reported success with use of spermatids in ICSI from patients with total lack of normal testicular sperm. Thirty-six males diagnosed with azoospermia underwent testicular biopsy; the spermatids thereby acquired from nine of these patients were used to fertilize oocytes by ICSI. Three of the procedures resulted in pregnancy with childbirth.

In veterinary medicine, testicular biopsy was first described in 1944 by Erb et al.[8] This group of investigators performed testicular biopsy by the open method to study vitamin A deficiency in bulls. The investigators did not assess the effect of testicular biopsy on the testicle. Testicular biopsy can lead to a decrease in sperm output secondary to sperm granuloma formation or intratesticular hemorrhage and an attendant increase in intratesticular pressure. Interference with spermatogenesis can occur. which can be permanent in some cases; in others, however, seminal values return to normal if given adequate time.[9]

Later in the 1940s, Sykes et al[10] investigated the consequences of testicular biopsy by the open method in bulls. They concluded that testicular biopsy in mature bulls led to a marked decrease in seminal sperm concentration. They also observed that further biopsies were associated with an increase in the number of abnormal spermatozoa and with morphologic changes in the tubules of the testis. Roberts,[11] who used the same method of biopsy in bulls, wrote in 1953 that testicular biopsy was of little use in veterinary medicine because it induced hemorrhage, making it difficult to perform. In the same year, Byers[12] concluded that the open method of testicular biopsy in bulls was in fact a useful technique and that it did not appreciably reduce the semen quality. He also suggested that testicular biopsy might be used to evaluate a bull's ability to produce high-quality semen. Veznik,[13] also using the open method in bulls, found it reliable provided that careful surgery and homeostasis were employed. However, he also observed a drop in sperm production on approximately day 23 after the testicular biopsy procedure. Heath et al[14] used a 14-gauge needle biopsy instrument in one testicle of six bulls and reported no changes in semen quality over a 90-day period.

In rams, Stipancevic[15] reported that the open method caused surgical trauma, which also affected spermatogenic function. Lunstra and Echternkamp[16] looked at the effects of repeated testicular biopsy in the ram during pubertal development. Unilateral testicular "open method" biopsy was performed, and bilateral castration was later performed. No difference was found in testicular development between control testes and the testes subjected to open biopsy. These investigators claimed that the success of their technique was due to avoidance of hemorrhage achieved with use of blunt dissection during biopsy to minimize damage to the vascular layer of the tunica albuginea.

Joshi et al[17] demonstrated a marked transient reduction in spermatozoal counts in men after unilateral or bilateral testicular biopsy. The reduction was observed in all patients, and normal values appeared after 4 weeks. These results are in contrast with the work of Rowley et al,[18] who observed a reduction in sperm count in only 39% of human beings, with a normal sperm count reappearing at 10 weeks after the initial procedure.

In 1971, Galina,[19] using the 12-gauge Vim-Silverman split needle biopsy method, performed testicular biopsy in boars, rams, bulls, and pony stallions. Clinical and histologic parameters were studied in all four species. In the boars, detailed weekly seminal examinations were made before and after testicular biopsy. No deleterious effects were observed. Paufler and Foote[20] studied the effect of repeated testicular biopsy (open method) of the same testis three times at 4-week intervals in rabbits and found that testis size, sperm output, and sperm motility and morphology did not differ from those in the controls.

The use of testicular biopsy in the horse was first discussed by Galina.[19] Smith[21] addressed the importance of defining a more precise site for the testicular biopsy in the stallion, to avoid the main branches of the testicular artery and thus the occurrence of undesirable hematomas. He concluded that testicular biopsy in stallions should be taken from the craniolateral quarter of the testicle to avoid damaging the lateral testicular artery. Many clinicians have alluded to the complications of testicular biopsy but have not presented adequate evidence to justify this concern. Cahill[22] reported that owners of famous Kentucky stallions with infertility problems did not consider that testicular biopsy aided in the diagnosis of the problem "for obvious reasons." Other investigators have found that testicular biopsy did not lead to deleterious effects. DelVento et al[23] evaluated the effects of unilateral testicular (open method) biopsy in stallions by recording changes in testicular width, gross appearance, and echogenicity from biopsied and nonbiopsied testes at 27 days. This group concluded that the open method of biopsy does not greatly alter the process of spermatogenesis or function of the testis in stallions. Threlfall and Lopate[24] found no histologic lesions after biopsy.

Hillman et al[25] reported for the first time the use of the Biopty gun procedure for testicular biopsy in stallions. No histopathologic or seminal changes due to the testicular biopsy procedure were identified. Faber and Roser[26] also reported that the use of the Biopty instrument to obtain biopsy samples was not detrimental to testicular function or spermatogenesis in the stallion. FNA currently is used successfully in veterinary medicine in dogs, mink, and horses[27-29] and appears to be the least invasive method.

TESTICULAR BIOPSY: TECHNIQUES, ADVANTAGES AND DISADVANTAGES

Several techniques to obtain a testicular biopsy specimen have been described: standard open surgical biopsy (or incisional biopsy), needle punch biopsy, Biopty gun needle biopsy, and FNA. All techniques provide material for study, but each approach has advantages and limitations.

Incisional or Open Biopsy

Incisional biopsy is performed with the patient under general anesthesia after surgical preparation and draping of the scrotum, inguinal areas, and posterior prepuce. The testicle is pushed forward as for castration, and a skin incision 1 to 2 cm in length is made, avoiding the area over the epididymis.[30] The testicle is gently forced toward the incision, subcutaneous tissues are incised, and the tunica vaginalis is grasped with the forceps so that an opening can be made to expose the testicle. A razor blade is used to incise the tunica albuginea. A wedge-shaped piece of testicular tissue that bulges through the incision is cut free with the razor blade. The tissue is placed immediately in Bouin's fixative. The tunica albuginea and the tunica vaginalis are sutured, as well as the skin. The biopsy tissue obtained by incision is less likely to contain artifacts associated with biopsy technique than are specimens obtained by punch or aspiration biopsy. Also, the size of the specimen is under the surgeon's control.[30,31] However, early reports of use of this technique in the bull indicated that incisional biopsy induced a decrease in sperm count, an increase in the number of abnormal sperm, tubular degenerative changes, adhesions between the tunics, and an increased risk of hemorrhage for 2 weeks to 4 months.[19]

Needle Punch Biopsy

Needle punch biopsies have been performed with the 14-gauge Vim-Silverman needle, the 14-gauge Franklin modified Vim-Silverman needle, the Tru-Cut needle, and the 16-gauge Jamshidi biopsy needle–syringe combination.[19,30-33] Needle punch biopsy may be done with the stallion under heavy sedation but in some cases may require the use of general anesthesia.[31] A small incision is made in the skin to facilitate introduction of the needle. The biopsy needle is manipulated in the conventional manner and is directed toward the center of the testicle as the cutting prongs are advanced. No sutures are required.[30,31]

The needle punch biopsy technique carries the risk of trauma to the inner portion of the testis, with the potential for significant permanent damage. Another disadvantage is that a specimen of size and quality sufficient for histologic examination is not obtained. Nevertheless, further studies comparing needle biopsies with standard surgical biopsies have indicated the presence of a high correlation between percutaneous and open surgical biopsy specimen analysis.[2] Kessaris et al[34] described a 95% correlation between percutaneous needle and open biopsy technique in 24 testes (19 patients) in whom both techniques were applied.

Spring-Loaded Split Needle Biopty Instrument

The Biopty gun (Bard Inc., Covington, GA) needle biopsy procedure has increased the ability of the clinician to obtain a consistently good core of tissue relatively painlessly without adjunctive anesthesia in an office setting. This instrument, with its spring trigger mechanism, has been widely used by urologists for transrectal prostate biopsy.[35]

Rajfer and Binder[36] described the use of this method for testicular biopsy in humans. Their procedure begins with infiltration of approximately 1 ml of lidocaine into the skin of the hemiscrotum. With one hand bracing the testis, the operator uses the tip of the biopsy needle (already loaded into the Biopty gun) to puncture the skin and then guides the needle to lie adjacent to the tunica albuginea of the testis, at which point the gun is fired. The needle is removed, and the tissue fragment characteristic of testicular parenchyma is placed into Bouin's solution. More than one pass of the needle may be made to obtain adequate tissue. The disposable 18-gauge needle is discarded after use. The depth of the biopsy with the standard Biopty gun is 22 mm. This method has been shown to be a cost-effective, simple, and reliable means of testicular biopsy in men and has replaced the traditional method of obtaining testicular tissue for histologic diagnosis.[36] Sufficient numbers of tubules for histopathologic diagnosis can be reliably obtained.[37,38]

The use of the Biopty gun for testicular biopsy in veterinary medicine was first reported by Hillman et al.[25] Testicular biopsy was performed in a total of 14 stallions. Seven of them were castrated 7 days after testicular biopsy, and no histopathologic changes due to the biopsy procedure were identified. Additionally, in 13 of the 14 post-castration testicular samples that were examined, the morphologic characteristics were similar to those of the biopsy sample. The other seven stallions had semen analysis performed pre- and post-testicular biopsy, and there was no significant decrease in any of the parameters measured.

A more recent report by Faber and Roser[26] describes in further detail the use of the Biopty instrument and its aftereffects in a group of 7 fertile stallions. The Biopty instrument was used to collect three samples from the left testis of each stallion. Each stallion was secured in a stanchion and sedated with detomidine HCL (Dormosedan; Norden/Smith Kline Animal Health, Exton, PA) intravenously (IV) at 20 to 40 µg/kg of body weight and butorphanol tartrate (Torbugesic; Fort Dodge, IA) IV at 0.1 mg/kg of body weight. The scrotum was aseptically prepared with iodine scrub and blocked with approximately 1 ml of a 2% lidocaine HCl solution (Abbott Laboratories, North Chicago, IL). A small incision was made through the scrotum in the center of the craniolateral quarter of the left testis. With the testis held down in the scrotum, a sterile 14-gauge split needle coupled to a spring-loaded Biopty instrument was placed through the incision against the tunica vaginalis (Figures 31-1 and 31-2). The Biopty instrument was subsequently fired into the testicular parenchyma and then removed. Two subsequent samples where collected through the same incision but at slightly different angles.

For this study, the testicular biopsy samples were processed as follows: Two punch specimens were individually placed in a 1.2-ml solution of phosphate-buffered saline (PBS), snap frozen immediately in liquid nitrogen, and stored at −70°C until processed for estradiol-17β, testosterone, and inhibin by RIA. Testicular extracts were analyzed for protein concentrations by the Bradford method (Bio-Rad). The third sample was placed in Bouin's solution for 6 hours, transferred to 50% alcohol, and then submitted to the University of California, Davis Veterinary Medical Teaching Hospital histopathology laboratory for preparation, hematoxylin and eosin (H&E) staining, and evaluation.

Semen was collected twice 1 hour apart before the biopsy and once a month after the biopsy for 9 consecutive months. The stallions were mated before and after the biopsy to 10 mares over two cycles. Six of the 7 stallions had slight edema, mainly around the site of injection, for 1 to 5 days after the biopsy procedure. The mean number of seminiferous tubules observed per biopsy specimen was 79 (Figure 31-3). Active spermatogenesis was evident in all histologic samples. The mean number of progressively motile morphologically normal sperm was not significantly different before and after the biopsy procedure. Pregnancy rates per estrous cycle before (50 ± 6%) and after (63 ± 9%) testicular biopsy were not significantly different. Total scrotal width was not different before and after biopsy. Testicular tissue hormone content was measured successfully by RIA, and plasma hormone concentrations fluctuated within normal ranges after biopsy in the expected seasonal patterns.

Testicular Fine Needle Aspiration

Testicular FNA also has been extensively described in both human and veterinary medicine.[4,28,29,38-42] This technique retrieves only cells, but the specimen acquired is sufficient to differentiate inflammatory diseases from noninflammatory diseases and also may allow diagnosis of neoplasia. Spermatogenic activity can be assessed by comparing the number of germinal cells with the number of Sertoli cells.[31,41]

Aspiration biopsy of the testis can be performed using a 22- or 23-gauge needle and a 5-ml syringe. The horse is sedated, and the scrotal skin is aseptically prepared with iodine scrub. The testicle is firmly immobilized, the needle is introduced into the substance of the testicle, and the syringe plunger is retracted as two or three passes are made into the testicle (see Figure 31-3). After careful release of the syringe plunger, the needle is withdrawn, and material obtained is ejected onto glass slides, air dried, smeared, and stained (Figure 31-4).[2,4,29-31] The smear is examined for Leydig cells, germ cells, and Sertoli cells under 1000× to 2000× magnification using light microscopy (Figure 31-5).

FNA has proved to be a simple, rapid, less painful, minimally invasive diagnostic procedure and an inexpensive method for evaluating the status of several organs.[43] Although no serious adverse effects of FNA have been described,[39] the method has not gained widespread acceptance in the evaluation of the infertile male, for numerous reasons. Many clinicians are afraid that FNA may cause severe trauma or hematoma, and experience in the field of clinical cytology is lacking among veterinarians in general. In addition, the amount of material obtained by FNA is far less than that obtained by open biopsy. Although cellular detail is excellent, FNA specimens do not provide information regarding peritubular fibrosis, the interstitial tissue, and the cellular arrangement.

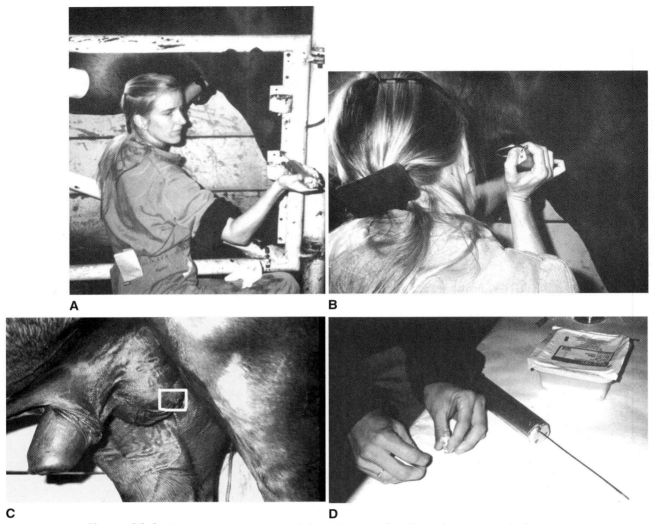

Figure 31-1   Testicular biopsy of the left testis using the Biopty instrument. **A,** Preparation; **B,** insertion; **C,** area of needle placement; **D,** storage of tissue. (Photo courtesy of
Janet F. Roser.)

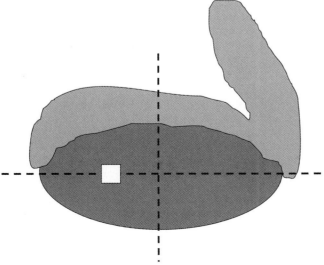

Figure 31-2   Biopsy incision in the craniolateral quarter of
the left testis.

EXAMINATION OF TESTICULAR BIOPSY SPECIMENS AND APPLICATIONS OF THE TECHNIQUE

Several available techniques allow for the evaluation of
the testicular specimen.[2] Cytologic evaluation provides a
rapid means of examining the cellular contents of the
seminiferous tubules. Histopathologic findings related to
infertility include abnormalities of tubular architecture
and those of cellular composition. Quantification of
histologic findings on testicular biopsy also may be
extremely useful. In general, the techniques use either
morphometric (tubular diameter or basement membrane
thickness) or cellular (number of cells or type of cells in
tubule) characteristics, or a combination of both.[2] Also,
extensive work has now been performed in assessing the
usefulness of DNA flow cytometry[44] and DNA image
analysis.[45] These modalities are becoming particularly relevant in the current era of sophisticated assisted reproductive technology applications, when the sensitive
detection of even minimal numbers of haploid cells in

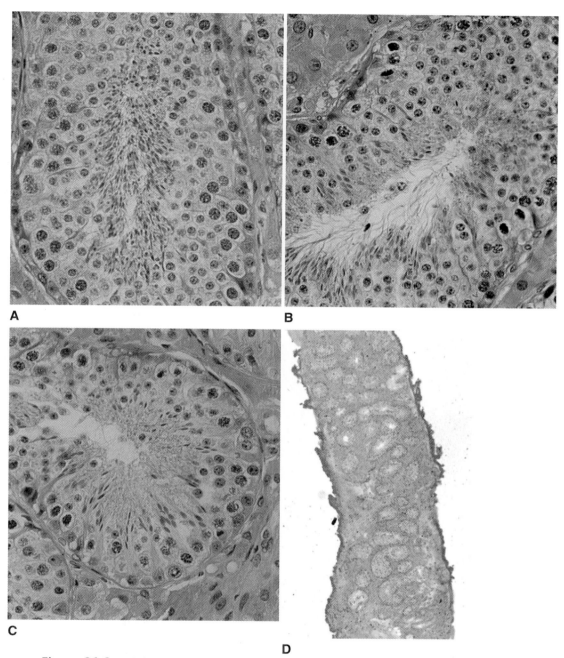

Figure 31-3   High-power (**A** to **C**) and low-power (**D**) views of histologic biopsy sections from individual stallions. Tissues sections illustrate seminiferous tubules with normal spermatogenesis. (Hematoxylin and eosin; 400×.) (Photo courtesy of Nathalie F. Faber.)

the biopsy specimen may have a great deal of significance. Immunocytochemistry studies of testicular biopsy samples have been used to evaluate spermatogenesis and Sertoli cell maturation status.[46] Molecular biology also may be applied to the analysis of testicular biopsy material. With use of Northern blot analysis, in situ hybridization, and transgenic mouse "knockout" studies, the quantitative documentation of expression of specific genes at various stages and under various abnormal states of spermatogenesis may be possible. The potential to intervene in such conditions through the developing tech-

nologies of gene therapy may someday open new avenues for the treatment of certain male infertility disorders.[2]

Another application using testicular biopsy analysis includes determination of intratesticular endocrine, paracrine, and autocrine factors. Morse et al[47] reported the testosterone concentrations in testes of normal men and the effects of testosterone propionate administration. This agent caused a decrease in testicular testosterone while producing the expected increase in plasma testosterone. Using testicular biopsy samples, Ruokonen et al[48] measured free and sulfate-conjugated neutral steroids in

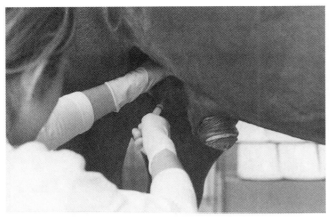

Figure 31-4 Testicular fine needle aspiration. The horse is sedated, and the scrotal skin has been aseptically prepared with iodine scrub. The testicle is firmly immobilized, and a 23-gauge needle attached to a 5-ml syringe is introduced into the parenchyma at the craniolateral quarter of the testis. The syringe plunger is retracted as two or three passes are made into the testicle. After careful release of the syringe plunger, the needle is withdrawn, and material obtained is ejected onto a glass slide, air dried, and stained with Giemsa stain. (Photo courtesy of Janet F. Roser.)

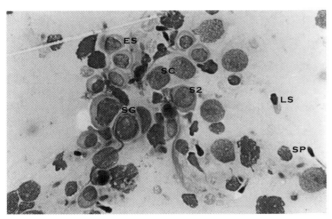

Figure 31-5 Testicular cell types by fine needle aspiration cytology (FNAC) in a horse. ES, early spermatid; LS, late spermatid; S2, secondary spermatocyte; SC, Sertoli cell; SG, spermatogonia; SP, spermatozoa. (Giemsa; 1000×.) (Photo courtesy of D.P. Leme.)

human testis tissue by gas-liquid chromatography and gas chromatography—mass spectrometry, adding more information about the role of sulfated precursors in the testicular biosynthesis of testosterone. Rodrigues-Rigau et al[49] studied the in vitro metabolism of pregnenolone in incubates of testicular tissue obtained by routine testicular biopsy in a number of infertile men. An abnormal distribution of metabolites was observed in at least 8 of the 26 patients studied. McCowen et al[50] performed testicular biopsies in 9 men with various degrees of subfertility who also had a left varicocele. Levels of testosterone and dihydrotestosterone (DHT) in the testicular tissue were measured. Although testicular tissue testosterone

and DHT levels varied greatly, levels measured from the left and the right testis were similar. The application of using testicular biopsy to measure testicular hormone concentrations has been described in the horse by Faber and Roser,[26] as presented earlier.

With the advent of assisted reproductive technology, testicular biopsy is now used therapeutically in human medicine to retrieve sperm for ICSI, with some degree of success.[5,6] Both FNA and needle punch biopsy methods are efficacious, but it appears that testicular open biopsy techniques constitute a more reliable method of retrieving sperm.[5] The ultimate choice of sperm retrieval method will depend not only on sperm availability but also on the physiologic consequences of the different techniques on testicular function. Whether these biopsy techniques will prove to be useful for ICSI in veterinary medicine is yet to be determined.

SUMMARY

Testicular biopsy is a promising method that, along with carefully performed history, physical examination, semen analyses, and appropriate assessment of endocrinologic variables, can afford the clinician the opportunity for more precise diagnosis and treatment of many male infertility disorders. The open surgical method was the first testicular biopsy technique described and appears to cause some deleterious effects in both humans and animals. In veterinary medicine, testicular biopsy procedures should be used with caution and discretion in conditions such as idiopathic subfertility, azoospermia, and suspected tumors because of the risk for testicular hemorrhage, inflammation, and swelling with consequent decline in spermatogenesis. At present, use of the Biopty gun is considered to be a cost-effective, simple, and reliable means of testicular biopsy, with little if any deleterious effects in the stallion on a short- or long-term basis.

Several available techniques allow for the evaluation of the testicular specimen, ranging from simple cytologic examination to the more sophisticated DNA image analysis and ICSI. The use of testicular biopsy samples to measure endocrine/paracrine/autocrine factors, along with morphologic evaluation, has proved successful in the stallion.[26]

With the advent of assisted reproductive technology, testicular biopsy is now used therapeutically in human medicine to retrieve sperm for ICSI, with some degree of success, but has yet to be tried in the stallion.

References

1. Charny CW: Testicular biopsy. JAMA 1940; 115:1429.
2. Coburn M, Kim ED, Wheeler TM: Testicular biopsy in the male infertility evaluation. In Lipshultz LI, Howards SS (eds): Infertility in the Male, New York, Churchill, pp 219-248, 1993.
3. Rowley MJ, O'Keefe KB, Heller CG: Decreases in sperm concentration due to testicular biopsy procedure in man. J Urol 1968; 101:347.
4. Mallidis C, Baker HWG: Fine needle tissue aspiration biopsy of the testis. Fertil Steril 1994; 61:367.

5. Chan PT, Schlegel PN: Diagnostic and therapeutic testis biopsy. Curr Urol Rep 2000; 1:266.

6. Safran A, Reubinoff BE, Porat-Katz et al: Assisted reproduction for the treatment of azoospermia. Hum Reprod Suppl 1998; 13(4):47.

7. Araki Y, Motoyama M, Yoshida A et al: Intracytoplasmic injection with late spermatids: a successful procedure in achieving childbirth for couples in which the male partner suffers from azoospermia due to deficient spermatogenesis. Fertil Steril 1997; 67:559.

8. Erb RE, Andrews FN, Bullard JF, Hilton JH: A technique for the simultaneous measurement of semen quality and testis histology in vitamin A studies of the dairy bull. J Dairy Sci 1994; 27:769.

9. Threlfall WR, Lopate C: Testicular biopsy. In Mckinnon AO, Voss JL (eds): Equine Reproduction, Philadelphia, Lea & Febiger, pp 943-949, 1993.

10. Sykes JF, Wrenn TR, Moore, LA et al: The effect of testis biopsy on semen characteristics of bulls. J Dairy Sci 1949; 32:327.

11. Roberts SJ: Testicular biopsy in bulls. Proceedings of the 1st World Congress on Fertility and Sterility 1953; 2:664.

12. Byers JH: The influence of testes biopsy on semen quality. J Dairy Sci 1953; 36:1165.

13. Veznik Z, Langer J: Testicular biopsy in bulls. Veti Med 1958; 31:575.

14. Heath AM, Carson RL, Purohit RC et al: Effects of testicular biopsy in clinically normal bulls. J Am Vet Med Assoc 2002; 220:507.

15. Stipancevic L: Biopsy of the testis in the ram: its application in diagnosing sterility and the effect of the operation on semen quality. Veterinarya Sarajevo 1966; 15:203.

16. Lunstra DD, Echternkamp SE: Repetitive testicular biopsy in the ram during pubertal development. Theriogenology 1988; 29:803.

17. Joshi KR, Purohit RC, Ramdeo IN: Effect of testicular biopsy on spermatozoal count. J Indian Med Assoc 1977; 69:277.

18. Rowley MJ, O'Keefe KB, Heller CG: Decreases in sperm concentration due to testicular biopsy procedure in man. J Urol 1968; 101:347.

19. Galina CS: An evaluation of testicular biopsy in farm animals. Vet Rec 1971; 88:628.

20. Paufler SK, Foote RH: Semen quality and testicular function in rabbits following repeated testicular biopsy and unilateral castration. Fertil Steril 1969; 20:618.

21. Smith JA: Biopsy and the testicular artery of the horse. Equine Vet J 1974; 6:81.

22. Cahill C: Immature spermatozoa in Thoroughbred stallions. Southwestern Vet 1975; 28:13.

23. DelVento VR, Amann RP, Trotter GW et al: Ultrasonographic and quantitative histologic assessment of sequelae to testicular biopsy in stallions. Am J Vet Res 1992; 53:2094.

24. Threlfall WR, Lopate C: Testicular biopsy. Proc Soc Theriogenol p 65, 1987.

25. Hillman RB, Casey PJ, Kennedy PC et al: Testicular biopsy in stallions. Proceedings of the 6th International Symposium on Equine Reproduction, Caxambu, MG, Brazil, p 145, 1994.

26. Faber NF, Roser JF: Testicular biopsy in stallions: diagnostic potential and effects on prospective fertility. J Reprod Fertil Suppl 2000; 56:31.

27. Sundqvist C, Toppari J, Parvinen M et al: Elimination of infertile male mink from breeding using sperm test, testicular palpation, testosterone test and fine-needle aspiration biopsy of the testis. Anim Reprod Sci 1986; 11:295.

28. Dahlbom M, Makinen A, Suominen J: Testicular fine needle aspiration cytology as a diagnostic tool in dog infertility. J Small Anim Pract 1997; 38:506.

29. Papa FO, Leme LP: Testicular fine needle aspiration cytology from a stallion with testicular degeneration after external genitalia trauma. J Equine Vet Sci 2002; 22:121.

30. Larssen RE: Testicular biopsy in the dog. Vet Clin North Am 1977; 7:747.

31. Finco DR: Biopsy of the testicle. Vet Clin North Am 1974; 4:377.

32. Netto NR: Needle method of testicular biopsy. Int Surg 1974; 59:172.

33. Carluccio A, Zedda MT, Schiaffino GM et al: Evaluations of testicular biopsy by Tru-Cut in the stallion. Vet Res Comm Suppl 2003; 27:211.

34. Kessaris DN, Wasserman P, Mellinger BC: Histopathological and cytopathological correlations of percutaneous testis biopsy and open testis biopsy in infertile man. J Urol 1995; 153:1151.

35. Marshall S: Prostatic needle biopsy: a simple technique for increasing accuracy. J Urol 1989; 142:1023.

36. Rajfer J, Binder S: Use of Biopty gun for transcutaneous testicular biopsies. J Urol 1989; 142:1021.

37. Morey AF, Deshon GE, Rozanski TA et al: Technique of Biopty gun testis needle biopsy. Urology 1993; 42:325.

38. Morey AF, Plymyer M, Rozanski TA et al: Biopty gun testis needle biopsy: a preliminary clinical experience. Br J Urol 1994; 74:366.

38. Papic Z, Katona G, Skrabalo Z: The cytology identification and quantification of testicular cell subtypes: reproducibility and relation to histologic findings in the diagnosis of male infertility. Acta Cytol 1988; 32:697.

39. Foresta C, Varotto A: Assessment of cytology by fine needle aspiration as a diagnostic parameter in the evaluation of the oligospermic subject. Fertil Steril 1992; 58:1028.

40. Gottschalk-Sabag S, Glick T, Bar-On E et al: Testicular fine needle aspiration as a diagnostic method. Fertil Steril 1993; 59:1129.

41. Leme DP, Papa FO: Cytological identification and quantification of testicular cell types using fine needle aspiration in horses. Equine Vet J 2000; 32:44.

42. Fasouliotis SJ, Safran A, Porat-Katz A et al: A high predictive value of the first testicular fine needle aspiration in patients with non-obstructive azoospermia for sperm recovery at the subsequent attempt. Hum Reprod 2002; 17:139.

43. Larkin HA: Veterinary cytology—fine needle aspiration of masses or swellings on animals. Ir Vet J 1994; 47:65.

44. Chang LS: Comparison between histopathology and DNA histogram of the testis. Proc Natl Sci Council Repub China 1991; 15:63.

45. Burger RA: Automated image analysis DNA cytometry in testicular cancer. Urol Res 1994; 22:17.

46. Bar-Shira Maymon B, Yavetz H, Schreiber L et al: Immunocytochemistry in the evaluation of spermatogenesis and Sertoli cell's maturation status. Clin Chem Lab Med 2002; 40:217.

47. Morse HC, Horike N, Rowley MJ et al: Testosterone concentrations in testes of normal men: effects of testosterone propionate administration. J Clin Endocrinol Metab 1973; 37:882.

48. Ruokonen A, Laatikainen T, Laitinen EA et al: Free and sulfate-conjugated neutral steroids in human testis tissue. Biochemistry 1972; 11:1411.

49. Rodrigues-Rigau LJ, Weiss DB, Smith KD et al: Suggestion of abnormal testicular steroidogenesis in some oligospermic men. Acta Endocrinol 1978; 87:400.

50. McCowen KD, Smith ML, Modarelli RO et al: Tissue testosterone and dihydrotestosterone from bilateral testis biopsies in males with varicocele. Fertil Steril 1979; 32:439.

CHAPTER 32

Spermatogenic Arrest (Testicular Degeneration)

ELIZABETH S. METCALF

Testicular degeneration is the most common cause of male infertility across species.[1] Because the seminiferous epithelium of the equine testis is highly susceptible to insult and injury, the resulting damage is at times reversible but is often irreversible.[2] Within the seminiferous tubules the dividing primary spermatocytes appear to be most sensitive to insult, followed in sensitivity by other differentiating germinal cells all the way to spermatids. Stem cells (type A spermatogonia), however, and Sertoli cells appear relatively resistant to injury and in many conditions will regenerate.[3] Therefore, the Sertoli-spermatic cell index can function as a useful measure of testicular degeneration.[4]

Testicular degeneration, which is acquired and potentially reversible, must be differentiated from testicular hypoplasia, which is irreversible and either congenital or, less likely, acquired.[5] Testicular degeneration can be further classified to differentiate between hypospermatogenesis (germ cell hypoplasia), which is characterized by a reduction in the number of germ cells per seminiferous tubule, and a maturation abnormality or arrest, which is manifested as a failure to complete spermatogenesis beyond a certain stage. Finally, testicular degeneration can also be associated with germ cell aplasia—a condition in which only Sertoli cells line the tubules.

CAUSES

Both intrinsic and extrinsic factors have been implicated as a cause of testicular degeneration. Intrinsic defects may exist in the germ cell or its supporting cells; this condition may perhaps have a hereditary basis. However, there are a large number of extrinsic factors that can influence spermatogenesis and cause degeneration of the seminiferous epithelium, thereby reducing fertility. These factors include (but are not limited to) temperature derangement, dietary deficiencies, vascular insults, androgenic compounds, other endocrine imbalances, heavy metals (cadmium and lead, in particular), toxins, radiation exposure, dioxin, alcohol, and infectious disease.

Thermoregulation of the testicle has received a great deal of attention with respect to testicular degeneration in the stallion. A temperature differential exists between the core body temperature and the intrascrotal testes. Thermal degeneration of the testicle occurs if temperature in the scrotum equals or exceeds core body temperature. This temperature derangement can occur in conditions of herniation, cryptorchid testicles, scrotal edema, heavy working conditions, scrotal dermatoses, and any cause of inflammation or orchitis (trauma, infectious agent, vascular disturbance) or periorchitis (secondary to peritonitis).[6]

An elevation of scrotal temperature, even as little as 2°C to 3°C, results in decreased concentration, motility, and total number of spermatozoa and an increase in morphologic abnormalities.[6] The damage is most apparent for 10 to 40 days following the insult in the stallion. Furthermore, adhesion formation following an acute episode of thermal damage can inhibit future movement of the testicles within scrotum, leading to a chronic condition.

Circulatory disturbances involving the testes, epididymides, and scrotum have also been associated with testicular degeneration. Occlusion of vessels may be caused by strongyle larvae migration, granuloma formation, vasculitis, and/or neoplasia. The formation of a varicocele may disturb the normal heat exchange mechanism of the testicle. Finally, spermatic cord torsion may damage the testicle by occluding vessels or causing an elevation of temperature secondary to inflammation.

Lastly, researchers have suspected that the development of antisperm antibodies may contribute to testicular degeneration in the stallion[7,8] as it has in other species.[9] They surmise that antisperm antibody production may be associated with many conditions that affect the testes—from obstructive disease to infection to thermal injury to physical injury (trauma, biopsy, even coitus)—and that it may be genetic. However, in the stallion, the association between antisperm antibody production and testicular degeneration appears less clear, perhaps at least in part due to the difficulty in developing an equine assay.

DIAGNOSIS

The effects of insult may not be readily apparent in semen quality. Indeed, there may be a lag time between testicular damage and changes in semen parameters. Therefore the clinical picture may range from a normal spermiogram to oligospermia to aspermia with changes in both the percentages of morphologically normal sperm and motile sperm. Although some researchers have associated testicular degeneration with the presence of a high percentage of immature germ cells in the ejaculate,[10] others caution assessment on this basis. Still, Blanchard and Johnson[11,12] reported an increased rate of germ cell loss during the phases of late meiosis and spermiogenesis in stallions with idiopathic testicular degeneration. Furthermore, they found that evidence of a low percentage of morphologically normal sperm, as well as a low percentage of progressively motile sperm, were good predictors of testicular degeneration.

The endocrine profile of stallions suffering from testicular degeneration may also show abnormalities. Motton and Roser[13] have demonstrated that although plasma luteinizing hormone (LH), follicle-stimulating hormone (FSH), estrogens (E), and testosterone (T) levels were not significantly different between subfertile and fertile stallions, LH and FSH levels tended to be higher and E, T, and inhibin levels tended to be lower in infertile versus subfertile and fertile stallions. These researchers suggest that endocrine dysfunction may actually occur at the postreceptor level in stallions with poor fertility.

On palpation this condition may appear unilateral or bilateral depending on the cause (local or general). In the early stages of degeneration, affected testes feel soft and flabby and lack turgor. A distinct wrinkling of the tunica albuginea may be felt. In later stages, testes are smaller and of firmer consistency due to a decrease in parenchyma. The epididymis may appear disproportionately large.

A testicular biopsy is necessary to differentiate between testicular degeneration and hypoplasia, especially in the young animal. In cases of degeneration, the cytology and pathology reports will likely contain evidence of cytoplasmic vacuoles, decreased thickness of the germinal epithelium, pyknosis of spermatocyte nuclei, giant cell formation, and fibrosis in cases of testicular degeneration. Further evidence of increased germ cell degeneration includes a decrease in number of the following types of cells: both A and B types of spermatogonia per testis, Sertoli cells per testis, late primary spermatocytes, round spermatids, and elongated spermatids per Sertoli cell. Certainly, a reduced germ cell:Sertoli cell ratio is associated with a low production of spermatozoa.

Finally, DNA microarray analysis of differential gene expression during spermatogenesis may aid in not only the diagnosis but also determining the etiology of subfertility and infertility.[14]

TREATMENT

In acute cases of testicular insult the removal of the inciting cause (torsion, occlusion of blood vessels, pyrexia, infection, etc.) may allow recovery and regeneration. In the acute cases, the use of antipyretic and antiinflammatory agents may prevent clinical signs. However, in idiopathic or chronic testicular degeneration it is unlikely that these agents will prove effective. It is postulated that hormonal therapy, particularly treatment with gonadotropin-releasing hormone (GnRH), may be beneficial in affected stallions that suffer from a defect in GnRH synthesis or release as long as the pituitary-testicular axis is intact. This area of treatment, however, remains controversial.

CONCLUSION

In summary, it appears that testicular degeneration is directly due to an intrinsic defect, either acquired or congenital, within the germ cells or indirectly due to a defect in or lack of supporting cells necessary for germ cell maturation and division.

References

1. Jubb KVF, Kennedy PPC, Palmer N: The male genital system. In Pathology of Domestic Animals, 3rd edition, vol 3, pp 428-432, Melbourne, Elsevier, 1985.
2. Parkinson TJ: Fertility and infertility in male animals. In Veterinary Reproduction and Obstetrics, 7th edition, pp 609-613, London, WB Saunders, 1996.
3. Johnson L, Blanchard TL, Varner DD et al: Factors affecting spermatogenesis in the stallion. Theriogenology 1997; 48(7):1199-1216.
4. Blanchard TL, Johnson L: Increased germ cell degeneration and reduced germ cell:Sertoli cell ratio in stallions with low sperm production. Theriogenology 1997; 47(3):665-677.
5. Cobern M, Kim ED, Wheeler TM: Testicular biopsy in male infertility evaluation. In Lipshultz LI, Howards SS (eds): Infertility in the Male, pp 219-248, St Louis, Mosby, 1997.
6. Friedman R, Scott M, Heath SE et al: The effects of increased testicular temperature on spermatogenesis in the stallion. J Reprod Fertil Suppl 1991; 444:127-134.
7. Zhang J, Ricketts SW, Tanner SJ: Antisperm antibodies in the semen of a stallion following testicular trauma. Equine Vet J 1990; 22:138-141.
8. Teuscher C, Kenney RM, Cummings MR, Catten M: Identification of two stallion sperm-specific proteins and their autoantibody response. Equine Vet J 1994; 26:148-151.
9. Turek PJ: Immunology and infertility. In Lipshultz LI, Howards SS (eds): Infertility in the Male, pp 305-325, St Louis, Mosby, 1997.
10. Long PL, Pickett BW, Sawyer HR et al: Identification of immature germ cells in semen of stallions. Equine Pract 1993; 15(5):29-33.
11. Blanchard TL, Johnson L: Increased germ cell loss rates and poor semen quality in stallions with idiopathic testicular degeneration. J Equine Vet Sci 2000; 20(14):362-365.
12. Blanchard TL, Johnson L, Varner DD et al: Low daily sperm output per ml of testis as a diagnostic criteria for testicular degeneration in stallions. J Equine Vet Sci 2001; 21(1):11.
13. Motton DD, Roser JF: HCG binding to the testicular LH receptor is similar in fertile, subfertile and infertile stallions. J Androl 1997; 18(4):411-416.
14. Laughlin AM, Forrest DW, Varner DD et al: DNA microarray analysis of gene expression in testicular tissue of stallions. Theriogenology 2002; 58(2-4):413-415.

CHAPTER 33

Endoscopy of the Reproductive Tract in the Stallion

AHMED TIBARY

Endoscopic or videoendoscopic examination of the reproductive tract is an important procedure for the diagnosis and treatment of some affections of the reproductive tract in stallions. This procedure is indicated with any disturbance in seminal quality, particularly hemospermia or pyospermia, in the absence of obvious lesions on the external genitalia. Endoscopy also should be considered in stallions with abnormalities of the internal accessory sex glands detected on transrectal palpation and ultrasonography.

Videoendoscopic examination of the urethra, colliculus seminalis, and bladder should be part of any workup for pyelonephritis, cystitis, cystic calculi, hematuria, hemospermia, pyospermia, urethral obstruction, urethritis, painful ejaculation, painful urination, dysuria, or unexplained infertility.[1-4] Videoendoscopy also is a valuable aid for direct access to accessory sex gland secretions for sampling or for direct instillation of drugs[3,5-8].

To perform a thorough examination, the practitioner should be familiar with the normal anatomy and appearance of the organs examined, as well as the proper choice of equipment and procedure to use.

ANATOMIC REVIEW

The anatomic structures of interest during endoscopic examination in the stallion are the urethra, the colliculus seminalis, the seminal vesicles, and the urinary bladder.

The urethra generally is subdivided anatomically into the penile urethra and the pelvic urethra. The *penile urethra* is enclosed ventrally within the corpus spongiosum penis. It ends in a urethral process that extends freely 1.5 to 3 cm within the glans penis. This area is a common site of traumatic injuries, infectious inflammation (particularly that associated with habronemiasis), and neoplasia (squamous cell carcinoma)

The *pelvic urethra* extends from the neck of the bladder to the ischiatic arch. The urethra is wider in the region of the seminal colliculus than near the bladder and ischiatic arch. The dilated pelvic portion of the urethra collects seminal fluid during emission. The stratum cavernosum, the primary contractile tissue surrounding the pelvic urethra, may be visible through the distended urethral mucosa during endoscopy. During ejaculation, the contents of the pelvic urethra collected during emission is evacuated by the rhythmic contractions of the urethralis muscle, which surrounds this area.

The *accessory sex glands* of the stallion include the vesicular glands (seminal vesicles), ampullae of the ductus deferens, prostate, and bulbourethral glands. All of these glands contribute secretions (seminal plasma) to the ejaculate volume. The anatomic feature most noticeable on videoendoscopy is the gland ducts or openings. Only the vesicular glands have a large enough opening for direct examination by endoscopy.

The openings (ejaculatory orifices) of the bulbourethral glands and urethral glands are located just cranial to the ischial arch. The ejaculatory orifices appear as almost vertical slits on either side of the colliculus seminalis. The prostatic duct openings are located on each side of the colliculus. They sometimes are very difficult to visualize endoscopically.

The bulbourethral and urethral gland openings are found on the dorsal and lateral walls of the pelvic urethra, respectively, approximately 3 to 4 cm caudal to the colliculus seminalis.

In many stallions, a remnant of the müllerian duct system, the uterus masculinus, is found between the ampullae as they converge under the isthmus of the prostate. This structure may be visualized ultrasonographically and appears as an elongated echolucent cyst. Occasionally, it is observed as a cyst at the colliculus seminalis, where it is referred to as the prostatic utricle.[9] Large cysts may interfere with emission, evacuation, or the passive loss of unejaculated sperm through the urethra.

PATIENT PREPARATION

Endoscopic examination is performed in the standing stallion after sedation to provide penile relaxation. Some authors suggest the use of intravenous xylazine (0.4 mg/kg); acetylpromazine (0.02 mg/kg given intravenously) has been used by others.[4] I prefer sedation with detomidine or a combination of xylazine and butorphanol.

The tail is wrapped, and transrectal palpation and ultrasonography may be performed before endoscopic examination. Sexual stimulation for 2 to 3 minutes (teasing) may increase secretion and dilation of the accessory sex gland.

Endoscopic examination requires at least three people: one person for direct manipulation of the endoscope into the urethra, one person at the controls of the endoscope "driver," and one person to help with stallion restraint. A fourth person may be needed for other manipulations such as rectal massage or insertion of other instruments (catheter or biopsy forceps) through the instrument channel of the endoscope.

The penis is grasped gently just above the glans and extended manually by gentle traction. The penis is then cleansed with warm water and soap. Some practitioners prefer the use of 1% povidone-iodine solution if the area is very dirty and oily. If an antiseptic solution is used, it should be rinsed off completely with sterile water before introduction of the endoscope. During the cleaning procedure, special attention is given to removal of smegma ("bean") from the urethral diverticulum, with careful examination of the urethral process for any lesion.

EQUIPMENT AND PROCEDURE

Equipment used for endoscopy of the stallion urogenital tract consists of flexible endoscopes or videoendoscopes. In general, the most commonly used types of endoscopes are either human gastroscopes or colonoscopes.[10-12] A flexible endoscope with a minimum length of 100 cm and maximum outer diameter of 10 mm is adequate for most light breeds of horses.[4,13,14] A pediatric gastroscope is necessary for the examination of small ponies and miniature horses. Use of a pediatric gastroscope with an outer diameter of 8 to 9 mm carries an added advantage in that it can be inserted into the lumen of the vesicular glands. Longer endoscopes (120 to 140 cm) may be necessary in large breeds of horses or if the penis becomes partially erect.

The equipment is sterilized before use and cleaned thoroughly after each endoscopic examination to avoid buildup of crystals in the various channels.[4,12] Cold disinfection in 2% glutaraldehyde or sterilization with ethylene oxide is adequate, but thereafter the instrument should be rinsed with sterile water before use.[15]

The endoscope is inserted aseptically into the urethral orifice after application of a sterile lubricant (I prefer use of a lubricant containing lidocaine). The operator inserts the endoscope with one hand while holding the glans penis tightly around it with the other hand (Figure 33-1). The close seal achieved in this manner allows the urethra to be distended by air if needed. Caution is required not to overdistend the urethra and bladder. If the stallion displays discomfort or assumes a urination posture, the operator's grip should be relaxed to allow urine flow.

The sterile flexible endoscope is advanced into the proximal urethral to allow visualization of the colliculus seminalis and associated duct openings. Momentary resistance may be encountered as the fiberscope passes through the ischial arch. After this landmark is passed, the image will change direction and become inverted.

CLINICAL FINDINGS

Examination of the Urethra

The normal urethral mucosa is pale pink with longitudinal folds (Figure 33-2). It may become slightly hyperemic and dark when it is distended with air (Figure 33-3), as a result of visualization of the corpus spongiosum blood vessels through the urethral mucosa.[4] The urethral lesions most commonly encountered include inflammation (urethritis), ulcerations, strictures, fissures, and varicosities in

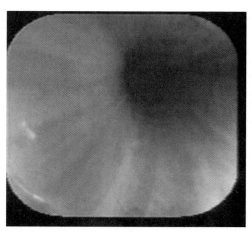

Figure 33-2 Normal urethral mucosa showing longitudinal folds.

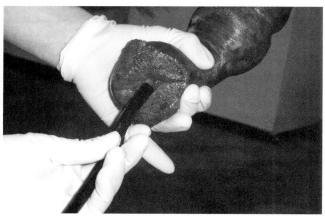

Figure 33-1 Insertion of the videoscope into the urethral orifice.

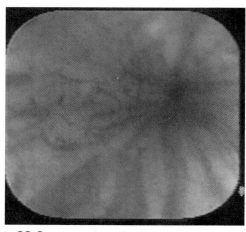

Figure 33-3 Normal urethral mucosa after distention.

the lumen, all of which should be relatively obvious to the trained eye.

As the endoscope is advanced past the ischial arch into the pelvic urethra, two rows of ducts are visualized on the dorsal aspect; these are the bulbourethral gland openings (Figure 33-4). This portion of the urethra also manifests two or more rows of ducts on its lateral aspect—the urethral gland ducts (Figure 33-5). Rectal massage or sometimes spontaneous rhythmic contractions may cause expression of bulbourethral gland secretions during examination (Figure 33-6).

Urethral defects or rents commonly are found in cases of hemospermia. Such rents generally are located at the level of the ischial arch or slightly cranial to it (Figure 33-7, *A* and *B*).

Hemospermia that appears or increases after belling of the glans penis suggests an ulcer or rent in the urethral mucosa that communicates with the erectile layer (stratum cavernosum).[4,13,16] Such rents may be single or multiple and typically range in size from 3 to 10 mm. They generally are linear and appear on the convex surface of the urethra near the level of the ischial arch.

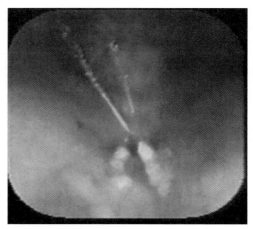

Figure 33-6   Bulbourethral secretion jet induced by rectal massage.

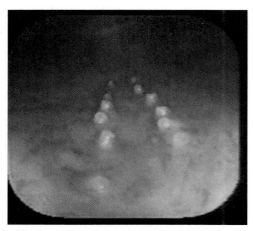

Figure 33-4   Bulbourethral gland orifices on the dorsal aspect of the pelvic urethra.

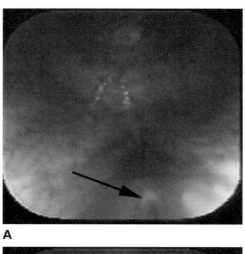

A

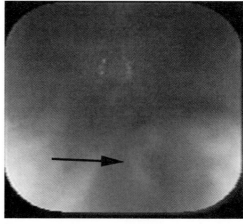

B

Figure 33-7   **A** and **B,** Urethral rent (*arrow*) located at the level of the ischial arch in a stallion presenting with hemospermia. Note the row of bulbourethral gland orifices and the colliculus seminalis, cranial to the lesions.

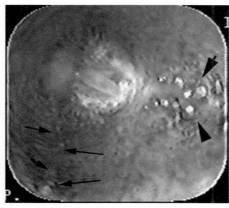

Figure 33-5   Urethral gland orifices (*thin arrows*), lateral to the dorsal bulbourethral gland ducts (*thick arrows*).

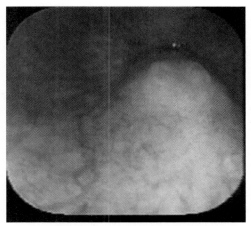

Figure 33-8 Normal colliculus seminalis.

Percutaneous placement of a hypodermic needle (20 gauge, 3.8 cm) into the lumen of the urethra may help determine the exact location of the defect externally.

These defects are thought to extend into the corpus spongiosum penis (CSP) and are believed to be due to an inherent wall weakness on the convex surface of the urethra at the level of the ischial arch.[13] Urethral rents have reportedly been resolved with subischial urethrostomy or laser surgery combined with supportive case and sexual rest.

Urethral strictures, growths, ulcers, and fissures and prolapsed subepithelial vessels also have been reported as visible urethral abnormalities.[7]

Examination of the Colliculus Seminalis

The colliculus seminalis is situated dorsally approximately 3 to 4 cm cranial to the ischial arch and is recognized as a prominent papilla.[4,14,15] The ejaculatory ducts can be identified on the lateral aspect of these structures and correspond to the area where both the ductus deferens and the vesicular gland open (Figure 33-8). Visualization of the ejaculatory ducts may be difficult initially if they are collapsed. Occasionally, the openings of the ductus deferens and the vesicular glands can be individually identified. Ejaculatory duct hyperplasia has been described in some stallions, but its significance is not clear.[15]

The prostatic ducts are smaller and disseminated laterally and proximally to the colliculus seminalis and are difficult to see unless the stallion has been stimulated. Rectal massage of the prostate may improve visualization of these ducts.[4,15]

The vesicular glands can be easily catheterized using a small-diameter (3 to 5 French), flexible polyethylene catheter or a stylet (Figure 33-9). The catheter is inserted into the instrument channel of the videoendoscope and serves as a route for direct aspiration of fluid or instillation of pharmacologic solutions for direct treatment.[1] It also helps to guide the scope head into the seminal vesicle (catheter diameter should be 8 to 9 mm) (Figures 33-10 and 33-11). Direct flushing of the vesicular gland is better accomplished by placing a catheter with an inflatable cuff.

Seminal vesiculitis (vesicular gland adenitis) sometimes is characterized by inflammation of the entire ejaculatory duct, which may appear red and swollen (Figure 33-12, *A* and *B*). Thick mucopurulent discharge or even some bloody discharge may be present (Figure 33-13). Catheterization may be difficult when inflammation is severe.[3,5,17]

Examination of the Bladder

The pelvic urethra continues past the colliculus seminalis for 2 to 3 cm and ends just caudal to the urinary bladder sphincter, also called the internal urethral orifice. Advancing the endoscope into the bladder requires some pressure and insufflation of air in order to dilate the sphincter. If an excessive amount of urine is present, it should be aspirated to allow a thorough examination of the bladder. If retrograde ejaculation is suspected, the urine should be collected for further cytologic evaluation, particularly if a semen collection attempt has been performed just before the endoscopic examination.

The lining of the bladder (mucosa) normally is pale or slightly reddened (Figure 33-14). In cases of cystitis, the mucosa may be very reddened and thickened. Irregular surface lesions may be biopsied using the biopsy channel of the endoscope. Excessive air dilation should be avoided, as it may cause embolism.

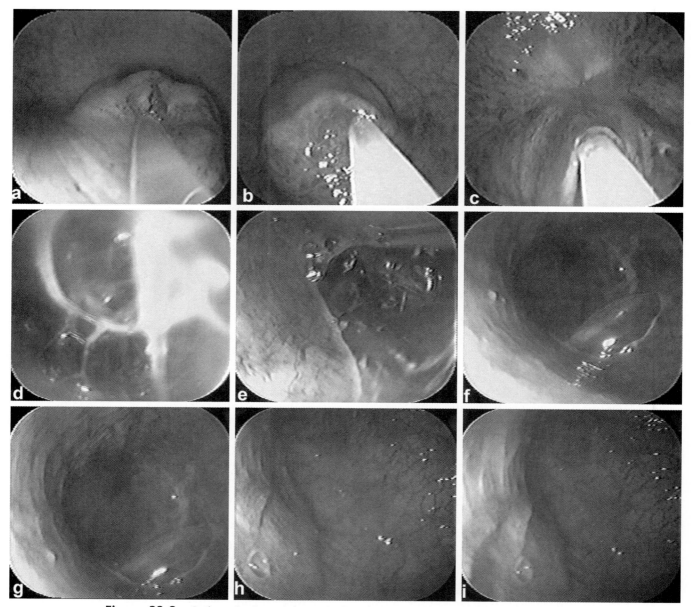

Figure 33-9   Catheterization of the vesicular gland using polyethylene tubing in a stallion with seminal vesiculitis (**A–C**). Note the thick mucopurulent contents of the gland (**D–F**). Gland lumen can be seen after flushing (**G–I**).

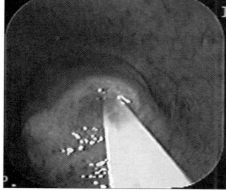

Figure 33-10   Insertion of the polyethylene tubing into the ejaculatory duct.

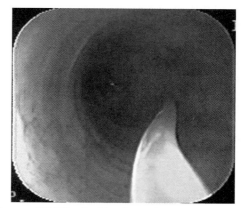

Figure 33-11   Inside view of a vesicular gland.

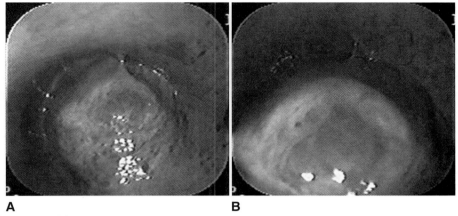

A   **B**

Figure 33-12 **A,** Swollen ejaculatory duct in a stallion with seminal vesiculitis. **B,** Close-up view of the duct.

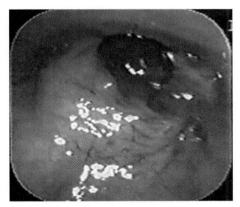

Figure 33-13   Severely inflamed ejaculatory duct.

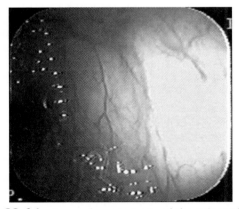

Figure 33-14   Normal appearance of the urinary bladder.

References

1. Varner DD, Blanchard TL, Brinsko SP et al: Techniques for evaluating selected reproductive disorders of stallions. Anim Reprod Sci 2000; 60/61:493-509.

2. Lloyd KCK, Wheat JD, Ryan AM, Matthews M: Ulceration in the proximal portion of the urethra as a cause of hematuria in horses: four cases (1978-1985). J Am Vet Med Assoc 1989; 194:1324-1326.

3. Freestone JF, Paccamonti DL, Eilts BE et al: Seminal vesiculitis as a cause of signs of colic in a stallion. J Am Vet Med Assoc 1993; 203:556-557.

4. Sullins KE, Traub-Dargatz JL: Endoscopic anatomy of the equine urinary tract. Compend Contin Educ Pract Vet 1984; 6:S663-S668.

5. Blanchard TL, Varner DD, Hurtgen JP et al: Bilateral seminal vesiculitis and ampullitis in a stallion. J Am Vet Med Assoc 1988; 192:525-526.

6. Holst WVD: Seminal vesiculitis in two stallions. Tijdschr Diergeneeskd 1976; 101:375-377.

7. McKinnon AO, Voss JL, Trotter GW et al: Hemospermia of the stallion. Equine Pract 1988; 10:17-23.

8. Voss JL, Pickett BW: Diagnosis and treatment of haemospermia in the stallion. J Reprod Fertil 1975; 23(Suppl):151-154.

9. Pozor MA, McDonnell SM: Ultrasonographic measurements of accessory sex glands, ampullae, and urethra of normal stallions of various size types. Theriogenology 2002; 58:1425-1433.

10. Burns J: Endoscopic instrumentation. In Slovis NM (ed): Atlas of Equine Endoscopy, St Louis, Mosby, 2004.

11. Murray MJ: Video Endoscopy. In: Traub-Dargatz JL, Brown CM (eds): Equine Endoscopy, St Louis, Mosby, 1997.

12. Lamar A: Standard fiberoptic equipment and its care. In Traub-Dargatz JL, Brown CM (eds): Equine Endoscopy, St Louis, Mosby, 1997.

13. Schumacher J, Varner DD, Schmitz DG, Blanchard TL: Urethral defects in geldings with hematuria and stallions with hemospermia. Vet Surg 1995; 24:250-254.

14. Slovis NM (ed): Atlas of Equine Endoscopy. St Louis, Mosby, 2004.

15. Steiner J: Stallion reproductive tract. In Slovis NM (ed): Atlas of Equine Endoscopy, St Louis, Mosby, 2004.

16. Sullins KE, Bertone JJ, Voss JL et al: Treatment of hemospermia in stallions: a discussion of 18 cases. Compend Continuing Educ Pract Vet 1988; 10:S1396-S1403.

17. Deegen E, Klug E, Lieske R et al: Surgical treatment of chronic purulent seminal vesiculitis in the stallion. Dtsche Tierarztl Wochensch 1979; 86:140-144.

CHAPTER 34
Penile Abnormalities

EARL M. GAUGHAN
PHILIP D. VAN HARREVELD

Congenital and developmental penile abnormalities are not common in horses. Several conditions have been recognized in horses; however, very few reports have been made of treatment options and related success. The most important aspect of management of penile anomalies is early detection and determination of the need for treatment. An understanding of the impact of a penile and/or preputial disorder on future breeding or urinary health may assist an owner in making decisions for treatment.

PREPUCE

Constriction or stenosis of the preputial ring is a narrowing of the preputial opening that inhibits the extrusion of the penis. This disorder is typically congenital; however, it may also result from local trauma. Congenital incidence of preputial stenosis may demonstrate clinical signs at birth or not until several months of age. Clinical signs are usually consistent with phimosis. Affected horses typically urinate within the prepuce, and in long-standing cases urine scalding and ulceration of preputial skin can be present.[1] Manual dilatation may be possible in some individuals; however, surgical correction is most often indicated. Transection of the dorsal aspect of the muscular ring through a stab incision in the skin of the preputial ring can release the penis from the prepuce. Simple closure of the skin with monofilament absorbable suture is recommended.[1] Topical hygiene and application of antibiotic ointments can successfully address any skin ulcers present.

Descriptions of congenital aplasia and hypoplasia of the prepuce have been discussed (Figure 34-1). Associations with other deformities have not been determined. Affected individuals are described as appearing paraphimotic without sufficient preputial tissue to manually replace the penis into the prepuce. The penile tissue appears to have sensory and motor innervation, but insufficient prepuce for normal positioning. No treatment has been described.[2]

PENIS

Congenital abnormalities of the equine penis are rare and include congenitally short penis, retroverted penis, aplasia or dysgenesis of the corpus spongiosum glandis, hypospadias (urethral orifice at the ventral aspect of the penis or in the perineal region), and epispadias (urethral orifice on the dorsal aspect of the penis).[1] One stallion with a congenitally short penis had a normal breeding career through between 5 and 10 years of age, when an inability to ejaculate developed.[3] Other conditions likely require close examination to determine if treatment is necessary or required. Partial or en bloc penile and preputial amputation may address severe abnormalities. Reconstruction of normal urethral anatomy can correct the disorders of hypospadias and epispadias in some individuals. It is typically advised and usually necessary to castrate affected horses if testicular tissue is present. Evaluation for intersex abnormalities is suggested when these penile abnormalities are identified.

INTERSEX

Several manifestations of abnormal male external genitalia have been described in horses.[1] The causes for these disorders are not completely understood; however, heritability and double fertilization or whole-body chimerism from fusion of early embryos have been postulated. True hermaphrodism (the presence of both male and female external genitalia, as well as both testicular and ovarian tissues) has been reported in some foals.[4,5] However, this is considered extremely rare. The male pseudohermaphrodite is considered more common.[1] Penilelike tissues have been observed as an exaggerated clitoris in association with normal- or abnormal-appearing vaginal structures (Figure 34-2). This may be located anywhere from the normal perineal location to the umbilicus. These individuals can demonstrate stallion-like behavior and often have cryptorchid testes in the abdomen or inguinal canal. True hermaphrodism is rare in horses and is marked by a poorly defined penis, absence of a scrotum, and the presence of ovotestes.[1] Female pseudohermaphrodism, ovaries associated with male external genitalia, is even more rare.

Treatment of intersex abnormalities in horses typically is directed at castration to address behavioral issues.[1] Testes are usually underdeveloped, perhaps even more so than the more typical cryptorchid testes found in the abdomen or inguinal canal. Some reconstructive surgery has been performed to change the appearance of the external genitalia of affected individuals.[6] Appropriate preplanning (i.e., whole blood for transfusion) and positioning should be considered. Attention to urinary outflow and castration are important as well, even though these individuals are typically sterile.

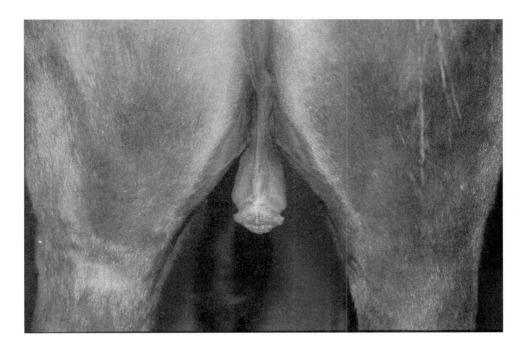

Figure 34-1 A weanling Quarter Horse with substantial hypoplasia of the prepuce exposing an underdeveloped distal penis.

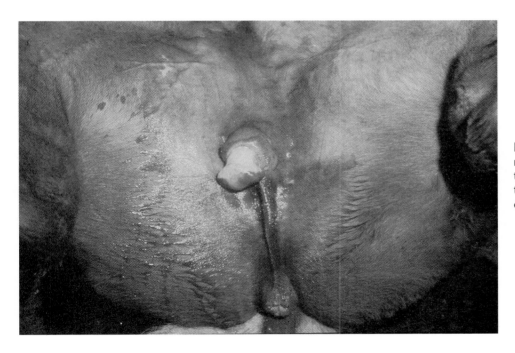

Figure 34-2 Male pseudohermaphrodism is demonstrated in this yearling Quarter Horse. Note the penilelike tissue at the ventral commissure of the vulva.

References

1. Vaughan JT: Surgery of the prepuce and penis. In McKinnon AO, Voss JL (eds): Equine Reproduction, Philadelphia, Lea & Febiger, 1993.
2. Vaughan JT: Surgery of the prepuce and penis. Proceedings of the 18th Annual Convention of the American Association of Equine Practitioners, pp 19-40, 1972.
3. Roberts SJ: Infertility in male animals. In Veterinary Obstetrics and Genital Diseases (Theriogenology), North Pomfret, Vt., David and Charles, 1986.
4. Dunn HO, Smiley D, McEntee K: Two equine true hermaphrodites with 64,XX/64,XY and 63,X/64,XY chimerism. Cornell Vet 1981; 71:123-135.
5. Walker DF, Vaughan JT: Bovine and Equine Urogenital Surgery, Philadelphia, Lea & Febiger, 1980.
6. Bracken FK, Wagner PC: Cosmetic surgery for equine pseudohermaphrodism. Vet Med Small Anim Clin 1983; 78:879-884.

CHAPTER 35

Penile Infections

EARL M. GAUGHAN
PHILIP D. VAN HARREVELD

Infectious disease of the equine penis is relatively uncommon. Sexually transmitted infectious disease is a concern for active stallions and can disrupt breeding use for extended periods of time. Other local infectious issues often are predisposed by parasitism, neoplasia, or trauma. Careful physical examination and appropriate laboratory-supported diagnostic efforts can lead to timely treatment and successful outcome. Delay in recognition and treatment can result in the need for aggressive surgical treatment, which can further interfere with or prevent a breeding career.

BACTERIAL INFECTION

Simple infection of the penis and/or prepuce by bacteria is not common.[1,2] Bacteria contaminants typically invade these tissues secondary to another cause. Typical bacterial infection complications are preceded by injury that opens the skin, neoplasia, or parasitism. Excessive washing with soap has resulted in coliform colonization, and excessive disinfection of the stallion's penis has been associated with removal of normal bacteria and colonization of potentially pathogenic bacteria such as *Pseudomonas*.[3] The microorganisms that are commonly identified are the bacteria that would be expected as local flora opportunists. *Streptococcus* spp., *Klebsiella* spp., and *Pseudomonas* spp. have been routinely implicated in penile and preputial infections.[2] It should be noted that these organisms have also been cultured from the equine penis and prepuce in routine screening of the skin when no lesions have been present.[2] Therefore culture results should be interpreted with strict attention to the clinical situation.

Treatment of bacterial infections should be directed at resolving the primary disease. In the unusual case of simple bacterial balanitis or balanoposthitis, topical treatment is usually successful in resolving the infection.[1,2] Close attention to hygiene with daily cleansing of the penis and prepuce is important. This can be accomplished with water alone or with a mild disinfecting soap. Care should be taken to ensure that all soap residues are removed after cleaning. Large volumes of water should be encouraged. If skin erosions are present or the infectious process appears advanced, application of local antibiotic ointments can help sterilize the tissues.[2] Ideally antibiotic selection should be based on culture and sensitivity results; however, systemic antibiotic administration is not commonly indicated. Sexual rest during treatment is necessary.

Prevention of bacterial infections may be possible through routine maintenance of hygiene practices. Monthly cleansing of the penis and prepuce with large volumes of water, water-based lubricants, or a mild soap can reduce smegma accumulation and associated skin irritation. Harsh soaps and antibiotic ointments should be avoided because the use of these agents can result in skin irritation/inflammation and potentially alter the normal skin flora such that infection may be more likely.[2]

VIRAL INFECTION

Viral infection of the penis and prepuce is also not very common in horses. Equine herpes virus 3 is the most common viral infection in male horses.[1,2] This virus is the cause of coital exanthema and is typically acquired through sexual transmission.[1-3] Vesicles and ulcers on the penile skin are common clinical signs, and the lesion sites are frequently invaded and infected secondarily by bacteria. Another name for this disease is genital horse pox due to the long-lasting, often depigmented healed ulcer sites.[1,2]

Coital exanthema is highly contagious, and sexual rest should be enforced during treatment. The lesions are painful, and affected stallions may avoid intromission during the acute phases of infection, although this may depend on an individual stallion's libido.[1,2] Treatment is typically directed at local hygiene and topical antibiotic application if bacterial contamination is considered a problem. Immune-competent horses will develop a successful immune response to help resolve the viral infection, yet the immunity is considered to be short-lived and perhaps only protective through the current breeding season.[2] This is typical for most herpes viruses.[2]

PROTOZOAL INFECTION

Dourine is a protozoal disease associated with *Trypanosoma equiperdum*.[1,2] This is a reportable disease considered to be currently eradicated in the United States.[2] Dourine is most commonly diagnosed in Africa, South America, and the Mediterranean regions.[1,2] This is a highly contagious, sexually transmitted disease apparently only affecting members of the horse family. Affected horses, weeks to months after exposure, develop swelling in the penis and prepuce as well as systemic signs of disease (i.e., fever, lethargy, anorexia).[2] Skin lesions are common at the penis, prepuce, and along the neck and shoulders. Lesions are erosive and often result in depigmented plaques. Mucopurulent exudate is often observed from the urethra and penile lesions.[2] Dourine is usually diagnosed by observation of the typical lesions and confirmation of trypanosomes in the discharge or by complement fixation examination.[2] Treatment is considered impractical, and isolation of infected individuals is highly recommended while disease confirmation efforts are conducted.[1,2]

PARASITISM

The most frequent parasitic considerations for lesions on the penis and prepuce of horses are *Habronema muscae*, *Habronema microstoma*, and *Draschia megastoma*.[2,4] These large stomach worms are most commonly found in warm, moist climates like the southeastern United States. Lesions of habronemiasis have been noted in many locations on the body. The penis and prepuce are common locations for infection as are wound sites on the limbs.[2] The larvae of the large stomach worms are typically delivered to these sites by flies. The preputial ring and the urethral process are common sites for habronemiasis lesions, which are also known as "summer sores." These lesions typically appear as granulomatous sites that can mimic granulation tissue secondary to wounding, squamous cell carcinoma, and verrucous type of equine sarcoid. Habronemiasis lesions may be pruritic, and affected horses may appear more aware of these lesions than the other similar-appearing lesions.

A final diagnosis of habronemiasis is based on impression smears, lesion scrapings, or biopsy. Impression smears may detect the sulfur granules typical of *Habronema* larvae presence. Scrapings of the granulating lesion may reveal larvae within the tissue. Biopsy results can further delineate the differences between the reactive lesion of habronemiasis and squamous cell carcinoma and equine sarcoid.[1,2] Eosinophilia, although commonly noted with this disorder, is not specific to the final diagnosis of habronemiasis.

Treatment of cutaneous habronemiasis of the penis and prepuce should be similar to that necessary at any other body lesion site. Systemic administration of ivermectin (0.2 mg/kg) may result in resolution of smaller lesions.[2] The need for follow-up treatment with a second dose 1 month after the first is not uncommon. Local treatment may be necessary for large or refractory lesions. Topical applications of antiinflammatory agents and larvicidal drugs have been beneficial.

Surgical debridement can assist antilarval treatment by reducing the bulk of the granulation tissue and potentially reducing parasite and microbial contaminant load. Debridement can be performed in the standing or anesthetized horse. General anesthesia and dorsal recumbency are suggested to address extensive lesions. Debridement can be accomplished with sharp instruments, lasers, or electrosurgical or cryosurgical applications. A combination of these techniques can also be successful. Wide margins of debridement into normal tissue are not necessary when treating *Habronema*. This allows local manipulations to be reasonably contained. Laser and cryogen application should be performed with attention to depth of tissue penetration, especially with penile lesions. Care should be exercised to avoid deep vascular and urethral tissues when these are not affected by the disease process.[5-7]

The urethral process is frequently infected by *Habronema* larvae, and surgical treatment is often required to resolve the infection in this site. The urethral process can be amputated without disrupting normal penile roles in breeding or urination. Urethral process resection can be performed in the standing horse; however, general anesthesia and dorsal recumbency can assist tissue manipulation. The urethral process can be excised with a scalpel blade, scissors, or laser. A urinary catheter should be placed. A circumferential incision is made from the skin through the corpus spongiosum penis and urethral mucosa. The skin is then apposed to the urethral mucosa with 2-0 or 3-0 monofilament absorbable suture material in a simple interrupted pattern. Up to 75% to 85% of the urethral process can be amputated.[5] This procedure can also be effective in the treatment of local neoplasia or sarcoid. The skin in the recess around the urethral process should be closely examined for additional lesions.

NEOPLASIA

Neoplastic disease of the penis and prepuce is well known in horses. Squamous cell carcinoma is by far the most commonly observed neoplastic disorder of male equine external genitalia.[1,2,5,6] Other mass-forming diseases include equine sarcoid, melanoma, mastocytoma, and hemangioma.[1,2]

Squamous cell carcinoma lesions can be observed on any skin surface of the penis and prepuce. There are numerous manifestations of these skin lesions. Close observation by the owner and veterinarian can help detect early lesion presence before substantial tissue destruction has occurred. Squamous cell carcinoma can appear as flat, pale plaques, ulcerated skin, nodular lesions underlying minimally abnormal-appearing skin lesions, pedunculated masses, small verrucous masses, or large granulomatous masses. Penile function may be normal or disrupted. Large masses of the penis or prepuce can be responsible for paraphimosis. Otherwise, squamous cell carcinoma lesions may go undetected for extended periods of time if urination or breeding are not observed.

Diagnosis of squamous cell carcinoma is based on clinical signs and the presence of one of the skin manifestations described. A thorough physical examination should include close visual and palpation investigation of local and regional lymphatic tissues. It is not common for squamous cell carcinoma to metastasize, because local extension and tissue destruction are more likely. However, extension to regional lymph nodes substantially reduces the prognosis and escalates the need for aggressive surgical treatment. Final diagnosis should be determined from histopathologic examination of biopsy samples.

Perhaps fortunately, there are a number of treatment approaches to penile and preputial squamous cell carcinoma that can be successful. Small, skin surface lesions will occasionally respond to topical chemotherapy with

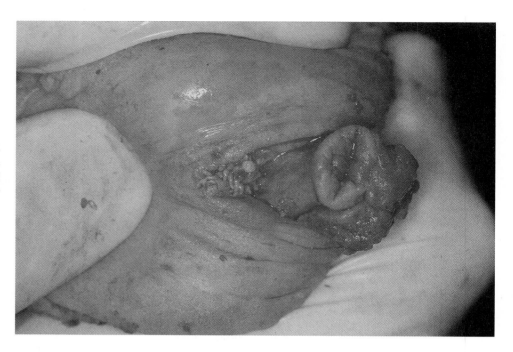

Figure 35-1 Close examination reveals squamous cell carcinoma lesions of the urethral process and recess in an older horse.

5-flourouracil ointment. Application of this ointment at 2-week intervals has been successful in resolving small lesions and maintaining larger lesions when surgical treatment was not elected. Care to avoid human skin contact with 5-flourouracil and excessive application to the horse should be standard. Radiation therapy with radon or iridium seed implants or radiation teletherapy have also been reported.[2] Systemic nonsteroidal anti-inflammatory drugs are recommended during any type of chemotherapy treatment.

There are several surgical options for the treatment of squamous cell carcinoma on the equine penis and prepuce.[5-7] Treatment selection is determined by the location and severity of the lesion. Local lesions can be excised and skin primarily closed with absorbable suture. There does not appear to be a critical need for large (1-cm) margins in the excision of these superficial masses. It is recommended to ensure that incisions reach normal skin; however, no specific guidelines have been determined, and successful resection without recurrence has been achieved with removal of minimal borders of normal tissue around simple squamous cell carcinoma lesions. Neoplastic lesions involving the urethral process can be managed much like habronemiasis lesions. Local resection of the mass lesion and urethral process can be successful (Figure 35-1). Local removal of neoplastic lesions can also be accomplished with laser techniques and cryosurgery.

Squamous cell carcinoma of the glans penis may be amenable to more aggressive local resection by partial posthioplasty or circumcision.[5,6] If normal skin margins can be reapposed, two circumferential skin incisions, one on each end of the lesion, can be created. The isolated skin can be circumferentially excised to remove the lesion. The skin margins should then be apposed with simple interrupted sutures using 2-0 monofilament absorbable material. With more extensive lesions, distal penile amputation of the glans penis should be considered. Several techniques have been described, including Scott's, Voinsot's, and Williams'.[5,8] Each technique removes the diseased aspect of the penis and creates a modified termination of the penis and urethra. Castration is typically recommended with partial penile amputation; however, newer collection techniques may allow a valuable stallion to continue to make semen available.

Advanced squamous cell carcinoma lesions involving the penis, prepuce, and regional lymphatic tissues can present discouraging potential (Figure 35-2). En bloc resection of all of these tissues may afford some affected horses an alternative to euthanasia.[8] This procedure requires general anesthesia and dorsal recumbency. Close examination is necessary to determine if resection can be accomplished and leave enough skin in place for complete closure. The author has completed this procedure on one horse in which the skin incision was left to heal by second intention. This was done to completely resect all detected neoplastic tissue. The horse had an extended recuperative period but ultimately returned to normal activity.

A urethral catheter should be placed when possible. An elliptical skin incision should be performed from the umbilicus to the distal perineum caudal to the scrotal region. Intact horses should be castrated. It has been suggested that castration be performed 3 to 4 weeks before penile and preputial resection; however, these procedures may be completed at the same time. The penile and preputial tissues, with regional lymphatics, should be elevated by a combination of sharp and blunt dissection. Numerous large vessels should be anticipated and ligated. Two options appear possible for management of the penile stump. Markel et al[9] described retroversion of the remaining penile stump to the ventral perineal region where the corpus cavernosum penis is secured to local subcutaneous tissue and the urethra sutured to skin.[5,9] Another option is to transect the penis just distal to the

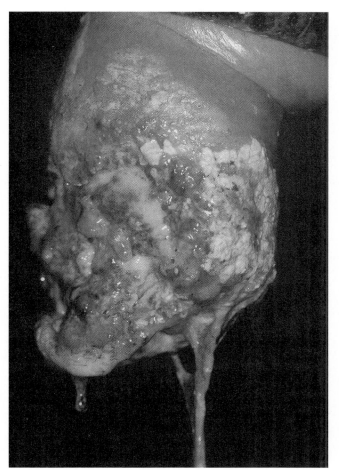

Figure 35-2 Severe, advanced squamous cell carcinoma in an older horse. Amputation of the glans penis and possibly the prepuce may be required for successful treatment.

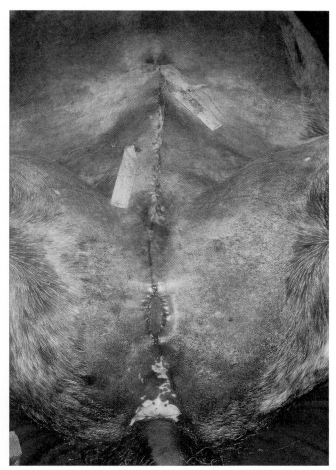

Figure 35-3 An aged horse in dorsal recumbency after en bloc resection of the penis, prepuce, and regional lymphatic tissues. A permanent perineal urethrostomy has been performed immediately dorsal to the penile amputation site.

site typical of a routine perineal urethrostomy. The corpus cavernosum penis is closed and secured to local fascia and subcutaneous tissue, and a permanent perineal urethrostomy is performed (Figure 35-3). This technique has worked well and appears to avoid the creation of a flexure in the penis.[8] Both of these procedures appear to provide an option for the treatment of advanced neoplastic destruction of the penis and prepuce.

Other neoplastic diseases of the penis and prepuce are far less common than squamous cell carcinoma. Treatment options are likely the same as for squamous cell carcinoma, and often surgical treatment is undertaken and completed before final histopathologic diagnosis is confirmed. The potential exception to this is equine melanoma. It may be advisable to reserve surgical treatment of melanoma until clinical signs associated with the mass indicate excision. Incomplete resection of melanoma has been associated with extension and metastasis, which should be avoided if possible.[2,4,5]

Equine sarcoid is occasionally diagnosed in the equine penis but is probably more likely in the prepuce. Both of these locations are not as likely for sarcoid occurrence as the head, limbs, and trunk. Local immunotherapy and chemotherapy can be successful with smaller lesions.

Larger masses typically require the same surgical considerations as squamous cell carcinoma. Once again, the mass lesion may provide the indication for surgical treatment, and the final diagnosis is determined by histopathologic results.[2]

Primary microbial infections, of the penis and prepuce are not common. Appropriate, routine health care and hygiene practices can avoid most opportunities for these diseases to occur. The incidence of neoplastic and parasitic disease of the penis and prepuce are much more common. The presence of these lesions can then predispose to secondary invasion of microorganisms, creating complicated disease situations. However, once again, with good owner compliance of regular visual and manual examination and hygiene practices, these disorders can be identified in their early stages when treatment is simpler and outcome success more likely.

References

1. Roberts SJ: Infertility in male animals. In Veterinary Obstetrics and Genital Diseases (Theriogenology), North Pomfret, Vt, David and Charles, pp 752-891, 1986.

2. De Vries PJ: Diseases of the testes, penis, and related structures. In McKinnon AO, Voss JL (eds): Equine Reproduction, Philadelphia, Lea & Febiger, pp 878-884, 1993.

3. Couto MA, Hughs JP: Sexually transmitted (venereal) diseases of horses. In McKinnon AO, Voss JL (eds): Equine Reproduction, Philadelphia, Lea & Febiger, pp 845-854, 1993.

4. Vaughan JT: Surgery of the prepuce and penis. In McKinnon AO, Voss JL (eds): Equine Reproduction, Philadelphia, Lea & Febiger, pp 933-942, 1993.

5. Schumacher J: The penis and prepuce. In Auer JA, Stick JA (eds): Equine Surgery, Philadelphia, WB Saunders, pp 540-557, 1999.

6. Vaughan JT: Penis and prepuce. In McKinnon AO, Voss JL (eds): Equine Reproduction, Philadelphia, Lea & Febiger, pp 885-894, 1993.

7. Vaughan JT: Surgery of the prepuce and penis. Proceedings of the 18th Annual Convention of the American Association of Equine Practitioners, pp 19-40, 1972.

8. van Harreveld PD, Gaughan EM et al: Penile surgery in horses. Comp Cont Educ Pract Vet 1998; 20:739-746.

9. Markel MD, Wheat JD, Jones K: Genital neoplasms treated by en bloc resection and penile retroversion in horses: 10 cases 1977-1986. J Am Vet Med Assoc 1988; 192(3):396-400.

CHAPTER 36

Trauma to the Penis

EARL M. GAUGHAN
PHILIP D. VAN HARREVELD

Traumatic injury of the penis in horses is not common.[1,2] Kick-related injury to the penis and prepuce of stallions and aggressive geldings by seasonal mares is likely the most frequent origin of trauma to this region.[1,2] Horses can also experience blunt trauma from obstacles or objects either in competitive pursuits or during playful activity. Lacerations and penetrating injury can also occur from a variety of sources.

Initial assessment of a horse with penile and/or preputial injury should include a complete physical examination, noting vital signs and detection of any systemic repercussions. Clinical signs of shock should be addressed with complete diagnostic efforts and aggressive medical treatment. Most commonly, penile/preputial trauma does not require exaggerated systemic support but concentrated local and systemic management of the local tissue lesions.

Close attention and observation should be directed at assessment of penile function and the horse's ability to position and maintain the penis in the normal preputial location. This may not be possible due to local tissue swelling; however, early signs of retraction efforts are encouraging for ultimate return to normal. It should be noted that an absence of obvious penile retraction does not rule out the final ability to return to normal function, especially when substantial penile and preputial swelling are present. Skin and deep tissues should be manually palpated and evaluated for warmth and possible sensation. Ultrasonographic examination may provide some information in regard to vascular blood flow and the nature of tissue swelling. Thermographic examination can also provide useful information relative to tissue perfusion and to establish a baseline from which to detect changes over the time of treatment.

TRAUMA WITHOUT OPEN WOUNDS

Blunt trauma to the penis/prepuce is likely the most common reason a veterinarian is asked to examine this region in an adult male horse. A complete physical examination should be performed with obvious attention to the external genitalia. Swelling that is marked in the acute phases after injury should be closely evaluated for the presence of a hematoma in which the hemorrhage is ongoing. The best detection method for this instance is likely ultrasonography.[3] It is not recommended to perform needle aspirates at this time due to the possibility of inoculating microorganisms into a potentially sterile site. Ultrasonography may also assist in the evaluation of established swelling because edema fluid will typically have a more echo-dense appearance than free fluid/blood.[3]

Acute hematoma formation should be treated as for any other episode of substantial hemorrhage.[1,2,4] Local tissue cooling with ice packs, cold running water, and local tissue pressure should be initiated at the earliest possible opportunity. The penis and prepuce should be compressed and elevated with a bandage or sling to approximate these tissues to the ventral body wall. If swelling is confined to the glans, a circumferential pressure bandage can assist in the reduction and resolution of bleeding and swelling. This should be maintained at all times other than when local, topical treatment is applied. The application of topical ointments, salves, and astringent agents should be approached carefully so that the skin is not irritated, which can exacerbate local swelling. Emollient ointments can assist some horses. Preparations with dimethyl sulfoxide (DMSO), lanolin, Furacin, petroleum jelly, and formulas for topical udder treatment in cattle can help keep penile and preputial skin protected from desiccation when retraction to normal position is not possible.[1]

Horses with penile and preputial hematomas should be treated with systemic antibiotics and nonsteroidal antiinflammatory drugs (NSAIDs). Substantial swelling may be more rapidly resolved with the administration of systemic DMSO (100 mg to 1.0 g/kg PO or IV once to twice per day for 3 days). Medication can be discontinued when swelling is reduced and normal function is resumed.

Blunt trauma can result in permanent penile dysfunction. Paraphimosis and priapism can both result from trauma to the penis and prepuce (Figure 36-1). Repositioning of the penis into the prepuce and return to normal function are the obvious goals of treatment for these disorders.[1,5-7]

If manual replacement of the penis into the sheath can be accomplished with little difficulty, a purse-string suture at the preputial orifice may successfully restrain the penis until swelling is resolved and function returned. This appears to be rarely successful, however. An alternative treatment for paraphimosis is the retraction and retention of the penis within the prepuce via a sutured, phallopexy procedure, the Bolz technique.[1,2] The retracted penis is fixed into position within the external lamina of the prepuce by making a longitudinal incision 10 cm caudal to the scrotum over the perineal raphae. The penis is dissected free of surrounding fascia and is

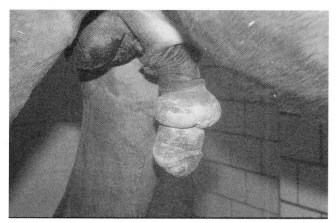

Figure 36-1 Paraphimosis is demonstrated in this middle-aged stallion that was kicked by a mare. A ring of fibrotic tissue resulted from the original tissue trauma. This lesion may be successfully treated with a partial posthioplasty.

retracted into the prepuce. This will create a sigmoid flexure to the penis, but this has not been associated with complications. The penis is secured into position with large (No. 2) nonabsorbable sutures or umbilical tape through the annular ring of the penis, which exit the skin 2 cm apart and 4 cm from the edge of the incision. The suture can be tied at the skin or secured over roll gauze. The penis should be retracted such that the rostral end of the glans is aligned with the preputial orifice. Sutures can be removed at 2 weeks after placement. If this technique fails to result in permanent return to normal penile position, more aggressive surgical treatment may be required.[1,2]

Occasionally horses with paraphimosis can be successfully managed with surgical treatment.[1,6] When paraphimosis is the result of trauma and resulting swelling and fibrosis, local resection of the redundant tissue can result in return of the penis to normal position in the prepuce. Partial posthioplasty (circumcision or "reefing") can remove the abnormal tissue and return the penis to normal function. This procedure is best performed with the affected horse under general anesthesia and in dorsal recumbency. A tourniquet is placed at the base of the penis, and the penile skin is aseptically prepared. Two parallel circumferential incisions, to the level of the subcutaneous tissue, are performed with substantial enough margins to completely remove the abnormal tissue. Before incision it is suggested that the practitioner determine if the penile skin can be adequately reapposed by tenting the skin with forceps under the lesion. The two skin incisions are connected sharply, and the subcutaneous tissue is undermined to remove the flap of skin (Figure 36-2). The incised skin edges are apposed with a simple interrupted pattern using 0-0 or 2-0 monofilament absorbable suture material. Several weeks of rest should be enforced after surgery to allow appropriate healing. This procedure can also be successful in the management of superficial dermal lesions of the penis.[1,2]

Priapism can result from trauma or after the administration of phenothiazine derivatives (acetylproma-

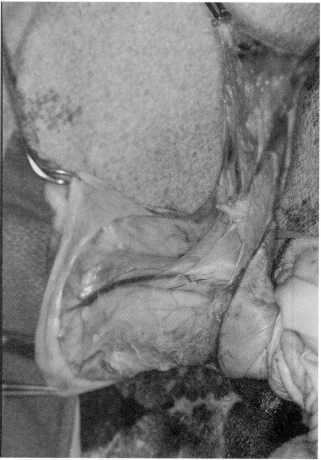

Figure 36-2 A partial posthioplasty or circumcision ("reefing") procedure is being performed. The circumferential flap of skin is elevated and removed to allow the penis to return to normal position. This procedure can also successfully resect local infectious and neoplastic lesions.

zine).[5,8-10] Although most commonly observed in stallions, geldings have also been affected. Perhaps the most important aspect of management of priapism is early diagnosis and initiation of aggressive treatment. The administration of benztropine mesylate (8 mg IV) has been associated with resolution of priapism that has occurred after phenothiazine tranquilization.[11] Early administration of the drug after recognition of the lesion is considered important for success. Other medical management attempts with NSAIDs, massage, slings, and diuretics have not met with good success. Any horse with refractory priapism, which is not immediately responsive to first treatment efforts, should be considered a candidate for lavage of the corpus cavernosum penis. This procedure attempts to remove clotting and sludged blood from the cavernosal tissue. The corpus cavernosum can be lavaged with the horse recumbent or standing. General anesthesia and dorsal recumbency appear to make the procedure easier and more likely to succeed. A 12- or 14-gauge hypodermic needle is inserted into the dorsal aspect of the corpus cavernosum proximal to the glans penis. A second needle is inserted into the corpus cavernosum about 10 to 15 cm caudal to the scrotum. Heparinized saline (10 units heparin per milliliter) is used to flush the corpus cavernosum. Typically the heparinized saline requires pressure to flush the cavernous tissue. This can be accomplished with a syringe-assisted drip set. A volume of heparinized saline sufficient to reach clear effluent or fresh blood should be used. This may require 2 to 4 L of lavage solution.[1] Typically, when the efflux is cleared, the penis will relax and can be positioned into the prepuce. A purse-string suture in the prepuce or a penile sling should then be placed to prevent recurrence. The lavage procedure can be repeated if necessary; however, more than two to three attempts typically indicates a refractory situation. Results are typically poor if the lavage is first attempted at greater than 24 hours from onset of priapism. If corpus cavernosum lavage fails to correct the condition, a shunt between the corpus cavernosum and corpus spongiosum or penile amputation should be considered.[1,9]

Blood can be diverted or allowed to escape the corpus cavernosum by creating a shunt between it and the corpus spongiosum, which is not involved with erection.[1,2] This procedure requires general anesthesia and dorsal recumbency. The penile shaft is exposed via a midline incision and blunt dissection approximately 15 cm caudal to the scrotum. The bulbospongiosus muscle is divided to expose the corpus cavernosum, which is incised (approximately 3 cm) in close proximity to the corpus spongiosum. The corpus cavernosum is lavaged with heparinized saline to clear the clotted blood. A parallel incision is made in the corpus spongiosum. The tunica albuginea of the corpus cavernosum is sutured (2-0 monofilament absorbable material) to the tunica albuginea of the corpus spongiosum to create a patent stoma between the two cavernous tissues. Subcutaneous tissue and skin should be routinely closed. This procedure is suggested early (4 to 6 hours) after occurrence of priapism if other methods fail to result in detumescence.[1,2]

Penile amputation or phallectomy is occasionally required for horses with refractory paraphimosis, priapism, or traumatic injury that renders the distal penile tissue irreparable in other manners. The same techniques are used to address aggressive local neoplastic disorders of the penis. This procedure should be undertaken for stallions only after careful consideration of postoperative expectations. Castration is typically indicated; however, semen from some individuals may be collectable with modern technological advances. If castration is selected, it is recommended to do so 3 to 4 weeks before the penis is amputated.[1,2,13]

Appropriate access and restraint for penile amputation is best obtained with general anesthesia and dorsal recumbency. A urethral catheter should be placed and a tourniquet positioned at the base of the penis when possible. The urethral catheter greatly assists identification of the ventral midline of the penis as well as the urethra itself. Several amputation techniques have been described for the penis. These include Scott's, Vinsot's, and Williams' techniques.[1]

The Scott technique involves a circumferential incision from the skin to the level of the urethra. A 4- to 5-cm length of urethra is preserved as the distal penis is

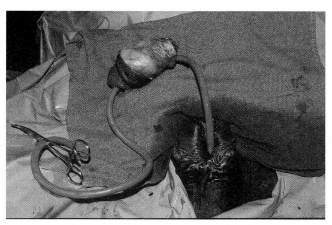

Figure 36-3 A partial penile amputation has been performed using the Williams technique. The stallion catheter simplifies identification of the urethra. Urethral mucosa is secured over the distal penile stump, which decreases complications.

transected and removed. The tunica albuginea of the corpus cavernosum is closed with a simple interrupted pattern using absorbable suture. The tunica albuginea of the corpus spongiosum is sutured to the submucosa of the urethra. The protruding urethral stump is sectioned into triangular segments as is the preputial skin. The urethral segments are then spatulated over the penile stump and sutured to the penile skin.[1]

The Vinsot technique uses a triangular incision at the ventral aspect of the penis with the triangle apex pointed distally. Incision is carried to the level of the urethra, which is then incised longitudinally. The urethral edges are sutured to the penile skin edge of the triangle with simple interrupted (2-0) absorbable suture. A large, nonabsorbable ligature is then placed around the penis distal to the apex of the triangle. The penis is transected distal to the ligature suture and the penile stump left to heal by second intention. Urethral stricture is a potential complication of this procedure.[1]

The Williams technique also uses a ventral triangular incision; however, the apex is directed proximally, not distally. The tissue within the triangle is excised, and a longitudinal incision is made to the urethral lumen. The urethral mucosa is then sutured to the skin in a simple interrupted pattern with absorbable (2-0) suture. The penis is then transected distal to the new urethral orifice. The tunica albuginea of the corpus cavernosum is closed with simple interrupted, absorbable suture. These sutures may also include the urethral mucosa. The penile stump is then covered by suture closure of the penile skin to urethral mucosa. This completely closes the penile tissues and appears less likely to result in urethral stricture[1] (Figure 36-3).

TRAUMA WITH OPEN WOUNDS

Abrasions and lacerations of the penis are not common. However, the same forces that traumatize the penis without opening the skin or deeper tissues can also result in open tissue disruption at the penis and prepuce. Stallions can be injured by tail hair or breeding sutures, mare kick trauma, or any number of miscellaneous sources. Physical examination is essential to understand what tissues have been injured and to what degree. After a thorough systemic examination, the penile and preputial tissues should be evaluated by external palpation, ultrasonography, and, potentially, urethral endoscopy. Although most lacerations are superficial and involve only the skin, marked hemorrhage may indicate involvement of the cavernous tissues. Blood loss and hematoma formation can be substantial. Treatment with systemic antibiotics and NSAIDs is suggested, as is tetanus prophylaxis.[1]

Small lacerations of penile and/or preputial skin can often be readily managed with the horse standing with sedation and local anesthesia. Thorough cleansing and disinfection of the injured site and surrounding skin should be performed. The skin should be apposed in the most straightforward manner possible. Simple interrupted and simple continuous patterns have been successful using either absorbable or nonabsorbable suture materials. If skin closure is not possible, second intention healing can result in a satisfactory outcome. Second intention healing through granulation and contracture is not the most desirable management method due to increased potential for penile deformation and local and ascending sepsis. If second intention management is necessary, daily attempts at maintaining good hygiene are suggested. Cleansing with a dilute antiseptic solution and topical application of antiseptic ointments can assist healing.[1]

Large and extensive wounds of the penis and prepuce are likely best managed with the horse under general anesthesia in dorsal recumbency. Lateral recumbency may be elected in some horses if access to the wound site it best accomplished in this manner. Wound closure is usually desirable. Delayed primary closure is often necessary to allow staged and thorough wound cleansing and debridement of contaminants and devitalized tissue. Preoperative attempts to reduce local swelling are also indicated. The urethra should be carefully reconstructed. The lacerated or torn urethral margins can be apposed with 3-0 or 2-0 absorbable material in a simple interrupted pattern. Linear, longitudinal lacerations of the urethra typically heal without stricture or complications with simple suture closure. With tissue loss or transverse wounds, a stallion catheter may help reduce structuring scar formation. As with all urinary tract closure, it is sug-

gested that the practitioner avoid placing suture material in the urethral lumen. After surgical repair of large wounds, continued medical treatment to reduce swelling and maintain good hygiene are important. Stallions should be rested and kept from mares for at least 2 weeks after wound repair.

Penile trauma can be devastating to a stallion's reproductive career. However, early assessment and detection of the extent of tissue damage and timely aggressive treatment can lead to successful return to normal activity. With loss of penile function and in situations with marked tissue disruption, several surgical options can be considered to return a horse to health and satisfactory hygiene.

References

1. van Harreveld PD, Gaughan EM et al: Penile surgery in horses. Comp Cont Educ Pract Vet 1998; 20(8):739-746.
2. Threlfall WR: Traumatic conditions of the penis and prepuce. In White NA II, Moore JM (eds): Current Practice of Equine Surgery, Philadelphia, JB Lippincott, pp 726-730, 1990.
3. Hyland J, Church S: The use of ultrasonography in the diagnosis and treatment of a haematoma in the corpus cavernosum penis of a stallion. 1995; Aust Vet J 72(12):468-469.
4. Perkins NR, Frazer GS: Reproductive emergencies in the stallion. Vet Clin North Am Equine Pract 1994; 10(3):671-683.
5. Wilson DV, Nickels FA, Williams MA: Pharmacologic treatment of priapism in two horses. J Am Vet Med Assoc 1991; 199(9):1183-1184.
6. Clem MF, DeBowes RM: Paraphimosis in horses, Part 2. Compend Contin Educ Pract Vet 1989; 11(2):184-188.
7. Simmons HA, Cox JE, Edwards GB et al: Paraphimosis in seven debilitated horses. Vet Rec 1985; 116:126-127.
8. Pearson H, Weaver BM: Priapism after sedation, neuroleptanalgesia and anaesthesia in the Horse. Equine Vet J 1978; 10(5):85-90.
9. Schumacher J, Hardin DK: Surgical treatment of priapism in a stallion. Vet Surg 1987; 16(3):193-196.
10. Lucke JN, Sansom J: Penile erection in the horse after acepromazine. Vet Rec 1979; 105(1):21-22.
11. Sharrock AG: Reversal of drug-induced priapism in a gelding by medication. Aust Vet J 1982; 58(1):39-40.
12. Gatewood DM, Cox JH, DeBowes RM: Diagnosis and treatment of acquired pathologic conditions of the equine penis and prepuce. Compend Contin Educ Pract Vet 1989; 11(12): 1498-1504.
13. Schumacher J, Vaughan JT: Surgery of the penis and prepuce. Vet Clin North Am Equine Pract 1988; 4(3):473-491.

CHAPTER 37

Significance of Bacteria Affecting the Stallion's Reproductive System

H. STEVE CONBOY

The stallion's genitalia and semen are often cultured as part of a breeding soundness examination, to satisfy import/export requirements, as a routine following breeding, or as part of a prepurchase examination. When bacteria are found on the external genitalia or in the semen it is important but often difficult to define the significance of such findings. The external genitalia of the stallion have a normal flora of bacteria that is thought to aid in resisting colonization of pathogens. The internal sex glands and associated urinary system are normally free of bacteria. It has been demonstrated that disturbing this flora of the external genitalia with chemical or antibacterial soaps can lead to the establishment of pathogenic organisms.[1-3]

Bacteria on the stallion's genitalia can be extremely significant in some cases and questionable to insignificant in others. The determining factors include the species of bacteria, the location of the bacteria, the relative number of bacteria, and the persistence of the bacteria. The presence of bacteria within the internal reproductive system of the stallion is associated with infection and is often quite difficult to treat.

Certain pathogenic bacteria are known to colonize the external genitalia and on occasion cause a true infection in the stallion, resulting in shedding of the bacteria during breeding or in the semen used for artificial insemination. Such bacteria reduce fertility and have the potential of infecting susceptible mares. Representatives of this group include the genus *Klebsiella* and *Pseudomonas*.[4] *Taylorella equigenitalis* colonizes the external genitalia of the stallion and is capable of causing severe endometritis in the mare but is not known to cause true genital infection in the stallion.[5] Other pathogenic bacteria that are known to colonize the external genitalia are *Streptococcus zooepidemicus* and *Escherichia coli*.[3] Special diagnostic features, treatment, and control measures of these bacteria will be discussed.

CULTURING THE STALLION

Culture samples should be taken from the unwashed, fully erect penis, the preejaculatory fluids, and an antiseptically collected semen sample. In the case of semen to be frozen, cultures should be taken from the extended semen just before being placed in the freezing straws.

Fresh cooled semen should be cultured periodically, if not on each shipment, to ensure that the extender antibiotics have killed all bacteria. The culture swabs should be placed in a transport media such as Amies and kept cool while being transported to the laboratory without delay. In the case of fastidious bacteria such as *T. equigenitalis,* cultures should be immediately refrigerated and sent to the laboratory as quickly as possible (ideally less than 24 hours). The stallion is presented to an estrous mare to stimulate erection, and the penis is rinsed with warm water and dried with a paper towel (soap and disinfectants will lessen the chance of bacterial isolation). Culture swabs are obtained from the fossa glandis, the urethral orifice, and the skin of the penis and the preputial folds. By briskly rubbing the glands of the penis, a preejaculatory fluid sample can be obtained from the distal urethra. Following semen collection, a postejaculation urethral sample is obtained by grasping the penis above the glands and inserting a sterile swab just inside the urethral orifice. A swab is then taken of the fresh semen. While semen samples are unavoidably contaminated with bacteria from the penis and prepuce,[6] the finding of large numbers of bacteria is highly suggestive of internal gland or urethral infection. This is particularly true if the semen isolates are inconsistent with the external genital cultures.[1,7]

TAYLORELLA EQUIGENITALIS (CONTAGIOUS EQUINE METRITIS ORGANISM)

Contagious equine metritis (CEM) was first reported from Newmarket, England, in 1977, where it caused a very serious outbreak of equine metritis. The causative organism was identified as a gram-negative microaerophilic coccobacillus that was named *Taylorella equigenitalis*. One year later two stallions imported from France were found to be asymptomatic carriers after initiating an outbreak of CEM on several breeding farms in Kentucky.[8] The significance of this outbreak is reflected by the imposed quarantine by the United States Department of Agriculture (USDA) that stopped the movement of all horses into and out of Kentucky until the disease was completely eradicated. A subsequent Code of Practice was developed by the State of Kentucky to prevent reintroduction of CEM. This code continues to be enforced 24 years later and has been adopted by several other states. The USDA also maintains stringent import requirements for mares and stallions desiring to enter the United States.[9]

Pathogenesis

The CEM organism (CEMO) is transmitted sexually between mares and stallions, but only the mare becomes infected. The stallion is considered an asymptomatic carrier. The organism may also be transmitted by contaminated instruments such as nondisposable vaginal speculums, rubber gloves, buckets, etc., and by contaminated frozen or fresh cooled semen.[8] The organism is capable of eroding the uterine epithelium, causing severe endometrial damage. A purulent discharge is commonly seen for up to 2 weeks followed by gradual healing and elimination of the organism. Fertility is greatly reduced, and, while uncommon, abortions have been reported.[10,11] Infected mares that carry to term have been known to have infected placentas.[12] The organism has been cultured from the vulva of fillies and the penis of colts from infected dams. These offspring are considered potential carriers of the CEMO.[13] Recovery is usually associated with restored fertility, but a significant number of recovered mares become chronic carriers and are capable of spreading the disease sexually. The organism can be recovered from the endometrium, clitoral fossa, and sinus of carrier mares. In the case of the stallion, the organism can be found in several locations on the penis (fossa glandis, urethral orifice, the skin of the penis, the preputial folds) and in preejaculatory fluids. All isolates of CEMO have been pathogenic to Thoroughbreds.[14]

Diagnosis

Bacterial isolation and serologic examination are used to confirm a diagnosis of CEM. Serologic evaluation is limited to the mare because there is no immune response in the stallion. Test breeding healthy mares is also used to identify carrier stallions.[15] This procedure is mandatory in the case of importing stallions into the United States. Following breeding, these mares are cultured and tested serologically at the appropriate time.

Culturing the organism from the stallion or the mare is the accepted method of diagnosing CEM.[16] In the case of the stallion, the unwashed erect penis is swabbed at the fossa glandis, the urethral orifice, the skin of the penis, the preputial folds, and preejaculatory fluid. If semen is available, it is also cultured. The mare's clitoral fossa and sinuses, as well as her endometrium, are swabbed. The culture swabs are placed in a transport media (Amies with charcoal) and refrigerated. They should be plated within 24 hours. The organism is fastidious, requiring special media and conditions for growth. Only a laboratory that is certified to culture *T. equigenitalis* should process samples. Suspect cases should be submitted to a reference laboratory for confirmation.[17]

The media of choice is chocolate agar with 10% horse blood and antibiotics to inhibit growth of contaminants. The plates are incubated at 37°C in 10% CO_2. Growth should occur by 48 hours, but negative samples should be held for 7 days. At 48 hours the colonies appear pinpoint,

grayish, and smooth bordered. At 72 hours the colonies are glossy, raised, and have elevated opaque centers.[18]

Smears from acute cases stained with Gram's or Giemsa reveal coccobacillus either free or inside of neutrophils. Diagnosis by this method should be confirmed by bacterial isolation.[19]

A complement fixation (CF) test is useful in monitoring mares bred to suspect stallions. This test is based on detecting antibodies resulting from exposure. The immune response requires 10 to 15 days after exposure before a positive test will occur, and then the antibodies are only reliable for 40 days. Therefore samples taken before 15 days post exposure may miss an infected mare, and those taken after 40 days may fail to identify a CEM carrier.[20,21] This test is routinely applied to mares between 15 and 40 days post breeding to imported stallions and to mares that follow the breeding of an imported mare.

A serum agglutination test (SAT) has been described that is reported to be very diagnostic in the acute phase of infection of the mare, but it also is not useful in the stallion.[22]

Other serologic tests that have been developed for diagnosing CEM include an enzyme-linked immunosorbent assay (ELISA), a passive hemagglutination (PHA), and an immunofluorescence test. But the CF test remains the serologic test of choice in the United States to date (2003).

Treatment

Stallions are treated by washing the erect penis and prepuce with a 4% chlorhexidine soap followed by coating the dried penis (including the fossa glandis) with an antimicrobial ointment such as nitrofurazone. When this treatment is administered for 5 consecutive days during sexual rest, it is usually successful.[14] Follow-up testing should include reculturing the stallion and breeding of test mares. The test mares are cultured and CF tested after being bred.[23]

Prevention

CEM is a reportable disease in the United States. The USDA has created measures to discourage the introduction of stallions and mares that are carriers of CEM. The greatest threat of introducing this disease is by horse owners who bring a mare or stallion into the United States for purposes other than breeding and circumvent the import test requirements for breeding animals. After these horses have completed their show or racing careers they are often used for breeding without thought of CEM testing. The results could be devastating to the equine industry. The second most likely source of acquiring this disease is from an improperly tested imported mare or stallion. Unfortunately, this situation has happened on more than one occasion, but, fortunately, the error has been quickly detected by regulatory tests within the United States.

Stallion and mare managers must be vigilant in screening mares and stallions in their breeding programs to prevent the introduction of this infection. The practice of requiring all imported mares and stallions to be CEM tested before breeding and CF testing at least the next three mares that follow the breeding of an imported mare greatly reduces the risk of introducing this bacterium into one's breeding operation. The use of antibiotic (gentamicin) semen extenders in an artificial insemination program will most likely prevent the spread of this organism.[8] Stringent hygienic practices that include the use of sterile or disposable equipment are essential to every breeding program. In countries where this disease has become endemic, the adoption of a well-designed code of practice has resulted in the signification reduction of CEM.

KLEBSIELLA PNEUMONIAE

Klebsiella pneumoniae is frequently found in the environment in soil and on vegetation (especially wood shavings and sawdust).[24] There are several pathogenic strains and many nonpathogenic strains, which makes assessing significance to positive cultures in the stallion difficult.

Pathogenesis

Klebsiella is frequently cultured from the feces, respiratory system, and reproductive system of the horse.[25] This organism is classified by its capsule type. There are 77 capsule types reported (K1-K72, K74, K79-K82).[26] Types K1, K2, and K5 have been most frequently associated with equine metritis.[27] Capsule type K1, which has been predominately isolated from equine metritis, is rarely found on the stallion's genitalia. Type K7 has been found to be less capable of causing metritis but along with K5 is the most frequent capsule type cultured from the stallion's genital tract. Capsule type K7 is thought to be part of the stallion's normal preputial flora.[28] One study found that in Draft breeds capsule type K39 was found to be the cause of metritis as opposed to type K1 in Thoroughbreds.[25] The same study found that following a period when CEM broke out in southwestern Japan (1980), there was an increase in equine metritis attributed to *K. pneumoniae* type K1 and a subsequent increased incidence of stallion isolations of *K. pneumoniae* type K1. This finding implies that the stallions became infected from the mares bred during this period. It is suggested that the increased incidence of *Klebsiella* metritis may be associated with the increased use of antibiotics to prevent the spread of CEM. *K. pneumoniae* is capable of causing genital infection,[1,29] but more frequently this organism establishes itself on the skin of the penis or the fossa glandis, where it is frequently found on routine culture.

Diagnosis

Stallions are cultured in the routine manner (see description in this chapter), and swabs are streaked onto blood agar, where under aerobic conditions it produces nonhemolytic mucoid colonies. When placed on MacConkey's agar, *K. pneumoniae* is seen as pink mucoid colonies. Gram's stain reveals gram-negative rods. Further biochemical tests are conducted to confirm the identification.[30] To identify the specific capsule type the isolate is subcultured for purity and then grown on Worfel-Ferguson medium to swell the capsules. An immunofluorescent stain with fluorescein isothiocyanate-labeled sera is used to differentiate the capsule type.[31]

After a positive culture of *K. pneumoniae* from the stallion's genitalia or semen is identified, a decision regarding the culture's significance must then be made. If the reason for culturing the stallion in the first place was because a number of his mares were suffering from poor fertility and demonstrated metritis associated with *K. pneumoniae*, it would be safe to assume that the isolate was indeed pathogenic. On the other hand, if the isolate was found on a routine culture, it would be prudent to determine the capsule type and its potential pathogenicity before initiating treatment or rejecting the stallion. If it is determined that the capsule type is indeed a pathogenic strain, test mares should be bred to the stallion to determine if in fact the stallion will infect mares. It has been reported that in many cases where both stallion and mares cultured positive for *K. pneumoniae* the capsule types were in fact different. In these cases the findings were considered unrelated.[32]

Treatment

Klebsiella infections are very resistant to treatment, and reoccurrence of contamination or infection is common. Antibiotic creams or ointments containing aminoglycosides have been advocated but can cause significant irritation to the skin and urethra. The sterilization affect of harsh treatments leave the penis susceptible to colonization by other pathogens.[33] Kenny and Cummings[34] have recommended the daily use of a genital rinse with a dilute solution of sodium hypochlorite for 2 weeks. This solution is made by adding 40 ml of bleach to 1 gallon of water. Smegma is removed before rinsing.[34] In refractory cases, sexual rest for 3 to 6 months may be effective therapy.[1]

Many stallions have been successfully managed by using the "minimum contamination technique" as developed by Kenny or through the use of artificial insemination. Each of these techniques uses antibiotics to kill the bacteria in the semen. In the case of the "minimum contamination technique" an antibiotic extender is placed in the mare's uterus just before natural cover. With artificial insemination, contaminated semen is allowed to incubate in an antibiotic extender for at least 20 minutes before insemination.[35] Postbreeding infusion with an aminoglycoside such as gentamicin has also been used. A formula containing 10 ml gentamicin, 10 ml sodium bicarbonate, and 10 ml physiologic saline can be safely infused into the uterus as soon as 4 hours post breeding.

Prevention

Proper hygiene is the most import factor in preventing the contamination or infection of the stallion's genitalia. Vigorous scrubbing with soaps or detergents destroys the normal flora of nonpathogenic bacteria on the penis, which allows the colonization of pathogens. Stallions should therefore be washed only occasionally and simply rinsed with clean water before and after mating.[33] Care must be taken to prevent an environment that is conducive to the growth of bacteria. Standing water and manure, as well as damp bedding (sawdust, straw, or shavings), create a perfect media for bacterial growth. Stallion managers should enforce a strict requirement of a negative uterine culture before each natural breeding. Microscopic examination of dismount samples will reveal neutrophils from infected mares, alerting managers to the possible exposure to pathogens. Stallions with heavy breeding schedules should be cultured routinely to detect a change in genital microflora that might indicate a pathogen.

PSEUDOMONAS AERUGINOSA

Pseudomonas aeruginosa is a gram-negative rod that is frequently found on the skin and external genitalia of both the mare and the stallion. The organism is found in warm damp locations and in standing water. Although *P. aeruginosa* can exist without causing infection, it is capable of infecting both stallions and mares.[36-38] This organism is classified by serotype and phage type and further classified by its ability to cause hemolysis. Those strains that produce hemolysins are considered infective, whereas those that do not are considered environmental.[39]

Pathogenesis

Like *Klebsiella*, *Pseudomonas* species can exist on both the mare and the stallion without causing pathologic conditions. Although it is quite common to isolate *Pseudomonas* from the stallion's penis without signs of infertility, the isolation of *P. aeruginosa* should be considered significant because, when the situation is right (skin or mucosal damage), the organism can become highly infective and very difficult to treat. *P. aeruginosa,* unlike other pseudomonads, is capable of producing damaging enzymes, as well as hemolysins, that enhance its ability to infect tissue. The pathologic effect is caused by extracellular toxins, and the production of these toxins is enhanced in the presence of damaged tissue.[40,41] Although there are numerous reports of groups of mares being infected (demonstrated by endometritis) by a stallion, mares that have genital trauma from foaling or mating are more susceptible than healthy mares.[37] Once infected, mares may develop a severe endometritis with a purulent discharge or frequently show only a mild metritis that is revealed on culture. Failure to conceive or early return to estrus is common.[42] Occasionally mares will conceive and abort from a placentitis later in gestation. In the case of abortion the organism can usually be recovered from the fetus and the placenta. Stallions that are mated to infected mares effectively transmit this organism to other mares.[43] Frequent washing of the stallion's penis destroys the normal skin flora and predisposes the penis to persistent colonization with *Pseudomonas* or other pathogens.[33]

Diagnosis

Aerobic culture is the diagnostic method of choice. Its fluorescent trait makes it visible under a Wood's light, but other nonpathogenic species of pseudomonads are also fluorescent, making this test unreliable.

P. aeruginosa produces greenish colonies on blood agar and pink colonies on MacConkey's agar. Its ability to grow at 41°C distinguishes it from the other pseudomonads, including *Pseudomonas fluorescens*. Some isolates take at least 48 hours to grow on blood agar, making it necessary to maintain plates for 48 hours or longer.[30] Serotyping and phage typing are more difficult and are not deemed necessary to justify treatment. Although both stallions and mares respond to a hemoagglutination test, results are too inconsistent for it to be useful.[43]

Treatment

Treating the stallion for *Pseudomonas* can be quite frustrating and prolonged. Apparent recovery is often followed by reoccurrence.[1] Aminoglycoside ointments are generally irritating to the skin and mucosa, and the transurethral infusion of even dilute solutions of aminoglycosides can cause severe irritation. One reported successful protocol uses an iodine-base surgical scrub followed by the application of a 1% silver sulfadiazine cream to the dried erect penis daily for 2 weeks.[44] Therapy can be monitored with a Wood's light. This therapy is followed by serial cultures to confirm success. Periodic cultures should be taken to detect reoccurrence. Another suggested treatment is to rinse the erect penis in a dilute solution of HCl that is made by adding 10 ml of HCl to a gallon of water. After the smegma has been removed from the penis, it is rinsed daily for 2 weeks, paying particular attention to the fossa glandis. If irritation occurs, the dilution is reduced by 20% increments until it is tolerated.[34] Once again, progress can be monitored with a Wood's light and cultures used to confirm success. A similar rinse can be used on a recovered stallion after each mating.

Stallions that fail to respond with a complete recovery can be managed with a "minimal contamination technique."[35]

Prevention

As in the case of preventing other bacterial infections, good hygiene is imperative. Strict enforcement of culture requirements for visiting mares should be mandatory. Instead of being washed, the stallion's penis should be rinsed with clear water before and after mating. The use of a dilute HCl rinse may be considered where infection has previously occurred.

OTHER POTENTIAL BACTERIAL PATHOGENS

The relationship of β-hemolytic streptococci (*S. zooepidemicus* and *Streptococcus equisimilis*) and *E. coli* to pathogenesis in the stallion is debatable. Some researchers do not place much significance on finding these bacteria on the stallion's external genitalia, and there is no evidence of their infecting the internal genital tissues.[37] Others list them as potential pathogens associated with reduced fertility.[1,6,25,30] It is interesting to note in a retrospective study of prebreeding cultures in Kentucky that the organisms most often cultured from the cervix and uterus are *S. zooepidemicus, E. coli,* and *S. equisimilis*.[45] Another study indicated that the clitoral fossa and vestibule of clinically normal mares frequently harbored large numbers of *S. zooepidemicus* and *E. coli*.[46] These bacteria could be a source of contamination and colonization of the stallion's penis. The increase of positive uterine cultures as the breeding season progresses could very likely result from the stallion pushing these bacteria up the mare's reproductive tract during breeding, as well as the continued exposure of the penis to these bacteria as it passes the vulva and vestibule during breeding.

Other bacteria that are considered potential pathogens include *Bordetella bronchiseptica, Citrobacter* spp., *Enterobacter* spp., *Proteus mirabilis, Proteus morganii, Proteus rettgeri, Proteus vulgaris, Providencia* spp., *Pseudomonas* spp. (not *P. aeruginosa*), and *Staphylococcus aureus*.[6]

NONPATHOGENIC BACTERIA

It is generally accepted that the stallion has a normal flora of microbes colonized on the external genitalia.[1,2,6,33] Bacteria included in this group are α-hemolytic streptococci, *Lactobacillus* spp., *Micrococcus* spp., *Bacillus* spp., *Alcaligenes* spp., *Flavobacterium* spp., *Serratia* spp. coagulase-negative staphylococci (*Staphylococcus lentiscus, Staphylococcus coptis, Staphylococcus haemolyticus, Staphylococcus xylous*), and nonhemolytic *Klebsiella*.

The importance of these bacteria cannot be overemphasized because they are essential to the general health of the integumentum of the external genitalia. Disturbing this flora will allow other bacteria that are potential pathogens to colonize the stallion's penis.

References

1. Dowsett DF: Seminal abnormalities. In Robinson NE (ed): Current Therapy in Equine Medicine, Philadelphia, WB Saunders, 1987.
2. Madsen M, Christensen P: Bacterial flora of semen collected from Danish Warmblood stallions by artificial vagina. Acta Vet Scand 1995; 36:1-7.
3. Bowen JM: Venereal diseases of stallions. In Robinson NE (ed): Current Therapy in Equine Medicine, Philadelphia, WB Saunders, 1987.
4. Squires EL, McGlothin DE, Bowen RA et al: Use of antibiotics in stallion semen for control of *Klebsiella pneumoniae* and *Pseudomonas aeruginosa*. J Equine Vet Sci 1981; 1:43-48.
5. Crowhurst RC: Genital infections of mares. Vet Rec 1977; 100:476.
6. Simpson RB, Burns SJ, Snell JR: Microflora in stallion semen and their control with semen extender. Proceedings of the 21st Annual Convention of the American Association of Equine Practitioners, p 255, 1975.
7. Varner DD, Taylor, TS Blanchard T: Seminal vesiculitis. In McKinnon AO, Voss JL (eds): Equine Reproduction, Philadelphia/London, Lea & Febiger, 1993.
8. Timoney PJ, Powell DG: Contagious equine metritis: epidemiology and control. Equine Vet Sci 1988; 8(1): 42-45.
9. Code of Federal Regulations 92.301, Nov 1995.
10. Fontijne P, Terlack EA, Hartman EC: *Taylorella equigenitalis* isolated from an aborted foal. Vet Rec 1989; 125:485.
11. Nakashiroh H, Naruse M, Sugimoto C et al: Isolation of *Haemophilus equigenitalis* from an aborted foetus. Natl Inst Anim Health Q Tokyo 1981; 21:184-185.
12. Powell DG, Whitwell K: The epidemiology of contagious equine metritis (CEM) in England 1977-1978. J Reprod Fertil Suppl 1979; 27:331-335.
13. Timoney PJ, Powell DG: Isolation of contagious equine metritis organism from colts and fillies in the United Kingdom and Ireland. Vet Rec 1982; 111:478-482.
14. Couto MA, Hughes JP: Sexually transmitted (venereal) diseases of horses. In McKinnon AO, Voss JL (eds): Equine Reproduction, Philadelphia/London, Lea & Febiger, 1993.
15. Knowels RC, Hendricks JB, King DD et al: Contagious equine metritis. Mod Vet Pract Nov 1978; 819-822.
16. Brown, BS, Timoney PJ: Contagious equine metritis and fluorescens. Vet Rec 1988; 123:39 (letter).
17. Biberstein EL: *Taylorella equigenitalis*. In Carter JR, Cole TR Jr (eds): Diagnostic Procedures in Veterinary Bacteriology and Mycology, San Diego, Academic Press, 1990.
18. Swerczek TW: Contagious equine metritis: outbreak of the disease in Kentucky and laboratory methods for diagnosing the disease. J Reprod Fertil Suppl 1979; 27:361-365.
19. Powell DD: Contagious equine metritis. In Morrow DA (ed): Current Therapy in Theriogenology 2, pp 786-792, Philadelphia, WB Saunders, 1986.
20. Croxton-Smith J, Benson JA, Dawson FLM: A complement fixation test for antibody to the contagious equine metritis organism. Vet Rec 1978; 103:270-278.
21. Cummow B, Herr S, Brett OL: A short reliable highly reproducible complement fixation test for the serological diagnosis of contagious equine metritis. Onderstepoort J Vet Res 1978; 53:241-243.
22. Brewer RA: Contagious equine metritis: a review/summary. Vet Bull 1983; 53:889-891.
23. Code of Federal Regulations 92.304:318, Jan 1,1991.
24. Duncan DW, Razzell WE: *Klebsiella* biotypes among coliforms isolated from forest environments and from produce. Appl Microbiol 1972; 24:933.
25. Kikuchi N, Iguchi I, Hiramune T: Capsule types of *Klebsiella pneumoniae* isolated from the genital tract of mares with metritis, extra-genital sites of healthy mares and the genital tract of stallions. Vet Microbiol 1987; 15:219-228.
26. Orskov I: Genus V *Klebsiella*. In Krieg N, Holt JC (eds): Bergey's Manual of Systematic Bacteriology, vol 1, pp 461-465, Baltimore, 1984.
27. Greenwood RES, Ellis DR: *Klebsiella aerogenes* in mares. Vet Rec 1976; 99:439.
28. Platt H, Atherton JG, Orskov I: *Klebsiella* and *Enterobacter* organisms isolated from horses. J Hyg 1976; 77:401-408.
29. Couch JRF, Atherton JG, Platt H: Venereal transmission of *Klebsiella pneumoniae* in a Thoroughbred stud from a persistently infected stallion. Vet Rec 1972; 90:21-24.
30. Ricketts SW, Young A, Medici EB: Uterine and clitoral cultures. In McKinnon AO, Voss JL (eds): Equine Reproduction, Philadelphia, Lea & Febiger, 1993.
31. Riser E, Noone P, Bonnet ML: A new serotyping method for *Klebsiella* species: development of the technique. J Clin Pathol 1976; 29:305-308.
32. Blanchard T, Kenney RM, Timoney PJ: Venereal diseases. Vet Clin North Am Equine Pract 1992; 8:191-203.
33. Jones RL: The effect of washing on the aerobic bacterial flora of the stallion's penis. Proceedings of the 30th Annual Convention of the American Association of Equine Practitioners, pp 9-16, 1984.
34. Kenny RM, Cummings MR: Potential control of stallion penile shedding of *Pseudomonas aeruginosa* and *Klebsiella pneumoniae*. Proceedings Symposium Vootplanting Pard, Gent, Belgium, 1990.
35. Kenny RM, Bergman RV, Cooper WL et al: Minimum contamination techniques for breeding mares: techniques and preliminary findings. Proceedings of the 21st Annual Convention of the American Association of Equine Practitioners, p 327, 1975.

36. Hughes JP, Asbury AC, Loy RG et al: The occurrence of *Pseudomonas* in the reproductive tract of stallions and its effect on fertility. Cornell Vet 1967; 57:53-69.

37. Hughes JP, Loy RG: The relationship of infection to infertility in the mare and stallion. Equine Vet J 1975; 7:157-159.

38. Hughes JP, Loy RG, Asbury AC et al: The occurrence of *Pseudomonas* in the reproductive tract of mares and its effect on fertility. Cornell Vet 1966; 56:595.

39. Al-Dujaili AH, Harris DM: *Pseudomonas aeruginosa* infections in hospitals: a comparison between "infective" and "environmental" strains. J Hyg (Lond) 1975; 75:195.

40. Liu PV: Factors that influence toxigenicity of *Pseudomonas aeruginosa*. J Bacteriol 1964; 88:1421-1427.

41. Liu PV: The roles of various fractions of *Pseudomonas aeruginosa* in pathogenesis: the effects of lecithinase and protease. J Infect Dis 1966; 116:112-116.

42. Simpson DJ: Venereal diseases of mares. In Robinson NE (ed): Current Therapy in Equine Medicine 2, Philadelphia, WB Saunders, 1987.

43. Atherton JG, Pitt TL: Types of *Pseudomonas aeruginosa* isolated from horses. Equine Vet J 1982; 14(4):329-332.

44. Johnson TL, Kenney RM, McGee WR et al: Pseudomonas infection in a stallion: a case report. Proceedings of the 26th Annual Convention of the American Association of Equine Practitioners, p 111, 1980.

45. Donahue M: Bacterial isolates from mares' reproductive tracts. Equine Dis Q 1994; 2:3-4.

46. Hindricks K, Cummings MR, Sertich PL et al: Clinical significance of aerobic bacterial flora of the uterus, vagina, vestibule and clitoral fossa of clinically normal mares. J Am Vet Med Assoc 1988; 193(1):72-75.

Chapter 38

The Subfertile Stallion

TERRY L. BLANCHARD

Suboptimal pregnancy rates remain a serious problem within the horse industry. When performing breeding soundness examinations on stallions intended for stud service, more than one third of prospective breeding stallions fail the evaluation, most commonly due to ejaculation of low numbers of normal, motile sperm.[1,2] Semen evaluations performed on stallions with lower than expected fertility often reveal similar findings. Unfortunately, the cause of ejaculation of low numbers of normal, motile sperm by stallions usually remains undetermined and, thus, is often medically untreatable.[3-5] Alteration in breeding management of stallions ejaculating low numbers of normal, motile sperm is therefore usually directed primarily at limiting the number of matings required of the stallion (i.e., number of mares booked to the stallion and number of matings per estrous cycle) to ensure that an optimal number of normal, motile sperm are used for each breeding.[4,6] Other methods of breeding management can also be tried in an attempt to improve fertility. Certainly there are many other factors that can contribute to lower than expected fertility in stallions in natural service mating programs. This chapter will discuss the economic impact of reduced stallion fertility, use of record analyses to assess the degree of subfertility, and some of the more commonly used management techniques used for stallions with suboptimal fertility in natural service mating programs.

ECONOMIC IMPACT OF LOWERED FERTILITY

A stallion with suboptimal pregnancy rates greatly increases the cost of producing foals from his book of mares. The increased costs associated with a stallion's lowered fertility arise from (1) increased mare expenses (e.g., extra covers, extra transport of mares to breeding sheds, extra veterinary examinations/treatments, and additional boarding fees required for mares left at a breeding farm/facility over repeated estrous cycles), (2) wasted maintenance costs associated with support of mares that do not produce foals; and (3) decreased income (e.g., from sale of penalized, late-born foals that arise from mares not becoming pregnant early in the year; lost income from failure to produce a foal; and lost income from nonproductive stud fees). Thus, the economic impact associated with breeding of a stallion with lowered fertility can be substantial.

The following example is used to further illustrate the magnitude of losses that can occur with just a 20% dif-ference in pregnancy rate. If a stallion bred a book of 100 mares (using only 1 cover per estrus) and achieved a 60% pregnancy rate per cycle over a total of 3 estrous cycles, the stallion would achieve a 93% seasonal pregnancy rate requiring a total of 156 covers. By contrast, if only a 40% pregnancy rate per cycle was achieved, the stallion would achieve a 78% seasonal pregnancy rate requiring a total of 196 covers (Box 38-1). The lower fertility would culminate in an extra 40 estrous cycles of breeding and their associated board and veterinary expenses over the course of the breeding season yet produce 15 fewer foals (assuming all pregnancies result in live foals), as well as an additional 15 years of nonproductive maintenance expense (15 additional barren mares). If the boarding fee at the breeding farm is $26 per day, the 40 extra estrous cycles of breeding (21 days/cycle) result in an extra cost of $21,840 compared to the cost for the higher level of fertility. If veterinary fees average $250 for examinations and treatments per cycle, the 40 extra estrous cycles of breeding result in increased veterinary fees of $10,000 over that for the higher level of fertility. The cost of the lower fertility in this example totals $31,840 and still does not include lost income from 15 stud fees, maintenance expense for 15 extra barren mares for 1 year, or lost income from 15 foals that will not be produced. While expenses, fees, and sale prices vary, this example serves to stress the importance of maximizing reproductive efficiency of the stallion.

SOME FACTORS THAT AFFECT STALLION FERTILITY

The veterinarian must remain cognizant that there are many factors that contribute to the overall fertility of a stallion, including inherent fertility of the stallion, inherent fertility of the mares bred by the stallion, and quality of management (e.g., nutrition and body condition, teasing and breeding management, level of veterinary care, etc.). Each contributing factor is capable of severely constraining the percentage and number of offspring produced each year by a given stallion. One should therefore not assume that lower than expected pregnancy outcome must be due to a problem with stallion fertility unless record analyses and examination findings, along with a thorough evaluation of mating practices, support this conclusion.

Investigation of suboptimal fertility in a stallion should be directed toward identifying and correcting contributing factors. In some cases, treatment of a disease condition (e.g., infection, ejaculatory dysfunction, etc.) may improve the stallion's fertility.[7] In other cases, no

Box   38-1

Influence of 2 (40%, 60%) Theoretical Pregnancy Rates per Cycle (PR/Cycle) on Number of Covers Required to Complete 3 Estrous Cycles of Breeding and Seasonal Pregnancy Rate (SPR) for a Stallion Mated to 100 Mares by Natural Cover

Fertility Achieved per Cycle and per Season with Theoretical 40% PR/cycle*
Lower Theoretical Fertility

100 mares bred 1st cycle × 40% PR/cycle = 40 mares pregnant on 1st cycle of breeding	100 covers
60 mares bred 2nd cycle × 40% PR/cycle = 24 mares pregnant on 2nd cycle of breeding	60 covers
36 mares bred 3rd cycle × 40% PR/cycle = 14 mares pregnant on 3rd cycle of breeding	36 covers
Total mares pregnant after 3 cycles of breeding	78
No. barren mares	22
Total no. covers for season	196

Higher Theoretical Fertility

100 mares bred 1st cycle × 60% PR/cycle = 60 mares pregnant on 1st cycle	100 covers
40 mares bred 2nd cycle × 60% PR/cycle = 24 mares pregnant on 2nd cycle	40 covers
16 mares bred 3rd cycle × 60% PR/cycle = 9 mares pregnant on 3rd cycle	16 covers
Total mares pregnant after 3 cycles of breeding	93
No. barren mares	7
Total no. covers for season	156

Assuming only 1 cover is required per estrus, and all pregnancies result in production of viable foals, the lower level of fertility would result in 40 extra covers throughout the season, yet produce 15 fewer foals (i.e., 15 more barren mares).
*No. mares bred per cycle × theoretical PR/cycle = no. mares pregnant.

treatment is indicated for the stallion, yet quality of the mare book will preclude significant improvement in fertility. More commonly, recommendations for altering breeding management practices can be made to improve the stallion's fertility. The following discussion is provided to aid the veterinarian in developing a breeding management plan that could maximize the fertility of a stallion with lower than expected pregnancy rates.

Historical Considerations

To assess potential changes in reproductive management in an effort to enhance fertility of a given stallion, it is important to first obtain a meaningful history. An assessment of past breeding performance (assuming the stallion has been bred previously) is a good place to start, since previous fertility is one of the best predictors of future fertility.[8] The number of seasons the stallion has been in service and whether/when any changes in fertility occurred provide useful historical information. Congenital problems that result in poor fertility are often evident from the first season the stallion is used for breeding, while acquired problems (trauma, deterioration in physical condition, occurrence of disease[s], or management changes) often result in a decline in fertility when compared to previous seasons or months within a given season. Age-related decline in a stallion's fertility is often gradual in onset, although the difference in pregnancy rates achieved from one year to the next can be dramatic if it is due to progressive testicular degeneration.[9]

Owners or managers of stallions may only provide impressions based on a few salient observations (e.g., a low seasonal pregnancy rate), which are usually insufficient to support meaningful conclusions about fertility. It is therefore incumbent on the veterinarian to thoroughly evaluate breeding records to characterize the fertility problem. If breeding records do not exist, meaningful evaluation can seldom be performed. Poorly organized records can make the task arduous or even impossible. Even the more modern computerized record systems will require some reorganization and summarizing of salient fertility endpoints to ensure a given stallion's fertility is adequately characterized.[10]

Do not hesitate to request records from previous years to substantiate whether a given stallion's fertility has changed or a decline in fertility occurred as a result of deteriorating quality of the mare book. It is common for first-year stallions to have a demanding book, with many high-quality mares. After the first or second season, and until/unless the stallion's offspring prove themselves, it becomes more difficult to fill his book. Thus, as the stallion's popularity declines, his book tends to accumulate fewer young, fertile mares and an increasing proportion of mares with lower fertility (Table 38-1). This changing quality of the mares in his book will many times explain a decline in fertility.[10]

The number of mares bred by the stallion in each season is another important consideration in assessing potential causes of lowered fertility. Pickett et al[6] estimated that a minimum of 40 mares must be bred in order to adequately evaluate the stallion's fertility. Many stallions do not breed a sufficient number of mares to adequately test their inherent fertility.[11] The veterinarian should be cautious in concluding that a stallion that breeds a limited number of mares does in fact have lowered fertility.

Table 38-1

Influence of Declining Quality of Mare Book on Fertility Achieved by a Thoroughbred Stallion in 2 Consecutive Years

Year	Class of Mare	No. Bred	No. Pregnant	No. Cycles	PR/Cycle	PR/Season
1	Barren	6	6	9	67%	100%
	Foaling	49	42	59	71%	86%
	Maiden	4	4	5	80%	100%
	Not bred	3	3	4	75%	100%
	Slipped	9	6	15	40%	67%
	Total	71	61	92	66%	86%
2	Barren	10	5	18	28%	50%
	Foaling	16	13	18	72%	81%
	Maiden	9	8	11	73%	89%
	Not bred	3	2	3	67%	67%
	Slipped	2	2	3	67%	100%
	Total	40	30	53	57%	75%

Seasonal pregnancy rate (PR/season) declined from 86% to 75%, and overall pregnancy rate/cycle (PR/cycle) declined from 66% to 57%. The lower than expected seasonal pregnancy rate in the second year was most likely due to 2 problems that are apparent from examining the records: (1) Low fertility in the barren mare group in year 2, which comprised one fourth of his book. Note that the PR/cycle was quite good in other classes of mares in year 2, and comparable in foaling and maiden mares (typically the most fertile classes of mares) both years. (2) Insufficient opportunity to rebreed mares that did not become pregnant. In this regard, note that only 53 cycles were used to cover the total book of 40 mares in year 2. The PR/cycle among other (than barren) classes of mares in year 2 varied from 67% to 73%; thus, if more opportunities had existed for covering those mares not becoming pregnant on the first cycle in those groups, seasonal pregnancy rate might not have been so low.

Regardless of the stallion's fertility level, in order to achieve a high seasonal pregnancy rate, it is important that the stallion has access to mares early in the season and that nonpregnant mares are returned for service in a timely manner (i.e., so that return service opportunities are not missed).[10] Few breeding operations consist entirely of highly fertile mares that will all become pregnant on 1 service. As a stallion's popularity declines, his stud fee usually follows. With less at stake, many mare owners are likely to take fewer precautions to ensure their mare is in good prebreeding condition, is having regular estrous cycles with no reproductive problems, is bred at the optimal time during estrus, has adequate prebreeding and postbreeding veterinary care in order to optimize establishment of pregnancy, and has early pregnancy diagnosis performed to ensure that if she fails to become pregnant, she is returned for service promptly at her next estrus. When a stallion's book of mares is afflicted with too many poorly managed mares, record analyses will reveal too many nonlactating (maiden, barren, slipped and not-bred) mares being bred only once, often quite late in the season. Additionally, breeding intervals between services for mares failing to become pregnant may be extended beyond the normal 3 week (18-24 day) inter-estrus interval. By contrast, a popular stallion with a high stud fee will begin breeding the majority of the nonlactating mares early in the breeding season.[11] This allows ample opportunity to get most of the nonlactating mares pregnant, even if mating on the first estrus is unsuccessful, and breeding intervals for the majority of

mares that fail to become pregnant on 1 service will mostly fall in a normal 18 to 24 day inter-estrus window. Finally, good veterinary care will ensure that mares are bred near to time of ovulation, thus resulting in a low percentage of mares in the book requiring multiple covers per estrus. If the number of covers per estrus is high, poor reproductive management (e.g., faulty teasing program, examinations performed too infrequently to reliably predict optimal time for mating, failure to use ovulation-inducing drugs to ensure ovulation near to time of mating, etc.) should be suspected as a problem contributing to lowered fertility of a stallion.

Mating Frequency

One question that often arises is whether diminishment of mating frequency would improve fertility of a stallion with suboptimal pregnancy rates. Because the influence of mating frequency on fertility achieved is a highly stallion-dependent phenomenon, no firm answer can be given without evaluation of the outcome achieved from a sufficient number of matings performed at different frequencies. Successful breeding seasons, in spite of the dramatic increase in Thoroughbred mare book sizes in the last decade, lead one to the conclusion that most stallions with normal testes size and semen quality can mate mares several times each day (assuming libido and mating ability are good) and still maintain good fertility. However, comparing pregnancy rates among days with differing numbers of covers may reveal whether breeding frequency

Table 38-2

Influence of Size of Mare Book and Frequency of Mating on Fertility (PR/Cycle) Achieved by 3 Thoroughbred Stallions during 1 Breeding Season

	STALLION		
	1	2	3
Book size	184	170	88
Seasonal PR	95%	95%	80%
Overall PR/cycle	64%	67%	49%
PR/cycle on days with 1 cover	80%	69%	48%
PR/cycle on days with 2 covers	60%	66%	65%
PR/cycles on days with 3 covers	67%	68%	44%
PR/cycle on days with 4 covers	72%	69%	41%
PR/cycle on 1st cover of day	72%	75%	49%
PR/cycle on 2nd cover of day	70%	60%	56%
PR/cycle on 3rd cover of day	60%	60%	44%
PR/cycle on 4th cover of day	65%	80%	20%
PR/cycle when ≥6 covers in preceding 3 days	67%	66%	43%
PR/cycle when ≥9 covers in preceding 3 days	59%	71%	29%

Stallion 3 (with a smaller book) appeared to suffer decline in pregnancy rates when more than 2 mares were covered per day, while high mating frequencies for stallions 1 and 2 (with larger books) did not appear to lower pregnancy rates to a level that would suggest they would benefit by constraining breeding frequency.

alters fertility of a given stallion (i.e., provide justification for limiting the number of covers per day to maximize opportunity for pregnancy establishment) (Table 38-2).

GENERAL MANAGEMENT STRATEGIES FOR STALLIONS WITH SUBOPTIMAL PREGNANCY RATES

Good breeding management practices, which should be common among all well-run breeding farms, become critical to the management of a stallion with suboptimal pregnancy rates if a substantial number of mares are to be bred. Mares should be in good body condition, free of genital infections, and have regular estrous cycles early in the breeding season so that nonlactating and early-foaling mares can become pregnant early, thus lessening the mating load later in the season when the preponderance of foaling mares are ready to breed. Frequent examinations (at least every other day initially, and once daily as the mare nears ovulation) and the use of ovulation-inducing hormones are essential in order to ensure that matings are not wasted and thus maximize the number of sperm that are available for each mare covered. The ascribed goal is to breed each mare as near to time of ovulation as possible. Postbreeding examination should be performed no later than the day after breeding to determine whether postbreeding endometritis/fluid accumulation is present and, if so, address it. Additionally, whether ovulation occurred or not should be recorded so that later record review can determine if mares were more likely to get pregnant when they ovulated sooner rather than later after breeding (e.g., 1 day, 2 days, etc.).

Management strategies employed with natural service mating programs using stallions with lowered fertility have included monitoring dismount samples for the presence of motile sperm and inflammatory cells to identify mares requiring a second cover or postbreeding treatment; infusion of semen extender into the uterus of the mare immediately prior to cover; impregnation (infusion of semen sample collected at dismount from the penis of the stallion immediately following cover); and purposeful multiple mating (doubling, tripling) of mares.

Monitoring of Dismount Semen Samples

Monitoring of dismount semen samples (collected as drippings from the stallion's urethra and appropriately diluted in a prewarmed semen extender) for the presence of motile sperm is a technique used to confirm that ejaculation occurred during a given cover. While it is rare for a stallion to exhibit behavioral and physiological signs of ejaculation yet fail to ejaculate, microscopic examination of the dismount semen sample will reveal few or no sperm present if ejaculation did not occur. In most instances, the stallion will promptly achieve another erection and cover the mare again within a few minutes. Repeating the mating sequence will thus improve the chance that the mare will become pregnant. The procedure is also useful for identifying incomplete ejaculates that some stallions occasionally deliver. Fortunately, the stallion that only occasionally incompletely ejaculates will likewise promptly achieve another erection and cover the mare again.

Routine examination of dismount samples is also useful for screening changing semen quality over the course of the season. If sperm concentration, motility, and morphology in dismount semen samples consistently declines, breeding soundness evaluation of the stallion may be in order, and potential treatment or changes in breeding management might then be considered. The reader is cautioned against making judgments based on examination of only 1 or 2 dismount samples, as poor sperm concentration or motility may be related more to the quality of the sample collected than to the ejaculate. In such cases, odds for development of pregnancy are just as good for the occasional cover with a poor quality dismount as with other covers for that stallion. It is the consistent decline in semen quality of dismount samples from a stallion that previously had good quality dismounts that should raise concern. Paying close attention to incoming reports of pregnancy outcome by date of cover will confirm whether concern is justified.

Monitoring of dismount samples for presence of inflammatory cells is also a useful undertaking. The occasional presence of a high number of neutrophils in a dismount semen sample suggests that the mare is the source of inflammation. Occasionally, a mare is identified that has an underlying genital infection that was not detected by routine prebreeding examination. The finding of a high number of neutrophils in dismount samples can therefore be used to alert the veterinarian to direct post-breeding treatment(s) for the affected mare. If there is a consistent increase in inflammatory cell numbers in virtually all dismount samples from a stallion mating mares of good reproductive quality, the possibility that the stallion has an internal genital infection should be considered and explored. Likewise, if semen collected in an artificial vagina has increased numbers of inflammatory cells, further diagnostic procedures should be performed to determine the location and extent of the infection and to arrive at appropriate treatment modalities.[7]

Brief mention is made here of routine scheduled culturing of swabs collected from the distal urethra, fossa glandis, and shaft of the penis of stallions used in natural service programs because potential venereal pathogens are commonly harbored on the external genitalia. Swabs should be collected before washing and prior to covering the first mare of the day. Some Thoroughbred farms perform these screening cultures weekly, bi-weekly, or even monthly. The reader is cautioned against incriminating the stallion for carrying a venereal pathogen simply because *Pseudomonas aeruginosa* or *Klebsiella pneumoniae* are recovered on culture, because these organisms are common environmental contaminants of soil, stall bedding, and breeding shed floors. There are many phage types of *Pseudomonas* and many capsule types of *Klebsiella* that are nonpathogenic, so the determination that a stallion is a carrier of a venereal pathogen should not be made based on recovering one of these organisms on culture without other confirmatory evidence.[12] Certainly any stallion from which these organisms are recovered should be reswabbed to determine whether true colonization of the external genitalia has occurred. The reader is referred elsewhere[12] for a discussion of diagnosis and treatment of venereal diseases in the stallion.

Prebreeding Infusion of Semen Extender

Infusion of semen extender containing antibiotics into the uterus of the mare immediately prior to cover has been proposed as a method to control/prevent endometritis, particularly when potentially pathogenic bacteria are being shed in the semen (dubbed the minimum contamination technique[13]). Results of one clinical trial confirmed the technique was beneficial in preventing postbreeding endometritis and improving pregnancy rates when a stallion with an internal genital infection caused by *Pseudomonas aeruginosa* (previously confirmed to be venereally transmitted) was mated to reproductively normal mares.[14] Though unproven, infusion of prewarmed semen extender immediately prior to cover may be of value when a given stallion's sperm are of short livability *in vitro* (e.g., longevity of sperm motility is short [minutes] when maintained at room temperature as raw semen), or when "hostile" fluid accumulations are present within a mare's genital tract (e.g., urine pooling, intrauterine fluid accumulation, presence of numerous neutrophils within the genital tract). In this respect, recent research by Troedsson[15] demonstrated that sperm are found bound to neutrophils in samples collected from mares with ongoing endometritis. It is common for sperm to be bound to neutrophils and for sperm motility to otherwise be poor

(perhaps also adversely affected by inflammatory cell products) when dismount samples are found to contain high numbers of neutrophils. If sufficient prewarmed extender is immediately added to the dismount sample, sperm binding will often decrease and sperm motility improve.

It is also possible that prebreeding infusion of extender might improve pregnancy rates when mares are mated on the first postpartum estrus. One recent study demonstrated a 10% improvement in foal-heat pregnancy rates in mares bred artificially with entire or half-ejaculates mixed with semen extender compared to mares bred by natural cover.[16] That study did not determine what factors might have contributed to this finding (e.g., improved sperm motility, beneficial factors of antibiotic-containing semen extender, decreased genital tract contamination, etc.).

The reader is cautioned that no scientific reports utilizing adequate numbers of mares and stallions exist that confirm prebreeding infusion of extender into the mare uterus can be beneficial to fertility of stallions. Additionally, determination of a suitable volume of extender for prebreeding infusions that would not be detrimental to fertility has not been made. Certainly use of an excess volume could be detrimental because fluid deposited into the uterus is rapidly expelled (within 20 minutes) following breeding[17] and because the act of mating itself results in substantial release of endogenous oxytocin with subsequent promotion of uterine contractions.[18] It seems logical that the volume of extender infused into the uterus should be limited for these reasons (e.g., perhaps to 35-50 ml), as larger volumes might result in premature expulsion of a significant portion of the ejaculate and prevent a significant number of ejaculated sperm from accessing the oviduct. Nevertheless, in clinical practice, the judicious use of this technique has sometimes been claimed to improve pregnancy rates.

Impregnation

Impregnation is a term used on central Kentucky Thoroughbred studs for a process whereby the dismount semen sample is collected following natural cover and then infused into the uterus of the mare that was just covered. Since debris from the mating process and breeding shed floor can get into dismount samples, it is wise to first filter the dismount semen sample to remove as much debris or dirt as possible, and then to immediately mix the dismount semen sample with a suitable volume of prewarmed extender prior to infusion into the uterus of the mare. The process has 2 potential advantages that might improve fertility: (1) it results in an increased number of sperm placed directly into the uterus; and (2) the extender provides some protection to sperm, which may improve their livability within the uterus until they can access the oviduct, where fertilization occurs.

Not all stallions will benefit from impregnations. Certainly some stallions that have a tendency to dismount early after ejaculation or that have difficulty remaining fully intromitted into the mare's vagina during mating are candidates that logically should benefit from the procedure (Table 38-3). Other stallion disorders that benefit from

Table **38-3**

Influence of Impregnations on Pregnancy Outcome (PR/Cycle) in 2 Stallions Used in Natural Service Programs

Stallion	No.	PR/Cycle without Impregnation	No.	PR/Cycle with Impregnation	Improvement
1	71	44%	114	66%	+22%
2	12	37%	56	64%	+27%

Both stallions tended to dismount prematurely. For impregnations, dismount semen samples were immediately filtered and mixed with prewarmed semen extender. After evaluating sperm concentration and motility, the extended semen (10-30 ml) was infused transcervically into the uterine body of the mare that was covered. Once impregnations were thought to result in improved fertility, attempts were made to utilize the protocol on all mares serviced by the stallions, regardless of cycle of cover.

impregnations include failure to ejaculate sufficient numbers of normal motile sperm (particularly if sperm motility rapidly declines *in vitro*), shedding of potential bacterial pathogens in semen, urospermia, and hemospermia. When an excessive amount of urine (regardless of whether the stallion or mare is the source of urine) is present in a dismount sample, addition of extender may not restore sperm motility, in which case impregnation with that sample is not indicated. One protocol employed by some farms is to impregnate all mares returning for mating on a second or later estrous cycle of the season (i.e., in nonimpregnated mares that failed to become pregnant on the first estrous cycle) (Table 38-4). Once a sufficient number of mares have been impregnated, pregnancy rates can be compared between impregnated and nonimpregnated mares. If fertility seems to be improved, impregnation may be justified as a standard protocol for that stallion.

In rare instances when a stallion ejaculates a low number of normal motile sperm of short longevity (i.e., sperm motility rapidly declines even when properly diluted in semen extender), managing his book of mares for multiple covers just prior to and immediately after ovulation may improve pregnancy rates. The strategy proposed is directed toward maximizing the number of live normal sperm that colonize the oviduct, increasing the number available near the time of expected fertilization.[19] By necessity, the number of mares in the stallion's book must be reduced as the stallion will be bred 2 or 3 times to a given mare in a 24-hour period. This mating strategy was found to improve pregnancy rates of one aged Thoroughbred stallion suffering from declining testes size and semen quality with very short livability of sperm *in vitro* (unpublished data: 0 pregnancies for 6 cycles [0% pregnancy rate (PR)/cycle] when only 1 cover per cycle; 7 pregnancies for 38 cycles [18% PR/cycle] when 2 covers per cycle; and 12 pregnancies for 28 cycles [43% PR/cycle] when 3 or more covers per cycle).

Summary

Investigation and management of suboptimal fertility achieved by a stallion should be directed toward identifying and correcting contributing factors. When routine reproductive management practices and veterinary care are good, there still remains a number of simple tech-

Table **38-4**

Influence of Impregnations on Pregnancy Outcome for Mares Mated on their Second Estrous Cycle (PR/2nd cycle) for 13 Stallions Used in Natural Service Programs

Stallion	PR/2nd Cycle without Impregnation	PR/2nd Cycle with Impregnation
1	5/10 (50%)	28/41 (68%)
2	7/13 (54%)	40/55 (73%)
3	1/3 (33%)	11/19 (58%)
4	4/8 (50%)	20/27 (74%)
5	1/2 (50%)	1/3 (33%)
6	3/6 (50%)	24/41 (59%)
7	6/9 (67%)	42/59 (71%)
8	1/4 (25%)	31/47 (70%)
9	3/12 (25%)	29/46 (63%)
10	4/9 (44%)	28/45 (62%)
11	1/2 (50%)	20/26 (77%)
12	6/9 (67%)	27/42 (64%)
13	0/3 (0%)	4/7 (57%)
Total	42/89 (47%)	305/458 (67%)

For impregnations, dismount semen samples were immediately filtered and mixed with prewarmed semen extender. After evaluating sperm concentration and motility, the extended semen (10-30 ml) was infused transcervically into the uterine body of the mare that was covered. Pregnancy rate per second cycle appeared to be improved in all but 2 stallions, although sufficient numbers of second cycle matings are lacking for some stallions.

niques that can be tried in an effort to improve pregnancy rates. The value gained from increased production of valuable foals, and collection of more stud fees, will more than pay for the increased management efforts required.

References

1. Pickett BW, Voss JL, Bowen RA et al: Seminal characteristics and total scrotal width (TSW) of normal and abnormal stallions. Proc Am Assoc Equine Pract 1987; 33:487.

2. Blanchard TL, Varner DD: Evaluating breeding soundness in stallions. 5. Predicting potential fertility. Vet Med Sept 1997; 815-818.

3. Roser JF: Idiopathic subfertility/infertility in stallions: new endocrine methods of diagnosis. Proc Soc Therio 1995; 136-146.

4. Blanchard TL, Varner DD: Testicular degeneration. In McKinnon AO, Voss JL (eds): Equine reproduction, Philadelphia, Lea and Febiger, 1993.

5. Blanchard TL, Johnson L, Roser AJ: Increased germ cell loss rates and poor semen quality in stallions with idiopathic testicular degeneration. J Eq Vet Sci 2000; 20:263.

6. Pickett BW, Squires EL, McKinnon AO: Influence of insemination volume and sperm number on fertility. In Pickett BW, Squires EL, McKinnon AO (eds). Procedures for collection, evaluation and utilization of stallion semen for artificial insemination, Fort Collins, Colorado State University Animal Reproduction Laboratory, Bulletin No. 03:51, 1989.

7. Varner DD, Schumacher J, Blanchard TL et al: Diseases and management of breeding stallions, Goleta, American Veterinary Publications, 1991.

8. Kenney RM, Hurtgen JP, Pierson RH et al: Clinical fertility evaluation of the stallion. Society for theriogenology manual 1983; 7.

9. Douglas RH, Umphenour N: Endocrine abnormalities and hormonal therapy. Vet Clin N Amer Equine Prac 1992; 8:237.

10. Love CL: Evaluation of breeding records. In Blanchard TL, Varner DD, Schumacher J et al (eds): Manual of equine reproduction, ed 2, St. Louis, Mosby, 2003.

11. Baker CB, Little TV, McDowell KJ: Studies of factors limiting reproductive success in horses and derivation of investigative strategies for identifying their causes. PhD dissertation, University of Kentucky, 1995.

12. Blanchard TL, Kenney RM, Timoney PJ: Venereal disease. Vet Clin N Amer Eq Prac 1992; 8:191.

13. Kenney RM, Bergman RV, Cooper WL et al: Minimal contamination techniques for breeding mares: techniques and preliminary findings. Proc Am Assoc Equine Practnr 1975; 21:327.

14. Blanchard TL, Varner DD, Love CL et al: Use of a semen extender containing antibiotic to improve the fertility of a stallion with seminal vesiculitis due to *Pseudomonas aeruginosa*. Theriogenology 1987; 28:541.

15. Troedsson MHT, Loset K, Alghamdi AM et al: Interaction between equine semen and the endometrium: the inflammatory response to semen. Animal Repro Sci 2001; 68: 273.

16. Blanchard TL, Thompson JA, Brinsko SP et al: Breeding mares on foal heat: a 5-year retrospective study. Proc Am Assoc Equine Practnr 2004; 50:525.

17. Katila T, Sankeri S, Makola O: Transport of spermatozoa in the genital tract of mares. J Reprod Fertil 2000; 56(Suppl):571.

18. Madill S, Troedsson MHT, Alexander SL et al: Simultaneous recording of pituitary oxytocin secretion and myometrial activity in estrous mares exposed to various breeding stimuli. Proc Int Symp Equine Reprod 1998; 7:93.

19. Liu I: Personal communication, 2002.

CHAPTER 39

Endocrine Diagnostics and Therapeutics for the Stallion with Declining Fertility

JANET F. ROSER

HORMONE REGULATION OF REPRODUCTIVE FUNCTION IN THE STALLION

In order to identify potential endocrine diagnostics and therapeutics for a stallion with declining fertility, it is first important to understand the endocrine, autocrine, and paracrine regulation of reproductive function in the stallion.

In most mammalian male species including the stallion, normal reproductive function is dependent upon a dynamic and integrative hypothalamic-pituitary-testicular axis (HPT) involving the classic hormone actions of gonadotropin-releasing hormone (GnRH), luteinizing hormone (LH), and follicle stimulating hormone (FSH), and the feedback mechanisms of steroids (androgens and estrogens) and proteins (inhibin and activin).[1-3] In the last decade it has become evident that other hormones such as prolactin, growth hormone (GH), thyroid hormone, vasopressin, opioids, and oxytocin regulate testicular function via the pituitary-testicular axis.[4,5] In addition, local testicular factors called paracrine/autocrine factors, such as growth factors, cytokines, and GnRH-like peptides, appear to modulate testicular cell function.[3,4,6] The presence of these local factors and the dynamic interactions with the endocrine system and fertility in the stallion are under investigation.[3] Specific endocrine tests measuring some of the above hormones are available as diagnostic tools for stallions presented with declining fertility,[7,8] but very few tests are available to measure paracrine/autocrine factors unless a testicular biopsy can be obtained so factors can be extracted from the tissue.[8] When an idiopathic subfertile stallion with testicular dysfunction and abnormal endocrine parameters is presented to a clinician, the first question asked is whether there are any endocrine therapies to prevent a further decline in spermatogenesis or to reverse the existing problem. This chapter presents an overview of the endocrine and possible paracrine and autocrine systems that regulate normal spermatogenesis in the stallion, the endocrine and possible paracrine and autocrine dynamics in idiopathic subfertile/infertile stallion, endocrine diagnostics for idiopathic subfertile/infertile stallions, and potential endocrine therapies.

Endocrine/Paracrine/Autocrine Systems

Endocrine System

The dynamic nature of the hormone interactions of the pineal gland and the HPT axis is constantly evolving (Figure 39-1). Studies in the stallion and other species demonstrate that hormones and local factors not previously considered to play a role in reproductive function may in fact be involved.[3,9-12] Since reviews on the classic endocrine system of the HPT axis in the stallion have been previously published,[1,3,13] only a brief discussion with updates will be presented herein.

Pineal gland and melatonin. The classic reproductive endocrine system in a seasonal breeder, such as the stallion, starts at the level of the pineal gland and the secretion of melatonin.[14] Melatonin is controlled by light signals received by the retina and transmitted via the optic nerve to the pineal gland.[14] With decreasing light, the pineal gland produces more melatonin, which inhibits the release of GnRH, resulting in a decrease in the gonadotropins, steroids, and testicular activity.[14] The endocrine events leading to maximum reproductive capacity in the stallion are initiated when day lengths are still short, albeit increasing.[15] The increase in day length (or light) is part of an external environmental rhythm or zeitgeber (time-giver) needed to stimulate recrudescence.[15] The fact that the stallion has an endogenous circannual cycle entrained by a zeitgeber should be kept in mind when sending breeding stallions from the northern to southern hemisphere. Without a period of short days (2-3 months) followed by increasing light, libido and sperm production could decline over time, particularly if the stallion is already a marginal breeder. Increasing the period of light suppresses melatonin synthesis by modulating the activity of its biosynthetic enzymes[16] and in turn, GnRH, LH, and FSH are released and testicular activity resumes.[17] Cleaver et al[18] reported that exposure of mares to constant light resulted in a marked decrease in circulating melatonin concentrations and an increase in hypothalamic GnRH content. It has been demonstrated that exogenous melatonin decreases plasma testosterone concentrations in stallions.[19]

HPT axis and feedback mechanisms. During the breeding season, when melatonin is low in seasonal

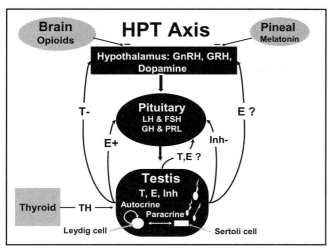

Figure 39-1 The equine hypothalamic-pituitary-testicular axis. Melatonin from the pineal gland regulates the production of gonadotropin-releasing hormone (*GnRH*) from the hypothalamus. GnRH regulates the release of luteinizing hormone (*LH*) and follicle stimulating hormone (*FSH*) from the pituitary. From the brain, opioids inhibit GnRH. From the hypothalamus, growth hormone releasing hormone (*GRH*) stimulates GH, and dopamine inhibits prolactin (*PRL*) in the pituitary. The pituitary hormones stimulate Leydig and Sertoli cells in the testis. Thyroid hormone (TH) from the thyroid gland stimulates testicular cells. Feedback mechanisms from the steroids, estrogen (*E*) and testosterone (*T*) and the protein inhibin are indicated as either positive (+) or negative (–) input on the hypothalamus or pituitary. Local autocrine and paracrine factors in the testis modulate the function of the Leydig and Sertoli cells.

breeders including the stallion, GnRH, in a pulsatile fashion, stimulates the gonadotroph cells in the anterior pituitary to produce LH and FSH.[20,21] These 2 gonadotropins are glycoproteins that are composed of 2 subunits, an α and β. The gonadotropins share the same α subunit but have different β subunits that designate the specificity of the hormone.[22] In the stallion, LH and FSH are episodically secreted[23,24] into the peripheral circulation where they travel to the testes to stimulate steroidogenesis and other actions in Leydig and Sertoli cells, respectively.[25,26] In the adult stallion, LH is responsible for stimulating androgens and estrogens from the Leydig cell,[25] whereas FSH stimulates estrogen, insulin-like growth factor (IGF-1), and transferrin from Sertoli cells.[3,26,27] It has been documented that FSH stimulates inhibin production from Sertoli cells in large domestic species,[28] and that inhibin is produced by the equine testis, specifically the Sertoli cells.[29,30] Studies are ongoing to show that FSH stimulates inhibin production from equine Sertoli cells.

A closed loop feedback system regulates the amounts of GnRH, LH, and FSH released from the hypothalamus and pituitary, respectively. This feedback system involves steroids and proteins from the testis in most mammalian species including the stallion.[1,13,31] In the stallion it has been shown that the major feedback mechanism of

testosterone appears to be at the level of the hypothalamus on GnRH to suppress LH.[32,33] In contrast, estradiol appears to increase the GnRH-induced LH release from the pituitary[32] and decrease baseline levels of FSH in serum.[33] The feedback effect of inhibin appears to be at the level of the pituitary on inhibiting FSH.[34] In addition to these classic reproductive hormones, other hormones such as prolactin, thyroid hormone, GH, and opioids have been investigated in the horse to determine if they play a role in reproductive function.

Prolactin, thyroid hormone, and GH. Prolactin, thyroid hormone, and GH have been reported to effect testicular function in other species. Prolactin appears to play a role in inducing transcription of the estrogen receptor.[35] Thyroid hormone in the adult rat is crucial to the onset of adult Leydig cell differentiation.[36] GH resistance is associated with reduced fertility in men.[37] GH may alter gametogenesis by affecting testosterone synthesis since testosterone is necessary for sperm production. GH increases basal or hCG-stimulated testosterone production in GH-deficient men.[38] Although prolactin and thyroid hormone fluctuate with the season in the horse,[39,40] the role of these hormones in reproductive function in the stallion is yet to be determined. Prolactin did not appear to stimulate testosterone production in equine Leydig cells in culture,[25] and the effects of thyroid hormone have not been investigated in the stallion. In the mare, thyroid function was not associated with infertility.[41] GH does not appear to fluctuate with season in the stallion.[42] However, treatment with a somatostatin analogue (GH inhibitor) caused a transient decrease in semen motility and hCG-induced testosterone release, suggesting a role of GH in the regulation of testicular function in stallions.[42] A direct effect of GH on Leydig cell steroidogenesis in culture was not observed.[43]

Opioids. In the stallion as well as other species, it appears that seasonal changes in GnRH/LH release are partly regulated by opioids. Opioids, secreted from the brain, travel to the hypothalamus and cause a decrease in GnRH release during the winter months.[44] Aurich et al[45] showed that treatment with an opioid antagonist naloxone caused an acute LH release in stallions outside of but not during the breeding season. The opioidioidergic regulation of LH release appears to require the presence of the gonads.[46]

Paracrine/Autocrine System
Although endocrine regulation of the testes is important to ensure that reproductive processes are synchronized with physiologic events, it has become increasingly apparent that it is probably the local paracrine/autocrine system that modulates the intricate network of cellular interactions in the stallion (Figure 39-2).[3] The roles of the paracrine and autocrine systems are to coordinate local functions between and within the 2 testicular compartments by modulating testicular actions of the endocrine system.[47] Paracrine factors are produced by one cell type and act on another cell type present in the same organ. Autocrine factors are substances that are produced by one cell type that act back on the same cell type.[47] Only a few of the relatively large group of paracrine/autocrine factors have been identified in the stallion testis: steroids,

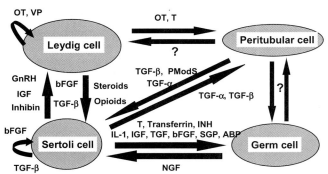

Figure 39-2 Paracrine-autocrine regulation of testicular function. Many of the local interactions in the equine testis are unknown. The figure presents a hypothetical paracrine-autocrine system based on what has been observed in other species. *GnRH,* Gonadotropin-releasing hormone; *IGF,* insulin-like growth factor; *bFGF,* basic fibroblast growth factor; *TGF,* transforming growth factor; *TGF-β,* transforming growth factor beta; *TGF-α,* transforming growth factor alpha; *IL-1,* interleukin-1; *SGP,* sulfated glycoprotein; *NGF,* nerve growth factor; *PModS,* a non-mitogenic paracrine factor produced by peritubular cells that modulates Sertoli cell function.

inhibin, IGF-I, and transferrin. IGF-I has been identified in testicular tissue in the stallion,[48] particularly in the Leydig and Sertoli cells.[3] Highest IGF-I production rates in Leydig cells appear to be during puberty, whereas highest production rates in Sertoli cells occur prior to puberty.[3] Although LH and GH do not appear to regulate IGF-I in Leydig cells, FSH does appear to stimulate IGF-I from Sertoli cells, but only prior to puberty.[3] However, IGF-I itself does not appear to stimulate a steroidogenic response from Leydig cells.[43]

In the stallion, transferrin, which has been postulated to deliver iron to developing germ cells,[49] is produced in Sertoli cells, with the highest production rate occurring at the time of puberty.[27] The levels of transferrin are proportional to sperm production in humans and cattle and may be an effective indicator of Sertoli cell function.[50]

Sertoli cells produce estrogen, with the highest production rate occurring during puberty.[51] Leydig cells appear to produce most of the estrogen in the adult stallion.[43,52] Testosterone is produced by the Leydig cells throughout development and into adulthood.[43] Recent evidence from our laboratory indicates that estrogen receptors are located on Leydig, Sertoli, and germ cells, depending on the stage of sexual development (personal observations). Androgen receptors are located on Sertoli, peritubular, and Leydig cells throughout development (personal observations). These data suggest that both estrogens and androgens are important locally in early testicular development and spermatogenesis in the stallion. Androgens have been reported to play a crucial role in the development of male reproductive organs and spermatogenesis.[53] In the last decade it has been demonstrated that estrogen is also important in regulating testicular function in the male.[54] Of interest is that estrogen has been reported to regulate inhibin production.[55]

When stallions were given an aromatase inhibitor to block estrogen production, inhibin levels decreased while FSH levels remained the same,[56] suggesting a local control of inhibin by estrogen. In other species it has been demonstrated that inhibin acts as a paracrine factor influencing Leydig cell steroidogenesis,[57-59] as well as spermatogenesis.[60,61]

The Endocrine, Paracrine, and Autocrine Dynamics in Idiopathic Subfertile/Infertile Stallions

Historically clinicians relied on baseline concentrations of reproductive hormones in the stallion to help diagnose breeding unsoundness. For example, low levels of testosterone were observed in azoospermic stallions.[62] Burns and Douglas[63] made the first association between elevated plasma concentrations of FSH and subfertility in stallions. Two studies indicated that circulating plasma levels of FSH and estrogens, and not LH and testosterone, could be good markers to predict future changes in fertility,[7,64] whereas another group of investigators suggested that measurement of serum levels of estrogens and testosterone may help in the diagnosis of infertile stallions when other methods are not available.[65] Whitcomb and coworkers[66] presented interesting data on the presence of what appears to be a circulating bioinactive LH isoform in stallions with poor breeding performance.

In addition to measuring basal levels of reproductive hormones in stallions with poor fertility, our laboratory has used the GnRH challenge test, whereby a bolus or intermittent infusion doses of synthetic GnRH were given to diagnostically assess pituitary and testicular responsiveness.[64,67] In human medicine, the GnRH challenge test appears to be of some value in revealing intrinsic differences in acute gonadotroph and Leydig cell stimulation between normal men and men with reproductive disorders.[68,69] When stallions were challenged with repetitive pulses of exogenous GnRH, different pituitary and testicular responses were observed between fertile and subfertile stallions and appeared to be dependent on season and gonadal status.[64,70] The pituitary and testes of fertile stallions appeared to be more responsive to pulsatile administration of GnRH in the nonbreeding season than the breeding season.[70] In contrast, the pituitary responsiveness to repetitive pulses of GnRH in subfertile stallions was significantly reduced during the nonbreeding season and not affected by seasonal changes.[70] When stallions were subject to a discrete dose of GnRH in a subsequent study, responsiveness was observed to be normal,[67] suggesting that a single dose is not enough to determine a pituitary disorder. "Priming" the pituitary with repetitive doses is a better measure of pituitary responsiveness. However, giving a single dose of GnRH, did show that the capacity of the Leydig cells to produce testosterone was significantly reduced in the subfertile stallions.[67]

The results of the above studies suggest that the low testicular response in subfertile stallions may be due to either a dysfunctional hypothalamic-pituitary axis producing bioactive LH or a primary testicular disorder. Further studies in our laboratory point to a primary

Effectors

(toxins, drugs, stress, steroids, nutrition, genetics)

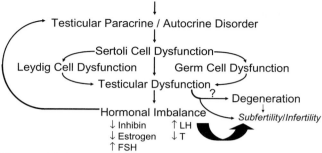

Figure 39-3 Hypothesis of events that may occur following a decline in testicular paracrine-autocrine factors owing to effectors such as toxins, drugs, stress, steroids, and nutrition or genentic abnormalities. Early hormonal changes in stallions with declining fertility are a decline in inhibin and estrogen with an increase in FSH. Moderate to severe testicular degeneration is associated with a decrease in testosterone and an increase in LH.

testicular problem. In one study, no significant differences were observed in pituitary function between fertile, subfertile, and infertile stallions 1 year after castration,[71] which points to a primary testicular dysfunction. In another study, a group of subfertile stallions had a significantly lower testosterone response to a challenge of hCG (10,000 IU) than did the fertile group,[72] suggesting an LH receptor disorder. A study by Motton and Roser[73] demonstrated that the LH receptors on Leydig cells were not affected in stallions with poor fertility, suggesting a post-receptor disorder. In the same laboratory it was shown that in subfertile stallions, testicular inhibin concentrations declined before changes in testicular steroid hormones were observed, suggesting that an early paracrine/autocrine dysfunction may occur at the level of the Sertoli cell[74] followed by the disruption of other cell types in the testis, hypothalamus, and pituitary. A low inhibin-Sertoli cell dysfunction could eventually lead to an increase in FSH that is seen in some stallions with declining fertility. In contrast, estrogen appears to be low.[7,64] Since estrogen is now known to be important in normal testicular function in other species,[54] low testicular estrogens, which come from both the Leydig and Sertoli cells in the stallion, may be another indicator of primary Sertoli cell dysfunction leading to poor spermatogenesis. Our hypothesis as to the etiology of idiopathic subfertility/infertility can be seen in Figure 39-3.

Endocrine Diagnostics

Certainly there are a number of problems that can affect stallion fertility that have nothing to do with the endocrine system, such as hemospermia, urospermia, venereal diseases, neoplasms, and viral and bacterial infections.[75] Endocrine diagnostics may not be useful in these cases. They can be useful in cases of idiopathic subfertility/infertility, testicular hypoplasia, or testicular

degeneration; particularly for identifying which component of the HPT axis is affected. It is important to remember that a change in the normal endocrine parameters does not necessarily mean that the problem is endocrine in nature; it may just be a result of an unrelated dysfunction. Endocrine tests have previously been reviewed.[8,76] Below is an overview.

Blood Sampling Procedures

When taking blood samples for measurement of reproductive hormones, the clinician should keep in mind the following.

- Secretion of hormones can be episodic throughout the day, so it is important to take more than one blood sample to get an average baseline. Six are recommended, once every hour on the same day between 10 AM and 3 PM. Alternatively, if only a rough estimate of baseline values is needed, a simpler approach is to take 3 blood samples, 1 each day for 3 days at the same time each day.
- Baseline concentrations of hormones can increase and decrease during the day, with some hormones, such as testosterone, reaching their highest levels during the middle of the day. It is important to be consistent in taking blood samples at a certain time of day for comparative purposes. The time of day is not as important as is the adherence to that time of day when taking multiple samples from the same animal or different animals.
- There is a large variation in concentrations among fertile stallions. The concentrations should be within the normal range. The normal range can be different from laboratory to laboratory because of the use of different reagents and different assays used to run the samples. Each laboratory should provide "in house" values for the normal range.
- A seasonal variation exists: highest levels of hormones are found during the breeding season (March to September) and lowest during the nonbreeding season (October to February) in the northern hemisphere. Of course, this is just the opposite for the southern hemisphere.
- Either plasma or serum samples can be used to evaluate endocrine parameters.
- Usually a 10-cc blood sample is adequate for the measurement of circulating levels of LH, FSH, testosterone, estradiol, and inhibin.

Baseline Concentrations of LH, FSH, Estradiol, Inhibin, and Testosterone

To obtain accurate baseline levels, 10 cc of venous blood is taken from the jugular once every hour from 10 AM to 3 PM on the same day. A less accurate measurement, but still useful and easier to obtain, would be to take 10 cc of venous blood every day for 3 days between 9 to 10 AM. Blood samples are kept at 4°C until processed. Plasma or serum is removed within a couple of hours and stored at −20°C until analyzed by radioimmunoassay (RIA) or enzyme immunoassay (EIA). Data from the 6 hourly samples will provide information relative to the occurrence of a midday rise in testosterone. A similar LH pattern should be observed. The association of LH and testosterone rising at the same time indicates that LH is appropriately stimulating the testes to produce testosterone. A subfertile stallion with testicular problems may show a rise in LH without a corresponding rise in testosterone. In general, based on previous research, a stallion with declining fertility usually shows changes in hormone levels in the following order: (1) increasing levels of FSH, (2) decreasing levels of estradiol and inhibin, (3) decreasing levels of LH, and finally, when the stallion is infertile, (4) decreasing levels of testosterone. These changes may take a few months or a few years, depending on the disorder. If the hourly blood sampling regime is not practical, the 3 daily blood samples regime can be used to adequately assess subfertility.

A Single Pulse GnRH Challenge Test

To assess pituitary and testicular responsiveness, a single dose of 25 μg of GnRH (Cystorelin, Merial Limited, Duluth, Ga.) is given intravenously (IV) at 9 AM. Blood samples are collected at 30 minutes (min) and 0 min prior to the injection and every 30 min after the injection, up to 120 min. Blood samples are kept at 4°C until processed. Plasma or serum is removed within a couple of hours and stored at –20°C until analyzed for LH and testosterone by RIA or EIA. An abnormal response to a single challenge may help in the diagnosis of a hypothalamic-pituitary disorder and/or a testicular disorder. Measurement of plasma hormone levels along with a GnRH challenge can be revealing.[67] For example, the stallion with low baseline levels of LH but good responsiveness to exogenous GnRH may have a problem at the hypothalamus (i.e., cannot produce or secrete normal levels of GnRH). This syndrome is referred to as hypogonadotropic hypogonadism. A stallion with normal baseline levels of LH but low testosterone may have a problem at the testicular level.

Three-Pulse GnRH Challenge Test

To assess pituitary responsiveness to endogenous GnRH, a series of small challenges using exogenous GnRH is necessary. This test can also be helpful in evaluating testicular input. Three small doses of GnRH (Cystorelin, 5 μg/dose) are given IV 1 hour apart in the nonbreeding season starting at 9 AM. The LH response from baseline is more pronounced in the nonbreeding season when HPT axis activity is at its lowest. Blood samples are taken every 10 min starting at 30 min prior to the first injection, 0 to 60 min after the first injection, 0 to 60 min after the second injection, and 0 to 60 min after the third injection. The entire process takes 210 min. Blood samples are kept at 4°C until processed. Plasma or serum is removed within a couple of hours and stored at –20°C until analyzed for LH. This test specifically evaluates the ability of the pituitary to be "primed" with a series of GnRH pulses. It also evaluates the testis for its ability to provide the necessary hormones, such as estrogen, for the "priming effect" to occur. A normal priming effect is observed when LH is released at a consistently higher level after each challenge. Compared to fertile stallions, subfertile stallions have a significantly lower response to the second and third injection of GnRH in the non-breeding season.[64]

A Challenge with hCG

To assess testicular responsiveness, a single dose of hCG (10,000 IU: Chorulon; Intervet, Millsboro, Delaware) is given IV at 9 AM. Blood samples are collected 30 min and 0 min prior to injection and every 30 min after the injection up to 3 hours posttreatment. Blood samples are kept at 4°C until processed. Plasma or serum is removed within a couple of hours and stored at –20°C until analyzed for testosterone. Since treating with hCG directly stimulates the testis, a poor testosterone response along with normal levels of LH and low levels of circulating testosterone would suggest that the problem is at the level of the testes. A study on fertile, subfertile, and infertile stallions indicated that only the infertile stallions had a poor testicular response to hCG.[72] HCG can also be used as a test for cryptorchidism.[77] The time regime for taking blood samples would be the same as above and blood samples would be analyzed for both testosterone and estrogen conjugates.[78]

Hormone Therapy

Attempts to develop an effective empirical hormonal method to treat stallions of all ages with fertility problems have so far been largely unsuccessful.[7,79] Hormone therapies that have been attempted are presented below.

GnRH

The use of GnRH as a "cure-all" for stallions with idiopathic subfertility has been highly overrated. Based on data published from trials treating idiopathic subfertile/infertile stallions with GnRH using various delivery systems, fertility did not appear to improve.[7,80,81,82] Although the evidence is equivocal, there is a possibility of down regulating the testis with GnRH,[79] as has recently been seen in stallions and geldings given Ovuplant (Peptech Limited, NSW, Australia), a GnRH agonist implant.[83] Hypogonadotropic hypogonadism (i.e., low levels of GnRH, LH, and FSH) has not been reported in stallions, so it is unlikely that giving more GnRH will improve fertility. In fact, many stallions have normal circulating concentrations of LH levels and testosterone but high concentrations of FSH, suggesting a problem in the feedback mechanism at the level of the testis. Thus the efficacy of GnRH therapy to increase sperm production or motility in stallions is questionable. However, a recent study carried out by Sieme et al[84] demonstrated that GnRH therapy during the nonbreeding season improved sexual behavior and increased the quality of frozen/thawed sperm in fertile stallions. However, in the same study, there were no observable motility changes found in the raw semen before freezing.[85] Immunization against GnRH caused a decrease in libido in adult stallions,[86,87] supporting the concept that GnRH and/or the gonadotropins either affect sexual behavior directly at the level of the brain or indirectly via testosterone release from the testis. GnRH has also been used to induce testicular descent in cryptorchids if one or both testes are already in the inguinal canal (personal communications). The success rate is variable. Treatments that have been suggested to help induce testicular descent in young colts (<2 years old) include 500 μg GnRH daily for up to 3 weeks.[88]

hCG

There are anecdotal reports that hCG has also been used to induce testicular descent in cryptorchids if one or both testes are already in the inguinal canal. There have not been any published controlled studies. Treatments that have been suggested to help induce testicular descent in young colts (<2 years old) include 2500 IU hCG twice a week for up to 6 weeks.[88] Theoretically hCG may stimulate testicular descent via testosterone release, but because hCG is a foreign protein to the horse, it can also stimulate an immune response.[89] Therefore its use as a therapeutic tool is not recommended.

GH

There is considerable evidence in mice, rats, and humans that GH affects testicular function by modulating gonadal steroid synthesis and gametogenesis.[90-93] In humans, a deficiency in GH can result in male infertility.[93] It appears that GH can increase plasma IGF-1 concentrations and restore sperm motility.[93] In the stallion, treatment with somatostatin (inhibitor of GH) twice daily for 10 days caused a transient decrease in semen motility and hCG-induced testosterone release, suggesting that GH may play an inhibitory role in the regulation of testicular function in the stallion.[42] However, GH treatment may improve fertility in the stallion with disturbances in GH output and impaired testicular function.

Steroids

It has been known for over 25 years that treatment with anabolic (androgens) steroids suppresses spermatogenesis in stallions,[94] most likely due to the negative feedback effects on LH.[95] It took about 90 days for stallions to recover (normal sperm count) from treatment when anabolic steroids were given daily for 88 days.[96] The therapeutic effect of treating stallions with estrogens has not been investigated. In some stallions with idiopathic subfertility/infertility, estrogens are low.[7,64] Estrogens have been shown to have a local effect on the testis of other species.[54] Estrogens have been shown to enhance the GnRH-induced LH release from equine pituitary cells in culture[32] but decrease circulating levels of FSH when given to geldings.[33] Estrogen may be a treatment of choice if given with eFSH.

Recombinant eLH and eFSH

In 1992 Douglas and Umphenour[7] suggested that equine gonadotropins may be beneficial in stallions with poor fertility, reporting that injection with a pituitary extract resulted in significant increases in LH. Treatment with pituitary extracts containing the gonadotropins have successfully induced superovulation in mares, but not consistently.[97] Unfortunately, there are not only a number of contaminants in preparations of pituitary extracts, but the material has a fixed ratio of eLH to eFSH that changes from batch to batch, decreasing the chances of manipulating a desired outcome. Pituitary extracts have not been tried in stallions with poor fertility. Recently, however, through a collaborative effort with Dr. Irv Boime (Washington University, St. Louis, Missouri) and Aspen-Bio Pharma (Dr. Mark Colgin), we have established clones for recombinant eLH and eFSH. The preparations of recombinant eLH and eFSH appear to work well in vitro using equine Leydig cells[26] or equine seminiferous tubules, respectively. Preliminary trials indicate that treatment with recombinant eLH appears to stimulate the production of testosterone in stallions and causes early induction of ovulation in mares.[98] Further, in vivo studies are planned for the future. Therapy with these 2 hormones may be beneficial in stallions with low gonadotropin levels or endogenous gonadotropins that may be bioinactive, as has been observed in infertile stallions.[66] The opportunity to treat with the individual gonadotropins enhances their manipulative power. Using cloned material ensures a constant and consistent supply of material to the clinician.

Summary

The reproductive function of the stallion is not only controlled by classic hormones such as LH, FSH, testosterone, estrogen, and inhibin, but appears to be modulated by other hormones such as prolactin, GH, thyroid hormone, and opioids. In addition, a paracrine/autocrine system appears to be important in local testicular function. There are several diagnostic tests to choose from to determine at what level of the reproductive axis there may be a primary dysfunction. Of course, there is no silver bullet, but as new therapeutic tools reach the marketplace, the veterinarian will be better prepared to manage the idiopathic subfertile/infertile stallion on a case by case basis.

References

1. Amann RP: Physiology and endocrinology. In Mckinnon AO, Voss JL (eds): Equine reproduction, Philadelphia, Lea & Febiger, pp 658-685, 1993.
2. McLachlan RI: The endocrine control of spermatogenesis. Baillieres Best Pract Res Clin Endocrinol Metab 2000; 14:345.
3. Roser JF: Endocrine and paracrine control of sperm production in stallions. Anim Reprod Sci 2001; 68:139.
4. Huhtaniemi I, Toppari J: Endocrine, paracrine and autocrine regulation of testicular steroidogenesis. In Mukhopadhyay AK, Raizada MK (eds): Tissue renin-angiotensin systems, New York, Plenum Press, pp 33-54, 1995.
5. Maran RR: Thyroid hormones: their role in testicular steroidogenesis. Arch Androl 2003; 49:375.
6. Huleihel M, Lunenfeld E: Regulation of spermatogenesis by paracrine/autocrine testicular factors. Asian J Androl 2004; 1:259.
7. Douglas RH, Umphenour N: Endocrine abnormalities and hormonal therapy. Vet Clin North Am (Equine Pract) 1992; 8:237.
8. Roser JF: Endocrine diagnostics for stallion subfertility. In Robinson NE (ed): Current therapy in equine medicine, London, WB Saunders, pp 257-263, 2003.
9. Skinner MK: Cell-cell interactions in the testis. Endocr Rev 1991; 12:45.
10. Gerlach T, Aurich JE: Regulation of seasonal reproductive activity in the stallion, ram and hamster. Anim Reprod Sci 2000; 58:197.
11. deKretser DM, Hedger MP, Loveland KI et al: Inhibins, activins and follistatin in reproduction. Hum Reprod Update 2002; 8:529.
12. Cooke PS, Holsberger DR, Witorsch RJ et al: Thyroid hormone, glucocorticoids, and prolactin at the nexus of

physiology, reproduction and toxicology. Tox Appl Pharm 2004; 194:309.

13. Roser JF: Reproductive endocrinology of the stallion. In Samper JC (ed): Equine breeding management and artificial insemination, Philadelphia, WB Saunders, pp 41-52, 2000.

14. Sharp DC, Cleaver BD: Melatonin. In Mckinnon AO, Voss JL (ed): Equine reproduction, Philadelphia, Lea & Febiger, pp 100-108, 1993.

15. Clay CM, Clay JN: Endocrine and testicular changes associated with season, artificial photoperiod and the peripubertal period in stallions. Vet Clin North Am (Equine Pract) 1992; 8:31.

16. Minneman KP, Wurtman RJ: Effects of pineal compounds on mammals. Life Sci 1975; 17:1189.

17. Fraschini F, Collu R, Martini L: Mechanisms of inhibitory action of pineal principles on gonadotropin secretion. In Walstenholm GEW, Knight J (eds): The pineal gland, London, Churchill Livingstone, pp 259-273, 1971.

18. Cleaver BD, Grubaugh WR, Davis SD et al: Effect of constant light exposure on circulating gonadotrophin levels and hypothalamic gonadotrophin-releasing hormone (GnRH) content in the ovariectomized pony mare. J Reprod Fert 1991; 44(Suppl):259.

19. Argo CM, Cox JE, Gray JL: Effect of oral melatonin treatment on the seasonal physiology of pony stallions. J Reprod Fert 1991; 44(Suppl):115.

20. Thiery JC, Chemineau P, Hernandez X et al: Neuroendocrine interactions and seasonality. Domest Anim Endocrinol 2002; 23:87.

21. Little TV, Holyoak GR: Reproductive anatomy and physiology of the stallion. Vet Clin N America 1992; 8:1.

22. Papkoff H, Sairam MR, Farmer SW et al: Studies on the structure and function of interstitial cell-stimulating hormone. Rec Prog Horm Res 1973; 29:563.

23. Irvine CHG: Gonadotropin-releasing hormone. J Equine Vet Sci 1983; 3:168.

24. Irvine CHG, Alexander SL: A novel technique for measuring hypothalamic and pituitary hormone secretion rates from collection of pituitary venous effluent in the normal horse. J Endocrinol 1986; 113:183.

25. Eisenhauer KM, Roser JF: Effects of lipoproteins, eLH, eFSH, and ePRL on equine testicular steroidogenesis in vitro. J Androl 1995; 16:18.

26. Roser JF, Sibley LE, Jablonka-Shariff A et al: Expression and bioactivity of single chain recombinant equine luteinizing hormone (eLH) and equine follicle stimulating hormone (eFSH). 15th ICAR, Brazil, Abstracts 2004; 2:572.

27. Bidstrup LA, Dean DJ, Pommer AC et al: Transferrin production in cultured Sertoli cells during testicular maturation in the stallion. Biol Reprod 2002; 66(Suppl):493.

28. Phillips DJ: Activins, inhibins and follistatins in the large domestic species. Dom Anim Endocrinol 2005; 28:1.

29. Roser JF, McCue P, Hoye E: Inhibin activity in the mare and stallion. Dom Anim Endocrinol 1994; 11:87.

30. Dean KJ, Roser JF: Inhibin and estradiol production by cultured equine Sertoli cells. Proceeding of the 16th Equine Nutrition and Physiology Symposium Abstract 1999; 190.

31. Matsumoto AM, Bremner WJ: Endocrinology of the hypothalamic-pituitary testicular axis with particular reference to the hormone control of spermatogenesis. Baillieres Clin Endocrinol Metab 1987; 1:71.

32. Muyan M, Roser JF, Dybdal N et al: Modulation of gonadotropin-releasing hormone-stimulated luteinizing hormone release in cultured male equine anterior pituitary cells by gonadal steroids. Biol Reprod 1993; 49:340.

33. Thompson DL Jr, Pickett BW, Squires EL et al: Effect of testosterone and estradiol-17β alone and in combination on LH and FSH concentrations in blood serum and pituitary of

34. Nagata S, Miyake YI, Nambo Y et al: Inhibin secretion in the stallion. Equine Vet J 1998; 30:98.

35. Frasor J, Gibori G: Prolactin regulation of estrogen receptor expression. Trends Endocrinol Metab 2003; 14:118.

36. Mendis-Handagama C, Ariyaratne S: Prolonged and transient neonatal hypothyroidism on Leydig cell differentiation in the postnatal rat testis. Arch Androl 2004; 50:347.

37. Laron Z, Klinger B: Effect of insulin-like growth factor-I treatment on serum androgens and testicular penile size in males with Laron syndrome (primary growth hormone resistance). Eur J Endocrinol 1998; 138:176.

38. Shoham Z, Conway GS, Ostergaard H et al: Cotreatment with growth hormone for induction of spermatogenesis in patients with hypogonadotropic hypogonadism. Fertil Steril 1992; 57:1044.

39. Thompson DL Jr, Johnson L, Wiest JJ: Effects of month and age on prolactin concentrations in stallion serum. J Reprod Fert 1987; 35(Suppl):67.

40. Johnson AL: Serum concentrations of prolactin, thyroxine and triiodothyronine relative to season and the estrous cycle in the nonpregnant mare. J Anim Sci 1986; 62:1012.

41. Meredith TB, Dobrinski I: Thyroid function and pregnancy status in broodmares. J Am Vet Med Assoc 2004; 224:892.

42. Aurich JE, Kranski S, Parvizi N: Somatostatin treatment affects testicular function in stallions. Therigenology 2003; 60:263.

43. Hess MF, Roser JF: A comparison of the effects of equine luteinizing hormone (eLH), equine growth hormone (eGH) and human recombinant insulin-like growth factor (hrIGF-I) on cultured equine Leydig cells during sexual maturation. Anim Reprod Sci, in press.

44. Gerlach T, Aurich JE: Regulation of seasonal reproductive activity in the stallion, ram and hamster. Anim Reprod Sci 2000; 58:197.

45. Aurich C, Schlote S, Hoppen H-O: Effects of the opioid antagonist naloxone on release of luteinizing hormone in mares during the anovulatory season. J Endocrinol 1994; 142:139.

46. Aurich C, Sieme H, Hoppe H: Involvement of endogenous opioids in the regulation of LH and testosterone release in the male horse. J Reprod Fertil 1994; 102:327.

47. Heindel JL, Treinen KS: Physiology of the male reproductive system: endocrine, paracrine and autocrine regulation. Tox Pathol 1989; 17:411.

48. Hess MF, Roser JF: The effects of age, season and fertility status on plasma and intratesticular insulin-like growth factor I concentrations in stallions. Theriogenology 2001; 56:723.

49. Skinner MK, Griswold MD: Sertoli cells synthesize and secret transferring-like protein. J Biol Chem 1980; 255:9523.

50. Sylvester SR, Griswold MD: The testicular iron shuttle: a "nurse" function of the Sertoli cells. J Androl 1994; 15:381.

51. Dean KJ, Roser JF: Inhibin and estradiol production by cultured equine Sertoli cells. Proceeding of the 16th Equine Nutrition and Physiology Symposium 1999; 190.

52. Hess MF, Roser JF: Immunocytochemical localization of cytochrome P450 aromatase in the testis of prepubertal, pubertal and postpubertal horses. Theriogenology 2004; 61:293.

53. Dohle GR, Smit M, Weber RFA: Androgens and male fertility. World J Urol 2003; 21:341.

54. O'Donnell L, Robertson KM, Jones ME: Estrogen and spermatogenesis. Endocrine Rev 2001; 22:289.

55. Depuydt CE, Mahmoud AM, Dhooge WE: Hormonal regulation of inhibin B secretion by immature rat Sertoli cells in vitro: possible use as a bioassay for estrogen detection. J Androl 1999; 20:54.

56. Stein TA, Ball BA, Conley AS: The effects of an aromatase inhibitor (Letrozole) on hormone and sperm production in the stallion. Theriogenology 2002; 58:381.

57. Hsueh AJ, Dahl KD, Vaughan J et al: Heterodimers and homodimers of inhibin subunits have different paracrine action in the modulation of luteinizing hormone-stimulated androgen biosynthesis. Proc Natl Acad Sci USA 1987; 84:5082.

58. Lin T, Calkins JK, Morris PL et al: Regulation of Leydig cell function in primary culture by inhibin and activin. Endocrinology 1989; 125:2134.

59. Lejeune H, Chuzel F, Sanchez P: Stimulation of both recombinant inhibin A and activin A on immature Leydig cell function in vitro. Endocrinology 1997; 138:4783.

60. Van Dissel-Emiliani FMF, Grootenhuis AJ, de Jong FH: Inhibin reduces spermatogonial numbers in testes of adult mice and Chinese hamsters. Endocrinology 1989; 125:1666.

61. Hakovirta H, Kaipia A, Soder O: Effects of activin-A, inhibin-A, and transforming growth factor-beta 1 on stage specific deoxyribonucleic acid synthesis during rat seminiferous epithelial cycle. Endocrinology 1993; 133:1664.

62. Sato K, Miyake M, Tunoda N et al: Relationship between the semen characteristics and serum testosterone and estrogen levels in three-year-old colts. Jap J Zootech Sci 1981; 52:447.

63. Burns PJ, Douglas RH: Reproductive hormone concentrations in stallions with breeding problems: case studies. J Equine Vet Sci 1985; 5:40.

64. Roser JF, Hughes JP: Seasonal effects on seminal quality, plasma hormone concentrations and GnRH-induced LH response in fertile and subfertile stallions. J Androl 1992; 13:214.

65. Inoue J, Cerbito WA, Oguri N et al: Serum levels of testosterone and oestrogens in normal and infertile stallions. Int J Androl 1993; 16:155.

66. Whitcomb RW, Schneyer AL, Roser JF et al: Circulating antagonist of luteinizing hormone associated with infertility in stallions. Endocrinology 1991; 128:2497.

67. Roser JF, Hughes JP: Dose-response effects of GnRH on gonadotropins and testicular steroids in fertile and subfertile stallions. J Androl 1992; 13:543.

68. Bain J, Moskowitz JP, Clapp JJ: LH and FSH response to gonadotropin releasing hormone (GnRH) in normospermic, oligospermic and azoospermic men. Arch Androl 1978; 1:147.

69. Dony JMJ, Smals AGH, Rolland R et al: Differential effect of luteinizing hormone-releasing hormone infusion on testicular steroids in normal men and patients with idiopathic oligospermia. Fert Steril 1984; 42:274.

70. Roser JF, Hughes JP: Prolonged pulsatile administration of gonadotropin-releasing hormone (GnRH) to fertile stallions. J. Reprod Fert 1991; 44(Suppl):155.

71. Bellanger JM, Roser JF: Gonadotropin levels and pituitary responsiveness in fertile, subfertile and infertile stallions prior to and after castration. Proc 14th Equine Nut Phys Symp 1995; 177.

72. Roser JF: Endocrine profiles in fertile, subfertile and infertile stallions: Testicular response to hCG in infertile stallions. Biol Reprod Monograph 1995; 1:661.

73. Motton DD, Roser JF: HCG binding to the testicular LH receptor is similar in fertile, subfertile and infertile stallions. J Androl 1997; 18:411.

74. Stewart BL, Roser JF: Effects of age, season and fertility status on plasma and intratesticular immunoreactive (IR) inhibin concentrations in stallions. Dom Anim Endocrinol 1998; 15:129.

75. McKinnon AO, Voss JL: Diseases of the stallion's reproductive tract. In McKinnon AO, Voss JL (eds): Philadelphia, Lea Febiger, pp 845-895, 1993.

76. Nett TM: Reproductive endocrine function testing in stallions. In McKinnon AO, Voss JL (eds): Philadelphia, Lea Febiger, pp 821-824, 1993.

77. Cox JE: Experiences with a diagnostic test for equine cryptorchidism. Equine Vet J 1975; 7:179.

78. Cox JE, Redhead PH, Dawson FE: Comparison of the measurement of plasma testosterone and plasma oestrogens for the diagnosis of cryptorchidism in the horse. Equine Vet J 1986; 18:179.

79. Brinsko SP: GnRH therapy for subfertile stallions. Vet Clin North Am (Equine Pract) 1996; 12:149.

80. Evans JW, Finley M: GnRH therapy in a stallion of low fertility. J Equine Vet Sci 1990; 10:182.

81. Blue BJ, Picket BW, Squires EL et al: Effect of pulsatile or continuous administration of GnRH on reproductive function of stallions. J Reprod Fertil 1991; 44(Suppl):145.

82. Roser JF, Hughes JP: Use of GnRH in stallions with poor fertility: A review. Proc 40th Annual AAEP Convention. 1994; 23.

83. Johnson CA, Thompson DL Jr, Carmill JA: Effects of deslorelin acetate implants in horses: single implants in stallions and steroid-treated geldings and multiple implants in mares. J Anim Sci 2003; 81:1300.

84. Sieme H, Troedsson MHT, Weinrich S et al: Influence of exogenous GnRH on sexual behavior and frozen/thawed semen viability in stallions during the non-breeding season. Theriogenology 2004; 61:159.

85. Personal communications with Dr. Mats Troedsson.

86. Malmgren L, Andresen O, Dalin AM: Effects of GnRH immunisation on hormone levels, sexual behaviour semen quality and testicular morphology in mature stallions. Equine Vet J 2001; 33:75.

87. Turkstra JA, van der Meer FJ, Knaap J et al: Effects of GnRH immunization in sexually mature pony stallions. Anim Reprod Sci 2005; 86:247.

88. Ptaszynska M: In Ptaszynska M (ed): Compendium of animal reproduction, ed 7, Boxmeer, Intervet International BV, pp 96-97, 2002.

89. Roser JF, Kiefer BL, Evans JW et al: The development of antibodies to human chorionic gonadotropin following its repeated injection in the cycling mare. J Reprod Fert Suppl 1979; 27(Suppl):173.

90. Zachman M: Interrelations between growth hormone and sex hormones-physiology and therapeutic consequences. Horm Res 1992; 38:1.

91. Chandrashekar V, Bartke A: The role of growth hormone in pituitary and testicular function in adult mice. Biol Reprod 1998; 58(Suppl):98.

92. Hull KL, Harvey S: Growth hormone: a reproductive endocrine-paracrine regulator. Rev Reprod 2000; 5:175.

93. Breier BH, Vickers MH, Gravance CG et al: Therapy with growth hormone: major prospects for the treatment of male subfertility? Endocr J 1998; 45(Suppl):S53.

94. Berndston WE, Hoyer JH, Squires EL et al: Influence of exogenous testosterone on sperm production, seminal quality and libido of stallions. J Reprod Fertil 1979; 27(Suppl):19.

95. Squires EL, Todter GE, Berndston WE et al: Effect of anabolic steroids on reproductive function of young stallions. J Anim Sci 1982; 54:576.

96. Squires EL, Berndston WE, Hoyer JH et al: Restoration of reproductive capacity of stallions after suppression with exogenous testosterone. J Anim Sci 1981; 53:1351.

97. Scoggin CF, Meira C, McCue PM et al: Strategies to improve the ovarian response to Whitcomb RW, Schneyer AL, Roser JF et al: Circulating antagonist of luteinizing hormone associated with infertility in stallions. Endocrinology 1991; 128:2497.

98. Roser JF, Boime I, Colgin M, Niswender KD: Development and efficacy of recombinant eLH and eFSH. Proceedings of the West Coast Equine Reproduction Symposium II: Limited Distribution pp 39-52, 2005.

SECTION V

Semen Collection and Evaluation

CHAPTER **40**

Evaluation of Raw Semen

ANDRÉS J. ESTRADA
JUAN C. SAMPER

With the fast growth of artificial insemination (AI) throughout the horse industry, and the acceptance of using shipped semen by almost all equine associations, the evaluation of raw semen for either immediate use or shipping has become a mandatory part of the elemental knowledge of veterinarians who are involved with equine reproduction. This chapter summarizes updated techniques to evaluate all features of a stallion's semen that help the clinician estimate the potential fertility of a particular ejaculate.

Although still used, traditional tests have had many detractors because of the lack of objectivity in the results obtained after semen evaluation. There is no single evaluation, parameter, or assay that can be used individually to determine the degree of fertility or infertility of a stallion,[1] so it is strongly recommended to use more than one test to evaluate a sample. There is still no test as good as pregnancy itself to predict fertility from a certain ejaculate; therefore the more tests used, the more accurate the estimates. A single assay does not generate confidence because only a small amount of sperm are tested and because a single sperm contains within it a multiple of subcellular compartments with completely different functions that must be intact for successful in vivo fertilization.[2]

WHEN RAW SEMEN SHOULD BE EVALUATED

There are many situations in which raw semen should be evaluated, including the following:

- Always after collection and before shipping
- As a part of the prepurchase evaluation
- Before the breeding season starts and at least one time during the season
- As an assessment for a certain stallion to be included in a breeding program as a sire
- As a part of the breeding soundness evaluation
- When fertility problems are suspected

- When low percentages of pregnancy are achieved or when they are not as high as expected
- To predict the ability of a certain stallion's semen to withstand cooling and freezing

To get a better idea of the current quality of a certain ejaculate, it should be evaluated both macroscopically and microscopically. The most popular means to perform these examinations are outlined below.

MACROSCOPIC EVALUATION

Color and Appearance

Once the semen is collected, it should be filtered if this was not done during the collection itself. General inspection of the ejaculate should be performed with the naked eye to rule out differences in color or appearance. Semen should be white or grayish-white; other types of colors are supportive of disorders. A semen sample that is blood-tinged and flocculent, with clumps of purulent material, may lead the clinician to suspect possible seminal vesiculitis.[3]

Samples with a urinelike smell and a yellowish color mean urospermia, defined as the presence of urine in the ejaculate. This disorder can be diminished by centrifuging the extended sample. Hemospermia refers to contamination of ejaculates with blood, and hemospermic ejaculates are reddish in color. Hemospermia can result from a variety of conditions. Trauma to the penis may result in injuries such as bruising, lacerations, and hemorrhage and most commonly involves the urethral process, and the application of rings or brushes to prevent masturbation may also lead to penile/urethral bruising. Tumors can also be considered a cause of hemospermia. Profuse arterial hemorrhage in ejaculates usually results from an idiopathic defect in the urethra that communicates with surrounding corpus spongiosum penis.[4] As with urospermia, hemospermia can be diminished by centrifugation of the extended sample.

Volume

After collection, the semen should be filtered and poured into a warm and sterile container such as a graduated cylinder or a baby bottle. The receptacle should be able to hold at least 100 ml, but when collecting Draft horses a bigger container may be needed.

The average volume produced by a stallion can be affected by different factors. One such factor is the effect of season. Differences of up to 50% have been reported between the height of the breeding season and the non-breeding season due to changes in the volume of gel production.[5] The frequency of collection can also affect volume, because stallions collected too frequently may show a decrease in volume produced. No significant effect should be seen in the great majority of stallions with a collection frequency of less than one ejaculate per 24 hours.[6] Age affects volume, which will increase from 2 to 16 years of age,[7] and the length of time that a stallion is teased before ejaculation has also been shown to have an effect on the volume of seminal plasma produced due to an increase of the gel-free fraction.[8] Clinical conditions such as urospermia, pyospermia, and hemospermia will increase the total volume as well.

MICROSCOPIC EVALUATION

Motility

Proper dilution cannot be done if motility is not calculated, because 500 million motile spermatozoa are needed for an insemination. The accuracy of motility determination is enhanced when a proper semen extender is added to the sample before evaluation.[9] As stated before in this chapter, it is of great importance to have warm all the devices that are going to be in contact with the semen, because any change (cold or warm) can affect motility and lead to inaccurate calculations. All equipment should be clean (disposable if possible). A good microscope is necessary for this evaluation and can be hooked up to a monitor to facilitate visualization. A drop of 5 to10 µl should be placed on a slide for calculation. Thick samples have more than one layer and cannot be reliably estimated. Samples of a higher concentration are usually judged by the human eye as having higher motility;[10] therefore semen should be extended to 25 to 50 × 10^6 spermatozoa per milliliter.

Motility at the edges of the coverslip declines more rapidly than in the center as a result of drying and exposure to air.[6] Therefore all readings should be taken at the center of the sample. The clinician should also make sure that all fields are free of debris and air bubbles, because they can also affect the outcome. Raw semen should not be used, because agglutination or sticking of sperm cells to the glass will give inaccurate results.[11]

Concentration

The number of spermatozoa produced by a normal stallion is a function of the testicular size. One gram of testicular parenchyma during the breeding season produces approximately 19 million spermatozoa per day, which decreases to 15 million during the nonbreeding season.[12] The total scrotal width is highly correlated with the testicular weight, size, and sperm production and is therefore regarded as an important consideration when evaluating the potential fertility of a certain stallion's ejaculate.[12] The amount of sperm produced by a stallion increases with age[13] because the total length of the seminiferous tubules becomes larger and increases by more than 30% during the life of the stallion.[6] Most stallions older than 4 years seem to have a similar sperm production per day per gram of testicular parenchyma during the breeding season.[6] Therefore, because daily sperm production is one factor affecting the number of spermatozoa available for ejaculation, usually more sperm will be ejaculated by older than younger stallions.

Hemocytometer

The hemocytometer, or counting chamber, is a direct method of counting sperm cells. Although it is more time-consuming than some of the other available methods of counting, it is considered the most accurate and reliable way to count spermatozoa. Most hemocytometers available from AI supply firms are accompanied by specific instructions. It is very important to read the instructions and to fully understand proper techniques of preparing the diluted sample and counting the sperm in the grid area. These systems are usually accompanied by a Unopette diluting system which, when properly used, allows one to accurately dilute the semen sample for counting in the hemocytometer chamber.[14] Box 40-1 provides a basic method for using a standard hemocytometer, but any specific instructions that accompany a hemocytometer should be followed.

Densimeters

A densimeter functions by passing a beam of light through the sample and then measuring the amount of light transmitted through the sample by a phototube. The result is then displayed on a meter (either analog or digital). The amount of light transmitted through the sample is inversely correlated with sperm concentration in the sample.[7]

In a standard spectrophotometer, a meter reading (optical density or percent transmittance) is converted to a chart with a corresponding sperm cell concentration. In the case of the SpermaCue (Minitub, Tiefenbach, Germany), the Animal Reproduction Systems (ARS) densimeter (Animal Reproduction Systems, Chino, Calif.), and some other spectrophotometers, the instrument itself further converts this meter reading directly to sperm per milliliter. The main difference between these two systems is that although raw semen can be used with the SpermaCue, a 1:20 dilution with formal saline must be made to use the densimeter manufactured by ARS.

Morphology

The high influence of normal morphologic characteristics of the viable sperm on first-cycle no-return rates indicates that this semen evaluation test is predictive of a stallion's future breeding performance, and breeding facilities should take this into consideration in their deci-

Box 40-1

Hemocytometer Instructions

1. Gently mix the ejaculate so that a representative sample is obtained.
2. Use only coverslips specifically designed for hemocytometer chambers. They are slightly thicker than regular disposable coverslips and are perfectly flat.
3. Dilute the semen. To make a 1:100 dilution, 0.1 ml of semen is added to 9.9 ml of formalin or a 1:200 dilution using an Unopette device.
4. Carefully clean and dry the chamber and coverslip after each use. Avoid scratching them.
5. Load the hemocytometer chamber without overflowing it.
6. Wait 2 minutes until sperm settle down. This will help avoid an incorrect count.
7. Count the sperm in both chambers. Use the average number of the two for the calculations. If the two numbers obtained vary by more that 10%, prepare another diluted sample and repeat the counting procedure.
8. Once the average number is obtained, the following formula should be used:

Sperm/ml (millions) =
Number counted × Dilution ratio × 10,000

9. Calculation of the total number of sperm is done by multiplying sperm concentration per milliliter by the total volume of the ejaculate.

Total number of sperm (10^9) =
Sperm/ml (millions) × Volume (ml)

Box 40-2

Most Common Stallion Sperm Abnormalities

An accurate evaluation of the percentage of normal/abnormal sperm can be done by counting 100 cells and sorting each cell into one of the following categories:

1. Normal
2. Abnormal head
3. Detached head
4. Abnormal/broken neck
5. Abnormal midpiece
6. Proximal droplet
7. Distal droplet
8. Coiled tail
9. Kinked tail

genesis, testicular degeneration, orchitis, and epididymitis, can be detected in some cases.[18]

Cytology

Cytologic examination is a very useful and quick way of evaluating whether or not the semen is contaminated with bacteria. After collection, a drop of raw semen should be placed on a slide (which does not have to be warm) and spread along the slide using a second, clean slide. Once the smear dries, it must be immersed for three consecutive times in a methanol fixative (usually blue or green in color), followed by one immersion in a xanthene dye (red) and one immersion in a thiazine dye (purple). This dye is commercially known as Diff Quick (Fischer Scientific Co., LLC, Middletown, Va.). Finally, the slide should be gently rinsed with deionized water and dried for evaluation. A count of more than six neutrophils per field is an indication of infection.

Membrane Evaluation

In recent years more attention has been given to evaluating sperm membrane integrity, because it is of fundamental importance in the fertilization process. The next two techniques will demonstrate how the evaluation of the sperm membrane can be used as a tool to evaluate equine semen quality.

Hypoosmotic Swelling

In a hypoosmotic solution, fluid is transported into the cell across the spermatozoal plasma membrane. While attempting to reach osmotic equilibrium between the inside and the outside of the cell, a functionally intact membrane swells away from the spermatozoal tail fibers, causing the tail to bend. Under a microscope, these sperm with functional membranes are easily recognized by their coiled tails, whereas sperm with damaged membranes will have straight tails.

To perform an hypoosmotic swelling (HOS) test, a sample of raw semen (100 µl) is incubated for 30 minutes

sion to accept a stallion for breeding.[15] The collector and the handler (if different) of the semen should be careful that every piece of equipment that makes contact with the ejaculate is at 37°C (98.6°F), because any change in temperature, even subtle, can affect the spermatozoa and lead to outcomes that are not realistic. The sample should be diluted in a 1:10 ratio to fixate the sperm, and the sorting can then be performed later because this is not a time-affected feature. A drop should be placed on a slide, covered with a coverslip, and mounted on the microscope with immersion oil under a 100× objective. If possible, a phase-contrast microscope should be used because it eliminates artifacts seen in stained smears.[16] A very accurate evaluation of the percentage of normal/abnormal sperm can be done by counting 100 cells and sorting each cell into one of the categories listed in Box 40-2.

Highly fertile stallions have more than 60% morphologically normal spermatozoa and less than 5% abnormalities of the acrosome and midpiece.[17] In conclusion, even though the relationship between sperm morphologic characteristics and fertility is far from clear, the sperm morphologic characteristics should be examined routinely because problems, such as aberrant spermato-

at 37°C in 900 µl of a sucrose solution (17.12 g in 50 ml of distilled, deionized water) adjusted to 100 mOsm. Evaluation is accomplished using bright field microscopy (100×). A minimum of 100 spermatozoa are evaluated per slide, and the percentage of them that show the typical coiled tail abnormality indicative of swelling are counted.[19]

Dead and Live

This technique is based on the capacity of the sperm membrane to absorb an eosin stain. Integrity of the plasma membrane is demonstrated by the ability of a viable (live) cell to exclude the dye, whereas the dye will diffuse passively into sperm cells that are dead and therefore have nonfunctional plasma membranes.[20]

A drop of eosin stain is placed on the edge of a clean slide. A previously diluted sample of semen (about 10 µl) is then placed next to the eosin, and the two are mixed. A second slide is held against the mixed droplet at a 45-degree angle, and the suspension is spread along the slide. Once the smear is dry, immersion oil should be added and the sample should be examined at 100× magnification. Sperm that have a damaged membrane will take up the dye and appear purple, whereas intact, live cells will appear white. One hundred cells should be counted and the amount of dead and live converted into percentages.

pH

Although pH measurement is not the most popular of the techniques used to evaluate semen, a clinician can gather some valuable information that, added to other data, will lead him or her to assess the fertility of a certain semen sample. Optimal pH is about 7.7, and alterations in this value negatively affect stallion sperm motility.[21] Among the reasons that a stallion's semen can have a low pH are urospermia and pyospermia.

Although little research has been done on the effects of pH on stallion semen, human sperm exhibit a greater reduction in motility in response to acidic conditions than alkaline conditions. Spermatozoa immobilized by acidic conditions are able to regain motility after the pH is returned to normal, but the effects of alkaline conditions are not reversible.[22] There is a reported negative correlation between seminal volume and pH and between the number of spermatozoa and pH[23] that suggests that samples with a high pH may have low spermatozoa concentrations.

Longevity

Although it is time consuming, longevity assay is a vital component of any stallion's semen that is destined to be cooled and shipped. Knowing the longevity of such a sample allows the clinician to predict the time that a certain ejaculate can withstand cooling when shipping semen is attempted and therefore the window available for successful insemination. The assay involves leaving a certain amount of diluted semen with a known concentration (between 25 and 50 million sperm per milliliter is recommended) in an Equitainer (Hamilton Thorn,

Louisville, Ky.)[1] and performing successive evaluations of the motility at 6, 12, 24, and 48 hours afterwards. The evaluations can be done with a light microscope, making sure that the sample to be evaluated is warmed before the observations are done.

CONCLUSION

With the very noticeable worldwide rise in acceptance of AI, the clinician who is involved in equine reproduction is routinely obligated to perform evaluations of raw semen. There are several techniques available for evaluating semen that are simple enough for any clinician or breeding manager to perform; however, for best results in pregnancy rates, a skilled clinician with greater knowledge of the mare and stallion reproductive tracts and experience in reproductive physiology is preferable.

Although not a complicated task, evaluation of raw semen needs to be performed by a skilled clinician, who possesses a basic kit of tools such as a good light microscope, dyes, and glassware that is preferably disposable. The application of the traditional techniques (volume, concentration, motility, and morphologic characteristics) to other, less used evaluations mentioned in this chapter will increase the chances of a very accurate assessment of the quality of a given semen sample.

References

1. Magistrini M: Semen evaluation. In Samper JC (ed): Equine Breeding Management and Artificial Insemination, pp 91-108, Philadelphia, Saunders, 1999.
2. Amann RP, Graham JK: Spermatozoal function. In McKinnon AO, Voss JL (eds): Equine Reproduction, pp 715-745, Philadelphia, Lea & Febiger, 1993.
3. Varner DD, Blanchard TL, Brinsko SP et al: Techniques for evaluating selected reproductive disorders of stallions. Anim Reprod Sci 2000; 60-61: 493-509.
4. Schumacher J, Varner DD, Schmitz DJ et al: Urethral defects in geldings with hematuria and stallions with hemospermia. Vet Surg 1995; 24:250-254.
5. Picket BW, Shiner KA: Recent developments in AI in horses. Livest Prod Sci 1994; 40:31-36.
6. Davies Morel MCG: Semen evaluation. In Morel MCG (ed): Equine Artificial Insemination, pp 190-233, Wallingford, UK, CABI, 1999.
7. Squires EL, Pickett BW, Amann RP: Effect of successive ejaculation on stallion seminal characteristics. J Reprod Fertil Suppl 1979; 27:7-12.
8. Ionata LM, Anderson TM, Pickett BW et al: Effect of supplementary sexual preparation on semen characteristics of stallions. Theriogenology 1991; 36(6):923-937.
9. Samper JC: Artificial insemination. In Samper JC (ed): Equine Breeding Management and Artificial Insemination, pp 109-131, Saunders, 1999.
10. Jasko DJ: Evaluation of stallion semen. Vet Clin North Am Equine Pract 1992; 8:129-148.
11. Colembrander B, Puyk H, Zandee AR et al: Evaluation of the stallion for breeding. Acta Vet Scand Suppl 1992; 88:29-37.
12. Rodriguez-Martinez H: Sperm production in the stallion. Acta Vet Scand Suppl 1992; 88:9-28.
13. Johnson L, Neaves WB: Age-related changes in the Leydig cell population, seminiferous tubules, and sperm production in stallions. Biol Reprod 1981; 24:703-712.

14. Singleton WL: Stimulating sperm concentration. December 31, 2002 (accessed) [http://web.ics.purdue.edu/~wsinglet/estimating.html].

15. Parlevliet JM, Colembrander B: Prediction of first season stallion fertility of 3-year-old Dutch Warmbloods with pre-breeding assessment of percentage of morphological normal live sperm. Equine Vet J 1999; 31:248-251.

16. Lock TF: Artifical insemination and semen handling. In Morrow DA (ed): Current Therapy in Theriogenology 2, pp 652-653, Philadelphia, WB Saunders, 1986.

17. Hurtgen JP: Evaluation of stallion for breeding soundness. Vet Clin North Am Equine Pract 1992; 8:149-162.

18. Mamlgrem L: Sperm morphology in stallions in relation to fertility. Acta Vet Scand 1992; 88:39-47.

19. Neild DM, Chaves MG, Flores M et al: The HOS test and its relationship to fertility in the stallion. Andrologia 2000; 32:351-355.

20. Colembrander B, Fazeli AR, van Buiten A et al: Assessment of sperm cell membrane integrity in the horse. Acta Vet Scand Suppl 1992; 88:49-58.

21. Griggers S, Paccamonti DL, Thompson RA: The effects of pH, osmolarity and urine contamination on equine spermatozoal motility. Theriogenology 2000; 56:613-622.

22. Makler A, David R, Blumenfeld Z et al: Factors affecting sperm motility. Part 7. Sperm viability is affected by change of pH and osmolarity of semen and urine specimens. Fertil Steril 1981; 36:507-511.

23. Pickett BW, Voss JL, Bowen RA et al: Comparison of seminal characteristics of stallions that passed or failed seminal evaluation. Proceedings of the 11th International Congress on Animal Reproduction and Artificial Insemination, vol 3, pp 380, 1998.

CHAPTER 41

Urospermia and Hemospermia

REGINA M. O. TURNER

UROSPERMIA

Urospermia is defined as the presence of urine in the seminal fluid. The condition is reported infrequently in stallions,[1] and little information is available on its pathogenesis and treatment. However, in one report, 36% of all cases of ejaculatory dysfunction in stallions involved urospermia.[2] Thus the condition may be more common than was previously believed, particularly in stallions with ejaculatory problems.

Physiology of Urine Voiding and Ejaculation

Emission, defined as the release of sperm and accessory gland fluids into the pelvic urethra, and ejaculation, defined as the forceful expulsion of the combined fluids from the urethra, are reflex actions that also involve nervous pathways from the cerebral cortex. Emission occurs as the result of a thoracolumbar reflex arc that causes contraction of the smooth muscle of the ductus deferens and accessory glands. This same reflex arc also is responsible for the simultaneous contraction of the smooth muscle of the bladder trigone, thus preventing urine voiding during emission and subsequent ejaculation. Both emission and bladder neck closure primarily involve α-adrenergic, sympathetic fibers (Figure 17.2-1). Similarly, ejaculation is predominantly an α-adrenergic, sympathetic event and is mediated primarily by a sacral reflex involving the pudendal nerve. The reflex initiates rhythmic contractions of the bulbocavernosus, ischiocavernosus, and urethralis muscles.[2,3] Sensory stimulation of the penis, usually together with psychic input from the brain, are the physiologic triggers for the ejaculatory reflex. However, both emission and ejaculation also can occur without prior sensory stimulation (e.g., pharmacologically induced).[4,5]

Pathophysiology

Any disease process that interferes with the normal synchronization of emission/ejaculation and bladder neck closure theoretically could result in urospermia. Reported causes of urospermia in stallions include neuritis of the cauda equina, equine herpesvirus 1, and sorghum toxicosis. In addition, urospermia can arise secondary to fractures, osteomyelitis, and neoplasias that impinge on the normal nervous pathways of the lumbosacral region.[1,6-8] Urospermia also has been reported in association with hyperkalemic periodic paralysis.[9] All of these problems typically result in multiple neurologic deficits, and so clinical signs may not be limited to those involving bladder neck closure.

However, in the author's experience, the majority of cases of urospermia in stallions are idiopathic, and the only apparent clinical sign is inappropriate urination during ejaculation. If carefully examined, some of these animals also may demonstrate mild urinary incontinence and/or subtle bladder dysfunction (e.g., an inability to completely void the bladder during voluntary urination) outside of the breeding situation. However, because the signs in breeding stallions are most dramatic at the moment of ejaculation, urospermia is often the only presenting complaint. In cases of idiopathic urospermia, the cause is typically attributed to some unidentified dysfunction of the emission and/or ejaculatory reflexes that permits a varying degree of bladder neck laxity at the moment of ejaculation, thus allowing for anterograde passage of urine through the urethra and resulting urine contamination of the ejaculate.

In men, incomplete bladder neck closure more typically is associated with retrograde ejaculation. During emission and ejaculation, semen passes in a retrograde fashion through the lax bladder neck and into the bladder, rather than moving anterograde through the penile urethra and urethral orifice.[10] Although a case of retrograde ejaculation has been documented in a stallion,[11] this condition appears to be a much less common manifestation of incomplete bladder neck closure in the horse than is urospermia.

Regardless of the pathophysiology of urospermia, it has been documented that urine contamination of the equine ejaculate negatively affects sperm motility.[12] This effect is most likely the result of changes in pH and osmolarity caused by the presence of urine in the ejaculate. The more urine present and the more concentrated the urine in the ejaculate, the more profound will be its negative impact on sperm motility and subsequent fertility.

Clinical Signs and Diagnosis

Stallions breeding by natural cover whose semen is not evaluated on a regular basis may present for infertility.[13] An accurate diagnosis of urospermia generally can readily be made in most stallions by collecting semen into an artificial vagina (AV) and observing gross urine contamination of the ejaculate. In more mild cases, the presence of urine in the semen may not be grossly apparent. Because sperm motility is severely adversely affected by

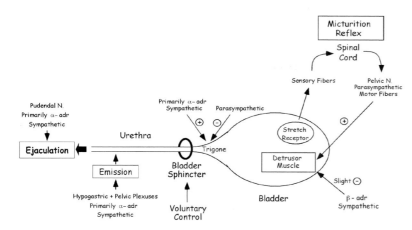

Figure 41-1 Schematic diagram showing the relevant nervous pathways involved in micturition, bladder neck closure, emission, and ejaculation. The micturition reflex is responsible for stimulating contraction of the detrusor muscle in response to bladder filling. Involuntary sympathetic and parasympathetic pathways control closure of the bladder trigone. Skeletal muscle control of the bladder sphincter is responsible for voluntary control of urination, although this voluntary control can be overridden by a reflex arc if bladder fill becomes excessive. Emission and ejaculation are primarily initiated by α-adrenergic fibers originating from the thoracic, lumbar, and sacral regions of the spinal cord.

the presence of urine,[12] reduced sperm motility may be the most apparent problem in more mildly affected animals. Microscopic examination of the ejaculate may reveal a large number of urine crystals. Even when urine contamination is not visibly evident, the presence of small amounts of urine often will alter the odor of the ejaculate. Urine also may increase the pH of the ejaculate.[14]

In cases in which small, grossly undetectable amounts of urine are suspected to be contaminating the ejaculate, creatinine or urea nitrogen levels can be run on a sample of whole ejaculate. A creatinine level of over 2.0 mg/dl or a urea nitrogen level of over 30 mg/dl is suggestive of urospermia.[15] These are simple tests that readily can detect the presence of even small amounts of urine contamination. As an alternative, commercially available test strips for the semiquantitative detection of urea nitrogen (Azostix, Miles, Inc.,) or nitrite (Multistix, Miles, Inc.) also can be used. However, care must be taken when using these stall-side tests because false positives are common when the appropriate protocol is not strictly followed. Specifically, when using the Azostix test to detect urospermia, it is recommended that the reagent pad be rinsed with distilled water after only 10 seconds horizontal exposure to the sample. After rinsing, the result can be read. A change in color of the test pad from yellow to green indicates the presence of urine. When using the Multistix test, the test pad should be placed in a horizontal position and exposed to the sample for $3^1/_2$ minutes before the test is read. A color change of the test pad from yellow to orange indicates the presence of urine.[15]

Urospermia can vary in severity from one ejaculate to another and often is sporadic. Thus collection of a single, urine-free ejaculate does not rule out the possibility of this condition. If urospermia is suspected, multiple semen collections, preferably when the stallion has a full bladder, are recommended to determine whether or not the disorder is present.

Observation and/or videotaping of the stallion in a box stall also may reveal some clinical signs. Affected animals may show evidence of neurologic or infectious disorders of the urinary system including dysuria, polyuria, and/or stranguria. In addition, videotaping of

the stallion allows for ready evaluation of masturbation activity and penis control. Abnormalities in either of these areas may suggest the presence of either a localized or systemic neurologic problem involving the reproductive tract.

Once a diagnosis of urospermia is made, it is recommended that the stallion have a full neurologic examination, including examination of cranial nerve function, limb function, anal tone, anal reflex, tail tone, and defecation pattern and frequency. Standard neurologic evaluations may reveal subtle deficits in other areas of the body, thus suggesting a more systemic cause for the urospermia. In addition, the urinary tract should be carefully examined. Palpation and ultrasonographic examination of the bladder before and after voluntary urination may reveal an incomplete ability to fully evacuate the bladder contents. In addition, the bladder wall and contents can be evaluated for lesions or for the presence of uroliths. An attempt can be made to express the bladder by palpation per rectum. The amount of pressure that is required to expel urine from the bladder can be used as an indirect measure of bladder sphincter and neck control. To evaluate the ability of the detrusor muscle to contract, bethanechol chloride, a cholinergic agent that normally causes evacuation of the bladder within 15 minutes of subcutaneous administration, can be given at a dose of 0.07 mg/kg body weight. Following urination, the bladder can be reexamined to determine if complete evacuation has occurred. A urinalysis and culture and sensitivity of a catheterized urine sample also should be performed to rule out possible infectious causes of bladder irritation. If a problem is identified, it should be addressed directly (e.g., systemic antibiotic administration for cases of bacterial cystitis) in hopes that correction of the underlying problem will improve or eliminate the urospermia.

Treatment

Limited therapeutic options are available for the treatment of idiopathic urospermia in stallions. And of these, none has been consistently effective. The nonspecific nature of most treatments for urospermia in the stallion reflects our poor understanding of the pathophysiology of the disease. In reality, urospermia is generally managed, rather than treated. Most management changes designed to minimize or eliminate urospermia focus on minimizing the amount of urine present in the bladder at the time of semen collection or natural breeding. Treatments addressed at correcting the suspected underlying cause(s) of the problem (e.g., a neurologic condition) could in theory be more effective. However, because most cases of urospermia are idiopathic, this generally is not an option.

The simplest and most established method for the management of urospermia is to encourage the stallion to completely empty the bladder immediately before semen collection or natural breeding.[16] This can usually be accomplished by moving the animal to a freshly bedded stall before he is taken to the breeding shed. Alternatively, fresh feces from another stallion can be placed in the subject stallion's stall. Most stallions will be stimulated to urinate with either one or both of these techniques. As a final option, diuretics can be used.[17] In the author's experience, these techniques can be quite helpful in reducing the frequency and severity of urospermia; however, they do not always result in a urine-free ejaculate. Many horses retain some variable amount of residual urine in the bladder after voluntary voiding, and this urine still can be expelled and adversely affect sperm quality. Nonetheless, practices such as these remain the mainstays of management of urospermia.

In animals in which voluntary voiding is not sufficient, or in cases in which a urine-free ejaculate must be obtained in a single session, the stallion's bladder can be completely emptied by passing a urinary catheter into the bladder to facilitate complete drainage.[18] The bladder then can be lavaged with several liters of sterile physiologic saline to insure that any residual bladder contents will not be harmful to the sperm should they be expelled during ejaculation. If a sufficient number of trained personnel are available, the bladder can be manually expressed completely per rectum following the final lavage and before the urinary catheter is removed. This more extreme method of emptying the bladder has been reported to be highly successful and reliably resulted in urine-free ejaculates.[8] In highly tractable animals, the procedure can be performed in the breeding shed, after the stallion has obtained an erection, thus avoiding the need for sedatives or tranquilizers and thus allowing for semen collection to proceed as soon as the bladder is fully evacuated. It should be kept in mind that repeated use of urinary bladder catheterization will predispose the stallion to urethritis and bacterial cystitis.[18] The owners should be informed of the risk before using this technique, and it may be advantageous to place the stallion on a prophylactic course of an appropriate antibiotic if catheterization is to be performed routinely.

Stallions typically ejaculate in a series of seven or eight pulses of semen.[19] Methods for separating an ejaculate by collecting individual pulses (fractions) have been described.[20] Theoretically, by fractionating the ejaculate, it should be possible to collect only the urine-free portions of the ejaculate, thus avoiding the problem of urine contamination.[17,18,21] However, in practice, the pattern of urine contamination of the ejaculate can vary from one ejaculate to the next.[21] Some ejaculates may be urine-free, whereas in other instances, urine contamination may precede, coincide with, or follow ejaculation. Even within the same stallion, the frequency and pattern of urospermia can vary from one ejaculate to the next. Nonetheless, collection of the ejaculate into different fractions may allow one to at least sporadically separate the urine-free fractions from the urine-contaminated fractions. The variable pattern of urine contamination seen in most stallions can make this approach frustrating and only occasionally successful.

Depending on the amount of urine contamination present in an individual ejaculate, it may be possible to improve the longevity of sperm motility by immediately diluting the raw ejaculate with a standard semen extender. In one study the addition of semen extender to urine-contaminated semen restored sperm motility to values similar to uncontaminated control ejaculates.[12] However, motility was followed only for 1 hour post contamination, and no fertility trials were performed. It is possible that, even with immediate extension and with minimal urine contamination, the longer-term longevity of sperm motility in extended, urine-contaminated ejaculates still will be of significantly lower quality than comparable urine-free ejaculates, particularly when urine contamination is moderate to heavy.

Recall that bladder neck (trigone) closure in the stallion is predominantly an α-adrenergic–controlled event (see Figure 41-1).[2] Because of this, there are several reports of α-adrenergic agonists being used to treat urospermia. The hypothesis is that increased α-adrenergic tone will increase bladder neck tone and so minimize urine leakage during ejaculation. In general, these agents are not particularly useful in themselves.[22] However, when combined with management practices aimed at evacuating the bladder as much as possible before ejaculation, these agents may be helpful. Examples of α-adrenergic agents that have been used to treat urospermia in stallions include imipramine hydrochloride (0.8 mg/kg PO 2 to 4 hours before semen collection), phenylpropanolamine (0.35 mg/kg PO twice daily), and noradrenaline.[8,16] We reported that imipramine, combined with the use of management changes designed to evacuate the bladder before ejaculation, was successful at managing severe urospermia in a breeding stallion for a period of 2 years.[8] However, this agent must be used with caution and with careful attention to dosage because, in men, higher doses have been implicated as causes of ejaculatory failure, erectile dysfunction, and impotence.[23,24]

Bethanechol chloride, a muscarinic parasympathetic receptor agonist, and flavoxate hydrochloride, a muscarinic parasympathetic antagonist, have been used for the treatment of urospermia with mixed or poor results.[18,22] Oxytocin also has been suggested as a means of constricting the bladder neck. However, results are reportedly poor.[25] Beta-blocking agents also have been employed but with little or no beneficial effects.[16]

Pharmacologic induction of ejaculation[4] has been suggested as a possible means of obtaining a urine-free ejaculate.[8] Ejaculation induced in this manner does not involve an increase in abdominal or intravesicular pressure and thus may minimize pressure on the urethral sphincter and bladder neck at the point of ejaculation.

When breed registries permit, it is worth considering the use of frozen semen for stallions severely affected by urospermia. One reasonable management technique is to use more aggressive treatment modalities (e.g., bladder catheterization, lavage, α-adrenergic agonists) for a period of time sufficient to collect, freeze, and bank a large volume of urine-free semen. Mares then can be bred when needed with frozen-thawed semen without the need for the stallion to produce a urine-free ejaculate on short notice or when labor or time are in short supply. This type of management may decrease the pressure and frustration associated with intermittent semen collection for immediate use or cooled transport.

Prognosis

The prognosis for complete resolution of idiopathic urospermia is poor. In most, if not all, reported cases the condition is intermittent but chronic. Because the underlying pathophysiology of the disease is not clear, treatments are generally palliative, rather than curative. However, the prognosis for the successful management of urospermia can be good if all involved parties are committed to the increased time and effort that is involved in handling the disorder. With meticulous management, and with a willingness to sometimes employ more aggressive treatment modalities (e.g., bladder catheterization and lavage), good pregnancy rates can be achieved even with severely affected stallions. However, before committing to the care and management of affected animals, all parties involved should be informed of the long-term and often frustrating nature of this condition. In cases in which a cause for the urospermia can be identified, the prognosis for resolution of the urospermia is related to the prognosis for the treatment and cure of the underlying cause.

HEMOSPERMIA

Hemospermia is defined as the presence of blood in the seminal fluid. The source of the blood can be anywhere in the reproductive tract, but the blood most commonly originates from lesions in the urethra, on the urethral process, or on the penis itself. Depending on the nature of the lesion, hemospermia may be present in all ejaculates or may be intermittent.

Etiology

The causes of hemospermia in the stallion are varied. The condition can result from bleeding or ulcerated lesions anywhere in the reproductive tract from the epididymis to the external surface of the penis. Some potential causes of hemospermia include epididymitis, blocked ampullae, seminal vesiculitis, urethral strictures, urethritis, urethral varicosities, neoplasia, and skin or mucosal surface lesions of the urethra, urethral process, glans penis, or penile shaft (Figure 41-2).[18,26-31] The average age of onset of horses with hemospermia varies greatly. Although any breed can be affected, the condition may be more common in Quarter Horses.[27]

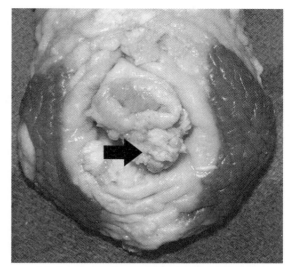

Figure 41-2 Squamous cell carcinoma of the urethral process of a stallion *(black arrow)*. During semen collection or natural cover this lesion readily ulcerated, resulting in mild to moderate hemospermia.

Trauma resulting in bleeding from the skin or mucosa of the reproductive tract is a relatively common cause of hemospermia. Often the urethral process is the site of injury.[32] The source of the trauma varies, but some of the more common causes include kicks from a mare during breeding, lacerations of the penis or urethral process from tail hairs of the mare during breeding, and urethral strictures or skin lesions caused by the use of stallion rings. Iatrogenic traumatic hemospermia can occur following urinary bladder catheterization or urethroscopy.

Before the widespread use of ivermectin-based anthelminthics, cutaneous habronemiasis was a commonly reported cause of hemospermia (Figure 41-3). Lesions caused by *Habronema* spp. are seen uncommonly in animals that are on proper anthelminthic programs. Stallions with blocked ampullae may exhibit hemospermia before or immediately following relief of the blockage.[33] It is likely that the discharge of chronically inspissated material from the ampullae results in trauma to the ampullary mucosa and subsequent hemorrhage into the ejaculate.

Infectious causes of hemospermia also have been reported. These include bacterial seminal vesiculitis, epididymitis, and urethritis. In addition, active equine herpesvirus 3 infections can result in ulcerations on the skin surface of the penile shaft and glans penis. These ulcerations readily bleed during breeding, resulting in hemospermia. Bacterial urethritis has been reported to be a relatively common cause of hemospermia in stallions. The most common organisms associated with bacterial urethritis include *Streptococcus* spp., *Escherichia coli,* and *Pseudomonas aeurogenosa,*[27] and the condition is seen more commonly in the pelvic urethra from the ischial arch to the colliculus seminalis, rather than in the penile urethra. Viral urethritis also has been suspected as a possible cause of hemospermia.[34]

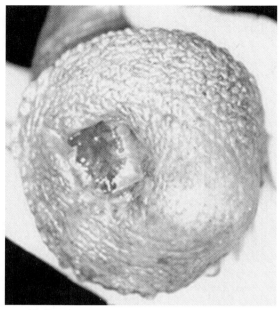

Figure 41-3 Ulcerations of the urethral process caused by cutaneous habronemiasis. This condition can readily be treated with ivermectin-based anthelminthics.

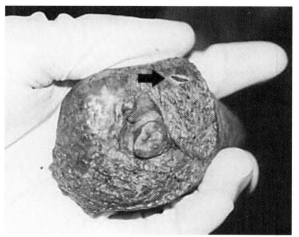

Figure 41-4 Small laceration of the glans penis *(black arrow)*. This lesion was difficult to identify on the stallion's nonerect penis. However, at the point of ejaculation, the wound opened dramatically and bled profusely, resulting in severe hemospermia. It is likely that the wound communicated with the underlying corpus spongiosum. During maximum glans fill, the increased pressure in the cavernous space forced the wound to open and allowed for significant and dramatic hemorrhage. This lesion was closed surgically after debridement of the wound's edges.

Regardless of the cause of the lesion, bleeding from the urethra, penile skin, or cavernous tissues typically is not seen when the stallion is at sexual rest. However, during breeding, the cavernous spaces of the penis engorge with blood, and blood pressure in the penile vessels increases. In association with this, the penile shaft, glans, and urethral process enlarge significantly. In addition, friction of the surface of the penis with an AV or with the mare's reproductive tract can cause irritation. All of these occurrences can combine to result in acute exacerbation of an existing lesion during intromission and at the moment of ejaculation. In some instances, hemospermia can be relatively mild, resulting only in a faint pink tinge to the ejaculate. However, in other cases (for example, a puncture wound or laceration to the glans penis that communicates with the underlying cavernous tissue), erection and ejaculation can acutely open an existing lesion and result in a sudden and sometimes dramatic hemorrhage into the ejaculate.

Clinical Signs and Diagnosis

Stallions breeding by natural cover whose semen is not evaluated on a regular basis may present for infertility because it has been documented that significant whole blood contamination of the ejaculate will reduce pregnancy rates.[35] The exact mechanism by which blood in the ejaculate reduces fertility is unclear because sperm motility, morphologic characteristics, and numbers generally are not affected by the presence of blood. In addition to infertility, blood may be seen at the mare's vulva following breeding, or it may be noted in the postejaculatory drippings.[30] An accurate diagnosis of hemospermia generally can readily be made by collecting semen into an AV and observing blood in the ejaculate. The amount of blood

contamination can vary dramatically, and thus the gross appearance of the ejaculate can range from pale pink (slight blood contamination) to that of frank blood (significant blood contamination). In some cases, profuse hemorrhage may be seen, usually in association with skin or urethral lesions that communicate with the underlying cavernous tissues.[31] In milder cases, microscopic examination of the ejaculate may aid in the diagnosis by revealing the presence of red blood cells. Some affected stallions may exhibit pain when they obtain a full erection or ejaculate.[27]

Hemospermia, like urospermia, can vary in severity from one ejaculate to another and often is sporadic. Thus collection of a single, blood-free ejaculate does not rule out a diagnosis of hemospermia. If hemospermia is suspected, multiple semen collections may be required to detect the condition. In particular, animals who are being examined following a period of sexual rest may not exhibit hemospermia in their first few ejaculates. Repeated ejaculations within a relatively narrow window of time (days) may be required to aggravate an old lesion sufficiently to cause recurrence of the condition.

Careful physical examination of the external surfaces of the penis and urethral process should be performed on both the nonerect and fully erect penis. Some superficial lesions are apparent on visual inspection. If a lesion is not identified, it may be helpful to collect semen and/or to fractionate semen using an open-ended AV. When properly filled, an open-ended AV allows the glans penis to fully extend out the end of the AV. This permits clear visualization of the glans during thrusting and during glans flare ("belling") and ejaculation. Some lesions that are not obvious in the nonerect penis become very apparent during maximum glans fill (Figure 41-4). In addition, fractionation of the ejaculate may help to localize the source of the bleeding. Bleeding from the skin surface may be present in all jets of the ejaculate. Blood in only the first few jets could suggest a testicular or epididymal lesion (because the first few sperm-rich jets originate largely from the testicles and epididymis) whereas blood in the later jets might suggest a problem with the accessory sex glands. These observations are rules of thumb and should be used in conjunction with multiple examination techniques to diagnose the source of the bleeding.

If the skin or urethral process is not identified as the source of the bleeding, then other diagnostic techniques can be employed to examine other areas of the reproductive tract. Palpation and ultrasonography of the scrotal contents may reveal abnormalities of the epididymis or spermatic cord. To the author's knowledge, testicular lesions have not been reported as causes of hemospermia. Nonetheless, examination of the testicles is recommended as part of a complete evaluation. Transrectal palpation and ultrasonography of the internal accessory glands also may identify pathologic conditions (e.g., blocked ampullae, seminal vesiculitis). Finally, urethroscopy with a flexible fiberoptic endoscope can be performed to fully examine the penile and pelvic urethra and to rule out the presence of mucosal lesions that could be contributing to the hemospermia. Idiopathic lesions in the urethra that communicate with the underlying corpus spongiosum penis have been reported as causes of sometimes profuse hemospermia.[31] These lesions most commonly are found near the pelvic ischium, but their small size can make them difficult to identify. It has been suggested that urethroscopy immediately following ejaculation may make the diagnosis more straightforward because blood may still be present in and around the lesion at this time.[32] When performing urethroscopy, the clinician should keep in mind that the procedure itself can readily cause secondary urethral hyperemia. Therefore one must use caution before using endoscopy to decide that urethral hyperemia is a cause for the hemospermia.

Contrast radiography has been suggested as another method of evaluating the urethra. Retrograde infusion of a contrast material into the urethra, followed by a series of radiographs may help to identify strictures, masses, fistulas, and other similar urethral lesions.[30] This method is used less commonly now that flexible endoscopy is readily available.

Treatment

The approach to treatment depends largely on the source of the hemorrhage, and so every effort should be made to accurately identify the cause of the hemospermia before initiating therapy. For example, the treatment of hemospermia originating from blocked ampullae would be handled quite differently than that originating from seminal vesiculitis. For the purposes of this chapter, only the most common and most general causes of hemospermia will be discussed. These are localized bacterial infections and skin or mucosal rents, lacerations, and ulcerations.

If an infectious cause is suspected, the source of the infection first should be determined. Swabs of the affected area should be obtained for bacteriologic culture and sensitivity testing. After choosing an appropriate antibiotic, the affected area should be treated locally (if it is accessible) or systemically (if not accessible). In some cases it is possible that bacterial contamination of a lesion might have developed secondary to the lesion, rather than be the cause of the lesion.[27] Another component of treatment for infectious hemospermia may or may not involve sexual rest. Some infected lesions benefit from sexual rest. For example, infected mucosal lesions often heal more rapidly if they are not repeatedly exposed to the friction and increases in pressure that occur during erection and ejaculation. On the other hand, one component of treatment of seminal vesiculitis can include frequent semen collections designed to help "flush out" the seminal vesicles and so more rapidly clear the problem.

In cases of traumatic or idiopathic rents, lacerations, and ulcerations, sexual rest is almost always the central component of a treatment plan. A minimum of several weeks and often several months of sexual rest are required. However, even with very prolonged periods of sexual rest, hemospermia may recur once the stallion returns to an active breeding program.[27] Note that sexual rest should not include discouraging normal spontaneous erections and penile movements (also called masturbation). These actions are physiologic, and it has been well documented that aggressive methods of discouraging their occurrence can be harmful to the animal.[36]

As an alternative to conservative treatment with sexual rest alone, surgical approaches may be combined with sexual rest to help encourage resolution of hemospermia resulting from traumatic or idiopathic lesions. Suturing of lacerations may be indicated. In the case of internal urethral lesions, the author has attempted laser ablation of the ulcerated area with mixed results. A more aggressive method of treatment is to perform a temporary (approximately 10 weeks' duration) subischial urethrotomy, thus allowing urine to bypass the distal aspects of the urethra entirely and also potentially reducing pressure in the corpus spongiosum penis at the end of urination.[27,31] Temporary subischial urethrotomy may result in a higher percentage of resolution of hemospermia than does sexual rest alone, especially when it is combined with daily topical placement of antimicrobials and anti-inflammatories into the urethral lumen.[27] However, this procedure is more costly and is associated with more side effects, including urethral strictures and fistulas.[27,37]

If the degree of hemospermia is mild, immediate extension of blood-contaminated ejaculates may be sufficient to allow pregnancies to occur.[29] Alternatively, if a stallion is breeding by natural cover, extender can be placed into the mare's uterus before breeding so that the stallion ejaculates into the extender and any blood contamination is diluted.

As a result of the underlying lesion, some animals may experience discomfort associated with ejaculation. If the pain is significant, it may eventually lead to ejaculatory problems and/or loss of libido. As such, animals exhibiting signs of pain in association with hemospermia may benefit from treatment with anti-inflammatory medications.

Other reported treatments for hemospermia include intravenous formalin administration and urine acidification.[34,38] However, neither of these methods resulted in long-term cures for the hemospermia, and so their use is questionable.

Prognosis

The prognosis for recovery, like the approach to treatment, varies based on the source of the hemospermia. Simple lacerations may heal with only rest. Puncture wounds may be more difficult to manage and may require surgical intervention. However, in general, in cases of acute trauma, the prognosis for full recovery is good if the animal is given an appropriate period of sexual rest. If rest alone is insufficient, the edges of the wound may need to be freshened and the wound sutured closed to allow for first intention healing.

Idiopathic ulcerated or rentlike lesions of the urethra can be more frustrating to deal with. Surgical correction and/or laser ablation may or may not be helpful, and it is not uncommon for hemospermia to recur in these cases even after extended periods of sexual rest. In many cases the healed area is very prone to reinjury once the animal returns to active breeding. Temporary subischial urethrotomy may increase the chances of a permanent resolution; however, even when this treatment is used, recurrence is not uncommon.

References

1. Blanchard TL, Varner DD, Bretzlaff KN: Diseases of the reproductive system: male reproductive disorders. In Smith B (ed): Large Animal Internal Medicine, p 1424, St Louis, Mosby, 1990.
2. McDonnell SM: Ejaculation: physiology and dysfunction. Vet Clin North Am Equine Pract 1992; 8:57-70.
3. Guyton AC: Textbook of Medical Physiology, Philadelphia, WB Saunders, 2000.
4. McDonnell SM, Love CC: Xylazine-induced ex copula ejaculation in stallions. Theriogenology 1991; 36:73.
5. McDonnell SM: Oral imipramine and intravenous xylazine for pharmacologically-induced ex copula ejaculation in stallions. Anim Reprod Sci 2001; 68:153-159.
6. McClure JJ: Paralytic bladder. In Robinson NE (ed): Current Therapy in Equine Medicine, pp 712-713, Philadelphia, WB Saunders, 1987.
7. Mayhew IG: Neurologic aspects of urospermia in the horse. Equine Vet Educ 1990; 2:68-69.
8. Turner RM, Love CC, McDonnell SM et al: Use of imipramine hydrochloride for treatment of urospermia in a stallion with a dysfunctional bladder. J Am Vet Med Assoc 1995, 207:1602-1606.
9. Naylor J, Nickel DD, Trimino G et al: Hyperkalemic periodic paralysis in homozygous and heterozygous horses: a co-dominant genetic condition. Equine Vet J 1999; 31: 153-159.
10. Lakin MM: Diagnostic assessment of disorders of male sexual function. In Montague DK (ed): Disorders of Male Sexual Dysfunction, p 26, Chicago, Yearbook Medical, 1988.
11. Brinsko SP: Retrograde ejaculation in a stallion. J Am Vet Med Assoc 2001; 218:551-553.
12. Griggers S, Paccamonti D, Thompson RA et al: The effects of pH, osmolarity and urine contamination on equine spermatozoal motility. Theriogenology 2001; 56:613-622.
13. Lowe JN: Diagnosis and management of urospermia in a commercial Thoroughbred stallion. Equine Vet Educ 2001; 13:4-7.
14. Hurtgen J: Evaluation of the stallion for breeding soundness. Vet Clin North Am 1992; 8:149-168.
15. Althouse GC, Seager SWJ, Varner DD et al: Diagnostic aids for the detection of urine in the equine ejaculate. Theriogenology 1989; 31:1141-1148.
16. Leendertse IP, Asbury AC, Boening KJ et al: Successful management of persistent urination during ejaculation in a Thoroughbred stallion. Equine Vet Educ 1990; 2:62-65.
17. Hurtgen J: Stallion genital abnormalities. In Robinson NE (ed): Current Therapy in Equine Medicine, p 561, Philadelphia, WB Saunders, 1987.
18. Varner D, Schumacher J, Blanchard T et al: Diseases and management of breeding stallions, Goleta, Calif, American Veterinary Publications, 1991.
19. Tischner M, Kosiniak K, Bielanski W: Analysis of the pattern of ejaculation in stallions. J Reprod Fertil 1974; 41:329-335.
20. Ellery JC: A modified equine artificial vagina for the collection of gel-free semen. J Am Vet Med Assoc 1971; 158: 765-766.
21. Nash JG Jr, Voss JL, Squires EL: Urination during ejaculation in a stallion. J Am Vet Med Assoc 1980; 176:224-227.
22. Hoyos Sepulveda ML, Quiroz Rocha GF, Brumbaugh GW et al: Lack of beneficial effects of bethanechol, imipramine or furosemide on seminal plasma of three stallions with urospermia. Reprod Domest Anim 1999; 34:489-493.
23. Segraves RT: Sexual side-effects of psychiatric drugs. Int J Psychiatry Med 1988; 18:243-252.
24. Segraves RT: Effects of psychiatric drugs on human erection and ejaculation. Arch Gen Psychiatry 1989; 46:275-284.
25. Voss JL, McKinnon AO: Hemospermia and urospermia. In McKinnon AO, Voss JL (eds): Equine Reproduction, pp 864-870, Philadelphia/London, Lea & Febiger, 1993.
26. Sojka JE, Carter GK: Hemospermia and seminal vesicle enlargement in a stallion. Compend Contin Educ Pract Vet 1985; 7:S587-S588.
27. Sullins KE, Bertone JJ, Voss JL et al: Treatment of hemospermia in stallions: a discussion of 18 cases. Compend Contin Educ Pract Vet 1988; 10:1396-1403.
28. Bedford SJ, McDonnell SM, Tulleners E et al: Squamous cell carcinoma of the urethral process in a horse with hemospermia and self-mutilation behavior. J Am Vet Med Assoc 2000; 216:551-553.
29. Blanchard TL: Use of a semen extender containing antibiotics to improve the fertility of a stallion with seminal vesiculitis due to *Pseudomonas aeruginosa*. Theriogenology 1987; 28:541-546.
30. McKinnon AO, Voss JL, Trotter GW et al: Hemospermia of the stallion. Equine Pract 1988; 10:17-23.
31. Schumacher J, Varner DD, Schmitz DG et al: Urethral defects in geldings with hematuria and stallions with hemospermia. Vet Surg 1995; 24:250-254.
32. Varner DD, Blanchard TL, Brinsko SP et al: Techniques for evaluating selected reproductive disorders of stallions. Anim Reprod Sci 2000; 60-61:493-509.
33. Love CC, Riera FL, Oristaglio (Turner) RM: Sperm occluded (plugged) ampullae in the stallion. Proceedings of the Annual Meeting of the Society for Theriogenology, pp 117-125, 1992.

34. Voss JL, Pickett BW: Diagnosis and treatment of hemospermia in the stallion. J Reprod Fertil Suppl 1975; 23:151-154.

35. Voss JL, Pickett BW, Shideler RK: The effect of hemospermia on fertility in horses. Proceedings of the 8th International Congress of Animal Reproduction and Artificial Insemination, pp 1093-1095, 1976.

36. McDonnell SM, Henry M, Bristol F: Spontaneous erection and masturbation in equids. Proceedings of the 5th International Symposium on Equine Reproduction, pp 664-665, 1991.

37. Laverty S, Pascoe JR, Ling GV et al: Urolithiasis in 68 horses. Vet Surg 1992; 21:56-62.

38. Voss JL, Wotowey JL: Hemospermia. Proceedings of the 18th Annual Convention of the American Association of Equine Practitioners, pp 103-112, 1973.

CHAPTER 42

Transmission of Diseases Through Semen

JAMES L. N. WOOD
JACQUELINE M. CARDWELL
JAVIER CASTILLO-OLIVARES
VIVIENNE IRWIN

It has been noted in clinical texts for more than 100 years that disease can be transmitted from apparently healthy stallions to mares at covering.[1,2] It is now known that in the horse, as in other species, various infections may be transmitted at covering through semen. In some cases these cause serious clinical disease, whereas in others the greatest impact is through reduced fertility and the subsequent economic or commercial impact.

This chapter reviews the infections that can be transmitted through equine semen or at covering between the stallion and mare. Although full sections are provided for common infections where venereal spread is fully characterized, attention is also drawn to less common infections or other diseases where the organism can be detected in semen, but where any role of venereal transmission has not been fully elucidated. For each infection, brief descriptions of the organism, signs of disease, its epidemiology, the detection of the organism, and the prevention of its spread through semen or natural covering are provided.

EQUINE ARTERITIS VIRUS

Equine arteritis virus (EAV) is the prototype member of the family Arteriviridae, which includes porcine reproductive and respiratory syndrome virus (PRRSV), lactate dehydrogenase elevating virus of mice (LDV), and simian hemorrhagic fever virus (SHFV). EAV is a small, enveloped, single-stranded RNA virus that is inactivated by most disinfectants. The endothelium of the small blood vessels and macrophages are the primary targets of EAV, but the virus can also replicate in different cell types in vivo and in vitro. It is transmitted by venereal and respiratory routes.[3,4] EAV can infect horses, donkeys, and mules, but natural infection in zebras has not been demonstrated.[5]

Clinical Signs

Symptoms of EAV vary widely in severity and range and depend on the virus strain and other factors such as age, breed, and immune status of the host.[6] The range of clinical signs varies between individuals within and between outbreaks, with breed appearing to be an important determinant of symptoms. In particular, susceptibility to infection appears to be the same for Standardbreds and Throroughbreds, but clinical disease is less frequently reported in the former, despite their high seroprevalence.

Infected horses may or may not present, after an incubation period of 3 to 14 day,[7] any combination of the possible clinical signs, the most common of which are fever (lasting up to 7 days and reaching up to 41°C); depression; lethargy; anorexia; conjunctivitis; rhinitis with serous nasal discharge; palpebral, periorbital, and / or supraorbital edema; edema of mammary glands, prepuce, ventral abdomen, and/or legs; and urticarial skin rash. Other signs include weakness, ataxia, congestion or petechia of mucosal membranes, respiratory distress, diarrhea, and abortion in the pregnant mare.

The two features of the disease that make its control important are its ability to cause both abortion in pregnant mares and persistent infections in stallions. Detailed study of the disease indicates that the venereal route, particularly stallion to mare, plays a critical role in the maintenance of the infection in the horse population.[8-10]

Infection of pregnant mares can result in abortion, which has a serious economic impact for the horse breeding industry. It usually occurs 10 to 33 days post infection and can occur without the mare displaying any clinical signs.[7] Abortions have been reported in mares between 3 and 10 months of gestation. Mares do not appear to suffer fertility problems after EAV infection, but stallions experience a reduction in the quality and quantity of the sperm during the acute phase of the disease. In contrast, no fertility problems have been observed in persistent carrier stallions.[11]

A proportion of stallions become chronically infected with EAV after the acute phase and can continue to excrete virus in the semen for months or years without displaying any signs of disease. EAV localizes in cells of the entire male urogenital tract, and it has been recovered from the epididymis, vas deferens, ampulla, seminal vesicle, bulbourethral gland, prostate, urinary bladder, and proximal urethra in persistently infected stallions.[12] Such persistent infection is testosterone dependent; castration results in cessation of virus excretion in semen after castration, although it can be maintained through administration of testosterone.[13] Persistent infections do not occur in colts infected before puberty.[14] Results from recently reported attempts to stop shedding by temporary chemical castration have been interesting,[15] but more work is required before this can be recommended as an effective procedure.

EAV is well preserved in both frozen and chilled equine semen and so can be transmitted most effectively through the use of natural covering and artificial insemination (AI),[3,4] whether the semen has been preserved by chilling or freezing.

Immune Responses

EAV infection in the horse induces virus-neutralizing antibody (VNAb) and cytotoxic T-lymphocyte responses.[16] Experimental infections indicate that VNAb in serum appears within the first week after infection[17-22] and remains at high levels for months or years. The appearance of VNAb in serum coincides with clinical recovery in experimentally infected animals.[18] Passively acquired maternal antibodies, which last between 2 and 8 months in foals,[23,24] prevented or moderated EAV infection, and horses vaccinated with formalin-inactivated vaccine showed various degrees of protection, which correlated to the VNAb at the time of challenge.[25,26] Although infection with EAV results in a long-lasting, if not lifelong, immunity and recovered horses do not show signs of disease, they are rarely protected from reinfection, and sterile immunity may not be achieved reliably with either inactivated or live vaccines.[21,27,28]

Diagnosis of Equine Viral Arteritis (EVA) and Detection of EAV in Carrier Stallions

Due to the asymptomatic nature of many natural EAV infections and the fact that several of the clinical signs of EVA are nonspecific, it is always necessary to confirm suspected EAV cases by laboratory testing.

Retrospective serologic diagnosis of EAV infection is made by detection of virus-specific antibodies in serum from convalescent horses. The most widely used serologic test and the one prescribed for international trade by the Office International des Epizooties (OIE) is the virus neutralization test (VNT) performed on microtiter plates as described by Senne et al.[29] The test, despite being widely used and suitable for large sample screening, can present problems in its performance, and discrepant results have been obtained by different laboratories.[30]

In specialist laboratories conversant with the use of the VNT, *VNAb has been demonstrated in all persistently infected stallions*. Thus the VNT is a useful screening assay for all stallions to help determine infection status. Nonspecific cytotoxicity of equine sera obtained from horses vaccinated with tissue culture–derived vaccines can, however, complicate the use of the VNT.[31] Use of enzyme-linked immunosorbent assay (ELISA) tests to replace the VNT has been investigated for some time.[32-34] The diagnostic ELISA test developed by Nugent et al[35] appears useful but has not yet become available commercially.

Virus isolation from clinical specimens appears most sensitive when RK-13 cells are used.[36] Isolation of EAV from clinical material is difficult and time consuming, for both semen and samples collected during the acute phase of the disease.[37]

All unvaccinated stallions with VNAb may be persistently infected semen shedders, and their semen should be examined for the presence of EAV. Detection of infected stallions can also be made indirectly by test mating. The suspected stallion is mated to two seronegative mares on two consecutive days, and detection of a rise in VNAb titer of the mares is taken as an indication of the shedding status of the stallion. Although slow and expensive, this is a safe method for determining the shedding status of a stallion.

Due to these inconveniences, molecular diagnostic methods have become increasingly popular in the last 10 years for the detection of EAV from clinical samples. The potential of these techniques for EAV diagnosis was demonstrated by Chirnside and Spaan,[38] and their methods provide the basis for molecular diagnostic protocols.[39,40] Modern real-time polymerase chain reaction (PCR) methods have facilitated high sample throughput, while minimizing cross contamination.[11,41]

Vaccination Against EAV

Currently there are two commercially available vaccines for the prevention of EVA, a live attenuated vaccine and a killed virus adjuvanted vaccine. The live vaccine, used extensively in some parts of the United States,[42,43] prevents clinical disease and significantly reduces viremia and virus excretion. However, its use is not recommended in pregnant mares. Recently a virus with an identical sequence to the vaccine strain was derived from an aborted fetus whose dam was vaccinated a few days earlier with the live vaccine.[44]

Inactivated vaccines were first developed in Japan and consisted of concentrated preparations of formalin-inactivated whole virus formulated without adjuvant. These vaccines stimulate neutralizing antibodies after an initial two-dose course. The antibody levels decline over a period of 6 months, and revaccination is recommended to sustain protective immunity. This immunity correlates with circulating neutralizing antibody levels.[25,26,28,45] The commercial inactivated vaccine (Artervac, Southampton, UK) is currently licensed in Germany and available in the United Kingdom (UK) and other European states under test certificates, although only limited data on efficacy and duration of immunity exist. The vaccine claims to stimulate VNAb after two doses, but some field studies and experimental observations showed that detectable titers may not be achieved even after three or more inoculations,[46] although higher titers were usually achieved after multiple doses.

The available vaccines do not allow discrimination of infected from vaccinated animals, which is necessary to allow serologic surveillance in nonendemic areas. The lack of serologic discrimination also hugely complicates international trade in vaccinated stallions and their semen. All stallions being vaccinated should be shown to be seronegative in an accredited laboratory on the day of vaccination, and thereafter serologic titers should be monitored. The induction of protective immune responses that can be differentiated from natural infections by using "marker" vaccines would overcome the problems mentioned above.[47,48]

Prevention of EAV Transmission at Covering or Insemination

Control relies on combining serologic surveillance, vaccination, and sound animal management practices. Special emphasis is put on detection of persistent shedding in stallions and prevention of the carrier state developing. However, the policies vary widely between different countries, being motivated in part by the differences in disease prevalence. There are various codes of practice that exist to prevent transmission of EAV on stud farms in Europe, including a Common Code of Practice used in many European states[49] and the British Equine Veterinary Association's Code of Practice for artificial insemination.[50] European Community directives cover the intracommunity trade in semen.[51]

In contrast to these European protocols, the American Horse Council Protocol on EAV bases its recommendations for the control of EAV on the extensive use of the live vaccine in stallions, permitting the breeding of immune or immunized mares to shedding stallions. The control measures implemented in the UK and Ireland, where prevalence is low, contrast to these; recommendations are based on serologic screening of mares and stallions before covering to ensure that infectious animals are restricted from the breeding population. Stallions vaccinated with the whole virus killed vaccine should also be serologically monitored annually. EVA is notifiable in stallions in several European states, including the UK and Ireland.

European legislation requires that stallions used for frozen semen collection should be demonstrated to be seronegative for EAV 14 days after collection of semen and that horses used for chilled semen production should be seronegative before entry into a licensed collection center.[51]

The use of AI is probably the best means of protecting stallions from becoming infected as a result of covering acutely infected, visiting mares. If stallions, such as Thoroughbreds, need to cover mares naturally, then they should be vaccinated and care exercised to ensure that mares are not acutely infected before covering. Serosurveillance of mare bands immediately before covering is useful in achieving this, but is not foolproof.[52]

CONTAGIOUS EQUINE METRITIS

Contagious equine metritis (CEM) is caused by infection with *Taylorella equigenitalis*, a microaerophilic bacterium also referred to as contagious equine metritis organism (CEMO). Two biotypes of the organism, distinguished by streptomycin sensitivity, have been characterized.[53] Infection in naïve animals causes an acute endometritis in most naïve mares, following a latent period of 2 to 12 days.[53] Primary infection in the mare usually results in short-term infertility, and this is the major impact of the disease. Infection is usually asymptomatic in stallions. It is spread venereally between mares and stallions and between infected mares and their offspring at parturition. It can also be spread mechanically.[54-57]

CEM is endemic in non-Thoroughbreds in several European countries but is largely absent from most Thoroughbred populations, including in Ireland, Britain, and France. Horses in the United States and Canada are thought to be free from infection, although there is some evidence of infection of donkeys with a related organism, *Taylorella asinigenitalis*.[54,58,59]

There is a wide range of opinions as to the clinical significance of the infection, in particular in Europe. Although some countries, including Ireland, Britain, the United States, and Canada, regard the infection as highly significant, others such as Belgium and the Netherlands regard the organism as an occasionally pathogenic commensal. It is clear that the major impact of the infection is economic, both through reduction of high levels of fertility now expected in intensive breeding operations and through stringent international controls on the movement of infected animals and germplasm.[51]

Outbreaks in the UK and Ireland have been controlled highly effectively by implementation of the recommendations of the Horserace Betting Levy Board's Codes of Practice.[49] A small number of cases of CEM have been diagnosed recently in the UK, but these have occurred in recently imported non-Thoroughbred animals and their contacts.[60] Recent cases have not been diagnosed in Ireland.

Long-term male and female carriers of the infection play a key role in the dissemination and maintenance of infection,[53] and the vast majority of persistently infected mares harbor *T. equigenitalis* on the mucous membrane surfaces of the clitoral sinuses and fossa.[53] It was noted around 25 years ago that available methods for the detection of CEMO in mares were not capable of detecting all infected mares.[61] The methods in common use today have not altered in substance since that time, even though more sensitive methods have become available.[62-66]

Diagnosis of CEM and Detection of CEMO

Clinical signs of CEM in mares include irregular return to service and a vulval discharge, which may range from very mild to extremely profuse. After the acute phase, infection in mares becomes asymptomatic, while the bacteria reside on the mucosal surface of the clitoris, particularly the clitoral fossa and sinuses. Signs of disease are not usually seen in infected stallions, although the organism can sometimes invade the accessory sex glands, causing inflammatory cells and bacteria to contaminate the semen.[53]

Laboratory diagnosis is essential to confirm the presence of *T. equigenitalis* infection in both mares and stallions. The bacteria are fastidious and require specific conditions for growth, including specialist media and a microaerophilic environment. Swabs used in the mare must be small enough to sample the clitoral sinuses.[53] All swabs should be placed immediately into Amies charcoal transport media and refrigerated if not immediately received by the diagnostic laboratory. Laboratories used for detection of *T. equigenitalis* should be experienced in the detection of the organism and appropriately accredited.

The authors have undertaken a systematic literature review[67] to estimate the sensitivity of detecting *T. equigenitalis* in different specimens at different times following infection. The results of this review were that around 95%

of mares infected more than 8 weeks previously should be detected through culture of a single clitoral swab. The organism was found in cervical swabs in only 30% of such chronically infected mares, although it was found in cervical swabs in nearly 85% of acutely infected mares.

Prevention of CEMO Transmission at Covering or Insemination

In order to prevent CEMO being transmitted from stallion to mare at covering or through AI in areas such as Europe where the infection may occur, care needs to be taken to ensure that neither animal is infected for natural covering and that the semen is not infected in the case of AI. Methods to ensure that neither animal is infected are described in the Code of Practice for CEM (operational in many European countries)[49] and also in North American texts.[57]

Briefly, swabs should be collected from stallions from the urethra, the urethral fossa, and the penile sheath, as well as from preejaculatory fluid, before covering and should be cultured for the presence of *T. equigenitalis*. A swab from the clitoris, including clitoral fossae, should be collected before covering from mares derived from populations where *T. equigenitalis* is endemic. For mares known to have been previously infected or from populations where the organism is not endemic, at least two sets of swabs from clitoris, as above, and from the cervix and endometrium at estrus are recommended to be cultured for CEMO before covering.

As for EVA, detection of the carrier state in stallions, particularly in first-season stallions infected with *T. equigenitalis* by their dams at birth, test mating of negative test mares can increase the sensitivity of detection of the infection.

Although AI can be expected to dramatically reduce the transmission of venereal pathogens by minimizing the contact between mares and stallions, care needs to be taken to ensure that stallions are not infected. Although some antibiotics used in semen extenders, particularly gentamicin, can markedly reduce the numbers of *T. equigenitalis* in contaminated semen,[68] the infection is not reliably eliminated even by this treatment. There are no published data that suggest that ceftiofur, now frequently used in many semen extenders, can eliminate the infection. Thus, whatever antibiotic is used in semen extenders, it is essential to ensure that stallions used for semen collection are not infected with *T. equigenitalis*.

COITAL EXANTHEMA

Coital exanthema is a mild, usually self-resolving disease caused by equine herpesvirus-3 (EHV-3). EHV-3 is an alphaherpesvirus, distinct from EHV-1 and EHV-4. Systemic illness is not usually seen with this infection, although local secondary bacterial infections can increase the severity of the clinical presentation. Many cases go unobserved because direct examination of either the vaginal mucosa or the penis and prepuce is usually required to see the lesions. However, there have been cases where lesions on the perineum and edema of the vulva labia have also been reported.[69] Infection in naïve animals is associated with the development of multiple raised nodules covered by crusty scabs.[70] The scabs rub off easily, leaving shallow erosions with irregular but sharply defined margins and hyperemia. The erosions enlarge peripherally and can become confluent before filling with exudate. These lesions generally resolve in 10 to 14 days, often leaving areas of depigmented epithelium.[71] In some cases the stallion will show no loss of libido when teased.[69]

It has yet to be proven that the EHV-3 virus can cause a latent infection. However, there is circumstantial evidence from field outbreaks of latency and reactivation. The epidemiology often suggests that the source of infection during EHV-3 outbreaks within closed breeding herds is most likely to have been an asymptomatic carrier in which the disease has been reactivated following coitus. Immediate early genes have also been identified that link EHV-3 with the latent state.[72] Severity of disease seems to vary between outbreaks, and some animals appear to carry particularly virulent strains of virus. However, it seems likely that infections with the less virulent strains may frequently go undetected because the prevalence of antibody in sexually active, mature horses is 50%, considerably higher than that expected from observations of the frequency of clinical disease.[73]

EHV-3 is spread venereally between mares and stallions. Following coitus the incubation period may be as long as 10 days, though in experimental conditions the period is about 48 hours.[73] Often the first symptom noted in mares is a vulval discharge following the onset of a secondary bacterial infection.

This disease does not tend to affect fertility.[74] However, abortion has been induced in the experimental situation following intrauterine inoculation of a mare at 7 months' gestation with EHV-3.[75] A lesion on the nostril of a 2-month-old foal from which EHV-3 was isolated has been reported following contact with an affected mare.[76] Similar lesions have also been induced experimentally following intranasal inoculation.[77]

Diagnosis of Coital Exanthema and EHV-3 infection

In animals demonstrating typical signs of acute coital exanthema, diagnosis may be made by demonstration of virus in samples collected from lesions or through demonstration of a seroconversion. Virus can be isolated by inoculation of clinical material onto cell cultures of equine origin, and negative-staining electron microscopy (EM) can be used to examine vesicular fluid or lesion scrapings to provide a rapid provisional diagnosis. Serologic diagnosis is usually made using a VNT. A PCR test is also available now for EHV-3 and is particularly used to enhance existing procedures,[78] due to its rapidity compared to virus isolation. In many cases, animals have seroconverted by the time lesions are detected and diagnoses are made presumptively on observation of spread of typical lesions at coitus, combined with demonstration of high circulating antibody titers.

Prevention of EHV-3 Transmission at Covering or Insemination

Currently there is no test to show which animals are latently infected with EHV-3 before covering. Latent infection may reactivate in some animals after the start of covering, and in some stallions transmission occurs in most covering seasons.[79] However, because EHV-3 causes a characteristic depigmentation of the affected pigmented skin, a retrospective study has suggested that these spots could be used to identify previously affected and hence likely carrier animals.[73]

When an animal develops signs of coital exanthema, natural covering should cease and the animal should be rested until a clinical recovery is made. Clinical diagnosis should be supported by laboratory testing to rule out other differential diagnoses, including CEM and EHV-1, which can cause similar lesions in some cases.

It is not clear whether EHV-3 can be transmitted by artificial insemination, but it is recommended that, unless otherwise shown to be safe, semen should not be collected from stallions where clinical signs or epidemiologic evidence exists suggestive of active EHV-3 infection. Although EHV-3 is primarily transmitted through coitus, infected fomites have also been implicated in its spread. Therefore it is possible that the virus can potentially be transmitted to the ejaculate through penile contact with an artificial vagina or sleeve.[80] However, the pain associated with active infection may discourage the stallion from service.

At present there is no vaccination available. Although EHV-3 is documented to be present in many regions such as the United States, Europe, and Australia, they have not implemented control or eradication programs because the disease is relatively mild and not of great economic significance.

DOURINE

Dourine is a severe, usually fatal disease caused by infection with *Trypanosoma equiperdum*. This is the only known trypanosome not transmitted by insect vectors. The incubation period and clinical signs (including severity and duration) vary widely. Although most cases are fatal, some recoveries do occur.[81] Clinical signs of dourine include periodic episodes of fever, local edema of genitals or mammary glands, vaginal discharge, incoordination, facial paralysis, anemia, emaciation, and edematous cutaneous plaques (up to 5 to 8 cm in diameter and 1 cm thick). The latter are often referred to as "silver dollar plaques" and are considered by some to be pathognomonic.[81] Neurologic signs also develop in some animals.

The infection is thought to be spread almost exclusively at coitus between mares and stallions,[82] being more readily spread from stallion to mare than vice versa.[81] It can also be spread by blood transfusion,[82] and there are some reports of infections in animals before sexual maturity,[83,84] consistent with mares' milk being infectious.[81]

The trypanosome is unusual in that it is a tissue rather than a blood parasite, but it is found in the seminal fluid and mucous exudate of the penis and sheath as well as in vaginal mucus.[81]

There was a large international epidemic of the disease after the Second World War, but infection has largely been eliminated from Europe and North America. It has been recently reported in Botswana, Namibia, Pakistan, Russia, South Africa, Brazil, Senegal, Uzbekistan, and Kyrgyzstan, with a single case diagnosed in Germany in 2002.[85]

Diagnosis of Dourine

In animals demonstrating signs suggestive of dourine, or those that have been in contact with animals with dourine, the infection is best confirmed by the use of serologic tests. Detection or demonstration of *T. equiperdum* in tissues or samples from clinical cases is difficult due to the very small numbers of organisms usually present. In general, direct observation of trypanosomes is not reliable when there are less than 10^6 parasites per milliliter of sample,[86] and although they are not routinely used for dourine, PCR techniques can markedly improve the detection of the organism *T. equiperdum*.[87]

The most widely used test for dourine and probably the most reliable is the complement fixation (CF) test.[81] Research on the use of ELISA tests has been performed,[88] but these tests are not in routine use. In most developed countries, dourine is notifiable, and suspicion of the disease must be reported to the appropriate regulatory authorities. Furthermore, it is a usual condition of importation from dourine endemic areas (and many others) that horses should be seronegative for dourine in the CF test before movement; a long history suggests that this is an effective means of excluding infected animals.

Prevention of Dourine Transmission

Nearly all transmission occurs by the venereal route, and because the infection is present in seminal plasma, it must be assumed that AI would be as effective at transmitting dourine as natural covering. If breeding is not being undertaken in a country certified free from dourine, all animals should be seronegative for dourine by the CF test before their use in breeding or semen collection.

OTHER INFECTIONS

Klebsiella pneumoniae and *Pseudomonas aeruginosa*

There are many different capsule types of *Klebsiella pneumoniae,* and most have never been associated with venereal disease in the horse. However, there is clinical evidence that *K. pneumoniae* capsule types 1, 2, and 5[49,89] and possibly type 7[90] may be transmitted venereally and may be associated with endometritis in the mare. Disease has not been reported in the stallion. Experimental induction of cytologically and histologically apparent endometritis in one mare has been demonstrated using capsule type 1, although this was not clinically apparent.[91] Capsule type 5 has been demonstrated in semen samples,[92] and so it must be assumed that *K. pneumoniae* can be transmitted equally well by AI as by natural covering.

Outbreaks of infection associated with venereal infection and natural covering with *Pseudomonas aeruginosa* have been reported.[89,92-97] Not all strains of the bacteria cause disease, and available laboratory tests have not been able to differentiate between pathogenic and apathogenic strains.[96]

Compared to *T. equigenitalis*, the seat of infection of mares with *K. pneumoniae* and *P. aeruginosa* is less well defined, with both infections being occasionally present in the bladder and urethra.[49]

Mares and stallions should be screened before covering or semen collection for the presence of venereally transmissible strains of *K. pneumoniae* and *P. aeruginosa* by aerobic culture for the presence of the organisms of clitoral and endometrial or cervical swabs. Covering and collection is not recommended when infection is present.[49] Although treatment of *K. pneumoniae* infections may be undertaken with appropriate antibiotic therapy, infection with *P. aeruginosa* can be harder to manage; generally, antibiotic treatment is not recommended, but washing of the penis and other external genitalia with mild disinfectant and the use of lactobacilli have been reported to be successful.

Streptococcus zooepidemicus

Streptococcus zooepidemicus is not usually regarded as a primary venereal pathogen in the horse, although it is associated with endometritis in the predisposed mare[97] (see other chapters in this volume) and it is a common infection of equine genitalia and semen, for example.[92,95] Fertility rates may therefore be increased in mares predisposed to endometritis if infection with this organism is reduced through intrauterine antibiotic therapy or through the use of antibiotics in semen extenders when AI is being used.

Miscellaneous Viral Infections

There are several viral infections in which the widespread viremia known to occur suggests that semen is likely to be infected during acute infections. These include equine infectious anemia (EIA), African horse sickness (AHS), and West Nile virus (WNV). In the case of AHS, animals would be expected to be too ill to allow semen collection, but individuals with EIA and WNV might be only subclinically infected. Thus care should be taken to ensure that stallions being used for natural covering or AI are not infected with these viruses.

Equine Herpesvirus-1

Venereal transmission of EHV-1 from stallion to mare at covering has never been demonstrated, but scrotal edema has been noted in severe outbreaks of EHV-1 during outbreaks of paralytic EHV-1 on stud farms[98] and virus has been demonstrated to be present in semen following experimental infection with one strain of EHV-1.[99] Thus it follows, in line with current recommendations for control of disease during such outbreaks,[49] that covering and semen collection should cease during outbreaks of paralytic EHV-1 infection.

Mycoplasmas

Mycoplasmas are common inhabitants of the genital tracts, as well as the upper respiratory tracts, of a wide range of mammalian species, and mycoplasmas and acholeplasmas have been isolated from both mares and stallions,[100] as well as from aborted equine fetuses.[101,102]

Species commonly isolated from the genital tracts of horses include *Mycoplasma equigenitalium* and *Mycoplasma subdolum*.[103,104] The epidemiology and transmission of these infections have not been characterized, although they can be isolated from semen and penile swabs,[100,105] as well as the clitoral fossa[104] and may well be transmitted at covering.

Mycoplasma infections have been associated with some cases of infertility in both mares and stallions, and some strains of *M. equigenitalium* can cause cytopathic effects in equine uterine tube cell explants and are likely to play a role in reproductive failure.[106] Although this association requires considerable further investigation,[103] it does not appear to have received recent attention in the literature or in general clinical work. Mycoplasma infections should be considered in cases of infertility in the horse, particularly where other infections and causes have been ruled out.

Piroplasmosis or Babesiosis

Equine piroplasmosis or babesiosis is caused by infection with the protozoan parasites *Babesia equi* and *Babesia caballi*.[107] The infections are transmitted by tick vectors and cause acute, subacute, or chronic diseases. Other than tick-borne infection, the only modes of transmission are iatrogenic or, rarely, intrauterine.[107,108] Transmission of the parasites with semen has never been reported[108] and can probably be assumed not to occur.

SUMMARY

Several infections, including EAV, CEMO, EHV-3, dourine, *K. pneumoniae,* and other bacteria, can be transmitted at covering or during AI. However, the spread of most infections can be prevented by appropriate sanitary measures, outlined here.

References

1. Pottie A: The propagation of influenza from stallions to mares. J Comp Pathol 1888; 1:37-38.
2. Clark I: Transmission of pink-eye from apparently healthy stallions to mares. J Comp Pathol 1892; 5:261.
3. Wood JLN, Chirnside ED, Mumford JA et al: First recorded outbreak of equine viral arteritis in the United Kingdom. Vet Rec 1995; 136:381.
4. Timoney PJ, McCollum WH: Equine viral arteritis: further characterisation of the carrier state in stallions. J Reprod Fertil Suppl 2000; 56:3.
5. Paweska JT, Binns MM, Woods PS et al: A survey for antibodies to equine arteritis virus in donkeys, mules and zebra using virus neutralisation (VN) and enzyme linked immunosorbent assay (ELISA). Equine Vet J 1997; 29:40.
6. Timoney PJ, McCollum WH: Equine viral arteritis. Vet Clin North Am Equine Pract 1993; 9:295.
7. Timoney PJ: Equine Viral Arteritis, International Veterinary Information Service, Ithaca, NY, 2002.
8. Timoney PJ, McCollum WH, Roberts AW et al: Demonstration of the carrier state in naturally acquired equine arteritis virus infection in the stallion. Res Vet Sci 1986; 41:279.
9. Holyoak GR, Giles RC, McCollum WH et al: Pathological changes associated with equine arteritis virus infection of

the reproductive tract in prepubertal and peripubertal colts. J Comp Pathol 1993; 109:281.

10. Timoney PJ, McCollum WH, Murphy TW et al: The carrier state in equine arteritis virus infection in the stallion with specific emphasis on the venereal mode of virus transmission. J Reprod Fertil Suppl 1987; 35:95.

11. Balasuriya UB, Leutenegger CM, Topol JB et al: Detection of equine arteritis virus by real-time TaqMan reverse transcription-PCR assay. J Virol Methods 2002; 101:21.

12. Neu SM, Timoney PJ, McCollum WH: Persistent infection of the reproductive tract in stallions experimentally infected with equine arteritis virus. Proceedings of the 5th International Conference on Equine Infectious Diseases, p 149, 1988.

13. Little TV, Holyoak GR, McCollum WH et al: Output of equine arteritis virus from persistently infected stallions is testosterone-dependent. Equine Infectious Diseases VI: Proceedings of the 6th International Conference on Equine Infectious Diseases, p 225, 1992.

14. Holyoak GR, Little TV, McCollam WH et al: Relationship between onset of puberty and establishment of persistent infection with equine arteritis virus in the experimentally infected colt. J Comp Pathol 1993; 109:29.

15. Fortier G, Vidament M, DeCraene F et al: The effect of GnRH antagonist on testosterone secretion, spermatogenesis and viral excretion in EVA-virus excreting stallions. Equine reproduction VIII: Proceedings of the Eighth International Symposium on Equine Reproduction. Theriogenology 2002; 58:24.

16. Castillo-Olivares J, Tearle JP, Montesso F et al: Detection of equine arteritis virus (EAV)-specific cytotoxic CD8+ T lymphocyte precursors from EAV-infected ponies. J Gen Virol 2003; 84:2745-2753.

17. Fukunaga Y, McCollum WH: Complement-fixation reactions in equine viral arteritis. Am J Vet Res 1977; 38:2043.

18. Fukunaga Y, Imagawa H, Tabuchi E et al: Clinical and virological findings on experimental equine viral arteritis in horses. Bull Equine Res Inst Japan 1981; 18:110-118.

19. McCollum WH: Development of a modified virus strain and vaccine for equine viral arteritis. J Am Vet Med Assoc 1969; 155:318.

20. McCollum WH: Vaccination for equine arteritis virus. Proceedings of the 2nd International Conference on Equine Infectious Diseases, p 143, 1970.

21. McCollum WH. Responses of horses vaccinated with a virulent modified-live equine arteritis virus propagated in the E. Derm (NBL-6) cell line to nasal inoculation with virulent virus. Am J Vet Res 1986, 47:1931.

22. Paweska JT, Volkmann DH, Barnard BJ et al: Sexual and in-contact transmission of asinine strain of equine arteritis virus among donkeys. J Clin Microbiol 1995; 33:3296.

23. McCollum WH. Studies of passive immunity in foals to equine viral arteritis. Vet Microbiol 1976; 1:45.

24. Hullinger PJ, Wilson WD, Rossitto PV et al: Passive transfer, rate of decay, and protein specificity of antibodies against equine arteritis virus in horses from a Standardbred herd with high seroprevalence. J Am Vet Med Assoc 1998; 213:839.

25. Fukunaga Y, Wada R, Matsumura T et al: Induction of immune response and protection from equine viral arteritis (EVA) by formalin inactivated-virus vaccine for EVA in horses. Zentralbl Veterinarmed B 1990; 37:135.

26. Fukunaga Y, Wada R, Matsumura T et al: An attempt to protect against persistent infection of equine viral arteritis in the reproductive tract of stallions using formalin inactivated-virus vaccine. Equine Infectious Diseases VI: Proceedings of the 6th International Conference on Equine Infectious Diseases, p 239, 1992.

27. McCollum WH, Timoney PJ, Roberts AW et al: Response of vaccinated and non-vaccinated mares to artificial insemination with semen from stallions persistently infected with equine arteritis virus. Proceedings of the 5th International Conference on Equine Infectious Diseases, p 13, 1987.

28. Fukunaga Y, Wada R, Imagawa H et al: Venereal infection of mares by equine arteritis virus and use of killed vaccine against the infection. J Comp Pathol 1997; 117:201.

29. Senne DA, Pearson JE, Carbrey EA: Equine viral arteritis: a standard procedure for the virus neutralization test and comparison of results of a proficiency test performed at five laboratories. Proceedings of the United States Animal Health Association, p 89, 1985.

30. Edwards S, Castillo-Olivares J, Cullinane A et al: International harmonisation of laboratory diagnostic tests for equine viral arteritis. Proceedings of the 8th International Conference on Equine Infectious Diseases, 1998.

31. Geraghty RJ, Newton JR, Castillo-Olivares J et al: Testing for equine arteritis virus. Vet Rec 2003; 152:755.

32. Lang G, Mitchell WR: A serosurvey by ELISA for antibodies to equine arteritis virus in Ontario racehorses. J Equine Vet Sci 1984; 4:153.

33. Chirnside ED, de Vries AA, Mumford JA et al: Equine arteritis virus-neutralizing antibody in the horse is induced by a determinant on the large envelope glycoprotein GL. J Gen Virol 1995; 76(Pt 8), 1989-1998.

34. MacLachlan NJ, Balasuriya UB, Hedges JF et al: Serologic response of horses to the structural proteins of equine arteritis virus. J Vet Diagn Invest 1998; 10:229.

35. Nugent J, Sinclair R, deVries AA et al: Development and evaluation of ELISA procedures to detect antibodies against the major envelope protein (G(L)) of equine arteritis virus. J Virol Methods 2000; 90:167.

36. Timoney PJ: Equine Viral Arteritis. In Commission OS (ed): Office International des Epizooties: Manual of Standards Diagnostic Tests and Vaccines, p 582, Paris, Office International des Epizooties, 2000.

37. Monreal L, Villatoro AJ, Hooghuis H et al: Clinical features of the 1992 outbreak of equine viral arteritis in Spain. Equine Vet J 1995; 27:301.

38. Chirnside ED, Spaan WJ: Reverse transcription and cDNA amplification by the polymerase chain reaction of equine arteritis virus (EAV). J Virol Methods 1990; 30:133.

39. Belak S, Ballagi Pordany A, Timoney PJ et al: Evaluation of a nested PCR assay for the detection of equine arteritis virus. Equine Infectious Diseases VII: Proceedings of the 7th International Conference, 1994.

40. Sekiguchi K, Sugita S, Fukunaga Y et al: Detection of equine arteritis virus (EAV) by polymerase chain reaction (PCR) and differentiation of EAV strains by restriction enzyme analysis of PCR products. Arch Virol 1995; 140:1483.

41. Westcott DG, King DP, Drew TW et al: Use of an internal standard in a closed one-tube RT-PCR for the detection of equine arteritis virus RNA with fluorescent probes. Vet Res 2003; 34:165.

42. Timoney PJ, McCollum WH: Equine viral arteritis-epidemiology and control. J Equine Vet Sci 1988; 8:54.

43. Timoney PJ, Castro AE, Heuschele WP: Equine viral arteritis. In Castro AE, Heuschele WP (eds): Veterinary Diagnostic Virology: a Practitioners Guide, St Louis, 1992, Mosby.

44. Moore BD, Balasuriya UB, Nurton JP et al: Differentiation of strains of equine arteritis virus of differing virulence to horses by growth in equine endothelial cells. Am J Vet Res 2003; 64:779.

45. Fukunaga Y, Wada R, Kanemaru T et al: Immune potency of lyophilized, killed vaccine for equine viral arteritis and its protection against abortion in pregnant mares. J Equine Vet Sci 1996; 16:217.

46. Cardwell JM, Newton JR, Wood JLN: Serological response to equine arteritis virus vaccination of stallions. British Equine Veterinary Association 41st Congress Equine Veterinary Journal, p 202, 2002.

47. Castillo-Olivares J, de Vries AA, Raamsman MJ et al: Evaluation of a prototype sub-unit vaccine against equine arteritis virus comprising the entire ectodomain of the virus large envelope glycoprotein (G(L)): induction of virus-neutralizing antibody and assessment of protection in ponies. J Gen Virol 2001; 82:2425.

48. Castillo-Olivares J, Wieringa R, Bakonyi T et al: Generation of a candidate live marker vaccine for equine arteritis virus by deletion of the major virus neutralization domain. J Virol 2003; 77:8470.

49. Archer L, Wade JF: Codes of practice on contagious equine metritis (CEM), equine viral arteritis (EVA), equine herpesvirus (EHV) and guidelines on strangles. Horserace Betting Levy Board, Newmarket, UK, 2003, R&W Publications.

50. British Equine Veterinary Association code of practice for the use of artificial insemination in horse breeding, Cambridge, UK, British Equine Veterinary Association, 2002.

51. Trade and importation of semen, ova and embryos. Directive 92/65/EC, 1992.

52. Cullinane A: Equine arteritis virus in Irish thoroughbreds. Vet Rec 2003; 153:570.

53. Timoney PJ: Contagious equine metritis. Comp Immunol Microbiol Infect Dis 1996; 19:199.

54. Powell DG: Contagious equine metritis. Equine Vet J 1978; 10:1.

55. Simpson DJ, Eaton Evans WE: Isolation of the CEM organism from the clitoris of the mare. Vet Rec 1978; 102:19.

56. Taylor CED: A recently recognised venereal disease of horses and its causative organism. J Infect 1979; 1:81.

57. Timoney PJ, Powell DG: Contagious equine metritis: epidemiology and control. J Equine Vet Sci 1988; 8:42.

58. Moore JE, Millar BC, Buckley TC: Potential misidentification of *Taylorella asinigenitalis* as *Taylorella equigenitalis*: implications for the epidemiology of CEM. J Equine Vet Sci 2000; 20:479.

59. Jang SS, Donahue JM, Arata AB et al: *Taylorella asinigenitalis* sp. nov., a bacterium isolated from the genital tract of male donkeys (*Equus asinus*). Int J Syst Evol Microbiol 2001; 51:971.

60. Jackson G, Carson T, Heath P et al: CEMO in a UK stallion. Vet Rec 2002; 151:582.

61. Timoney PJ: Contagious equine metritis in Ireland. Vet Rec 1979; 105:172.

62. Anzai T, Eguchi M, Sekizaki T et al: Development of a PCR test for rapid diagnosis of contagious equine metritis. J Vet Med Sci 1999; 61:1287.

63. Anzai T, Wada R, Okuda T et al: Evaluation of the field application of PCR in the eradication of contagious equine metritis from Japan. J Vet Med Sci 2002; 64:999.

64. Chanter N, Vigano F, Collin NC et al: Use of a PCR assay for *Taylorella equigenitalis* applied to samples from the United Kingdom. Vet Rec 1998; 143:225.

65. Matsuda M, Moore JE: Recent advances in molecular epidemiology and detection of *Taylorella equigenitalis* associated with contagious equine metritis (CEM). Vet Microbiol 2003; 97:111.

66. Premanandh J, George LV, Wernery U et al: Evaluation of a newly developed real-time PCR for the detection of *Taylorella equigenitalis* and discrimination from *T. asinigenitalis*. Vet Microbiol 2003; 95:229.

67. Wood JLN, Cardwell J, Park AW: Results of a quantitative risk assessment of the risks of reducing swabbing requirements for the detection of *Taylorella equigenitalis*. Veterinary Record 2005; 157:41-46.

68. Timoney PJ, O'Reilly PJ, Harrington AM et al: Survival of *Haemophilus equigenitalis* in different antibiotic-containing semen extenders. J Reprod Fertil Suppl 1979; 27:377-381.

69. Gibbs E, Roberts M: Equine coital exanthema in the United Kingdom. Equine Vet J 1972; 4:74.

70. Bryans JT, Allen GP, Bryans JT et al: In vitro and in vivo studies of equine "coital" exanthema. In Equine Infectious Diseases III, Proceedings of the 3rd International Conference on Equine Infectious Diseases, pp 322-336, Basel, S. Karger, 1973.

71. Smith KC: Herpesviral abortion in domestic animals. Vet J 1997; 153:253.

72. Edington N: Latency of equine herpesviruses. Equine Infectious Diseases VI: Proceedings of the 6th International Conference on Equine Infectious Diseases, p 195, 1992.

73. Studdert MJ: Equine coital exanthema. In Studdert MJ (ed): Virus Infections of Vertebrates, vol 6, p 39, Amsterdam, Elsevier Science, 1996.

74. Pascoe RR: Effect of equine coital exanthema on the fertility of mares covered by stallions exhibiting the clinical disease. Aust Vet J 1981; 57:111.

75. Gleeson LJ, Sullivan ND, Studdert MJ: Equine herpesviruses type 3 as an abortigenic agent. Aust Vet J 1976; 52:349.

76. Crandell RA, Davis ER: Isolation of equine coital exanthema virus (equine herpesvirus 3) from the nostril of a foal. J Am Vet Med Assoc 1985; 187:503.

77. Burki F, Lorin D, Sibalin M et al: (Experimental genital and nasal infection of horses with the virus of equine coital exanthema). Zentralbl Veterinarmed B 1974; 21:362.

78. Dynon K, Varrasso A, Ficorilli N et al: Identification of equine herpesvirus 3 (equine coital exanthema virus), equine gammaherpesviruses 2 and 5, equine adenoviruses 1 and 2, equine arteritis virus and equine rhinitis A virus by polymerase chain reaction. Aust Vet J 2001; 79:695.

79. Wood JLN, Newton JR: Unpublished observations, 2005.

80. Metcalf ES: The role of international transport of equine semen on disease transmission. Anim Reprod Sci 2001; 68:229.

81. Dourine. In Manual of standards, diagnostic tests and vaccines, Chapter 2.5.2, Office International des Epizooties, 2000.

82. Parkin BS: The demonstration and transmission of the South African strain of *Trypanosoma equiperdum* of horses. Onderstepoort J Vet Sci Anim Industry 1948; 23:41.

83. Caporale VP, Battelli G, and Semproni G: Epidemiology of dourine in the equine population of the Abruzzi region. Zentralbl Veterinarmed B 1980; 27:489.

84. Robinson EM: Dourine infection in young equines. Onderstepoort J Vet Sci Anim Industry 1948; 23:39.

85. Office International des Epizooties: Handistatus II: annual animal disease status reports, vol 2003, Office International des Epizooties, 2003.

86. Paris J, Murray M, McOdimba F: A comparative evaluation of the parasitological techniques currently available for the diagnosis of African trypanosomiasis in cattle. Acta Tropica 1982; 39:307.

87. Clausen PH, Gebreselassie G, Abditcho S et al: Detection of trypanosome DNA in serologically positive but aparasitaemic horses suspected of dourine in Ethiopia. Tokai J Exp Clin Med 1998; 23:303.

88. Bishop S, Rae PF, Phipps LP et al: *Trypanosoma equiperdum*: detection of trypanosomal antibodies and antigen by enzyme-linked immunosorbent assay. Br Vet J 1995; 151:715.

89. Timoney PJ: Incidence of certain equine venereal diseases in Ireland for 1978/1979. International Symposium on Equine Venereal Diseases, pp 18-19, 1980.

90. Weiss R, Bohm KH, Merkt H et al: Examination of the bacterial flora of prepuce and nose of horses, especially breeding stallions, with special reference to *Klebsiella*. Part 3.

Serological investigations on *Klebsiella* strains. Berl Munch Tierarztl Wochenschr 1976; 89:193.

91. Ricketts SW: Endometrial biopsy studies of mares experimentally infected with *Haemophilus equigenitalis* and *Klebsiella aerogenes* capsule type 1. International Symposium on Equine Venereal Diseases, pp 27-36, 1980.

92. Madsen M, Christensen P: Bacterial flora of semen collected from Danish warmblood stallions by artificial vagina. Acta Vet Scand 1995; 36:1.

93. Rossdale PD: Control of equine venereal diseases, *Pseudomonas* and *Klebsiella*. International Symposium on Equine Venereal Diseases, pp 48-50, 1980.

94. Merkt H, Klug E, Gunzel AR: Control of equine venereal diseases, *Klebsiella* and *Pseudomonas*. International Symposium on Equine Venereal Diseases, pp 50-53, 1980.

95. Aurich C, Spergser J, Nowotny N et al: Prevalence of venereal transmissible diseases and relevant potentially pathogenic bacteria in Austrian Noriker draught horse stallions. Wien Tierarztl Monatsschr 2003; 90:124.

96. Atherton JG, Pitt TL: Types of *Pseudomonas aeruginosa* isolated from horses. Equine Vet J 1982; 14:329.

97. Allen WE, Newcombe JR: Aspects of genital infection and swabbing techniques in the mare. Vet Rec 1979; 104:228.

98. McCartan CG, Russell MM, Wood JL et al: Clinical, serological and virological characteristics of an outbreak of paresis and neonatal foal disease due to equine herpesvirus-1 on a stud farm. Vet Rec 1995; 136:7.

99. Tearle JP, Smith KC, Boyle MS et al: Replication of equid herpesvirus-1 (EHV-1) in the testes and epididymides of ponies and venereal shedding of infectious virus. J Comp Pathol 1996; 115:385.

100. Moorthy ARS, Spradbrow PB, Eisler MED: Isolation of mycoplasmas from the genital tract of horses. Aust Vet J 1977; 53:167.

101. Moorthy ARS, Spradbrow PB, McEvoy T: Isolation of mycoplasmas from an aborted equine foetus. Aust Vet J 1976; 52:385.

102. Heitmann J, Kirchhoff K, Petzoldt K et al: Isolation of acholeplasmas and mycoplasmas from aborted horse fetuses. Vet Rec 1979; 104:350.

103. Bermudez VM, Miller RB, Johnson WH et al. The prevalence of *Mycoplasma* spp. and their relationship to reproductive performance in selected equine herds in Southern Ontario. J Reprod Fertil Suppl 1987; 35:671.

104. Bermudez VM, Miller RB, Johnson WH et al: Effect of sample freezing on the isolation of *Mycoplasma* spp. from the clitoral fossa of the mare. Can J Vet Res 1988; 52:147.

105. Lemcke RM, Kirchhoff H: *Mycoplasma subdolum,* a new species isolated from horses. Int J Syst Bacteriol 1979; 29:42.

106. Bermudez VM, Miller RB, Rosendal S et al: Measurement of the cytotoxic effects of different strains of *Mycoplasma equigenitalium* on the equine uterine tube using a calmodulin assay. Can J Vet Res 1992; 56:331.

107. Phipps LP: Equine piroplasmosis. Equine Vet Educ 1996; 8:33.

108. Friedhoff KT, Soulé C: An account on equine babesioses. Rev Sci. Tech 1996; 15:1191.

CHAPTER 43

Advanced Semen Tests for Stallions

STUART A. MEYERS

Evaluation of male fertility in horses has been primarily limited to mare cycle and seasonal pregnancy rates, foaling rate, and nonreturn to estrus.[1] In certain countries and on some farms, identification and culling of subfertile males that have been associated with lowered fertility serves as the most economic solution to problems of sire infertility. However, when the value of an individual stallion is high, further investigations into the nature of the subfertility may be warranted. A test for prediction of fertility in unproven sires has been elusive because an array of factors contribute to the interaction between male and female that results in "good fertility."

In most cases of male subfertility the underlying causes are largely unknown; reduced fertility occurs with a variety of causes and numerous contributory factors. Identifiable factors that can contribute to a male's decreased fertility include inadequate numbers of morphologically normal, progressively motile sperm; suboptimal management systems; testicular degeneration and genital tract trauma; poor overall health and body condition; and psychologic or behavioral problems. The role of other factors such as environmental toxin exposure; endocrine, autocrine, and paracrine control of spermatogenesis; epididymal dysfunction; and the function of sperm cells is less clearly defined. The objective of this presentation is to discuss several recently developed methods of assessing spermatozoal function and dysfunction as might occur during toxicologic exposure, trauma, or subfertility.

CONVENTIONAL SEMEN EVALUATION

Indirect evaluation of stallion fertility, defined as the ability to cause conception, pregnancy, and the birth of live young, has been performed traditionally by assessment of ejaculated semen. Adjunctive evaluation of testicular parameters such as size, shape, volume, ultrasonographic appearance, and total scrotal width has also been routinely performed. Conventional semen evaluation is not considered to be a direct measure of fertility and consists of measurements of sperm morphologic and movement characteristics and seminal fluid characteristics, including pH, turbidity, color, and presence of immature germ cells or somatic cells. Many of these parameters are relatively well correlated to fertility in most males evaluated; however, few have been able to account fully for decreased fertility in some males.

Clearly, males with extremely low numbers of motile, morphologically normal sperm in their ejaculates are typically incapable of causing conceptions and may be justifiably considered to be infertile. However, some males that have normal to moderately low numbers of morphologically normal, motile sperm in their ejaculates either fail to cause conceptions or cause a decreased conception rate under good breeding management schemes. The subfertility in this latter population is not well defined by conventional semen evaluation. Diagnostic tests, which probe sperm function, are needed to determine the potential causes and explore treatments for this type of subfertility. This would provide diagnostic information about sperm function that would otherwise not be available for males in which conventional semen evaluation fails to identify a cause for diminished fertility. Several laboratories are developing tests for sperm integrity and function based on subcellular mechanisms in differing spermatozoal compartments, including sperm lipid composition, DNA integrity, membrane integrity, resistance to osmotic stress, sperm-zona or sperm-oolemmal binding, signal transduction, and numerous others. It should be mentioned that clinical relevance has not been worked out for many of the following parameters because of small sample populations, but the cell physiologic background should provide rationale to include a number of these assessments on a clinical basis.

EVALUATION OF SPERM FUNCTION

For a single spermatozoon to fertilize an oocyte and develop into an embryo, sufficient numbers of motile sperm must ascend the female genital tract, become capacitated, acquire hyperactivated motility, undergo the acrosome reaction, penetrate the oocyte extracellular investing layers (which include the cumulus oophorus and zona pellucida), and initiate fusion with the oocyte's plasma membrane. Fertilization also includes sperm nuclear decondensation, male pronucleus formation, and syngamy of male and female pronuclei. Many of these crucial steps in the fertilization process may be artificially isolated as demonstrated by the success of in vitro fertilization in several species. In human medicine the ability to undergo acrosome reactions, to bind and penetrate human ova, and to fuse with zona-free hamster ova have proven to be clinically useful as predictors of in vitro fertilization success and infertility in men. Such function tests have also been performed in livestock species but have not become routinely useful in equine medicine possibly because much subfertility results from conventionally diagnosable sperm deficits such as diminished total numbers of morphologically normal, progressively motile sperm in ejaculates.

Clinical evaluation of fertilization-based sperm function has been applied most widely in human andrology and has included end points such as measurements of total and progressive motility, hypoosmotic swell test, cervical mucus penetration, hyperactivated motility, sperm fusion with zona-free hamster oocytes, or homologous in vitro fertilization. Measures of capacitation and acrosomal physiology have proven to be useful adjuncts to motility and morphologic end points for diagnosis and treatment of human male factor infertility.

In veterinary medicine, bull fertility has been correlated to acrosome reaction inducibility by chondroitin sulfates and dilauroylphosphatidylcholine liposomes.[2] Other than evaluation of sperm motility, which has not been highly correlated to stallion fertility, there are presently few clinically available indices of sperm function in equine reproduction. For assessment of subfertility, evaluation of sperm function at end points more finitely defined than "fertility" may be appropriate.

CAPACITATION AND ACROSOME REACTION

It has been shown for several species that sperm must undergo the process of capacitation as a prerequisite for most events of fertilization, including cumulus penetration, zona binding and penetration, the acrosome reaction (acrosomal exocytosis), and fusion with the oocyte. Sperm capacitation has been suggested to include increases in intracellular calcium, phosphorylation of protein tyrosine residues, and reversible changes in the sperm plasma membrane, including removal of cholesterol and cholesteryl esters by cholesterol acceptor molecules in the female genital tract or in artificial media. Capacitation in vivo occurs within the female genital tract but can be induced artificially in vitro for sperm of many species, including the horse. The acrosome reaction can occur only following completion of capacitation and can be induced by a variety of chemical and biologic agents. Cytologic techniques for quantitation of acrosome reactions have been applied in several species, including stallions, bulls, and boars. Sperm that are nonviable experience a "false" acrosome reaction, which must be differentiated from the true exocytotic acrosome reaction in order to reflect capacitational changes. Supravital stains, such as Hoechst 33258 or propidium iodide, accomplish this task efficiently. Consequently, the acrosome reaction in live sperm may be considered a rational end point for evaluation of sperm function because it can be used to evaluate a complex set of cell behaviors.

Progesterone has been evaluated for its ability to stimulate acrosome reactions because in some species, including horses, the preovulatory follicle has been reported to secrete progesterone before ovulation and luteinization.

Therefore progesterone is likely to be present in oviductal fluids and within the cumulus of ovulated oocytes. Differences have been reported for efficiency of progesterone-induced acrosome reactions in sperm of human fertile and subfertile patients, and this has been attributed to the lack of progesterone receptor on sperm or to a nonfunctional receptor. It is not known whether these subfertile patients had a congenital absence of progesterone receptor, or whether an acquired condition resulted in the loss of functional receptor or receptor subunit. The author and others have reported similar results for fertile and subfertile stallions.[3,4] It has been determined that bull and stallion sperm have receptors for progesterone.

Acrosome reaction status in stallion sperm has been evaluated using various staining methods. These include immunofluorescence methods with specific antibodies, both monoclonal and polyclonal,[3,5,6] labeling with fluoresceinated lectins,[6,7-9] chlortetracycline labeling (CTC) and transmission electron microscopy[10] (TEM), and nonfluorescence methods.[11,12] Electron microscopy offers direct imaging of the acrosome-associated membranes and is considered to be the "gold standard" but is the most costly and requires the most skill in comparison to other methods. Few methods offer significant advantages over others; however, the lectin-staining methods generally offer speed and ease of use, although a fluorescence microscope is required. Nonfluorescence methods have also been used, but few staining methods have been validated against TEM. Pratt et al[13] demonstrated the use of a Coomassie Blue method that was validated for use in canids, but this has not been reported for stallion sperm.

Several additional sperm function tests based on isolated steps in fertilization have been developed for livestock species. It has been demonstrated that sperm binding to the equine zona pellucida and subsequent acrosome reaction rates in bound sperm are higher for fertile stallions in comparison with subfertile stallions.[3,8,14,15] Similar results have been reported for rams, boars, and bulls. The ability of motile sperm from subfertile men to bind to the zona is correlated with their ability to complete fertilization in vitro.

SPERM-OVIDUCTAL BINDING

Studies of stallion sperm capacitation under coculture conditions have suggested that the ability to bind to and release from oviductal epithelial cells (OEC) in culture is associated with sperm function.[16,17] Sperm oviductal binding has great potential as an adjunct function test regarding cryopreserved sperm. Dobrinski et al[17] reported that the ability of cryopreserved equine spermatozoa to attach to equine OEC in vitro is reduced compared with fresh extended spermatozoa and suggested that this could be due to changes other than a reduction in postthaw motility or membrane integrity. The authors also indicated that the decreased ability of frozen-thawed spermatozoa to attach to OEC could explain in part the reduced fertility of cryopreserved sperm in the horse. Although the mechanisms are unclear concerning the cell biology of sperm-oviductal adhesion, these studies of sperm cell functions could eventually reveal cellular functions and molecular mechanisms that sperm must acquire to attain successful fertilizing capacity.

SPERM DNA AND CHROMATIN INTEGRITY

The nature of sperm DNA damage has not been clearly determined. It is known that a relationship exists between males with poor sperm parameters and spermatozoal DNA damage. Two broad theories have been advanced to explain the appearance of DNA anomalies in ejaculated sperm. The first theory suggests that endogenous nicks in DNA occur during specific stages of spermiogenesis. It has been demonstrated that the presence of nicks in the DNA is greatest during the transition from round to elongated spermatids in rodents. An alternative theory has been proposed in which the presence of endogenous DNA nicks is characteristic of programmed cell death, or apoptosis, followed by elimination of defective germ cells.

Sperm DNA has been analyzed by a number of laboratories using a variety of techniques. The nick translation assay directly assesses DNA nicks. High levels of nicks have been related to reduced fertility in men. The terminal deoxynucleotidyl transferase (TUNEL) assay has been used to evaluate DNA fragmentation and strand breaks, and these breaks have been correlated with abnormal chromatin packaging and protamination, as well as abnormal sperm morphologic characteristics and motility in human sperm. The sperm chromatin structure assay (SCSA), which measures DNA susceptibility to acid- or heat-induced denaturation, has been effectively used to identify males with poor fertility in a variety of species, including stallions.[18] The single-cell gel electrophoresis method (SCGE, or Comet, assay) is one of the most sensitive methods of detecting DNA fragmentation/strand breaks and has been well correlated to the SCSA and TUNEL assays. Of these techniques, the Comet assay can be used to detect DNA damage in individual sperm cells with the highest sensitivity; the SCSA cannot be used to evaluate individual cell DNA damage. In addition to factors that affect sperm survival, it is increasingly evident that "sublethal" damage to sperm is an important limitation to successful cryopreservation in the horse. For stallion sperm, there is little experimental or clinical data demonstrating any mechanisms for the described decrease in sperm fertility associated with cryopreservation of sperm. Recent research from the author's laboratory suggests that equine sperm undergoing low-temperature storage experience characteristics of premature capacitation, osmotic damage, and DNA damage.[19-22] Our data suggest that the initial cooling of equine semen to 4°C that occurs before cryopreservation, as well as during cooling of transported semen, is capable of inducing significant fragmentation of sperm DNA. Further, recent studies have extended the occurrence of DNA damage to that of cryopreservation, suggesting that conventional cryopreservation is capable of inducing significant DNA fragmentation of stallion sperm.[23] The observed degree of sperm DNA damage could influence the fertility of certain stallions, although sperm populations are significantly heterogeneous with regard to sperm morphologic characteristics and biochemical function.

CELL SIGNALING PATHWAYS: INTRACELLULAR CALCIUM AND TYROSINE PHOSPHORYLATION

The initial event in sperm capacitation is a rise in intracellular calcium, bicarbonate, and hydrogen peroxide, which collectively activate adenylyl cyclase to produce cyclic adenosine monophosphate (cAMP). The stimulation of cAMP then activates protein kinase A (PKA), which in turn phosphorylates a number of proteins. Visconti and Kopf[24] have correlated mouse, human, and bovine sperm capacitation with an increase in protein tyrosine phosphorylation of a variety of protein substrates of Mr 40,000-120,000. The authors suggest that protein tyrosine phosphorylation mediates a variety of cellular functions such as growth regulation, cell cycle control, cytoskeleton assembly, ionic current regulation, and receptor regulation and is an essential downstream component of capacitation. Recent studies suggest that reactive oxygen species (ROS) and osmotic stress may contribute to membrane leakiness and subsequent increases in intracellular calcium concentration and downstream phosphorylation cascades.[23,25] The assays can be performed using fluorescence microscopy or flow cytometry using a variety of calcium-sensitive dyes including Fura-2AM and Fluo-3. This author and others have also demonstrated that one consequence of cryoinjury to sperm is excessive levels of protein tyrosine phosphorylation within the sperm tail region.[20,25-27]

MITOCHONDRIAL MEMBRANE POTENTIAL

Changes in mitochondrial membrane potential (MMP), particularly notable in the sperm's midpiece region, has also been reported as a consequence of osmotic and oxidative cellular stress.[28] The assays used to determine MMP have been largely flow cytometric evaluations using the commercially available cationic fluorescence dyes JC-1[29] and Mito-Tracker[30]; however, fluorescence microscopy can also be useful. The dyes are excellent indicators of mitochondrial membrane depolarization and fluoresce at varying wavelengths dependent on high or low membrane potential. Individual cells (microscopy) or cell populations (flow cytometry) can be tracked for changes in red or green fluorescence relative to various cellular stressors. It may also be useful to combine multiple fluorophores with affinities to various cellular compartments and determine MMP, acrosomal and calcium status, cell viability/membrane permeability, and phosphorylation simultaneously in single cells using fluorescence microscopy or flow cytometry.

SPERM CELL MEMBRANE FUNCTION

Lipid Composition

The plasma membrane of sperm is unique within species with regard to phospholipid composition (approximately 70% phospholipids, 25% neutral lipids, and 5% glycolipids). Variation among species in susceptibility to cold shock appears to be correlated with membrane lipid composition.[31] Cold-shock resistance is generally greater for species with sperm membranes characterized by high sterol-to-phospholipid ratio and a high degree of saturation of phospholipid-bound acyl moieties. Stallion sperm displayed a low sterol-phospholipid relationship compared to bull sperm but slightly higher than the highly cold-shock sensitive sperm of the boar, suggesting that stallion sperm should have different requirements for low-temperature storage than that of bull and boar sperm.[31] Resistance to toxic insult could also be reflected by plasma membrane integrity and phospholipid composition. Membrane fluidity can be assessed by measuring the fluorescence polarization anisotropy or differential scanning calorimetry of sperm and is also indicative of ability to withstand freezing-thawing. Fluidity is largely dependent on cholesterol-phospholipid molar ratio and ratio of saturated to unsaturated lipids. A marked increase in these two indices of fluidity indicates a significant decrease in fluidity of plasma membrane measured at physiologic temperature.

Thermotropic Lipid Phase Transitions

Plasma membranes respond to temperature changes through lipid phase transitions. Liquid, crystalline, and gel phases can coexist in individual cells during freezing and thawing. The sperm of most mammalian species undergo thermotropic lipid phase transitions in the temperature range of 17° to 36°C.[31,32] Evidence that cold-shock damage to mammalian and invertebrate sperm cells is mediated by lipid phase transitions has been reported. Although subfertility based on abnormal lipid phase behavior has not been reported, it is possible that genetic or acquired lipid group defects could be detectable using lipid phase transition activity. Boar sperm exhibits a cooperative phase transition compared to human sperm, which displays a minor transition, an indication that sperm susceptible to cold shock display distinct phase transition behavior. Sperm from most species are susceptible to varying degrees of cold shock in which rapid cooling above 0°C confers major structural and functional damage to sperm. In addition to physical membrane disruption, cooling sperm below the lipid phase transition temperature may disrupt membrane enzyme systems including adenosinetriphosphatase (ATPase). Several studies have demonstrated that thawed sperm display increased intracellular calcium concentration, and this is indicative of poor control of calcium regulation. Lipid membrane phase transitions of equine and nonhuman primate sperm have been studied in the author's laboratory using Fourier Transform Infrared Spectroscopy (FTIR). This method provides a sensitive, noninvasive probe of lipid packing within the cell membrane and is detected by melting trends of membrane lipids. Although there exists little clinical data on membrane lipid phase transitions, this assay could be applied on a clinical basis in the future as more becomes known regarding this biophysical phenomenon.

Cellular Response to Oxidative Stress

Within the past several years, clinicians and basic scientists have gained a wider understanding about the impor-tance of oxidative stress in sperm. Recent studies have indicated that ROS play an important role in normal sperm function and that an imbalance in the production or degradation of ROS may have serious adverse effects on sperm. Reactive oxygen species may be generated during oxidative metabolism, and increased generation of ROS has also been attributed to both abnormal and damaged sperm. Damage to equine sperm by freezing and thawing has been demonstrated to increase ROS generation, and this effect could be stallion dependent.[33] Because equine sperm contain a relatively high content of polyunsaturated fatty acids, their susceptibility to oxidative damage is increased. Subsequent membrane lipid peroxidation by ROS results in decreased membrane fluidity—a parameter that is essential to sperm for the fusogenic functions of acrosome reactions and sperm fusion to the oocyte plasma membrane during fertilization, as well as motility and resistance to osmotic and thermal stress. Several laboratories have developed methods to detect the degree of ROS generation in sperm and seminal fluid and sperm lipid peroxidation, and these tests could become clinically useful as a routine sperm function evaluation method. Detection of lipid peroxidation using the fluorescent dye C_{11}-BODIPY has been reported as a microplate assay,[34] and these authors demonstrated an increase in lipid peroxidation during cooled storage of stallion sperm.

Cellular Response to Osmotic Stress

The hypoosmotic swelling test (HOS) has been used for sperm membrane responsiveness from a variety of species, including boar, human, bull, and stallion and has been related to sperm function and subfertility.[35-39] The main principle is based on water transport across the sperm tail membrane under hypotonic conditions. When cellular water transport mechanisms are adequate, water is able to flow down its concentration gradient and cause swelling of the plasma membrane over the sperm tail. The sperm tail develops a characteristic distal coil, and cell populations can be counted manually or automatically. This fundamental measure is simple to perform and could gain more clinical application as further understanding of stallion sperm water transport becomes available. Water transport biophysical modeling has recently been reported for stallion sperm.[40]

The rate at which osmotic volume regulation, and hence cooling, warming, or response to stressors, may take place is highly dependent upon the cell's hydraulic conductivity (water permeability), Lp. Water permeability has been shown to be dependent on temperature, cryopreservative, and ice crystal formation, and there is evidence that plasma membrane permeability is regionally variable in sperm. Lipid packing structure has been suggested to be altered by intramembranous cryoprotectants and may be a mechanism whereby Lp and signal transduction processing could be altered during cooling. Studies in the author's laboratory have suggested that exposure of sperm to variations in temperature and medium resulted in differences in the ability of stallion sperm to volume-regulate.[25] This suggests that sperm survival in the female genital tract, as well as following cryopreservation, is dependent on the quality of the fluid extracellular environment and may be ultimately stallion dependent. Using the Coulter counter method, sperm cell volume can be accurately measured in response to hypoosmotic conditions, as in the HOS test, but precise measurements can be taken for target cell populations.

CONCLUSION

In recent years, advances in cell function have become increasingly applicable to sperm, and methods to assess functional capacity of sperm are in various stages of development and application. Much of the recent literature regarding sperm has focused on male subfertility and cryoinjury as avenues for improvement and further understanding of sperm function. Consequently, as more knowledge is acquired pertaining to stallion sperm, new applications of the associated technologies will be increasingly applied to clinical situations.

References

1. van Buiten A, van den Broek J, Schukken YH et al: Validation of non-return rate as a parameter for stallion fertility. Livest Prod Sci 1999; 60(1):13-19.
2. Ax RL, Dickson K, Lenz RW: Induction of acrosome reactions by chondroitin sulfates in vitro corresponds to nonreturn rates of dairy bulls. *J Dairy Sci* 1985; 68:387-390.
3. Meyers SA, Overstreet JW, Liu IKM et al: Capacitation in vitro of stallion spermatozoa: comparison of progesterone-induced acrosome reactions in fertile and subfertile males. J Androl 1995; 16:47-54.
4. Rathi R, Colenbrander B, Stout TAE et al: Progesterone induces acrosome reaction in stallion spermatozoa via a protein tyrosine kinase dependent pathway. Mol Reprod Dev 2003; 64(1):120-128.
5. Zhang J, Boyle MS, Smith CA et al: Acrosome reaction of stallion spermatozoa evaluated with monoclonal antibody and zona-free hamster eggs. Mol Reprod Dev 1990; 27:152-158.
6. Cross NL, Morales P, Overstreet JW, Hanson FW: Two simple methods for detecting acrosome-reacted human sperm. Gamete Res, 1986; 15:213-226.
7. Casey PJ, Hillman RB, Robertson KR et al: Validation of an acrosomal stain for equine sperm that differentiates between living and dead sperm. J Androl 1993; 14(4):289-297.
8. Cheng FP, Fazeli A, Voorhout WF et al: Use of peanut agglutinin to assess the acrosomal status and the zona pellucida-induced acrosome reaction in stallion spermatozoa. J Androl 1996; 17(6):674-682.
9. Cheng FP, Gadella BM, Voorhout WF et al: Progesterone-induced acrosome reaction in stallion spermatozoa is mediated by a plasma membrane progesterone receptor. Biol Reprod 1998; 59(4):733-742.
10. Varner DD, Ward CR, Storey BT et al: Induction and characterization of acrosome reaction in equine spermatozoa. Am J Vet Res 1987; 48(9):1383-1389.
11. Didion BA, Dobrinsky JR, Giles JR et al: Staining procedure to detect viability and the true acrosome reaction in spermatozoa of various species. Gamete Res 1989; 22(1):1-7.
12. Christensen P, Whitfield CH, Parkinson TJ: In vitro induction of acrosome reactions in stallion spermatozoa by heparin and A23187. Theriogenology 1996; 45(6):1201-1210.
13. Pratt NC, Patton ML, Durrant BS et al: Verification of the Coomassie acrosome stain with transmission electron-microscopy. Biol Reprod 50(Suppl 1):105-105, 1994.
14. Meyers SA, Liu IKM, Overstreet JW et al: Sperm-zona pellucida binding and zona-induced acrosome reactions in the horse: comparisons between fertile and subfertile males. Theriogenology 1996; 46(7):1277-1288.
15. Pantke P, Hyland JH, Galloway DB et al: Development of a zona pellucida-sperm binding assay for the assessment of stallion fertility. Biol Reprod Mono 1:681-688, 1995.
16. Ellington JE, Ignotz GG, Varner DD et al: In vitro interaction between oviduct epithelial and equine sperm. Arch Androl 1993; 31(2):79-86.
17. Dobrinski I, Thomas PG, Ball BA: Cryopreservation reduces the ability of equine spermatozoa to attach to oviductal epithelial cells and zonae pellucidae in vitro. J Androl 1995; 16(6):536-542.
18. Kenney RM, Evenson DP, Garcia MC et al: Relationships between sperm chromatin structure, motility, and morphology of ejaculated sperm, and seasonal pregnancy rate. Biol Reprod Mono 1:647-653, 1995.
19. Bedford SJ, Meyers SA, Varner DD: Acrosomal status of fresh, cooled and cryopreserved stallion spermatozoa. J Reprod Fertil Suppl 2000; 56:133-140.
20. Linfor J, Pommer A, Meyers S: Osmotic stress induces tyrosine phosphorylation of equine sperm. Theriogenology 2002; 58:349-352.
21. Pommer AC, Meyers SA: Tyrosine phosphorylation is an indicator of capacitation status in fresh and cryopreserved stallion spermatozoa. Theriogenology 2002; 58:345-348.
22. Linfor JJ, Meyers SA: Detection of DNA damage in response to cooling injury in equine spermatozoa using single-cell gel electrophoresis. J Androl 2002; 23(1):107-113.
23. Baumber J, Ball BA, Linfor JJ: Reactive oxygen species and cryopreservation promote deoxyribonucleic acid (DNA) damage in equine sperm. Theriogenology 58(2-4):301-302, 2002.
24. Visconti PE, Kopf GS: Regulation of protein phosphorylation during sperm capacitation. Biol Reprod 1998; 59:1-6.
25. Pommer AC, Rutllant J, Meyers SA: The role of osmotic resistance on equine spermatozoal function. Theriogenology 2002; 58:1373-1384.
26. Cormier N, Sirard MA, Bailey JL: Premature capacitation of bovine spermatozoa is initiated by cryopreservation. J Androl 1997; 18:461-468.
27. Bailey J, Bilodeau JC, Cormier N: Semen cryopreservation in domestic animals: a damaging and capacitating phenomenon. J Androl 2000; 21:1-7.
28. Ball BA, Vo A: Osmotic tolerance of equine spermatozoa and the effects of soluble cryoprotectants on equine sperm motility, viability, and mitochondrial membrane potential. J Androl 2001; 22:1061-1069.
29. Gravance C, Garner D, Baumber J: Assessment of equine sperm mitochondrial function using JC-1. Theriogenology 2000; 53:1691-1703.
30. Garner DL, Thomas CA, Joerg HW et al: Fluorometric assessments of mitochondrial function and viability in cryopreserved bovine spermatozoa. Biol Reprod 1997; 57:1401-1406.
31. Parks J, Lynch D: Lipid composition and thermotropic phase behavior of boar, bull, stallion, and rooster sperm membranes. Cryobiology 1992; 29:255-266.
32. Drobnis EZ, Crowe LM, Berger T et al: Cold shock damage is due to lipid phase transitions in cell membranes: a demonstration using sperm as a model. J Exp Zool 265:432-437, 1993.
33. Ball BA, Vo AT, Baumber J: Generation of reactive oxygen species by equine spermatozoa. Am J Vet Res 2001; 62:508-515.
34. Ball BA, Vo AT: Detection of lipid peroxidation in equine spermatozoa based upon the lipophilic fluorescent dye C11-BODIPY581/591. J Androl 2002; 23:259-269.

35. Lechniak D, Kedzierski A, Stanislawski D: The use of HOS test to evaluate membrane functionality of boar sperm capacitated in vitro. Reprod Domest Anim 2002; 37(6):79-80.
36. Tartagni M, Schonauer MM, Cicinelli E et al: Usefulness of the hypo-osmotic swelling test in predicting pregnancy rate and outcome in couples undergoing intrauterine insemination. J Androl 2002; 23(4):498-502.
37. Rota A, Penzo N, Vincenti L et al: Hypoosmotic swelling (HOS) as a screening. Theriogenology 2000; 53(7):415-420.
38. Neild DM, Chaves MG, Flores M et al: The HOS test and its relationship to fertility in the stallion. Andrologia 2000; 32(6):51-55.
39. Neild DM, Gadella BM, Chaves MG et al: Membrane changes during different stages of a freeze-thaw protocol for equine semen cryopreservation. Theriogenology 59(8):1693-1705, 2003.
40. Devireddy RV, Swanlund DJ, Olin T et al: Cryopreservation of equine sperm: optimal cooling rates in the presence and absence of cryoprotective agents determined using differential scanning calorimetry. Biol Reprod 2002; 66:222-231.

Preservation of Genetics from Dead or Dying Stallions

J A M E S   K .   G R A H A M
C L A I R E   C A R D

PRESENTATION OF CLINICAL CASES

The most practical method of genetic preservation of valuable stallions is the cryopreservation of sperm cells. Veterinary practitioners are frequently contacted in emergency situations regarding the preservation of material from valuable stallions that are diagnosed with medical conditions carrying a grave prognosis, suffer life-threatening illness or injury, or are found dead. Medical conditions that may carry a grave prognosis include advanced renal failure, peritonitis, salmonellosis, pleuropneumonia, disseminated neoplasia (lymphosarcoma, seminoma, melanosarcoma, adenocarcinoma), primary or secondary heart failure, progressive neurologic disease, encephalitis, hepatic encephalopathy, and severe founder. Surgical conditions such as colic related to gastrointestinal torsion, volvulus, and strangulation may carry a poor prognosis for survival. The surgical prognosis depends on a number of factors such as the nature of the gastrointestinal problem, time to referral, and condition of the bowel at surgery. Fatal injuries to stallions may include the following conditions: irreparable cranial, pelvic, limb, or vertebral fractures; chest trauma; diaphragmatic hernias; lacerations causing fatal hemorrhage; and rupture of the suspensory apparatus. Death may be imminent in some cases, or euthanasia may be the only acceptable option. Unfortunately, there is incomplete data on the effect of chemical euthanasia on the viability of samples taken for genetic preservation. Trailer accidents, entrapment, lightning strike, smoke inhalation, predation, poisoning, anaphylactic reactions, electrocution, and drowning account for a small proportion of death losses. Colic in older stallions accounts for the largest percentage of deaths.

DIAGNOSTICS

A physical examination of a disabled or dying stallion is required to determine the prognosis and time frame available for preservation of genetic material. A complete evaluation may include clinical pathologic evaluations of blood, serum, urine, joint fluid, cerebral spinal fluid, and abdominal fluid. Fecal examinations, culture and sensitivity of specimens, radiographs, ultrasonographic examination, neurologic examination, exploratory surgery, or biopsy may be required. In the case of a deceased stallion it is important to determine the approximate time of death, based on history or physical features such as body temperature, and presence or absence of rigor mortis. Breed association approval for using semen from deceased stallions should be checked by the owner.

PROGNOSIS

Semen quality is influenced by stress, fever, and illness in the stallion. The duration of the stress affects semen quality because of the impact on the spermatogenic cycle; therefore the longer the duration of the problem, the greater the effect on the spermiogram. The ability to collect semen from terminally disabled or dying stallions is influenced by humane welfare aspects in terms of minimizing pain and stress in the individual. The stallion's pain should be managed with nonsteroidal anti-inflammatory drugs; opioid or morphine derivatives administered orally, intravenously (IV), transdermally, or through an epidural approach. Chemical ejaculation is a viable option for stallions that are no longer able to complete the breeding act or those that have musculoskeletal problems such as limb fractures that prevent the stallion from breeding.

Chemical ejaculation protocols appear to be less successful in stallions that are diseased or highly stressed. This may be due in part to the overall deteriorated health condition of the stallion, medications he is receiving, effects of endogenous epinephrine and cortisol, or a combination of factors.

For this procedure the stallion is fitted with a bag around his prepuce that is secured around his girth. The bag is used for semen collection and needs to be large enough to accommodate the erect penis, because imipramine hydrochloride causes spontaneous erection. Combinations of oral imipramine hydrochloride 0.5 mg/kg followed in 2 hours with xylazine, 0.4 mg/kg IV, have given the best results. The xylazine dose should be titrated to cause good sedation over a 2-minute period. Ejaculation typically occurs either shortly after xylazine administration or after 20 minutes of sedation. The semen is usually emitted in a concentrated state. It should be processed immediately to avoid cold shock.

PRESERVATION OF GENETIC MATERIAL

Options in terminally ill or dying stallions include chemical ejaculation, electroejaculation, epididymal sperm collection, intracytoplasmic sperm injection (ICSI), spermatogonial stem cell transplantation, and harvesting material for cloning.

Electroejaculation

Electroejaculation has been reported in sedated and anesthetized stallions and standing zebra stallions. The quality of the ejaculate obtained by this method has not been reported to be as satisfactory as that obtained by chemical ejaculation or epididymal flushing. An advantage of electroejaculation is that it may be repeated more than once.[1]

The stallion should be heavily sedated or placed under general anesthesia. Manure should be removed from the rectum. The stallion should be positioned in lateral recumbency. The semen collector should be positioned along the back of the stallion reaching over to steady the penis. A yearling bull–sized probe should be lubricated and placed in the rectum with the electrical contacts facing ventrally. Beginning at the lowest power setting, intermittent electrical stimulation of 3 seconds on, 3 seconds off, using three repetitions at each power setting should be performed until a semen sample is obtained. There will be involuntary leg movement associated with the periods of stimulation. The penis will become erect.

This procedure may be coupled with castration to obtain viable sperm just before euthanasia. The procedure carries the risk of rectal injury or rupture. Samples may not be obtained from all stallions.

Epididymal Sperm Collection

Micropuncture of the epididymis or fine-needle aspiration may be performed to obtain a small sample of sperm cells for in vitro use, low-dose insemination, or cryopreservation. Other options include the surgical removal of the epididymal and testicular tissue along with a portion of the vas deferens from a stallion. Halothane anesthesia did not have detrimental effects on epididymal sperm cell viability.[2] The epididymal tissue may be recovered from a stallion at euthanasia or taken from a stallion that has been deceased for less than 4 hours. If longer periods of time have elapsed since death, then the sperm cells may decrease in viability. Excessively hot or cold weather will also influence the viability of the sperm cells. Epididymal tissue stored cooled at 4°C for 24 hours yielded spermatozoa that could be cryopreserved.[3] In other species storage for a number of days at 4°C was performed, and viable sperm were obtained.

It is important to recover a long piece of the vas deferens by performing a modification of the open castration technique. The tunica vaginalis is opened, and traction is placed on the testicle. In the surgical approach the spermatic cord is identified, and it is followed and transected as it enters the inguinal ring. Therefore the epididymis and testes are removed with as much of the spermatic cord attached as possible. If the stallion is deceased, the vas deferens in the spermatic cord may be followed through the inguinal ring into the abdomen. The abdomen should be opened through a flank approach, and the vas may be dissected free near the entrance into the ampulla. The vas deferens should be ligated or clamped where it is cut. If the tissue is being sent to a laboratory for processing, the shipper should contact the laboratory for their current recommended shipping conditions. Many laboratories suggest the tissue should be shipped moistened in saline at 4°C.

The vas deferens should be dissected free of the spermatic chord and the deferent artery. The end of a tomcat catheter or blunt 22-gauge needle may be introduced into the end of the vas deferens; a hemostat or ligature may be applied to the end around the catheter or needle. A small volume of extender (<10 ml) should be flushed through the vas. The injection will occur under pressure, and the end of the vas should be steadied over a collection tube or Petri dish. The first few drops will contain the most sperm. Care should be taken not to contaminate the sample with blood. Once flushed, the vas deferens should be sectioned into small pieces and soaked in extender for at least 15 minutes. The epididymides should be removed from the testis. Multiple cuts into the tissue or minces of the tissue should be performed and the tissue soaked in extender. Processing samples through glass wool or adding seminal plasma did show a beneficial effect when performed before cryopreservation.[4] The extended sperm cell samples that have little debris should be processed similarly to neat semen. Extended sperm cell samples containing cellular debris or blood should be processed through a discontinuous 40/90 Percoll or silica particle gradient to remove debris and then the pelleted sperm cells rinsed before freezing. The sperm cells may be then processed for freezing or used fresh with artificial insemination or low-dose insemination techniques. The number of sperm cells used for low-dose insemination may be as few as 5 million sperm cells.

Motility of the sperm cells is achieved by the addition of accessory sex gland fluid at ejaculation. Therefore sperm cell samples obtained from the vas deferens generally have higher motility than those cells recovered from the epididymides, and although the percentage of sperm cells with progressive motility may be acceptable, the sperm cells usually have a slow velocity, despite a high proportion having intact membranes using the eosin nigrosin preparation.

Intracytoplasmic Sperm Injection

ICSI, spermatogonial stem cell preservation, and cloning are low-yield experimental techniques for assisted reproduction in horses. In ICSI the tail is removed from a sperm cell, and the nucleus is injected into an oocyte. A pulse of electric current is used to activate the development of the embryo. This technique has been used with limited success in horses because of problems culturing equine embryos. Freezing epididymal sperm cells before ICSI did not have a detrimental effect on the outcome in humans when thawed motile sperm cells were compared with fresh sperm cells.[5]

Spermatogonial Stem Cell Preservation

Xenotransplantation of stallion spermatogonial stem cells into immunocompromised mice whose spermatogenesis had been destroyed did not result in sperm cell production but was reported to produce germ cells and served as a bioassay of germ cell function.[6] Spermatogonial stem cells have been successfully transplanted from goat bucks to immune-competent unrelated prepubertal recipient bucks; such an approach may be used in stallions in the future.[7]

The cells are removed from the testis by fine-needle aspiration or by surgical removal. The spermatogonial stem cells may be used fresh, cultured, or cryopreserved. The spermatogonial stem cells are then injected into the testis of a prepubertal male. The spermatogonia colonize the seminiferous epithelium, and in a proportion of the treated recipients the sperm produced after puberty will be a mixture of the donor and recipient animals. This is also a technique that may be used to propagate a transgene from one male individual into a larger population of males.

Cloning

Mules

Nuclear transfer and somatic cell cloning has been successful in producing three identical male mule clones and male and female horse clones. Sheep, mice, cattle, rabbits, goats, rats, pigs, cats, dogs, mules, white-tailed deer, and horses have produced live offspring using this technique. Initial studies showed that the transfer of nuclei of fetal origin were more successful in cloning research. A nucleus from fetal mule skin was injected into an enucleated horse oocyte. Oocytes were collected by transvaginal aspiration. Calcium activation was used to initiate embryonic development. The authors used elevated extracellular calcium concentrations in the activation and culture phase, which they report may have contributed to competent nuclear transfer. The authors showed that mule somatic cells have developmental competence and that horse oocytes may reprogram equine somatic cell nuclei, resulting in embryonic and full-term fetal development. Sterility in the mule is likely due to a number of factors such as the failure to produce viable oocytes and sperm cells, thus effectively blocking normal estrous cycles, spermatogenesis, and fertilization because the odd chromosome number (mules, n = 63; donkey, n = 62; horse, n = 64) does support development using nuclear transfer technology.

Horses

Equine fibroblast cell lines from skin biopsies were established for one stallion and one mare. Abattoir ovaries were used, and oocytes were matured in vitro. The nucleus and zona were removed from the oocytes. Cell fusion between oocyte and fibroblast cells resulted in 513 male-derived and 328 female-derived embryos. Most of the fused embryos (97%) activated and were cultured in vitro. Twenty-two blastocysts (8 male, 14 female) resulted. A nonsurgical embryo transfer was performed using 17 embryos, and 4 pregnancies resulted. One fetus went to term, and its mother was the donor of the skin cells. Therefore this is the first report of a live birth from a donor acting as its own recipient. The authors show that

immunologic recognition by the mother of the fetus as foreign is not necessary for a successful pregnancy. Presently equine clones have been produced using geldings as sires. In the future studies may be performed to verify the reproducibility of traits such as character and sporting performances using clones.[8,9] Equine cloning is now being offered by private enterprises.

Sample Collection

Successful storage of a DNA sample depends on time, temperature, tissue handling, and laboratory techniques. There are many commercial companies that supply kits to collect skin cells from a variety of species. The companies store cultured skin fibroblasts as a means of preserving genetic material. Skin from stallions may be stored and cultured for fibroblast storage at any time from a live horse as a means of preserving genetic material. The skin sample is collected using sterile technique and shipped in sterile containers for overnight delivery.

The skin from deceased stallions may be harvested post mortem. The exact time frame for a viable collection is not known; however, viable cells are less likely to be obtained the longer the time from death. Some companies report successful storage of cells from animals that have been deceased for 14 days but also failures in animals that have been deceased for 1 day. The animal's body should be kept cool but not frozen if there is a time lapse from death to sample collection. The clones produced from this gene-banked DNA would be genetically identical to the donor except for their mitochondrial DNA. The mitochondrial DNA is provided by the oocyte, and mitochondria are essential for energy production in cells; hence if the mitochondrial DNA are not optimal, this may be a limiting factor in cloned performance animals.

There was a recent report on identical quadruplicate bulls obtained by embryo splitting. The bulls were therefore identical in mitochondrial and somatic cell DNA. The sperm cell production was satisfactory in three of the four adult quadruplicate bulls, suggesting that environmental factors influenced the production of one bull. Similarly, environmental effect, differences in mitochondrial DNA, epigenetic reprogramming, and other factors would be expected to influence the productivity and fertility of cloned horses or mules. Prospective owners considering this technology should consider the moral and ethical issues involved and need to be aware that cloning is a reproductive technique, not a tool for resurrection of an individual.

References

1. Card CE, Manning ST, Bowman PA et al: Pregnancies from imipramine xylazine chemically induced ex copula ejaculation in a disabled stallion. Can Vet J 1996; 37:91.
2. Schulman ML, Gerber D, Nurton J et al: Effects of halothane anaesthesia on the cryopreservation of epididymal spermatozoa in pony stallions. Equine Vet J 2003; 35:93.
3. Bruemmer JE, Reger H, Zibinski G et al: The effect of storage at 5°C on the motility and cryopreservation of stallion epididymal spermatozoa. Theriogenology 2002; 58:405.

4. Tiplady CA, Morris LH, Allen WR et al: Stallion epididymal spermatozoa: pre freeze and post-thaw motility and viability after three treatments. Theriogenology 2002; 58:225.

5. Cayan S, Lee D, Conaghan J et al: A comparison of ICSI outcomes with fresh and cryopreserved epididymal spermatozoa from the same couples. Hum Reprod 2001; 16:495.

6. Dobrinski I, Avarbock MR, Brinster RL: Germ cell transplantation from large domestic animals into mouse testis. Mol Reprod Dev 2000; 57:270.

7. Honaramooz A, Behboodi E, Megee SO et al: Fertility and germline transmission of donor haplotype following germ cell transplantation in immunocompetent goats. Biol Reprod 2003; 69:1260.

8. Galli C, Lagutina I, Crotti G et al: Pregnancy: a cloned horse born to its dam twin. Nature 2003; 464:635.

9. Hinrichs K: Update on ICSI and equine cloning. Theriogenology 2005; 64:535.

CHAPTER 45

Insemination with Frozen Semen

JUAN C. SAMPER

ANDRÉS J. ESTRADA

ANGUS O. MCKINNON

Artificial insemination (AI) with frozen semen involves the timely introduction of an adequate number of sperm into the mare's uterus. To ensure success in an AI program with frozen semen, knowledge of the reproductive tract of the mare is very important. Mare selection, as well as close monitoring of the cycle, are key factors that will determine the success of this kind of program (see Suggested Readings at the end of this chapter).

In the equine industry (especially in some breeds), artificial insemination with frozen semen is not well understood, and that makes many owners and breeders approach the subject with skepticism. Cryopreservation of spermatozoa remained an enigma until the serendipitous discovery of glycerol in 1948 by scientists in Cambridge, England.[1,2] Regretfully, there is still much progress needed in processes of successful cryopreservation of equine spermatozoa (see Suggested Readings).

Since 1957, when the first foal born from frozen semen was reported,[3] many attempts have been made to maximize this reproductive technique. In spite of these efforts, the technique has not developed as quickly as it has in bovine semen. Reasons for this include a lack of research, a lack of funds available, the relatively small number of mares bred with frozen semen,[4] and little selection pressure for equine fertility because performance, not fertility, is the prime determinate for breeding.[5] Successful pregnancies can be difficult to achieve with frozen stallion semen. Important factors that affect pregnancy rates with frozen semen are (1) the stallion, (2) semen processing and handling, (3) mare's status, and (4) experience of the inseminator.[6]

As with many reproductive techniques, the use of AI with frozen semen has advantages and disadvantages.

ADVANTAGES

- There should be no requirement to schedule shipments of semen to fit the mares' ovulation.
- The stallion does not have to be taken out of competition to breed or have his competitive attitude possibly upset by having to be bred, apart from time necessary to collect semen for freezing.
- The market of semen is global, because there is no limitation on duration of delivery time.

- There is an "insurance factor" should the stallion become ill or die and be unable to fulfill his breeding commitments.
- Transport costs are decreased.
- There are decreased stress and risk to mare and foal.

DISADVANTAGES

- Not all stallions will have semen that freezes well.
- Pregnancy rates for artificial insemination with frozen semen are typically a little lower than those seen with fresh or cooled semen.
- Freezing semen is more expensive per breeding dose than preparing cooled semen.
- There is currently no standardized method for freezing and thawing stallion semen.
- Frozen semen has a shorter life span in the mare's uterus than fresh semen; hence veterinarians have to provide more intense mare management.
- Selection of mares must be stricter when inseminating with frozen semen than with fresh diluted or shipped semen.
- There is an apparent higher percentage of early embryonic death.

SELECTING THE PROPER MARE FOR ARTIFICIAL INSEMINATION WITH FROZEN SEMEN

Although all mares theoretically could be bred with frozen semen, the recognized lower pregnancy rate per cycle suggests only mares that are reproductively normal would be good candidates. To be considered reproductively normal, the mare should have a uterine biopsy of either I or IIA. Mares with biopsies ranked IIB or III have a very low expected foaling rate.[7] Mares with known delayed uterine clearance should be avoided, as well as breeding during the foal heat. Other poor choices include mares not in good body condition and, in general, old mares or mares that have not been able to get pregnant under good management conditions.

The mare should be examined manually and with ultrasonography to identify any anatomic malformations, fluid accumulation, or any other abnormalities.

Uterine cysts should be recorded in order to avoid confusion when evaluating for pregnancy. All mares (except maiden mares) should be cultured, and cytologic evaluation is strongly recommended, especially in older mares or mares that have not had foals for long time. When culturing a mare, it should be ensured that the swab enters the uterus and collects bacteria only from the body of the uterus.[8] If required, Caslick's procedure should be performed to avoid contamination of the reproductive tract.

TIMING OF THE INSEMINATION WITH FROZEN SEMEN

It is critical when inseminating with frozen semen to know when the mare is going to ovulate in order to deposit the semen as close as possible to the time of ovulation, preferably before ovulation. Synchronization of ovulation obviously has many advantages in a breeding program. Because the follicular status of the mares can be predetermined, mares can be mated at a more precise time, increasing the chances of pregnancy and decreasing embryonic loss.[9] Currently there are two available products that help the clinician induce a reliable ovulation time and thus increase the success of insemination with frozen semen. Human chorionic gonadotrophin (hCG) (Chorulon, Intervet Inc., Holland) is a glycoprotein hormone with luteinizing hormone (LH) activity. More recently a biodegradable short-term implant of a gonadotropin-releasing hormone (GnRH) analogue, deslorelin (Ovuplant, Fort Dodge), has been given to mares to hasten ovulation.[10] Although both products have been reported to control the time of ovulation in the mare, it has been suggested that Ovuplant has fewer complications such as failure to respond.

hCG reliably induces ovulation at 36 plus or minus 4 hours and Ovuplant at 41 plus or minus 3 hours.[11] Among the disadvantages that synchronization with hCG has are inconsistencies in response between and within mares and antibody formation, which may or may not cause refractoriness and impair fertility.[12] Ovulation induction with deslorelin has been associated with increased interovulatory intervals in some mares.[13] However, a recent study confirmed that removing the deslorelin implant 48 hours after administration prevented the suppression of follicle-stimulating hormone (FSH) secretion and subsequent follicular development.[14]

There are two approaches currently used for insemination of frozen semen. Firstly and most commonly mares are inseminated immediately before, during, or after ovulation. This approach requires considerable effort and multiple examinations using palpation/ultrasonography. The principal advantages of this regimen are firstly, it decreases to only one the number of times a mare is bred during an individual estrous cycle, and secondly, it should avoid breeding mares with abnormal ovulations such as anovulatory hemorrhagic follicles.[5] The other approach that appears to be gaining favor is to breed two times approximately 24 hours apart. The first insemination is at 24 hours after hCG or Ovuplant, and the second either 12 or 16 hours later, respectively. Because frozen semen is thought to survive in the mare's reproductive tract for up to 12 hours and current recom-

mendations are to breed mares within 12 hours before ovulation to 6 hours post ovulation, these two inseminations cover the period of recommended breeding with less requirement for examination and no reported decrease in fertility. The major disadvantage of the latter technique is the potential for semen wastage or at least usage. The inflammatory response post insemination may be a problem in some mares.

THAWING AND EVALUATION OF THE SEMEN

Frozen semen straws (the most common method of storage) may be thawed in a variety of ways, either at a lower temperature for a longer period of time or at higher temperature for a shorter period of time. In general, 0.5-ml straws may be thawed at 37° C for at least 30 seconds. Larger straws do not thaw as effectively at 37° C for short periods; therefore thawing at 50°C is highly recommended.[15] It is important to be sure that if more than one straw is thawed, the straws are separated from each other to avoid differences in thawing temperatures in the places where two or more straws are making contact.

Frozen semen can also be kept in containers other than straws. These include plastic bags made out of polypropylene, pellets, and aluminum packages, but their popularity has been overridden by the different sizes of straws.[16,17]

To summarize this step, Table 45-1 gives clear instructions for current recommendations for thawing equine semen.

Some protocols for thawing semen involve the addition of warmed thawing extender to aid the thawing process. The extender may also increase the volume and/or aid in preservation of spermatozoa viability.[18]

In a survey made by Samper and Morris[19] in 1998, it was evident that the criteria and methods for thawing semen are far from standardized, making horse breeders lose faith in insemination with frozen semen. Although there are several methods recommended for thawing of equine frozen semen, it is strongly advised to follow the thawing instructions that accompany the semen from the storage facility or the freezer when shipped. Regardless of the thawing procedure or packing system, it is well

Table 45-1

Thawing Protocols for Frozen Stallion Semen Presented in Different Packages

Type of Package	Thawing Temperature	Thawing Time (seconds)
Single 0.5-ml straw	7°C/167°F	7
Multiple 0.5-ml straws	37°C/99°F	At least 30
2.5-ml straws	50°C/122°F	45
4.0-ml straws	50°C/122°F	45
5.0-ml straws	50°C/122°F	45
0.1-ml pellets	37°C/99°F	At least 15
Polyethylene bags	20°C/68°F	30

accepted that once semen has been thawed, it should be used for insemination almost immediately.[20]

Although motility is not a predictor of fertility, the percentage of motile progressive sperm could be taken as a good indicator of the number of viable sperm.[21] Motility may be assessed either visually (with the help of a microscope) or using a computerized motility analysis system.[22] Morphologic characteristics can be checked with samples fixed in formal saline or by staining a sample with the aid of a dye. General-purpose cellular stains (Wright's, Giemsa, hematoxylin-eosin, India ink) can be used,[23] but live-dead stains (aniline-eosin, eosin-nigrosin, eosin-fast green) are more widely used for the determination of cell viability.[24] Integrity of the plasma membrane is shown by the ability of a viable cell to exclude the dye, whereas the dye will diffuse passively into cells with damaged plasma membranes.[25]

INSEMINATION PROCEDURE

Once the veterinarian decides that the mare is ready to be bred with frozen semen, the mare should be placed in stocks and her tail wrapped and held by somebody else or by a piece of rope attached to the stocks. If the person in charge of the AI anticipates rectal manipulation may be necessary, the feces should be removed from the rectum before cleaning the perineum. The perineal area should be washed (using Ivory soap, Betadine scrub, or a dilute chlorhexidine solution) and rinsed with water at least three times. If the mare is being rinsed with a hose instead of a bucket, the water stream should not be pointed against the vulva in order to avoid forcing water into the vagina or vestibule.[26]

The inseminator should wear a plastic sleeve (turned inside-out if it is not sterile) and should place a *small amount* of lubricating gel onto the glove. The gel should be *nonspermicidal* due to its deleterious effects on longevity, motility, or viability of the sperm.[27] The insemination pipette, with the syringe loaded with semen attached to the end, should be kept as clean as possible, avoiding any contact with any structures except the inseminator's glove, and the tip should be protected by being held between the thumb and the palm of the inseminator.[28] The two lips of the vulva must be separated to let the inseminator insert the arm surrounding the pipette across the vagina and the vestibule so that the tip of the pipette can be inserted through the cervix and into either the body or one of the horns of the uterus. In a study using an insemination dose of 500 million sperm, Rigby et al[29] reported a bigger recovery of sperm in the oviducts when they inseminated close to the uterotubal junction than when they inseminated in the uterine body. In either case, once the tip of the pipette has reached its destination, the plunger of the syringe should be depressed completely to deposit the semen. A 21-inch pipette holds almost 5 ml of fluid, so the syringe should include at least 5 ml of air to ensure that all semen has been expelled into the uterus. Caslick's procedure should be performed as required.

Although some authors advise multiple inseminations until ovulation takes place, others recommend that the breeder inseminate only one time, before ovulation, to avoid the inflammatory response that previous ovulations can trigger.[30,31] It is also recommended to inseminate before the ovulation rather than after because the high levels of estrogen present enhance the ability of the uterus to remove polymorphonuclears (PMNs) and excess fluids after insemination.[32] However, as noted above, this may inadvertently result in mares being bred before an anovulatory hemorrhagic follicle is identified.

POSTINSEMINATION PROCEDURE

After the insemination has been performed, the clinician must perform an ultrasonographic examination of the mare and check for fluids, which if present should be removed with lavages made with lactated solution and some applications of oxytocin (Vedco). These lavages can be done between 4 hours and 3 days after ovulation, 1 day before the egg (if fertilized) reaches the uterus. A normal pregnancy diagnostic ultrasonographic examination should be performed 14 to 16 days after ovulation.

CONCLUSION

Although more expensive than inseminations with fresh extended and shipped semen and more demanding of skills from the clinician, AI with frozen semen is a technique that should not be underestimated as an outstanding equine reproductive tool. Insemination with frozen semen, although a challenging technique, provides benefits for mare and stallion owners, as well as veterinarians. Although frozen semen has been successfully used in the bovine and porcine industries, there is still a significant lack of research in the freezing and thawing of stallion semen specifically. More research will enhance the advantages of using frozen stallion semen and will play a crucial role with the quickly increasing demand for this technique. As the use of frozen semen is accepted by more and more horse associations around the world, it will become an increasingly frequent part of the daily labor for equine practitioners.

Suggested Reading

AUTHOR'S NOTE: These articles were still available online at the compilation of this chapter but may or may not be at the publication of this book.

Leopold S: Artificial insemination with frozen semen. November 20, 2002 (accessed) [http://www.equinecentre.comau/health_repro_ai.shtm1].

Pycock J: Technique for AI with frozen semen. November 30, 2002 (accessed) [http://www.pycock.co.uk/article8.htm].

References

1. Polge C: Functional survival of fowl spermatozoa after freezing at -79 degrees C. Nature 1951; 167(4258):949-950.
2. Smith AU, Polge C: Survival of spermatozoa at low temperatures. Nature 1950; 166(4225):668-669.
3. Barker CAV, Gandier JCC: Pregnancy in a mare from frozen epididymal spermatozoa. Can J Comp Med Vet Sci 1957; 21:47.

4. Samper JC: Artificial insemination. In Samper JC (ed): Equine Breeding Management and Artificial Insemination, p 122, WB Saunders, 2000.

5. McKinnon AO: Artificial insemination of cooled, transported and frozen semen. In Equine Stud Medicine, pp 319-337, Sydney, Australia, Post Graduate Foundation in Veterinary Science, 1996.

6. Metcalf EJ: Maximizing reproductive efficiency in private practice: the management of mares and the use of cryopreserved semen. Proceedings of the Annual Meeting of the Society for Theriogenology, p 155, 1955.

7. Kenney RM, Doig PA: Equine endometrial biopsy. In Morrow DA (ed): Current Therapy in Theriogenology 2, pp 723-729, Philadelphia, WB Saunders, 1986.

8. Pycock J: Breeding management of the problem mare. In Samper JC (ed): Equine Breeding Management and Artificial Insemination, pp 195-228, Philadelphia, WB Saunders, 2000.

9. Voss JL: Human chorionic gonadotropin. In McKinnon AO, Voss JL (eds): Equine Reproduction, pp 325-328, Philadelphia, Lea & Febiger, 1993.

10. McKinnon AO, Nobelius AM, Figueroa STD et al: Predictable ovulation in mares treated with an implant of the GnRH analog deslorelin. Equine Vet J 1993; 25:321-323.

11. McKinnon AO, Perriam WJ, Lescun TB et al: Effect of a GnRH analogue (Ovuplant), hCG and dexamethasone on time to ovulation in cycling mares. World Equine Vet Rev 1997; 2(3):16-18.

12. Roser JF, Keifer BL, Evans JW et al: The development of antibodies to human chorionic gonadotrophin following its repeated injection in the cycle mare. J Reprod Fertil Suppl 1979; 27:173.

13. McCue PM, Farquhar EM, Carnevale EM et al: Removal of deslorelin (Ovuplant) implant 48 hours after administration results in normal interovulatory intervals in mares. Theriogenology 58:865-870, 2002.

14. Farquhar VJ, McCue PM, Carnevale EM et al: Deslorelin acetate (Ovuplant) therapy in cycling mares: effect of implant removal on FSH secretion and ovarian function. Equine Vet J 2001.

15. Martin JC, Klug E, Gunzel AR: Centrifugation of stallion semen and its storage in large volume straws. J Reprod Fertil 27:47-51, 1979.

16. Amann RP, Pickett BW: An Overview of Frozen Equine Semen: Procedures for Thawing and Insemination of Frozen Spermatozoa, Experimental Station Animal Reproduction Laboratory.

17. Love CC, Loch WL, Bristol F et al: Comparison of pregnancy rates achieved with frozen semen using two packaging methods. Theriogenology 1989; 31:613-622.

18. Davies Morel MCG: Semen Storage and Transportation in Equine Artificial Insemination, p 295, CABI, 1999.

19. Samper JC, Morris CA: Current methods for stallion semen cryopreservation: a survey. Theriogenology 1998; 49:895-903.

20. Samper JC: Techniques for Artificial Insemination in Current Therapy in Large Animal Theriogenology, p 39, Philadelphia, WB Saunders, 1997.

21. Long PL, Picket BW, Sawyer HR et al: Relationship between morphologic and seminal characteristics of equine spermatozoa. J Vet Sci 1993; 10:298-300.

22. Davies Morel MCG: Semen evaluation. In Morel MCG (ed): Equine artificial insemination, pp 190-233, CABI, 1999.

23. Varner DD, Schumacher J, Blanchard TL et al: Diseases and Management of Breeding Stallions, Goleta, Calif, American Veterinary Publications, 1991.

24. Katilla T: In vitro evaluation of frozen-thawed stallion semen: a review. Acta Vet Scand 2001; 42:199-217.

25. Colembrander B, Fazeli AR, van Buiten A et al: Assessment of sperm cell membrane integrity in the horse. Acta Vet Scand Suppl 1992; 88:49-58.

26. Brinsko SP, Varner DD: Artificial insemination. In McKinnon AO, Voss JL (eds): Equine Reproduction, pp 790-797, Philadelphia, Lea & Febiger, 1993.

27. Froman DP, Amann RP: Inhibition of motility of bovine, canine and equine spermatozoa by artificial vagina lubricants. Theriogenology 1983; 20(3):357-361.

28. Metcalf ES: Insemination and breeding management. In Samper JC (ed): Equine Breeding Management and Artificial Insemination, pp 179-194, Philadelphia, WB Saunders, 2000.

29. Rigby S, Derczo S, Brinsko SP et al: Oviductal sperm numbers following proximal uterine horn or uterine body insemination. Proceedings of the 46th Annual Convention of the American Association of Equine Practitioners, pp 332-334, 2000.

30. Troedsson MHT, Loset K, Alghamdi AM et al: Interaction between equine semen and the endometrium: the inflammatory response to semen. Anim Reprod Sci 2001; 68:273-278.

31. Katila T: Sperm-uterine interactions: a review. Anim Reprod Sci 2001; 68:267-272.

32. Katila T: Uterine defense mechanisms in the mare. Anim Reprod Sci 1996; 42:197-204.

Assisted Reproductive Techniques

CHAPTER 46

Collection and Transfer of Oocytes in Mares

ELAINE M. CARNEVALE

Methods to successfully collect and transfer equine oocytes have resulted in new reproductive technologies. Because oocytes are collected directly from the follicles, various reproductive pathologic conditions of donors can be avoided, and offspring can be obtained from mares that are considered infertile using standard breeding techniques or embryo transfer.

COLLECTION AND TRANSFER OF THE PREOVULATORY OOCYTE

Commercial Use of Oocyte Transfer

Oocyte transfer has been used to obtain pregnancies from mares that are unsuccessful embryo donors because of various reproductive pathologic conditions.[1] Because fertilization, embryo development, and fetal development occur within the recipient, pathologic conditions associated with ovulation or the tubular genitalia of donors are avoided. Although the first foal after an oocyte transfer was obtained in 1988,[2] the technique was not used for commercial transfers until the late 1990s.[1,3] A number of factors could affect the development or survival of embryos before they are recovered from the uterus between 6 and 8 days after ovulation.

The effects of pathologic conditions associated with ovulation and the oviduct on fertility are not well defined. However, results of studies suggest that reductions in fertility occur before the embryo enters the uterus, especially in older mares. The oviducts of old mares ($\geq$20 years) and young mares (2 to 9 years) were flushed between 1 and 4 days after ovulation. Recovery rates of recently ovulated oocytes or embryos were significantly lower for old compared with young mares (17/29, 59%, and 26/27, 96%, respectively).[4] Results of the study suggest that either ovulation does not occur or that the oocyte does not enter the oviduct in some older mares. The incidence of ovulation failure increased with aging in mares and during the autumn months.[5,6]

In addition to collection and movement of the oocyte, the oviduct functions in the selection and storage of sperm. Scott et al[7] compared numbers and motility of sperm in the oviducts of fertile and subfertile mares. Few sperm in the oviducts of subfertile mares were motile, but highly motile sperm were found in the oviducts of normal mares. Oviductal pathologic conditions could be associated with failure of sperm transport and fertilization in subfertile mares. Globular masses, composed of type I collagen, were found more frequently in the oviducts of older than younger mares.[8] The effect that these masses have on fertility is not known. Further research is needed to define the extent that follicular and oviductal pathologic conditions affect fertility in the mare.

Uterine causes of reduced fertility are frequently diagnosed in the mare. Infectious and/or inflammatory changes within the uterus are easily diagnosed and are harmful to the sperm and embryo. Mares with severe or persistent endometritis are expensive to treat and frequently do not provide embryos. Cervical lacerations, cervical or uterine adhesions, or urine pooling will also prevent mares from being successful embryo donors. In some mares, repeated embryo collection attempts are unsuccessful, although the cause of infertility is not diagnosed.

When oocytes are collected and transferred, pathologic conditions of the donor's tubular genitalia are avoided. Donors that do not ovulate properly can still be acceptable oocyte donors if they develop a normal preovulatory follicle from which the oocyte can be collected. Therefore the collection and transfer of oocytes allows offspring to be produced from mares with a variety of reproductive pathologic conditions that would otherwise prevent the production of embryos or foals.

The Oocyte Donor

For commercial transfers, oocytes are often collected from maturing follicles between 0 and 16 hours before anticipated ovulation. The collection of oocytes from preovulatory follicles has the disadvantage that only one or two oocytes are collected per cycle. However, collection of oocytes from preovulatory follicles has many advantages. The equine cumulus complex in the immature follicle has a broad base of attachment and cellular projections into the theca interna.[9] Therefore collection of oocytes from immature follicles, before the luteinizing hormone (LH) surge, is difficult, and collection rates are low. In addition, the maturation in vitro of immature oocytes is more difficult than in vitro culture of preovulatory (maturing) oocytes. Immature oocytes are matured in a complex medium containing additions of hormones and, potentially, growth factors for approximately 30 hours; in contrast, culture of preovulatory oocytes can be accomplished in a relatively simple medium within 12 hours. After maturation, competence of oocytes matured in vitro is probably reduced when compared with oocytes collected from the preovulatory follicle. Therefore, in this author's laboratory, oocytes for commercial transfers are usually collected within 16 hours before the anticipated ovulation of the dominant follicle.

Requirements for oocyte donors are minimal. The donor needs to grow a preovulatory follicle containing a viable oocyte. In general, oocytes from young donors (3 to 13 years) are considered more viable than oocytes from older donors. When oocytes were collected from the preovulatory follicles of young donors (6 to 10 years) and old donors (20 to 26 years) and transferred into the oviducts of young recipients (3 to 7 years), significantly more oocytes from young compared with old donors developed into embryonic vesicles (11/12, 92%, versus 8/26, 31%).[10] Oocytes from old versus young mares had more morphologic anomalies, such as large vesicles or irregular shapes, when imaged using light and electron microscopy.[11] However, pregnancies were obtained from old (≥20 years) mares in this author's commercial oocyte transfer programs,[1] although more transfers were required to produce a pregnancy when oocytes were collected from older mares.

Oocyte Collection

Induction of follicle and oocyte maturation occurs through the administration of human chorionic gonadotropin (hCG) or a gonadotropin-releasing hormone (GnRH) analogue to the donor. In this author's laboratory, criteria for hCG administration are: (1) a follicle >35 mm in diameter, (2) relaxed cervical and uterine tone, and (3) uterine edema or estrous behavior for a minimum of 2 days. Oocytes are usually collected from preovulatory follicles between 22 and 36 hours after administration of hCG (1500 to 2500 IU, IV) to donors. Therefore ovulation would be anticipated to occur within 0 to 14 hours. Some mares appear to be refractory to hCG, and administration of hCG will not be adequate to time ovulation. In these cases the author administers a GnRH agonist (deslorelin acetate, 2.1 mg SQ; Ovuplant, Peptech Limited, NSW, Australia) and hCG (2000 IU, IV) between 4 and 5 hours later. When collected, oocytes are probably in the metaphase I or II stages of development.

Oocytes have been collected from the follicles of mares using laparotomies,[12] colpotomies,[13,14] flank punctures,[15]

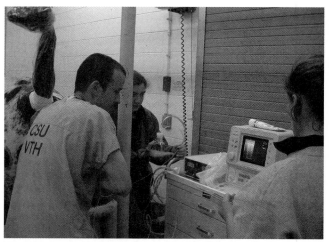

Figure 46-1 Follicle aspiration using the transvaginal, ultrasound-guided technique. The ultrasonographic image is viewed while flush medium is injected *(syringe on right)* and follicular fluid and medium are collected into a sterile bottle *(center)*.

and transvaginal, ultrasound-guided, follicular aspirations.[16,17] In this author's laboratory, oocytes are usually collected by ultrasound-guided punctures through the vaginal wall. For some mares, aspirations through the vagina can be difficult because of pathologic conditions such as melanomas or severe uterine discharge. In these instances we use flank punctures to collect oocytes.

Collection of oocytes using flank puncture involves the placement of a trocar through the flank, ipsilateral to the preovulatory follicle, at the approximate position of the ovary. The ovary is manipulated per rectum, and the preovulatory follicle is positioned against the end of the cannula. While the ovary is stabilized per rectum, a needle (12- to 17-gauge) is placed through the cannula and into the follicular antrum. Follicular contents are removed by gentle lavage and aspiration.

Transvaginal, ultrasound-guided follicular aspirations require use of an ultrasound machine and a transducer casing with a needle guide (Figure 46-1). Linear, curvilinear, and sector transducers have been used. The rectum is evacuated, and the vulva is cleaned. The mare is sedated and twitched. Rectal contractions have been minimized through the administration of propantheline bromide (0.04 mg/kg IV)[1] or the intrarectal deposition of lidocaine. A nontoxic lubricant is applied to the transducer to improve contact with the vaginal wall. The transducer is positioned within the anterior vagina, lateral to the posterior cervix and ipsilateral to the preovulatory follicle. Transrectal manipulations are used to position the follicle with the follicular apex juxtaposed to the needle guide. A needle is advanced through the needle guide to puncture the vaginal and follicular walls. In the author's laboratory, a 12-gauge, double-lumen needle is used (Cook Veterinary Products, New Buffalo, Mich.). The follicular fluid is aspirated from the follicle using a pump (Cook Veterinary Products, New Buffalo, Mich.) set at 150 mm Hg. As the follicular fluid is aspirated from the follicle, the lumen is lavaged with between 50 and 100 ml of

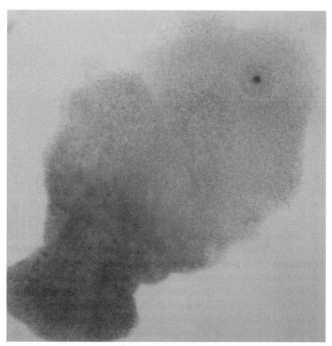

Figure 46-2 Cumulus oocyte complex collected from a follicle 24 hours after the donor received hCG. The oocyte is the dark circular area *(top right)* surrounded by cumulus cells. The darker cells *(bottom left)* are granulosa cells.

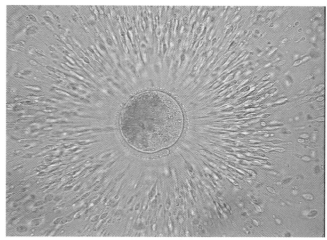

Figure 46-3 A mature equine oocyte. Note expansion of cumulus cells and a polar body at the 5 o'clock position.

flush, typically modified Dulbecco's Phosphate buffered solution or an embryo flush solution (emCare, ICP, Auckland, New Zealand) with additives of fetal calf serum (1%) or bovine serum albumin (0.4%) and heparin (10 IU/ml).

Media and equipment are warmed to 38.5° C before aspirations. Care is taken to prevent cooling of the oocyte during the collection or search procedures. Upon collection, the recovered media and follicular fluid is poured into large search dishes and examined under a dissecting microscope to locate the oocyte. We do not filter the medium, because the cumulus oocyte complex is sticky and could adhere to the filter. Aspirations of preovulatory follicles are frequently tinged with blood because the maturing follicle is highly vascular.

The equine oocyte is slightly greater than 100 µm in diameter; however, it is surrounded by a mass of cumulus cells that is often greater than 1 mm in diameter (Figures 46-2 and 46-3). The cumulus complex appears translucent in the bloody flush solution and usually can be seen with the naked eye. After identification, the cumulus oocyte complex should be washed in medium to remove attached blood and debris.

Oocyte Culture and Transfer

Different scenarios can be used for timing oocyte collections and transfers. However, the complete interval between administration of hCG and transfer is usually between 36 and 40 hours. In one study the time of oocyte collection (24 versus 36 hours after administration of hCG to donors) did not affect pregnancy rates.[18] Similar results have been obtained in this author's laboratory, with good pregnancy rates for oocytes collected at different intervals after administration of hCG.[19]

If oocytes are collected more than 30 hours from hCG administration or if the follicle appears to be within a few hours from ovulation, oocytes are transferred immediately into a recipient's oviduct. The cumulus complex of oocytes directly before ovulation is sticky; and the cumulus cells, including the cells directly surrounding the oocyte, are expanded. Oocytes collected approximately 24 hours after hCG administration are cultured in vitro between 12 and 16 hours before transfer. Most oocytes are cultured in medium similar to that first described by Carnevale and Ginther[10] (Tissue Culture Medium 199 with additions of 10% fetal calf serum, 0.2 mM pyruvate, and 50 µg/ml gentamicin). An incubator is used to maintain an atmosphere of 5% or 6% CO_2 and air and a temperature between 38° and 39° C. In one study,[20] oocytes were collected approximately 24 hours after hCG administration. Oocytes were immediately transferred into recipient's oviducts, and oocyte maturation was completed within the oviduct. The recipients were inseminated approximately 16 hours after transfer, when maturation of oocytes should have been completed. Pregnancy rates were not significantly different for oocytes cultured in the oviduct or for a second group of oocytes that were cultured within an incubator (43% and 57%, respectively). Therefore it is feasible that an oocyte could be collected at any time after 24 hours from the time of administration of hCG to the donor and transferred directly into the recipient's oviduct. This scenario eliminates the equipment and expertise required for oocyte culture, making the procedure more practical in a clinical setting. The best time to inseminate the recipient is probably between 32 and 36 hours after the donor received hCG. This should allow the oocyte to mature to metaphase II before fertilization.

In this author's laboratory, recipients for oocyte transfer are between 3 and 10 years of age. The recipient's reproductive tract provides the environment for sperm transport, fertilization, and embryo development. Reproductive tracts of recipients are examined using transrectal palpation and ultrasonography to confirm that the recipient's uterus and cervix are normal. Oocytes are transferred through a surgical procedure with exposure of the ovary through the recipient's flank. Mares with short, thick flanks and short broad ligaments are not good candidates for recipients. Length of the ligament can be examined by transrectal manipulation of the ovary, determining the distance between the dorsal abdominal wall and the ovary, and determining the extent that the ovary can be moved in a medial direction. In mares with short broad ligaments and thick flanks, exposure of the ovary and oviduct can be difficult and can result in poor transfer conditions.

Because recipients will be inseminated, recipients should be in a natural or induced estrus with endometrial edema and an open cervix. Cyclic and noncyclic, hormone-treated mares have been used as oocyte recipients. Cyclic recipients are synchronized with donors. The recipient's own oocyte must be aspirated before transfer of the donor's oocyte to prevent fertilization of the recipient's oocyte. Therefore we usually administer hCG to recipients and donors at the same time. If an oocyte is successfully collected from the donor, the recipient's oocyte is also collected. Aspiration of the recipient's oocyte can be attempted through the surgical incision at the time of transfer. However, preovulatory follicles are large and flaccid and could be ruptured when attempting to expose the follicle during surgery. Collapse or aspiration of a recipient's follicle does not guarantee that the recipient's oocyte will not be fertilized.[21] If an oocyte is not collected from the recipient's follicle, an alternate recipient should be used.

Noncyclic mares or mares with reduced follicular activity can be used as oocyte recipients, eliminating the need to collect the recipient's oocyte. Anestrus and early transitional mares have been successfully used as recipients during the nonovulatory season.[1,22] During the breeding season, a high dose of a GnRH agonist (4.2 mg deslorelin acetate) has been used to reduce ovarian follicular activity.[23] The mares are then treated as noncyclic recipients. An alternative method to obtain mares with small follicles is to administer progesterone and estrogen (150 mg progesterone and 10 mg estradiol daily)[3] to cyclic mares. The treatment will cause a transient follicular regression, allowing the recipient to be treated as a noncyclic mare.

Before oocyte transfers, estradiol (2 to 5 mg daily for 3 to 7 days) is administered to noncyclic recipients. The reproductive tract of a noncyclic recipient is examined to confirm that the uterus has endometrial edema and that the cervix is open. After transfer, progesterone (150 to 200 mg daily) or progestins (altrenogest, 0.44 mg/kg PO; Regumate, Intervet, Millsboro, Del.) are administered daily. Pregnancies were maintained through the administration of exogenous progesterone or progestins.[1]

Oocytes are transferred into the recipient's oviduct during a standing flank laparotomy. Before surgery, recipients are placed in a stock. The surgical area is clipped and scrubbed, and a presurgical sedative (xylazine HCl, 0.3 mg/kg, and butorphanol tartrate, 0.01 mg/kg, IV) is

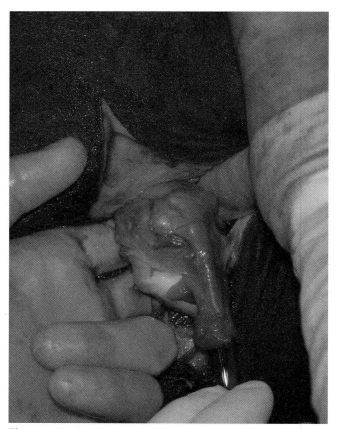

Figure 46-4 Exposure of the ovary and placement of a pipette into the infundibular region of the oviduct.

administered. A line block is done using approximately 100 ml of 2% lidocaine. Directly before surgery, additional sedation is administered (detomidine HCl, 9 μg/kg, and butorphanol tartrate, 0.01 mg/kg, IV). A dorsalventral incision, approximately 8 cm in length, is made midway between the last rib and tuber coxae. Muscle layers are separated using blunt dissection.

Although tranquilization, preparation, closure, and aftercare of recipients are similar to previously described methods for embryo transfer,[24] the incision is made slightly more dorsal and posterior to the preferred incision for embryo transfer. Once the peritoneum is punctured, the ovary is exteriorized through the incision without unnecessary manipulation of the ovary or oviduct. The ovary is rotated gently to expose the oviduct.

Within 5 minutes of transfer, the oocyte is removed from the incubator and placed into transfer medium that has been warmed (38° to 39° C). Plastic and glassware are also warmed. The author uses a fire-polished, glass pipette for transfers. The oviductal os is located by following the outline of the oviduct along the external surface of the infundibulum. The infundibulum is identified, and the pipette containing the oocyte is inserted into the os and carefully advanced 2 to 3 cm (Figure 46-4). The oocyte and less than 0.1 ml of medium are released into the oviduct. The ovary is returned to the abdominal cavity, and the surgical site is closed.

Insemination of Recipients

Use of stallions with good fertility is essential to maximize the success of oocyte transfer. In this author's commercial program, most semen is cooled and transported. Semen is provided from numerous stallions of variable fertility.[1,19]

The equine oocyte remains viable for approximately 12 hours after ovulation.[25] Oocytes should be mature at the time of transfer; therefore recipients are inseminated before and/or directly after transfer. Single inseminations before[26,27] or after[20] oocyte transfer have resulted in pregnancies. During most experimental transfers, recipients were inseminated approximately 12 hours before and 2 hours after transfers with a total of 2×10^9 progressively motile sperm. In a commercial program with older donors and cooled semen from numerous stallions of variable fertility, pregnancy rates were significantly higher when recipients were inseminated before or before and after oocyte transfer than when recipients were inseminated only after transfer (18/45, 40%; 27/53, 51%; and 0/10, respectively).[19] Although not significantly different, when recipients were inseminated before and after versus only after transfer, pregnancy rates were 11% higher. The results suggest that insemination of a recipient before oocyte transfer with a minimum of 1×10^9 progressively motile sperm (PMS) from a fertile stallion is sufficient. If fertility of the stallion is not optimal, insemination of the recipient before and after transfer could be beneficial.

After insemination and transfer, the recipient's uterus is examined with ultrasonography to detect intrauterine fluid collections. If fluid is detected, recipients are aggressively treated to resolve uterine inflammation or infection. Treatments are similar to those used for natural cycles and include oxytocin or prostaglandin to stimulate uterine clearance or lavage and antibiotic infusions.

Success of Oocyte Collection and Transfer

The anticipated success of oocyte transfer is dependent on the quality of oocytes and sperm and on expertise of personnel. Collection rates of oocytes from preovulatory follicles vary with experience of the clinician. With experience, collection rates between 70% and 80% are anticipated. Embryo development rates after the experimental transfers of oocytes from young, fertile donors have ranged from less than 20% to greater than 90%, but rates between 60% and 80% are probable. In a recent experiment, this author's laboratory transferred oocytes into the oviduct contralateral to the recipient's own ovulation. Parentage testing was done on embryos recovered at day 16 from recipients' uteri. In the study, embryo development rates were not different for ovulated or transferred oocytes (9/13, 69%, and 32/44, 73%, respectively),[28] suggesting that the viability of ovulated oocytes and of transferred oocytes is not different.

In this author's commercial program for oocyte transfer, we have older, subfertile mares and use cooled, transported semen from numerous stallions with variable fertility. Pregnancy rates per transfer were 27% during the first year of the program.[1] However, pregnancy rates have continued to increase to greater than 40% per transfer.

ADDITIONAL USES FOR OOCYTE TRANSFER

Transported Ovaries

The development of methods to handle and transfer equine oocytes has resulted in new assisted reproductive techniques with clinical significance.

When a mare dies, her genetic potential is contained within the oocytes remaining in her ovaries. Oocytes from the ovaries of valuable mares that have died or have been euthanized can be collected and transferred. Ovaries can be collected from mares immediately after death and shipped to a facility for oocyte recovery, maturation, and transfer. This technique was first attempted in 1999[1]; a pregnancy was established, which later underwent embryonic death. In 2002 the first foal was produced after the shipment of ovaries across the country before oocyte collection, maturation, and transfer.[29] In the study, oocytes were transferred from five mares that were euthanized because of medical conditions with poor prognoses. Although four pregnancies were established after the transfers, only one pregnancy was maintained through gestation, and a healthy foal was produced. During 2002 in this author's laboratory, oocytes were collected from the transported ovaries of four mares that were euthanized; two pregnancies were established and are ongoing. Although further work is needed to establish the best protocol for transport of ovaries and maturation of oocytes, the recent studies suggest that this procedure can be successfully used to produce limited offspring after the death of a valuable mare.

Oocyte Cryopreservation

Oocyte transfer has the potential to be used with cryopreserved oocytes. Cryopreservation of the oocyte is difficult, because the oocyte is a single cell with a high surface-to-volume ratio, limiting rates that cryoprotectants and water can move in and out of the oocyte.[30] Successful fertilization of oocytes that were cryopreserved has been documented.[31,32] In 2001 the first foals were born after cryopreservation of equine oocytes.[27] The oocytes were vitrified (rapid freeze), warmed, and transferred into the oviducts of inseminated recipients. Twenty-six oocytes were vitrified, three oocytes developed into embryonic vesicles, and two foals were born. Although further research is needed to determine the optimal conditions for oocyte cryopreservation, this technique could provide a valuable method for the preservation of female genetics.

Gamete Intrafallopian Transfer

Techniques used for oocyte transfer can also be used to obtain pregnancies when sperm availability is limited. Maximum fertility was obtained when mares were inseminated with 500×10^6 PMS every other day during estrus.[33] However, assisted reproductive techniques are being developed that reduce the minimum number of motile sperm required for inseminations. Gamete intrafallopian transfer (GIFT) involves the placement of oocytes and a low number of sperm into the recipient's oviduct. The first successful GIFT was reported in 1998.[22] Since the first GIFT, fresh sperm has been repeatedly used with success for GIFT. After collection, raw semen was centrifuged through a density gradient to obtain a high percentage of motile sperm that was free of debris and seminal plasma. PMS (2×10^5) were placed in medium containing oocytes, and gametes were transferred into the oviducts of recipients. Pregnancy rates obtained with GIFT ranged from 27% to 82%.[20,34,35]

In humans, GIFT has been used extensively for subfertile couples, including cases of male subfertility. In the horse, because a low number of sperm is used and because sperm are placed near the site of fertilization, GIFT could be used to produce pregnancies from subfertile stallions, frozen semen, and sex-sorted sperm. Recent studies in this author's laboratory using cooled and frozen semen for GIFT resulted in pregnancy rates of 25% and 8%, respectively.[35] Reasons for lower pregnancy rates, when cooled or frozen semen versus fresh semen is used for GIFT, are being investigated.

Intracytoplasmic Sperm Injection

Because in vitro fertilization has not been repeatable in the horse, intracytoplasmic sperm injection (ICSI) has received attention as an assisted reproductive technique for the subfertile male. During ICSI one sperm is aspirated into a fine-bore needle and injected into a mature oocyte. The injected oocyte can be cultured in vitro or transferred into a recipient's oviduct. Squires et al[36] reported the first successful ICSI of an equine oocyte that was matured in vitro. Foals have been produced by ICSI using oocytes matured in vivo or in vitro,[37,38] but pregnancy rates per transferred oocyte were low (6% to 13%). Recently several investigators reported the in vitro production of blastocysts with increased efficiency,[39-41] increasing the expectations of establishing ICSI as a practical assisted reproductive technique for the horse.

CONCLUSION

With the development of methods to handle and transfer equine oocytes, new reproductive technologies have been developed. With increasing research and expertise, the clinical use of oocyte technologies will continue to advance. Oocyte transfer has the potential to be used for obtaining pregnancies from subfertile mares and stallions, mares that have died, and cryopreserved oocytes. Use of oocyte transfer presents the equine owner and clinician with new possibilities for obtaining foals.

References

1. Carnevale EM, Squires EL, Maclellan LJ et al: Use of oocyte transfer in a commercial breeding program for mares with reproductive abnormalities. J Am Vet Med Assoc 2001; 218:87-91.
2. McKinnon AO, Carnevale EM, Squires EL et al: Heterogenous and xenogenous fertilization of in vivo matured equine oocytes. J Equine Vet Sci 1988; 8:143-147.
3. Hinrichs K, Provost PJ, Torello EM: Treatments resulting in pregnancy in nonovulating, hormone-treated oocyte recipient mares. Theriogenology 2000; 54:1285-1293.
4. Carnevale EM, Griffin PG, Ginther OJ: Age-associated subfertility before entry of embryos into the uterus in mares. Equine Vet J Suppl 1993; 15:31-35.
5. Carnevale EM, Bergfelt DR, Ginther OJ: Follicular activity and concentrations of FSH and LH associated with senescence in mares. Anim Reprod Sci 1994; 35:231-246.
6. Carnevale EM: Folliculogenesis and ovulation. In Rantanen NW, McKinnon AO (eds): Equine Diagnostic Ultrasonography, pp 201-211, Baltimore, Williams & Wilkins, 1998.
7. Scott MA, Liu IKM, Overstreet JW: Sperm transport to the oviducts: abnormalities and their clinical implications. Proceedings of the 41st Annual Convention of the American Association of Equine Practitioners, pp 1-2, 1995.
8. Liu IKM, Lantz KC, Schlafke S et al: Clinical observations of oviductal masses in the mare. Proceedings of the 30th Annual Convention of the American Association of Equine Practitioners, pp 41-45, 1990.
9. Hawley LR, Enders AC, Hinrichs K: Comparison of equine and bovine oocyte-cumulus morphology within the ovarian follicle. Biol Reprod 1995; 1:243-252.
10. Carnevale EM, Ginther OJ: Defective oocytes as a cause of subfertility in old mares. Biol Reprod 1995; 1:209-214.
11. Carnevale EM, Uson M, Bozzola JJ et al: Comparison of oocytes from young and old mares with light and electron microscopy. Theriogenology 1999; 51:299.
12. Vogelsang MM, Kraemer DC, Bowen MJ et al: Recovery of equine follicular oocytes by surgical and non-surgical techniques. Theriogenology 1986; 25:208.
13. Hinrichs K, Kenney RM: A colpotomy procedure to increase oocyte recovery rates on aspiration of equine preovulatory follicles. Theriogenology 1987; 27:237.
14. Hinrichs K, Kenney DF, Kenney RM: Aspiration of oocytes from mature and immature preovulatory follicles in the mare. Theriogenology 1990; 34:107-112.
15. Palmer E, Duchamp G, Bezard J et al: Recovery of follicular fluid and oocytes of mares by non-surgical puncture of the preovulatory follicle. Theriogenology 1986; 25:178.
16. Cook NL, Squires EL, Ray BS et al: Transvaginal ultrasound-guided follicular aspiration of equine oocytes. J Equine Vet Sci 1993; 15:71-74.
17. Carnevale EM, Ginther OJ: Use of a linear ultrasonic transducer for the transvaginal aspiration and transfer of oocytes in the mare. J Equine Vet Sci 1993; 13:331-333.
18. Hinrichs K, Betschart RW, McCue PM et al: Effect of time of follicle aspiration on pregnancy rate after oocyte transfer in the mare. J Reprod Fertil Suppl 2000; 56:493-498.
19. Carnevale EM, Maclellan LJ, Coutinho da Silva MA et al: Equine sperm-oocyte interaction: results after intraoviductal and intrauterine inseminations of recipients for oocyte transfer. Anim Reprod Sci 2001; 68:305-314.
20. Carnevale EM, Maclellan LJ, Coutinho da Silva MA et al: Comparison of culture and insemination techniques for equine oocyte transfer. Theriogenology 2000; 54:982-987.
21. Coutinho da Silva MA, Carnevale EM, Maclellan LJ et al: Injection of blood into preovulatory follicles of equine oocyte transfer recipients does not prevent fertilization of the recipient's oocyte. Theriogenology 2002; 57:538.
22. Carnevale EM, Alvarenga MA, Squires EL et al: Use of non-cycling mares as recipients for oocyte transfer and GIFT. Proceedings of the Annual Conference of the Society for Theriogenology, p 44, 1999.
23. Carnevale EM, Checura CH, Coutinho da Silva MA et al: Use of deslorelin acetate to suppress follicular activity in mares used as recipients for oocyte transfer. Theriogenology 2001; 55:358.

24. Squires EL, Seidel GE: Collection and Transfer of Equine Embryos. Animal Reproduction and Biotechnology Laboratory Bulletin No. 08, pp 24-26, Fort Collins, Colorado State University, 1995.

25. Ginther OJ: Reproductive Biology of the Mare, 2nd edition, pp 299-300, Cross Plains, Wis, Equiservices, 1992.

26. Scott TJ, Carnevale EM, Maclellan LJ et al: Embryo development rates after transfer of oocytes matured in vivo, in vitro, or within oviducts of mares. Theriogenology 2001; 55:705-715.

27. Maclellan LJ, Carnevale EM, Coutinho da Silva MA et al: Pregnancies from vitrified equine oocytes collected from superstimulated and non-stimulated mares. Theriogenology 2002; 58:911-919.

28. Carnevale, EM, Coutinho da Silva MA, Maclellan LJ et al: Effects of culture media and time of insemination on oocyte transfer. Theriogenology 2002; 58:759-762.

29. Carnevale EM, Maclellan LJ, Coutinho da Silva MA et al: Pregnancies attained after collection and transfer of oocytes from ovaries of five euthanatized mares. J Am Vet Med Assoc 2003; 222:60-62.

30. Vatja G: Vitrification of oocytes and embryos of domestic animals. Anim Reprod Sci 2000; 60-61:357-364.

31. Maclellan LJ, Lane M, Sims MM et al: Effect of sucrose or trehalose on vitrification of equine oocytes 12 h or 24 h after the onset of maturation, evaluated after ICSI. Theriogenology 2001; 55:310.

32. Hochi S, Fujimoto T, Choi Y et al: Cryopreservation of equine oocytes by 2-step freezing. Theriogenology 1994; 42:1085-1094.

33. Householder DD, Pickett BW, Voss JL et al: Effect of extender, number of spermatozoa and hCG on equine fertility. J Equine Vet Sci 1981; 1:9-13.

34. Coutinho da Silva MA, Carnevale EM, Maclellan LJ et al: Embryo development rates after oocyte transfer comparing intrauterine or intraoviductal insemination and fresh or frozen semen in mares. Theriogenology 2001; 55:359.

35. Coutinho da Silva MA, Carnevale EM, Maclellan KA et al: Use of fresh, cooled and frozen semen during gamete intrafallopian transfer in mares. Proceedings of the 8th International Symposium on Equine Reproduction. Theriogenology 2002; 58:763-766.

36. Squires EL, Wilson JM, Kato H: A pregnancy after intracytoplasmic sperm injection into equine oocyte matured in vitro. Theriogenology 1996; 45:306.

37. Cochran R, Meintjes M, Reggio B et al: Live foals produced from sperm-injected oocytes derived from pregnant mares. J Equine Vet Sci 1998; 18:736-741.

38. McKinnon AO, Lacham-Kaplan O, Trounson AO: Pregnancies produced from fertile and infertile stallions by intracytoplasmic sperm injection (ICSI) of single frozen/thawed spermatozoa into in vivo matured mare oocytes. J Reprod Fertil Suppl 2000; 56:513-517.

39. Galli C, Maclellan LJ, Crotti G et al: Development of equine oocytes matured in vitro in different media and fertilised by ICSI. Theriogenology 2002; 57:719.

40. Li X, Morris LHA, Allen WR: The development of blastocysts after intracytoplasmic sperm injection of equine oocytes. Havemeyer Foundation Monograph Series No. 3: Equine Embryo Transfer, pp 30-31, 2000.

41. Maclellan LJ, Sims MM, Squires EL: Effect of invasive adenylate cyclase during oocyte maturation on the development of equine embryos following ICSI. Havemeyer Foundation Monograph Series No. 3: Equine Embryo Transfer, pp 35-36, 2000.

CHAPTER 47

Intracytoplasmic Sperm Injection

ANGUS O. MCKINNON
ALAN O. TROUNSON
SHERMAN J. SILBER

An examination of the procedures, opportunities, and some of the ethical issues of human assisted reproductive techniques (ART) would appear relevant to this discussion of equine intracytoplasmic sperm injection (ICSI). The reasons for use of human ART often are different from those in domestic animals, and especially ICSI. For instance, the most common reason for human ICSI is male factor infertility, because standard in vitro fertilization (IVF) works well with normal fertile men. In horses, ICSI is used primarily to obtain embryos from mares that fail to provide them in routine reproductive procedures or as a research tool for embryo production. In the future, equine ICSI use is expected to parallel the developments seen in the human field. This is likely to result in similar technical and even ethical issues. Human ART and ICSI rely on multiple oocyte collection and transfer, as well as embryo culture and cryopreservation. Equine ICSI is just starting to address these issues, and currently the best pregnancy rates are reported after in vivo–matured single oocyte collection and ICSI coupled with immediate embryo transfer performed before confirmation of the fertilization result (Figure 47-1).[1]

HUMAN STUDIES AND ISSUES

Collection and Preparation of Gametes

Oocytes

Human ICSI commonly involves collection of multiple in vivo matured oocytes after ovarian superovulation induced by pituitary gonadotropins. Stimulation protocols typically involve either gonadotropin-releasing hormone (GnRH) agonists or antagonists to suppress release of luteinizing hormone (LH), which can cause premature ovulation. Follicle-stimulating hormone (FSH) is used to stimulate multiple follicles, and human chorionic gonadotropin (hCG) may be used for final maturation of oocytes. The drug, dose and timing of gonadotropin administration will vary according to individual decisions of the clinician and the specifics of the patient's case. For instance, some women are over suppressed by long duration administration of the GnRH agonists, and others may respond rapidly to initial stimulation. Some women respond better to LH suppression with antagonists of

GnRH, rather than agonists. In addition, approximately 0.5% to 2% of superovulation treatments result in **ovarian hyperstimulation syndrome**, which may be very painful for the patient.[2]

Most commonly, multiple in vivo–matured oocytes are utilized. Collection is facilitated by either ultrasonographically guided transvaginal aspiration or laparoscopic retrieval. "Ultrasonically guided follicular aspiration is shown to be superior to laparoscopic oocyte recovery as far as ovarian accessibility and complication rate are concerned."[3]

Spermatozoa

If spermatozoa cannot be harvested by ejaculation, then surgical extraction must be performed. Spermatozoa blocked by obstructive azoospermia can be removed by various microsurgical approaches, such as testicular sperm extraction (TESE). TESE is the most common technique to diagnose the cause of azoospermia and to obtain sufficient tissue for sperm extraction to be used either fresh or as a cryopreserved specimen. It involves one or multiple small biopsies of testis tissue and therefore is called **testicular fine needle aspiration** (TFNA). When a needle and syringe are used to puncture the skin to aspirate a sperm specimen, the procedure is called **percutaneous epididymal sperm aspiration** (PESA). PESA is popular because it can be performed repeatedly at low cost. PESA, like TFNA, can be completed without a surgical incision; however, it may not yield a suitable sample. **Microsurgical epididymal sperm aspiration** (MESA) involves direct retrieval of sperm from individual epididymal tubules and is performed under a microscope. It is completed by isolating the tubes and then aspirating the fluid. MESA limits damage to the epididymis while avoiding blood contamination of its fluid and yields high quantities of motile sperm that can be readily frozen and thawed for subsequent IVF treatments.

There no longer seem to be any categories of male factor infertility that cannot be treated with ICSI. Even for men with azoospermia caused either by obstruction or by germinal failure, ICSI may be performed successfully. The only failures will be in azoospermic men who have neither spermatozoa nor spermatids retrievable from the testis, but these men comprise a small percentage of the cases with severe male factor. The source of the spermatozoa and the

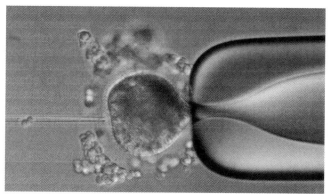

Figure 47-1 Injection of the spermatozoa into an in vivo–matured equine oocyte.

cause of the sperm defect appear to have no effect on the success of the procedure, whether the spermatozoon is epididymal, fresh or frozen, testicular, ejaculated, or from the testicles of men with severe defects in spermatogenesis. Maturation arrest, Sertoli cell-only, cryptorchidism, chemotherapy and mumps do not appear to have a major impact on the pregnancy rate. Of all the factors studied in couples where the male is severely infertile or azoospermic, the only factor that seems to matter (as long as spermatozoa are retrieved) is the age of the wife and, to a considerably lesser extent, her ovarian reserve. Extensive genetic and paediatric follow-up studies of ICSI pregnancies have revealed no increased risk of congenital malformation (2.6%), no increased risk of de-novo autosomal abnormalities, and a 1.0% risk of sex chromosomal abnormalities.[4]

Fertilization

Fertilization can be achieved through a number of means, including "classical" IVF, gamete intrafallopian transfer (GIFT), intracytoplasmic sperm injection (ICSI), and various other methods of micro-manipulation.

Classical IVF relies on laboratory fertilization, and GIFT relies on normal physiologic fertilization in vivo. With both techniques, normal spermatozoa with the ability to swim, penetrate, decondense, and fertilize the oocyte are needed. Techniques of zona manipulation—zona drilling, zona dissection, and subzonal injection (SUZI)—all carry the risk of poorer embryonic development and/or the potential for multiple sperm fertilization of the one oocyte (polyspermy) but were developed to address the poor results with IVF and GIFT in cases of severe male factor infertility.[5]

ICSI was developed by Gianpiero Palermo in Belgium,[6] resulting in the birth of the first child in 1992.[7] Subsequently, a large amount of experimental and clinical data have been amassed. ICSI involves injection of a single spermatozoon into the cytoplasm of the oocyte. The oocyte is held in position by suction through a fine, rounded glass pipette. A single spermatozoon is immobilized by tail crushing or chemical retardation before aspiration into an extremely fine, sharp glass pipette and then insertion though the zona pellucida. Concerns were expressed initially about the potential to produce offspring from "inferior" sperm and the opportunity to transmit genetic abnormalities.

There is an ongoing discussion regarding conflicting data on malformation rate in children born after intracytoplasmic sperm injection (ICSI). A prospective, multicentric, control cohort study was done in Germany. Fifty-nine centres prospectively recruited pregnancies before the 16th week of gestation, which were included in the study if they were ongoing beyond this time. Children were examined according to a standardized procedure. A control cohort of children conceived spontaneously was taken from a prospective birth registry (Mainzer Modell), where children were examined according to the exact same criteria as the ICSI cohort. Major malformation rate was calculated, based on data of all liveborn and stillborn children, as well as on all spontaneous and induced abortions, beginning with the 16th week of gestation. In the ICSI cohort, 8.6% of infants (291/3372), and in the control cohort 6.9% of infants (2140/30940), had a major malformation. This resulted in a crude relative risk (RR) of 1.25 (95% confidence interval 1.11-1.40). There was no influence of sperm origin on major malformation rate in children born after ICSI. There is an increased risk for a child born after ICSI to have a major malformation compared with a child that has been spontaneously conceived. Based on knowledge of the early developmental steps following ICSI, as well as on data of conventional IVF in general, it is assumed that this increased risk is due to parental factors causing the infertility, which has led to ICSI in the first place.[8]

Other studies have not supported these findings and are discussed later in this chapter.

The growing popularity of this technique reflects an ability to increase the control over and success rates for fertilization. ICSI, unlike standard IVF, guarantees the entrance of a single sperm directly into a single egg.

After micro-manipulation (i.e., ICSI and other techniques), the oocytes are cultured in vitro using defined medium and observed for early embryonic development. Developing embryos are graded, sorted, and transferred either fresh or frozen, or discarded.

The use of cytoplasmic transfer as an assisted reproductive technique has generated much attention and criticism. The technique involves the injection of cytoplasm from a healthy oocyte into a recipient oocyte considered unviable and includes the transfer of donor mitochondria. The consequences are the possible transmission of two mitochondrial (mt)DNA populations to the offspring. This pattern of inheritance is in contrast with the strictly maternal manner in which mtDNA is transmitted after natural fertilization and ICSI.[9]

Embryo Culture

With human ART, embryo culture and cryopreservation have resulted in an increased efficiency and flexibility. Commonly early-cleavage-stage embryos are transferred into the uterus despite the recognition that the embryo would not be expected in the uterine environment for at least 2 or 3 more days. This may result in a uterine environment that is not ideal for the embryo, perhaps associated with poor uterine clearance or an abnormal hormonal milieu. In addition, synchrony between the embryo and the uterus is poor. Oocytes fertilized and then cultured in vitro may be subjected to culture conditions that have affected the ability of the embryo to grow, and the technique also assumes that all oocytes, fertilized and in vitro–matured, have a similar ability to develop.

Pregnancy rates are three times higher when in vivo–derived blastocysts (obtained by uterine flushes in fertile women) are transferred, compared with in vitro–derived early-cleavage-stage embryos (as with IVF for infertile women).[10] Culturing embryos to the blastocyst stage in vitro has recently been associated with significant advantages. First, embryo morphology at the blastocyst stage is a predictor of pregnancy rates.[10] Second, the most viable embryo within the group of cultured embryos may be selected.[10] Third, the problems of multiple pregnancies may be addressed by examination of the probability that a single embryo will be transferred successfully before the transfer is performed. It also has been hypothesized that the uterine environment may not be as hostile to a blastocyst as to an earlier-cleavage-stage embryo.[10]

Furthermore, as the score of the blastocysts obtained using sequential media is directly related to implantation and pregnancy rates, it is possible to determine which patients should be offered a single blastocyst transfer, thereby addressing the issue of twins conceived through ART.[11]

Transfer

Embryos commonly are transferred at the 4- to 8-cell stage (day 2 or 3 after fertilization), although a current trend is for embryo culture and transfer at the blastocyst stage[11] because this approach could be expected to improve implantation rates. In addition, embryo grade is correlated with pregnancy rates.[12]

Embryos are mostly transferred through the vagina in a non–embryo-toxic catheter, through the cervix and into the uterus. The number of embryos transferred depends on embryo quality and age of the woman. More embryos are transferred into older women, with less success.[13-15]

Preimplantation genetic diagnosis (PGD) to identify chromosomally normal embryos has recently become a development applied to embryos before transfer. This technique involves the biopsy of a blastomere from an 8- to 16-cell embryo. Gender, genetic disorders, and chromosomal number and structure are commonly evaluated.

Despite its novelty, preimplantation genetic diagnosis has become an alternative to traditional prenatal diagnosis, allowing the establishment of only unaffected pregnancies and avoiding the risk of pregnancy termination. In addition, preimplantation genetic diagnosis is presently applied for much wider indications than prenatal diagnosis, including common diseases with genetic predisposition and preimplantation human leukocyte antigen typing, with the purpose of establishing potential donor progeny for stem cell treatment of siblings. Many hundreds of apparently healthy, unaffected children have been born after preimplantation genetic diagnosis, presenting evidence of its accuracy, reliability and safety. Preimplantation genetic diagnosis appears to be of special value for avoiding age-related aneuploidies in patients of advanced reproductive age, improving reproductive outcome, particularly obvious from their reproductive history, and is presently an extremely attractive option for carriers of balanced translocations to have unaffected children of their own.[16]

On occasion, zona-assisted hatching may be employed to help the embryo break out of the zona pellucida. Previous implantation failure in otherwise normal patients may suggest this problem. Chemicals, lasers, and mechanical manipulation all have been used to create a breach in the zona.[17]

Assisted hatching entails the opening or thinning of the zona pellucida before embryo transfer in order to improve the results of in vitro fertilization (IVF) and intracytoplasmic sperm injection (ICSI). The technique can be performed mechanically, chemically or with a laser beam. A piezoelectric method has also been described. Meta-analyses of randomised trials have shown that assisted hatching increases the clinical pregnancy, implantation and on-going pregnancy rates in patients with poor prognosis for IVF and ICSI, particularly those with repeated implantation failure. The technique is not without risks, and has been associated with an increased incidence of monozygotic twinning. Nevertheless, it remains an invaluable tool in assisted reproductive technology.[18]

This may be even more relevant in cases of in vitro maturation of oocytes.

Immature oocyte recovery followed by in-vitro oocyte maturation and in-vitro fertilization is a promising new technology for the treatment of human infertility. The technology is attractive to potential oocyte donors and infertile couples because of its reduced treatment intervention. Immature oocytes were recovered by ultrasound-guided transvaginal follicular aspiration. Oocytes were matured in vitro for 36-48 h followed by intracytoplasmic sperm injection (ICSI). Embryos were cultured in vitro for 3 or 5 days before replacement. Assisted hatching was performed on a day 5 blastocyst stage embryo. Embryo and uterine synchrony were potentially enhanced by luteinization of the dominant follicle at the time of immature oocyte recovery. Mature oocyte and embryo production from immature oocyte recovery were similar to the previous IVF results of the patients. A blastocyst stage embryo, produced as a result of in-vitro maturation, ICSI, in-vitro culture and assisted hatching, resulted in the birth of a healthy baby girl at 39 weeks of gestation.[19]

Pregnancy

Approximately 30% of IVF pregnancies produce twins, 5% triplets, and less than 1% more than three children. Multiple pregnancies carry high risks for the woman and the fetuses.

Multiple gestation pregnancy rates are high in assisted reproductive treatment cycles because of the perceived need to stimulate excess follicles and transfer excess embryos in order to achieve reasonable pregnancy rates. Perinatal mortality rates are, however, 4-fold higher for twins and 6-fold higher for triplets than for singletons. Since the goal of infertility therapy is a healthy child, and multiple gestation puts that goal at risk, multiple pregnancy must be regarded as a serious complication of assisted reproductive treatment cycles. The 1999 ESHRE Capri Workshop addressed the psychological, medical, social and financial implications of multiple pregnancy and discussed how it might be prevented. Multiple gestations are high risk pregnancies which may be complicated by prematurity, low birthweight, pre-eclampsia, anaemia, postpartum haemorrhage, intrauterine growth restriction, neonatal morbidity and high neonatal and infant mortality. Multiple gestation children may suffer long-term consequences of perinatal complications, including cerebral palsy and learning disabilities. Even when the babies are healthy they must share their parents' attention and may experience slow language development and behavioural problems. Current data indicate that the average hospital cost per multiple gestation delivery is greater than the average cost of in-vitro fertilization (IVF) and intracytoplasmic sperm injection (ICSI) cycles. Prevention is the most important means of decreasing multiple gestation rates. Multiple gestation rates in ovulation induction and superovulation cycles can be reduced by using lower dosage gonadotrophin regimens. If there are more than three mature follicles, the cycle should be converted to an IVF cycle, or it should be cancelled and intercourse should be avoided. In IVF cycles two embryos can be transferred without reducing birth rates in most circumstances. Embryo reduction involves extremely difficult decisions for infertile couples and should be used only as a last resort. Assisted reproductive treatment centres and registries should express cycle results as the proportion of singleton live births; twin and triplet rates should be reported separately as complications of the procedures. Reducing the multiple gestation pregnancy rate should be a high priority for assisted reproductive treatment programmes, despite the pressure from some patients to transfer more embryos in order to improve success. If nothing is done, public concern may lead to legislation in many countries, a step that would be unnecessary if assisted reproductive treatment programmes and registries took suitable steps to reduce multiple pregnancy rates.[20]

There are data regarding the possible influences of extended embryo culture to the blastocyst stage as well as zona pellucida manipulation on the incidence of monozygotic multiples. This is interesting, as one aim of extended culture with embryo selection is to minimize the multiple pregnancy rate. We report, to our knowledge, on the first case of monozygotic twins and monozygotic triplets after ICSI and the transfer of two blastocysts. Monozygotic multiples after ICSI and blastocyst transfer and the resulting problems are another reason to encourage the transfer of only one blastocyst. In our opinion, the incidence of 5.9-8.9% monozygotic multiple occurrence after ICSI and blastocyst transfer reported in the literature requires that patients are informed of the uncertainties until this phenomenon and its risk factors are better understood.[21]

Current Status of Human Intracytoplasmic Sperm Injection

Since the publication of the first papers on the use of ICSI for oligozoospermia in 1992 and 1993, much scientific work has been applied to extending its application to virtually every type of male infertility.[4,7,22,23] In 1995 Nagy[24] confirmed that the most severe cases of oligoasthenoteratozoospermia produced the same pregnancy rates as for mild cases of male factor infertility, which were no different from those for men with normal spermatozoa undergoing conventional IVF. Then it was demonstrated that the way in which the spermatozoa are pretreated before ICSI is immaterial, and that any method for aspirating the spermatozoa into an injection pipette and transferring them into the oocytes is adequate.[25] It also was reported that fertilization failure was always related either to poor egg quality or to sperm nonviability.[26] It appeared that no matter how severe morphologic defect, or with the most severe motility defect or the smallest number of spermatozoa in the ejaculate (pseudoazoospermia), no negative effect on the pregnancy rate was observed with ICSI. Only absolute immotility of ejaculated or epididymal spermatozoa lowered the fertilization

rate, and this was found to be not due to the immotility of the spermatozoon but rather to its nonviability. Completely nonmotile spermatozoa that were viable were still capable of normal fertilization and pregnancy rates.[27]

ICSI then took another leap forward with the development of sperm aspiration and extraction techniques, which allowed couples in which the male was absolutely azoospermic to achieve pregnancy rates no different from those in which the male had a normal sperm count.[28] The first successful attempts at sperm aspiration combined with ICSI were reported in 1994.[29] Conventional IVF with aspirated epididymal spermatozoa yielded a pregnancy rate of only 9% and a delivery rate of only 4.5%, whereas ICSI with aspirated epididymal spermatozoa in men with congenital absence of the vas deferens (CAVD) yielded a pregnancy rate of 47% and a delivery rate of 33%. Furthermore, no difference in pregnancy rates was found with use of epididymal spermatozoa retrieved for any cause of obstruction, whether it was failed vasoepididymostomy, CAVD, or simply irreparable obstruction.[30]

However, this breakthrough for men with CAVD brought with it a serious problem. It was soon discovered that CAVD is caused by mutations on the cystic fibrosis transmembrane conductance regular gene (CFTR) located on chromosome 7. Although now this is taken for granted, in 1992 it was a startling discovery. . . . This discovery meant that all patients and their wives undergoing sperm aspiration with ICSI for CAVD required careful genetic screening for cystic fibrosis, and if the wife was a carrier (4% risk of carrier status in the general population), then the embryos should undergo preimplantation genetic diagnosis using polymerase chain reaction, so that only healthy embryos would be replaced.[27]

The first case of successful preimplantation embryo biopsy for cystic fibrosis, on the embryo of a man who had undergone MESA and ICSI for CAVD, was reported in 1994.[31] "The use of MESA and ICSI for CAVD led to intense molecular study of the genetic mystery of how the condition of CAVD is transmitted via defects in the cystic fibrosis gene."[27]

Soon after the MESA-ICSI procedure was developed in 1994, it was discovered that testicular spermatozoa could fertilize as efficiently as ejaculated spermatozoa and also result in normal pregnancies.

In this study (May 1 until August 31, 1994) a total of 15 azoospermic patients suffering from testicular failure were treated with a combination of testicular sperm extraction (TESE) and intracytoplasmic sperm injection (ICSI). Spermatozoa were available for ICSI in 13 of the patients. Out of 182 metaphase II injected oocytes, two-pronuclear fertilization was observed in 87 (47.80%); 57 embryos (65.51%) were obtained for either transfer or cryopreservation. Three ongoing pregnancies out of 12 replacements (25%) were established, including one singleton, one twin and one triplet gestation. The ongoing implantation rate was 18% (six fetal hearts out of 32 embryos replaced).[32]

TESE truly revolutionized the treatment of infertile couples with azoospermia. The development of TESE meant that even patients with zero motility of the epididymal spermatozoa or of ejaculated spermatozoa, or even men with no epididymis, could still have their own genetic child, so long as there was normal spermatogenesis. It also meant that surgeons could easily perform a testicle biopsy, enabling the retrieved spermatozoa to be used for ICSI without the need for the microsurgical expertise required to perform a conventional MESA procedure.[27]

It also was demonstrated that epididymal spermatozoa, despite fairly weak motility, could be frozen and, after thawing, yield pregnancy rates no different from those obtained with freshly retrieved epididymal spermatozoa.

In seven patients who did not become pregnant following microsurgical epididymal sperm aspiration (MESA) and intracytoplasmic sperm injection (ICSI), a subsequent ICSI was performed using previously cryopreserved supernumerary epididymal spermatozoa without re-operating on the husband. During the original MESA procedure a mean sperm concentration of 12.3 × 10(6)/ml was achieved. The supernumerary spermatozoa were cryopreserved for later use. After thawing frozen epididymal spermatozoa a mean concentration of 1.9 × 10(6) spermatozoa/ml was obtained in straws containing a total volume of sperm suspension of 250 microliters. From 68 intact oocytes injected with frozen-thawed epididymal spermatozoa, a two pronuclear fertilization rate of 45% and a cleavage rate of 82% were obtained. A total of 17 embryos were replaced in the seven patients, resulting in two ongoing singleton pregnancies and one twin delivery. Six embryos were cryopreserved. In conclusion, it would appear mandatory to cryopreserve supernumerary spermatozoa during a MESA in order to avoid subsequent further scrotal surgery.[33]

Because of the remarkable success with the freezing of very-poor-quality epididymal spermatozoa for subsequent ICSI, couples did not have to time the MESA exactly with the partner's egg retrieval. This also meant that men about to undergo chemotherapy and/or radiotherapy for cancer could have a single ejaculate frozen, causing no delay in treatment of the cancer, and this one ejaculate would be sufficient for almost an infinite number of IVF-ICSI cycles.[27]

Finally, in a majority of patients with testicular failure (caused either by maturation arrest, Sertoli cell–only syndrome, cryptorchid testicular atrophy, post-chemotherapy azoospermia, or even Klinefelter's syndrome), a very tiny number of spermatozoa or spermatids usually can be extracted from extensive testicular biopsy specimens and used for ICSI.[32,34]

Early studies of the kinetics of spermatogenesis in the testicle demonstrated that often a tiny amount of spermatogenesis was present if one examined quantitatively and carefully the testicle biopsy of men who were azoospermic from non-obstructive testicular failure. However, the significance of this 'threshold' phenomenon was not appreciated until the era of ICSI, when it was realized that these spermatids could be harvested, and normal pregnancy rates achieved, in the ~60% of such patients who possessed this minuscule degree of spermatogenesis in otherwise completely deficient testicles.[27]

There has been some excitement generated over the possibility of using 'round cells' derived from testicular tissue (or even from the ejaculate), which are presumably early spermatids, for ICSI in the absence of elongated spermatozoa. Infertility clinics around the world are now endeavoring to use this technique, which may have unfortunate implications. . . . The problems with this approach are: (i) in human spermatogenesis, it is widely known that matu-

ration arrest is a problem associated with meiosis, and not with sperm maturation. Wherever there are early round spermatids, there will also be elongated mature spermatids with a tail; and (ii) clinics not aware of this reality are tempted to inject 'round cells' when they cannot retrieve spermatozoa. The truth is, that if those round cells were genuinely spermatids, then a better search would have revealed the presence of mature spermatozoa. On the other hand, it is extremely difficult, using Hoffman optics, to distinguish with certainty a round spermatid from a Sertoli cell nucleus with its prominent nucleolus, or even from some spermatocytes. Where there are truly no spermatozoa, there may be many 'round cells' either with Sertoli cell only, or with maturation arrest, that are not round spermatids.[27]

The current ability of most men to father a child, regardless of the quality of the sperm count, even if there are apparently no mature spermatozoa at all, is dramatic. It appears that the results of ICSI are not related to the source of the spermatozoa (whether ejaculated, testicular, or epididymal), or to the quality of the spermatozoa (with regard to morphology or motility). ICSI results are not influenced by whether the spermatozoon has been frozen or is fresh, whether it is retrieved with ease (as in the case of normal spermatogenesis or with ejaculated spermatozoa), or whether the spermatozoon was extracted directly from the Sertoli cell after hours of painstaking searching of a testis sample.[27] With regard to the infertile or azoospermic male and ICSI, none of these factors has had any significant influence on fertilization, cleavage, or pregnancy rate. In fact, the only significant factor in the success of ICSI appears to be the age of the female partner.[27,30]

Are the Offspring Normal? The Genetics of Intracytoplasmic Sperm injection

A major development in 1996 was the detailed follow-up study of ICSI-conceived children and the information it provided about the genetics of infertility.

A prospective follow-up study of 877 children born after ICSI was carried out. The aim of this study was to compile data on karyotypes, congenital malformations, growth parameters and developmental milestones so as to evaluate the safety of this new technique. The follow-up study included agreement to genetic counselling and prenatal diagnosis and was based on a physical examination at the Centre for Medical Genetics (Dutch-speaking Brussels Free University, Brussels, Belgium) at 2 months, 1 year and 2 years, when major and minor malformations and a psychomotor evolution were recorded. Between April 1991 and July 1995, 904 pregnancies obtained after intracytoplasmic sperm injection (ICSI) led to the birth of 877 children (465 singletons, 379 twins and 33 triplets). Prenatal diagnosis determined a total of 486 karyotypes, of which six were abnormal (1.2%) and six (1.2%) were familial structural aberrations, all transmitted from the father. This slight increase in de-novo chromosomal aberrations and the higher frequency of transmitted chromosomal aberrations are probably linked directly to the characteristics of the infertile men treated rather than to the ICSI procedure itself. In all, 23 (2.6%) major malformations were observed in the children born, defined as those causing functional impairment or requiring surgical correction. No particular malformation was disproportionately frequent. Compared with most registers of children born after assisted reproduction and with registers of malformation in the general population, the figure of 2.6% was within the expected range. These observations should be further completed by others and by collaborative efforts. In the meantime, patients should be counselled about the available data before any treatment: the risk of transmitted chromosomal aberrations, the risk of de-novo, mainly sex chromosomal, aberrations and the risk of transmitting fertility problems to the offspring. Patients should also be reassured that there seems to be no higher incidence of congenital malformations in children born after ICSI.[35]

Since the introduction of ICSI in 1991, medical outcome studies on ICSI children have been performed, but few have addressed developmental outcome. Hence, this outcome was assessed by performing a standard developmental test on children born after ICSI as compared with children born after IVF, at the age of 2 years.

METHODS: In a prospective study, the medical and developmental outcomes of 439 children born after ICSI (378 singletons, 61 twins) were compared with those of 207 children born after IVF (138 singletons, 69 twins), at the age of 24-28 months. These children were part of a cohort of children followed since birth. Of children reaching the age of 24-28 months between May 1995 and March 2002, 44.3% (2375/5356) were examined by a paediatrician who was unaware of the type of treatment used for each couple. Of all the children born, 12.2% (439/3618) in the ICSI group and 11.9% (207/1738) in the IVF group underwent a formal developmental assessment using the Bayley Scale of Infant Development (mental scale) by a paediatrician blinded to the type of treatment. RESULTS: There was no significant difference in maternal educational level, maternal age, gestational age, parity, birthweight, neonatal complication rate or malformation rate at 2 years between ICSI and IVF singletons, or between ICSI and IVF twins. No significant difference was observed in the developmental outcome using the Bayley scale at the age of 24-28 months (raw scores or test age) between ICSI children or IVF children. A multivariate regression analysis for the singleton children indicated that parity, sex (boys had lower scores than girls) and age had a significant influence on the test result, but that the fertility procedure (ICSI versus IVF) did not influence the test result. ICSI children from fathers with low sperm concentration, low sperm motility or poor morphology had a similar developmental outcome to that of children from fathers with normal sperm parameters. There were no significant differences between the initial cohort and the group lost to follow-up, nor between the psychologically tested and the non-tested group for a number of variables such as maternal educational level, birthweight in singletons and neonatal malformation rate. Although only some of the cohort of ICSI children were evaluated, a representative sample of both ICSI and IVF children was compared. CONCLUSIONS: There is no indication that ICSI children have a lower psychomotor development than IVF children. Paternal risk factors associated with male-factor infertility were found not to play a role in developmental outcome.[36]

Genetic Basis for Infertility

There is now abundant evidence in a wide range of mammalian and non-mammalian species to show that the relative size of the testis and the morphology of the spermatozoa are infallible predictors of the mating system. Species with the largest testis/body weight ratios and the best spermatozoa have a multi-male or promiscuous mating system in which sperm competition operates. Judged by these criteria,

men were not designed to be promiscuous. There is increasing evidence in humans to show that most spontaneous mutations of the germ line occur in the testis. Because these provide the variability on which natural selection can operate, the testis holds the key to evolution. Genes on the Y chromosome that control male fertility are particularly prone to mutations, perhaps because of the mutagenic metabolites produced by the metabolically active testis. Testicular descent into a scrotum, and cooling by countercurrent heat exchange between the spermatic artery and vein may have evolved as a way of holding the mutation rate in check. The hormones secreted by the testis, which control libido and aggression, ensure that these male mutations are disseminated as widely as possible throughout the population.[37,38]

This led us to speculate that perhaps deficient spermatogenesis, despite a variety of so-called causes is in most cases genetically determined (excluding, of course, mumps, orchitis, post-cryptorchidism testicular atrophy, postchemotherapy azoospermia, etc.).[39]

The first phase of this genetic control of male fertility came from Professor Roger Short's analysis of infertility in the three types of great apes, i.e., gorilla, orangutan and chimpanzee. Chimpanzees travel together in troops of about 40 males and females, and whenever anyone of the females in the troop goes into heat, every single male in the troop has intercourse with her. Consequently, one would expect that the male with the highest sperm count and the best quality sperm is most likely to be the father of any child born to any female who has had sex with multiple partners. The extensive sperm competition among the sperm of all the chimpanzees who have mounted her has resulted in male offspring that have inherited the best sperm count. Therefore, chimpanzees would be expected to have high sperm counts because of their promiscuous mating behavior if we assume that sperm production, both quantitative and qualitative, is genetically transmitted. In fact, this is the case. Chimpanzees, who are extremely promiscuous, have gigantic testicles and huge sperm counts, and gorillas who are faithful to their mates, and in whom there is no sperm competition because the female is only having sex with one given mate for her entire lifetime, have very small testicles and extremely low sperm counts. Professor Short concluded from this that male fertility was a genetically transmitted trait.[39]

The next suggestion from studies of exotic species came with the cheetah. All cheetahs in the world are so genetically inbred and identical that even skin grafts from one cheetah to another never reject. This inbreeding has resulted in all male cheetahs having an extremely poor sperm count with 90% abnormal forms and very low numbers. The infertility of the inbred male cheetah clearly demonstrates a genetic cause of the very same types of semen abnormalities that we see in the infertile human. Therefore, we had speculated for the last eleven years that there may be a genetic cause for the majority of cases of oligospermia and azoospermia.[39]

The common domestic cat is an important research model for endangered felids, as well as for studying genetic dysfunctions, infectious diseases and infertility in humans. Especially significant is the trait of teratospermia (ejaculation of <40% morphologically normal spermatozoa) that commonly occurs in about 70% of the felid species or subspecies studied to date. Teratospermia, discovered more than two decades ago in the cheetah, is important: (i) for understanding the significance of sperm form and function; and (ii) because this condition is common in human males. It is apparent from IVF that deformed spermatozoa from teratospermic felids do not fertilize oocytes. However, the *inability of spermatozoa from teratospermic males to bind, penetrate and decondense in the cytoplasm of the oocyte is not limited to malformed cells alone. Normal shaped spermatozoa from teratospermic males have reduced functional capacity. IVF results have consistently revealed a direct correlation between teratospermia and compromised sperm function across felid species and populations. The most significant differences between normospermic (>60% normal spermatozoa per ejaculate) and teratospermic felids include: (i) the time required for sperm capacitation and the acrosome reaction to occur in vitro; (ii) culture media requirements for capacitation in vitro; (iii) phosphorylation patterns of tyrosine residues on sperm membrane proteins during capacitation; (iv) susceptibility to chilling-induced sperm membrane damage; (v) sensitivity to osmotic stress; (vi) stability of sperm DNA; (vii) sperm protamine composition; and (viii) fertilizing ability after intracytoplasmic sperm injection. In conclusion, (i) the felids (including wild species) are valuable for studying the functional significance of both pleiomorphic and normally formed spermatozoa from teratospermic donors, and (ii) the impact of teratospermia is expressed at both macrocellular and subcellular levels.* [39,40]

Now, in a collaborative study with the human genome project and the Massachusetts Institute of Technology, we have indeed found that about 11% of men with either azoospermia or severe oligospermia consistently are found to have deletions in the Y chromosome in a specific region we have called the AZF loci (short for "azoospermia factor"), and the first specific gene candidate localized to this area has been called DAZ (deleted in azoospermia). Deletion I of this DAZ gene is always associated with azoospermia or severe oligospermia, and thus far no normal fertile men have been found to have a deletion of this gene candidate. Furthermore, there is a homolog copy of this DAZ gene not only on the Y chromosome in men, but on chromosome 3 in both men and women, indicating it may even tell us something about female infertility. There are undoubtedly many other genes and loci that affect sperm production, and we have only just begun the search. Furthermore, we know that about 1.3% of azoospermic or severely oligospermic men have chromosomal abnormalities, usually balanced translocation, that can give us other clues and doorways to explore with our molecular tools many other possibilities for genetic causes of male infertility. [39]

HORSE STUDIES

Live Foals from Horse ART

Only two foals have been reported from conventional IVF in the horse. [41]

The results of in vitro fertilization (IVF) in the mare are less advanced than in most of the other domestic mammals. The different steps which have contributed to the success of IVF with the birth of two foals are shown: the preparation of oocytes and capacitated spermatozoa, the fertilization technique, the embryo culture and transfer. After induction of ovulation in the mare with equine pituitary extract, the preovulatory follicles are punctured just before ovulation. The oocytes matured in vivo are in vitro inseminated with fresh semen treated by Ionophore A23187. The embryos are cultured until their transfer to the oviduct of a recipient mare by a surgical technique. The development of in vitro maturation of immature oocytes from slaughtered ovaries will give a larger number of oocytes for IVF attempts. The development of the embryo culture to obtain the blastocyst

stage will allow a non surgical transfer in the uterus of a mare. [41]

Both foals were born from fertilization of in vivo matured oocytes. Despite much interest and some promising results,[42] further success has not been forthcoming, casting doubt on the usefulness of the technique as an infertility treatment.

The reason for such poor results of IVF in the horse is unknown but has been suggested to be inability of the horse oocyte to allow penetration of spermatozoa. This was not associated with zona pellucida hardening (ZPH).

In vitro fertilization (IVF) has had poor success in the horse, a situation related to low rates of sperm penetration through the zona pellucida (ZP). Zona pellucida hardening (ZPH) is seen in mouse and rat oocytes cultured in serum-free medium. The hardened ZP is refractory to sperm penetration. Fetuin, a component of fetal calf serum, inhibits ZPH and allows normal fertilization rates in oocytes cultured in the absence of serum. We evaluated whether fetuin is present in horse serum and follicular fluid (FF) and whether fetuin could inhibit ZPH in equine oocytes matured in vitro, thus increasing sperm penetration during IVF. The presence of fetuin in equine serum and FF was confirmed by immunoblotting. Oocytes submitted to in vitro maturation (IVM) in medium containing fetuin were used for ZPH assay or IVF. Intracytoplasmic sperm injection (ICSI) was carried out as a control procedure, The presence of fetuin during IVM did not affect the rate of maturation to metaphase II. Maturation of oocytes in the presence of fetuin reduced ZPH in a dose-dependent manner. After both IVF and ICSI, there was no significant difference in oocyte fertilization between fetuin-treated and untreated oocytes. The fertilization rate was significantly higher after ICSI than after IVF, both in fetuin-treated and in untreated oocytes. In conclusion, fetuin reduced ZPH in equine oocytes but did not improve sperm penetration during IVF. This implies that, in the horse, "spontaneous" ZPH is unlikely to be the major factor responsible for inhibiting sperm penetration in vitro. [43]

The birth of the first ICSI foal was reported in 1996.[44] A technique relevant to a commercial application was reported with birth of live foals from in vivo–matured oocytes using ICSI with frozen spermatozoa from fertile and infertile stallions.[1] The study examined the use of ICSI for in vitro fertilization of equine oocytes and their developmental potential when transferred to the fallopian tubes of synchronized mares. Oocytes were aspirated from mature follicles 39 hours after a GnRH analogue injection and transported 190 kilometers at 39°C. Semen from both a fertile and an infertile stallion was frozen and later prepared for injection. Successfully injected oocytes were surgically transferred into the ampulla of the fallopian tube either (1) 4 to 8 hours after injection or (2) were cultured for 24 to 48 hours before transfer. Twenty-six oocytes were treated by ICSI. Three oocytes fragmented after injection (12%). Eight oocytes were returned for immediate transfer to recipient mares. Of the 15 cultured oocytes, 8 (53%) had two polar bodies and cleaved to 2 cells at 24 hours after injection. Pregnancies were identified on days 12 to14 after transfer in 4 of the 16 (25%) recipients that had either transferred embryos (1/8) or freshly injected oocytes (3/8). Two of the four pregnancies did not progress beyond 30 days, and two mares had foals. There was no apparent difference in the establishment of pregnancies from oocytes injected with frozen/thawed sperm of the fertile (3/14) and the infertile stallion (1/2).[1]

Subsequently, foals were born from follicles aspirated from pregnant mares.[45] These oocytes, as in the work of Squires,[44] were matured in vitro. A total of 263 follicles were punctured in 20 aspiration procedures, and 174 oocytes were retrieved in one of two experiments. Eighty-six (49%) were classified as mature after culture in TCM-199. A cleavage rate of 55% (47/86) occurred after ICSI. A total of 31 embryos were transferred into the oviducts of recipient mares, resulting in the birth of two foals. Four pregnancies in total were established (one pregnancy per eight oocytes transferred); however, two underwent early embryonic death, and two subsequently foaled.[45]

An important development that increased the applicability of equine ICSI to clinical situations was the report of live foals from embryos cultured to the blastocyst stage.[46] Success with this technique means that oocytes and semen can be shipped to remote locations that are skilled in ICSI techniques and then transferred nonsurgically after demonstration of normal blastocyst development.

The influence of coculture with either oviduct epithelial cells or fetal fibroblast cells on in vitro maturation of equine oocytes and their potential for development to blastocysts and fetuses after intracytoplasmic sperm injection (ICSI) was investigated. The oocytes were obtained from ovaries from abattoirs and were matured in vitro for 2-30 h in TCM199 only, or in TCM199 coculture with oviduct epithelial cells or fetal fibroblast cells. Metaphase II oocytes were subjected to ICSI with an ionomycin treated spermatozoon. The injected oocytes were cultured for 79 days in Dulbecco's modified Eagle's medium. Morphologically normal early blastocysts were transferred to the uteri of recipient mares. Nuclear maturation rates and the rates of cleavage to the two cell stage for injected oocytes were similar in the groups of oocytes that were matured in TCM 199 (49 and 63%), in coculture with oviduct epithelial cells (53 and 65%) or in coculture with fetal fibroblasts (51 and 57%). There were no significant differences in the proportions of blastocysts that developed from the two cell embryos derived from oocytes matured by coculture with either oviduct epithelial cells (30%) or fetal fibroblasts (17%). However, significantly higher proportions of blastocysts were produced from both these coculture groups than from the groups of oocytes matured in TCM199 only (P < 0.05). Six of the blastocysts that had developed from oocytes cocultured with oviduct epithelial cells were transferred into recipient mares and four pregnancies resulted. These results demonstrate a beneficial influence of coculture with either oviduct epithelial cells or fetal fibroblasts for maturation of oocytes in vitro.[46] A report from Italy highlighted the production of pregnancies from embryos that were frozen and thawed and successfully transferred into recipients. The technique combined transvaginal collection of immature oocytes, in vitro maturation, ICSI and culture of the early embryos in vitro or in vivo (sheep oviduct). The efficiency of the procedure was higher when in vivo culture was used.[47]

Sperm/Oocyte Interactions

Classically it has been suggested that sperm need to activate the oocyte after ICSI. This would appear to be less important for human ICSI than for bovine ICSI.[48]

In the human and the mouse, intracytoplasmic sperm injection (ICSI) apparently triggers normal fertilization and may result in offspring. In the bovine, injection of spermatozoa must be accompanied by artificial methods of oocyte activation in order to achieve normal fertilization events (e.g., pronuclear formation). In this study, different methods of oocyte activation were tested following ICSI of in vitro-matured bovine oocytes. Bovine oocytes were centrifuged to facilitate sperm injection, and spermatozoa were pretreated with 5 mM dithiothreitol (DTT) to promote decondensation. Sperm-injected or sham-injected oocytes were activated with 5 mu M ionomycin (A23187). Three hours after activation, oocytes with second polar bodies were selected and treated with 1.9 mM 6-dimethylaminopurine (DMAP). The cleavage rate of sperm-injected oocytes treated with ionomycin and DMAP was higher than with ionomycin alone (62 vs 27%, P less than or equal to 0.05). Blastocysts (2 of 41 cleaved) were obtained only from the sperm-injected, ionomycin + DMAP-treated oocytes. Upon examination 16 h after ICSI, pronuclear formation was observed in 33 of 47 (70%) DMAP-treated oocytes. Two pronuclei were present in 18 of 33 (55%), while 1 and 3 pronuclei were seen in 8 of 33 (24%) and 7 of 33 (21%) oocytes, respectively. In sham-injected oocytes, pronuclear formation was observed in 15 of 38 (39%) with 9 (60%) having 2 pronuclei. As a single calcium stimulation was insufficient and DMAP treatment could result in triploidy, activation by multiple calcium stimulations was tested. Three calcium stimulations (5 mu M ionomycin) were given at 30-min intervals following ICSI. Two pronuclei were found in 12 of 41 (29%) injected oocytes. Increasing the concentration of ionomycin from 5 to 50 mu M resulted in a higher rate of activation (41 vs 26%). The rate of metaphase III arrest was lower while the rate of pronuclear formation and cleavage development was higher in sperm-injected than sham-injected oocytes, suggesting that spermatozoa contribute to the activation process. Further improvements in oocyte activation following ICSI in the bovine are necessary.[48]

The need for horse oocyte activation is less apparent. Conflicting results are reported with use of fresh, chilled, or frozen semen, suggesting that the type of sperm preparation influences the need to activate the oocyte.[49]

Studies involving frozen spermatozoa and ICSI reported good cleavage rates without sperm activation.[1,43,50-53]

The effects of four reagents on the activation and subsequent fertilization of equine oocytes, and the development of these after intracytoplasmic sperm injection, were investigated. Cumulus-oocyte complexes collected from equine ovaries obtained from an abattoir were matured in vitro for 40-44 h in TCM199 medium before being injected, when in metaphase II, with an immobilized stallion spermatozoon. The cumulus-oocyte complexes were then subjected to one of five activation treatments: (a) 10 mu mol ionomycin l(-1) for 10 min; Co) 7% (v/v) ethanol for 10 min; (c) 100 mu mol thimerosal l(-1) for 10 min; (d) 250 mu mol inositol 1,4,5-triphosphate l(-1) injection; and (e) no treatment (control). After 18-20 h further culture, the cumulus-oocyte complexes were assessed for activation by observing whether they had progressed through second anaphase-telophase and had formed a female pronucleus. The proportions of oocytes activated after each treatment were: 16/27 (59%) for ionomycin; 14/25 (56%) for ethanol; 22/28 (79%) for thimerosal; 15/27 (56%) for inositol 1,4,5-triphosphate; and 0/20 (0%) for the untreated controls. Thus, significantly more oocytes (P < 0.05) were acti-

vated by treatment with thimerosal than by the other four treatments. The proportions of oocytes that cleaved to the two-cell stage at 24-30 h after sperm injection in the groups treated with ionomycin, ethanol and thimerosal were 7/20 (35%), 5/19 (26%) and 11/ 23 (48%), respectively. No cleavage was observed in any of the control oocytes or those treated with inositol 1,4,5-triphosphate, Furthermore, evidence of normal fertilization was observed in 2/7 (29%), 2/5 (40%) and 7/11 (64%) of the oocytes treated with ionomycin, ethanol and thimerosal, respectively. These results demonstrated that: (a) it is possible to activate equine oocytes with the chemical stimulants, ionomycin, ethanol, thimerosal and inositol 1,4,5-triphosphate; (b) thimerosal is more effective than the other three reagents in facilitating both meiotic activation and normal fertilization of equine oocytes; and (c) chemical activation may also stimulate parthenogenetic cleavage of oocytes without concurrent changes in the head of the spermatozoon.[54]

Intracytoplasmic sperm injection (ICSI) is the method of choice for fertilizing horse oocytes in vitro. Nevertheless, for reasons that are not yet clear, embryo development rates are low. The aims of this study were to examine cytoskeletal and chromatin reorganization in horse oocytes fertilized by ICSI or activated parthenogenetically. Additional oocytes were injected with a sperm labeled with a mitochondrion-specific vital dye to help identify the contribution of the sperm to zygotic structures, in particular the centrosome. Oocytes were fixed at set intervals after sperm injection and examined by confocal laser scanning microscopy. In unfertilized oocytes, microtubules were present only in the metaphase-arrested second meiotic spindle and the first polar body. After sperm injection, an aster of microtubules formed adjacent to the sperm head and subsequently enlarged such that at the time of pronucleus migration and apposition it filled the entire cytoplasm. During syngamy, the microtubule matrix reorganized to form a mitotic spindle on which the chromatin of both parents aligned. Finally, after nuclear and cellular cleavage were complete, the microtubule asters dispersed into the interphase daughter cells. Sham injection induced parthenogenetic activation of 76% of oocytes, marked by the formation of multiple cytoplasmic microtubular foci that later developed into a dense microtubule network surrounding the female pronucleus. The finding that a parthenote alone can produce a microtubule aster, whereas the aster invariably forms at the base of the sperm head during normal fertilization, indicates that both gametes contribute to the formation of the zygotic centrosome in the horse. Finally, 25% of sperm-injected oocytes failed to complete fertilization, mostly due to absence of oocyte activation (65%), which was often accompanied by failure of sperm decondensation. In conclusion, this study demonstrated that union of the parental genomes in horse zygotes is accompanied by a series of integrated cytoskeleton-mediated events, failure of which results in developmental arrest.[55]

In oocytes from all mammalian species studied to date, fertilization by a spermatozoon induces intracellular calcium $[Ca^{2+}]i$ oscillations that are crucial for appropriate oocyte activation and embryonic development. Such patterns are species-specific and have not yet been elucidated in horses; it is also not known whether equine oocytes respond with transient $[Ca^{2+}]i$ oscillations when fertilized or treated with parthenogenetic agents. Therefore, the aims of this study were: (i) to characterize the activity of equine sperm extracts microinjected into mouse oocytes; (ii) to ascertain in horse oocytes the $[Ca^{2+}]i$ -releasing activity and activating capacity of equine sperm extracts corresponding to the activity present in a single stallion spermatozoon;

and (iii) to determine whether equine oocytes respond with $[Ca^{2+}]i$ transients and activation when fertilized using the intracytoplasmic sperm injection (ICSI) procedure. The results of this study indicate that equine sperm extracts are able to induce $[Ca^{2+}]i$ oscillations, activation and embryo development in mouse oocytes. Furthermore, in horse oocytes, injection of sperm extracts induced persistent $[Ca^{2+}]i$ oscillations that lasted for >60 min and initiated oocyte activation. Nevertheless, injection of a single stallion spermatozoon did not consistently initiate $[Ca^{2+}]i$ oscillations in horse oocytes. It is concluded that stallion sperm extracts can efficiently induce $[Ca^{2+}]i$ responses and parthenogenesis in horse oocytes, and can be used to elucidate the signalling mechanism of fertilization in horses. Conversely, the inconsistent $[Ca^{2+}]i$ responses obtained with sperm injection in horse oocytes may explain, at least in part, the low developmental success obtained using ICSI in large animal species.[56]

In all species studied, fertilization induces intracellular Ca2+ $[Ca^{2+}]i$ oscillations required for oocyte activation and embryonic development. This species-specific pattern has not been studied in the equine, partly due to the difficulties linked to in vitro fertilization in this species. Therefore, the objective of this study was to use intracytoplasmic sperm injection (ICSI) to investigate fertilization-induced $[Ca^{2+}]i$ signaling and, possibly, ascertain problems linked to the success of this technology in the horse. In vivo- and in vitro-matured mare oocytes were injected with a single motile stallion sperm. Few oocytes displayed $[Ca^{2+}]i$ responses regardless of oocyte source and we hypothesized that this may result from insufficient release of the sperm-borne active molecule (sperm factor) into the oocyte. However, permeabilization of sperm membranes with Triton-X or by sonication did not alleviate the deficient $[Ca^{2+}]i$ responses in mare oocytes. Thus, we hypothesized that a step downstream of release, possibly required for sperm factor function, is not appropriately accomplished in horse oocytes. To test this, ICSI-fertilized horse oocytes were fused to unfertilized mouse oocytes, which are known to respond with $[Ca^{2+}]i$ oscillations to injection of stallion sperm, and $[Ca2+]i$ monitoring was performed. Such pairs consistently displayed $[Ca^{2+}]i$ responses demonstrating that the sperm factor is appropriately released into the ooplasm of horse oocytes, but that these are unable to activate and/or provide the appropriate substrate that is required for the sperm factor delivered by ICSI to initiate oscillations. These findings may have implications to improve the success of ICSI in the equine and other livestock species.[57]

ICSI Used for Studying Developmental Competence of In Vivo and In Vitro Matured Oocytes

In vitro versus in vivo oocyte maturation usually has resulted in reduced embryonic development and lower pregnancy rates after ICSI and culture and/or embryo transfer. This difference also has been demonstrated with in vitro culture systems for embryonic development compared with in vivo systems (e.g., the sheep oviduct), regardless of method of oocyte collection.

Blastocyst formation rates during horse embryo in vitro production (IVP) are disappointing, and embryos that blastulate in culture fail to produce the characteristic and vital glycoprotein capsule. The aim of this study was to evaluate the impact of IVP on horse embryo development and capsule formation. IVP embryos were produced by intracytoplasmic sperm injection of in vitro matured oocytes and either culture in synthetic oviduct fluid (SOF) or temporary transfer to the oviduct of a ewe. Control embryos were flushed from the uterus of mares 6-9 days after ovulation. Embryo morphology was evaluated with light microscopy, and multiphoton scanning confocal microscopy was used to examine the distribution of microfilaments (AlexaFluor-Phalloidin stained) and the rate of apoptosis (cells with fragmented or terminal deoxynucleotidyl transferase-mediated dUTP nick end-labeling-positive nuclei). To examine the influence of culture on capsule formation, conceptuses were stained with a monoclonal antibody specific for capsular glycoproteins (OC-1). The blastocyst rate was higher for zygotes transferred to a sheep's oviduct (16%) than for those cultured in SOF (6.3%). Day 7 IVP embryos were small and compact with relatively few cells, little or no blastocoele, and an indistinct inner cell mass. IVP embryos had high percentages of apoptotic cells (10% versus 0.3% for in vivo embryos) and irregularly distributed microfilaments. Although they secreted capsular glycoproteins, the latter did not form a normal capsule but instead permeated into the zona pellucida or remained in patches on the trophectodermal surface. These results demonstrate that the initial layer of capsule is composed of OC-1-reactive glycoproteins and that embryo development ex vivo is retarded and aberrant, with capsule formation failing as a result of failed glycoprotein aggregation.[58]

This study was conducted to evaluate in vivo and in vitro development of in vitro-matured equine oocytes fertilized by intracytoplasmic sperm injection. Oocytes were collected from slaughterhouse-derived ovaries, matured in vitro, and injected with frozen-thawed stallion sperm. In vivo development was assessed after transfer of injected oocytes to the oviducts of recipient mares. Mares were killed 7.5-8.5 days after transfer and the uterus and oviducts flushed for embryo recovery. Of 132 injected oocytes transferred, 69 (52%) were recovered; of these, 25 (36%) were blastocysts with a blastocoele and capsule. In vitro development was assessed in three culture systems. Culture of zygotes in modified Chatot, Ziomek, Bavister medium with BSA containing either 5.5 mM glucose for 7.5 days or 0.55 mM glucose for 3 days, followed by 3 mM glucose for 2 days, then 4.3 mM glucose for 2.5 days, did not result in blastocyst formation. Culture of zygotes in Dulbecco modified Eagle medium (DMEM)/F-12 with 10% fetal bovine serum with and without coculture with equine oviductal epithelial explants yielded 16% and 15% blastocyst development, respectively. Development to blastocyst was significantly lower in G1.3/2.3/BSA than in DMEM/F-12/BSA or in either medium with 10% added serum (2% vs. 18%, 18% or 20%; P < 0.05), suggesting that requirements for equine embryo development differ from those for other species. These results indicate that in vitro-matured equine oocytes are sufficiently competent to form 36% blastocysts in an optimal environment (in vivo). While we identified an in vitro culture system that provided repeatable blastocyst development without coculture, this yielded only half the rate of development achieved in vivo.[59]

Follicle atresia and granulosa cell apoptosis may be related to oocyte meiotic and developmental competence. We analyzed the relationships among granulosa cell apoptosis, initial cumulus morphology, oocyte nuclear maturation in vitro, and pronucleus formation after intracytoplasmic sperm injection (ICSI) in the horse. For each follicle, the size was measured and granulosa cells were used for DNA laddering analysis. Oocytes were evaluated for cumulus morphology, cultured for in vitro maturation, and submitted to ICSI. Apoptosis was categorized as absent, intermediate, or advanced according to the relative concentrations of two DNA fragments at 900 and 360 base pairs (bp). In 98 oocyte-follicle pairs, 52 oocytes were classified as expanded (Exp), 39 as compact (Cp), and 7 as having a partial (P) cumulus. Advanced apoptosis was detected in 55% (54/98) of follicles; 37% (36/98) of follicles showed an intermediate level of apoptosis; and 8 follicles (8%) were nonapoptotic. Follicle size was not significantly correlated with granulosa cell apoptosis (P > 0.05). Significantly more Exp than Cp oocytes originated from follicles with advanced apoptosis (P < 0.001). The proportion of oocytes maturing in vitro was significantly higher in oocytes issuing from apoptotic follicles than in oocytes issuing from healthy follicles (P < 0.05). The proportion of normally (two pronuclei) or abnormally fertilized oocytes (one or greater than two pronuclei, or partially decondensed sperm) did not differ in relation to granulosa cell apoptosis. We conclude that, in the mare, granulosa cell apoptosis is related to cumulus expansion and an increase in oocyte meiotic competence but has no effect on the proportion of meiotically competent oocytes that activate after ICSI. These results provide selection criteria for horse oocytes used in assisted reproductive techniques so that embryo production may be maximized.[60]

This study was conducted to evaluate the effect of initial cumulus morphology (expanded or compact) and duration of in vitro maturation (24, 30 or 42 h) on the developmental competence of equine oocytes after intracytoplasmic sperm injection (ICSI). The effect of manipulation temperature (room temperature vs 37 degrees C) at the time of ICSI and concentration of glucose (0.55 vs 5.5 mM) during embryo culture was also investigated. The nuclear maturation rates of expanded (Ex) oocytes were significantly (P < 0.001) higher than those of compact (Cp) oocytes at all maturation times (61-72 vs 23-25% respectively). Forty-eight hours after ICSI of mature Ex oocytes, the rate of cleavage with normal nuclei was significantly (P < 0.05) higher for oocytes matured for 24 h than for those matured for 30 or 42 h (73 vs 57-59% respectively). For Cp oocytes, the morphologic cleavage rates for oocytes matured for 30 h were significantly (P < 0.05) higher than for those matured for 24 or 42 h (86 vs 55-61% respectively). The overall proportion of embryos having more than four normal nuclei at 48 h culture was significantly higher (P < 0.05) for Cp than for Ex oocytes. Manipulation temperature did not affect development of embryos from Ex or Cp oocytes at 96 h after ICSI. Culture in high-glucose medium significantly increased morphologic cleavage of Cp, but not Ex, oocytes (P < 0.05). Embryos from Cp oocytes had a significantly higher average nucleus number after 96-h culture than did embryos from Ex oocytes. These data indicate that developmental competence differs between Ex and Cp equine oocytes, and is differentially affected by the duration of maturation and by composition of embryo culture media.[61]

The foregoing studies emphasize the importance of media capable of optimal culture conditions for both nuclear and cytoplasmic maturation of any oocytes to be used in ART. To date in vivo matured and ICSI injected equine oocytes have been better at providing normal development (per embryo) and live foal rate (per embryo transferred). Techniques to culture in vitro–matured and ICSI-fertilized oocytes to the blastocyst stage and resultant pregnancy, however, have provided much encouragement for continued development of co-culture with oviductal epithelial cells.

The future of equine ICSI from a commercial standpoint will revolve around the ability to consistently provide embryos that can develop to an age that they can be transferred nonsurgically into the uterus—from morula to expanding blastocyst.

References

1. McKinnon AO, Lacham-Kaplan O, Trounson AO: Pregnancies produced from fertile and infertile stallions by intracytoplasmic sperm injection (ICSI) of single frozen-thawed spermatozoa into in-vivo matured oocytes. J Reprod Fertil Suppl 2000; 56:513.
2. Duckitt K: Infertility and subfertility. Clin Evid 2003; 9:2044-2073.
3. Feichtinger W, Kemeter P: Laparoscopic or ultrasonically guided follicle aspiration for in vitro fertilization? J In Vitro Fertil Embryo Transf 1984; 1:244.
4. Silber SJ: Intracytoplasmic sperm injection today: a personal review. Hum Reprod 1998; 13(Suppl 1):208.
5. Laws-King A, Trounson A, Sathananthan H, Kola I: Fertilization of human oocytes by microinjection of a single spermatozoon under the zona pellucida. Fertil Steril 1987; 48:637.
6. Palermo G, Joris H, Devroey P, Van Steirteghem AC: Pregnancies after intracytoplasmic injection of single spermatozoon into an oocyte. Lancet 1992; 340:17.
7. Van Steirteghem AC, Liu J, Joris H et al: Higher success rate by intracytoplasmic sperm injection than by subzonal insemination. Report of a second series of 300 consecutive treatment cycles. Hum Reprod 1993; 8:1055.
8. Ludwig M, Katalinic A: Malformation rate in fetuses and children conceived after ICSI: results of a prospective cohort study. Reprod Biomed Online 2002; 5:171.
9. St John JC: Ooplasm donation in humans: the need to investigate the transmission of mitochondrial DNA following cytoplasmic transfer. Hum Reprod 2002; 17:1954.
10. Jones GM: Growth and viability of human blastocysts in vitro. Reprod Med Rev 2001; 8:241.
11. Gardner DK, Lane M, Schoolcraft WB: Culture and transfer of viable blastocysts: a feasible proposition for human IVF. Hum Reprod 2000; 15(Suppl 6): 9.
12. Scott RT Jr, Hofmann GE, Veeck LL et al: Embryo quality and pregnancy rates in patients attempting pregnancy through in vitro fertilization. Fertil Steril 1991; 55:426.
13. George SS, Fernandes HA, Irwin C et al: Factors predicting the outcome of intracytoplasmic sperm injection for infertility. Natl Med J India 2003; 16:13.
14. Giannini P, Piscitelli C, Giallonardo A et al: Number of embryos transferred and implantation. Ann N Y Acad Sci 2004; 1034:278.
15. Lahav-Baratz S, Koifman M, Shiloh H et al: Analyzing factors affecting the success rate of frozen-thawed embryos. J Assist Reprod Genet 2003; 20:444.
16. Kuliev A, Verlinsky Y: Preimplantation genetic diagnosis in assisted reproduction. Expert Rev Mol Diagn 2005; 5:499.
17. Petersen CG, Mauri AL, Baruffi RL et al: Implantation failures: success of assisted hatching with quarter-laser zona thinning. Reprod Biomed Online 2005; 10:224.
18. Sallam HN: Assisted hatching. Minerva Ginecol 2004; 56:223.
19. Barnes FL, Crombie A, Gardner DK et al: Blastocyst development and birth after in-vitro maturation of human primary oocytes, intracytoplasmic sperm injection and assisted hatching. Hum Reprod 1995; 10:3243.
20. Multiple gestation pregnancy. The ESHRE Capri Workshop Group. Hum Reprod 2000; 15:1856.
21. Unger S, Hoopmann M, Bald R et al: Monozygotic triplets and monozygotic twins after ICSI and transfer of two blastocysts: case report. Hum Reprod 2004; 19:110.
22. Palermo GD, Cohen J, Alikani M et al: Development and implementation of intracytoplasmic sperm injection (ICSI). Reprod Fertil Dev 1995; 7:211.
23. Van der EJ, Van den AE, Vitrier S et al: Selective transfer of cryopreserved human embryos with further cleavage after thawing increases delivery and implantation rates. Hum Reprod 1997; 12:1513.
24. Nagy ZP, Liu J, Joris H et al: The result of intracytoplasmic sperm injection is not related to any of the three basic sperm parameters. Hum Reprod 1995; 10:1123.
25. Liu J, Nagy Z, Joris H et al: Intracytoplasmic sperm injection does not require special treatment of the spermatozoa. Hum Reprod 1994; 9:1127.
26. Liu J, Nagy Z, Joris H et al: Analysis of 76 total fertilization failure cycles out of 2732 intracytoplasmic sperm injection cycles. Hum Reprod 1995b; 10:2630.
27. Silber SJ: 2005b. [http://www.infertile.com/treatmnt/treats/icsirev/icsirev.htm]. Accessed June 2005.
28. Silber SJ, Devroey P, Tournaye H, Van Steirteghem AC: Fertilizing capacity of epididymal and testicular sperm using intracytoplasmic sperm injection (ICSI). Reprod Fertil Dev 1995a; 7:281.
29. Silber SJ, Nagy ZP, Liu J et al: Conventional in-vitro fertilization versus intracytoplasmic sperm injection for patients requiring microsurgical sperm aspiration. Hum Reprod 1994; 9:1705.
30. Silber SJ, Nagy Z, Liu J et al: The use of epididymal and testicular spermatozoa for intracytoplasmic sperm injection: the genetic implications for male infertility. Hum Reprod 1995b; 10:2031.
31. Liu J, Nagy Z, Joris H et al: Successful fertilization and establishment of pregnancies after intracytoplasmic sperm injection in patients with globozoospermia. Hum Reprod 1995a; 10:626.
32. Devroey P, Liu J, Nagy Z et al: Pregnancies after testicular sperm extraction and intracytoplasmic sperm injection in non-obstructive azoospermia. Hum Reprod 1995a; 10: 1457.
33. Devroey P, Silber S, Nagy Z et al: Ongoing pregnancies and birth after intracytoplasmic sperm injection with frozen-thawed epididymal spermatozoa. Hum Reprod 1995b; 10:903.
34. Silber SJ, Van Steirteghem A, Nagy Z et al: Normal pregnancies resulting from testicular sperm extraction and intracytoplasmic sperm injection for azoospermia due to maturation arrest. Fertil Steril 1996; 66:110.
35. Bonduelle M, Wilikens A, Buysse A et al: Prospective follow-up study of 877 children born after intracytoplasmic sperm injection (ICSI), with ejaculated epididymal and testicular spermatozoa and after replacement of cryopreserved embryos obtained after ICSI. Hum Reprod 1996; 11(Suppl 4):131.
36. Bonduelle M, Ponjaert I, Steirteghem AV et al: Developmental outcome at 2 years of age for children born after ICSI compared with children born after IVF. Hum Reprod 2003; 18:342.
37. Short RV: Human reproduction in an evolutionary context. Ann N Y Acad Sci 1994; 709:416.
38. Short RV: The testis: the witness of the mating system, the site of mutation and the engine of desire, Acta Paediatr Suppl 1997; 422:3.
39. Silber SJ: 2005a. [http://www.infertile.com/inthenew/sci/modern.htm.] Accessed June 2005.
40. Pukazhenthi BS, Wildt DE, Howard JG: The phenomenon and significance of teratospermia in felids. J Reprod Fertil Suppl 2001; 57:423.

41. Bezard J, Magistrini M, Battut I et al: In vitro fertilization in the mare. Recueil De Med Veterinaire De L'Ecole D'Alfort 1992; 168:993.

42. Palmer E, Bezard J, Magistrini M, Duchamp G: In vitro fertilization in the horse. A retrospective study. J Reprod Fertil Suppl 1991; 44:375.

43. Dellaquila ME, DeFelici M, Massari S et al: Effects of fetuin on zona pellucida hardening and fertilizability of equine oocytes matured in vitro. Biol Reprod 1999; 61:533.

44. Squires EL, Wilson JM, Kato H, Blaszczyk A: A pregnancy after intracytoplasmic sperm injection into equine oocytes matured in vitro. Theriogenology 1996; 45:306.

45. Cochran R, Meintjes M, Reggio B et al: Production of live foals from sperm-injected oocytes harvested from pregnant mares. J Reprod Fertil Suppl 2000; 56:503.

46. Li XH, Morris LHA, Allen WR: Influence of co-culture during maturation on the developmental potential of equine oocytes fertilized by intracytoplasmic sperm injection (ICSI). Reproduction 2001; 121:925.

47. Galli C, Crotti G, Turini P et al: Frozen-thawed embryos produced by ovum pick up of immature oocytes and ICSI are capable to establish pregnancies in the horse. Theriogenology 2002; 58:705.

48. Chung JT, Keefer CL, Downey BR: Activation of bovine oocytes following intracytoplasmic sperm injection (ICSI). Theriogenology 2000; 53:1273.

49. Choi YH, Love CC, Love LB et al: Developmental competence in vivo and in vitro of in vitro-matured equine oocytes fertilized by intracytoplasmic sperm injection with fresh or frozen-thawed spermatozoa. Reproduction 2002; 123:455.

50. Dellaquila ME, Cho YS, Minoia P et al: Effects of follicular-fluid supplementation of in-vitro maturation medium on the fertilization and development of equine oocytes after in-vitro fertilization or intracytoplasmic sperm injection. Hum Reprod 1997b; 12:2766.

51. Dellaquila ME, Cho YS, Minoia P et al: Intracytoplasmic sperm injection (ICSI) versus conventional IVF on abattoir-derived and in vitro-matured equine oocytes. Theriogenology 1997a; 47:1139.

52. Grondahl C, Hansen TH, Hossaini A et al: Intracytoplasmic sperm injection of in-vitro matured equine oocytes. Biol Reprod 1997; 57:1495.

53. Tremoleda JL, Colenbrander B, Stout TAE, Bevers MM: Reorganisation of the cytoskeleton and chromatin in horse oocytes following intracytoplasmic sperm injection. Theriogenology 2002; 58:697.

54. Li XH, Morris LH, Allen WR: Effects of different activation treatments on fertilization of horse oocytes by intracytoplasmic sperm injection. J Reprod Fertil 2000; 119:253.

55. Tremoleda JL, Van Haeften T, Stout TA et al: Cytoskeleton and chromatin reorganization in horse oocytes following intracytoplasmic sperm injection: patterns associated with normal and defective fertilization. Biol Reprod 2003b; 69:186.

56. Bedford SJ, Kurokawa M, Hinrichs K, Fissore RA: Intracellular calcium oscillations and activation in horse oocytes injected with stallion sperm extracts or spermatozoa. Reproduction 2003; 126:489.

57. Bedford SJ, Kurokawa M, Hinrichs K, Fissore RA: Patterns of intracellular calcium oscillations in horse oocytes fertilized by intracytoplasmic sperm injection: possible explanations for the low success of this assisted reproduction technique in the horse. Biol Reprod 2004; 70:936.

58. Tremoleda JL, Stout TAE, Lagutina I et al: Effects of in vitro production on horse embryo morphology, cytoskeletal characteristics, and blastocyst capsule formation. Biol Reprod 2003a; 69:1895.

59. Choi YH, Roasa LM, Love CC et al: Blastocyst formation rates in vivo and in vitro of in vitro-matured equine oocytes fertilized by intracytoplasmic sperm injection. Biol Reprod 2004b; 70:1231.

60. Dell'Aquila ME, Albrizio M, Maritato F et al: Meiotic competence of equine oocytes and pronucleus formation after intracytoplasmic sperm injection (ICSI) as related to granulosa cell apoptosis. Biol Reprod 2003; 68:2065.

61. Choi YH, Love LB, Varner DD, Hinrichs K: Factors affecting developmental competence of equine oocytes after intracytoplasmic sperm injection. Reproduction 2004a; 127:187.

CHAPTER 48

In Vitro Fertilization

KATRIN HINRICHS

In vitro fertilization (IVF) is used clinically in cattle and humans. In cattle, oocytes are recovered from cows in vivo up to twice weekly by transvaginal ultrasound-guided follicular puncture. The recovered oocytes are subjected to in vitro maturation then fertilized in vitro, and the resulting embryos are cultured in vitro to the blastocyst stage, at which point they are transferred transcervically to the uteri of recipient cows. The procedure of in vitro embryo production is commercially successful in cattle and allows progeny to be obtained from cows that cannot themselves provide embryos for transfer.

Although the clinical demand for similar protocols in the horse is high, a major obstacle to employing in vitro embryo production in horses has been the failure of IVF to be repeatably successful. As of this writing, only two foals have been born from IVF, both in France, in 1990 and 1991.[1,2] Both foals were a result of IVF of oocytes that were recovered from mature follicles of mares ex vivo. Many laboratories have worked on equine IVF over the ensuing years, but an effective and repeatable technique has still not been established.

The major difficulty associated with IVF in the horse appears to be penetration of the zona pellucida, because fertilization rates are greatly increased if a breach is made in the zona pellucida before sperm are coincubated with the oocytes.[3,4] This has been done by removing a portion of the zona pellucida under micromanipulation or by dissolving a hole in the zona using a directed jet of acidic solution, again under micromanipulation. Although high fertilization rates (>80%) were obtained with these procedures, polyspermy (fertilization of the oocytes by more than one sperm) also resulted,[4] because the main barrier to polyspermy (i.e., change of the character of the zona pellucida after fertilization) was bypassed. Although the proportion of oocytes that undergo polyspermy can be decreased by manipulation of sperm numbers, some risk remains and these methods cannot be recommended for IVF. In addition, because these techniques both require micromanipulation, they entail equipment and labor similar to intracytoplasmic sperm injection (ICSI). ICSI has been shown to be a repeatable and efficient method for fertilization of horse oocytes in vitro[5,6] and so has become the method of choice (see chapter on ICSI).

Although ICSI provides a method for fertilization of horse oocytes in vitro, it is labor-intensive and is applicable only to laboratories having specialized equipment and trained personnel. Therefore work on standard IVF continues. Most work has concentrated on methods for capacitating equine sperm so that they may successfully penetrate the zona pellucida. It has been suggested that the equine zona may be at fault, perhaps becoming hardened when oocytes are cultured in vitro. However, when in vitro–matured equine oocytes are transferred to the oviduct of an inseminated mare, over 70% of the oocytes become normally fertilized, indicating that the oocytes are capable of being penetrated.[7]

Methods that have been used to successfully induce capacitation of equine sperm (i.e., that resulted in some oocytes becoming fertilized in vitro) are essentially limited to treatment with calcium ionophore or with heparin. In one study it was shown that calcium ionophore treatment was superior to heparin treatment for fresh sperm but that only heparin treatment was effective with frozen-thawed sperm.[8] Calcium ionophore induces capacitation by localizing in the plasma membrane and allowing calcium influx into the sperm. It is possible that membrane changes induced by freezing cause frozen-thawed sperm to be susceptible to damage during this process.

Clinically, use of frozen sperm for IVF would be more efficient than use of fresh sperm: there is no need to collect semen from the stallion each time IVF is performed, many more IVF procedures may be performed with one ejaculate, and it allows use of a stallion that is not at the same location as the laboratory. Therefore it would seem prudent when considering use of IVF clinically to explore methods involving frozen sperm. Currently the most repeatable method apparent is that used by workers in Germany, who have published two papers reporting similar penetration and fertilization rates (up to 46% and 29%, respectively).[8,9] This method entails thawing the semen and performing "swim up," in which the semen is layered under fresh medium and incubated to allow motile sperm to migrate up into the fresh medium. The medium is then aspirated and centrifuged to concentrate the sperm. The sperm pellet is added to an equal volume of medium containing 200 µg/ml heparin and is incubated for 10 minutes. This is then diluted with fresh medium without heparin and an aliquot of this suspension is added to the droplet containing the oocytes to obtain a final concentration of 1 million motile sperm per milliliter. However, other laboratories have not yet repeated these results. When it is established that a basal level of fertilization may be repeatably achieved with this system, further work may concentrate on factors that affect fertilization rate when it is used. Major factors that may affect the efficiency of IVF using this technique include the composition of the media used for capacitation and fertilization (including presence or absence of calcium, glucose, and sperm motility enhancers such as epinephrine), the amount and type of heparin used, and the amount of heparin present in the final fertilization droplet.

Now that oocyte recovery from valuable mares is a commonplace technique associated with oocyte transfer, the potential of IVF for clinical use has become more apparent. Hopefully, methods for efficient equine IVF will soon be developed and, in conjunction with in vitro embryo culture and transcervical transfer, will allow foals to be produced from isolated oocytes without need for micromanipulation or surgery.

References

1. Palmer E, Bézard J, Magistrini M et al: In vitro fertilisation in the horse: a retrospective study. J Reprod Fertil Supp 1991; 44:375-384.
2. Bézard J: In vitro fertilization in the mare. Proceedings of the International Scientific Conference on Biotechnics in Horse Reproduction, p 12, 1992.
3. Li LY, Meintjes M, Graff KJ et al: In vitro fertilization and development of in vitro-matured oocytes aspirated from pregnant mares. Biol Reprod 1995; 1:309.
4. Choi YH, Okada Y, Hochi S et al: In vitro fertilization rate of horse oocytes with partially removed zonae. Theriogenology 1994; 42:795.
5. Choi YH, Love CC, Love LB et al: Developmental competence in vivo and in vitro of in vitro-matured equine oocytes fertilized by intracytoplasmic sperm injection with fresh or frozen-thawed sperm. Reproduction 2002; 123:455.
6. Galli C, Crotti G, Turini R et al: Frozen-thawed embryos produced by ovum pickup of immature oocytes and ICSI are capable to establish pregnancies in the horse. Theriogenology 2002; 58:705.
7. Hinrichs K, Love CC, Brinsko SP et al: In vitro fertilization of in vitro-matured equine oocytes: effect of maturation medium, duration of maturation, and sperm calcium ionophore treatment, and comparison with rates of fertilization in vivo after oviductal transfer. Biol Reprod 2002; 67:256.
8. Alm H, Torner H, Blottner S et al: Effect of sperm cryopreservation and treatment with calcium ionophore or heparin on in vitro fertilization of horse oocytes. Theriogenology 2001; 56:817.
9. Torner H, Alm H, Mlodawska W et al: Determination of development in horse zygotes and spermatozoa during fertilization in vitro. Theriogenology 2002; 58:693.

CHAPTER 49

In Vitro Oocyte Maturation

KATRIN HINRICHS

Recovery of immature oocytes from excised ovaries, followed by maturation of these oocytes in vitro, may be done to obtain foals after the death of a valuable mare[1] or to conduct research on oocyte physiology and fertilization. Methods for recovery and classification of horse oocytes vary substantially from those for oocytes of other species, and veterinarians working in this area should familiarize themselves with methods specific to the horse.

OOCYTE RECOVERY

The oocyte of the horse is difficult to dislodge from the follicle wall. In cattle follicles the oocyte and its surrounding cumulus cells protrude into the follicle lumen on a narrow "neck," which is easily broken; however, in the horse the oocyte is imbedded within the granulosa layer that lines the follicle.[2] In addition, the equine cumulus is firmly anchored to the ovarian stroma (theca) beneath it by numerous projections. For these reasons, aspiration of follicles with a needle and syringe or vacuum apparatus, as done for bovine oocytes, results in a low yield of oocytes in the horse. In addition, aspiration preferentially recovers oocytes from partially atretic follicles, in which the granulosa is starting to degenerate and is losing integrity.[3] Therefore the preferred method for recovery of oocytes from horse ovaries is to slice open the follicles and to scrape the entire granulosa cell layer from the follicle to recover the oocyte.

Excess tissue (mesentery and oviduct) is trimmed away from the ovary with scissors, and the ovary is examined to locate follicles on the surface. Once located, a follicle is opened completely (so that the interiors of both halves are visible) with a scalpel blade. The granulosa layer is scraped from the wall of the follicle using a bone curette. A 0.5-cm curette works for most follicles; however, if large volumes of ovaries are to be processed, larger and smaller curettes are useful for larger and smaller follicles. The curette should be passed over one swath of the follicle wall, then the contents of the curette washed into a dish before passing the curette over another swath. This avoids losing tissue from the curette into the fluid within the follicle, as might occur if numerous back-and-forth motions are made. The tissue is washed from the curette into a 35-mm Petri dish, using a stream of medium from an 18- to 20-gauge needle attached to a 10-ml syringe. The medium typically used is Hepes-buffered TCM199 with Hank's salts (Gibco Life Technologies, Inc., Grand Island, N.Y.) plus ticarcillin (0.1 mg/ml, SmithKline Beecham Pharmaceuticals, Philadelphia, Pa.). Phosphate-buffered saline solution may also be used for a wash solution, but it is more likely to undergo pH changes than is the complete medium.

The contents of each follicle are washed into a separate dish. Once all of the visible follicles on the surface of the ovary have been processed, the ovary is sliced in 0.5-cm slices to visualize any follicles within the ovary. All follicles on the ovary may be processed; although the maturation rate for oocytes from small follicles is lower than that for large follicles, they still have the potential to perform successfully.[4]

Each Petri dish is examined under a dissection microscope at 10× to 40× to locate the oocyte. The character of the mural granulosa cells within the dish should be evaluated at this time. Compact granulosa appears as sheets of tissue (Figure 49-1). These sheets may have ragged edges where they are torn but when viewed from the side have a smooth surface without evidence of protruding cells. The smoothness of the granulosa is best evaluated by examining the edge of a fold of tissue. Expanded granulosa ranges from sheets of tissue with uneven granularity and cells protruding from the surface (Figure 49-2, A), to shards of slightly puffy tissue, to completely expanded, cloudlike masses of cells (Figure 49-2, B), often with a yellow coloring.

The oocyte may be difficult to locate because it may be imbedded within a sheet of tissue (see Figures 49-1 and 49-2, A) or be in the middle of a large mass of expanded cells (see Figure 49-2, B). As opposed to an embryo, which is completely spherical, the oocyte may appear to be irregular in shape (see Figure 49-2, B). This may be due to asymmetrical distribution of the dark granules within the oocyte cytoplasm (Figure 49-3). In cattle such oocytes are discarded because they do not have a homogenous cytoplasm; however, in horses this asymmetrical distribution of granules actually indicates that the oocyte is meiotically competent.[5]

Once the oocyte is located, the character of the cumulus should be evaluated. The cumulus may best be examined by evaluating the smoothness of the surface of the granulosa that forms the hillock over the oocyte (Figure 49-4); it may be necessary to turn the oocyte on its side in order to evaluate this. In this author's laboratory, only oocytes that have a compact cumulus and compact mural granulosa are classified as compact (Cp); oocytes having either expansion of the cumulus or expansion of the mural granulosa, or both, are classified as expanded (Ex). Classification of the oocyte is important because the two groups have different requirements for optimum maturation.

Although the cumulus of Ex oocytes is expanded, this does not indicate that they are preovulatory. Finding preovulatory follicles in excised ovaries collected from mares at random stages of the cycle is rare; only 1 ovary in 1 of 21 mares would be expected to have a follicle that is within 24 hours of ovulation; because the average number of follicles per ovary is about 7, only 1 follicle in 294 (2 ovaries per mare × 21 mares × 7 follicles per ovary) would be preovulatory. Cumulus expansion in Ex oocytes is instead a sign of follicle atresia. For this reason, Ex oocytes are typically discarded in other species. However, in the horse early follicle atresia appears to allow prematurational changes within the oocyte that increase its

ability to mature in vitro.[5] In contrast, Cp oocytes come from viable follicles but are largely juvenile and may fail to mature in vitro. Only those Cp oocytes from large follicles (>20 mm in diameter) have maximal meiotic competence.

Oocytes showing obvious signs of degeneration should be discarded. Typically these have a cumulus that is extremely expanded with little cellularity or is sparse or absent, and the oocyte cytoplasm when viewed at 40× or higher is obviously shrunken, misshapen, or dense with no visible cytoplasmic membrane. Oocytes that are completely denuded of cumulus should also be discarded. Typically in this author's laboratory, about 60% of oocytes are classified as Ex, 30% as Cp, and 10% or less as degenerated.

Once the oocyte has been located and classified, if necessary it (including the cumulus immediately surrounding it) is cut out from the sheet of granulosa cells or mass of expanded granulosa using two 18- to 20-gauge 1.5-inch needles. A simple method for transferring oocytes from one dish to another is use of a sterile glass Pasteur pipette and bulb; however, any sterile pipette system may be used. Oocytes are placed together in a holding dish (containing the same medium used for oocyte recovery) that has been labeled with the oocyte type. The holding dish is kept at room temperature (22° to 25°C) until all oocytes have been collected. Oocytes may be held for up to 4 hours in the M199 holding medium without an effect on maturation rate.[6]

CULTURE FOR MATURATION

After all of the oocytes have been recovered, they are transferred to maturation medium. Ex and Cp oocytes should be cultured separately. Media used for maturation

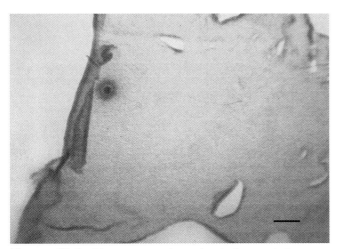

Figure 49-1 Horse oocyte in a sheet of compact granulosa, as recovered from the follicle by scraping with a bone curette. Bar = 500 μm.

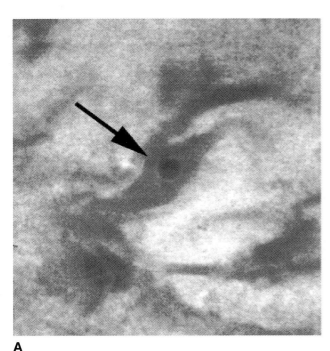

A

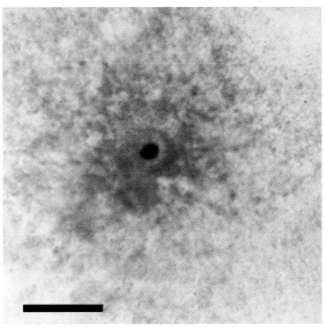

B

Figure 49-2 **A,** Horse oocyte *(arrow)* in a sheet of expanded granulosa cells. **B,** Horse oocyte in an expanded cumulus mass. Bar = 500 μm.

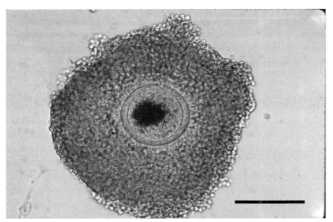

Figure 49-3 Horse oocyte showing uneven color to cytoplasm; this is normal and is associated with potential to mature in vitro. Bar = 200 μm.

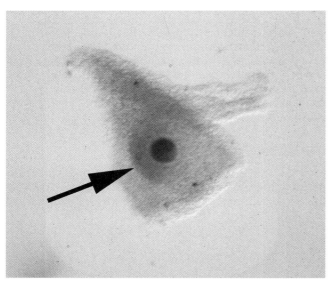

Figure 49-4 Horse oocyte dissected from a sheet of granulosa. The cut edges around the oocyte appear ragged because they have been torn; the smoothness of the cumulus hillock *(arrow)* indicates that the granulosa is compact.

of horse oocytes have not been critically tested for effects on subsequent embryo viability; however, two studies comparing M199/Earle's salts-based medium (given below) and a more complicated medium based on synthetic oviductal fluid with additional growth factors, steroid hormones, and luteinizing hormone (EMM1[7]) showed no difference in embryo growth in vitro. Both of these media are buffered to maintain pH in 5% CO_2, requiring a CO_2 incubator. Medium that does not require CO_2 incubation (M199 with Hank's salts and 25 mM Hepes, with 5 μU/ml FSH [Sioux Biochemicals Inc., Sioux Center, Iowa], 10% fetal bovine serum [Gibco], and 25 μg/ml gentamicin [Gibco]) has been used successfully for oocyte maturation,[8] but subsequent embryo development has not been evaluated.

In this author's laboratory, we use the fairly simple maturation medium of M199 with Earle's salts (Gibco) with 5 μU/ml FSH, 10% fetal bovine serum, and 25 μg/ml gentamicin. Care should be taken with all media that medical preparations of components (e.g., gentamicin for injection) are not used in media because they may contain preservatives that will compromise oocyte viability. Only embryo-quality components from a reputable supply company should be used.

Because the maturation medium is buffered to maintain a pH of 7.4 when exposed to 5% CO_2, it should be prepared before oocyte recovery and equilibrated in a 5% CO_2 incubator for at least 2 hours before it is used. Both the maturation medium and the holding medium (which is buffered to pH 7.4 in room atmosphere) contain phenol red, a pH indicator that is brick red at pH 7.4, turns yellow when acidic, and purple when basic. Oocytes should not be placed in the medium if it is not the appropriate color. The color may be used to determine whether the media has equilibrated adequately with the CO_2 environment. Typically, this author's laboratory equilibrates 3 to 4 ml of medium in several 35-mm Petri dishes within the incubator for several hours. We then use this medium to prepare 150-μl droplets for culture, several hours before oocyte recovery.

Microdroplets are prepared using a calibrated pipette with disposable tips; if none is available, an all-plastic tuberculin syringe with a small-gauge needle attached may be used to measure the approximate amount of medium. To prepare three 150-μl droplets, 75 μl of medium is placed in each of three drops on the floor of a 35-mm Petri dish. The drops are then covered with light white mineral oil (Sigma), which has been previously equilibrated in the CO_2 incubator (this may be done by pouring oil into a 100-ml Petri dish or a 50-ml conical tube left with the top ajar and placing these in the incubator). Approximately 3.5 ml of oil will be needed per Petri dish; the droplets should be completely covered. After the droplets are covered with oil, 75 μl additional medium is added to each droplet. This results in a droplet that has a smaller footprint in the dish and is more spherical than if all 150 μl was added at once.

When transferring the recovered oocytes from the holding dish to the culture droplets, a narrow pipette should be used to limit the amount of medium transferred along with the oocytes. For each culture dish 15 oocytes are taken from the holding dish and placed in one of the three droplets in the culture dish. They are then washed by transferring them to the second and then the third droplet in the dish. Once they are in the third droplet, the dish is placed in the incubator in a humidified atmosphere of 5% CO_2 at 38.2°C.

Oocytes classified as Ex should be cultured for 24 hours and those classified as Cp should be cultured for 30 hours before being used for oocyte transfer or other fertilization methods.[9]

If oocytes are to be transported to another laboratory, they may be transferred from the holding dish to 1 ml of equilibrated maturation medium in a 1-ml borosilicate glass tube and placed into a commercial portable incubator at 39° to 38.5°C. The oocytes will mature during transport.[8] On arrival at the destination laboratory the oocytes may be transferred to equilibrated droplets of maturation medium as above, or the top of the tube they are in may be loosened and the tube placed in a CO_2 incubator, or theoretically they may be left to complete maturation within the portable incubator. Transported oocytes mature successfully, but their potential for embryo development has not been evaluated.

EVALUATION OF MATURE OOCYTES

In this author's laboratory, typically 60% to 70% of Ex oocytes and 20% to 30% of Cp oocytes will mature to MII in culture. However, the author's laboratory transports ovaries from abattoirs located 3 to 4 hours from the laboratory, and it may be 5 to 9 hours from the time of the mare's death to the time the oocytes are recovered from the ovary. The proportion of Cp oocytes maturing in vitro is dependent upon the time of recovery of the oocytes from the ovaries. If oocytes are recovered within 1 hour of the mare's death or ovary excision, the maturation rate for Cp oocytes is over 60%.[10] This is because the more juvenile chromatin of the Cp oocytes degenerates over time when held within the ovary, but some of these oocytes will mature in vitro if recovered immediately. There is a slight improvement (10%) in maturation rate for Ex oocytes when recovered immediately after excision of the ovaries.

Evaluation of oocytes for maturation to MII is done by examining them under high power (>40×) for presence of a polar body. This can be done only after removal of the majority of the cumulus cells. If oocytes are to be used for oviductal oocyte transfer, it may not be advantageous to remove cumulus cells because this may interfere with the ability of the oocyte to stay within the oviduct after transfer.

After maturation the cumulus of both Ex and Cp oocytes should appear to be expanded. To denude the cumulus while keeping the oocyte viable, the oocytes are placed into a solution of 0.05% hyaluronidase in holding medium (Hepes-buffered TCM199 as used for oocyte collection). Oocytes are denuded by repeatedly pulling them in and out of smaller and smaller diameter pipettes (Pasteur pipettes pulled over an open flame). The smallest diameter pipette should allow the zona-enclosed oocyte to enter while becoming slightly deformed. In this way the cumulus cells are scraped from the surface of the zona. Horse oocytes have remarkably extensive processes of the cumulus cells through the zona; this makes the cumulus more tightly bound to the zona and thus much harder to denude than are oocytes of other species. Care should be taken to maintain the oocytes at incubator temperature during handling.

If oocyte viability is unimportant (e.g., the oocyte will be fixed for examination), then denuding may be performed by pipetting in a solution of 0.25% trypsin and 1 mM EDTA in Hank's salts without $CaCl_2$, $MgCl_2$, or $MgSO_4$ (Gibco). This solution interferes with cell-to-cell communication among cumulus cells and simplifies their removal.

Denuded oocytes may be selected for presence of a polar body. The oocyte is rolled with a needle or fine pipette while being observed under 40× to 100×. The polar body is seen as a small membrane-covered sphere within the perivitelline space (the area between the oocyte membrane and the inner surface of the zona pellucida). The polar body of horse oocytes may be small (Figure 49-5) in comparison with that of bovine or murine oocytes but can be located with good precision once the operator is familiar with the technique. If oocytes

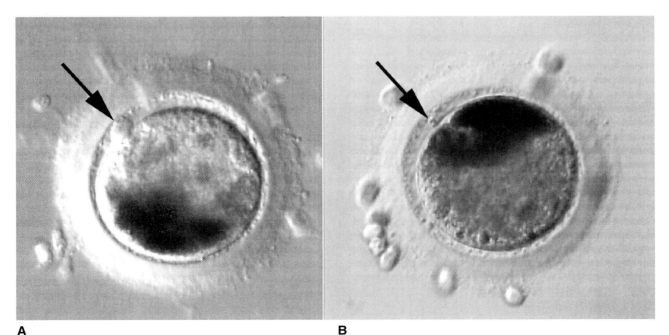

A   **B**

Figure 49-5 Mature (metaphase II) horse oocytes showing (**A**) large and (**B**) small polar bodies *(arrows)*. Both are within normal limits. These oocytes were recovered from the preovulatory follicles of mares ex vivo.

are not completely denuded of cumulus, the polar body may not be visible, but the integrity of the oocyte membrane is closely associated with successful maturation and may be used as a criterion to eliminate degenerating oocytes. The mature, viable horse oocyte usually has a bicolored cytoplasm with separate light and dark areas, and the cytoplasmic membrane is easily visible, giving a noticeable perivitelline space (see Figure 49-5).

If oocytes are to be sacrificed to evaluate their chromatin configuration, they may be fixed in buffered formol saline (as prepared for stallion sperm fixation) briefly and placed on a slide with the minimum amount of fluid. Mounting medium (6.5 µl of 9:1 glycerol:PBS containing 2.5 µg/ml Hoechst 33258) is divided in three droplets placed around the oocyte, and this is covered with a coverslip. The viscosity of the glycerol keeps the cover slip from crushing the oocytes. The slide is left at room temperature overnight or longer (or may be incubated for ≈2 hours or longer) and examined using fluorescence microscopy to determine the chromatin configuration.[4,5] If a fluorescence microscope is not available, then the oocytes may be fixed in a solution of acetic acid and absolute alcohol (1:3) overnight. The oocytes are then placed on a slide, and a coverslip with small amounts of paraffin placed on each corner (to keep the coverslip from crushing the oocytes) is pressed over the droplet until the oocytes are slightly flattened. Stain of 2% orcein in 60% acetic acid is then introduced under the coverslip while the oocytes are viewed under 400×. The orcein stains the chromatin, and it becomes slightly refractory; however, the results are much less vivid than with fluorescent staining and are short-lived.

References

1. Carnevale EM, Maclellan LJ, Coutinho da Silva MA et al: Pregnancies attained after collection and transfer of oocytes from ovaries of five euthanatized mares. J Am Vet Med Assoc 2003; 222:60.
2. Hawley LR, Enders AC, Hinrichs K: Comparison of equine and bovine oocyte-cumulus morphology within the ovarian follicle. Biol Reprod 1995; 1:243.
3. Dell'Aquila ME, Masterson M, Maritato F et al: Influence of oocyte collection technique on initial chromatin configuration, meiotic competence and male pronucleus formation after intracytoplasmic sperm injection (ICSI) of equine oocytes. Mol Reprod Dev 2001; 60:79.
4. Hinrichs K, Schmidt AL: Meiotic competence in horse oocytes: interactions among chromatin configuration, follicle size, cumulus morphology, and season. Biol Reprod 2000; 62:1402.
5. Hinrichs K, Williams KA: Relationships among oocyte-cumulus morphology, follicular atresia, initial chromatin configuration, and oocyte meiotic competence in the horse. Biol Reprod 1997; 57:377.
6. Love CC, Love LB, Varner DD et al: Effect of holding at room temperature after recovery on initial chromatin configuration and in vitro maturation rate of equine oocytes. Theriogenology 2002; 57:1973.
7. Maclellan LJ, Lane M, Sims MM et al: Effect of sucrose or trehalose on vitrification of equine oocytes 12 h or 24 h after the onset of maturation. Theriogenology 2001; 55:310.
8. Love LB, Choi YH, Love CC et al: Effect of ovary storage and oocyte transport method on maturation rate of horse oocytes. Theriogenology 2003; 59:765.
9. Choi YH, Hinrichs K: Unpublished data.
10. Hinrichs K, Choi YH: Unpublished data.

CHAPTER 50

Low-Dose Insemination Techniques

PHIL MATTHEWS
LEE MORRIS

BACKGROUND

To obtain acceptable per cycle pregnancy rates, the minimum recommended number of spermatozoa contained within a conventional insemination dose is generally >300 × 10[6] progressively motile spermatozoa for fresh semen[1-4] and >200 × 10[6] progressively motile spermatozoa for frozen semen.[5] It has been shown that conventional insemination of mares with ≤100 × 10[6] spermatozoa results in unsatisfactory per cycle pregnancy rates.[6,7]

Since the advent of fluorescence-activated cell separation technology[8] to sort spermatozoa into their X- and Y-chromosome-bearing populations at flow rates of 1000 to 5000 spermatozoa per second,[9,10] there has been renewed interest in the fertility of low numbers of spermatozoa. Consequently, this interest in low-dose insemination has fueled research and clinical trials aimed to reduce the minimum recommended dose of conventionally frozen stallion spermatozoa. Scott et al[11] observed that there is an aggregation of spermatozoa on the uterine side of the uterotubal junction, and subsequent research has focused on how few sperm may actually be necessary to result in fertilization when placed onto the papilla of the oviduct or within the oviduct.[12,13] These fertility investigations and novel methods of low-dose insemination have contributed to the investigation of the fertility of epididymal spermatozoa[14] and the potential to improve the fertility of subfertile stallions and mares.[15]

Several studies have explored different low-dose insemination techniques, which can be grouped into two general methods: rectally guided insemination techniques[13,16] and hysteroscopic techniques in which the papilla of the oviduct is actually visualized and becomes the target for semen deposition.[12,17,18] Both insemination techniques have been developed to minimize sperm wastage and deposit a small number of spermatozoa closer to the site of the sperm reservoir in the mare. These techniques have been used to examine the fertility of fresh, chilled or frozen, and sorted and nonsorted spermatozoa. The sperm numbers have varied dramatically but have always been lower than the conventional insemination dose of 200 to 500 ×10[6] spermatozoa.

For practical reasons and based on the insemination regimens outlined in the preliminary studies,[12,19] most practitioners have used a "timed insemination" technique that is aimed at depositing the spermatozoa deep within the uterus before ovulation. This has been made possible by the use of ovulation-induction agents that facilitate the ability to predict ovulation in estrous mares and optimize fertility.[20]

HYSTEROSCOPIC INSEMINATION PROCEDURE

Equipment

Expensive endoscopic equipment and a minimum of two people are required to perform the hysteroscopic insemination procedure. A variety of endoscopes are available for veterinary use that are suitable for hysteroscopic insemination. The researchers of the original studies[9,12,19,21] used a Pentax EPM 3000 videoendoscope. Since then Minitube (Germany) has designed a purpose-built hysteroscope for mares. For hysteroscopic insemination, the scope should have a diameter of 11 to 13 mm, a channel for the insemination catheter, and a channel to allow the insufflation of the uterus with air. One of these channels should allow extraction of air from the uterus at the end of the procedure. A wider diameter scope (11 to 13 mm) is preferable over one that is more narrow (7 to 9 mm) to minimize the risk of the scope "doubling-back" on itself during its advancement through the uterine lumen. The ideal scope length is 1.4 to 1.6 m to facilitate the insemination of larger breed mares. To minimize the duration of the procedure and improve the accuracy of semen deposition directly onto the uterotubal junction, it is desirable to visualize the images on a monitor through either a videoendoscope or a camera attached to a normal endoscope.

Insufflation of the uterine lumen with air during passage of the scope reduces any damage to the endometrium and minimizes the duration of the procedure. Most videoendoscopes pump sufficient air through an air channel, but a nonvideoendoscope requires an auxiliary pump to supply air through the working channel. By simple reversal of the hosing, surgical suction pumps have been employed successfully for this purpose. These same pumps can be used to aspirate the air from the uterine lumen after the semen has been deposited.

An insemination catheter must be made out of a nonspermicidal material, be of sufficient length to pass through the endoscope, and include an appropriate attachment on one end for a syringe. The original double-lumen catheter was made from polythene (V-EFIS-2-200, COOK, Brisbane, Australia), and since then suitable single-lumen endoscopy catheters, 1.7 m long and with a 2.6 mm diameter, have been used (Product 64835, Har-Vet, Spring Valley, USA). A 5 to 60 ml syringe is attached to the proximal end of the catheter. The syringe is used to draw semen into the catheter, and sufficient air is needed within the syringe to push the semen from the catheter. During the insemination procedure it is important to ensure that the semen remains located in the distal end of the catheter.

Proper cleaning or sterilization of the endoscope is required after use and between mares to remove infectious organisms and to prevent cross-contamination of spermatozoa. However, the cleaning solution or disinfectant must be well rinsed from the exterior of the scope, as well as from the flush and biopsy channels, so that it does not provide a source of irritation to the endometrium. Water, detergent, or disinfectant solutions are spermicidal and need to be rinsed and removed from the scope. Ideally, disinfectants that contain glutaraldehyde should be avoided unless they can be thoroughly removed from the scope. Once any protein material has been rinsed from the scope, the working channels should be rinsed with 70% alcohol before being air-dried. Sterilization of the scope with ethylene oxide is also possible, but this process takes time and severely limits the number of procedures that can be performed in a given time frame.

Insemination Procedure

Before the commencement of the insemination, the mare should be sedated to minimize any movement or discomfort. The mare should be restrained in stocks, her tail tied out of the way, her rectum evacuated, and her vulva and perineal area washed and rinsed thoroughly with a gentle soap.

Once the mare is ready, the semen is prepared. The endoscopic catheter is extruded from the distal end of the scope, and the insemination dose is aspirated into the distal end of the catheter. The catheter is withdrawn into the scope and the scope protected in the gloved palm of the operator's hand. The distal end of the scope is introduced into the vagina of the mare and guided through the mare's cervix into the uterus. A minimal amount of air is used to insufflate the uterus to facilitate the visualization of the uterine lumen. Introduction of too much air into the uterus results in a rigid pipelike consistency of the uterine wall. If the uterus is overinflated, the small insemination dose tends to run away from the site of deposition, the papilla of the uterotubal junction. Ideally, some endometrial folds remain after insufflation of the uterus; they help trap the semen at the site of deposition in the cranial uterine horn.

Once the end of the scope is in the uterine body, the cervix is held closed around the scope to prevent the escape of air through the soft, estrous cervix. The scope is advanced into the uterine body until the bifurcation of the uterine horns is visualized, and then it is advanced carefully within the lumen of the horn ipsilateral to impending ovulation until the papilla of the uterotubal junction is visualized in the cranial tip of the uterine horn. It is important to be certain that the scope has not turned during this process; if there is the slightest doubt about the scope's location, then it should be withdrawn or the mare's reproductive tract can be palpated per rectum to confirm that the scope is in the correct horn. Morris et al[19] demonstrated that if a low dose of frozen semen were deposited in the horn contralateral to the side of ovulation, only 8% (1/12) mares conceived.

Once the papilla is identified, the catheter can be advanced through the working channel of the scope until the tip of the catheter is visible. The tip of the endoscope can be controlled so that the catheter can be pointed directly at, or just above, the uterotubal papilla and then the semen is deposited. To optimize the viability of the spermatozoa, the small volume of semen (≤ 0.5 ml) should be deposited gently onto the papilla in an attempt to trap the sperm cells within the bubbles that form and attach to the papilla.[12,19] Manning et al[17] described a technique for directly depositing sperm into the oviduct with a 3.5 g French catheter, with disappointing results. In clinical practice, the volumes of an insemination dose are typically 0.5 to 1 ml and contain 50 to 200 $\times$ 10^6 spermatozoa. When this larger volume is deposited on the papilla a high proportion of the insemination dose runs away from the papilla. For these larger volumes, a single-lumen catheter is preferred to the double-lumen catheter, and the insemination dose should be evacuated quickly from the catheter to maximize the number of spermatozoa deposited onto the papilla. In both cases the aim is to deposit and retain a high proportion of the insemination dose at the uterotubal junction and prevent it from being washed caudally into the uterine body.

Any air should be removed immediately after deposition of the insemination dose. This can be achieved by pressing the hand ventrally on the uterus per rectum to force the air out through the open cervix or it can be accomplished more slowly, but potentially more thoroughly, by suction through the scope itself upon its withdrawal from the uterine lumen. Whichever technique is used, it is thought to be beneficial, if not imperative, to evacuate as much air as possible.

DEEP UTERINE INSEMINATION PROCEDURE

Equipment

At the same time that endoscopic insemination was being pioneered, the ultrasound-guided, deep uterine insemination procedure was developed for sex-sorted spermatozoa.[16] This technique is relatively simple and less time consuming than the endoscopic insemination procedure.

During the early development of the deep uterine insemination method, Buchanan et al[16] used a disposable artificial insemination pipette (IMV, France) to deposit the small volume of semen into the cranial uterine horn. This pipette was not flexible enough to negotiate the bifurcation of the uterine horns without causing some discomfort or superficial damage to the endometrium. Since then, long (>55 cm), flexible pipettes have been developed by Minitube (Germany) and IMV (France). They are designed to facilitate the advancement of the pipette through the uterine lumen with minimal trauma. The end of the Minitube pipette has a round "bulb" that aids progress through the lumen and is easy to palpate per rectum at the cranial end of the uterine horn. Furthermore, this pipette has an internal stylette that can evacuate the semen from a 0.5 ml straw and then withdraw the straw from the lumen of the pipette. It is possible to bend the tip of the IMV flexible catheter to aid its progress past the uterine bifurcation.

Insemination Procedure

The mare should be prepared in a manner similar to that described for endoscopic insemination. However, most mares do not require sedation for this deep uterine insemination procedure. The technique involves the introduction of a flexible catheter or pipette, per vaginum, through the cervix and into the body of the uterus. In some cases the inseminator's hand is then withdrawn from the vagina and introduced rectally. The pipette is palpated within the uterine lumen, and by manipulating the uterus while pushing the catheter with the other hand, the catheter is introduced into the uterine horn ipsilateral to the preovulatory follicle. This procedure is aided by manipulating the uterine horn of choice into a more cranial position to "straighten" the bifurcation and align the entrance of the uterine horn with the uterine body longitudinally. The aim is to deposit the spermatozoa at the cranial tip of the uterine horn in close proximity to the papilla.

DISCUSSION

Several reviews of the literature have compared the pregnancy results obtained from either hysteroscopic or deep uterine insemination.[22-24] Overall, it appears that there were no differences in the pregnancy results obtained from either insemination method when more than 5×10^6 fresh spermatozoa were contained within the insemination dose. For frozen semen, Morris et al[19] demonstrated that hysteroscopic insemination produced a higher pregnancy rate when the insemination dose was reduced from 14×10^6 to 3×10^6 motile, frozen-thawed spermatozoa than conventional insemination. However, there was no difference in the fertility of 14×10^6 spermatozoa deposited by either conventional insemination into the uterine body or by hysteroscopic insemination at the uterotubal junction. More work is required to describe any differences reported in the fertility of conventional versus low dose-hysteroscopic insemination within commercially available stallions.[22] To date there have been no reports of a direct comparison of the efficacy of hysteroscopic, deep and conventional uterine insemination with low doses of frozen semen from within the same stallion.

In practice, a single 0.5 ml straw of commercially frozen semen usually contains at least 50 to 100×10^6 spermatozoa. This is far in excess of the low sperm numbers evaluated under research conditions, and these relatively high sperm numbers should compensate for variation in stallion fertility when deposited deep within the uterus by either insemination method. Indeed, the hysteroscopic insemination procedure may represent "overkill" for the insemination of such high numbers and volume (0.5 ml) of commercially frozen stallion spermatozoa. If the insemination volume is greater than 0.25 ml,

then there may be no advantage obtained by depositing it hysteroscopically at the uterotubal junction because a high proportion of the inseminate will not be retained at the uterotubal junction as it moves away via the uterine folds. The ability of only 0.6 ml semen to be effectively distributed throughout the uterus after conventional insemination and for sufficient spermatozoa to migrate into the oviduct for fertilization to occur was demonstrated by Allen et al.[25] Since then, elegant scintigraphy studies have revealed the passage of a 5 ml insemination bolus throughout the entire uterus of the mare.[26] Moreover, it is possible for sufficient chilled[13] or frozen-thawed spermatozoa in only 0.1 to 0.2 ml to migrate from the contralateral to ipsilateral uterotubal papilla.[19]

On the other hand, hysteroscopic insemination is indicated in preference to deep uterine insemination when the sperm numbers are significantly reduced, such as after FACS separation during the sex-preselection process[21,27] or for insemination with epididymal spermatozoa when the motility is reduced. Insemination of frozen-thawed epididymal spermatozoa has produced acceptable pregnancy rates only after hysteroscopic insemination, but not conventional insemination.[12]

In the early studies there were few cases of uterine fluid accumulation detected ultrasonographically 15 hours after hysteroscopic insemination with either fresh (1%) or frozen (3%) semen.[12] Sieme et al[15] investigated the value of hysteroscopic insemination in problem mares. The results from this study revealed that problem mares benefited from conventional insemination into the uterine body when compared to hysteroscopic insemination, whereas the converse was true for fertile mares. Further investigation of the effects of hysteroscopic insemination on the uterine health of normal mares revealed that post breeding endometritis was more likely to persist in excess of 48 hours if the insemination procedure took more than 7 minutes.[24] Buchanan et al[16] reported a high embryonic loss rate (38%) between days 16 and 60 of gestation after ultrasound-guided deep uterine insemination. This study was performed using a relatively inflexible pipette, which may have induced sufficient uterine trauma to cause uterine inflammation and subsequent embryonic loss. Since this study, more flexible pipettes have been developed, and significant pregnancy loss has not been reported.

Low-dose insemination techniques may be useful to manage the physiologic and logistical problems of inadequate sperm numbers. The practitioner can use this technique with fresh semen if a stallion is overbooked on a particular collection day. The semen can be extended and centrifuged to create pellets that contain a minimum number of spermatozoa for either deep uterine or hysteroscopic insemination to effectively increase the number of doses available without jeopardizing stallion fertility.

The value of hysteroscopic insemination over deep uterine insemination has been described for very low numbers (5×10^6) of morphologically normal, sex-sorted spermatozoa.[27] However, if there are defects in the sperm morphology or defects in the fertilizing capacity in addition to the low numbers of spermatozoa available for insemination, then neither hysteroscopic nor deep uterine insemination improves the pregnancy rates. In an attempt to overcome the limitations of poor quality ejaculates, Alvarenga and Leão[28] observed no beneficial effects after washing frozen-thawed spermatozoa through a density gradient to select a more motile population of spermatozoa for hysteroscopic insemination. Similarly, pregnancy rates did not improve when Nie and Johnson[29] processed spermatozoa through glass wool-Sephadex, Percoll, or by swim up before deep uterine horn insemination. Nor did pregnancy rates improve after washing frozen-thawed epididymal spermatozoa through a density gradient before hysteroscopic insemination.[14]

CONCLUSION

Further study is required to determine the optimal number of spermatozoa and method of insemination for individual stallions. It may then be beneficial to freeze the low doses of spermatozoa in 0.25 ml straws to maximize the use of particular stallions in a hysteroscopic insemination program. The beneficial effects of hysteroscopic insemination over deep uterine insemination are only realized when the inseminate contains less than 5×10^6 spermatozoa and the volume of the inseminate is less than 0.5 ml. In practice, deep uterine insemination of 50 to 100×10^6 from a fertile stallion should produce pregnancy rates equivalent to those obtained with higher doses of semen used for conventional insemination for the same stallion. The interaction of the fertility of any mare and stallion combination will need to be assessed to ultimately determine the optimal method of insemination to maximize their fertility.

References

1. Householder DD, Pickett BW, Voss JL, Olar TT: Effect of extender, numbers of spermatozoa, and hCG on equine fertility. Equine Vet Sci 1981; 1:9-13.
2. Pickett BW, Voss JL: The effect of semen extenders and sperm number on mare fertility. J Reprod Fertil Supp 1975; 23:95-98.
3. Gahne S, Ganheim A, Malmagren L: Effect of insemination dose on pregnancy rate in mares. Theriogenology 1998; 49:1071-1074.
4. Vidament M, Dupere AM, Julienne P et al: Equine frozen semen freezability and fertility field results. Theriogenology 1997; 48:907-917.
5. Pickett BW, Voss JL, Squires EL et al: Collection, preparation and insemination of stallion semen. Colorado State University, Fort Collins, CO, Animal Reproduction Laboratory Bulletin No10, 2000.
6. Pace MM, Sullivan JJ: Effect of timing of insemination, numbers of spermatozoa, and extender components on the pregnancy rates in mares inseminated with frozen stallion semen. J Reprod Fertil Suppl 1975; 15-121.
7. Voss JL, Wallace RA, Squires EL et al: Effects of synchronization and frequency of insemination on fertility. J Reprod Fertil Suppl 1979; 27:257-261.
8. Johnson LA, Flook JP, Hawk HW: Sex preselection in rabbits: live birth from X and Y sperm separated by DNA and cell sorting. Biol Reprod 1989; 41:199-203.
9. Lindsey AC, Morris LH, Allen WR et al: Hysteroscopic insemination of mares with low numbers of nonsorted or flow sorted spermatozoa. Equine Vet J 2002; 34:128-132.
10. Hollinshead FK, O'Brien JK, Maxwell WMC, Evans G: Production of lambs of predetermined sex after the insemina-

11. Scott MA, Liu IKM, Overstreet JW, Enders AC: The structural morphology and epithelial association of spermatozoa at the utero-tubal junction: a descriptive study of equine spermatozoa in situ using scanning electron microscopy. J Reprod Fertil Suppl 2002; 56:415-421.
12. Morris LHA, Hunter RHF, Allen WR: Hysteroscopic insemination of small numbers of spermatozoa at the uterotubal junction of preovulatory mares. J Reprod Fertil 2000; 118:95-100.
13. Brinsko SP, Rigby SL, Lindsey AC et al: Pregnancy rates in mares following hysteroscopically or transrectally guided insemination with low sperm numbers at the utero-tubal papilla. Theriogenology 2003; 59:1001-1009.
14. Morris LHA, Tiplady CA, Allen WR: The in vivo fertility of caudal epididymal spermatozoa in the horse. Theriogenology 2002; 58:643-646.
15. Sieme H, Bonk A, Hamann H et al: Effects of different artificial insemination techniques and sperm doses on fertility of normal mares and mares with abnormal reproductive history. Theriogenology 2004; 62:915-928.
16. Buchanan BR, Seidel GE Jr, McCue PM et al: Insemination of mares with low numbers of either unsexed or sexed spermatozoa. Theriogenology 2000; 53:1333-1344.
17. Manning ST, Bowman PA, Fraser M, Card C: Development of hysteroscopic insemination of the uterine tube in the mare. In Proceedings of the Annual Meeting of the Society for Theriogenology, pp 84-85, 1998.
18. Vazquez JJ, Medina VM, Liu IKM et al: Nonsurgical uterotubal insemination in the mare. In Proceedings of the Annual Meeting of the Society for Theriogenology, pp 82-83, 1998.
19. Morris LHA, Tiplady CA, Allen WR: Pregnancy rates in mares after a single fixed time hysteroscopic insemination with low numbers of frozen-thawed spermatozoa onto the uterotubal junction. Equine Vet J 2003; 35:197-201.
20. Barbacini S, Zavaglia G, Gulden P et al: Retrospective study on the efficiency of hCG in an equine artificial insemination programme using frozen semen. Equine Vet Educ 2000; 12:312-317.
21. Lindsey AC, Schenk JL, Graham JK et al: Hysteroscopic insemination of low numbers of flow sorted fresh and frozen thawed stallion spermatozoa. Equine Vet J 2002; 34:121-127.
22. Morris LHA, Allen WR: An overview of low dose insemination in the mare. Reprod Domest Anim 2002; 37:206-210.
23. Morris LHA: Low-dose insemination in the mare: an update. Anim Reprod Sci 2004; 82:625-632.
24. Lyle SK, Ferrer MS: Low-dose insemination—why, when, and how. Theriogenology 2005; 64:572-579.
25. Allen WR, Bowen JM, Frank CJ et al: The current position of AI in horse breeding. Equine Vet J 1976; 8:72-74.
26. Katila T, Sankari S, Mäkelä O: Transport of spermatozoa in the genital tracts of mares. J Reprod Fertil Suppl 2000; 56:571-578.
27. Lindsey AC, Varner DD, Seidel GE Jr et al: Hysteroscopic or rectally guided, deep uterine insemination of mares with spermatozoa stored 18h at either 5° C or 15° C prior to flow cytometric sorting. Anim Reprod Sci 2005; 85:125-130.
28. Alvarenga MA, Leao KM: Hysteroscopic insemination of mares with low number of frozen-thawed spermatozoa selected by Percoll gradient. Theriogenology 2002; 58:651-653.
29. Nie GJ, Johnson KE: Pregnancy rate in mares following insemination with a low-dose of progressively motile or filtered sperm cells deep in the uterine horn. Proceedings of the Equine Symposium and Society for Theriogenology Annual Conference, San Antonio, Tex, p 303, 2000.

CHAPTER 51

Embryo Transfer and Related Technologies

ANGUS O. MCKINNON
EDWARD L. SQUIRES

Embryo transfer (ET) in horses was first described in 1972[1-2] and has been performed commercially since the 1980s.[3-6]

The development of equine ET has lagged behind other domestic species due to the limitation of one embryo transfer per year imposed by most of the major breed registries. In 2002 the American Quarter Horse Association (AQHA), acting on legal advice, withdrew the rule governing the number of embryos transferred per mare per year and retrospectively allowed registration of multiple ET-derived foals from the beginning of the introduction of ET to the AQHA legislation. This is expected to have significant implications for the number of ETs performed in the coming years.

ET has traditionally been most widely used in the older mare that fails to get pregnant or that conceives, establishes a pregnancy, and then undergoes early embryonic death (EED) or abortion. This limits the technology because these mares are less likely to provide embryos for transfer than normal, reproductively healthy mares.[7,8] More recently ET has been used in performance mares (racing, showing, polo, cutting, etc.) and has been combined with newer technologies such as breeding with frozen semen, low dose insemination techniques, and other assisted reproductive techniques (ART) such as oocyte transfer and intracytoplasmic sperm injection (ICSI). Adoption of these techniques places pressure on researchers to develop methods of superovulation and better cryopreservation of larger embryos and even oocytes.

ET can be performed on yearling[9] or 2-year-old mares as a method to get them into production 1 or 2 years earlier than traditional breeding. In addition, ET has been used to produce offspring from endangered equids such as the Przewalski's horse, zebras,[10] and the endangered Poitou donkey[11] (Figure 51-1).

MANAGEMENT OF DONORS AND RECIPIENTS

Embryos are usually collected on day 6, 7, or 8 (day 0 is day of ovulation) from naturally single or occasionally multiple ovulations. Embryos are collected 1 day later if the mare has been bred to frozen semen rather than fresh or cooled semen. There is an extremely rapid growth that occurs in the horse embryo from a morula to an expanding blastocyst (day 5 to day 7)[12,13] that results in special characteristics defining embryo development (Figure 51-2).

Day 6 embryos are smaller, harder to harvest, and are the best developmental age for micromanipulation such as bisection[14] or for freezing.[15,16] Day 8 embryos are the largest size that can comfortably fit into a 0.25 ml pipette for transfer.

Factors that affect embryo recovery are age of the mare, semen quality, semen type (fresh, cooled, or frozen), and number of ovulations of the mare.[4]

Mares with a history of establishing pregnancies and then aborting are better candidates than those with a history of repeatedly returning to estrus after breeding, as they most likely will not provide a fertilized egg for recovery from the uterus. We have demonstrated a significantly lower recovery of embryos from mares with a history of infertility compared to normal experimental mares.[4] This is not believed to be due to failure to identify the embryo or differences in fluid recovery. Apparently the poor recovery rates from infertile mares is due to absence of fertilization and/or altered gamete transport (which either prevents spermatozoa from reaching the egg or the fertilized egg from reaching the uterus) or an increased incidence of early embryonic death.[8,17-20] Also, in our experience, multiple embryos per cycle are more frequently recovered from Thoroughbred and Warmblood mares compared to Quarter Horses or Arabian mares. In one study conducted over a total of 59 estrous cycles, a spontaneous multiple ovulation (>2 ovulations) was detected in 56% of cycles. The majority of ovulations occurred the same day (68.6%) or 1 day apart (27%). Embryo recovery 7 days after a single ovulation was 52.8% compared to 10.6% for spontaneously double ovulating mares ($P < 0.001$).[21] Recovery rates for days 7, 8, and 9 post-ovulation were similar, but recovery of embryos on day 6 was slightly lower.[22-25] The lower embryo recovery rate on day 6 may be attributed to (1) failure to identify the embryo in the recovery medium, (2) loss of the embryo during recovery procedure due to its small size, (3) failure to obtain the embryo in the uterine flush because of its greater specific gravity, or (4) failure of some embryos to enter the uterus by day 6. More than likely the latter 2 reasons are of greater significance. In one study involving 27 mares that failed to provide an embryo on day 6.5, 9 established a pregnancy without subsequently being rebred.[26] Some of these pregnancies may have originated from a second ovulation that was not detected and occurred after cessation of palpation at the end of estrus. In another study, 143 embryo recovery attempts were performed on day 6. Ninety-two mares (64%) failed to provide an embryo. Eighty-three mares that failed to provide an embryo were subjected to embryo recovery again on day 7 post-ovulation. The recovery of 18 embryos on day 7 (22%), whose mean development stage (early blastocyst) and size (330 μm) were not significantly different from embryos recovered on day 6, suggested that failure of recovery on day 6 was due to delayed oviductal transport, not flushing technique.[26] Embryo recovery 6.5 days after ovulation in superovulated mares was 1.5 versus 2.6 when these same mares were flushed 7.5 days after ovulation.[27]

Embryo Recovery

Methods of recovery have not varied much from the original description of Imel.[3] A catheter is introduced into the vagina through the cervix and approximately 5 cm into the uterine body. Once in position, the cuff of the catheter is inflated with 60 ml of sterile saline or air. The catheter is then drawn back against the internal os of the cervix to assure a tight seal. A buffered solution (e.g., Dulbeccos phosphate buffered saline) is infused into the uterus (1 to 2 liters at a time) and recovered by gravity through a 75 micron filter. The procedure is repeated at least 3 times but commonly more often (up to 6). A study of how to improve embryo recovery demonstrated that embryos were recovered on the first 3 liters in 31.6% of attempts from 209 client mares. A total of 32 additional embryos were subsequently recovered during the extra flush attempt with 2 additional liters of medium.[28] If the media is clear it may be reused immediately on the same mare. The filtered media is tipped into a search dish and is then examined under 7 to 15× magnification with a stereo dissection microscope.

Occasionally it may be necessary to perform the flush in a mare with her cervix fully dilated and a hand inserted in the uterus. In these cases fluids are difficult to contain

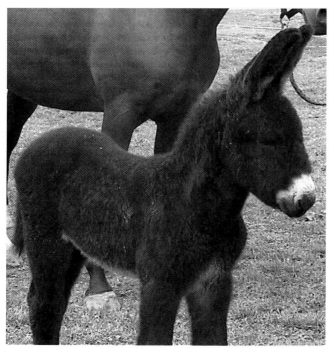

Figure 51-1   The birth of an endangered donkey (Poitou) from ET into a mare.

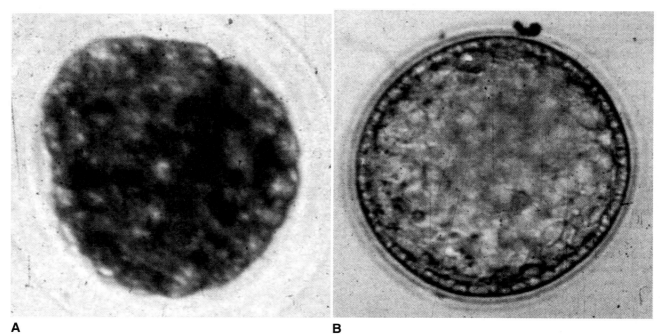

A   **B**

Figure 51-2   **A,** An equine morula. **B,** A day 6.5 equine embryo (expanding blastocyst).

within the uterus. It has been suggested that embryo recovery rates will be improved by allowing some time (3 minutes) from infusion of the first flushing solution until recovery[29] and also after administering oxytocin.

If enough people are available, a considerable time saving may be introduced by searching as the flushing is performed. Ideally the filtered fluids are examined after every 2 liters. Usually the larger embryos (day 8 and 9) can be seen with the naked eye, but the younger embryos (day <8) require use of the microscope. The recovered embryos are washed and graded and then maintained in the culture dish at room temperature until transferred.

Recipient Mares

Proper selection and management of recipient mares is probably the most important factor affecting success of an equine embryo transfer program. Maiden mares or young mares that have a history of producing 1 or 2 foals are preferred as recipients. Clients have a right to expect quiet and well-handled mares as recipients. We prefer recipient mares that weigh 450 to 550 kg, and are 3 to 10 years of age and halter broken. The method of matching recipients with donors in our embryo transfer program may be unique because of the large number of recipient mares we maintain. Usually a donor can be matched with a recipient that has ovulated spontaneously, without using hormones to synchronize their cycle. Where large numbers of recipient mares are not available, synchronization of ovulation can be provided by hormonal therapy (see Chapter 3). It is preferable that at least 2 recipients are available for each donor mare. A full reproductive exam is performed on all mares. Recipient mares should be fed to maintain good body weight and condition. An effort is made to use only those recipients that have experienced 2 or more normal cycles. Recipients are selected that have ovulated 1 day prior (+1) or 0 to 3 days after (0, −1, −2, −3) the donor mare.

Mares that receive an embryo nonsurgically are treated with antibiotics and Regumate for 5 days after transfer. Recipients may be examined with ultrasonography at 11 to 12 days of gestation (4 to 5 days post-transfer).[26,30,31] Mares are reexamined on days 15, 25, 35, 45, and 60 of pregnancy. Embryonic death between day 15 and 60 of gestation appears to be no greater in embryo transfer recipients than in mares inseminated with fresh semen.[32] The influence of the size of the recipient on the ease of foaling and the subsequent size of the foal is an unresolved issue. It certainly is important from the client's perspective that he or she receive a recipient that is big enough to let the foal be born a normal size. The experiments reported of Walton and Hammond[33] and of Tischner[34] are indicative of our philosophy, in that the size and health of the uterus determine the size of the foal at term. This was also supported by work from Newmarket:

The influence of maternal size on foal birthweights and the total microscopic area of fetomaternal contact at the placental interface was studied by comparing placentae from normal Thoroughbred-in-Thoroughbred and Pony-in-Pony control pregnancies with those from between-breed Thoroughbred-in-Pony (deprived in utero environment) and Pony-in-Thoroughbred (luxurious in utero environment) pregnancies created by embryo transfer. Strong positive correlations were revealed between foal birthweight and both the gross area of the placenta and the total microscopic area of fetomaternal contact via the microcotyledons. The results highlight the importance of the intrauterine environment for the growth and development of the equine fetal foal.[35]

A development in the late 1980s in equine embryo transfer was the use of ovariectomized steroid-treated mares as recipients.[36-38] It is necessary before transfer of the embryo to treat the ovariectomized mare with progesterone or progestins (synthetic progesterone-like compounds) for 4 to 7 days before transfer until between day 100 and day 140 of pregnancy (when placental progestogens will maintain pregnancy).[39] Pregnancy rates after surgical transfer into ovariectomized progestin treated mares were similar to intact controls (70%).[38] Parturition and lactation of ovariectomized embryo transfer recipients have been reported to be normal.[40] The use of ovariectomized steroid-treated mares as recipients eliminates the need for synchrony of ovulation between donor and recipient and reduces the number of recipients per donor; however, the need for daily administration of progestins reduces its appeal dramatically. To further demonstrate that the uterus and progesterone were all that were necessary to nourish an equine pregnancy, it was reported that foals were born after ET into mares with gonadal dysgenesis.[41] Early in the breeding season, when mares are not cycling naturally, intact mares can be used as recipients by supplementation with a progestin.

Embryo Transfer

In earlier publications on ET we advocated the use of surgical transfer of equine embryos[4] as various studies on nonsurgical transfer of equine embryos have been attempted by others[7,42-44] with extremely variable results (12.5%-71% pregnancy rates). Currently we restrict the use of surgical transfer to ART (such as ICSI, GIFT, or oocyte transfer) because pregnancy rates have been greater than 75% per embryo transferred at day 15 for more than 8 years using nonsurgical transfer. Many variations of nonsurgical transfer have been reported[45,46]; however, careful management of delicate tissues in standard nonsurgical ET will result in consistent pregnancy rates without the need to grasp novel procedures. Our equipment preference is the Cassou (IMV, L'Aigle, France) ET transfer pipette (0.25 ml straw), which has a sterile disposable outer sheath and a thin plastic wrap (sanitary sleeve) that the transfer pipette pushes through as the cervix is penetrated.

Factors Affecting Pregnancy Rates

The majority of embryo transfers have been performed 6 to 8 days post-ovulation. Limited studies are available addressing the effect of embryo age on pregnancy rate. From results of experiments[22,23,25,47] it appears that the older, larger embryos are less viable in nonsurgical transfer and possibly even surgical transfer. The older embryos

(>8 days), with their increased fluid-volume-to-surface ratio, may not withstand the shock of recovery and transfer to recipients as well as smaller embryos. Despite this, we have produced foals transferring embryos at 10 days of age (Figure 51-3). Once we identify the mare is pregnant using ultrasonography, we then harvest and transfer the embryo. No expensive identification equipment is necessary; however, the catheter used to flush the mare is necessarily large. The first foal from this technique was born at the Goulburn Valley Equine Hospital (GVEH) in 1993. To date the 10-day nonsurgical transferred pregnancy rates are not very encouraging.

As the morphology of the embryo becomes more abnormal, the possibility of a pregnancy resulting from transfer of the embryo decreases.[4] Also interesting is the reported lower pregnancy rates and higher embryonic loss after ET from older mares.[16]

A total of 638 embryo transfers conducted over 3 years was retrospectively examined to determine which factors (recipient, embryo, and/or transfer) significantly influenced pregnancy and embryo loss rates and to determine how rates could be improved:

On Day 7 or 8 after ovulation, embryos (fresh or cooled/transported) were transferred by surgical or nonsurgical techniques into recipients ovulating from 5 to 9 d before transfer. At 12 and 50 d of gestation (Day 0 = day of ovulation), pregnancy rates were 65.7% (419 of 638) and 55.5% (354 of 638). Pregnancy rates on Day 50 were significantly higher for recipients that had excellent to good uterine tone or were graded as "acceptable" during a pretransfer examination, usually performed 5 d after ovulation, versus recipients that had fair to poor uterine tone or were graded "marginally acceptable." Embryonic factors that significantly affected pregnancy rates were morphology grade, diameter and stage of development. The incidence of early embryonic death was 15.5% (65 of 419) from Days 12 to 50. Embryo loss rates were significantly higher in recipients used 7 or 9 d vs 5 or 6 d after ovulation. Embryos with minor morphological changes (Grade 2) resulted in more (P < 0.05) embryo death than embryos with no morphological abnormalities (Grade 1). Between Days 12 and 50, the highest incidence of embryo death occurred during the interval from Days 17 to 25 of gestation. Embryonic vesicles that were imaged with ultrasound during the first pregnancy exam (5 d after transfer) resulted in significantly fewer embryonic deaths than vesicles not imaged until subsequent exams. In the present study, embryo morphology was predictive of the potential for an embryo to result in a viable pregnancy. Delayed development of the embryo upon collection from the donor or delayed development of the embryonic vesicle within the recipient's uterus was associated with a higher incidence of pregnancy failure. Recipient selection (age, day after ovulation, quality on Day 5) significantly affected pregnancy and embryo loss rates.[48]

RELEVANT TECHNOLOGICAL ADVANCES

Embryo Storage

Cooled, transported embryos increase the flexibility of equine ET by allowing major centers to maintain large numbers of recipients for transfer of embryos collected from remote locations.[49] This means that experienced personnel can perform the transfer and that the expenses of maintaining a herd for a small population of donor mares are eliminated. The procedures for cooling and transporting equine embryos were first described in 1987.[50] Originally the transport media described was Ham's F10 with a 5% CO_2 gas mixture to buffer it.[50] The main drawback to this media was the inability to maintain the media in a state ready for use. Preparation of media for cooling or transport of embryos under field conditions would be more practical with the use of a nongassed medium such as Ham's F10 with Hepes buffer. However, day 14 pregnancy rates for embryos transferred surgically after storage in Ham's F10 plus 10% fetal calf serum plus 5% CO_2, 5% O_2, and 90% N_2 for 24 hours at 5°C were better (P < 0.05) (14/20, 70%) than embryos maintained identically but with Hepes buffering of the Ham's F10 media (4/20, 20%).[51] Results from more recent work suggest that other media (EmCare, ICP, Auckland, New Zealand, or Vigro Holding Plus, A-B Technology, Pullman, WA) are also useable.[52-55] These aforementioned commercial media do not have to be gassed and come in small, disposable vials, making them attractive for commercial use.

Embryos are cooled to 5°C in an Equitainer or other form of passive cooling device. Embryos are generally packaged in 4 ml plastic tubes or 0.25 ml straws, sealed, and placed into a larger volume of media to minimize temperature variations.

Pregnancy rates from embryos cooled and transported are similar to transfer of embryos immediately.[56]

The number of embryos transferred after cooling and transport at both our ET centers has been steadily increasing.

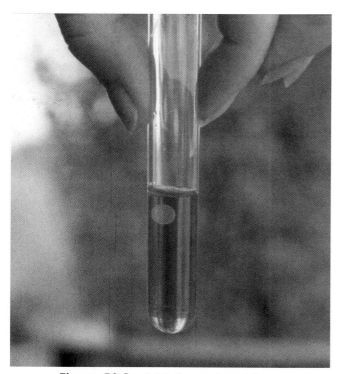

Figure 51-3   A 10-day equine embryo.

Frozen embryo technology has lagged behind other equine ET developments. This may be due in part to a perceived lack of applicability due to the inability to repeatedly harvest multiple embryos and in part to breed registry restrictions on transferring frozen embryos. Technical difficulties with freezing larger embryos may also be a contributing factor. Advantages of freezing embryos include (1) embryos can be stored indefinitely, thus preserving important genetic lines; (2) embryos can be collected from donors and transferred into recipients at a later time, thus minimizing the number of recipients; and (3) embryos can be transported within and exported from countries at our convenience without regard to matching of recipient cycles. Cryopreservation of equine embryos[15,57,58] resulted in reasonable pregnancy rates. Results can be improved further if only embryos at the morula or early blastocyst stage of development are frozen. An interesting development that nicely demonstrates the flexibility of ET is the freezing of equine embryos in the breeding season and successful establishment of pregnancies after transfer in the nonbreeding season into ovariectomized mares treated for 6 days with Regumate before transfer.[59] In these cases, recipients need to be kept on Regumate treatment until at least 100 days of pregnancy.[60]

Techniques involve addition of glycerol in 1 or 2 steps to a final concentration of 10%. Other cryoprotectants such as 1,2-propanediol and ethylene glycol have been examined.[61,62] Numerous studies have been published with the following general conclusions consistently reported.[59,61-64] Success from cryopreservation of larger embryos is still not commercially viable. The protocol first reported by Slade et al[15] is quite efficacious for embryos less than 200 μm and can be modified to remove glycerol in 3 steps (inclusive of 10% sucrose).

Expected pregnancy rates from smaller embryos (late morulas and early blastocysts, i.e., <300 microns) after freeze-thaw is around 70%.[15,65,66] Success with larger, expanded blastocysts (>300 microns) is much less, at around 10% to 20%.[15,58,59] One study reported good pregnancy rates from larger embryos at 57%.[66] The exact reason for failure of large embryos to survive the freeze-thaw process is not currently known, although it possibly relates to differences in permeability to cryoprotectants at different embryo ages,[61] which is probably related to the capsule[64,67] and the recognition that the inner cell mass cells are more susceptible to damage during cryopreservation than the trophectoderm.[68]

Recent research on equine embryo preservation has concentrated on vitrification of embryos.[69] Vitrification is explained well by the following quotation.

The failure of complex mammalian organs, such as the kidney, to function following freezing to low temperatures is thought to be due largely to mechanical disruption of the intercellular architecture by the formation of extracellular ice. Classical approaches to the avoidance of ice formation through the imposition of ultra-rapid cooling and warming rates or by gradual depression of the equilibrium freezing point during cooling to −80 degrees C have not been adequate. An alternative approach relies on the ability of highly concentrated aqueous solutions of cryoprotective agents to supercool to very low temperatures. At sufficiently low temperatures, these solutions become so viscous that they solidify without the formation of ice, a process termed vitrification. When embryo suspensions are cryopreserved using conventional procedures, this supercooling behaviour allows intracellular vitrification, even in the presence of extracellular ice. We have therefore used mouse embryos to examine the feasibility of obtaining high survival following vitrification of both the intra- and extracellular solutions and report here that in properly controlled conditions embryos seem to survive in high proportions after cryopreservation in the absence of ice.[70]

Theoretically, vitrification will result in more time efficiency and does not involve expensive computer-controlled freezing rate equipment.[69] Initial studies with vitrification were quite promising, with demonstration of similar pregnancy rates from open pulled straw systems and a cryoloop versus conventional techniques:

The open pulled straw (OPS) and cryoloop have been used for very rapid cooling and warming rates. The objective of this experiment was to compare efficacy of vitrification of embryos in OPS and the cryoloop to conventional slow cool procedures using 0.25 mL straws. Grade 1 or 2 morulae and early blastocysts (< or = 300 microm in diameter) were recovered from mares on Day 6 or 7 post ovulation. Twenty-seven embryos were assigned to three cryopreservation treatments: (1) conventional slow cooling (0.5 degrees C/min) with 1.8 M ethylene glycol (EG) and 0.1 M sucrose, (4) vitrification in OPS in 16.5% EG, 16.5% DMSO and 0.5 M sucrose, or (3) vitrification with a cryoloop in 17.5% EG, 17.5% DMSO, 1 M sucrose and 0.25 microM ficoll. Embryos were evaluated for size and morphological quality (Grade 1 to 4) before freezing, after thawing, and after culture for 20 h. In addition, propidium iodide (PI) and Hoechst 33342 staining were used to assess percent live cells after culture. There were no differences (P > 0.1) in morphological grade or percent live cells among methods. Mean grades for embryos after culture were 2.9 +/− 0.2, 3.1 +/− 0.1, and 3.3 +/− 0.2 for conventional slow cooling, OPS and cryoloop methods, respectively. Embryo grade and percent live cells were correlated, r = 0.66 (P < 0.004). Thus OPS and the cryoloop were similarly effective to conventional slow-cooling procedures for cryopreserving small equine embryos.[71]

This and other studies have utilized embryo culture and laboratory techniques to assess embryo viability.[71-73]

A more recent report has demonstrated the applicability of vitrification to early equine embryos by transferring embryos into recipients:

In a preliminary study (Experiment 1), embryos were exposed in three steps to vitrification solutions containing increasing concentrations of ethylene glycol and glycerol (EG/G); the final vitrification solution was 3.4 M glycerol + 4.6 M ethylene glycol in a base medium of phosphate-buffered saline. Embryos were warmed in a two-step dilution and transferred into uteri of recipients. No pregnancies were observed after transfer of *blastocysts >300 μm (n = 3). Transfer of morulae or blastocysts <= 300 μm resulted in four embryonic vesicles (4/6, 67%). In a second experiment, embryo recovery per ovulation was similar for collections on Day 6 (28/36, 78%) versus Days 7 and 8 (30/48, 62%). Embryos <= 300 and >300 μm were vitrified, thawed and transferred as in Experiment 1. Some embryos <300 μm were also transferred using a direct-transfer procedure (DT). Embryo development rates to Day 16 were not different for embryos <= 300 μm that were treated as in Experiment 1 (10/22, 46%) or transferred by DT (16/26, 62%). Embryos >300 μm (n = 19) did not produce embryonic vesicles.[69]*

Recently, 20 embryos were transferred that had been cooled for 12 to 19 hours, then vitrified. Thirteen of 20 (65%) mares became pregnant compared to 15 of 20 pregnancies from embryos vitrified immediately after collection.[28] Clearly this study has supported the potential of on-farm embryo collection followed by transport to a facility capable of handling vitrification.

Superovulation

Some of the advantages of superovulation would be (1) the possibility for collection of multiple embryos, (2) higher pregnancy rates per embryo recovery attempt, (3) an increase in the number of embryos available to freeze, and (4) an increase in the number of preovulatory follicles that may enable harvesting of more in vivo matured oocytes. Other benefits not strictly related to ET would be improving pregnancy rate from problem breeders and better pregnancy rates from subfertile stallions[74] or from frozen semen from some stallions. Even an increase in the number of pregnancies per cycle would be a huge boon to the breeding industry, providing sophisticated techniques of twin or multiple vesicle elimination where available.[74] Some of the problems are (1) inconsistency in number of mares responding to superovulation treatments, (2) lack of availability of commercial superovulatory drugs, (3) considerable cost of the superovulation treatment, and (4) possible lowered viability of multiple embryos.

In cattle, sheep, and a variety of nondomestic species, treatment with equine chorionic gonadotropin (eCG, initially known as pregnant mare serum gonadotropin [PMSG]) or FSH reliably induces multiple ovulation and has improved the efficiency of ET. The horse is extremely refractory to stimulation with eCG. Some treatments attempted to induce superovulation in horses, and their results are listed below.

Gonadotropin-Releasing Hormone (GnRH)
GnRH has been reported to induce ovulation in seasonally anestrus mares[75-77]; however it has been demonstrated to be ineffective in cycling mares during the regular breeding season for induction of multiple ovulation.[78,79]

Equine Pituitary Extract (EPE)
EPE is a crude pituitary extract obtained from extraction[80] of abattoir-derived pituitaries containing 6% to 10% LH and 2% to 4% FSH. It has been clearly demonstrated that multiple ovulation can be induced in both seasonally anovulatory and cycling mares with EPE.[81-85] However, the induction of ovulation in the seasonally anovulatory mare is impractical because a large number of those mares fail to continue to cycle after the induced ovulation and if they become pregnant fail to maintain the corpus luteum (CL). In addition, effective doses of pituitary extract for induction of multiple ovulation are higher in anovulatory mares. Pituitary extract administered during diestrus for a period of approximately 1 week appears to be an effective means of inducing multiple ovulation in cycling mares. However, ovulation rates are quite low in comparison to those obtained in cattle, usually ranging from 2 to 4 ovulations per mare. A more refined form of EPE has just become available (see FSH below). There are two questions, however, that have not been adequately resolved. Are multiple ovulations associated with a reduced number of embryos per ovulation? Are they reduced in viability? It is most likely that the reduced number of embryos (embryos/ovulation) is related to those mares that have multiple ovulations on the same ovary. In relation to viability, although it was suggested that reduction in viability of multiple embryos occurred by one group,[84,85] much of this was recorded before ultrasonography. Subsequent experiments[21] refuted earlier work and encouraged the use of embryos collected from superovulatory programs. One study[86] was able to show that fertilization rates and embryonic development from oviductal embryos collected from either EPE-treated mares or controls were identical. Purification of EPE by removing luteinizing hormone (LH) has not resulted in an improvement in ovulations or embryo recovery rate.[87,88] A pregnancy rate of 70% was reported for embryos collected from superovulated mares after vitrification and transfer.[28] The superovulation response was increased by increasing the frequency of administration,[89] and this was subsequently shown to be associated with the total dose of EPE:

Mares receiving 50 mg of EPE once daily developed a greater number (P = 0.008) of preovulatory follicles than the remaining groups of EPE-treated mares, and more (P = 0.06) ovulations were detected for mares receiving 25 mg EPE twice daily compared to those receiving either 25 mg EPE once daily and 12.5 mg EPE twice daily.[90]

Although the response is much lower than seen in cattle, sheep, and humans, the horse does have the ability to respond to FSH (in the form of EPE). On average it can be expected that the response will be approximately 3 to 4 times the normal ovulation rate.

FSH
Early studies on the use of FSH[91] demonstrated a mean ovulation rate for FSH-P (porcine FSH) treated mares of 1.7 ± 0.6 versus 1.0 for controls. Another study found that FSH-P was not as efficient as equine pituitary extract (EPE), with ovulation rates of 2.2 for EPE, 1.6 for FSH, and 1.0 for controls.[92] Dosages of FSH were between 150 and 200 mg as often as twice daily in mid to late diestrus. A study from Cornell University[92] showed an ovulation rate of 1.80, 1.54, and 1.50 for mares treated with 8, 16, or 32 mg purified porcine FSH (Folltropin) compared to 1.2

for the controls. Injections were given twice daily from day 6 (PGF$_{2\alpha}$ on day 6) until follicles greater than or equal to 40 mm were detected. Unfortunately, the next season the ovulation rates for the lowest effective dose, when studied in more detail, were not different from controls.[93]

Recently a commercial form of equine FSH has been released onto the market as eFSH (Bioniche Animal Health USA, Inc., Athens, GA). It has already been demonstrated as useful in increasing ovulation and embryo recovery rates:

The objective of this study was to evaluate the efficacy of purified equine follicle stimulating hormone (eFSH) in inducing superovulation in cycling mares. In the first experiment, 49 normal, cycling mares were used in a study at Colorado State University. Mares were assigned to 1 of 3 groups: group 1, controls (n = 29) and groups 2 and 3, eFSH-treated (n = 10/group). Treated mares were administered 25 mg of eFSH twice daily beginning 5 or 6 days after ovulation (group 2). Mares received 250 cloprostenol on the second day of eFSH treatment. Administration of eFSH continued until the majority of follicles reached a diameter of 35 rum, at which time a deslorelin implant was administered. Group 3 mares (n = 10) received 12 mg of eFSH twice daily starting on day 5 or 6. The treatment regimen was identical to that of group 2. Mares in all 3 groups were bred with semen from 1 of 4 stallions. Pregnancy status was determined at 14 to 16 days after ovulation. In experiment 2, 16 light-horse mares were used during the physiologic breeding season in Brazil. On the first cycle, mares served as controls, and on the second cycle, mares were administered 12 mg of eFSH twice daily until a majority of follicles were 35 turn in diameter, at which time human chorionic gonadotropin (hCG) was administered. Mares were inseminated on both cycles, and embryo collection attempts were performed 7 or 8 days after ovulation. Mares treated with 25 mg of eFSH developed a greater number of follicles (35 mm) and ovulated a greater number of follicles than control mares. However, the number of pregnancies obtained per mare was not different between control mares and those receiving 25 mg of eFSH twice daily. Mares treated with 12 mg of eFSH and administered either hCG or deslorelin also developed more follicles than untreated controls. Mares receiving eFSH followed by hCG ovulated a greater number of follicles than control mares, whereas the number of ovulations from mares receiving eFSH followed by deslorelin was similar to that of control mares. Pregnancy rate for mares induced to ovulate with hCG was higher than that of control mares, whereas the pregnancy rate for eFSH-treated mares induced to ovulate with deslorelin did not differ from that of the controls. Overall, 80% of mares administered eFSH had multiple ovulations compared with 10.3% of the control mares. In experiment 2, the number of large follicles was greater in the eFSH-treated cycle than the previous untreated cycle. In addition, the number of ovulations during the cycle in which mares were treated with eFSH was greater (3.6) than for the control cycle (1.0). The average number of embryos recovered per mare for the eFSH cycle (1.9 +/- 0.3) was greater than the embryo recovery rate

for the control cycle (0.5 +/- 0.3). In summary, the highest ovulation and the highest pregnancy and embryo recovery rates were obtained after administration of 12 mg of eFSH twice daily followed by 2500 IU of hCG. Superovulation with eFSH increased pregnancy rate and embryo recovery rate and, thus, the efficiency of the embryo transfer program.[94]

Another study with eFSH showed consistent embryo recovery and multiple ovulation:

Administration of 12.5 mg of eFSH twice daily until follicles were = 33 mm followed by hCG 30 hr later, provided the highest ovulation rate and embryo recovery. Averaged across both cycles, 85% of mares had = 2 ovulations/cycle and the average embryo recovery per flush was 2.0 embryos. Embryo recovery per ovulation was similar to that obtained in untreated experimental mares (55 to 65% per ovulation). Thus, embryo recovery from eFSH-treated mares was 3 to 4 times higher than what one would expect from untreated, single-ovulating mares.[27]

Similarly, no matter how treatments were administered, eFSH has provided good ovulation rates:

Cycling mares (n = 40) were randomly assigned to 1 of 4 groups 7 days after ovulation: (1) 12.5 mg eFSH twice daily until half the cohort of follicles were greater than 35 mm; (2) 12.5 mg eFSH twice daily until half the cohort of follicles were greater than 32 mm; (3) 12.5 mg eFSH twice daily for 3.5 days followed by 12.5 mg eFSH enriched with LH twice daily until half the cohort of follicles was greater than 35 mm; (4) 25 mg eFSH once daily until half the cohort of follicles were greater than 32 mm. Mares in groups 1 and 3 were injected with hCG (2500 IU intravenously) at the end of eFSH treatment, while mares in groups 2 and 4 were administered hCG approximately 42 and 54 hr following the last eFSH treatment, respectively. Each mare experienced a non-treated estrous cycle before being randomly re-assigned to a second treatment. Ovulation rate for the pre-treatment control was 1.1 ± 0.2 and for mares in treatment groups 1 to 4 3.3 ± 1.3, 4.1 ± 1.9, 3.5 ± 2.0, and 2.8 ± 1.4, respectively. Overall, ovulation rate in eFSH treated mares was 3.4 ± 1.7 ovulations per cycle. One or more embryos were recovered from >80% of mares in each treatment group, and embryo recovery rate per flush was similar among treatment groups (1.9 ± 1.2, 2.6 ± 1.9, 1.9 ± 1.4 and 1.8 ± 1.5, respectively; P > 0.05). The overall embryo recovery rate was 2.1 ± 1.5 embryos per flush. In summary, ovulation rate was higher for mares treated with eFSH compared to non-treated controls. Ovulation rate in mares in which hCG was delayed (follicle coasting) was higher (P<0.05) when treatments were given twice a day versus once per day. There were no differences in embryo recovery rates among treatment groups. Administration of eLH in conjunction with eFSH did not have an advantage over mares treated with only eFSH.[95]

eFSH has also been demonstrated efficacious for hastening the transition period in mares,[96] although studies on maintenance of the CL still must be performed.

Inhibin Vaccination

Inhibin is produced by the granulosa cells of the dominant follicle. It serves to suppress FSH production. It is inversely related to FSH at all stages of the cycle. Increasing FSH through inhibin immunisation has increased ovulation rates in cattle and sheep vaccinated against either the ovine or bovine alpha subunit of inhibin, respectively. The GVEH were first to report on using inhibin immunisation to increase ovulation rates in mares.[74] Mares were immunized on day 0 and 35. Ovulation rates preimmunization and in the control groups were 1.2 per cycle. Between the 2 vaccinations, ovulations were 1.86 and rose to 2.29 in the cycle after immunization. All mares either double or triple ovulated.[74] This observation was confirmed by workers in California[97] who vaccinated normally cycling mares at 3-week intervals, 5 times. Similar results occurred, and, in addition, embryos were recovered at the rate of 1.6 versus 0.7 per cycle in immunized versus control mares, respectively. In a later study, passive immunization against inhibin did increase ovulation rate; however, it was not as high as active immunization and had other attendant side effects such as hypersensitivity and, on one occasion, death.[98] Although immunization against inhibin has been successful, it was not able to produce large numbers of ovulations. To our knowledge it is not being actively researched.

Embryo or Gamete Manipulations

Embryo Splitting

Embryo bisection to create identical twins is useful for research into diseases that have an inherited basis with an environmental predisposition such as osteochondritis dessicans (OCD) and other forms of developmental orthopedic disease (DOD). Matched full siblings would remove much of the inherent genetic variation. Commonly 1 twin is used as a control, and the other is assigned to a specific treatment. The reduction in numbers of experimental animals decreases costs and unnecessary animal experimentation. Another reason to bisect equine embryos is the production of almost perfectly matched twins as show or carriage animals. A further reason would be to improve the overall number of pregnancies from a given number of embryos. In cattle the technique results in approximately 50% more pregnancies than transfer of single, nonmanipulated embryos with approximately 20% production of identical (monozygotic) twins.[98] Early attempts to create identical twins were successful, with embryos recovered from the oviduct, but were quite time and labor intensive.[99] Two pairs of identical twins were obtained from 13 demi and 17 quarter embryos.[99] Workers at Colorado State University were first to obtain identical twin pregnancies from nonsurgically recovered day 5.5 or 6 embryos.[24] Another study at CSU[14] demonstrated that the zona pellucida was not necessary for the continuing development of bisected embryos in vivo and the complex, expensive, and sophisticated micro-manipulation equipment was not necessary. These workers showed that pregnancy rates per original embryo were decreased (14/30) compared to the nonmanipulated embryos (12/15) and that 5 pairs of identical twins could be obtained from 30 embryos (1:6 ratio). Only morulae and early blastocysts were split in this experiment. In England, 2 sets of identical twins were obtained from 14 embryos bisected.[100] It was interesting to note that 0/16 demi embryos from blastocysts established a pregnancy compared to 8/12 demi embryos from morulae. To our knowledge the successes reported above have not been improved upon, and this is probably responsible for the limited usefulness of the technique.

Oocyte Retrieval

For a variety of reasons, gamete research in the horse has lagged behind species such as cattle. Equine researchers have thus benefited from the information explosion associated with other species, including human programs. In cattle, the in vitro maturation of oocytes from immature follicles harvested from either slaughterhouse-collected ovaries or by trans-vaginal ultrasonographic guided ovum pick up (OPU) has become a routine procedure. A recent report on OPU in cattle demonstrated that over a 6-month period it was possible for 16% of immature oocytes to develop to a transferable embryo stage, and a pregnancy rate of 40% was obtained. This was associated with the production of about 50 calves in a 6-month period, which is a 4-fold increase over the expected annual production with standard ET techniques.

Initial studies in the horse concentrated on in vivo matured oocyte collection, and most were performed through the flank in the standing mare by aspiration through large bore needles of follicular fluid while the follicle was held in situ per rectum.[101-104] Oocyte recovery rates of 6/18 (33.3%),[101] 45/63 (71.4%),[102] 11/36 (30.5%),[104] and 9/16 (56.3%)[103] were reported, respectively. Other techniques such as colpotomy were also described[105] but were not associated with an improved recovery (9/13 in hCG-stimulated mares compared to 15/21 in nonstimulated follicles) and were abandoned.

Subsequently, mature oocyte collection has been performed with a transvaginal ultrasound-guided approach.[106-109] At CSU, 99 preovulatory follicles yielded a total of 62 oocytes (63%). The best results were obtained from use of a 12 gauge double lumen continuous flushing device (36/43, 84%).[108] During diestrus recovery rates were low (71/323, 22%) and were not affected by the type of needle.[108] The procedure has also been successful in recovering oocytes from mares that have been superovulated[108] and early pregnant mares.[110] Immature oocytes are much more difficult to obtain due to their close association to the granulosa cells.[108] They are best obtained from slaughterhouse ovaries by dissection of the follicle and gentle scraping of the surface[111,112]; however, there are numerous reports of their recovery with OPU.[113,114]

Oocyte Transfer

Old mares that fail to provide embryos for transfer are ideal candidates for techniques wherein fertilization occurs elsewhere (i.e., in the oviduct of another mare). Oocyte transfer (OT) involves collection of an oocyte from a donor mare and transfer of the oocyte into a recipient mare's oviduct. The oocyte is either matured in vivo and collected from a preovulatory follicle or collected during diestrus and matured in vitro. The recipient is inseminated so that fertilization and embryonic development occur within the oviduct and uterus. Transfer of in vivo matured oocytes into the oviduct of a recipient mare already bred was first reported in 1988.[102] Fifteen oocytes were transferred, and 2 days later, 3 fertilized oocytes were identified from a total of 10 recovered (30%). These were transferred, and 2 established pregnancies, with 1 producing a live foal.[102] The technique has numerous advantages for those mares that fail to provide embryos by standard methods. Because it involves more physiological techniques than IVF, it is commercially applicable[102] and the equipment necessary is much less sophisticated.[101] The main drawback is the need to recover the recipient's own oocyte that she may have ovulated. In cases where this is not possible, the identity of the foal will be in question until confirmed with blood or DNA typing. A variation was reported in England,[115] with in vitro maturation of immature oocytes before transferring them into oviducts of bred recipients. The ability of in vivo matured oocytes to be fertilized in oviducts of young fertile mares was compared for young fertile mares and old infertile mares.[8] They found that more ($P < 0.005$) oocytes were fertilized and developed from young mares (11/12, 92%) compared to old mares (8/26, 31%) and hypothesized that it was the oocyte of the older mare, not the oviduct, that caused the problem of infertility.[8] Another study reported lower pregnancy rates (2/26, 7.7%).[116] However, it has been proposed that a commercial application for OT should be forthcoming[117] based on 6 of 8 transferred oocytes establishing a pregnancy.

Generally in vivo matured oocytes are harvested within a few hours of ovulation. Two studies, however, confirmed that collection at 24 hours after stimulation with hCG (i.e., 12 hours from the expected time of ovulation) was capable of providing normal pregnancy rates.[118,119] This may be a better technique because it is less likely that the follicle will have ovulated compared to the technique that calls for waiting close to the expected ovulation time (36 ± 4 hours with hCG and 41 ± 3 hours with Ovuplant).[119]

Many studies attest to the benefit of transferring in vivo versus in vitro matured oocytes:

Objectives of the present study were to use oocyte transfer: 1) to compare the developmental ability of oocytes collected from ovaries of live mares with those collected from slaughterhouse ovaries; and 2) to compare the viability of oocytes matured in vivo, in vitro, or within the oviduct. Oocytes were collected by transvaginal, ultrasound-guided follicular aspiration (TVA) from live mares or from slicing slaughterhouse ovaries. Four groups of oocytes were transferred into the oviducts of recipients that were inseminated: 1) oocytes matured in vivo and collected by TVA from preovulatory follicles of estrous mares 32 to 36 h after administration of hCG; 2) immature oocytes collected from diestrous mares between 5 and 10 d after aspiration/ovulation by TVA and matured in vitro for 36 to 38 h; 3) immature oocytes collected from diestrous mares between 5 and 10 d after aspiration/ovulation by TVA and transferred into a recipient's oviduct <1 h after collection; and 4) immature oocytes collected from slaughterhouse ovaries containing a corpus luteum and matured in vitro for 36 to 38 hours. Embryo development rates were higher (P < 0.001) for oocytes matured in vivo (82%) than for oocytes matured in vitro (9%) or within the oviduct (0%). However, neither the method of maturation nor the source of oocytes affected (P > 0.1) embryo development rates after the transfer of immature oocytes.[114]

A summary of the current applications to oocyte transfer appears below:

In some mares with lesions of the reproductive tract, embryo collection and survival rates are low or collection of embryos is not feasible. For these mares, oocyte transfer has been proposed as a method to induce pregnancies. In this report, a method for oocyte transfer in mares and results of oocyte transfer performed over 2 breeding seasons, using mares with long histories of subfertility and various reproductive lesions, are described. Human chorionic gonadotropin or an implant containing a gonadotropin-releasing hormone analog was used to initiate follicular and oocyte maturation. Oocytes were collected by means of transvaginal ultrasound-guided follicular aspiration. Following follicular aspiration, cumulus oocyte complexes were evaluated for cumulus expansion and signs of atresia; immature oocytes were cultured in vitro to allow maturation. The recipient's ovary and uterine tube (oviduct) were exposed through a flank laparotomy with the horse standing, and the oocyte was slowly deposited within the oviduct. Oocyte transfer was attempted in 38 mares between 9 and 30 years old during 2 successive breeding seasons. All mares had a history of reproductive failure while in breeding and embryo transfer programs. Twenty pregnancies were induced. Fourteen of the pregnant mares delivered live foals. Results suggest that oocyte transfer can be a successful method for inducing pregnancy in subfertile mares in a commercial setting.[120]

Oocyte transfer is a potential method to produce offspring from valuable mares that cannot carry a pregnancy or produce embryos. From 2000 through 2004, 86 mares, 19.2 +/– 0.4 yr of age (mean +/– S.E.M.), were used as oocyte donors in a clinical program at Colorado State University. Oocytes were collected from 77% (548/710) of preovulatory follicles and during 96% (548/570) of cycles. Oocytes were collected 21.0 +/– 0.1h after administration of hCG to estrous donors and cultured 16.4 +/– 0.2h prior to transfer into recipients' oviducts. At 16 and 50 d after transfer, pregnancies were detected in 201 of 504 (40%) and 159 of 504 (32%) of recipients, respectively, with an embryo-loss rate of 21% (42/201). Pregnancy rates were similar (P > 0.05) for cyclic and noncyclic recipients and for recipients inseminated with cooled, fresh or frozen semen. One or more recipients were detected pregnant at 16 and 50 d, respectively, for 80% (69/86) and 71% (61/86) of donors. More donors <20 than >/=20 yr (mean ages +/– S.E.M. of 15.5 +/– 0.4 and 23.0 +/– 0.3 yr, respectively) tended (P=0.1) to have one or more pregnant recipients at 50 d (36/45, 80%; 28/45, 62%, respectively). Results of the program confirm that pregnancies can consistently be obtained from older, subfertile mares using oocyte transfer.[121]

Another application for oocyte transfer is the production of foals after in vitro maturation of immature oocytes from mares that have died.[122]

In Vitro Oocyte Maturation

Immature oocytes for maturation studies have traditionally been recovered from slaughterhouses or ovariectomy, until the advent of equine OPU.[112] It is possible that the future of equine IVF in the horse will be related to in vitro maturation (IVM) studies because in vivo matured oocytes are expensive (one per cycle) and time consuming to obtain. Fertilization but not pregnancy has been obtained from IVM oocytes[115,123-125] subjected to IVF. The problem may be associated with the culture of the oocytes or capacitation of the spermatozoa (necessary for penetration and fertilization).[126,127] ICSI replaces the current techniques involving difficult capacitation procedures and will ultimately result in embryos developed from infertile stallions and infertile mares.[128] In time it is expected that in vitro matured oocytes will be routinely fertilized and transferred, resulting in multiple pregnancies per oocyte collection attempt.

In Vitro Fertilization

The first foal born from IVF was born in France on June 14, 1990.[129] A few years later the same laboratory repeated the feat. Unfortunately another foal has not been forthcoming in any laboratory anywhere in the world. This highlights the difficulty of obtaining IVF foals in the horse.[130] The procedure is well documented in humans and cattle. The horse has a zona pellucida that seems very resistant to sperm penetration or spermatozoa that are very difficult to capacitate. Most successful fertilization under IVF conditions in the horse has revolved around the use of a toxic agent, calcium ionophore A23187.[126] This ionophore dramatically reduces the life of spermatozoa. Another difficulty that holds back progress in this area is the lack of a suitable number of in vivo matured oocytes. The two major barriers to successful in vitro fertilization are oocyte maturation and sperm capacitation.

Intracytoplasmic Sperm Injection

Successful ICSI has been reported in the horse.[131] In this experiment, 4 injected eggs from slaughterhouse oocytes were transferred into the oviduct of recipient mares and 1 pregnancy established and resulted in the first ICSI foal. More recently we have obtained foals from ICSI with a different approach.[128] We obtained in vivo matured oocytes and injected them with a single frozen sperm. Two foals were born from this procedure in 1998. The most important demonstration of the later technique was that the procedure has been shown to be repeatable and the eggs were collected from live cycling mares. After the report of foals from ICSI by CSU and GVEH, other foals were born.[132] This is quite exciting because it bypasses capacitation procedures to help the sperm penetrate the zona pellucida. We expect the immediate future of IVF to involve ICSI of either in vitro or in vivo matured oocytes.

Recently some interesting things have happened with ICSI. First is the following report that activation of the oocyte may improve fertilization rates:

The effects of four reagents on the activation and subsequent fertilization of equine oocytes, and the development of these after intracytoplasmic sperm injection, were investigated. Cumulus-oocyte complexes collected from equine ovaries obtained from an abattoir were matured in vitro for 40-44 h in TCM199 medium before being injected, when in metaphase II, with an immobilized stallion spermatozoon. The cumulus-oocyte complexes were then subjected to one of five activation treatments: (a) 10 μ mol ionomycin l(-1) for 10 min; Co) 7% (v/v) ethanol for 10 min; (c) 100 μ mol thimerosal l(-1) for 10 min; (d) 250 μ mol inositol 1,4,5-triphosphate l(-1) injection; and (e) no treatment (control). After 18-20 h further culture, the cumulus-oocyte complexes were assessed for activation by observing whether they had progressed through second anaphase-telophase and had formed a female pronucleus. The proportions of oocytes activated after each treatment were: 16/27 (59%) for ionomycin; 14/25 (56%) for ethanol; 22/28 (79%) for thimerosal; 15/27 (56%) for inositol 1,4,5-triphosphate; and 0/20 (0%) for the untreated controls. Thus, significantly more oocytes (P < 0.05) were activated by treatment with thimerosal than by the other four treatments. The proportions of oocytes that cleaved to the two-cell stage at 24-30 h after sperm injection in the groups treated with ionomycin, ethanol and thimerosal were 7/20 (35%), 5/19 (26%) and 11/23 (48%), respectively. No cleavage was observed in any of the control oocytes or those treated with inositol 1,4,5-triphosphate. Furthermore, evidence of normal fertilization was observed in 2/7 (29%), 2/5 (40%) and 7/11 (64%) of the oocytes treated with ionomycin, ethanol and thimerosal, respectively. These results demonstrated that: (a) it is possible to activate equine oocytes with the chemical stimulants, ionomycin, ethanol, thimerosal and inositol 1,4,5-triphosphate; (b) thimerosal is more effective than the other three reagents in facilitating both meiotic activation and normal fertilization of equine oocytes; and (c) chemical activation may also stimulate parthenogenetic cleavage of oocytes without concurrent changes in the head of the spermatozoon.[133]

Second is a report again from Newmarket that ICSI of IVM oocytes that are then cultured to the blastocyst stage can result in pregnancies:

The influence of co-culture with either oviduct epithelial cells or fetal fibroblast cells on in vitro maturation of equine oocytes and their potential for development to blastocysts and fetuses after intracytoplasmic sperm injection (ICSI) was investigated. The oocytes were obtained from ovaries from abattoirs and were matured in vitro for 2~30 h in TCM199 only, or in TCM199 co-culture with oviduct epithelial cells or fetal fibroblast cells. Metaphase II oocytes were subjected to ICSI with an ionomycin-treated spermatozoon. The injected oocytes were cultured for 7-9 days in Dulbecco's modified Eagle's medium. Morphologically normal early blastocysts were transferred to the uteri of recipient mares. Nuclear maturation rates and the rates of cleavage to the two cell stage for injected oocytes were similar in the groups of oocytes that were matured in TCM 199 (49 and 63%), *in co-culture with oviduct epithelial cells (53 and 65%) or in co-culture with fetal fibroblasts (51 and 57%). There were no significant differences in the proportions of blastocysts that developed from the two cell embryos derived from oocytes matured by co-culture with either oviduct epithelial cells (30%) or fetal fibroblasts (17%). However, significantly higher proportions of blastocysts were produced from both these co-culture groups than from the groups of oocytes matured in TCM199 only (P< 0.05). Six of the blastocysts that had developed from oocytes co-cultured with oviduct epithelial cells were transferred into recipient mares and four pregnancies resulted. These results demonstrate a beneficial influence of co-culture with either oviduct epithelial cells or fetal fibroblasts for maturation of oocytes in vitro.[134]*

Xenogenous Fertilization

Apparently, attempted fertilization in the oviduct of another species of animal has only been reported twice.[102,135] Transfer of in vivo matured oocytes and equine semen into rabbits was not reported to be successful; however, the techniques were crude and the numbers performed quite small.[136] Transfer of in vitro matured oocytes with spermatozoa has resulted in fertilization:

The in vitro production (IVP) of equine embryos using currently available protocols has met limited success; therefore investigations into alternative approaches to IVP are justified. The objective of this study was to evaluate the feasibility of xenogenous fertilization and early embryo development of in vitro matured (IVM) equine oocytes. Follicular aspirations followed by slicing of ovarian tissue were performed on 202 equine ovaries obtained from an abattoir. A total of 667 oocytes (3.3 per ovary) were recovered from 1023 follicles (recovery rate, 65%). Oocytes underwent IVM for 41 +/- 2 h (mean +/- S.D.), before being subjected to xenogenous gamete intrafallopian transfer (XGIFT). An average of 13 +/- 0.8 oocytes and 40 × 10(3) spermatozoa per oocyte were transferred into 20 oviducts of ewes. Fourteen percent of transferred oocytes (36/259) were recovered between 2 and 7 days post-XGIFT and 36% of those recovered displayed embryonic development ranging from the 2-cell to the blastocyst stage. Fertilization following XGIFT was also demonstrated by the detection of zinc finger protein Y (ZFY) loci. Ligation of the uterotubal junction (UTJ), ovarian structures, or the duration of oviductal incubation did not significantly affect the frequency of embryonic development or recovery of oocytes/embryos after XGIFT. In conclusion, equine embryos can be produced in a smaller non-equine species that is easier for handling.[135]

Intrafollicular Transfer of Immature Equine Oocytes

Instead of transferring the oocytes to the oviduct as in oocyte transfer, another technique reported is to transfer immature oocytes to the follicle of another horse. If this horse is bred, then the possibility exists to collect multiple embryos from the recipient mare and then transfer them into subsequent recipients. The genetics of the foals can be sorted out at a later date. The first embryos produced by this technique were reported from Tufts University.[137] They transferred 146 oocytes into 12 mares and recovered 18 embryos from 6 mares and no embryos from 6 mares. Embryos in excess of the number of ovulations were obtained in four mares (excess embryos of 1, 2, 3, and 6). It was interesting to note that most (127) oocytes were immature and that the only recipient to receive expanded oocytes (n = 6) was the one that provided the 6 excess embryos. The relatively low success as a method to mature immature oocytes suggests that oocytes may need more time in the follicle before ovulation (most mares ovulated around 40 hours after transfer) or that they had been collected from atretic follicles.

Low Dose Insemination

The recent work in Newmarket[138] on pregnancies from extremely low numbers of spermatozoa is quite exciting. Pregnancies have been obtained routinely with as little as 1 million sperm.

Mares were inseminated with motile spermatozoa suspended in 30-150 mu l Tyrode's medium directly onto the uterotubal papilla at the anterior tip of the uterine horn, ipsilateral to the ovary containing a dominant pre-ovulatory follicle of greater than or equal to 35 mm in diameter, by means of a fine gamete intrafallopian transfer (GIFT) catheter passed through the working channel of a strobed light videoendoscope. Insemination of 10, 8, 25, 14, 11 and 10 mares with, respectively, 10.0, 5.0, 1.0, 0.5, 0.1 or 0.001 × 10(6) motile spermatozoa resulted in conception rates of, respectively, 60, 75, 64, 29, 22 and 10%. Deposition of $1.0 × 10^6$ motile spermatozoa onto the uterotubal papilla began to approach the limit of successful fertilization. These doses are far lower than the 3-15 × 10(9) spermatozoa normally ejaculated by fertile stallions during mating, and the accepted minimum dose of 500 × 10(6) spermatozoa used for conventional uterine body insemination in mares. The simplicity of the technique offers a practical means of exploiting new breeding technologies that require very small numbers of spermatozoa in horse breeding.[138]

Readers should be aware that pregnancy rates per cycle are unlikely to be increased with this technique; however, the potential to breed a large number of mares with a limited number of spermatozoa is enhanced.

Techniques to Influence the Sex of Offspring

Embryos

Sexing embryos by staining has been possible (see below), but it is time consuming and reduces viability of embryos:

This experiment was designed (1) to determine if H-Y antigen is expressed on the cell surface of pre-implantation equine blastocyst stage embryos, (2) if so, to identify differences in expression on inner cell mass (ICM) versus trophectoderm cells and (3) to evaluate whether the detection of this glycoprotein would aid in the identification of equine embryonic sex. A total of 33 blastocyst stage horse embryos were collected 6-7 days post-ovulation by trans-cervical flush and were immediately evaluated for the presence of H-Y antigen. Additionally, 17 embryos, collected at similar stages and cultured for 72 h, were similarly evaluated. Embryos were recovered and evaluated by use of a dissecting microscope and then washed for 5 min in phosphate buffered saline supplemented with 1 g/l glucose, 36 mg/l pyruvate, 1% antibiotic-antimycotic and 10% fetal calf serum (FCS) (PBS-2). Embryos were placed in the primary antibody medium and cultured for 60 min. The primary antibody medium consisted of monoclonal antibodies to H-Y antigen (previously determined to have male-specific activity) dilute 1/5 (v/v) with PBS-2 (without FCS, PBS- 1). Following an additional wash, embryos were cultured in PBS-1 containing 1/10 (v/v) fluorescein isothiocyanate conjugated goat anti-mouse or rabbit anti-mouse IgM Fc specific antiserum. Embryos were evaluated at 200-400 times to identify cell specific fluorescence of either trophectoderm or ICM cells. Following evaluation, embryonic sex was independently verified with karyotypes to identify sex chromosomes. Of the 50 embryos evaluated, 29 were evaluated as non-fluorescent and 21 fluorescent. Expression of H-Y antigen was detected on both trophectoderm and ICM cell types in those embryos classified as fluorescent. Ninety-one percent (11/12) of fluorescent and 75% (12/16) of non-fluorescent embryos from readable karyotypes corresponded to the predicted sex as determined by detection of H-Y antigen (overall, 23/28, 82%). These results indicate detection of H-Y antigen to be an accurate method of predicting the sex of equine embryos.[139]

Sexing embryos by biopsy offers a better alternative:

Embryo biopsy has been used to detect inherited disorders and to improve the phenotype by analyzing of linkages between marker loci and the desired characteristics. Unfortunately, early procedures required the removal of a large portion (one-half) of the embryo for analysis, and the transfer of bisected equine embryos has not been particularly successful. Recent discovery of the polymerase chain reaction (PCR) has made possible the detection of specific DNA sequences from only a few cells. We investigated whether the removal of a small biopsy would allow for successful PCR and normal embryonic development. In the study reported here, 14 microblade-biopsied Day 6 to 7 equine embryos were transferred nonsurgically into recipient mares. The sex of each embryo was determined from the biopsy by means of restriction fragment length polymorphism analysis of the ZFY/ZFX loci after PCR amplification. The embryos were sexed as 8 females and 6 males on the basis of PCR assay results. Two embryos were biopsied using a needle aspiration technique, but no PCR amplification products resulted from these attempts. Eight intact control embryos were transferred to recipient mares using the same method. Pregnancy rates were 3/14 and 6/8 for the microblade biopsy and control groups, respectively. All of the microblade biopsy group pregnancies were females. One was aborted for cytogenetic analysis. Two were born after normal gestation. With improved pregnancy rates, this technique could be used for pre-implantation diagnostics of equine embryos. As gene mapping advances and associations between particular

DNA sequences and inherited traits become established, a rapid PCR technique could be used to select embryos before transfer.[140]

Sperm

Recently, Flow Cytometry has been used for evaluating sperm viability[141] as well as to sex equine sperm. Foals have now been born from sex-selected sperm.[142-144] The current problem with accurate sex selection is the low number of sperm that can be sorted in a reasonable time frame. The first pregnancy resulted from surgical insemination of 150,000 X bearing sex-selected sperm. Clearly this ushers in an exciting new era in reproductive techniques. It probably will not be long before we can routinely obtain foals from sex-selected frozen-thawed sperm by ICSI.

References

1. Oguri N, Tsutsumi Y: Nonsurgical recovery of equine eggs, and an attempt at nonsurgical egg transfer in horses. J Reprod Fertil 1972; 31:187-195.
2. Oguri N, Tsutsumi Y: Nonsurgical egg transfer in mares. J Reprod Fertil 1974; 41:313-320.
3. Imel KJ, Squires EL, Elsden RP et al: Collection and transfer of equine embryos. J Am Vet Med Assoc 1981; 179:987-991.
4. McKinnon AO, Squires EL: Equine embryo transfer. Vet Clin North Am Equine Pract 1988; 4:305-333.
5. Squires EL, Imel KJ, Shideler RK et al: Recent advances in equine embryo transfer. Proceedings of the American Association of Equine Practitioners, pp, 161-172, 1980.
6. Squires EL, Imel KJ, Iuliano MF et al: Factors affecting reproductive efficiency in an equine embryo transfer programme. J Reprod Fertil 1982; 32(Suppl):409-414.
7. Vogelsang SG, Sorensen AM Jr, Potter GD et al: Fertility of donor mares following nonsurgical collection of embryos. J Reprod Fertil 1979; (Suppl):383-386.
8. Carnevale EM, Ginther OJ: Defective oocytes as a cause of subfertility in old mares. Bio Reprod Mono Ser 1995; 1:209-214.
9. Camillo F, Vannozzi I, Rota A et al: Age at puberty, cyclicity, clinical response to PGF2 alpha, hCG and GnRH and embryo recovery rate in yearling mares. Theriogenology 2002; 58:627-630.
10. Summers PM, Shephard AM, Hodges JK et al: Successful transfer of the embryos of Przewalski's horses (*Equus przewalskii*) and Grant's zebra (*Equus burchelli*) to domestic mares (*Equus caballus*). J Reprod Fertil 1987; 80:13-20.
11. McKinnon AO. Embryo Transfer with an endangered species of donkey. 2005 (accessed) [www.gvequine.com.au].
12. Betteridge KJ, Eaglesome MD, Mitchell D et al: Development of horse embryos up to twenty-two days after ovulation:observations on fresh specimens. J Anat 1982; 135:191-209.
13. McKinnon AO, Squires EL: Morphologic assessment of the equine embryo. J Am Vet Med Assoc 1988; 192:401-406.
14. McKinnon AO, Carnevale EM, Squires EL et al: Bisection of equine embryos. Equine Vet J 1989; 8(Suppl):129-133.
15. Slade NP, Takeda T, Squires EL et al: A new procedure for the cryopreservation of equine embryos. Theriogenology 1985; 24:45-58.
16. Squires EL, Carnevale EM, McCue PM et al: Embryo technologies in the horse. Theriogenology 2003; 59:151-170.

17. Ball BA, Little TV, Hillman RB et al: Embryonic loss in normal and barren mares. Proceedings of the American Association of Equine Practitioners 1985; 535-543.

18. Ball BA, Little TV, Hillman RB et al: Pregnancy rates at days 2 and 14 and estimated embryonic loss rates prior to day 14 in normal and subfertile mares. Theriogenology 1986; 26:611-620.

19. Ball BA, Hillman RB, Woods GL: Survival of equine embryos transferred to normal and subfertile mares. Theriogenology 1987; 28:167-174.

20. Ball BA, Little TV, Weber JA et al: Survival of day-4 embryos from young, normal mares and aged, subfertile mares after transfer to normal recipient mares. J Reprod Fertil 1989; 85:187-194.

21. Squires EL, McKinnon AO, Carnevale EM et al: Reproductive characteristics of spontaneous single and double ovulating mares and superovulated mares. J Reprod Fertil 1987; 35(Suppl):399-403.

22. Iuliano MF. The effect of age of the equine embryo and method of transfer on pregnancy rate, Colorado State University, 1983.

23. Iuliano MF, Squires EL, Cook VM: Effect of age of equine embryos and method of transfer on pregnancy rate. J Anim Sci 1985; 60:258-263.

24. Slade NP, Williams TJ, Squires EL et al: Production of identical twin pregnancies by microsurgical bisection of equine embryo. Proceeding of the International Congress on Animal Reproduction and Artificial Insemination 1984; 10:241-243.

25. Steffenhagen WP, Pineda MH, Ginther OJ: Retention of unfertilized ova in uterine tubes of mares. Am J Vet Res 1972; 33:2391-2398.

26. McKinnon AO, Squires EL, Voss JL: Ultrasonic evaluation of the mare's reproductive tract: Part II. Compend Cont Educ Pract Vet 1987; 9:472-482.

27. Squires EL, Welch SA, Denniston DJ et al: Evaluation of several eFSH treatments for superovulation in mares. Theriogenology 2005; 64:791.

28. Hudson JJ, McCue PM: How to increase embryo recovery rates and transfer success. Proc AAEP 2004; 50:406-408.

29. Hinrichs K: A simple technique that may improve the rate of embryo recovery on uterine flushing in mares. Theriogenology 1990; 33:937-942.

30. McKinnon AO, Voss JL, Squires EL et al: Diagnostic ultrasonography. In McKinnon AO, Voss JL (eds): Equine Reproduction, Philadelphia, Lea & Febiger, pp 266-302, 1993.

31. Squires EL, Voss JL, Villahoz MD et al: Use of ultrasound in broodmare reproduction. Proceedings of the American Association of Equine Practitioners, pp 27-43, 1983.

32. Villahoz MD, Squires EL, Voss JL et al: Some observations on early embryonic death in mares. Theriogenology 1985; 23:915-924.

33. Walton A, Hammond J: The maternal effects on growth and conformation in Shire horse-Shetland pony crosses. Proceedings Royal Society of Biology 1938; 125:311-335.

34. Tischner M: Development of Polish-pony foals born after embryo transfer to large mares. J Reprod Fertil 1987; 35(Suppl):705-709.

35. Wilsher S, Ball M, Allen WR: The influence of maternal size on placental area and foal birthweights in the mare. Pferdeheilkunde 1999; 15:599-602.

36. Hinrichs K, Sertich PL, Kenney RM: Use of Altrenogest to prepare ovariectomized mares as embryo transfer recipients. Theriogenology 1986; 26:455-460.

37. Hinrichs K, Kenney RM: Effect of timing of progesterone administration on pregnancy rate after embryo transfer in ovariectomized mares. J Reprod Fertil 987; 35(Suppl):439-443.

38. McKinnon AO, Squires EL, Carnevale EM et al: Ovariectomized steroid-treated mares as embryo transfer recipients and as a model to study the role of progestins in pregnancy maintenance. Theriogenology 1988; 29:1055-1064.

39. Anderson GF: Evaluation of the hoof and foot relevant to purchase. Vet Clin North Am Equine Pract 1992; 8:303-318.

40. Hinrichs K, Sertich PL, Cumings NR et al: Pregnancy in ovariectomized mares achieved by embryo transfer: a preliminary study. Equine Vet J 1985; 3(Suppl):74-75.

41. Hinrichs K, Riera FL, Klunder LR: Establishment of pregnancy after embryo transfer in mares with gonadaldysgenesis. J In Vitro Fert Embryo Transf 1989; 6:305-309.

42. Castleberry RS, Schneider HJ, Griffin JL: Recovery and transfer of equine embryos. Theriogenology 1980; 13:90.

43. Douglas RH: Some aspects of equine embryo transfer. J Reprod Fertil 1982; 32(Suppl):405-408.

44. Oguri N, Tsutsumi Y: Nonsurgical transfer of equine embryos [abstract]. Arch Androl 1980; 5:108.

45. Silva LA, Gastal EL, Gastal MO et al: A new alternative for embryo transfer and artificial insemination in mares: Ultrasound-guided intrauterine injection. J Equine Vet Sci 2004; 24:324-332.

46. Wilsher S, Allen WR. An improved method for nonsurgical embryo transfer in the mare. Equine Vet Edu 2004; 16:39-44.

47. Allen WR, Stewart F, Trounson AO et al: Viability of horse embryos after storage and long-distance transport in the rabbit. J Reprod Fertil 1976; 47:387-390.

48. Carnevale EM, Ramirez RJ, Squires EL et al: Factors affecting pregnancy rates and early embryonic death after equine embryo transfer. Theriogenology 2000; 54:965-979.

49. Cook VM, Squires EL, McKinnon AO et al: Pregnancy rates of cooled, transported equine embryos. Equine Veterinary Journal 1989; 8(Suppl):80-81.

50. Carnevale EM, Squires EL, McKinnon AO: Comparison of Ham's F10 with carbon dioxide or Hepes buffer for storage of equine embryos at 5 C for 24 h. J Anim Sci 1987; 65:1775-1781.

51. Carnevale EM, Squires EL, McKinnon AO: Comparison of Ham's F10 with CO2 or Hepes buffer for storage of equine embryos at 5 C for 24 H. J Anim Sci 1987; 65:1775-1781.

52. McCue PM, Scoggin CF, Meira C et al: Pregnancy rates from equine embryos cooled for 24 hours in Ham's F-10 vs EmCare embryo holding solution. Proc Ann Meet Soc Therio, San Antonio, 2000; 147.

53. Moussa M, Duchamp G, Mahla R et al: Comparison of pregnancy rates for equine embryos cooled for 24 h in Ham's F-10 and emcare holding solutions. Theriogenology 2002; 58:755-757.

54. Moussa M, Duchamp G, Mahla R et al: In vitro and in vivo comparison of Ham's F-10, Emcare holding solution and ViGro holding plus for the cooled storage of equine embryos. Theriogenology 2003; 59:1615-1625.

55. Moussa M, Tremoleda JL, Duchamp G et al: Evaluation of viability and apoptosis in horse embryos stored under different conditions at 5 degrees C. Theriogenology 2004; 61:921-932.

56. Carney NJ, Squires EL, Cook VM et al: Comparison of pregnancy rates from transfer of fresh versus cooled, transported equine embryos. Theriogenology 1991; 36:23-32.

57. Slade NP. Cryopreservation of the equine embryo, Colorado State University, 1984.

58. Takeda T, Elsden RP, Squires EL: In vitro and in vivo development of frozen-thawed equine embryos. Proceedings of the International Congress on Animal Reproduction and Artificial Insemination 1984; 10:246-250.

59. Squires EL, Seidel GE Jr, McKinnon AO: Transfer of cryo-preserved embryos to progestin-treated ovariectomised mares. Equine Vet J 1989; 8(Suppl):89-91.

60. Shideler RK, Squires EL, Voss JL et al: Exogenous progestin therapy for maintenance of pregnancy in ovariectomized mares. Proceedings of the American Association of Equine Practitioners, 1981; 27:211-219.

61. Pfaff RT: Effetcs of cryoprotectants on viability of equine embryos, Colorado State University, 1994.

62. Seidel GE Jr, Squires EL, McKinnon AO et al: Cryopresevation of equine embryos in 1, 2 propanediol. Equine Vet J 1989; 8(Suppl):87-88.

63. Czlonkowska M, Boyle MS, Allen WR: Deep freezing of horse embryos. J Reprod Fertil 1985; 75:485-490.

64. Seidel GE: Cryopreservation of equine embryos. Vet Clin N Am: Equine Pract 1996; 12:85.

65. Hochi S, Maruyama K, Oguri N: Direct transfer of equine blastocysts frozen-thawed in the presence of ethylene-glycol and sucrose. Theriogenology 1996; 46:1217-1224.

66. Maclellan LJ, Carnevale EM, daSilva MAC et al: Cryo-preservation of small and large equine embryos pre-treated with cytochalasin-B and/or trypsin. Theriogenology 2002; 58:717-720.

67. Legrand E, Bencharif D, BarrierBattut I et al: Comparison of pregnancy rates for days 7-8 equine embryos frozen in glyc-erol with or without previous enzymatic treatment of their capsule. Theriogenology 2002; 58:721-723.

68. Wilson JM, Caceci T, Potter GD et al: Ultrastructure of cryo-preserved horse embryos. J Reprod Fertil 1987; 35(Suppl): 405-417.

69. EldridgePanuska WD, diBrienza VC, Seidel GE et al: Estab-lishment of pregnancies after serial dilution or direct trans-fer by vitrified equine embryos. Theriogenology 2005; 63:1308-1319.

70. Rall WF, Fahy GM: Ice-free cryopreservation of mouse embryos at -196 degrees C by vitrification. Nature 1985; 313:573-575.

71. Oberstein N, O'Donovan MK, Bruemmer JE et al: Cryo-preservation of equine embryos by open pulled straw, cryoloop, or conventional slow cooling methods. Theri-ogenology 2001; 55:607-613.

72. Hochi S, Fujimoto T, Oguri N: Large equine blastocysts are damaged by vitrification procedures. Reprod Fertil Dev 1995; 7:113-117.

73. Young CA, Squires EL, Seidel GE et al: Cryopreservation pro-cedures for Day 7-8 equine embryos. Equine Vet J 1997; (Suppl):98-102.

74. McKinnon AO, Brown RW, Pashen RL et al: Increased ovu-lation rates in mares after immunisation against recombi-nant bovine inhibin alpha-subunit. Equine Vet J 1992; 24:144-146.

75. Ginther OJ, Bergfelt DR: Effect of GnRH treatment during the anovulatory season on multiple ovulation rate and on follicular development during the ensuing pregnancy in mares. J Reprod Fertil 1990; 88:119-126.

76. Johnson AL: Induction of ovulation in anestrous mares with pulsatile administration of gonadotropin-releasing hormone. Am J Vet Res 1986; 47:983-986.

77. Johnson AL: Gonadotropin-releasing hormone treatment induces follicular growth and ovulation in seasonally ane-strous mares. Bio Reprod 1987; 36:1199-1206.

78. Harrison LA, Squires EL, Nett TM et al: Use of gonadotropin-releasing hormone for hastening ovulation in transitional mares. J Anim Sci 1990; 68:690-699.

79. Harrison LA, Squires EL, McKinnon AO: Comparison of hCG, Burserelin and Luprostiol for induction of ovula-tion in cycling mares. J Equine Vet Sci 1991; 11:163-166.

80. Guillou F, Combarnous Y: Purification of equine gonado-tropins and comparative study of their acid-dissociation and receptor-binding specificity. Biochim Biophys Acta 1983; 755:229-236.

81. Douglas RH, Nuti L, Ginther OJ: Induction of ovulation and multiple ovulation in seasonally-anovulatory mares with equine pituitary fractions. Theriogenology 1974; 2:133-142.

82. Douglas RH: Review of induction of superovulation and embryo transfer in the equine. Theriogenology 1979; 11:33-46.

83. Lapin DR, Ginther OJ: Induction of ovulation and multiple ovulations in seasonally anovulatory and ovulatory mares with an equine pituitary extract. J Anim Sci 1977; 44:834-842.

84. Woods GL, Scraba ST, Ginther OJ: Prospect for induction of multiple ovulations and collection of multiple embryos in the mare. Theriogenology 1982; 17:61-72.

85. Woods GL, Ginther OJ: Ovarian response, pregnancy rate, and incidence of multiple fetuses in mares treated with an equine pituitary extract. J Reprod Fertil 1982; 32(Suppl): 415-421.

86. Dippert KD, Jasko DJ, Seidel GE et al: Fertilization rates in superovulated and spontaneously ovulating mares. Theri-ogenology 1994; 41:1411-1423.

87. Hofferer S, Lecompte F, Magallon T et al: Induction of ovu-lation and superovulation in mares using equine LH and FSH separated by hydrophobic interaction chromatogra-phy. J Reprod Fertil 1993; 98:597-602.

88. Rosas CA, Alberio RH, Baranao JL et al: Evaluation of 2 treat-ments in superovulation of mares. Theriogenology 1998; 49:1257-1264.

89. Alvarenga MA, McCue PM, Bruemmer J et al: Ovarian super-stimulatory response and embryo production in mares treated with equine pituitary extract twice daily. Theri-ogenology 2001; 56:879-887.

90. Scoggin CF, Meira C, McCue PM et al: Strategies to improve the ovarian response to equine pituitary extract in cyclic mares. Theriogenology 2002; 58:151-164.

91. Irvine CHG: Endocrinology of the estrous cycle of the mare: applications to embryo transfer. Theriogenology 1981; 15:85-104.

92. Squires EL, Garcia RH, Ginther OJ et al: Comparison of equine pituitary extract and follicle stimulating hormone for superovulating mares. Theriogenology 1986; 26:661-670.

93. Fortune JE, Kimmich TL: Purified pig FSH increases the rate of double ovulation in mares. Equine Vet J 1993; 15(Suppl):95-98.

94. Niswender KD, Alvarenga MA, McCue PM et al: Superovu-lation in cycling mares using equine follicle stimulating hormone (EFSH). J Equine Vet Sci 2003; 23:497-500.

95. Welch SA, Denniston DJ, Hudson JJ et al: The effect of "coasting" on eFSH-induced superovulation in mares. The-riogenology 2005 (in press).

96. Niswender KD, McCue PM, Squires EL: Effect of purified equine follicle-stimulating hormone on follicular develop-ment and ovulation in transitional mares. J Equine Vet Sci 2004; 24:37-39.

97. McCue PM, Carney NJ, Hughes JP et al: Ovulation and embryo recovery rates following immunization of mares against an inhibin alpha-subunit fragment. Theriogenology 1992; 38:823-831.

98. McCue PM, Hughes JP, Lasley BL: Effect on ovulation rate of passive immunization of mares against inhibin. Equine Vet J 1993; 15(Suppl):103-106.

99. Allen WR, Pashen RL: Production of monozygotic (identi-cal) horse twins by embryo micromanipulation. J Reprod Fertil 1984; 71:607-613.

100. Skidmore J, Boyle MS, Cran D et al: Micromanipulation of equine embryos to produce monozygotic twins. Equine Vet J 1989; 8(Suppl):126-128.

101. McKinnon AO, Wheeler M, Carnevale EM et al: Oocyte transfer in the mare: preliminary observations. J Equine Vet Sci 1986; 6:306-309.

102. McKinnon AO, Carnevale EM, Squires EL et al: Heterogenous and xenogenous fertilization of in vivo matured equine oocytes. J Equine Vet Sci 1988; 8:143-147.

103. Palmer E, Duchamp G, Bezard J et al: Recovery of equine follicular fluid and oocytes of mares by non-surgical puncture of preovulatory follicles [abstract]. Theriogenology 1986; 25:178.

104. Vogelsang MM, Kraemer DC, Bowen MJ et al: Recovery of equine follicular oocytes by surgical and nonsurgical techniques. Theriogenology 1986; 25:208.

105. Hinrichs K, Kenney RM: A colpotomy procedure to increase oocyte recovery rates on aspiration of equine preovulatory follicles. Theriogenology 1987; 27:237.

106. Bruck I, Raun K, Synnestvedt B et al: Follicle aspiration in the mare using a transvaginal ultrasound-guided technique. Equine Vet J 1992; 24:58-59.

107. Bruck I, Synnestvedt B, Greve T: Repeated transvaginal oocyte aspiration in unstimulated and FSH-treated mares. Theriogenology 1997; 47:1157-1167.

108. Cook NL, Squires EL, Ray BS et al: Transvaginal ultrasound-guided follicular aspiration of equine oocytes. Equine Vet J 1993; 15(Suppl):71-74.

109. Squires EL, Cook NL: Ultrasound-guided follicular aspiration. Equine Diagn Ultrasonogr 1998; 213-220.

110. Meintjes M, Bellow MS, Paul JB et al: Transvaginal ultrasound-guided oocyte retrieval in cyclic and pregnant horse and pony mares for in vitro fertilization. Biol Reprod Mono 1995; 1:273-279.

111. Franz LC, Squires EL, ODonovan MK et al: Collection and in vitro maturation of equine oocytes from estrus, diestrus and pregnant mares. J Equine Vet Sci 2001; 21:26-32.

112. Shabpareh V, Squires EL, Seidel GE et al: Methods for collecting and maturing equine oocytes in-vitro. Theriogenology 1993; 40:1161-1175.

113. Dellaquila ME, Masterson M, Maritato F et al: Influence of oocyte collection technique on initial chromatin configuration, meiotic competence, and male pronucleus formation after intracytoplasmic sperm injection (ICSI) of equine oocytes. Mol Reprod Dev 2001; 60:79-88.

114. Scott TJ, Carnevale EM, Maclellan LJ et al: Embryo development rates after transfer of oocytes matured in vivo, in vitro, or within oviducts of mares. Theriogenology 2001; 55:705-715.

115. Zhang JJ, Boyle MS, Allen WR: Recent studies on in vivo fertilisation of in vitro matures horse oocytes. Equine Vet J 1989; 8(Suppl):101-104.

116. Ray BS, Squires EL, Cook NL et al: Pregnancy following gamete intrafallopian transfer in the mare. J Equine Vet Sci 1994; 14:27-30.

117. Hinrichs K, Matthews GL, Freeman DA et al: Oocyte transfer in mares. J Am Vet Med Assn 1998; 212:982-986.

118. Carnevale EM, Maclellan LJ, daSilva MA et al: Comparison of culture and insemination techniques for equine oocyte transfer. Theriogenology 2000; 54:981-987.

119. McKinnon AO, Perriam WJ, Lescun TB et al: Effect of a GnRH analogue (Ovuplant), hCG and dexamethasone on time to ovulation in cycling mares. World Equine Vet Rev 1997; 2:16-18.

120. Carnevale EM, Squires EL, Maclellan LJ et al: Use of oocyte transfer in a commercial breeding program for mares with reproductive abnormalities. J Am Vet Med Assn 2001; 218:87.

121. Carnevale EM, Coutinho da Silva MA, Panzani D et al: Factors affecting the success of oocyte transfer in a clinical program for subfertile mares. Theriogenology 2005; 64:519-527.

122. Carnevale EM, Maclellan LJ, daSilva MAC et al: Pregnancies attained after collection and transfer of oocytes from ovaries of five euthanatized mares. J Am Vet Med Assn 2003; 222:60-62.

123. Delcampo MR, Donoso X, Parrish JJ et al: Selection of follicles, preculture oocyte evaluation, and duration of culture for in-vitro maturation of equine oocytes. Theriogenology 1995; 43:1141-1153.

124. Zhang JJ, Muzs LZ, Boyle MS: In vitro fertilization of horse follicular oocytes matured in vitro. Mol Reprod Devel 1990; 26:361-365.

125. Zhang JJ, Muzs LZ, Boyle MS: Variations in structural and functional changes of stallion spermatozoa in response to calcium ionophore A23187. J Reprod Fertil 1991; 44(Suppl): 199-205.

126. Blue BJ, McKinnon AO, Squires EL et al: Capacitation of stallion spermatozoa and fertilisation of equine oocytes in vitro. Equine Vet J 1989; 8(Suppl):111-116.

127. Ellington JE, Ball BA, Blue BJ et al: Capacitation-like membrane-changes and prolonged viability in-vitro of equine spermatozoa cultured with uterine tube epithelial-cells. Am J Vet Res 1993; 54:1505-1510.

128. McKinnon AO, Lacham-Kaplan O, Trounson AO: Pregnancies produced from fertile and infertile stallions by intracytoplasmic sperm injection (ICSI) of single frozen-thawed spermatozoa into in-vivo matured oocytes. J Reprod Fertil 2000; 56(Suppl):513-517.

129. Palmer E, Bezard J, Magistrini M et al: In vitro fertilization in the horse. A retrospective study. J Reprod Fertil 1991; 44(Suppl):375-384.

130. Bezard J, Magistrini M, Battut I et al: In vitro fertilization in the mare. Recueil De Medecine Veterinaire De L'Ecole D'Alfort 1992; 168:993-1003.

131. Squires EL, Wilson JM, Kato H et al: A pregnancy after intracytoplasmic sperm injection into equine oocytes matured in vitro. Theriogenology 1996; 45:306.

132. Cochran R, Meintjes M, Reggio B et al: Production of live foals from sperm-injected oocytes harvested from pregnant mares. J Reprod Fert Suppl 2000; 56:503-512.

133. Li XH, Morris LH-A, Allen WR: Effects of different activation treatments on fertilization of horse oocytes by intracytoplasmic sperm injection. J Reprod Fertil 2000; 119: 253-260.

134. Li XH, Morris LHA, Allen WR: Influence of coculture during maturation on the developmental potential of equine oocytes fertilised by intracytoplasmic sperm injection (ICSI). Reproduction 2001; 121:925-932.

135. Wirtu G, Bailey TL, Chauhan MS et al: Xenogenous fertilization of equine oocytes following recovery from slaughterhouse ovaries and in vitro maturation. Theriogenology 2004; 61:381-391.

136. McKinnon AO, Squires EL, Carnevale EM et al: Heterogenous and xenogenous fertilization of equine oocytes [abstract]. Theriogenology 1988; 29:278.

137. Hinrichs K, DiGiorgio LM: Embryonic development after intra-follicular transfer of horse oocytes. J Reprod Fertil 1991; 44(Suppl):369-374.

138. Morris LA, Hunter RF, Allen WR: Hysteroscopic insemination of small numbers of spermatozoa at the uterotubal junction of preovulatory mares. J Reprod Fertil 2000; 118:95-100.

139. Wood TC, White KL, Thompson DLJ et al: Evaluation of the expression of a male-specific antigen on cells of equine blastocysts. J Reprod Immunol 1988; 14:1-8.

140. Huhtinen M, Peippo J, Bredbacka P: Successful transfer of biopsied equine embryos. Theriogenology 1997; 48:361-367.

141. Merkies K, Chenier T, Plante C et al: Assessment of stallion spermatozoa viability by flow cytometry and light microscope analysis. Theriogenology 2000; 54:1215-1224.

142. Lindsey AC, Bruemmer JE, Squires EL: Low dose insemination of mares using non-sorted and sex-sorted sperm. Anim Reprod Sci 1902; 68:279-289.

143. Lindsey AC, Schenk JL, Graham JR et al: Hysteroscopic insemination of low numbers of flow sorted fresh and frozen/thawed stallion spermatozoa. Equine Vet J 2002; 34:121-127.

144. Lindsey AC, Varner DD, Seidel GE et al: Hysteroscopic or rectally guided, deep-uterine insemination of mares with spermatozoa stored 18 h at either 5 or 15 degrees C prior to flow-cytometric sorting. Theriogenology 2002; 58:659-662.

SECTION VII

The Pregnant Mare: Diagnosis and Management

CHAPTER 52

Pregnancy Diagnosis in the Mare*

JONATHAN F. PYCOCK

FERTILIZATION

The uterine tube has the ability to transport sperm toward the ovary while transporting the ovum in the opposite direction. Fertilization of the ovum occurs in the oviduct in mares. The fertilized egg or conceptus then takes 5 to 6 days to reach the uterus.

EMBRYONIC AND FETAL DEVELOPMENT

The conceptus is highly mobile throughout the entire uterus until day 16 after ovulation. The early movement of the conceptus is thought to play a key role in the physiologic event known as *maternal recognition of pregnancy*. The mobility phase ends when the conceptus becomes stationary and "fixation" occurs at the base of the right or left uterine horn. Fixation in postpartum mares tends to occur in the previously nongravid horn. Implantation occurs gradually and relatively late in the mare, beginning around day 40. It is not complete until approximately day 140. By convention, the term *embryo* is used up to day 40 and the term **fetus** after day 40.

Endometrial cups are a unique feature of the equine placenta. On or about day 28 of gestation, the chorionic girdle begins to form at the junction of the yolk sac and allantoic membranes. Specialized cells from the chorionic girdle invade the underlying uterine epithelium between days 36 and 38. Once in the endometrium, they enlarge and become clumped together to form the endometrial cups. The cups are arranged in a circle at the base of the gravid uterine horn. Endometrial cups produce equine chorionic gonadotropin (eCG), which stimulates the primary corpus luteum (CL) and causes induced second-

ary follicles to ovulate and/or luteinize. Because progesterone production remains high, mares do not show signs of estrus at the time of these secondary ovulations. This is independent from the presence of a fetus, so once the endometrial cups are formed, eCG production will proceed even in instances in which embryonic or fetal loss occurs.

ROUTINE PREGNANCY DIAGNOSIS

It is important to be able to tell if a mare is pregnant for management and husbandry reasons: Pregnant mares should be managed differently from nonpregnant mares. They should have further examinations to monitor the development of the pregnancy, confirm the absence of twin pregnancies, and monitor for early embryonic or fetal death. Twin pregnancies are bad news in the mare, and if the pregnancy is diagnosed early enough, appropriate intervention is possible (see Chapter 54).

It is just as important to identify the nonpregnant mare as soon as possible. Some mares have prolonged luteal activity (previously termed "persistent corpus luteum"), and the maintenance of circulating progesterone concentrations in these nonpregnant mares means that they do not spontaneously return to estrus. Persistence of luteal activity in the nonpregnant mare is a major cause of subfertility and is the main cause of anestrus during the breeding season. Traditionally, the term "prolonged diestrus" has been used to describe a condition in which the function of the CL continues beyond its normal cyclic lifespan of 15 to 16 days, resulting in the maintenance of elevated circulating progesterone concentrations for longer than expected. The term *prolonged luteal activity* is preferred, because "persistent diestrus" implies that the CL persists, whereas it is possible that other CLs are formed sequentially from diestrous

*Used by permission from UK VET: Volume 9, No. 4, May 2004.

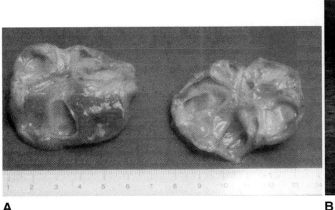
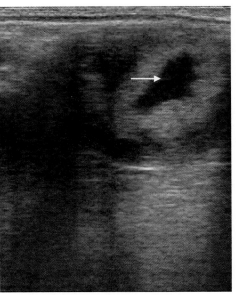

A   **B**

Figure 52-1 **A,** Gross specimen of left and right ovaries cut in half, showing a corpus luteum visible in the left ovary. A small central space can be seen in the corpus luteum. **B,** An ultrasound image of the equine corpus luteum with a centrally located anechoic area (*arrow*). The equine corpus luteum may remain uniformly echoic throughout its period of detection, or as in this image, an anechoic area may develop. In fact, a continuous distribution from uniformly echoic through to almost completely anechoic can be appreciated, with only a small border of luteal tissue.

ovulations. Prolonged luteal activity occurs in up to 20% of estrous cycles and are not accompanied by estrus; the cervix will remain pale in color, dry, and tightly closed. If diestrous ovulations occur late in the luteal phase, they will be refractory to the effect of endogenous luteolysins, resulting in a persistent luteal phase. Such abnormal luteal activity is associated with significant problems in reproductive management because affected mares may erroneously be assumed to be pregnant.

Plasma progesterone profiles are indistinguishable from those of pregnant animals. The uterus becomes firm and tubular (tonic) and the cervix is typical of that of pregnancy. Transrectal ultrasound imaging fails to detect a conceptus, but a CL can be detected in the ovary (Fig. 52-1, *A* and *B*). The ability to detect the CL throughout diestrus represents a profound diagnostic advantage of ultrasonography over rectal palpation.

Failure of synthesis and/or release of prostaglandin $F_{2\alpha}$ ($PGF_{2\alpha}$) at the end of diestrus and failure of the corpus luteum to respond to $PGF_{2\alpha}$ are the most likely causes of persistence of the CL. Treatment is by injection of a luteolytic dose of $PGF_{2\alpha}$ or a synthetic analogue. The interval between treatment and ovulation varies considerably depending on the size of follicles at the time of treatment. Therefore, ultrasonographic examination of the mare before such treatment is always advisable in order to assess the status of folliculogenesis.

A clinical examination by a veterinary surgeon involving rectal palpation and ultrasound evaluation of the internal organs is the most accurate and useful method of pregnancy diagnosis. Nonetheless, several potential pitfalls have been recognized, including the confusion of uterine cysts for conceptuses and the presence of multiple conceptuses.

Speculum Examination of the Cervix

The vagina and cervix of the early pregnant mare are covered in pale, dry mucous membranes. The cervix is closed and resembles exactly the cervix of the mare in diestrus. As the pregnancy progresses, the external opening of the cervix becomes covered in tacky, dry mucus. Later in pregnancy (after 6 months), the cervix can be very relaxed.

Rectal Examination

Cervix
In early pregnancy (16 to 30 days), the cervix can be palpated on the floor of the pelvis as a rigid, firm structure (as during diestrus).

Ovaries
Both ovaries should be palpated, although ovarian palpation contributes little to pregnancy diagnosis. This is because both ovaries usually are enlarged from 18 to 40 days as a result of follicular development and the CL is not palpable. From 40 to 120 days, extensive ovarian activity with ovulations, luteinization, and development of secondary corpora lutea is evident. Follicular activity decreases from 120 days to term, and the ovaries become small and inactive. The position of the ovaries up to 60

days of pregnancy is as for the nonpregnant mare. From then on, they are drawn cranially and medially but remain dorsal to the uterus. From 5 months of pregnancy onward, the ovaries usually are not palpable.

Uterus

Both uterine horns and body should be palpated. Pregnancy diagnosis is based on tone and location of uterus and contents.

15 to 24 Days. The uterus becomes more tubular and turgid from 15 to 24 days after ovulation and is readily palpable. It is not possible to feel the conceptual swelling. The uterus may be tonic in mares in a prolonged luteal phase and in nonpregnant mares bred at the foal heat, which are still undergoing uterine involution.

24 to 28 Days. At about 26 days, the conceptual swelling develops at the uterine horn-body junction but can be difficult to palpate except in maiden mares. The swelling is 3 to 4 cm in diameter (about the size of a golf ball) and bulges ventrally.

28 to 35 Days. The uterus is still turgid, and the conceptual bulge is more obvious. The uterine wall over the conceptus begins to feel thin.

35 to 60 Days. As the conceptus grows, the swelling becomes larger and spherical and feels more like a fluid sac. By 42 days it is about 5 by 7 cm in size (the size of a tennis ball). The uterine tone around the bulge begins to decrease so that the swelling becomes less tense.

60 to 90 Days. By 60 days, the conceptus swelling is approximately 12 cm in diameter and fills the pregnant horn. After 60 days, the pregnancy is like an elongated football and starts to involve the uterine body. The examiner must be careful not to confuse it with the bladder or a case of pyometra. The uterus migrates cranially.

Between days 60 and 100, the uterus is low within the abdomen, and the fetus usually cannot be palpated. From 4 to 5 months onward, the fetus usually can be palpated.

Ultrasound Examination

Rectal examination should always precede ultrasound examination. An initial rectal examination ensures removal of all fecal material, facilitates rapid location of the tract during scanning, and provides information on texture of structures.

Diagnosis of Early Pregnancy

Day 10. The equine embryonic vesicle can first be detected at day 10 (day 0 = day of ovulation), when sufficient anechoic yolk sac fluid has developed. In Figure 52-2, the black yolk sac fluid is enclosed within the trophoblast, resulting in a spherical outline with a diameter of 4 to 6 mm.

Day 12. The vesicle grows slowly (around 1.5 mm/day) until day 12, when the vesicle is ~8 mm in size. In Figure 52-3, the two hyperechoic short lines on the dorsal and ventral borders of the conceptus are known as *specular reflections.* Although they may aid location of the early embryonic vesicle, they are not indicative of pregnancy but represent a physical phenomenon arising from the reflection of the ultrasound beam; cysts tend to cause nonspecular reflections. The anechoic vesicle is highly mobile at this stage and found in either horn or in the body. It is important to examine both uterine horns and the body thoroughly.

Mares usually are not scanned as early as day 12 because it is possible to miss the conceptus if scanning conditions are not ideal and the ovulation date is not accurately known. If an ovulation occurred 1 or 2 days after the first ovulation, any pregnancy arising from this later ovulation would be too small to be detected.

Day 14. The 14-day conceptus is 14 to 18 mm in diameter. In Figure 52-4, the day 14 conceptus is 16 mm across and lies centrally in the uterine body. Note the spherical shape and increase in size over that of the day 11 conceptus. The embryonic vesicle grows at a rate of

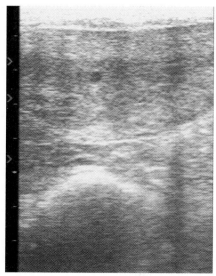

Figure 52-2 Equine conceptus at day 10 of pregnancy. (Courtesy of Dr. Juan Samper.)

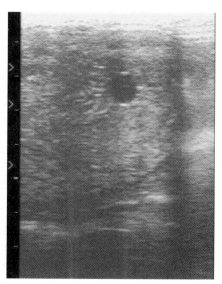

Figure 52-3 Equine conceptus at day 12 of pregnancy. (Courtesy of Dr. Juan Samper.)

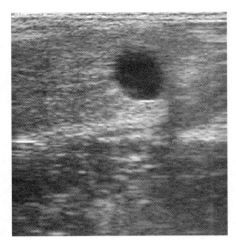

Figure 52-4   Equine conceptus at day 14 of pregnancy. (Courtesy of Dr. Juan Samper.)

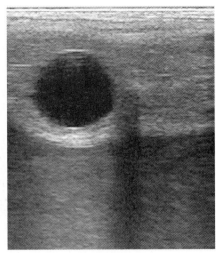

Figure 52-6   Equine conceptus at day 17 of pregnancy.

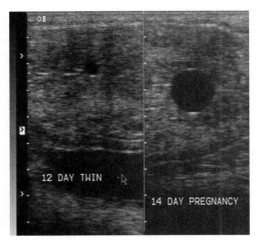

Figure 52-5   Twin pregnancy in the mare, with one conceptus 14 days and the other 12 days from ovulation. The disparity in age is the reason for the difference in size between the vesicles. The smaller vesicle should be crushed.

approximately 3.5 m/day between days 12 and 16 of pregnancy and remains highly mobile, making thorough examination of all parts of the uterus important.

In the event of twin pregnancies, both vesicles usually can be seen at 14 days, even if the second co-twin arose from a later ovulation (Fig. 52-5). This fact, together with the mobility and relatively small size of the conceptuses, makes 14 to 15 days the optimal time during pregnancy for diagnosis and intervention in twin pregnancies. It is important to realize that if twin pregnancies arise from asynchronous ovulations, one conceptus is likely to be larger than the other. This is not an indication to leave the smaller conceptus; manual crushing should still be performed.

Although pregnancy diagnosis is highly accurate even at this early stage, an important consideration is the possibility of confusing uterine cysts and the presence of twin conceptuses. Ideally, the practitioner will already have performed an ultrasound examination before the

mare is bred, but this is not always possible. If the first scan is performed at day 14 or 15, then a second examination can be done the next day in cases of confusion, to see if the pregnancy has changed position or the conceptus has grown in size. This strategy should allow differentiation from a cyst before unilateral fixation of twin conceptuses has occurred.

Some veterinarians point out that it may be better to delay the first examination until day 18, when nonpregnant mares have had the opportunity to return to estrus, to identify the optimal time for the next breeding. By then, however, correction of unilateral twins will be very difficult. Although undoubtedly a natural mechanism exists for reduction of twin pregnancies to singletons in mares, I believe that the effectiveness of this mechanism has been exaggerated and that it is not as successful as manual crushing of one twin at day 15, which has a 95% success rate in my experience.

Day 17.   By day 17 the vesicle normally is fixed at the base of either the left or the right horn (Fig. 52-6). The shape is still regular but more ovoid than strictly spherical. The vesicle is approximately 25 mm in size.

Day 21.   At day 21 of pregnancy, the conceptus is no longer spherical but is irregular in outline, as seen in Figure 52-7. This irregular shape is normal and is not an indication of imminent pregnancy loss. The appearance can be so irregular that it can be confused with a collection of intraluminal uterine fluid, particularly because no embryo is likely to be visible at this stage. Therefore, a single pregnancy scan at day 21 is a bad idea. In Figure 52-7, note the thickened dorsal wall of the uterus and the presence of a slight edema pattern above the conceptus. These features may be due to estrogen production by the conceptus or the follicular development typical of this stage of pregnancy. If the pregnancy is normal, the primary corpus luteum also should be visible. If the edema pattern of the uterus becomes widespread, this may be an indicator of early embryonic death. In such cases, it is important to reschedule subsequent pregnancy examinations at more frequent intervals than normal,

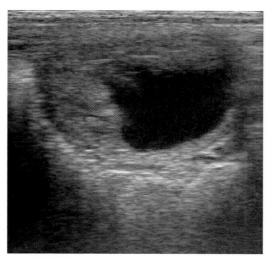

Figure 52-7 Equine conceptus at day 21 of pregnancy.

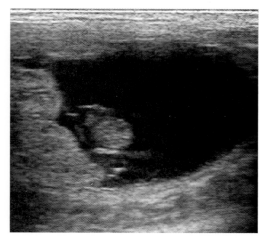

Figure 52-9 Equine conceptus at day 26 of pregnancy.

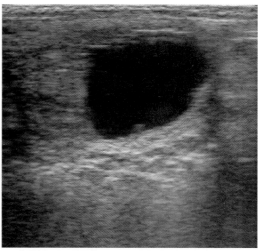

Figure 52-8 Equine conceptus with a 3-mm embryo at day 21 of pregnancy.

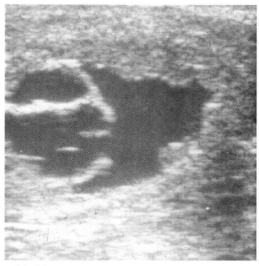

Figure 52-10 Ultrasound image of the uterus showing an irregularly shaped uterine cyst (*left-hand half* of the image) adjacent to a 24-day conceptus (*right-hand half* of the image) with an embryo 4 mm in length visible on the ventral surface of the conceptus in the 4 o'clock position (*arrow*).

and the first reexamination should be in 3 or 4 days to monitor the pregnancy.

Figure 52-8 shows an image from another day 21 pregnancy. As expected, the conceptus is irregular in outline, but here the embryo is seen as a 3-mm, echoic oval structure found in its normal site ventrally within the trophoblast vesicle. Rarely the embryo is first detected at a different site, and while the reason for this is not known, such pregnancies appear to develop normally. At this stage, the embryo has not lifted itself off the trophoblast wall and can therefore be very easy to miss.

The detection of an embryo in this image, but not in the day 21 image in Figure 52-7, indicates that some variation in appearance of features is normal. In addition, if the mare was examined daily during breeding, the true age of the conceptus can vary within a range of 0 to 24 hours. This variability alone may account for considerable difference in appearance of embryos at known gestation lengths. All embryos should be detectable by day 24, however. Failure to detect an embryo after that time is an indication that the pregnancy will ultimately fail.

Day 26. By day 26 of pregnancy, the embryo is approximately 8 mm in length. In Figure 52-9, the embryo has developed in the seven o'clock position within the trophoblast. This is perfectly normal. The heartbeat normally can be detected as a flickering movement in the middle of the echoic embryo around this stage of pregnancy. With the high-quality ultrasound machines now available, the heartbeat often can be detected a few days earlier, around day 23. It is important to recognize the embryo and identify a heartbeat, because the irregularly shaped vesicle may be confused with an endometrial cyst (Fig. 52-10) or intrauterine fluid accumulation (Fig. 52-11).

Uterine cysts are fluid-filled and are immobile, anechoic structures with an obvious border. They can be

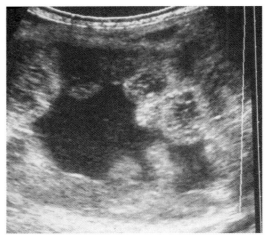

Figure 52-11   The uterine body in longitudinal section on an ultrasound study. The two most obvious features are endometrial edema and free luminal fluid. The edema usually is physiologically normal. Free fluid certainly is not normal in early diestrus or pregnancy. In early estrus, small collections of fluid sometimes are seen. In this mare, the depth of fluid is more than 2 cm, which should be considered excessive, even during estrus.

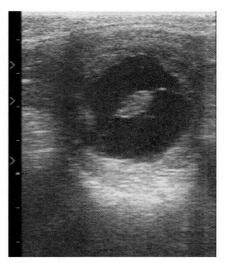

Figure 52-12   Equine conceptus at day 30 of pregnancy: Typical appearance.

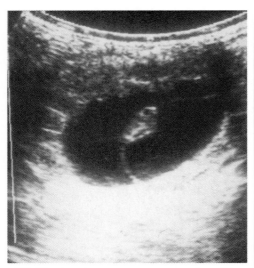

Figure 52-13   Equine conceptus at day 30 of pregnancy: Atypical appearance. In this image, the yolk sac is to the *left* and the allantois to the *right*.

The allantoic sac emerges as a small anechoic area from beneath the embryo. Over the next few days, the development of the allantois will lift the embryo dorsally, and the yolk sac gradually will reduce in size. This change in ratio of the yolk sac to allantois is an important feature in aging pregnancies.

Day 30. By day 30 of pregnancy, the developing allantois, the regressing yolk sac and the associated dorsal "ascent" of the embryo can be visualized on the ultrasound scan. In Figure 52-12, the allantois has enlarged in such a manner that the two sacs are approximately equal in size. The apposition of yolk sac and allantois results in an ultrasonically visible thin line normally oriented horizontally. The embryo is highly echogenic and is clearly visible on the line separating the allantoic and yolk sacs. The heartbeat can be readily detected during the real-time ultrasound examination.

In normal pregnancies, by day 30 the echoic line representing the apposed walls of the yolk sac and allantois sometimes can be aligned vertically, rather than horizontally (Fig. 52-13). Caution in interpretation of findings is advised, however, because this appearance also can be confused with that of twin pregnancies of earlier gestation when the breeding history is unknown.

Day 32. At day 32 of pregnancy, the embryo usually is in the dorsal part of the vesicle, at a 12 o'clock position in Figure 52-14. The embryo is approximately 12 mm in length. The volume of the allantois exceeds that of the yolk sac. The aim of examination at this stage of pregnancy is to confirm that a single conceptus is developing normally. If failure of normal development is noted or if twins are detected, it usually is possible to terminate the pregnancy and re-breed the mare. If examination is delayed until after day 33, however, the endometrial cups may have developed, and even if pregnancy is terminated, eCG production may continue for a variable time, sometimes preventing normal estrous

located anywhere in the uterus, and although their precise relationship to subfertility is not clear, they are the structures most likely to confound the diagnosis of early pregnancy. Differentiation is easiest on the basis of previous mapping of cysts before the mare has been bred and also can be based on the characteristic mobility and rapid growth rate of the early pregnancy. Some cysts remain difficult to distinguish, and previous cyst mapping is vital. Uterine cysts can be single or multiple, or small or large and often compartmentalized. Large cysts may impede movement of the early conceptus, but their importance is that they are easily confused with embryonic vesicles.

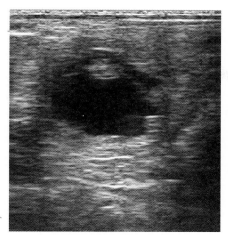

Figure 52-14 Equine conceptus at day 32 of pregnancy.

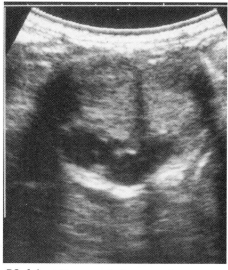

Figure 52-16 Ultrasound image of ovary with two corpora lutea.

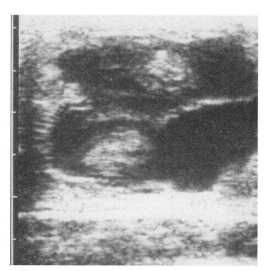

Figure 52-15 Ultrasound image showing unilateral fixation of twin conceptuses at day 33 of pregnancy.

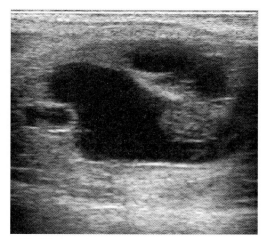

Figure 52-17 Equine conceptus at day 45 of pregnancy.

cycles for the rest of the breeding season. In Figure 52-15, showing a set of twins at 31 days of pregnancy, two embryonic masses can be clearly detected. The conceptuses have become fixed at the base of the same horn—a feature termed *unilateral fixation*. Although they are very close together, they have not developed within the same trophoblast. If this mare had been scanned at an earlier stage of pregnancy, the co-twins would almost certainly have been seen as two separate vesicles. Almost all twins in mares are dizygotic, arising from two separate ovulations. Examination of the ovaries is important at every examination for pregnancy to provide information on the number and appearance of the corpora lutea.

Mares with twins almost always have two corpora lutea. In Figure 52-16, the primary CL is visible as a uniformly echoic area. A CL readily detectable on ultrasound images usually is producing progesterone. Ultrasonographic assessment of the CL may be useful in assisting a decision to provide exogenous progesterone or progestogen supplementation. Note the presence of several folli-

cles in the figure; this is quite normal for early pregnant mares.

Day 45. By day 45, the envelopment of the yolk sac by the allantochorion placenta is almost complete, and the membranes of the allantois have converged on it to form the umbilical cord, clearly visible in Figure 52-17. The yolk sac is still visible as a small anechoic area within the developing umbilical cord. As the fetus grows, it descends from its position proximal to the mesometrium, and the umbilicus lengthens accordingly. The fetus has descended approximately two thirds of the way toward the ventral part of the allantois. A circular uterine cyst can be seen to the left of the fetus in the 9 o'clock position.

Day 60. By day 60 of pregnancy, the diameter of the conceptus exceeds the scanning width of the ultrasound probe, as seen in Figure 52-18. Several features of the fetus are readily detectable.

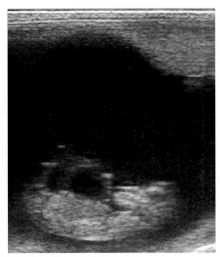

Figure 52-18   Equine conceptus at day 60 of pregnancy.

Timing of Routine Ultrasound Scans in Pregnancy

The first ultrasound examination should be performed around 15 days after covering, to diagnose pregnancy early and provide appropriate intervention in twin pregnancies. A second examination around 26 to 30 days after covering allows the veterinarian to check for normal development of the pregnancy and to rule out the presence of twins. Although these timings are arbitrary, if examination is delayed until after day 33, endometrial cup activity may prevent normal estrous cycles for the rest of the breeding season, as described previously. In addition, much time may be lost if early embryonic death has occurred (earlier scanning will allow earlier detection of such losses).

Additional scans may be needed in mares that are prone to twinning, have many cysts, or have lost pregnancies before. Cost is an important consideration, as with many aspects of horse breeding, and a compromise must be struck between what is best and what is practical in economic terms. If, on economic grounds, a mare can be scanned only once, this examination should be

Box   52-1

Protocol for Ultrasound Diagnosis/Evaluation of Pregnancy*

First examination	Day 14 to 15
Second examination	Day 24 to 27
Third examination	Day 33 to 35
Autumn examination	October
Day of ovulation is day 0.	

*When ovulation time is known.

performed around day 26, when an obvious embryo with heartbeat should be visible. All mares scanned in foal in the breeding season should be checked in autumn by internal examination to make sure that they are still pregnant. A recommended protocol for timing of ultrasonographic scans for pregnancy diagnosis and monitoring is summarized in Box 52-1.

Multiple Ovulation

Double ovulations occur during 8% to 30% of estrous cycles, the frequency depending on the breed and type of the mare (Thoroughbreds have the highest rate; ponies the lowest). Accurate detection of double ovulation is important because twinning is undesirable for at least two reasons: First, it accounts for 10% to 30% of abortions, and second, even if both fetuses survive and are carried to term, many are dysmature, resulting in a high neonatal mortality rate. The reason for the low survival rate of twins is due to competition for placental space. A further complication is that if embryonic or fetal death occurs after the formation of the endometrial cups, these latter structures persist until they spontaneously regress as if pregnancy had been maintained, resulting in pseudopregnancy.

Effective twin management is a vital part of maximizing fertility on the stud farm and is the subject of an excellent review in the next chapter.

CHAPTER 53

Fetal Sex Determination

RICHARD D. HOLDER

Equine fetal sexing is the determination of sex of an equine fetus after 55 days of gestation. Different techniques for determination are required for the different stages of gestation. Technique 1, performed between 55 and 90 days of gestation, involves finding the genital tubercle (precursor to the penis in the male and precursor to the clitoris in the female) and determining its location relative to other fetal structures. The genital tubercle appears as a hyperechoic bilobulated "equals" sign 2 to 3 mm in length and develops between the hind legs on the ventral midline of both sexes at 50 to 55 days. Migrations of the tubercle that indicate the sex of the fetus begin about day 54 to 55. A determination cannot be made before 55 days because the migration toward the umbilical cord in the male or toward the anus in the female has not yet occurred. Using technique number one, the veterinarian should be able to make a diagnosis 95% of the time on the first examination with 99% accuracy. The examination should take from a few seconds to 5 minutes to perform.

Technique 2, performed between 90 days and 150 days of gestation, involves finding the external genitalia of the fetus (penis, glans penis, prepuce, and gonads in the male and mammary gland, teats, clitoris, and gonads in the female). At this stage (90 to 150 days) the veterinarian should be able to formulate a diagnosis 90% of the time on one examination with 99% accuracy. It should take from a few seconds to 10 minutes to perform the examination depending on the experience of the practitioner.

Around 150 days of gestation the fetus begins to assume an anterior presentation. This means that the head will be easily accessible, but the pelvic area will be out of reach. The fetus is much larger now and does not change positions often. Therefore rectal scanning for the determination of sex after 150 days is very difficult. The percentage of accurate diagnoses between 150 and 200 days would be very low (5% to 25% of attempts made by rectal examination).

Technique 3 involves performing a transabdominal scan and finding external genitalia after 150 days of gestation. In the author's experience, determining sex transabdominally has a very low percentage of diagnosis and is very time consuming. In addition, clipping of the abdomen is sometimes required, and access to a more powerful ultrasound machine is helpful. Because of the low percentage of diagnosis, the extra amount of time required and clipping and ultrasound machine requirements, the author strongly recommends that techniques 1 and 2 be used for determination of sex in the equine.

The information obtained from the fetal sexing procedure is simply a management tool to be used by the owner or manager. Depending on the sire, the dam, or both, the fetal gender may affect the value of the foal. Consequently, this affects the value of the mare. (For example, if the value of the mare changes depending on the gender of the foal, then appraisals, sales reserves, insurance coverage, and collateral limits for loans could all be affected.) This knowledge of the fetal gender could affect various management decisions such as where to foal the mare. (If you want to race a New York–bred colt, it is impractical to send a mare carrying a filly to New York to foal.) Some other considerations include cash flow predictions that could be determined earlier. Is the owner going to have a certain individual for sale (income) or an individual to race (expense)? Perhaps an owner wants a particular sex from a particular cross; if that breeding was successful, the owner could breed the following year to a different stallion, or the owner could try again to the same stallion if the desired sex did not result from the first mating. In this way the mating list could be determined much earlier. Perhaps if a mare is carrying a colt, the size of the fetus may be of some concern and precautions at foaling may be taken. Each year as the demand for fetal sex determination increases, there seem to be more new reasons for owners' wanting to know the sex of the fetus.

If a practitioner is the only one in his or her area able to accurately perform a sexual determination, the procedure can develop into a new worthwhile profit center for the practice. Figure 53-1 is a graph of increasing demand when fetal sex determination was introduced into the area.

MATERIALS NEEDED FOR FETAL SEX DETERMINATION

1. Quality ultrasound machine with a 5-MHz linear array rectal transducer (ALOKA 500 SSD [Aloka Co., Ltd., Wallingford, Conn] or equivalent).
   A. Settings: If the overall gain, near gain, or far gains are set too high, the contrast between the fetus and background is less and the tubercle is more difficult to see.
2. Rectal palpation essentials:
   A. Lubricant, sleeves.
   B. Restraint: stocks, lip chain, twitch, etc.
   C. Tranquilizers: Depending on the situation, tranquilization is acceptable, but this may cause the uterus to relax and drop away from

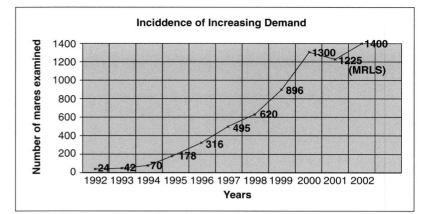

Figure 53-1 Graph of increasing demand when fetal sex determination was introduced into the area.

Table **53-1**

Fetal Anatomical Development Chart

Days	Visualization
55-60	Fetus is very small; genital tubercle is difficult to see and may or may not be fully migrated.
60-70	Fetus is easily accessible; tubercle is distinct and fully migrated. **(Easiest and most ideal time for fetal sex determination)**
70-80	Fetal tubercle is distinct but slightly more difficult to reach.
80-90*	Difficult to access fetus; tubercle is less distinct; genitalia development is just beginning. **(Most difficult time)** (Figure 10-2)
90-100	Fetus is generally accessible; genitalia are not very well developed. (Difficult to differentiate genitalia at times)
100-110	Genitalia becoming more evident.
110-120	Fetus is very accessible, and genitalia is well developed. **(Ideal time in technique 2 for determination)**
120-140	Genitalia are well developed, but posterior of fetus may be difficult to access at times.
140-150†	At times fetus has anterior presentation with posterior out of reach.
150+	Usually the fetus has anterior presentation, and posterior of fetus is out of reach. Transrectally this stage is difficult, with a low percentage diagnosis of 5-25%.
150 to Term	Transabdominal—low percentage diagnosis, time consuming, need to clip abdomen, more powerful ultrasound machine is helpful.

*At 80 to 90 days the fetus is often difficult to reach due to the position of the uterus in the posterior abdomen. At approximately 80 days the allantoic fluid of the pregnancy pulls the uterus over the rim of the pelvis. The fetus is small, falls to the most ventral portion of the uterus, and is very difficult to reach. As the uterine contents (fetus and fluids) increase in size, the uterus actually elevates more in the abdominal cavity and becomes easier to reach and view the fetus.
†Mares that are 130 to 150 days that are out of reach should be viewed again for possible position change.

the examiner, making it more difficult to reach. The author uses 200 mg of xylazine and 10 mg of butorphanol tartrate mixed intravenously (IV).

    D. Propantheline bromide may be used to prevent rectal straining—30 mg IV.

3. Ultrasound stand on wheels—for close eye-level viewing.
4. Subdued lighting—for good screen visualization.
5. Hat—to remove surrounding glare.
6. Fly spray (if needed) —to keep mare movement to a minimum.
7. Video or printers are helpful to verify the diagnosis and for record keeping.

FETAL DEVELOPMENT

See Tables 53-1 and 53-2 and Figure 53-2.

PROCEDURE—TECHNIQUE 1

- The procedure involves a thorough evacuation of the feces from the rectum to allow easy manipulation of the transducer.
- Determine positioning of the fetus by scanning the entire fetus (see Figures 53-3, 53-7, *A*, and 53-13):
  The skull is a good anterior marker.
  The heart is a good ventral marker.

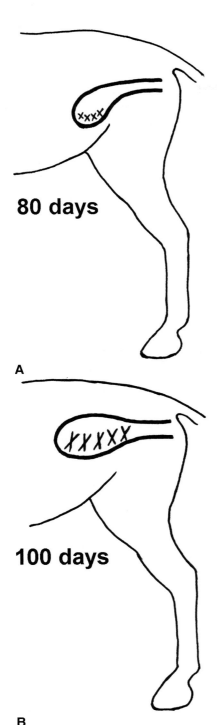

Figure 53-2 **A,** At 80 to 90 days it is the most difficult time to access fetus, tubercle is less distinct, and genitalia development is just beginning. **B,** At 100 days genitalia are becoming more evident.

Ribs coming off vertebrae and base of tail are good dorsal markers.

The tail is a good posterior marker (see Figure 53-20).

- When the position of the fetus has been determined, proceed to the posterior part of fetus until the transducer has gone completely off the posterior part of the fetus (see Figure 53-7, *A*).

- Gradually ease back on the fetus with the transducer cutting a plane perpendicular to the axis of the spine of the fetus (see Figure 53-7, *A, B*).

- A cross section of the tailhead should be picked up on the dorsal aspect of the fetus. It will appear as a hyperechoic round mass with very little muscle tissue around it (see Figures 53-9, *E,* 53-10, *A,* and 53-18).

- Ventrally, two tibias (hyperechoic round structures, with no muscle mass) should be seen forming a triangle with the tailhead (see Figure 53-9, *A* to *E*).

- If the fetus is a female, there will be a hyperechoic tubercle within the tibia-tailhead triangle with the tubercle slightly toward the tailhead. The female tubercle is difficult to consistently identify other than within the tibia-tailhead triangle (see Figure 53-9, *B* to *E*).

- If the fetus is a male, nothing will be seen within the tibia-tailhead triangle.

- If nothing is seen in the triangle, move the transducer gradually anteriorly along the fetus, keeping the same perpendicular plane (Plane II or III) to the axis of the spine of the fetus (see Figure 53-7, *A* and *B*).

- A hyperechoic equals sign should appear between the two tibias (the tibias moving anteriorly change to the stifles or femurs) (see Figure 53-8, *A* and *B*).

- TIP: Remember tibias have no muscle mass around them, and femurs do have muscle mass around them.

- Moving further anteriorly, the large round abdomen will be seen. In the male the tubercle can often be seen on the outside ventral wall of the abdomen just posterior to the urachus, which is seen as a dark hole 4 to 5 mm in diameter (see Figures 53-13 to 53-15).

- Moving the transducer back and forth over the posterior area in this plane usually exhibits a visible tubercle.

- The male tubercle can also be readily seen from a frontal plane (Plane I) (see Figure 53-3). This plane exhibits the front legs, ventral abdomen, and hind legs, with the tubercle appearing slightly anterior to a line drawn between the hind legs (usually femurs or stifles) (see Figure 53-4, *A* to *C*).

PROCEDURE—TECHNIQUE 2

- After 90+ days of gestation, the tubercle is less distinct.

- Proceed to the posterior aspect of the fetus. Find where the posterior muscles of the buttocks come together and form a definite cleavage on the ventral midline (see Figure 53-18).

- Follow the cleavage posteriorly to the tailhead.

- If the fetus is a female, a clitoris will appear as a small round structure in the cleavage shortly before the tailhead is reached (see Figure 53-10, *A*).

Table 53-2

Ultrasonic Cross Sectional Anatomy Found in Planes I, II, and III

Plane I	Plane II	Plane III
Ultrasound cuts a frontal plane	Ultrasound cuts a plane perpendicular to axis of spine in pelvic area	Ultrasound cuts a plane perpendicular to axis of spine in posterior abdominal area
Figure 53-3 Plane I	**Figure 53-6, A** Anus near tail	**Figure 53-13** Plane III
Figure 53-4, A to C Slide of 60-day male, frontal plane	**Figure 53-6, B** Clitoris in cleavage	**Figure 53-14** 60-Day male tubercle
Figure 53-5 134-Day female mammary gland	**Figure 53-7, A, B** Plane II	**Figure 53-15** 65-Day male tubercle
	Figure 53-8, A 60-Day male	**Figure 53-16, A** 140-Day male prepuce
	Figure 53-8, B 65-Day male	**Figure 53-16, B** 145-Day prepuce and urachus
	Figure 53-9, A to E Tibia-tailhead (T-T) triangle	**Figure 53-17, A** 94-Day prepuce and penis
	Figure 53-10, A 80-Day clitoris	**Figure 53-17, B** 95-Day prepuce and penis
	Figure 53-10, B 90-Day mammary gland	**Figure 53-17, C** 117-Day prepuce and penis
	Figure 53-11 124-Day mammary gland	**Figure 53-21** Female gonads at 119 days
	Figure 53-12, A to D Shaft of penis	**Figure 53-22, A, B** Male gonads at 125 days
	Figure 53-18 113-Day posterior midline	**Figure 53-19** Flank view 109-day shaft and glans penis
	Figure 53-20 153-Day tail	
	Figure 53-23 Bones of hindlimbs and pelvis	

- TIP: Caution: If the small round structure is too close to the tailhead, it could be the anus (see Figure 53-6, A).
- Follow the midline or cleavage line anteriorly to encounter the mammary gland in the female (see Figure 53-10, B and C, and 53-11) or the prepuce and penis in the male (see Figure 53-12, A to D).
- A mammary gland appears as a triangular structure with slightly denser tissue than surrounding muscle tissue. It may have two bright hyperechogenic teats and slightly dense areas in each half of the mammary gland; it may also have a translucent division between halves of the mammary gland (see Figure 53-11).
- In the male, the prepuce may appear as a cone-shaped structure with a hyperechoic area within the cone. The hyperechoic area is the penis itself (see Figures 53-16, A to C, and 53-17, A to C).
- Sometimes the actual shaft of the penis can be seen with a hyperechoic distal segment (see Figure 53-12, A to D).
- Occasionally the shaft and glans penis can be seen on a flank view (see Figure 53-19).
- If the prepuce is viewed from a cross section across the posterior ventral abdomen, it will appear as a cone-shaped structure off of the ventral abdominal wall just posterior to the urachus (see Figures 53-16, A, B, and 53-17, A to C).
- The gonads can be viewed from a plane III view of the posterior abdomen near the urachus (male, see Figure 53-22; female, see Figure 53-21).

Text continued on p. 356

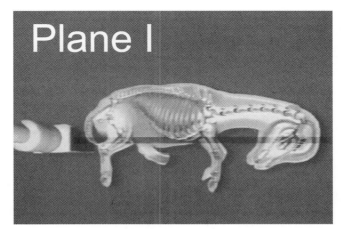

Figure 53-3   Plane I.

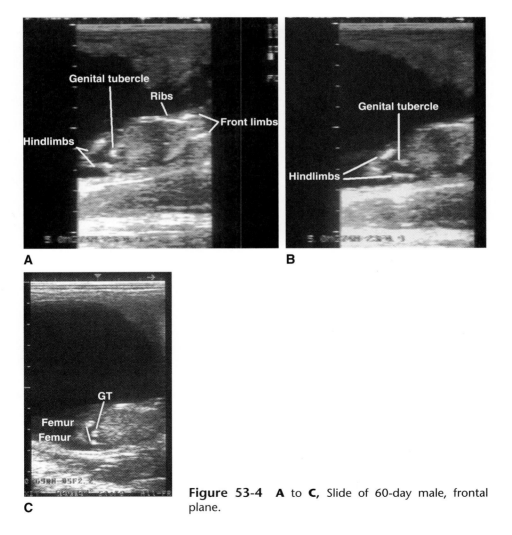

Figure 53-4   **A** to **C,** Slide of 60-day male, frontal plane.

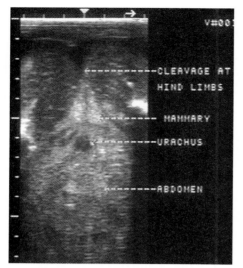

Figure 53-5 134-Day female mammary gland.

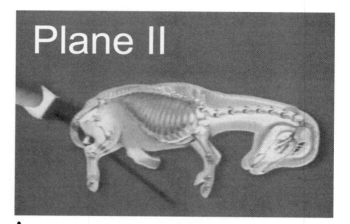

Plane II

A

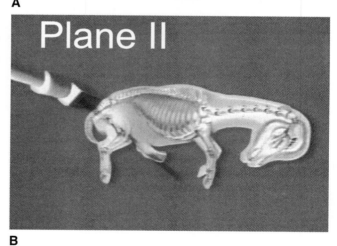

Plane II

B

Figure 53-7 **A** and **B,** Plane II.

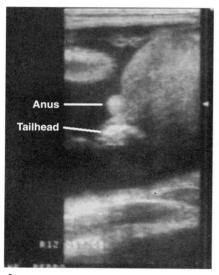

A

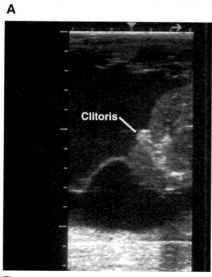

B

Figure 53-6 **A,** Anus near tail. **B,** Clitoris in cleavage.

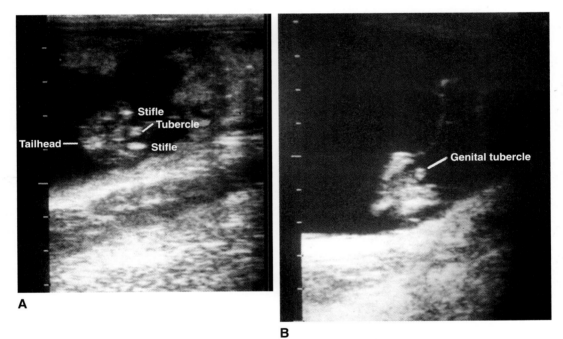

A

B

Figure 53-8 **A,** 60-Day male. **B,** 65-Day male.

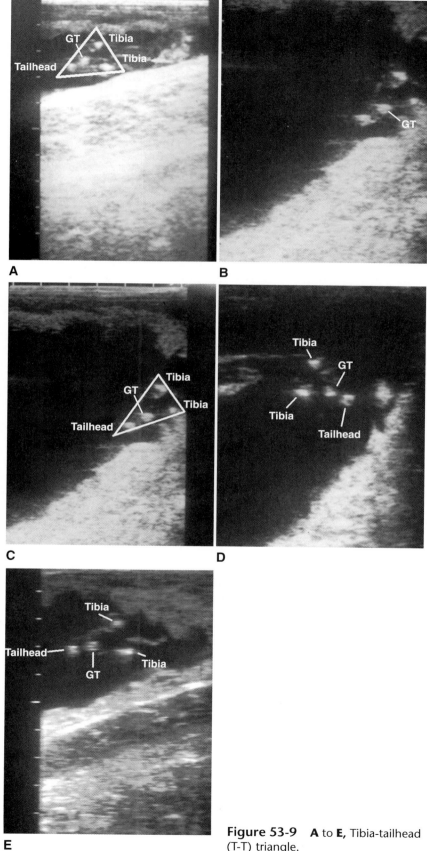

Figure 53-9   **A** to **E,** Tibia-tailhead (T-T) triangle.

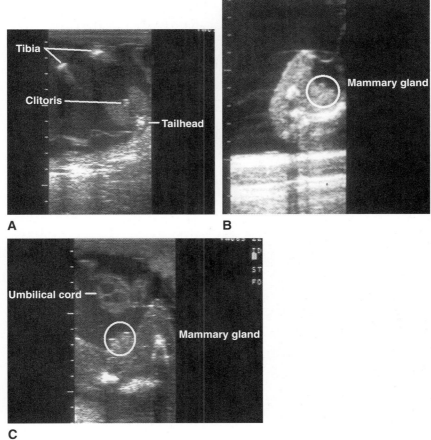

Figure 53-10 **A,** 80-Day clitoris. **B,** 90-Day mammary gland. **C,** 95-Day mammary gland.

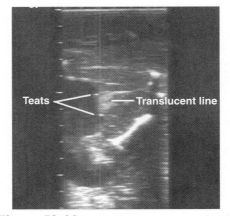

Figure 53-11 124-Day mammary gland.

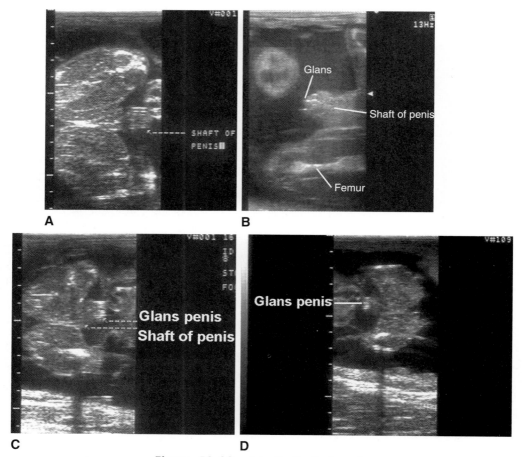

Figure 53-12   **A** to **D,** Shaft of penis.

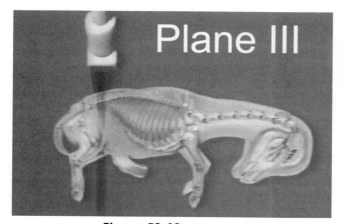

Figure 53-13   Plane III.

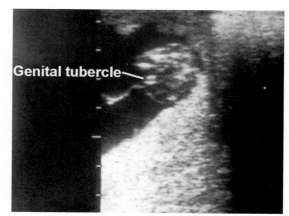

Figure 53-14   60-Day male tubercle.

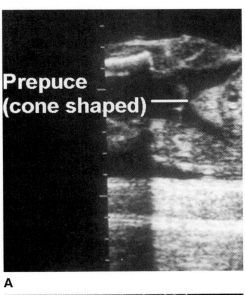

A

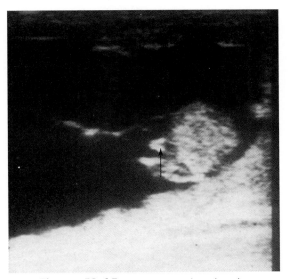

Figure 53-15   65-Day male tubercle.

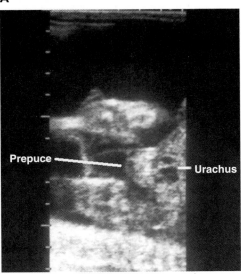

B

Figure 53-16 A, 140-Day male prepuce. **B,** 145-Day prepuce and urachus.

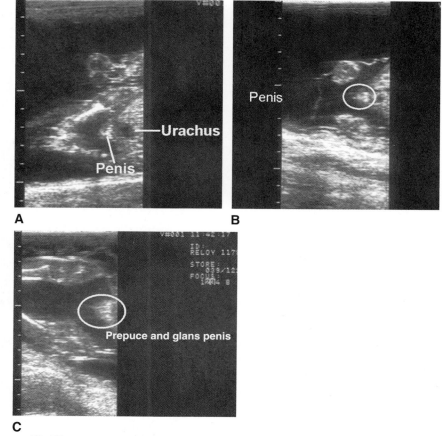

Figure 53-17   A, 94-Day prepuce and penis. **B,** 95-Day prepuce and penis. **C,** 117-Day prepuce and penis.

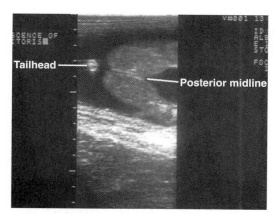

Figure 53-18   113-Day posterior midline.

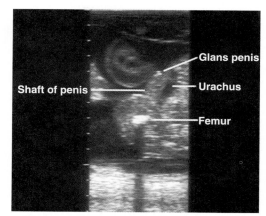

Figure 53-19   Flank view 109-day shaft and glans penis.

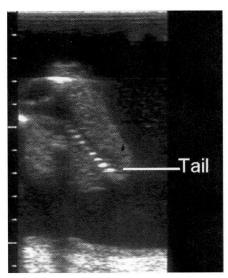

Figure 53-20   110-Day tail.

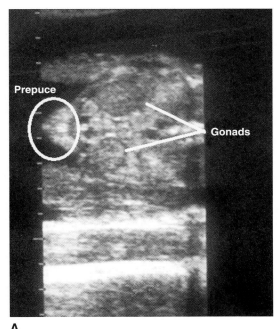

A

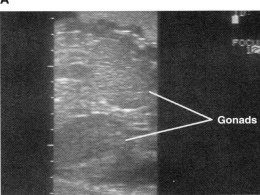

B

Figure 53-22   Homogenous structures. **A** and **B,** Male gonads at 125 days.

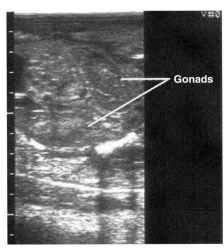

Figure 53-21   Female gonads at 119 days. Translucent horseshoe within gonad.

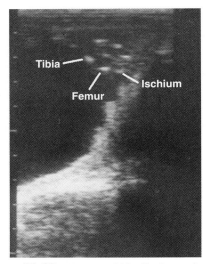

Figure 53-23   Bones of hindlimbs and pelvis.

- As the fetus gets older, the genitalia become more developed and more easily differentiated from surrounding tissue. However, as the fetus develops, it becomes more difficult to access the posterior area. After day 150, the fetus begins to have an anterior presentation, which puts the posterior pelvic area out of reach. Also, because of its size, the fetus is less mobile and less frequently rotates the posterior pelvic area to a more accessible position. A fetal sex determination has been diagnosed at 194 days on transrectal examination, but this is very unusual and possibly not a good sign if the fetus is in a posterior presentation this late in gestation.

CONCLUSION

There are a few precautions to consider:

1. It is mandatory to keep good records of determination.
2. Do not guess—guessing leads to errors; errors lead to lack of confidence in procedure.
3. Certificates can be given, but there are no guarantees given.

It should be emphasized that these techniques are for gender identification only and not for gender control. It would be difficult to have a mare successfully pregnant at 60 days, terminate the pregnancy, and have the mare successfully remated that season.

Learning these sex determination techniques provides a worthwhile service to clients but requires many hours of actual ultrasonographic visualization of the equine fetus between 55 and 150 days of gestation. Only when the ultrasonographic cross-sectional anatomy of the fetus is learned will confidence of an accurate sexual determination be achieved.

Supplemental Reading

Ginther OJ: Ultrasonic Imaging and Animal Reproduction: Horses Book 2, Cross Plains, Wis, Equiservices, 1995.

Ginther OJ, Curran S, Ginther M: Fetal Gender Determination in Cattle and Horses [instructional video], Cross Plains, Wis, Equiservices, 2002.

Holder RD: A Guide to Equine Fetal Sexing (55-150 days) 2002 [instructional video], Wallingford, Conn, Aloka, 2002,.

Holder RD: Fetal sex determination in the mare between 55 and 150 days gestation. Proceedings of the 46th Annual Convention of the American Association of Equine Practitioners, pp 321-324, 2001.

Renaudin CD, Gillis CL, Tarantal AL: Transabdominal Ultrasonographic Determination of Fetal Gender in the Horse During Mid-Gestation [instructional video], Davis, Calif, University of California, Davis, School of Veterinary Medicine.

CHAPTER 54

Twin Reduction Techniques

ANGUS O. MCKINNON

We have known three things about twins for a long time. First, twins are repeatable within the same mare. Second, the twinning rate varies according to breed. Third, the more fertile the stallion, the more twins he is expected to achieve.

Twins are avoidable and should not occur on well-managed breeding farms. Clients understand this and are demanding the most sophisticated management programs available. Presented below are the management techniques in use at the Goulburn Valley Equine Hospital. The hospital is a major referral center and each year is expected to handle multiple referral cases of twin pregnancy that are diagnosed after cessation of the mobility phase.

Historically twins have been the single most important cause of abortion in Thoroughbreds.[1,2] Because most twin pregnancies terminate in early fetal resorption or loss, late term abortions, or the birth of small growth retarded foals, and because mares aborting twins in late gestation frequently have foaling difficulties, damage their reproductive tracts, and are difficult to rebreed, twins are disastrous financially. If foals are born alive they are frequently small, have intra-uterine growth retardation, and a poor survival rate, with many needing expensive, sophisticated, critical care.

Origin, associations, and a general overview of twinning in the horse have been published elsewhere.[3,4]

It is our responsibility to successfully manage early pregnancies such that no mare delivers or aborts twin foals. In consultation with farm managers, owners, and clients, we must utilize available equipment and technology commensurate with economic constraints and other owner/manager preferences to diagnose twin pregnancies as early as practically possible. It is also the responsibility of a veterinary profession to adequately inform owners/managers/clients of reasons why twins may be not diagnosed.

Twins are still occasionally missed despite multiple examinations. Reasons why twins may not be detected, despite repeated examination are (1) difficulty distinguishing structures (this may be related to a poor examination environment, i.e., too much light, poor display characteristics of the ultrasonographic unit, mare movement and/or lack of restraint), (2) variable growth patterns, (3) inability to detect heart beats of adjacent embryos, (4) operator experience, and (5) resolution of the equipment. The most common cause of misdiagnosing the presence of twin pregnancies is examination before the time period that a second pregnancy (asynchronous ovulation) may be reasonably expected to be detected. Another reason appears to be scanning too quickly.

The incidence of abortion has been reported as decreasing,[5] and in the German Thoroughbred industry it has almost halved since the advent of ultrasonography.[6]

ORIGIN OF TWINS

Twins in the horse are unlikely to be identical. Almost all cases of twin pregnancy are expected to be related to multiple ovulation, although at least two occurrences of monozygotic twin pregnancies have been suspected.[7,8] The reason for lack of identical twin formation in the horse is probably related to the capsule.[9] The capsule forms in equine embryos aged around 6 days, shortly after their entry into the uterus.[10,11] When embryos were cultured before the formation of the capsule, hatching occurred in a manner similar to that which occurs in the bovine[11]; however, when embryos were cultured after formation of the capsule, the zona pellucida continued to become progressively thinner and finally fell away from the developing conceptus. Other species that do not have a capsule, such as sheep, cattle, and humans, all have the ability to routinely give birth to identical twins, which apparently form from pinching of a hatching embryo by the zona pellucida.

It has been shown that twins in mares are as likely to result from synchronous versus asynchronous ovulation[12] and that pregnancy rate per follicle was identical for double ovulations on opposite ovaries to that obtained from single ovulations per cycle, but was higher than the pregnancy rate per follicle when double ovulations occurred on the same ovary.[13]

THE OUTCOME OF TWIN PREGNANCIES

Understanding the outcome of twin pregnancies allowed to develop is of great importance to veterinarians, farm managers, and owners. Also important is when to intervene and what probability of success such interventions may be expected to achieve.

WHAT HAPPENS IF WE DO NOTHING?

The mare is very efficient at reducing twins to a single pregnancy. This is done by a competitive absorption of nutrients that is related to size and position of the early pregnancy and later to orientation of the embryo proper within the developing conceptus.[14] However, the initiation of any nonintervention program depends on the age of identification, the orientation of the vesicles, and any disparity in size.

Recognition = 16 Days from Ovulation

Embryo reduction before or on the day of fixation is not considered an important aspect of the natural correction of twins.[15] The probability of a mare losing one or both vesicles of a set of twins from identification before fixation is minimal and approximates that of early embryonic death for the same time period (per vesicle). The recognition of twin pregnancies before fixation day (day 16) is dependent on the day of examination relative to the day of ovulation. Asynchronous ovulations occasionally result in a gross disparity in vesicle size, sometimes as much as 4 to 5 days (i.e., identification of a day 11-12 and a day 16 vesicle concurrently) (Figure 54-1, *A*). In instances such as this, examination one day earlier may have failed to detect the younger of the 2 pregnancies. Recognition that all twin pregnancies occur from multiple ovulations dictates mandatory reexamination of all mares that have 2 corpora lutea (CL) and only a single vesicle detected before fixation (day 16). Recognition before fixation is also dependent on operator experience, resolution of the equipment (= 5 MHZ preferred), monitor capabilities, restraint, other facilities (ability to darken the environment), the presence of uterine cysts, and the skill of the examiner.

Recognition after Fixation (after Day 16)

The recognition of unilaterally fixed twins from day 17 through to 21 (before clear recognition of the developing fetus within the vesicle) may be the most difficult time to determine whether there are twins present. Ultrasonic-graphically, all that is detectable is a thin line (the apposition of the 2 yolk sacs) running approximately in the middle of a slightly over-sized vesicle (Figure 54-1, *B*). Recognition of the fetus(es) within the vesicle a few days later makes differentiation easier (Figure 54-2). Occasionally an inexperienced operator may confuse an abnormally orientated 28 to 30 day single pregnancy with 17 to 20 day unilaterally fixed twins (Figure 54-3). From days 22 to 60 the presence of multiple fetuses, umbilical cords, and general excess in the number of visible membranes should alert the practitioner to the likelihood of more than 1 pregnancy (Figure 54-4). The junction between 2 developing fetuses (after 30 days) between the 2 allantochorions results in a common membrane from the area of apposition. This common membrane has been referred to as the *twin membrane* (see Figure 54-4)[16] and has diagnostic potential, particularly late in pregnancy when it might not be possible to view both fetuses transrectally (>100 days). After 100 days, careful transabdominal ultrasonography may be necessary to determine the presence of twins.

Days 17 to 40

The outcome of pregnancies post fixation is dependent upon their size (diameter) and the nature of their fixation. *Unilateral* (both fixed together at the same corpus cornual junction) fixation reduction is much higher than *bilateral* (one on each side) fixation reduction. Fortunately, unilateral fixation is much higher (approximately 70%) compared to bilateral (30%).[14] In 28 mares with known ovulatory patterns, synchronous ovulations did not affect the type of fixation (9/17 unilateral, 8/17 bilateral). However, for asynchronous ovulation, the frequency of unilateral fixation (10/11) was greater ($P < 0.01$)

Figure 54-1 **A,** Twins with a large disparity in age (~day 10 and day 15). **B,** Twins at approximately day 15. Note the indentation of the corpus cornual junction and the horizontal line that is lower and marks the junction between the 2 vesicles.

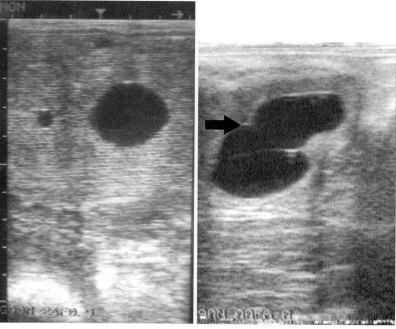

A   B

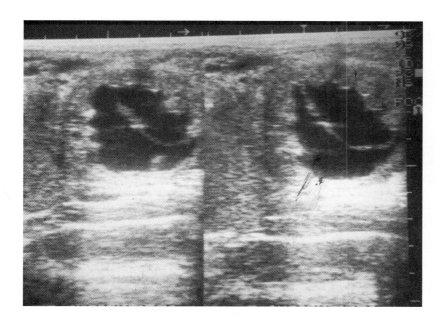

Figure 54-2 Recognition of a fetus in each vesicle at or around day 20 to 22 helps identification of some twins.

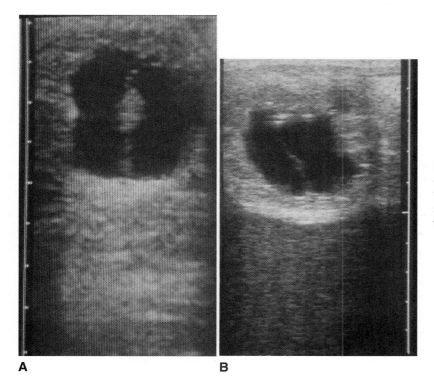

A   B

Figure 54-3 A, An abnormally orientated ~30 day pregnancy should not be confused with twins wherein the vesicle has coalesced into a single vesicle with an ultrasonically visible line within (B).

than the frequency of bilateral fixation (1/11). The incidence of embryo reduction was greater ($P < 0.01$) for unilateral fixation (14/19) than for bilateral fixation (0/9) and was greater ($P < 0.05$) for asynchronous ovulation (9/11) than for synchronous ovulation (5/17).[14] Practically speaking this means that if asynchronous ovulations have resulted in significant age differences between vesicles (i.e., >3 mm diameter at day 15), then rate of embryonic reduction is very high.[14] In cases of unilateral fixation, 22 of 22 mares with vesicles of dissimilar size

had reduction compared to 19 of 26 (73%) with vesicles of similar size.[17] As a result of work studying reduction of unilateral versus bilateral twin pregnancies in mares from days 17 to 40, Ginther proposed that the nutrient intake from the larger vesicle (before the fetus was present) prevented adequate nutrition of the smaller vesicle. Later the position of the fetus proper and its emerging allantoic sac seemed to determine whether a given conceptus survived or underwent late reduction. The fetus, the vascularized wall of the yolk sac adjacent to the fetus, and the emerg-

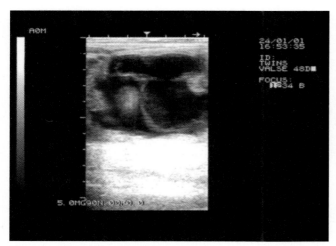

Figure 54-4 Two 48-day pregnancies can be seen with the twin membrane in between.

ing allantoic sac were exposed to the endometrium (uterine lumen) in the surviving vesicles. In the vesicles that underwent reduction, much of the corresponding area of the vesicle wall was covered by the wall of the adjacent survivor and was thus deprived of adequate embryonal-maternal exchange and therefore regressed.

In summary, dissimilarity in diameter increases the likelihood of unilateral fixation, increases the incidence of reduction for unilateral fixed vesicles, hastens the day of occurrence of reduction and shortens the interval from initiation to completion of reduction.[14]

The incidence of reduction for *bilaterally fixed vesicles* is negligible and approximates that of standard early embryonic death in this period.

Of the 85% of reductions by day 40 in cases of unilateral fixed twin pregnancies, 59% of reductions occurred between days 17 and 20, 27% between days 21 and 30, and 14% between days 31 and 38. The majority of early reductions occurred spontaneously, by day 20, compared to reductions after day 20, which were preceded by a gradual decrease in size of the eliminated vesicle. In addition, when twins were dissimilar in diameter (4 mm or more), they were more likely to undergo reduction by day 20.[17] Other studies have demonstrated similar results. The hypothesis of an early embryonic reduction mechanism for elimination of excess embryo in mares is not new and was suggested as early as 1982. However, ultrasonography was necessary to adequately document the occurrence and nature of the reduction.[18]

Day 40 Onward

Ginther and Griffin[16] examined the natural outcome of bilateral twins (one in each horn) that were viable on day 40 in 15 pony mares. Readers should be aware that pony mares are not necessarily a good model for larger breeds, as the incidence of twins is low and evidence suggests that the larger the breed (Draught, Thoroughbred and Warmblood), the higher the probability of maintaining twins.

Fifteen pony mares were monitored by ultrasonography until the outcome of the pregnancy was determined. Sixty-six percent (10/15) of the pregnancies resulted in either death of both (80%) or death of one (20%) during months 2 or 3. Nothing occurred from then until month 8. Between months 8 and 11, 2 mares lost 1 fetus (fetal death was associated with mummification) and 2 mares lost both. The 2 mares that lost 1 pregnancy both delivered undersized, weak foals at birth. One mare (7%) delivered live twins at term, and 2 normal foals were born from mares losing the 1 pregnancy (absorption of the fetus rather than mummification) in month 2. In this study, 6 live foals were born (2 of normal size) from a total of 15 mares and 30 fetuses. This incidence is similar to a previous report wherein, of 130 pregnant mares with twins, only 17 live foals (13%) were produced.[19] An interesting observation from the latter report was that from the 102 mares that delivered live or dead twins in the previous year, only 37 produced live foals the next seasons, and thus over 2 seasons there was an average of 23% producing live foals.[19] An earlier study[20] was extremely useful in categorizing outcome of twins that managed to survive to later pregnancy. Twinning accounted for 22% of the cases of abortion and stillbirth between 1967 and 1970. Sixty-two sets of twins and their placentas were examined from Thoroughbred mares. All were considered to be dizygous. Abortion or stillbirth of both twins from 3 months of gestation to term occurred in 64.5% of mares, although most (72.6%) slipped from 8 months to term. In the remaining cases 1 twin (21%) or both twins (14.5%) were born alive. Most foals at term were stunted and emaciated, and of the 31 alive at birth, only 18 survived to 2 weeks of age.[20] In this study, twin placentation was divided into 3 morphological groups according to the disposition of the chorionic sacks within the uterus. Type A placentation was seen in 79% of cases (48 sets of twins). One fetus occupied 1 horn and most of the body (mean 68% of the total functional surface area), while the other twin occupied only 1 horn and usually only a small part of the adjacent body. Where the chorions abutted there was a variable degree of invagination of the smaller chorion into the allantoic cavity of the larger twin. These pregnancies frequently ended in abortion or stillbirth of 1 or both twins. In this group, 31 of 48 mares lost their pregnancies between 3 and 9 months (64.5%). The gestation length in this group was frequently shorter, and at birth the larger twin had a much greater chance of survival than the smaller one. In this group, only 6 foals of 48 sets were born alive. Of the 6 fetuses born alive, 5 were the larger twin. Type B placentation occurred in 11% of cases (7 sets), and the placentas were orientated such that the villous surface areas were more or less equally divided and each fetus occupied 1 horn and half of the body. Both foals were usually similar in size and were usually born alive. Nine foals survived to 2 weeks from 6 sets of twins that made it to term. In this group (7 total), 1 was aborted at 7 months. Type C placentation was seen in 10% of cases (6 sets of twins). In this group there was a greater disparity between the surface area of the 2 chorions. The smaller twin occupying only part of one horn died earlier on and became mummified. The larger twin was usually born alive and had a fair chance of survival. In this group, 3 foals were born alive from 6 pregnancies at term.[21] The authors attributed the loss of twin fetuses and poor survival rates to placental insufficiency.

It should be clear that our philosophy is that nonintervention is only acceptable when twins are diagnosed as a unilateral occurrence between days 17 and 40, and then the decision depends on factors such as the value of the foal, the potential for rebreeding, and the ability of the veterinarian to manually intervene. Intervention in twin pregnancies is strongly recommended in all other circumstances (see below).

WHEN AND HOW SHOULD WE INTERVENE?

Recognition at or before 16 Days from Ovulation

The first technique for manual crush of the conceptus during the mobility phase utilized manual reduction with good results[21] and was a variation on previously reported techniques for twin pregnancies.[22,23] The technique involved gentle manipulation of the embryonic vesicle to the tip of 1 uterine horn and manual rupture. When applied to single pregnancies it resulted in pseudopregnancy, and when applied to twin pregnancies it resulted in a single pregnancy in 7 of 8 attempts.[21] Later, utilizing the same techniques, mares were treated with single or multiple progestagen administration (hydroxyprogesterone caproate), an anti-prostaglandin (flunixin meglumine) plus progestagen, or given no treatment before manual embryonic rupture in the mobility phase.[24,25] The technique resulted in 10 of 10 (100%) mares maintaining pregnancy in the control group (no treatment, just manual rupture) and 37 of 40 (92.5%) in the treated mares group. The amount of $PGF_{2\alpha}$ released was directly correlated with the pressure required to cause embryonic rupture. Flunixin meglumine inhibited $PGF_{2\alpha}$ release after embryonic rupture. Treatment with progestagen plus flunixin meglumine or progestagen singly or multiply was not better than no treatment at all (although it was subsequently shown that the progestagen chosen had no ability to maintain pregnancy in ovariectomized mares and did not bind to progesterone receptors in the horse).[26] Another report[27] demonstrated that 60 of 66 mares (90.9%) maintained a single vesicle after manual reduction was attempted prior to fixation. Five of the 6 mares in which the procedure was not successful subsequently conceived. Since 1984,[28] we have used a modification[4] of the technique described originally.[21] With this technique, the ultrasound probe is used to manipulate the vesicles while keeping one or both vesicles in view during the manipulation and, more importantly, the crushing or rupture of the vesicle (Figure 54-5). Utilizing this technique it is possible to more accurately and quickly separate vesicles. It was originally proposed[21] that when vesicles were in apposition mares be reexamined approximately 1 hour later. By utilizing the probe to manipulate vesicles, separation is achieved (prefixation) very quickly in most instances. Commonly, the smaller fetus is destroyed despite the lack of evidence to support pre-fixation reduction. On occasion it is necessary to revisit the mare 24 to 48 hours after the original evaluation if the smaller of the two vesicles is less than 1 cm in diameter, as sometimes these can be more difficult to destroy.

Separation of vesicles should always be possible if the vesicles are still able to be identified as 2 spherical, noncoalesced structures. Briefly, the technique involves separation of the vesicles using the probe. A finger is placed on either side of the probe to help stabilize the vesicle to be moved. Gentle back and forth movement of the probe with pressure results in the 2 vesicles becoming separated (Figure 54-6). The separation is identified by lack of a vesicle under the probe. The vesicle can be crushed as close as 0.5 cm from the other, but it is generally best to separate them at least 2 cm, in case the mare moves at the time of increasing pressure. The vesicle is crushed by gradually increasing the pressure using the probe. Occasionally, refractory cases may need a sudden increase in pressure much like a quick flick of the end of the probe. This latter technique is quite useful for smaller (day 11-13) vesicles.

When the vesicle is crushed it is not uncommon for fluid to surround the other. This is not a problem at this stage of pregnancy. Later (day 25), fluid surrounding the other vesicle is thought to be a potential problem.

At the GVEH (www.gvequine.com.au/breeding_efficiency.htm), records were evaluated for 1716 Thoroughbred (TB) mare cycles and 1294 Standardbred (St B) mare cycles. Twins were diagnosed in 245 of 1716 cycles in TB mares (14.3%) and 46 of 1294 of St B cycles (3.5%). After twin reduction, mares are not routinely examined until the next scheduled examination (i.e., 21-25 days post ovulation [detection of the fetus]). When mares were reexamined after prefixation embryonic reduction, 10 of 245 TB mares (4%) had lost the remaining pregnancy and 8 of 46 St B mares (17.4%) were empty. The number of TB mares losing the remaining pregnancy (4.0%) is similar to 3.7% (63/1716), which was the calculated rate of early embryonic death (EED) on the same farms for mares with a single pregnancy diagnosed at day 13 to 15 and then subsequently found to be empty at the next scan. Interestingly, the number of St B pregnancies lost was much higher after twin reduction (8/46, 17.4%) compared to the calculated rate of EED (7.1%). This, we believe, was likely related to economics, wherein the St B clients are unwilling to scan too early. Thus twins, when detected, are likely to be closer to final fixation or fixed already and harder to manage.

It is our contention that the procedure has developed to the stage that it is *always expected* that a single pregnancy will exist after prefixation embryo reduction is attempted. Unless a mistake occurs and the other vesicle is ruptured at the time of initial manipulation, we feel that any failure to survive the procedure is more likely a result of uterine inflammatory changes and infection rather than a result of the procedure. We believe that this is the most reliable technique available but feel it is important to highlight the experience of the personnel involved. From discussions with farm managers and other veterinarians it is clear that only veterinarians involved with sophisticated reproductive management, such as the routine use of ultrasonography, can expect to achieve these types of results. Our strong recommendation to vet-

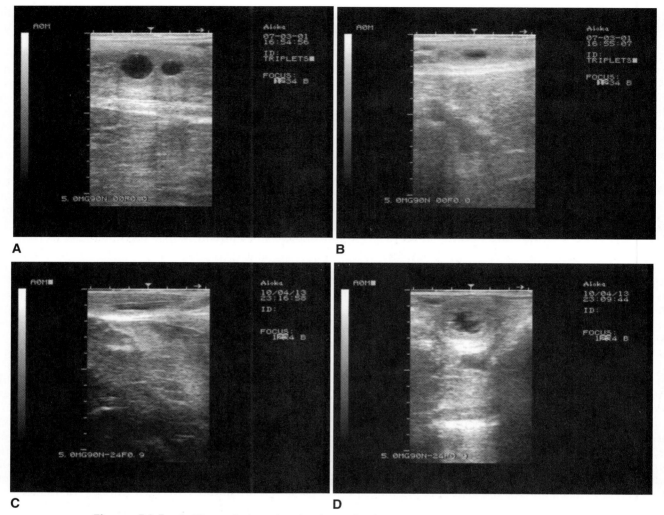

Figure 54-5 **A,** The technique for simple crush of a vesicle prefixation. The vesicles to be separated are identified. **B,** Frequent back and forth scanning may be necessary to continually confirm the location of each vesicle, and then gentle pressure is used to separate it from the other. **C,** As pressure is gradually increased, the vesicle changes shape and starts to flatten. At the appropriate moment, a little quick extra pressure completes ablation. **D,** It is quite common to see fluid immediately after the crush.

erinarians and clients is that all mares be examined within 14 to 16 days of breeding. Expected time to ovulation after breeding will depend on frequency of examination and use of ovulation induction agents such as hCG or GnRH. Factors that may modify this decision are breed, mare value, ability of the stud master or owner to facilitate examination of the mare, and, on occasion, education of the owner.

Recognition after Fixation (after Day 16)

Days 17 to 20
In all cases of *bilaterally fixed* twins, 1 is destroyed immediately. The mare has an extremely efficient biological embryo reduction mechanism that operates when twins are in apposition (*unilaterally fixed*).[14,18,29] Reduction occurred in 100% of 22 mares with asynchronous ovula-

tion (differences in vesicle sizes of >4 mm in diameter) and in 19 of 26 mares (73%) with a vesicle size difference of 0 to 3 mm. Because the rate of embryo reduction between day 17 and 20 is so high for unilateral fixation, equine practitioners frequently elect to leave these developing pregnancies and determine their outcome later. Our philosophy is that if the 2 vesicles have coalesced into one larger vesicle with an ultrasonographically visible line in division (see Figure 54-3, *B*), they are left totally alone; however, if the individual vesicles have still retained a spherical orientation or a spherical shape (like a figure 8), then they can be separated gently with the probe and crushed either in situ or after being manipulated apart (Figure 54-6). Due to the nature of our practice, few mares present with this configuration in the Thoroughbred population; however, it is not uncommon in the Standardbred population, wherein economics

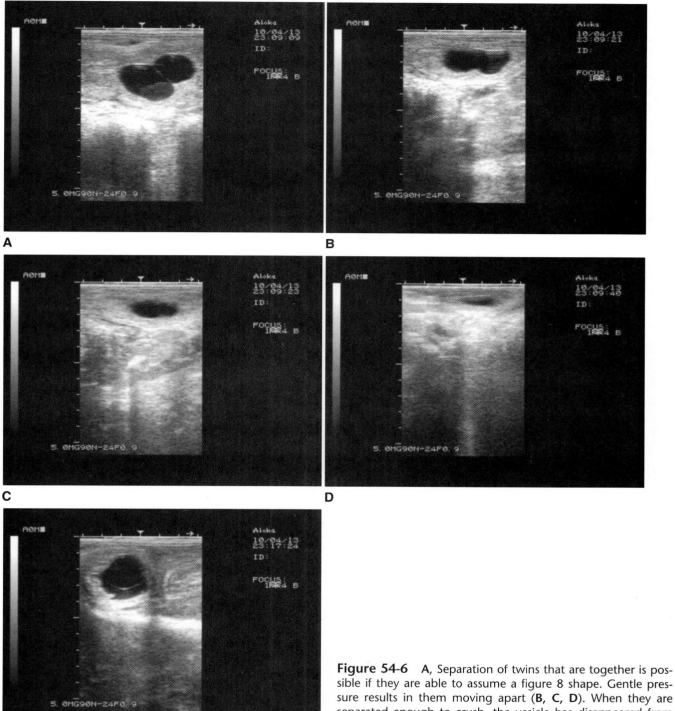

Figure 54-6 **A**, Separation of twins that are together is possible if they are able to assume a figure 8 shape. Gentle pressure results in them moving apart (**B, C, D**). When they are separated enough to crush, the vesicle has disappeared from the screen. **E**, When vesicles are in close proximity to each other at the time of the crush, it is quite common for fluid from the crushed vesicle to surround the other.

dictate that pregnancy diagnosis is often delayed past the time the mobility phase has ended. Results from our practice with twins in this configuration are reduced compared to prefixation intervention procedures. Others have reported good results postfixation. One group reported success in 49 of 50 cases post fixation.[24] The work of Bowman (1986)[27] more closely parallels our experiences. With bilateral embryo fixation and intervention, he reported almost no losses with 40 of 44 mares from day 16 to day 30 (90.9%), having a single pregnancy detected on day 45. With unilateral fixation the results were the following: days 16 to 17, 16 of 18 (89%); days 18 to 19, 23 of 24 (95.8%); days 20 to 21, 8 of 13 (61.5%); days 22 to 24, 4 of 9 (47.4%); days 25 to 30, 1 of 4 (25%). Because of the high incidence of embryo reduction with unilateral fixation and the low incidence with bilateral fixation, we have clear recommendations with twins in the day 17 to 20 period. Those that have rounded (figure 8 shaped) twins, still retaining their vesicle turgidity, that can be separated are crushed either in situ or after being manipulated apart. In all cases where the vesicles have appar-ently coalesced into a larger vesicle with an ultrasonic-graphically single line dividing the two, we leave them alone, more particularly so if there is any unevenness in vesicle size. In all cases of bilaterally fixed twins, one is destroyed immediately.

Days 21 to 30

All cases of bilaterally fixed twins of this age group are manipulated, and one is destroyed immediately (Figure 54-7). In most cases we do not attempt to manually destroy one vesicle with unilaterally fixed twins (Figure 54-8) of this age group until after day 30 and before day 35. At this age it is too easy to rupture both vesicles, and the maximum success we believe we can expect is 50% (see previous section), which is less than or similar to the mares' own biological reduction mechanism.

Days 30 to 35

During the period before the formation of endometrial cups, gentle pressure may be placed on one vesicle. We do not attempt total ablation at this time as resulting

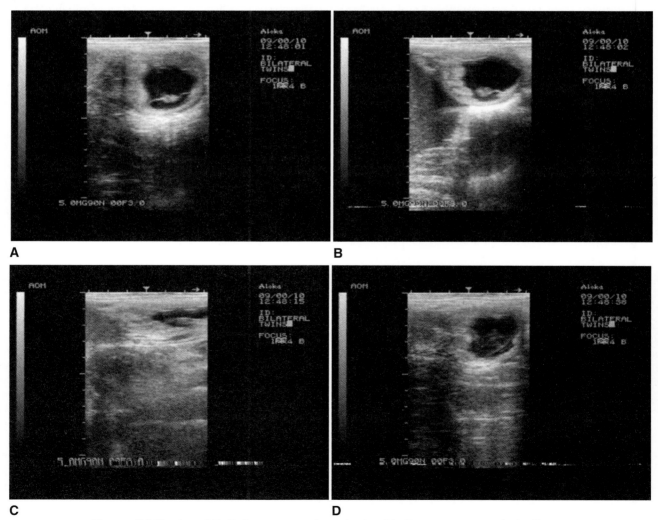

Figure 54-7 **A** and **B**, Twins at approximately day 24. Firm pressure results in flattening of the vesicle (**C**) and, ultimately, rupture (**D**).

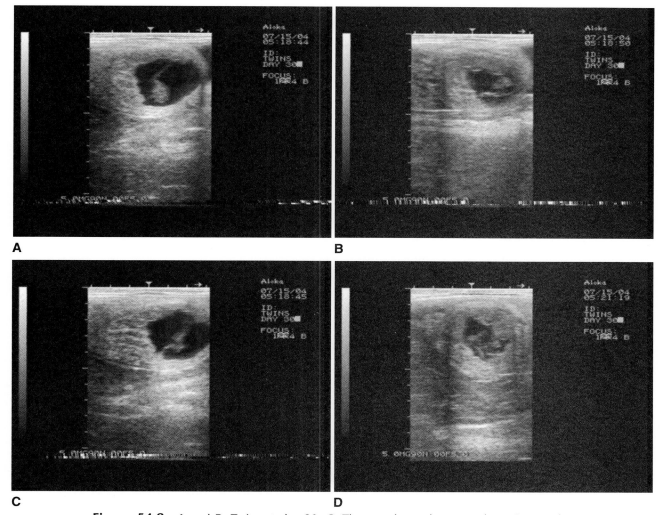

Figure 54-8 **A** and **B**, Twins at day 30. **C**, The membrane between the twins can be clearly detected. **D**, Rupture of the vesicle is demonstrated by multiple membranes. It is not ideal to rupture membranes in unilateral pregnancies or bilateral pregnancies after approximately day 35.

fluid sometimes surrounds the other fetus and effectively separates placental (chorionic girdle/trophoblast cells) attachments to the uterus. In these cases (total rupture of the vesicle), death of the remaining vesicle is very common. Between days 30 and 35 we attempt to pinch one vesicle and create a "snow flake" effect, which is the shedding of cells from the membranes. Demonstration of this effect almost always results in gradual loss of the affected conceptus. The pinching of the vesicle can be likened to membrane slipping of a bovine pregnancy except that we use the probe to produce the effect. Occasionally, in mares with multiple cysts, twins may be missed and then identified at a later time. In general, if they are unilateral, it is best to leave them to the mare's natural embryonic reduction method; however, ablation can be attempted (Figure 54-9).

Days 36 to 60

From day 36 onward it is a reasonable assumption that endometrial cup formation and subsequent eCG secre-

tion will prevent many mares from returning to heat after early embryonic death. Abortion after 35 days is commonly associated with difficulties recycling the mare.[30,31] In one study[32] in which mares were aborted either between days 26 and 31 or between days 30 and 50, 8 of 11 became pregnant versus 2 of 7, respectively. This is similar to the work of Pascoe,[19] who concluded that the administration of a prostaglandin analogue less than 35 days from gestation was outstandingly successful as a method of treatment for twin pregnancy.

Manual intervention at this time is, in our experience, very good in bilateral twin pregnancies (<45 days), but only approximately 50% successful in unilateral twin pregnancies. Success improves with use of more subtle pressure and damage to the chorioallantoic membrane rather than complete rupture in one attempt. Demonstration of the snowflake effect without vesicle rupture consistently results in a gradual (48 hour) stress of the fetus and ultimate loss of heartbeat for the conceptus. These pregnancies have the fetal fluids that become

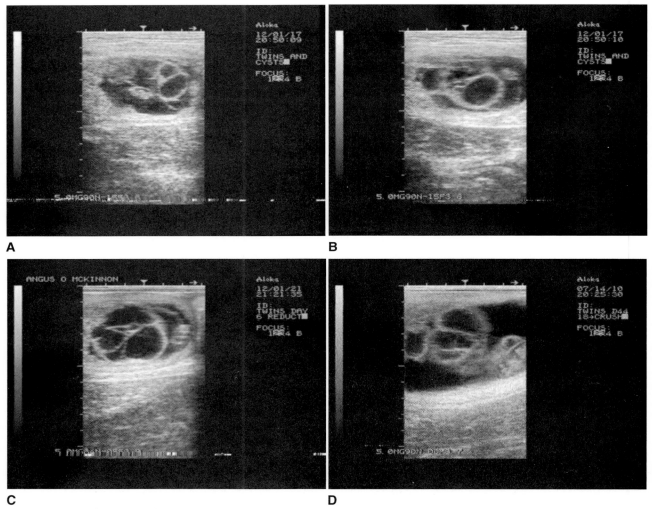

Figure 54-9   Twins identified with multiple cysts. **A,** The fetus is visible in the lower left hand corner. **B,** The other twin is visible in the upper right hand corner. **C,** A single pregnancy is present 6 days after manipulation. **D,** A single pregnancy is detected 18 days after manipulation.

progressively more hyperechoic and reduce in size without interfering with the survival of the other fetus (Figure 54-10). Early pregnancies tend to be resorbed without a major increase in echogenicity of the fetal fluids (Figure 54-11). It is important with these fetuses to always attempt to damage the same one. Multiple attempts (i.e., every day or every other day for 5 to 10 sessions) may be necessary to elicit the correct response (Figure 54-12); however, quite frequently we are unable to create sufficient damage for fetal destruction. In these cases, rather than creating major trauma (rupture of the vesicle), an alternative approach is sought after day 60. A combination of membrane slip and/or oscillation of the fetus is used. If we are unsuccessful in establishing a response at this stage, then the pregnancy is left until after day 100 (see below). Our anticipated success rates are 50% reduction, and approximately 50% of cases result in further examination after day 100. With careful

manipulation the demise of both fetuses should occur less than 5% of the time.

A variety of methods have reportedly been used to treat twins at this stage. Manual crushing was originally reported,[23] and results suggest that earlier crushing is better and, if possible, crushing should occur before day 31 because after day 35 manual rupture is sometimes not possible. The author quoted the following results between day 35 and 45: 60% resorption of both, 20% single foaling, and 20% survival of both. Pascoe[19] demonstrated that needle puncture of 1 twin combined with nonsteroidal antiinflammatory treatment (meclofenmic acid) resulted in no foals born. A more elaborate and invasive approach, such as intra-fetal injection with saline via a laparotomy, has been reported,[33] as has removal of 1 fetus via a video endoscope[34] (abandoned as being not practical). An interesting report was the surgical technique for removal of 1 conceptus from mares with twin

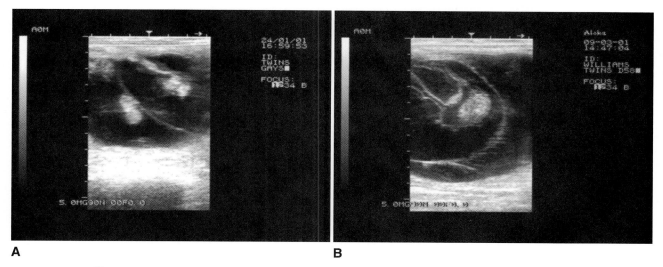

Figure 54-10   **A**, Identification of twin pregnancies at approximately day 45. **B**, Multiple traumas to the membranes/fetus have resulted in death of 1 fetus with increased echogenicity of the fetal fluids and lack of heart beat.

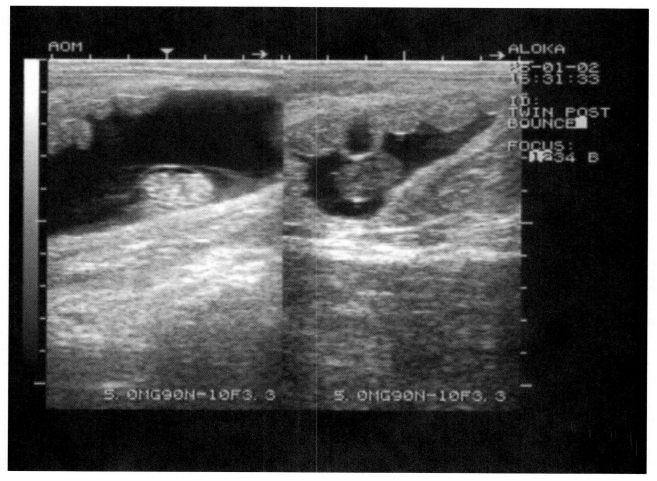

Figure 54-11   Normal 48-day pregnancy on the left and resorption of fluids and the fetus on the right.

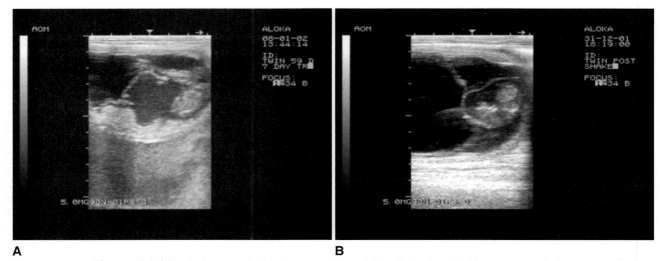

A

B

Figure 54-12 **A,** Increased debris and echogenicity of the fetal fluids are a good sign of fetal demise. **B,** Occasionally an increase in size of the amnionic cavity is observed with fetal demise.

concepti more than 35 days of gestational age.[35,36] Eight mares had bicornuate pregnancies, and 7 mares had uni-cornuate twin concepti. Five of 6 surviving mares with bicornuate twin concepti delivered a single viable foal, and none of the 7 mares originally with uni-cornuate twin concepti produced a foal. The poor survival rate of uni-cornuate twin concepti was attributed to disruption of the remaining chorioallantois during surgery. Trans-vaginal ultrasound guided fetal puncture for destruction of 1 of a set of twin pregnancies has been reported.[37] Fetal fluids from 1 fetus were aspirated while observing the relationship between the needle fetus yoke sac and allan-tochorion between days 20 and 45. Three of 4 bicornu-ate twin pregnancies resulted in a single pregnancy 10 days or greater after interference (similar to or less than our ability to manually destroy 1 conceptus in this con-figuration). Three of 9 (33%) still had a viable single preg-nancy after 10 days when twins were fixed together (between day 20 and 45). These results were disappoint-ing; however, they may be improved with experience and/or antibiotic therapy at the time of intervention. Ultrasound guided fluid withdrawal between day 50 and 65 was studied in single pregnancies[38]; however, the study did not involve any twins. Our experiences with trans-vaginal ultrasound-guided fetal reduction are small (n = 5); however, between 45 and 60 days, the fetus within the vesicle was difficult to position. We have only attempted to directly puncture the fetus, not aspirate fluid, and are unlikely to persevere with this technique (fetal puncture at this age) due to the difficulties involved. All cases ended in loss of both fetuses, usually within 3 days of interference. A more recent report suggested around 20% success with transvaginal procedures.[39]

Days 60 to 100
Between day 60 and 100 it becomes more difficult to damage the chorioallantois. In these cases we identify the most conveniently located (always the smallest) of the twins and repeatedly traumatize it by oscillation, or membrane slip, or attempt to damage the cranium with multiple attempts of single digit percussion. Similarly to the previous scenario, approximately 50% succumb to this procedure; however, it is tedious and time consum-ing, and thus we commonly avoid this time period.

Days 100 Onward
Probably the most common reason for being presented mares at this late stage of gestation with twins is failure of the aforementioned techniques. Less frequently twins have been missed in earlier diagnostic attempts, and more recently there has been an increase in diagnosis of twins at this stage due to the widespread use of fetal sexing procedures (R Holder, personal communication). Fre-quently mares have been identified with twins late in the breeding season, and the owner has adopted a noninter-vention approach. Because the possibility of fetal reduc-tion after 100 days is very low and the probability of abortion or stillbirth is extremely high, an approach was developed to eliminate 1 pregnancy at a later stage of ges-tation.[40] The technique involved transabdominal ultra-sonographic identification of the twins and intracardiac injection of a lethal substance. The smaller twin was always identified. Initial results with saline and air were unsuccessful, but when the solution was replaced with potassium chloride, 7 of 18 mares (39.9%) had a single live foal. We have been utilizing this technique since 1988 and can report similar experiences. Our initial success was not very promising (2/10 live foals) until the potassium chlo-ride solution was replaced with 10 to 20 ml of procaine penicillin,[4] which has resulted in a live foal rate of 56%. The current procedure at the GVEH is to tranquilize the mare with Detomidine[41] and identify the smaller fetus, or in the case of evenly sized fetuses, the one with more potential for placental expansion. A 6 to 10 inch, 16 needle with a tip designed for ultrasonographic enhance-ment (Cook, Australia) is passed through the needle guide biopsy channel into either the heart, lungs, or abdomen of the identified fetus (Figure 54-13). Penicillin is injected,

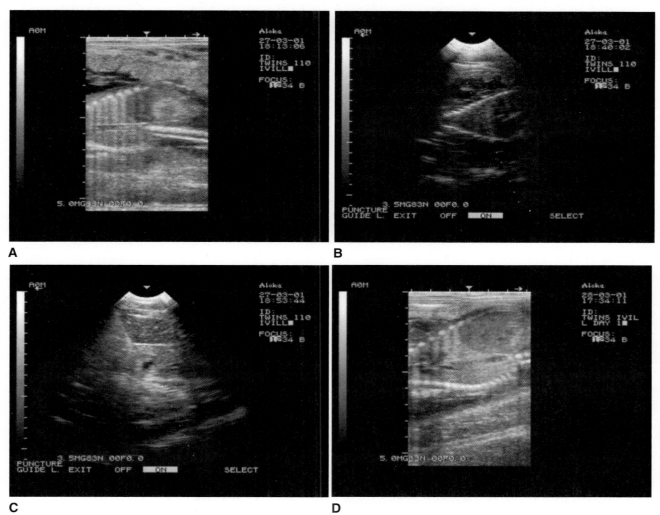

A **B**

C **D**

Figure 54-13 **A**, Twins at approximately 110 days (transrectal). The ribs, lungs, liver, aorta, and abdominal contents can be clearly identified. **B**, Transabdominal scan demonstrating the line of needle puncture. **C**, Immediately after injection of penicillin. The needle is visible to the left of the puncture line guide. The fetal chest is not as easy to see as it is filled with penicillin. In addition, some penicillin has escaped outside the chest. **D**, The surviving twin one day after injection. The fetal heart, lungs, liver, ribs, and aorta are all clearly visible.

Continued

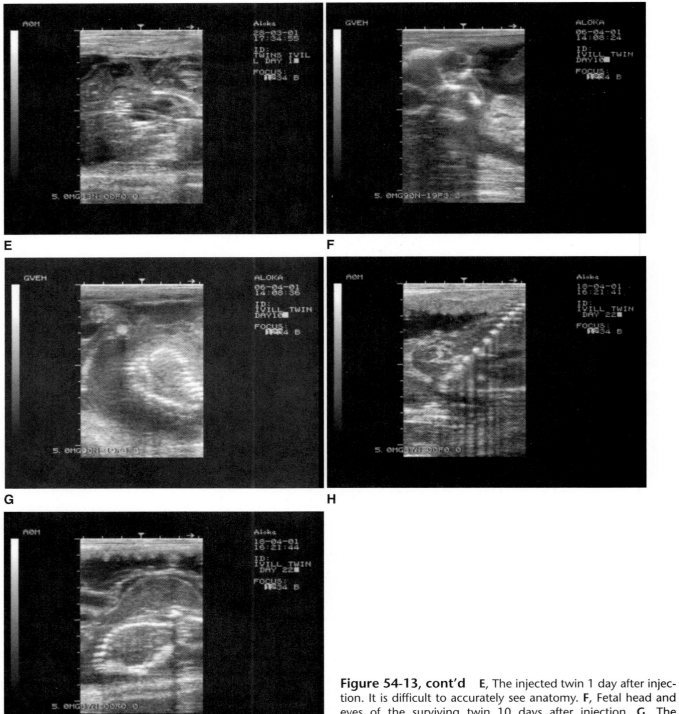

Figure 54-13, cont'd   **E,** The injected twin 1 day after injection. It is difficult to accurately see anatomy. **F,** Fetal head and eyes of the surviving twin 10 days after injection. **G,** The injected twin showing signs of advanced mummification at 10 days after injection. **H,** Same as **D** and **F** at 22 days after injection. **I,** Same as **E** and **G** at day 22 after injection.

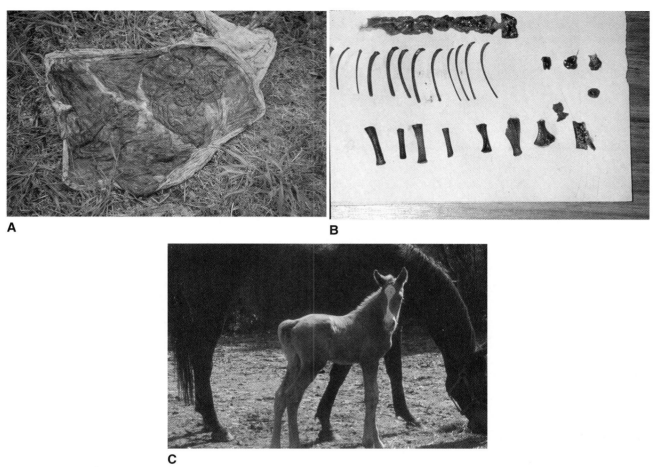

Figure 54-14 **A,** Membranes containing mummified bones. The client was kind enough to arrange the bones they collected (**B**) and the foal was of normal size at birth (**C**).

and the fetus is monitored for the next 5 to 10 minutes. If the needle is in the chest or abdomen, the demise of the fetus still occurs, though it takes a little longer (up to 5 minutes). The apparent advantages of penicillin as we see them are the following: (1) it reduces iatrogenic bacterial contamination, (2) it can be visualized ultrasonicgraphically as it is injected, and (3) fetal death can still be obtained without intracardiac needle placement. We have attempted to place mares on Regumate and long-term oral antibiotics but have found no difference in fetal survival rates with either treatment compared to no treatment. At the time of needle puncture mares are treated with systemic antibiotics for 3 days and intravenous phenylbutazone. There has been much discussion about the production of small, dysmature foals from successful use of this technique. While this occasionally does occur, care in correct fetus identification (biggest fetus with the most potential for placental expansion) has lowered the occurrence of this outcome dramatically. This is more readily possible when there have been multiple opportunities to observe fetal size, position with the pregnant horn(s), and uterine body and placental arrangements. After injection and death, the fetus gradually becomes mummified

(Figure 54-13, *G* and *I*). Commonly these fetal remnants can be detected within the placenta at birth (Figure 54-14).

Late in gestation twins may be difficult to recognize with transrectal ultrasonography except in those cases of observation of the twin membrane.[16] Abdominal ultrasonography is useful to diagnose twins.[40,42]

In the event of failure to diagnose twin pregnancies, abortion is occasionally heralded by lactation late in gestation (>7 months). There are reports of successful maintenance of pregnancy despite premature lactation (>1 month before foaling) in cases with twin gestation. Apparently the premature lactation is induced by fetal death and the beginning of mummification of 1 fetus, which thus threatens the remaining live fetus. Four mares with apparent impending twin abortion were able to deliver live single foals concurrent with a mummified twin after supplementation with progesterone was initiated upon recognition of inappropriate lactation late in gestation.[43,44] In these cases, although foals were born small, they survived and thrived normally. Further work will be necessary to determine which mares will respond best or even at all to supplementation with progesterone for initiation of premature lactation.

From all of the preceding discussion it should be obvious to readers that in our opinion the best method of handling twins is early identification and destruction of one (day 11 to 16).

After submission of the manuscript for publication, the author became aware of an additional technique described by Wolfsdorf and colleagues.[45] This technique offers a new approach to twins by manipulation between 65 to 110 days, which traditionally is a period that has usually been devoid of useful techniques. The technique is performed best in standing mares through a flank laparotomy. The clinician can feel each fetus and then separate the head of one from its neck by grasping the cranial cervical vertebrae and breaking the collateral ligaments to the skull. The technique has been consistent and rewarding with good results.

References

1. Acland HM: Abortion in mares. In McKinnon AO, Voss JL (eds): Equine Reproduction. Philadelphia, London, Lea & Febiger, pp 554-562, 1993.
2. Acland HM: Abortion in mares: diagnosis and prevention. Compend Cont Educ Pract Vet 1987; 9:318-326.
3. Ginther OJ. Reproductive biology of the mare: basic and applied aspects, ed 2, Cross Plains, Wisconsin, Equiservices, 1992.
4. McKinnon AO, Rantanen NW. Twins. In Rantanen NW, McKinnon AO (eds): Equine diagnostic ultrasonography. Philadelphia, Williams and Wilkins, pp 141-156, 1998.
5. Hong CB, Donahue JM, Giles RC et al: Equine abortion and stillbirth in central Kentucky during 1988 and 1989 foaling seasons. J Vet Diagn Invest 1993; 5:560-566.
6. Merkt H, Jochle W: Abortions and twin pregnancies in Thoroughbreds: rate of occurrence, treatment and prevention. J Equine Vet Sci 1993; 13:690-694.
7. Newcombe JR. The probable identification of monozygous twin embryos in mares. J Equine Vet Sci 2000; 20:269-274.
8. Rooney JR. The fetus and foal. In Rooney JR (ed): Autopsy of the horse. Philadelphia, Williams and Wilkins Co, pp 121-133, 1970.
9. McKinnon AO, Voss JL, Squires EL et al: Diagnostic ultrasonography. In McKinnon AO, Voss JL (eds): Equine Reproduction. Philadelphia, London, Lea & Febiger, pp 266-302, 1993.
10. Betteridge KJ, Eaglesome MD, Mitchell D et al: Development of horse embryos up to twenty two days after ovulation: observations on fresh specimens. J Anat 1982; 135:191-209.
11. McKinnon AO, Carnevale EM, Squires EL et al: Bisection of equine embryos. Equine Vet J 1989; 8(Suppl):129-133.
12. Ginther OJ. Relationships among number of days between multiple ovulations, number of embryos, and type of embryo fixation in mares. J Equine Vet Sci 1987; 7:82-88.
13. Ginther OJ, Bergfelt DR: Embryo reduction before day 11 in mares with twin conceptuses. J Anim Sci 1988; 66:1727-1731.
14. Ginther OJ: The nature of embryo reduction in mares with twin conceptuses: deprivation hypothesis. Am J Vet Res 1989; 50:45-53.
15. Ginther OJ: Twin embryos in mares. I: From ovulation to fixation. Equine Vet J 1989; 21:166-170.
16. Ginther OJ, Griffin PG: Natural outcome and ultrasonic identification of equine fetal twins. Theriogenology 1994; 41:1193-1199.
17. Ginther OJ: Twin embryos in mares. II: Post fixation embryo reduction. Equine Vet J 1989; 21:171-174.
18. Ginther OJ, Douglas RH, Woods GL: A biological embryo-reduction mechanism for elimination of excess embryos in mares. Theriogenology 1982; 18:475-485.
19. Pascoe RR: Methods for the treatment of twin pregnancy in the mare. Equine Vet J 1983; 15:40-42.
20. Jeffcott LB, Whitwell K: Twinning as a cause of foetal and neonatal loss in the Thoroughbred mare. J Comp Pathol 1973; 83:91-106.
21. Ginther OJ: The twinning problem: from breeding to day 16. Proc AAEP 1983; 29:11-26.
22. Pascoe RR: A possible new treatment for twin pregnancy in the mare. Equine Vet J 1979; 15:40-42.
23. Roberts CJ: Termination of twin gestation by blastocyst crush in the broodmare. J Reprod Fertil 1982; 32(Suppl):447-449.
24. Pascoe DR, Pascoe RR, Hughes JP et al: Management of twin conceptuses by manual embryonic reduction: comparison of two techniques and three hormone treatments [published erratum appears in Am J Vet Res 1988 Feb;49(2):273]. Am J Vet Res 1987; 48:1594-1599.
25. Pascoe DR, Pascoe RR, Hughes JP et al: Comparison of two techniques and three hormone therapies for management of twin conceptuses by manual embryonic reduction [abstract]. J Reprod Fertil 1987(Suppl); 35:701-702.
26. McKinnon AO, Figueroa STD, Nobelius AM et al: Failure of hydroxyprogesterone caproate to maintain pregnancy in ovariectomized mares. Equine Vet J 1993; 25:158-160.
27. Bowman T: Ultrasonic diagnosis and management of early twins in the mare. Proc AAEP 1986; 35-43.
28. McKinnon AO, Squires EL, Pickett BW: Equine diagnostic ultrasonography, ed 1, Colorado State University, Animal Reproduction Labroraty, 1988.
29. Ginther OJ: Postfixation embryo reduction in unilateral and bilateral twins in mares. Theriogenology 1984; 22:213-223.
30. Baucus KL, Squires EL, Morris R et al: The effect of stage of gestation and frequency of prostaglandin injection on induction of abortion in mares. Proc Eq Nut Phys Soc 1987;255-258.
31. Squires EL, Bosu WTK: Induction of abortion during early to mid gestation. In McKinnon AO, Voss JL (eds): Equine Reproduction. Philadelphia, London, Lea & Febiger, pp 563-566, 1993.
32. Penzhorn BL, Bertschinger HJ, Coubrough RI: Reconception of mares following termination of pregnancy with prostaglandinF2 alpha before and after day 35 of pregnancy. Equine Vet J 1986; 18:215-217.
33. Hyland JH, Maclean AA, Robertson-Smith GR et al: Attempted conversion of twin to singleton pregnancy in two mares with associated changes in plasma oestrone sulphate concentrations. Aust Vet J 1985; 62:406-409.
34. Allen WR, Bracher V: Videoendoscopic evaluation of the mare's uterus: III. Findings in the pregnant mare [see comments]. Equine Vet J 1992; 24:285-291.
35. Pascoe DR, Stover SM: Surgical removal of one conceptus from fifteen mares with twin concepti. Vet Surg 1989; 18:141-145.
36. Stover SM, Pascoe DR. Surgical removal of one conceptus from the mare with a twin pregnancy [abstract]. Vet Surg 1987; 16:87.

37. Bracher V, Parlevliet JM, Pieterse MC et al: Transvaginal ultrasound-guided twin reduction in the mare. Vet Rec 1993; 133:478-479.

38. Squires EL, Tarr SF, Shideler RK et al: Use of transvaginal ultrasound-guided puncture for elimination of equine pregnancies during days 50 to 65. J Equine Vet Sci 1994; 14:203-205.

39. Macpherson ML, Reimer JM: Twin reduction in the mare: current options. Anim Reprod Sci 2000; 60:233-244.

40. Rantanen NW, Kincaid B. Ultrasound guided fetal cardiac puncture: a method of twin reduction in the mare. Proc AAEP 1988; 173-179.

41. McKinnon AO, Carnevale EM, Squires EL et al: Clinical evaluation of detomidine hydrocholoride for equine reproductive surgery. Proc AAEP 1988; 563-568.

42. Pipers FS, Adams-Brendemuehl CS: Techniques and applications of transabdominal ultrasonography in the pregnant mare. J Am Vet Med Assoc 1984; 185:766-771.

43. Roberts SJ, Myhre G: A review of twinning in horses and the possible therapeutic value of supplemental progesterone to prevent abortion of equine twin fetuses the latter half of the gestation period. Cornell Vet 1983; 73:257-264.

44. Shideler RK: Prenatal lactation associated with twin pregnancy in the mare: a case report. J Equine Vet Sci 1987; 7:383-384.

45. Wolfsdorf KE, Rodgerson DH, Holder R: How to manually reduce twins between 60 and 120 days' gestation using cranio-cervical dislocation. Paper presented at the 51st Annual Convention of the American Association of Equine Practitioners, 2005.

CHAPTER 55

Early Embryonic Loss

DIRK K. VANDERWALL
JOHN R. NEWCOMBE

Although not a universal definition, early embryonic loss in the mare is generally defined as pregnancy failure that occurs up to day 40 of gestation, which corresponds to the time of transition from the embryo stage to the fetal stage of conceptus development.[1] The diagnosis of early embryonic loss and recognition of factors contributing to its occurrence have been dramatically improved by the widespread use of transrectal ultrasonography for early pregnancy diagnosis. Under field conditions, transrectal ultrasonography is used routinely for pregnancy diagnosis as early as day 12 to 14 postovulation, whereas under experimental conditions it may be used as early as day 10 or 11; therefore ultrasonography allows direct (and repeatable) assessment of the conceptus during approximately three quarters of the interval when early embryonic loss occurs. Before day 10 or 11 the conceptus is too small to be visualized with standard ultrasonographic equipment; therefore other techniques have been used to study embryonic loss during that interval. Specifically, assisted reproductive techniques such as embryo transfer, transvaginal ultrasound-guided follicle aspiration (TVA), and oocyte transfer and experimental techniques such as in vitro embryo culture and light/electron microscopy of oocytes/embryos have been used to study early embryonic development and embryonic loss before day 11.

INCIDENCE

Because of the practicality and accuracy of using transrectal ultrasonography for the diagnosis of pregnancy as early as day 10, a considerable amount of data has been generated on the incidence of embryonic loss after that time. Although it can be difficult to compare data across experiments because of variables such as differences in the interval studied and whether experiments were conducted under controlled conditions or under field conditions, based on serial examination with ultrasonography the incidence of embryonic loss has ranged from approximately 2.5% to 25%, with a weighted mean across studies of 7.7% (Table 55-1). The highest embryonic loss rates (25% to 30%) have been detected in mares greater than 18 years of age.[2,3]

The lack of a practical method of diagnosing pregnancy before day 10 makes detection of embryonic loss between fertilization and day 10 difficult. In addition, pregnancy loss before day 10 must be differentiated from fertilization failure. Data compiled from studies that used the recovery of cleaved ova on day 2 postovulation as an estimate of the fertilization rate indicate that fertilization rates were 91% in young mares and 85% in aged mares inseminated with fresh, fertile semen under experimental conditions (Table 55-2). In contrast, Carnevale and Ginther[4] reported that the estimated fertilization rate on day 1.5 was significantly higher in young versus aged mares (88% versus 45%, respectively); however, that difference may have been due to delayed embryonic development in the aged mares, because the cleavage rate on day 3 was not different for young and aged mares (100% for both groups), and the embryos from aged mares were about one cleavage division delayed in their development compared with the young mares. Therefore it appears fertilization rates are very high (>90%) in young mares and may be just slightly lower (85%) in aged mares. Although fertilization rates are high, embryo recovery rates between days 6 and 9 are markedly lower for aged versus young mares,[5,6] which implies a high rate of embryonic loss during the first week of gestation in the latter mares. That is further supported by reports that the estimated embryonic loss rate between fertilization and day 14 was less than 10% for young mares compared with 60% to 70% for aged mares.[7,8]

Based on the data described above, the cumulative incidence of early embryonic loss between fertilization and day 40 may be as low as 10% to 20% in young mares to more than 70% in aged mares. Under field conditions the detected incidence of embryonic loss between days 12 and 40 is on the order of 10% to 15% for young mares and 25% to 30% for aged mares. At those levels, early embryonic failure represents a considerable economic loss to the equine industry in the form of increased costs associated with additional breeding of mares and/or decreased foal production. This chapter will review our current understanding of the factors that cause and/or contribute to early embryonic loss in the mare. Although a considerable body of information about early embryonic loss was generated before the advent of transrectal ultrasonography (i.e., before approximately 1980), due to the limitations of such studies (accuracy, interval studied, etc.), this review will focus upon data obtained using transrectal ultrasonography.

ETIOLOGY

Factors that may contribute to the occurrence of embryonic loss in the mare have been classified as intrinsic, extrinsic, and embryonic.[9,10] Intrinsic factors include endometrial disease, progesterone deficiency, maternal age, lactation, foal-heat breeding, and time of insemination relative to ovulation. Extrinsic factors include stress;

Table 55-1

A Review of Studies* on Early Embryonic Loss in Mares Detected With Transrectal Ultrasonography

Reference	Interval Studied	No. Losses / No. Pregnancies	%
Chevalier and Palmer, 1982[86]	23 ± 6 to 43 ± 10	69/1295	5.3
Simpson et al, 1982[87]	14 to 63	13/326	4.0
Ginther et al, 1985[88†]	11 to 50	5/27	18.5
		37/154	24.0
Villahoz et al, 1985[89‡]	15 to 50	61/354	17.2
Woods et al, 1985[59§]	14 to 48	42/404	10.4
Woods et al, 1987[2§]	14 to 48	60/559	10.7
Forde et al, 1987[90]	18 to 42	13/437	3.0
Chevalier-Clement, 1989[36§]	22 ± 5 to 44 ± 12	165/2989	5.5
Vogelsang et al, 1989[79]	15 to 35	85/1085	7.8
Irvine et al, 1990[91]	17 to 42	17/179	9.5
Baucus et al, 1990[66†]	12 to 50	7/54	13.0
Woods et al, 1990[62‖]	11 to 40	20/85	23.5
Lowis and Hyland, 1991[92]	18 to 45	10/132	7.6
Meyers et al, 1991[60]	12 to 40	34/509	6.7
Bruck et al, 1993[93]	24 to end of season	103/1379	7.5
Tannus and Thun, 1995[37]	14 to 40	20/229	8.7
Pycock and Newcombe, 1996[41¶]	14 to 30	17/168	10.1
Newcombe, 1997[94§]	11 to 39	8/313	2.6
Barbacini et al, 1999[64]	14 to 50	31/349	8.9
Carnevale et al, 2000[95#]	12 to 50	65/419	15.5
Morris and Allen, 2002[61]	15 to 35	119/1144	10.4
Hemberg et al, 2004[3]	14 to foaling	49/391	12.5
Weighted-mean		936/12,171	7.7

*Only studies with at least 25 mares were included.
†Experimental mares.
‡Embryo recipient and experimental mares.
§Singleton pregnancies only.
‖Experimental mares inseminated before or after ovulation.
¶Only includes untreated control mares.
#Embryo recipient mares.

nutrition; season/climate; transrectal palpation/ultrasonography; sire and/or semen processing/handling; and gamete handling/manipulation for assisted reproductive techniques. Embryonic factors include chromosomal anomalies or other inherent characteristics of the embryo. Regardless of cause, indications of impending embryonic loss detectable with transrectal ultrasonography have included irregular shape of an embryonic vesicle, prolonged mobility of a vesicle, an undersized vesicle, loss of embryonic heartbeat, lack of development of the embryo proper, dislodgement of a vesicle with loss of fluid, and edema of the endometrial folds.[9]

Intrinsic Factors

Endometrial Disease
Endometrial disease is further classified as inflammatory or noninflammatory. Inflammatory forms of endometrial disease include acute and chronic endometritis, whereas noninflammatory forms include periglandular fibrosis and endometrial cysts. Acute endometritis is characterized

by an influx of neutrophils into the stroma of the endometrium and the uterine lumen. When discussing acute endometritis, it is important to note that a physiologic (i.e., normal) acute endometritis occurs in all mares after breeding as a result of deposition of semen in the uterine lumen,[11,12] and it is the spermatozoa and other components of the ejaculate/inseminate that are responsible for inducing the inflammatory response.[13] Reproductively sound mares clear this mating-induced uterine contamination/inflammation between 24 and 48 hours following mating,[11] whereas mares susceptible to endometritis do not,[14] which leads to a persistent mating-induced endometritis. Mares that develop persistent mating-induced endometritis accumulate fluid within the uterine lumen because of impaired (i.e., delayed) physical clearance of inflammatory material[14-16] exacerbated by increased fluid production. Factors that may contribute to the delayed uterine clearance in susceptible mares are (1) decreased myometrial activity,[16] (2) decreased lymphatic drainage from the uterus,[17] and/or (3) abnormal reproductive conformation (e.g., pendulous uterus located

Table 55-2

Estimated Fertilization Rates* in Young and Aged Mares

Reference	Young Mares (%)		Aged Mares (%)
Ball et al, 1986[7]	10/11 (91)		11/12 (92)
Woods et al, 1991[96]	35/39 (90)		14/16 (88)
	21/25 (84)		——————
Brinsko et al, 1994[97]	24/24 (100)	——— † ———	16/20 (80)
Total	90/99 (91)		41/48 (85)

*Determined at day 2 postovulation by number of cleaved ova / number of cleaved ova + number of recently ovulated unfertilized ova.
†P<0.05.

ventral to the pelvic brim)[18] or temporary/permanent dilation of uterine horn (e.g., post partum). Similarly, mares with an acute infectious endometritis accumulate inflammatory fluid in the uterine lumen as a consequence of the body's uterine defense mechanisms that are activated in an effort to eliminate the infectious agent.

The pathologic intrauterine fluid that accumulates during persistent mating-induced endometritis and infectious endometritis can adversely affect fertility by (1) impairing spermatozoal motility and/or viability if breeding/insemination is performed while the uterus is inflamed[19,20] or (2) inducing embryonic loss if the endometritis persists beyond day 5 postovulation, when the embryo enters the uterine lumen from the oviduct[21] and the corpus luteum becomes sensitive to prostaglandin $F_{2\alpha}$ (PGF$_{2\alpha}$).[22,23] It has been demonstrated that acute inflammation associated with intrauterine fluid collections during diestrus increases the incidence of embryonic loss.[23,24] Similarly, mares with a history of endometritis had significantly higher early embryonic loss rates compared with mares with no history of endometritis.[2] Therefore routine therapy for persistent mating-induced endometritis and infectious endometritis is directed at removing the fluid that has accumulated in the uterine lumen and in the case of infectious endometritis eliminating the inciting microbial agent(s). Treatment generally includes the use of ecbolic agents such as oxytocin[25] and PGF$_{2\alpha}$,[26] which may be used alone or in combination with large-volume uterine lavage[27]; in addition, appropriate antimicrobial agents are used to treat infectious endometritis.

In contrast with acute endometritis, chronic endometritis is characterized by an influx of lymphocytes into focalized areas of the endometrial stroma. Chronic inflammation appears to develop in response to any disturbance within the uterus, both normal (e.g., pregnancy) and abnormal (e.g., infectious endometritis), and is commonly identified in uterine biopsy specimens. Chronic inflammation does not appear to impair fertility, because mares with chronic inflammation can support and maintain early embryonic development.[28] Therefore no treatment is indicated specifically for chronic inflammation.

Clinically, noninfectious abnormalities of the endometrium such as periglandular fibrosis have been considered an important factor in the occurrence of both early embryonic loss and fetal death,[29] and because this type of pathologic change in the endometrium is generally more severe in aged mares,[30,31] it seemed to be a foregone conclusion that periglandular fibrosis caused higher embryonic loss rates in aged mares. However, when Ball et al[28] tested that hypothesis by transferring morphologically normal, day 7 or 8 blastocysts into the uterus of young (minimal pathologic conditions) and aged (extensive pathologic conditions) recipient mares, embryo survival rates (55% and 45% at day 12) and embryonic loss rates between days 12 and 28 (9% and 11%) were not different for the young and aged recipient mares. Their results indicated that the uterine abnormalities (periglandular fibrosis and chronic inflammation) present in the aged mare's uteri did not result in a higher incidence of early embryonic loss in those mares; therefore it appears that other factors are primarily responsible for the higher early embryonic loss rates observed in aged mares (see discussion below).

Another common form of noninflammatory endometrial abnormality is cystic dilation, which is characterized as being either glandular or lymphatic (for review see Stanton et al[32]). Essentially all cysts that are grossly or ultrasonographically detectable are lymphatic in origin[33] and range in size from a few millimeters to several centimeters in diameter. The incidence of endometrial cysts increases with mare age,[32] which is a potentially confounding factor when assessing the effect of cysts on fertility. There are two plausible mechanisms by which cysts could adversely affect fertility. Firstly, large cysts (>3 cm) might impair intrauterine mobility of the conceptus, which could lead to failure of maternal recognition of pregnancy caused by an inability of the conceptus to adequately block endometrial PGF secretion with subsequent regression of the corpus luteum.[34] Secondly, if a conceptus were to become fixed in direct contact with a cyst(s), the conceptus might be deprived of adequate nutrient exchange in a manner similar to adjacent twin conceptuses through the deprivation hypothesis proposed by Ginther.[35] Several reports have described an adverse effect of endometrial cysts on fertility (i.e., decreased pregnancy rates and/or increased early embryonic loss rates)[23,36,37];

however, when mare age was accounted for when analyzing the data, there was no evidence of an overall effect of endometrial cysts on embryonic loss rates in mares.[38]

Despite the lack of conclusive evidence that endometrial cysts have a detrimental effect on fertility, treatment may be pursued in mares that have large and/or numerous cysts in conjunction with a poor reproductive history.[32] Specific treatments that have been used to remove/eliminate cysts include manual rupture/ablation, drainage/aspiration, mechanical removal by ensnaring the cysts with obstetric wire, endoscopic electrocoagulation, and laser therapy (reviewed in Stanton et al[32]). Anecdotally, cyst removal may help some mares, because in a group of 39 aged mares (for which complete follow-up data was available) that had been barren for 1 year, 62% of the mares became pregnant after cyst removal using laser photoablation.[39]

Progesterone Deficiency

Despite a paucity of scientific evidence supporting its efficacy, prophylactic administration of exogenous progesterone to pregnant mares in an effort to enhance maintenance of pregnancy continues to be a widespread practice. Although low progesterone levels caused by primary corpora luteal insufficiency has been proposed as a cause of early embryonic loss in mares that could warrant administration of exogenous progesterone, its occurrence has not been clearly documented.[40] Without a specific indication (or contraindication) for its use, progesterone supplementation is often empirically performed in mares that have a history of repeated pregnancy failure when no specific factor causing pregnancy loss is identified. Despite the fact that there is no evidence that routine use of exogenous progesterone will decrease the incidence of early embryonic loss, preliminary studies using the gonadotropin-releasing hormone (GnRH) agonist buserelin in mares (40 µg administered on day 10 or 11 of pregnancy) have shown a reduction in embryonic loss rate before day 30,[41,42] which may be due to a beneficial effect of increased levels of endogenous progesterone.

Although primary luteal insufficiency has not been documented, it has been shown that some pregnant mares will undergo luteolysis on days 14 to 16 in spite of the presence of an embryo in the uterus.[43-45] This condition is characterized by distinct edema of the endometrial folds especially in the uterine body, the vesicle is more often in the body than the horns, and the mare may begin to show signs of estrous behavior. This situation can be confirmed retrospectively by a plasma progesterone concentration of less than 1 ng/ml. The condition is most commonly seen in pregnancies conceived in the immediate postpartum period[46] and raises the question of whether an abnormal embryo has failed to block luteolysis or whether spontaneous luteal regression is resulting in the loss of an otherwise viable pregnancy. The former possibility can be supported following the identification of small-for-age vesicles on days 12 to 15, which fail to block luteolysis at days 14 to 15; the mare returns to estrus and loses the vesicle. Such pregnancies may initially be saved by the timely administration of progesterone, but many of these fail to develop an embryo-proper. This is a clear example of natural elimination of a potentially nonviable preg-

nancy. In contrast, the clinician may sometimes find a normal size-for-age pregnancy in a mare that is returning to estrus. Prompt treatment with exogenous progesterone may prevent this impending pregnancy loss, but treatment must be continued until the mare forms an accessory corpus luteum. When the development of the vesicle and embryo appears normal, the pregnancy has a good chance of going to term.

If the decision is made to provide exogenous progesterone to a mare for maintenance of pregnancy, it is important to use one that is efficacious. Currently there are no commercially available formulations of progesterone labeled for use in pregnant mares; therefore the use of exogenous progesterone for maintenance of pregnancy is an "extra-label" use. Two preparations of progesterone commonly administered to pregnant mares are daily oral administration of the synthetic progestin altrenogest or daily intramuscular administration of progesterone in oil. Although both treatments have been shown to be efficacious by their ability to maintain pregnancy in mares without an endogenous source of progesterone,[47,48] the need for daily administration is a major drawback of these formulations. In an attempt to eliminate the need for daily administration of exogenous progesterone preparations, there has been interest in the use of long-acting formulations of progesterone that can be administered at weekly (or longer) intervals. There are anecdotal reports of the clinical use of long-acting synthetic progestins labeled for use in women for maintenance of pregnancy in mares; however, these formulations were unable to maintain pregnancy in mares after $PGF_{2\alpha}$-induced luteolysis.[49,50] Experimentally, progesterone-impregnated microspheres have been shown to provide sustained release of progesterone that will maintain pregnancy following $PGF_{2\alpha}$-induced luteolysis when administered every 10 days[51]; however, a commercially available preparation of this long-acting progesterone formulation is not available. Recently a compounded proprietary long-acting progesterone formulation was shown to be efficacious for pregnancy maintenance in mares in which endogenous progesterone secretion had been eliminated with treatment with exogenous $PGF_{2\alpha}$ on day 18 of gestation.[52] Administration of 1.5 g progesterone every 7 days provided sufficient progesterone levels to maintain pregnancy through day 45 of gestation, when the study was terminated.

In pregnant mares the fetal-placental unit begins secreting progesterone and related progestagens between days 80 and 100 of gestation,[53] the levels of which become sufficient to maintain pregnancy after day 100[54,55]; therefore progesterone supplementation is generally discontinued between days 100 and 120, because there is no physiologic basis for continued administration of exogenous progesterone after that time (for a pregnancy that is developing normally).

Maternal Age

Because the uterine environment of aged mares appeared suitable for the maintenance of pregnancy (previously discussed), Ball et al[8] then performed an experiment designed to compare the viability of embryos collected from young and aged mares following their transfer to the uterus of young recipient mares. Day 4 embryos were collected from the oviducts of young and aged mares and transferred to young recipient mares; the survival rate of embryos from young mares was significantly higher than those from aged mares (84% versus 25%, respectively). Because the embryos from the aged mares had lower survival rates after transfer to a normal uterine environment, and the embryos had never been exposed to the uterine environment of the aged mares, it suggested that adverse effects of the oviductal environment and/or inherent embryonic defects were responsible for the lower survival (i.e., higher embryonic loss) rate of the embryos from the aged mares.

In a subsequent experiment, Carnevale and Ginther[56] used TVA and oocyte transfer to compare the viability of oocytes/embryos from young and aged mares. Oocytes were collected from mares using TVA between 21 and 26 hours after administration of human chorionic gonadotropin (hCG); oocytes were then cultured in vitro for 16 to 20 hours and then surgically transferred to the oviducts of young recipient mares that were inseminated before and after transfer. The use of oocyte transfer allowed fertilization and embryonic development to occur in the recipient mare, avoiding potentially deleterious effects of the oviductal environment on the oocytes (i.e., in the aged mares). When pregnancy was diagnosed on day 12 with transrectal ultrasonography, significantly more oocytes from young versus aged mares resulted in embryonic vesicles (92% versus 31%, respectively). These results clearly implicated inherent defects within the oocytes of aged mares as an important cause for their reduced viability, because the oocytes were never exposed to the tubular genitalia of the donor mares.

To further investigate oocyte quality, Carnevale et al[57] used light and transmission electron microscopy to compare quantitative and qualitative differences in oocytes from young and aged mares. Oocytes were collected from mares using TVA between 20 and 26 hours after administration of hCG; immediately after collection, oocytes were fixed and processed for microscopy. When imaged with light microscopy, significantly more oocytes from aged versus young mares contained large intracellular vesicles. In addition, individual oocytes from aged mares had morphologic anomalies not imaged in oocytes from young mares, including large vesicles in the ooplasm or associated with the nucleus, oblong or irregular shapes, areas of ooplasm without organelles, and sections of oolemma with sparse microvilli. Quantification of cellular organelles using images from transmission electron microscopy resulted in no significant differences between oocytes from young and aged mares. These results indicated that degenerative and/or inherent morphologic defects are present in oocytes from aged mares and the extent and type of changes varies among individual oocytes; however, it remains to be determined whether the specific abnormalities observed in this study cause reduced oocyte viability.

Lactation

It is plausible the energy demands of lactation and/or hormonal changes associated with lactation could affect the incidence of early embryonic loss. For example, progesterone levels were found to be significantly lower in lactating mares compared with nonlactating mares[58]; however, two large field studies[2,59] did not detect any difference in embryonic loss rates between lactating and nonlactating mares.

Foal-Heat Breeding

There are conflicting data on the effect of foal-heat breeding on the incidence of early embryonic loss in mares. In a field study of Thoroughbred, Standardbred and Saddlebred mares,[2] there was no difference in embryonic loss rates between mares bred on foal heat versus those bred on subsequent cycles. In contrast, two other studies[60,61] that also examined Thoroughbred and Standardbred mares identified significantly higher embryonic loss rates in mares bred at foal heat compared with those bred at subsequent heats. It seems likely this discrepancy may be due to other factors such as management decisions, which could include such factors as determining which (if any) mares are bred on foal heat. Clearly, this is an area that warrants further study.

Time of Insemination Relative to Ovulation

Insemination of mares after ovulation has been associated with an increased incidence of early embryonic loss. Woods et al[62] found that embryonic loss rates between days 15 and 40 of gestation were significantly higher in mares inseminated within 24 hours postovulation compared with mares inseminated before ovulation with fresh semen (34% versus 14%, respectively). Similarly, Koskinen et al[63] reported that 5 of 13 mares (38.5%) inseminated postovulation lost their pregnancies between days 16 and 25 of gestation compared with no pregnancy losses in 15 mares inseminated before ovulation. The underlying cause of the observed higher incidence of embryonic loss in mares inseminated after ovulation is not known. One possibility is that oocyte quality is altered such that fertilization is not adversely affected, but that embryonic viability is. Another possibility is that the delayed timing of fertilization with a postovulation insemination causes proportional delay in embryonic development that could compromise the ability of the conceptus to block luteolysis. The latter possibility is supported by the finding that the embryos were significantly smaller in mares inseminated postovulation compared with mares inseminated before ovulation,[62] and that four of the five pregnancy losses that occurred in mares inseminated postovulation failed between days 16 and 21,[63] which corresponds with the time that progesterone levels would have decreased if the conceptus had not been able to block luteolysis. In contrast to the previous data, a more recent study[64] did not detect any difference in embryonic loss rates in mares inseminated within 6 hours postovulation and those inseminated before ovulation with frozen semen. Collectively, these results are not incompatible, in that it may simply reflect that the adverse effects of insemination after ovulation are not manifested unless insemination occurs more than 6 hours after ovulation.

Extrinsic Factors

Stress

It is plausible that maternal stress could contribute to the occurrence of early embryonic loss because it has been demonstrated that stress associated with severe pain (e.g., colic), infectious disease, and weaning resulted in a 30% to 50% decrease in circulating progesterone levels in pregnant mares.[65] The adverse effect of stress on progesterone levels is apparently mediated through adrenal corticosteroids, because administration of 150 mg of prednisolone to two pregnant mares resulted in a sharp, although transient, decrease (approximately 30% to 40%) in progesterone level.[65] A subsequent study[66] demonstrated that both cortisol levels and progesterone levels increased significantly when mares were transported for 9 hours during early gestation compared with nontransported control mares; in addition, there was no difference in early embryonic loss rates between the transported and nontransported mares.

Besides the potential for adverse effects of stressful conditions to be mediated through increased glucocorticoid levels, the deleterious effects of certain metabolic (e.g., enteritis) and/or infectious (e.g., metritis) diseases may be mediated through the systemic effects of bacterial endotoxin. Intravenous administration of bacterial endotoxin to 9 pregnant mares between days 23 and 55 of gestation resulted in pregnancy loss in 7 of the mares within 5 days of treatment; in contrast, infusion of endotoxin to 10 mares between 56 and 318 days of gestation did not induce any pregnancy losses.[67] Luteal activity was compromised in all mares by 9 hours after treatment with endotoxin, but progesterone concentrations were consistently lower in mares that lost their pregnancies (1 to 2 ng/ml) than those that did not lose their pregnancies. The adverse effect of the endotoxin on luteal function occurs due to release of endogenous $PGF_{2\alpha}$, and although the release of $PGF_{2\alpha}$ can be abrogated by the administration of flunixin meglumine, in order to be efficacious it must be administered at a very early stage of the endotoxemia, when clinical signs are often not yet apparent.[68] Another therapeutic option to prevent endotoxin-induced pregnancy loss is to administer exogenous progesterone, because daily administration of altrenogest prevented pregnancy loss associated with endotoxemia.[69]

Nutrition

A seminal study on the effect of nutrition on the fertility of mares was reported by Henneke et al[70] in 1984. They randomly assigned 32 foaling Quarter Horse mares to one of four dietary treatments designed to reach the following nutritional endpoints: (1) attain high body condition from 90 days prepartum to foaling and then maintain high body condition through 90 days postfoaling, (2) attain high body condition from 90 days prepartum to foaling then lose body condition to 90 days postfoaling, (3) lose body condition from 90 days prepartum to foaling then maintain low body condition until 90 days postfoaling, and (4) lose body condition from 90 days prepartum to foaling then gain weight after foaling to attain high body condition by 90 days postfoaling. Body condition scores were assessed as previously described.[71] At the start of the study, the average body condition score for all four groups of mares was between 6.0 and 6.7. At foaling, average body condition scores of groups 1 and 2 were 55 and 7.5, respectively, while the condition scores for groups 3 and 4 were 3.4 and 3.8, respectively. At 90

days postfoaling, the condition scores for groups 1 to 4 were 7.1, 4.7, 3.7, and 6.8, respectively. Mares were not bred at foal heat but were inseminated beginning with the second postpartum estrus; if mares did not become pregnant, they were bred a maximum of three cycles. The results demonstrated a profound effect of nutrition on fertility in group 3, the mares fed to lose condition prepartum and then maintain poor body condition through 90 days postfoaling. The overall per-cycle pregnancy rate was significantly lower for group 3 compared with the other groups, and the embryonic loss rate between days 30 and 90 was significantly higher for group 3 (75%) compared with the other groups (0 to 12%). In addition, when compared across treatment groups, mares in the study that foaled with a body condition score less than 5.0 had significantly lower pregnancy rates, and none of the mares that were maintained with a condition score of less than 5.0 after foaling was pregnant at 90 days of gestation.

In a subsequent report, van Niekerk and van Niekerk[72] examined the effect of total protein intake and protein quality on the incidence of early embryonic loss in lactating and nonlactating mares. They found that 5 of 14 mares (35.7%) receiving low-quality protein in their diet underwent embryonic loss between days 14 and 90 of gestation compared with only 3 of 41 mares (55%) that received higher-quality protein in their diets. Together with the results of Henneke et al,[70] it highlights the importance of nutrition for optimum fertility in the mare. All indications are that to maximize reproductive efficiency and minimize early embryonic loss, mares should receive good-quality feedstuffs in sufficient quantity to maintain optimum body condition.

In addition to nutritional effects of energy intake/body condition and/or nutrient content/quality on embryonic loss, ingestion of environmental toxicants may adversely affect embryonic development. For example, ingestion of endophyte-infected fescue has been implicated as a possible cause of early embryonic loss, because 3 of 6 mares consuming endophyte-infected fescue underwent early embryonic loss between days 16 and 35 of gestation compared with 0 of 8 and 0 of 7 mares consuming endophyte-free fescue or nontoxic endophyte fescue, respectively.[73] Another example of an apparent environmental effect on early embryonic loss is the association between ingestion of Eastern tent caterpillars and early embryonic loss as part of mare reproductive loss syndrome (MRLS) (see Chapter 56, Mare Reproductive Loss Syndrome).[74]

Season/Climate

In cattle it has been demonstrated that seasonal and/or climatic conditions such as heat stress can adversely affect early embryonic development, leading to higher embryonic loss rates.[75] However, in horses there is no clear-cut evidence of an environmental effect on early embryonic loss, because the date of ovulation/establishment of pregnancy was not different for mares that maintained pregnancies versus those that lost pregnancies.[59] Hearn et al[76] reported significantly higher early embryonic loss rates for mares bred in February and March versus those bred later in the season (in the Northern Hemisphere); however, rather than a true seasonal effect, it could reflect that a higher proportion of the mares bred early in the season were barren, which would likely include more aged mares, resulting in higher loss rates.

Transrectal Palpation/Ultrasonography

Although an early report[77] indicated an adverse effect of transrectal palpation on fertility in the mare, there is no evidence that routine performance of transrectal palpation[78] or transrectal ultrasonography[33,79] performed by an experienced clinician has any adverse effect on early pregnancy.

Sire and/or Semen Processing/Handling

Although an early (before ultrasound) study indicated that the stallion could influence the incidence of pregnancy loss after day 42 of gestation,[80] a more recent study of more than 3700 pregnant mares found that of 261 stallions examined, there was no effect of the stallion on pregnancy loss rates between days 22 and 44.[36] With the tremendous increase in the use of cooled-transported semen and frozen semen, it raises the possibility that semen processing and/or handling procedures (e.g., x-irradiation of shipped semen samples) could alter the spermatozoa in such a manner as to contribute to higher embryonic loss; of those possibilities, only x-irradiation has been studied in a controlled manner. England and Keane[81] found that the typical airport security screening system would expose semen samples to between 0.5 and 1.0 µSv. In a subsequent breeding trial, they bred three groups of 8 mares with semen from one stallion that had been exposed to x-irradiation doses of 0, 1.0, or 10.0 µSv; an entire ejaculate was irradiated and inseminated into each mare once during estrus within 48 hours before ovulation. The day 14 pregnancy rates for the three treatment groups were 0 µSv (7 mares), 1.0 µSv (8 mares), and 10.0 µSv (7 mares). Of the 22 pregnancies that were established, one was lost at day 65 (0 µSv group), whereas the remaining 21 mares delivered a foal at term (one died at parturition). Therefore there was no evidence of any effect of x-irradiation of the semen on early embryonic loss rates.

Gamete Handling/Manipulation

During the last 10 to 15 years there has been tremendous interest in the development of a wide range of new assisted reproductive techniques that may allow production of offspring from mares and/or stallions that otherwise may be incapable of reproducing. Techniques that are being developed include oocyte transfer, in vitro fertilization (IVF), intracytoplasmic sperm injection (ICSI), sexed semen, and nuclear transfer (i.e., cloning). The successful application of these procedures requires that equine gametes are collected and handled appropriately. For successful fertilization the oocyte must be viable and at the correct stage of maturation (meiotic and cytoplasmic). Oocytes "resting" in the ovary are in prophase of meiosis I and contain a distinct nucleus (germinal vesicle). During maturation in vivo, which occurs during the 36 hours before ovulation, the nuclear membrane breaks down, and meiosis resumes and progresses to metaphase II. At ovulation the oocyte has reached and is arrested in metaphase II,[82] the stage at which it is fertil-

izable. Metaphase II oocytes are characterized by the presence of the first polar body. Oocytes can be collected from mature preovulatory follicles or from immature follicles. Oocytes collected from small, immature follicles must undergo maturation in vitro. The development of successful culture systems for routine in vitro maturation of equine oocytes is currently an area of considerable research interest. Like the oocyte, sperm must be collected and handled appropriately for use with IVF, ICSI, and semen sexing procedures.

It is plausible that the handling and manipulation the oocyte and/or sperm undergo for use in these procedures could itself adversely affect fertilization and/or early embryonic development. Currently there is conclusive evidence that cloned equine embryos have a very high incidence of early embryonic loss (80% to 100%)[83] that is often characterized by lack of formation of an embryo-proper.[84] Similarly, McKinnon et al[85] observed that a high proportion (50%) of conceptuses produced using ICSI failed to develop an embryo-proper and did not develop beyond day 30, which suggests the ICSI procedure contributed to abnormal development, because only 4.4% of equine pregnancies typically fail to develop an embryo-proper.[45] Clearly, further work is needed to assess the potential impact of new assisted reproductive techniques on early embryonic development.

Embryonic Factors

As described earlier, increasing maternal age is clearly associated with decreased oocyte quality, which may reflect chromosomal and/or other inherent changes within the oocyte that apparently do not affect fertilization rates but dramatically increase the incidence of early embryonic loss in aged mares. Similarly, oocyte handling/manipulation for assisted reproductive techniques appears to affect oocyte quality, which likewise can adversely affect early embryonic development. Further research is indicated to identify the specific detrimental changes that occur in oocyte quality with increasing mare age and how to minimize or prevent impairment of oocyte/embryo quality when performing assisted reproductive techniques.

SUMMARY

As described, a multitude of factors can contribute to the occurrence of early embryonic loss in a mare. It is clear that some factors such as increasing maternal age are directly associated with higher embryonic loss rates, whereas other factors such as breeding at foal heat are less clearly linked to pregnancy loss. In addition, there may be interactions among the various factors (e.g., mare age, foal heat, lactation, nutrition) that may compound their effects on embryonic loss. As important as recognizing potential causes of embryonic loss is knowing whether anything can be done to decrease the incidence of early embryonic loss in mares. At this time, it is unlikely that anything can be done to overcome early embryonic loss in aged mares that is caused by inherently poor oocyte quality. In contrast, nutritional effects on embryonic loss can be minimized if not eliminated completely, as can the adverse effects of insemination after ovulation. Probably the most important aspect of the clinical management of early embryonic loss in the mare is to recognize that it will inevitably occur in some mares, and the most appropriate course of action is to diagnose its occurrence as early as possible in order to provide an opportunity for rebreeding the mare as soon as possible (if the loss occurs during the breeding season). Early detection of embryonic loss can best be accomplished by performing serial examinations with transrectal ultrasonography every 10 days to 2 weeks between days 14 and 40 of gestation.

References

1. Ginther OJ: Reproductive Biology of the Mare: Basic and Applied Aspects, 2nd edition, Cross Plains, Wis, Equiservices, 1992.
2. Woods GL, Baker CB, Baldwin JL: Early pregnancy loss in brood mares. J Reprod Fertil Suppl 1987; 35:455-459.
3. Hemberg E, Lundeheim N, Einarsson S: Reproductive performance of thoroughbred mares in Sweden. Reprod Domest Anim 2004; 39:81-85.
4. Carnevale EM, Griffin PG, Ginther OJ: Age-associated subfertility before entry of embryos into the uterus of mares. Equine Vet J 1993; 15(suppl):31-35.
5. Woods GL, Hillman RB, Schlafer DH: Recovery and evaluation of embryos from normal and infertile mares. Cornell Vet 1986; 76:386-394.
6. Vogelsang SG, Vogelsang MM: Influence of donor parity and age on the success of commercial equine embryo transfer. Equine Vet J 1989; 8(suppl):71-72.
7. Ball BA, Little TV, Hillman RB et al: Pregnancy rates at days 2 and 14 and estimated embryonic loss rates prior to day 14 in normal and subfertile mares. Theriogenology 1986; 26:611-619.
8. Ball BA, Little TV, Weber JA, Woods GL: Survival of day-4 embryos from young, normal mares and aged, subfertile mares after transfer to normal recipient mares. J Reprod Fertil 1989; 85:187-194.
9. Ball BA, Woods GL: Embryonic loss and early pregnancy loss in the mare. Compend Contin Educ Pract Vet 1987; 9:459-470.
10. Ball BA: Embryonic loss in mares: incidence, possible causes and diagnostic considerations. Vet Clin North Am Equine Pract 1988; 4:263-290.
11. Katila T: Onset and duration of uterine inflammatory response of mares after insemination with fresh semen. Biol Reprod 1995; 1:515-517.
12. Troedsson MHT: Uterine response to semen deposition in the mare. Proc Annu Mtg Soc Therio pp 130-135, 1995.
13. Kotilainen T, Huhtinen M, Katila T: Sperm-induced leukocytosis in the equine uterus. Theriogenology 1994; 41:629-636.
14. LeBlanc MM, Neuwirth L, Asbury AC et al: Scintigraphic measurement of uterine clearance in normal mares and mares with recurrent endometritis. Equine Vet J 1994; 26:109-113.
15. Troedsson MHT, Liu IKM: Uterine clearance of non-antigenic markers (^{51}Cr) in response to a bacterial challenge in mares potentially susceptible and resistant to chronic uterine infections. J Reprod Fertil 1991; 44(suppl):283-288.
16. Troedsson MHT, Liu IKM, Ing M et al: Multiple site electromyography recordings of uterine activity following an intrauterine bacterial challenge in mares susceptible and resistant to chronic uterine infection. J Reprod Fertil 1993; 99:307-313.
17. LeBlanc MM, Johnson RD, Calderwood Mays MB et al: Lymphatic clearance of India ink in reproductively normal mares and mares susceptible to endometritis. Biol Reprod 1995; 1:501-506.
18. LeBlanc MM: Recurrent endometritis: is oxytocin the answer? Proc Annu Conv Am Assoc Equine Practnr 1994; 40:17-18.
19. Squires EL, Barnes CK, Rowley HS et al: Effect of uterine fluid and volume of extender on fertility. Proc Annu Conv Am Assoc Equine Practnr 1989;25-30.
20. Troedsson MHT, Alghamdi A, Laschkewitsch T, Xue J-L: Sperm motility is altered in uterine secretions from mares with postbreeding endometritis. Proceedings of the 44th Annual Convention of the American Association of Equine Practitioners, pp 66-67, 1998.
21. Freeman DA, Weber JA, Geary RT et al: Time of embryo transport through the mare oviduct. Theriogenology 1991; 36:823-830.
22. Oxender WD, Noden PA, Bolenbaugh DL et al: Control of estrus with prostaglandin $F_{2\alpha}$ in mares: minimal effective dose and stage of estrous cycle. Am J Vet Res 1975; 36:1145-1147.
23. Adams GP, Kastelic JP, Bergfelt DR et al: Effect of uterine inflammation and ultrasonically-detected uterine pathology on fertility in the mare. J Reprod Fertil 1987; 35 (suppl):445-454.
24. Carnevale EM, Ginther OJ: Relationships of age to uterine function and reproductive efficiency in mares. Theriogenology 1992; 37:1101-1115.
25. LeBlanc MM, Neuwirth L, Mauragis D et al: Oxytocin enhances clearance of radiocolloid from the uterine lumen of reproductively normal mares and mares susceptible to endometritis. Equine Vet J 1994; 26:279-282.
26. Combs GB, LeBlanc MM, Neuwirth L et al: Effects of prostaglandin $F_{2\alpha}$, cloprostenol and fenprostalene on uterine clearance of radiocolloid in the mare. Theriogenology 1996; 45:1449-1455.
27. LeBlanc MM: Oxytocin—the new wonder drug for treatment of endometritis? Equine Vet Educ 1994; 6:39-43.
28. Ball BA, Hillman RB, Woods GL: Survival of equine embryos transferred to normal and subfertile mares. Theriogenology 1987; 28:167-174.
29. Kenney RM: Cyclic and pathologic changes of the mare endometrium as detected by biopsy, with a note on early embryonic death. J Am Vet Med Assoc 1978; 172:241-262.
30. Gordon LR, Sartin EM: Endometrial biopsy as an aid to diagnosis and prognosis in equine infertility. J Eq Med Surg 1978; 2:328-336.
31. Doig PA, McKnight JD, Miller RB: The use of endometrial biopsy in the infertile mare. Can Vet J 1981; 22:72-76.
32. Stanton MB, Steiner JV, Pugh DG: Endometrial cysts in the mare. J Equine Vet Sci 2004; 24:14-19.
33. McKinnon AO, Squires EL, Voss JL: Ultrasonic evaluation of the mare's reproductive tract, part 2. Compend Contin Educ Pract Vet 1987; 9:472-480.
34. McDowell KJ, Sharp DC, Grubaugh W et al: Restricted conceptus mobility results in failure of pregnancy maintenance in mares. Biol Reprod 1988; 39:340-348.
35. Ginther OJ: The nature of embryo reduction in mares with twin conceptuses: deprivation hypothesis. Am J Vet Res 1989; 50:45-53.
36. Chevalier-Clement F: Pregnancy loss in the mare. Anim Reprod Sci 1989; 20:231-244.
37. Tannus RJ, Thun R: Influence of endometrial cysts on conception rate of mares. Zentralbl Veterinarmed A 1995; 42:275-283.

38. Eilts BE, Scholl DT, Paccamonti DL et al: Prevalence of endometrial cysts and their effect on fertility. Biol Reprod 1995; 1:527-532.

39. Griffin RL, Bennett SD: Nd:YAG laser photoablation of endometrial cysts: a review of 55 cases (2000-2001). Proceedings of the 48th Annual Convention of the American Association of Equine Practitioners, pp 58-60, 2002.

40. Allen WR: Luteal deficiency and embryo mortality in the mare. Reprod Domest Anim 2001; 36:121-131.

41. Pycock JF, Newcombe JR: The effect of the gonadotrophin-releasing hormone analog, buserelin, administered in diestrus on pregnancy rates and pregnancy failure in mares. Theriogenology 1996; 46:1097-1101.

42. Newcombe JR, Martinez TA, Peters AR: The effect of the gonadotropin-releasing hormone analog, buserelin, on pregnancy rates in horse and pony mares. Theriogenology 2001; 55:1619-1631.

43. Ginther OJ: Embryonic loss in mares: incidence, time of occurrence, and hormonal involvement. Theriogenology 1985; 23:77-89.

44. Newcombe JR: Spontaneous oestrous behaviour during pregnancy associated with luteal regression, ovulation and birth of a live foal in a part Thoroughbred mare. Equine Vet Educ 2000; 2:111-114.

45. Vanderwall DK, Squires EL, Brinsko SP et al: Diagnosis and management of abnormal embryonic development characterized by formation of an embryonic vesicle without an embryo in mares. J Am Vet Med Assoc 2000; 217:58-63.

46. Newcombe JR: Unpublished data.

47. Shideler RK, Squires EL, Voss JL et al: Progestagen therapy of ovariectomized pregnant mares. J Reprod Fertil 1982; 32 (suppl):459-464.

48. Knowles JE, Squires EL, Shideler RK et al: Relationship of progesterone to early pregnancy loss in mares. J Equine Vet Sci 1993; 13:528-533.

49. McKinnon AO, Tarrida Del Marmol Figueroa S, Nobelius AM et al: Failure of hydroxyprogesterone caproate to maintain pregnancy in ovariectomized mares. Equine Vet J 1993; 25:158-160.

50. McKinnon AO, Lescun TB, Walker JH et al: The inability of some synthetic progestagens to maintain pregnancy in the mare. Equine Vet J 2000; 32:83-85.

51. Ball BA, Wilker C, Daels PF et al: Use of progesterone in microspheres for maintenance of pregnancy in mares. Am J Vet Res 1992; 53:1294-1297.

52. Vanderwall DK, Williams JL, Woods GL: Use of a compounded proprietary long-acting progesterone formulation for maintenance of pregnancy in mares. Proc Annu Mtg Soc Therio, p 8, 2003 (abstract).

53. Squires EL, Ginther OJ: Collection technique and progesterone concentration of ovarian and uterine venous blood in mares. J Anim Sci 1975; 40:275-281.

54. Holtan DW, Squires EL, Lapin DR et al: Effect of ovariectomy on pregnancy in mares. J Reprod Fertil Suppl 1979; 27:457-463.

55. Hinrichs K, Sertich PL, Palmer E et al: Establishment and maintenance of pregnancy after embryo transfer in ovariectomized mares treated with progesterone. J Reprod Fertil 1987; 80:395-401.

56. Carnevale EM, Ginther OJ: Defective oocytes as a cause of subfertility in old mares. Biol Reprod 1995; 1:209-214.

57. Carnevale EM, Uson M, Bozzola JJ et al: Comparison of oocytes from young and old mares with light and electron microscopy. Theriogenology 1999; 51:299 (abstract).

58. van Niekerk FE, Van Niekerk CH: The effect of dietary protein on reproduction in the mare. Part 6. Serum progestagen concentrations during pregnancy. J S Afr Vet Assoc 1998; 69:143-149.

59. Woods GL, Baker CB, Bilinski J et al: A field study on early pregnancy loss in Standardbred and Thoroughbred mares. J Equine Vet Sci 1985; 5:264-267.

60. Meyers PJ, Bonnett BN, Mckee SL: Quantifying the occurrence of early embryonic mortality on three equine breeding farms. Can Vet J 1991; 32:665-672 (abstract).

61. Morris LH, Allen WR: Reproductive efficiency of intensively managed Thoroughbred mares in Newmarket. Equine Vet J 2002; 34:51-60.

62. Woods J, Bergfelt DR, Ginther OJ: Effects of time of insemination relative to ovulation on pregnancy rate and embryonic loss rate in mares. Equine Vet J 1990; 22:410-415.

63. Koskinen E, Lindeberg H, Kuntsi H et al: Fertility of mares after postovulatory insemination. Zentralbl Veterinarmed A 1990; 37:77-80.

64. Barbacini S, Gulden P, Marchi V et al: Incidence of embryo loss in mares inseminated before or after ovulation. Equine Vet Educ 1999; 11:251-254.

65. Van Niekerk CH, Morgenthal JC: Fetal loss and the effect of stress on plasma progestagen levels in pregnant Thoroughbred mares. J Reprod Fertil Suppl 1982; 32:453-457.

66. Baucus KL, Ralston SL, Nockels CF et al: Effects of transportation on early embryonic death in mares. J Anim Sci 1990; 68:345-351.

67. Daels PF, Starr M, Kindahl H et al: Effect of *Salmonella typhimurium* endotoxin on PGF-2α release and fetal death in the mare. J Reprod Fertil Suppl 1987; 35:485-492.

68. Daels PF, Stabenfeldt GH, Hughes JP et al: Effects of flunixin meglumine on endotoxin-induced prostaglandin F2 alpha secretion during early pregnancy in mares. Am J Vet Res 1991; 52:276-281.

69. Daels PF, Stabenfeldt GH, Hughes JP et al: Evaluation of progesterone deficiency as a cause of fetal death in mares with experimentally induced endotoxemia. Am J Vet Res 1991; 52:282-288.

70. Henneke DR, Potter GD, Kreider JL: Body condition during pregnancy and lactation and reproductive efficiency of mares. Theriogenology 1984; 21:897-909.

71. Henneke DR, Potter GD, Kreider JL et al: Relationship between condition score, physical measurements and body fat percentage in mares. Equine Vet J 1983; 15:371-372.

72. van Niekerk FE, Van Niekerk CH: The effect of dietary protein on reproduction in the mare. Part 7. Embryonic development, early embryonic death, foetal losses and their relationship with serum progestagen. J S Afr Vet Assoc 1998; 69:150-155.

73. Christiansen DL, Hopper R, Hill NS et al: Early embryonic death in mares grazing endophyte infected fescue. Proc Annu Mtg Soc Therio p 43, 2003 (abstract).

74. Webb BA, Barney WE, Dahlman DL et al: Eastern tent caterpillars (*Malacosoma americanum*) cause mare reproductive loss syndrome. J Insect Physiol 2004; 50:185-193.

75. Rensis FD, Scaramuzzi RJ: Heat stress and seasonal effects on reproduction in the dairy cow—a review. Theriogenology 2003; 60:1139-1151.

76. Hearn P, Bonnet B, Samper J: Factors affecting pregnancy and pregnancy loss on one Thoroughbred farm. Proceedings of the 39th Annual Convention of the American Association of Equine Practitioners, pp 161-163, 1993.

77. Voss JL, Pickett BW, Back DG et al: Effect of rectal palpation on pregnancy rate of nonlactating, normally cycling mares. J Anim Sci 1975; 41:829-834.

78. Irwin CFP: Early pregnancy testing and its relationship to abortion. J Reprod Fertil Suppl 1975; 23:485-489.

79. Vogelsang MM, Vogelsang SG, Lindsey BR et al: Reproductive performance in mares subjected to examination by diagnostic ultrasound. Theriogenology 1989; 32:95-103.

80. Platt H: Aetiological aspects of abortion in the Thoroughbred mare. J Comp Pathol 1973; 83:199-205.

81. England GCW, Keane M: The effect of x-radiation upon the quality and fertility of stallion semen. Theriogenology 1996; 46:173-180.

82. King WA, Bezard J, Bousquet D et al: The meiotic stage of preovulatory oocytes in mares. Genome 1987; 29:679-682.

83. Woods GL, White KL, Vanderwall DK et al: A mule cloned from fetal cells by nuclear transfer. Science 2003; 301:1063.

84. Woods GL, White KL, Vanderwall DK et al: Cloned mule pregnancies produced using nuclear transfer. Theriogenology 2002; 58:779-782 (abstract).

85. McKinnon AO, Lacham-Kaplan O, Trounson AO: Pregnancies produced from fertile and infertile stallions by intracytoplasmic sperm injection (ICSI) of single frozen-thawed spermatozoa into *in vivo* matured mare oocytes. J Reprod Fertil Suppl 2000; 56:513-517.

86. Chevalier F, Palmer E: Ultrasonic echography in the mare. J Reprod Fertil Suppl 1982; 32:423-430.

87. Simpson DJ, Greenwood RES, Ricketts SW et al: Use of ultrasound echography for early diagnosis of single and twin pregnancy in the mare. J Reprod Fertil Suppl 1982; 32:431-439.

88. Ginther OJ, Bergfelt DR, Leith GS et al: Embryonic loss in mares: incidence and ultrasonic morphology. Theriogenology 1985; 24:73-86.

89. Villahoz MD, Squires EL, Voss JL et al: Some observations on early embryonic death in mares. Theriogenology 1985; 23:915-924.

90. Forde D, Keenan L, Wade J et al: Reproductive wastage in the mare and its relationship to progesterone in early pregnancy. J Reprod Fertil Suppl 1987; 35:493-495.

91. Irvine CHG, Sutton P, Turner JE et al: Changes in plasma progesterone concentrations from days 17 to 42 of gestation in mares maintaining or losing pregnancy. Equine Vet J 1990; 22:104-106.

92. Lowis TC, Hyland JH: Analysis of post-partum fertility in mares on a thoroughbred stud in southern Victoria. Aust Vet J 1991; 68:304-306.

93. Bruck I, Anderson GA, Hyland JH: Reproductive performance of thoroughbred mares on six commercial stud farms. Aust Vet J 1993; 70:299-303.

94. Newcombe JR: Observations on early pregnancy diagnosis and early embryonic loss in the mare. Ir Vet J 1997; 50:534-536.

95. Carnevale EM, Ramirez RJ, Squires EL et al: Factors affecting pregnancy rates and early embryonic death after equine embryo transfer. Theriogenology 2000; 54:965-979.

96. Woods GL, Weber JA, Vanderwall DK et al: Selective oviductal transport and fertilization rate of equine embryos. Proceedings of the 37th Annual Convention of the American Association of Equine Practitioners, pp 197-201, 1991.

97. Brinsko SP, Ball BA, Miller PG et al: In vitro development of day 2 embryos obtained from young, fertile mares and aged, subfertile mares. J Reprod Fertil 1994; 102:371-378.

CHAPTER 56

Mare Reproductive Loss Syndrome

W. THOMAS RIDDLE
MICHELLE M. LEBLANC

In the spring of 2001 and 2002, central Kentucky experienced large numbers of early- and late-term fetal losses in mares. In addition to the reproductive losses, a number of pericarditis and endophthalmitis cases were also identified. Together these reproductive and nonreproductive cases have been termed mare reproductive loss syndrome (MRLS). Other areas of Kentucky and neighboring states also reported smaller numbers of cases consistent with MRLS.

The economic impact to Kentucky was estimated to be nearly $336 million in 2001 and between $84 million and $100 million in 2002. In 2001 there were approximately 550 late-term losses, between 2000 and 3000 early fetal losses, approximately 30 endophthalmitis cases, and between 50 and 60 pericarditis cases. In 2002, fewer cases were seen, with 165 late-term losses, approximately 500 early fetal losses, 6 endophthalmitis cases, and 9 pericarditis cases being reported. The financial ramifications from MRLS will be felt for years following the actual cases. As an example, the 2002 Keeneland November Breeding Stock Sale was the smallest since 1993, with 864 foals entered, compared with 1063 in 2001 and 1379 in 2000. The 2003 Keeneland July Select Yearling Sale was cancelled with a primary reason being fewer yearlings available as a result of MRLS losses.

EARLY FETAL LOSSES*

MRLS was first observed in pregnant mares presented for fetal sexing between 60 and 70 days of gestation. Beginning on April 26, 2001, some of these mares had dead fetuses surrounded by allantoic and amniotic fluids containing hyperechoic material. In just a few short weeks the estimated fetal losses reached nearly 3000. These large numbers had never before been reported in central Kentucky or anywhere in the world. The only comparable experience in central Kentucky was in 1980 and 1981, when smaller numbers of early fetal losses, estimated to be 256 in 1980 and 162 in 1981, were seen. Breeding dates

*A portion of this section was presented at the First Workshop on Mare Reproductive Loss Syndrome, August 27-28, 2002, at the Maxwell H. Gluck Equine Research Center at the University of Kentucky, Lexington, Kentucky, and at the Annual Conference of the Society for Theriogenology, September 16-20, 2003, Columbus, Ohio.

and gestational ages were similar in the 1980-1981 and 2001-2002 losses; however, ultrasonography was not available in the early 1980s, so detailed comparisons could not be made. Another similarity was that mares occasionally retained the fetus and placental membranes after abortion, an uncommon finding at this stage of gestation. Interestingly, in the four years in which losses occurred (1980-81, 2001-02), entomologists reported the presence of a greater than normal number of eastern tent caterpillars (ETC). No cause was ever determined for the losses in 1980 and 1981.

Mares experiencing early fetal loss from MRLS typically presented with no outward signs. Occasionally the mare had a serosanguineous or purulent vulvar discharge. Some mares were found with membranes protruding from their vulvas with the fetus located either in the vagina or uterus. A small percentage (estimated at less than 5%) exhibited mild signs of colic, abdominal straining, or low-grade fevers (101° to 101.5°F) 1 to 3 days before early fetal loss.

Often with MRLS losses the mare appeared to be pregnant when examined by rectal palpation. The uterus would have normal to slightly less fluid distention expected for the stage of gestation, and it was only on ultrasonographic examination that the mare was found to have a compromised or dead fetus. Before the appearance of MRLS in 2001, ultrasound examinations were conducted only through 30 to 35 days of gestation to confirm pregnancy in Thoroughbred mares in central Kentucky, unless fetal sexing was requested. Since the MRLS outbreak, mares are scanned through 60 to 90 days of gestation to confirm that the fetus is viable. The typical ultrasonographic appearance of a pregnancy afflicted by MRLS is a dead fetus surrounded by echogenic allantoic and amnionic fluid, with amnionic fluid being more hyperechoic than allantoic fluid.

The majority of losses in the author's practice (Riddle) occurred between 40 and 80 days of gestation, with a range of 32 to 140 days (Table 56-1). In 2001 these mares were bred between February 10 and April 10, whereas in 2002 breedings ranged from February 15 to April 1. In 2001 losses were identified between April 26 and July 2, whereas losses in 2002 began on April 29 and ended on June 3.

Most losses in 2001 occurred over a 3-week period beginning April 26, whereas losses in 2002 were more

Table 56-1

Gestational Ages Represented

	2001	2002
30-39 days	3	0
40-49 days	8	5
50-59 days	11	0
60-69 days	12	5
70-79 days	11	6
80-89 days	4	0
90-99 days	4	1
100-140 days	3	1

evenly distributed over a 5-week period beginning April 29. In 2001 there were 56 losses on the seven farms managed by the practice (Riddle), whereas in 2002, 18 losses occurred on only two of the seven farms. These figures indicate a 68% decrease in MRLS losses from 2001 to 2002. The majority of equine practitioners in central Kentucky experienced a similar decrease.

Pregnancy rates between 15 and 35 days in 2001 and 2002 were not adversely affected by MRLS. In 2001 the status of the mares that aborted in the author's practice (Riddle) was equally represented with 19 barren mares (34%), 20 maiden mares (36%), and 17 foaling mares (30%) aborting. In 2002, maiden mares represented 56% of the losses (5 barren mares, 28%; 3 foaling mares, 16%). This finding is likely related to a heavy load of ETC in fields on one farm that housed the maiden mares. Of the 56 mares that aborted from MRLS in 2001, 31 remained in the care of the author (Riddle) in 2002. Thirty of these 31 conceived, and 1 mare remained barren. Two of the 30 pregnant mares were again affected by MRLS on their subsequent pregnancy in 2002.

A number of ancillary diagnostic tests were performed on aborting mares in an attempt to identify the cause. Serum progesterone concentrations were measured in 16 mares when fetal death was noted. Concentrations were adequate to maintain pregnancies in these mares (>4 ng/ml). Complete blood counts and blood chemistry values were within normal limits. In 2001 and 2002 uterine cultures were taken on all aborting mares in the author's practice. Bacteria isolated included alpha and beta streptococcus, *Escherichia coli,* and *Enterobacter cloacae.* Uterine cytologic findings within 7 days of abortion from 5 mares in 2001 showed moderate to severe inflammation. This inflammation was consistent with a recent abortion and was not unique to MRLS. Following abortion, all mares received uterine lavages and were treated for 5 days with the appropriate antibiotic based on culture and sensitivity. On subsequent heats uterine cytologic findings were within normal limits, and no bacteria were isolated on uterine culture in most mares. In 2001 uterine biopsies were performed on 10 mares 1 to 3 months after MRLS abortion. Histologic findings were mild, and those present could not be related to MRLS.

Hyperechoic allantoic and amniotic fluids were consistent findings in mares that aborted between 35 and 140

days from MRLS. Before 2001, echogenic fetal fluids were not reported during thousands of ultrasonographic examinations conducted to determine fetal sex between 58 and 75 days of gestation. In 2001 and 2002, hyperechoic fetal fluids were reported in all mares that retained a dead fetus and in many mares with a live fetus. In an attempt to determine the makeup of the hyperechoic fetal fluids, allantoic fluid aspirates were obtained from three mares that retained a dead fetus in utero in 2001. Culture of the fluid grew alpha *Streptococcus* in two cases and *E. coli* in the third. Cytologic examination of the fluid showed sheets of squamous epithelial cells, cocci or rods in chains, and a rare neutrophil. It was proposed that the hyperechoic material seen on ultrasonography of the uterus was squamous epithelial cells. The presence of hyperechoic fetal fluids in mares carrying a live fetus before 80 days of gestation was associated with a high risk of loss. In 2001, 8 of 29 mares (27.5%) identified via ultrasonography to have a live fetus and echogenic fluids between 40 and 80 days of gestation aborted within 30 days of examination. In 2002, only 5 of 69 mares (7%) that were between 40 and 80 days of gestation with a live fetus and echogenic fluids aborted. Differences between the two years may be related to exposure rates, development of immunologic resistance to the MRLS toxin, or to unknown causes.

In 2001, once veterinarians noted the relationship between early fetal loss and echogenic fetal fluids, mares were repeatedly examined between 40 and 120 days of gestation by ultrasonography to evaluate fetal fluid clarity. It was noted that fetal fluids appeared to become echogenic in all mares around 80 days of gestation. This clinical observation resulted in a study designed to determine when reproductively normal mares develop echogenic fluids and to determine if the fetal fluids of mares exposed to MRLS differed from the fetal fluids of mares not exposed.[1] Ultrasonographic examinations of the reproductive tract were conducted between July 30, 2001, and August 30, 2001, on 178 mares that were 55 to 176 days pregnant. One hundred and four mares resided in Kentucky, and 74 resided in Florida. Allantoic and amniotic fluids in both groups of mares were found to be anechoic before 85 days of gestation and hyperechoic after 85 days of gestation.

In 2001, when MRLS was first identified, there was an obvious desire to implement treatments or control measures aimed at preventing further abortions. It was difficult to make reasonable recommendations because the cause of the syndrome was not known. Many treatments were given to mares at risk of aborting but none prevented losses. Broad-spectrum antibiotics were given because bacteria had been isolated from aborted fetuses and placentas. Domperidone and mycotoxin binders were administered to mares in late gestation because some late-term abortions showed signs consistent with fescue toxicity (premature placental separation and thickened placentas). Flunixin meglumine was used for its antiinflammatory and antiendotoxin properties, and pentoxifylline was recommended by some practitioners for its reaginic properties.

Clinical impression in 2001 strongly supported the ETC as being associated with MRLS because massive numbers of ETC inundated central Kentucky and southern Indiana and Ohio that spring. Therefore efforts were made to restrict mares' contact with ETC and to restrict caterpillar numbers in the spring of 2002. The ETC has a natural resurgence about every 10 to 20 years, and it lasts for 2 to 3 seasons. The resurgence is then followed by a drastic decline in numbers. The ETC has a life span of about 5 to 8 weeks in central Kentucky. Caterpillars first hatch in mid-March, leave their tents in droves daily in search of food, and then return. During their short tenure they molt their skins approximately 5 times as they grow in length and diameter. Their preferred food is the leaves of cherry trees, one of the most common trees in central Kentucky. It is not uncommon to see trees defoliated by the caterpillars. In an attempt to reduce contact of pregnant mares with ETC in 2002, pasture turn-out was limited to 2 to 6 hours a day, and on some farms mares were muzzled when out in pasture. Limited turn-out successfully eliminated MRLS losses on some farms, whereas others experienced significant losses. Muzzling mares on pasture appeared to be close to 100% effective at preventing MRLS. Most farms attempted to control caterpillars by either spraying or cutting down cherry trees. When spraying was successful in eliminating caterpillars, MRLS was prevented; however, in many cases sprays were not effective in eliminating the caterpillars. Farms that cut down all cherry trees reported minimal losses to MRLS. In 2003 the number of caterpillars was greatly reduced because control measures were continued and a virus wiped out the majority of the population. No cases of MRLS were reported in 2003.

LATE-TERM LOSSES

In addition to early fetal losses, a smaller, but significant number of mares (approximately 550 in 2001 and 165 in 2002[2]) experienced late-term fetal loss during the same time period in late April and May. These losses occurred in the last trimester, with most mares within 30 days of the expected foaling date. The majority of these mares exhibited no signs of impending foaling or abortion. Labor was reported to be intense and was often characterized as explosive. Of the fetuses submitted to the Livestock Diagnostic Disease Center, 32% were from deliveries with premature separation of the placenta and dystocia was reported for 11%.[3]

The resulting foals from these late-term MRLS cases were either dead at birth or extremely compromised. Clinical signs were consistent with asphyxia, and most afflicted foals required resuscitation.[4] Surviving foals were referred to intensive care facilities. Upon admission, the foals were found to be dehydrated, hypothermic, and tachycardic, with irregular respiration. Leukopenia, hypoglycemia, and acidosis were consistently noted. Bilateral hyphema was noted in a significant number of foals. Therapy included resuscitation, supportive care, and antibiotics. Prognosis for survival was poor.

Pathologic findings in the late-term MRLS fetuses included inflammation of the amnionic segment of the umbilical cord (funisitis), inflammation of the amnion, pneumonia, fetal bacteremia, and occasionally placentitis.[5] The most remarkable finding was the appearance of the amnionic umbilical cord, which in many cases was edematous and grayish-yellow, with a roughened and hemorrhagic surface. Because there was no single laboratory test or necropsy finding that confirmed a diagnosis of MRLS in the late-term foal, diagnosis was made based on a combination of factors, which included history, time of year, bacteriologic findings, and pathologic findings.[5]

PERICARDITIS

Pericarditis was one of two nonreproductive syndromes associated with MRLS. In 2001 and 2002, outbreaks of fibrinous, effusive pericarditis were seen concurrent with the occurrence of early- and late-term fetal loss.[6] These cases occurred in all ages and genders and in multiple breeds. Epidemiologic studies that examined the cases of pericarditis and MRLS found that the two diseases were highly associated with each other.[7] However, mares with pericarditis were not at increased risk for experiencing fetal loss.[8] Pathologists found a fibrinous, effusive pericarditis with the epicardium covered by a thick, motheaten layer of fibrin. Pericardial fluid was cultured in 34 cases in 2001. Bacteria were recovered in 15 cases. Actinobacillus sp. was isolated in 11 of the 15 cases.

ENDOPHTHALMITIS

In addition to pericarditis, a second nonreproductive syndrome, endophthalmitis, was associated with MRLS. This condition was characterized by inflammatory debris in both the anterior and posterior segments and was seen in horses of all ages and genders and multiple breeds.[9] Most of the afflicted horses were less than 2 years of age. All cases were unilateral and were unresponsive to aggressive therapy. Without exception, all horses became blind in the affected eye.

MRLS RESEARCH

In the summer and autumn of 2001, numerous theories were proposed for the cause of MRLS. Some theories centered on the ingestion of toxic substances in pasture grasses, whereas others implicated the ETC. Theories associated with the grasses included electrolyte imbalances in grasses induced from repeated freeze-thaws in the spring, nitrate-nitrite toxicity, ingestion of poison hemlock, white clover, tall fescue alkaloids, grasses that contained mycotoxins, and ammonia toxicity. Ingestion or inhalation of the ETC was thought to be associated with the absorption of either a biologic (bacteria, virus, or parasite) or chemical toxin. In the winter of 2001, an epidemiologic survey conducted by the University of Kentucky identified four factors associated with increased MRLS: breeding date in February 2001, moderate to high concentration of ETC in mare areas, presence of wild cherry trees around pastures, and having more than 50 mares on the farm.[10] Two factors were associated with a low incidence or no incidence of MRLS: absence of caterpillars and feeding hay to mares in pasture.

Based on the above-mentioned risk factor of caterpillar exposure and MRLS, a trial feeding caterpillars and their excreta to pregnant mares was undertaken in the spring of 2002. Pregnant mares housed on pasture were exposed to either ETC with excreta or excreta alone. Ten mares housed under identical conditions were maintained as controls. Treatments were sprinkled on pasture to which mares were exposed for 6 hours per day. Seven of 10 mares aborted in both the ETC with excreta and excreta only groups. Three of 10 mares in the control group aborted.[11] Abortions in the control group were thought to be caused by caterpillars that wandered from the treatment to control pens.

A second study was designed to complement the previous study by removing the mares from exposure to grass and to more strictly control the treatments of ETC and their frass.[12] Frass is the feces of the caterpillar. Fifteen mares between 40 and 80 days of gestation were housed in stalls for a quarantine period of 12 days and then gavaged with either 2.5 g of frass, 50 g of starved ETC, or 500 ml of water for 10 days (five mares in each group). Physical examinations were conducted every 8 hours, and the reproductive tract was evaluated by ultrasonography once daily. Four of the 5 mares gavaged with ETC aborted on trial days 8, 10, and 13. No mares fed frass or gavaged with water aborted. Ultrasonographic findings were similar to that seen in clinical cases. The allantoic and amnionic fluids became hyperechoic before the fetus died, or the hyperechoic findings were associated with fetal death.

Feeding trials were also conducted in 2002 with ETC to determine if it was associated with late-term losses and to possibly identify the toxic principle or the portion of caterpillar associated with the syndrome. In one study mares in late gestation were gavaged with either 50 g of ETC or water daily.[13] Six of six mares fed caterpillars aborted, with the first abortion occurring 68 hours after the first treatment. None of the control mares aborted. Additional studies revealed that the integument and not the gastrointestinal contents induced abortion, that autoclaving the ETC rendered them nontoxic, and that freezing did not destroy the toxin.

Work in 2003 centered on identification of the toxin in ETC and development of experimental animal models. Sebastian et al fed irradiated ETC to five mares in late gestation to determine if the toxin associated with ETC was a biologic or chemical agent. Irradiation of caterpillars eliminated bacteria or viruses from the caterpillars. Three of the five mares aborted, indicating that the toxin responsible for MRLS may be a chemical and not a biologic toxin. McDowell et al[14] added ETC to the ration of five gilts in midgestation (40 g per gilt per day for 10 days) to determine if the domestic pig could be used as an animal model for MRLS. Two of five gilts fed ETC aborted their entire litter, while none of the five control gilts aborted. The two gilts fed ETC that aborted, along with their nontreated pairs, were euthanized, and necropsy was performed 1 to 3 days after the abortions. The remaining gilts were euthanized, and necropsy was performed 29 days after the onset of the trial. Streptococcus bacteria were isolated from fetuses of all gilts fed ETC, whether or not they aborted, and from fetuses of one control gilt. Bacteria isolated from the control fetuses were less numerous and of a different strain than those isolated from fetuses of ETC-treated gilts. Caterpillar

setae, the barbed, hairlike structures found on the outside of ETC, were found in the alimentary tracts of gilts fed ETC, and it was hypothesized that their presence may contribute to the syndrome. The experiment demonstrated for the first time that ETC could cause abortion in a nonequid in a manner consistent with MRLS and indicated that domestic pigs may be a useful model for studying the syndrome. In 2004, investigators at the University of Kentucky investigated whether setae were associated with abortions when fed to pregnant mares. Results of that work are not currently available.[15]

CONCLUSION

There are many lessons to be learned from central Kentucky's experience with MRLS:

1. As soon as there is a suspicion of a disease outbreak, whether a recognized disease or not, appropriate samples should be collected for laboratory analysis, including serum, whole blood, urine, uterine culture, cytologic specimens, and biopsy specimens. If mares are out on pasture, samples of grasses, other vegetation, soils, and water should be collected. If there is an overabundance of a specific arthropod or insect, specimens should be obtained and appropriate scientists or specialists notified. Samples should be stored frozen if immediate analysis is not possible. If samples prove to be unneeded, they can always be discarded. If they are needed and they were not collected, the opportunity has been missed.
2. A system should be established for reporting a suspected outbreak to a central body that will decide when to notify veterinarians and farm managers.
3. The veterinarian must work closely with the farm manager and farm workers in collecting information to determine the cause of the outbreak.
4. Open communication among veterinarians and among farm owners and managers is critical. A disease outbreak is not the time to be territorial or to conceal needed information.
5. Do not hesitate to seek outside expertise.

References

1. Vince KJ, Riddle WT, LeBlanc MM et al: Ultrasonographic appearance of fetal fluids between 55 and 176 days of gestation in the mare: effect of mare reproductive loss syndrome. Proceedings of the 27th Annual Convention of the American Association of Equine Practitioners, pp 350-351, 2002.
2. Powell D: An update on mare reproductive loss syndrome (MRLS) in Kentucky. Presented at Mare Reproductive Loss Syndrome Think Tank, Lexington, Ky, January 2003.
3. Williams N: Mare reproductive loss syndrome laboratory findings. Presented at Mare Reproductive Loss Syndrome Think Tank, Lexington, Ky, January 2003.
4. Byars TD, Seahorn TL: Clinical observations of mare reproductive loss syndrome foals presented for neonatal critical care. Proceedings of the First Workshop on Mare Reproductive Loss Syndrome (MRLS), pp 15-16, 2002.

5. Williams NM, Bolin DC, Donahue RC et al: Gross and histopathological correlates of mare reproductive loss syndrome. Proceedings of the First Workshop on Mare Reproductive Loss Syndrome (MRLS), pp 24-25, 2002.

6. Bolin DC, Harrison LR, Donahue JM et al: The pericarditis correlate of mare reproductive loss syndrome. Proceedings of the First Workshop on Mare Reproductive Loss Syndrome (MRLS), pp 25-26, 2002.

7. Cohen N, Carey J, Donahue J et al: Report of pericarditis cases—control study. Prepared for the Governor's Task Force on the Mare Reproductive Loss Syndrome, 2001.

8. Slovis NM: Clinical observations of the pericarditis syndrome. Proceedings of the First Workshop on Mare Reproductive Loss Syndrome (MRLS), pp 18-20, 2002.

9. Latimer C: Endophthalmitis: a syndrome associated with mare reproductive loss syndrome? Proceedings of the First Workshop on Mare Reproductive Loss Syndrome (MRLS), pp 17-18, 2002.

10. Dwyer RM, Garber L, Traub-Dargatz J et al: A case-control study of factors associated with excessive proportions of early fetal losses associated with mare reproductive loss syndrome in central Kentucky during 2001. J Am Vet Med Assoc 2003; 613-619.

11. Webb BA, Barney WE, Dahlman DL et al: Induction of MRLS by directed exposure of susceptible mares to eastern tent caterpillar larvae and frass. Proceedings of the First Workshop on Mare Reproductive Loss Syndrome (MRLS), pp 78-79, 2002.

12. Bernard WV, LeBlanc MM, Webb BA: Gavage of Eastern Tent Caterpillars is associated with early fetal loss in the mare. J Am Vet Med Assoc 2004; 225:717-721.

13. Sebastian M, Bernard W, Harrison L et al: Experimental induction of mare reproductive loss syndrome with irradiated eastern tent caterpillar to assess whether the primary pathogen in mare reproductive loss syndrome is a toxic molecule or a microorganism. In Powell DG, Furry D, Hala G (eds): *Proceedings of a Workshop on the Equine Placenta*, Lexington, KY, pp 27-28, Dec 2003.

14. McDowell KJ, Williams NM, Donahue JM, Poole L et al: Deductive investigations of the role of eastern tent caterpillars in mare reproductive loss syndrome. In Powell DG, Furry D, Hale G (eds): *Proceedings of a Workshop on the Equine Placenta*. Lexington, KY, pp 99-103, Dec 2003.

15. Adkins P: Tracking the source of mare reproductive loss syndrome. Equus, pp 44-49, Jan 2005.

CHAPTER 57

Maintenance of Pregnancy

ANGUS O. MCKINNON
JONATHAN F. PYCOCK

In order to properly evaluate possible therapies to help mares maintain pregnancy, we first need to understand some of the reasons why mares suffer from either early embryonic death (EED) or abortion.

EARLY EMBRYONIC DEATH

Improvement in ultrasonographic equipment has permitted initial investigation of early embryonic losses between days 10 and 20 of gestation.[1] This technique, combined with embryo recovery, permits investigation of embryo losses between day 6, which is the first time an embryo can be routinely recovered from the uterus, and day 11, which is the first time the vesicle can be consistently detected by ultrasonography. The real incidence of EED prior to day 6 is unknown. However, it was suggested that a major proportion of EED in infertile mares occurs in the oviduct.[2] Workers in Wisconsin have suggested that in aged, subfertile mares, the primary problem may actually be the oocyte.[3] In the future, much more clear delineation of the various incidences of problems from the different parts of the reproductive tract will be forthcoming. The incidence of EED has been reported to be between 5% and 30% of established pregnancies.[4,5] In earlier studies utilizing ultrasonography, it appeared that EED occurred in mares much earlier than previously reported.[1,6] Various causes and factors responsible for EED in mares, apart from presence of twins, have been suggested, including nutrition,[7,8] plant estrogens and photo-period,[9] endophyte infected tall fescue,[10] seminal treatments,[11] lactation stress, and foal-heat breeding,[12] genital infections,[4,5,12] chromosomal abnormalities, hormonal deficiencies,[8] anabolic steroids,[1] stress,[8] failure of maternal recognition and deficiency of pregnant mare serum gonadotropin (PMSG or eCG) production,[13] immunological factors,[14,15] and even a higher incidence from some individual stallions.[16] Migration of the conceptus was originally believed to be a contributing factor in EED; however, it is now known to be a normal characteristic of the horse conceptus.[17] Lactating mares and mares bred during foal heat have been reported to have a higher incidence of EED than non-lactating mares.[12,18,19] However, in a survey of 2,562 pregnancies in lactating and non-lactating mares, the incidence of EED was similar.[20] Prior to the advent of ultrasonography, recognition and timing of EED was difficult. From data collected over 2 breeding seasons[1] involving 356 mares diagnosed pregnant by ultrasonography, the overall incidence of EED through day 50 postovulation was 17.3%.

The majority (77.1%) of EED occurred prior to day 35 postovulation. During the period 15 to 35 days postovulation, a greater ($P < 0.05$) incidence of EED occurred between days 15 and 20 (26.2%) and 30 and 35 (29.5%) postovulation compared to other time periods. Maternal recognition of pregnancy has been reported to occur between 14 and 16 days postovulation.[21,22]

Embryo development and morphology was useful to predict EED in an embryo transfer program.[23]

638 embryo transfers conducted over 3 yr were retrospectively examined to determine which factors (recipient, embryo and transfer) significantly influenced pregnancy and embryo loss rates and to determine how rates could be improved. On Day 7 or 8 after ovulation, embryos (fresh or cooled/transported) were transferred by surgical or nonsurgical techniques into recipients ovulating from 5 to 9 d before transfer. At 12 and 50 d of gestation (Day 0 = day of ovulation), pregnancy rates were 65.7% (419 of 638) and 55.5% (354 of 638). Pregnancy rates on Day 50 were significantly higher for recipients that had excellent to good uterine tone or were graded as ''acceptable'' during a pretransfer examination, usually performed 5 d after ovulation, versus recipients that had fair to poor uterine tone or were graded ''marginally acceptable.'' Embryonic factors that significantly affected pregnancy rates were morphology grade, diameter and stage of development. The incidence of early embryonic death was 15.5% (65 of 419) from Days 12 to 50. Embryo loss rates were significantly higher in recipients used 7 or 9 d vs 5 or 6 d after ovulation. Embryos with minor morphological changes (Grade 2) resulted in more (P < 0.05) embryo death than embryos with no morphological abnormalities (Grade 1). Between Days 12 and 50, the highest incidence of embryo death occurred during the interval from Days 17 to 25 of gestation. Embryonic vesicles that were imaged with ultrasound during the first pregnancy exam (5 d after transfer) resulted in significantly fewer embryonic deaths than vesicles not imaged until subsequent exams. In the present study, embryo morphology was predictive of the potential for an embryo to result in a viable pregnancy. Delayed development of the embryo upon collection from the donor or delayed development of the embryonic vesicle within the recipient's uterus was associated with a higher incidence of pregnancy failure. Recipient selection (age, day after ovulation, quality on Day 5) significantly affected pregnancy and embryo loss rates.[23]

In addition, a higher rate of EED has been reported with delayed insemination that is either greater than 12 hours[24] or greater than 18 hours postovulation.[25]

It should be noted that formation of endometrial cups occurs on approximately day 35. EED is diagnosed when an embryonic vesicle seen previously is not observed on 2 consecutive ultrasonographic scans and/or when only remnants of a vesicle are observed. Ultrasonographic criteria for impending EED are an irregular and indented vesicle, fluid in the uterine lumen, and vesicular fluid that contains echogenic spots. EED is suspected, particularly after day 30, when no fetal heartbeat is observed, there is poor definition of fetal structure, fetal fluids are very echogenic, or the largest diameter of the fetal vesicle is 2 standard deviations smaller than the mean established for that specific day of age. Vesicles increasing in size more slowly than normal may also be characteristic of EED.[6] Indications obtained by ultrasonographic scanning of impending loss at later stages include failure of fixation, an echogenic ring within the vesicle, a mass floating in a collection of fluid, and a gradual decrease in volume of placental fluid with disorganization of placental membranes (Figure 57-1). On occasion EED may be anticipated by identification of endometrial folds in an early pregnant uterus with or without visible fluid (Figure 57-2). Ultrasonographic scanning during early pregnancy is an extremely useful management tool for pregnancy detection and determination of EED. However, if pregnancy rates are not reported until day 50, the discrepancy between pregnancy and foaling rates decreases. In one study, the risk of pregnancy loss decreased as gestation increased.

3740 mares were diagnosed pregnant by ultrasound around day 22 (± 5) (day 0 being the day of last service) and checked again around day 44 (± 12). Parturition or abortion was recorded for all mares which were still pregnant at the second test. Pregnancy loss between the two early pregnancy diagnoses was 8.9% (n = 3740). This rate was 5.5% (n = 2984) when one normal single pregnancy was diagnosed on the first test. It was increased when uterine endometrial cysts were present (24.4%; n = 86) or when the conceptus looked abnormal (34.8%; n = 279). Following 278 twin pregnancy tests, 9.7% of total resorptions of both twins and 61.5% of unilateral resorption of one of them were observed.

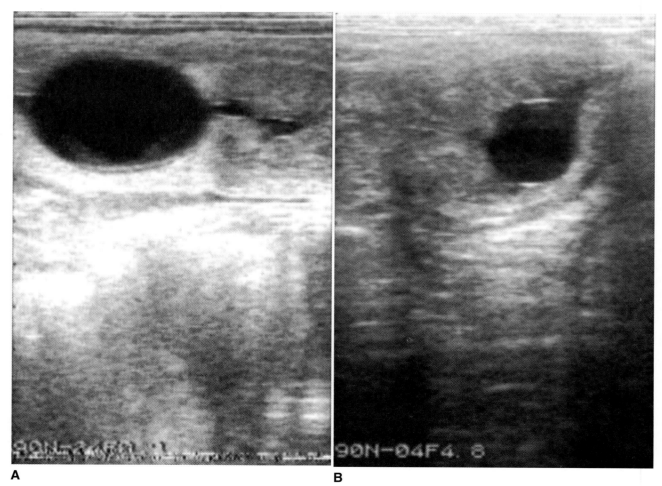

A   **B**

Figure 57-1   EED suspected due to association of free fluid around the vesicle (**A** and **B**) as well as edema of the endometrial folds (**B**).

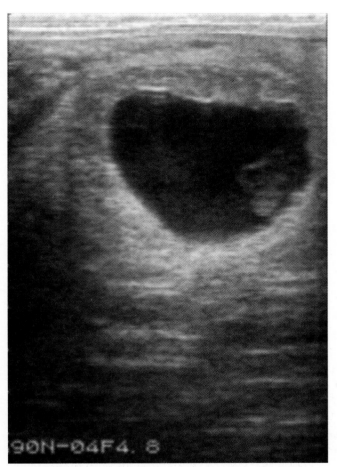

Figure 57-2   EED depicted by increased echogenicity of the fetal fluids and loss of fetal structure and clarity.

Following 113 crushings of one twin conceptus, 20.3% of resorption of the remaining twin conceptus was noted. Abortion rate between day 44 and day 310 was 9.1% (n = 2988). Abortions were more frequent in the case of twin pregnancies (52.8%; n = 53). A higher abortion rate of the remaining twin conceptus was observed after crushing (23.8%; n = 80) or after natural resorption of one of the twins (13.5; n = 148). Early and late pregnancy loss increased with the age of the mare. Resorption rate, but not abortion rate, increased with parity. Breed had no effect on pregnancy loss. Reproductive status was not linked with embryonic death frequencies, but abortion rate increased if the mare became pregnant during foal heat. Similar resorption rates were observed in 261 different stallion "harems" (groups of mares served by the same stallion). Similarly, the rate of abortion was not linked to the stallion (192 groups of mares). The day by day risk of pregnancy loss decreased steadily as pregnancy progressed.[26]

In this study, the higher than expected pregnancy loss from mares with twin pregnancies that either were assisted in elimination of or spontaneously eliminated one pregnancy was surprising and does not parallel our experiences.

ABORTION

Abortion can be *infectious* or *noninfectious*, and the subject has been well reviewed.[27] Many studies have been reported that implicate the relative importance of various causes. Unfortunately there are still many gaps in our knowledge, and the one concerning the common pathological diagnosis is "unable to determine the cause." This may on occasion be our fault for not providing adequate or suitable material in a sterile or even timely manner to the laboratory.

A total of 309 miscarried equine fetuses and foals were submitted for necropsy at the Institut de pathologie du cheval between May 1st, 1986 and April 30th, 1990. An infectious origin could be established in 34.6% of the cases, of which 79.0% were of bacterial aetiology and 21.0% of viral aetiology. Of the bacteria, 26.1% of the isolates were streptococci and 19.3% were Escherichia coli. The only virus involved was the equine rhinopneumonitis virus.[28]

Pathology case records of 3,514 aborted fetuses, stillborn foals, or foals that died < 24 hours after birth and of 13 placentas from mares whose foals were weak or unthrifty at birth were reviewed to determine the cause of abortion, death, or illness. Fetoplacental infection caused by bacteria (n = 628), equine herpesvirus (143), fungi (61), or placentitis (351), in which an etiologic agent could not be defined, was the most common diagnosis. Complications of birth, including neonatal asphyxia, dystocia, or trauma, were the second most common cause of mortality and were diagnosed in 19% of the cases (679). Other common diagnoses were placental edema or premature separation of placenta (249), development of twins (221), contracted foal syndrome (188), other congenital anomalies (160), and umbilical cord abnormalities (121). Less common conditions were placental villous atrophy or body pregnancy (81), fetal diarrhea syndrome (34), and neoplasms or miscellaneous conditions (26). A diagnosis was not established in 16% of the cases seen (585). The study revealed that leptospirosis (78) was an important cause of bacterial abortion in mares, and that infection by a nocardioform actinomycete (45) was an important cause of chronic placentitis.[29]

Pathologic and microbiologic examinations were performed on 1,211 aborted equine fetuses, stillborn foals, and placentas from premature foals in central Kentucky during the 1988 and 1989 foaling seasons to determine the causes of reproductive loss in the mare. Placentitis (19.4%) and dystocia-perinatal asphyxia (19.5%) were the 2 most important causes of equine reproductive loss. The other causes (in decreasing order) were contracted foal syndrome and other congenital anomalies (8.5%), twinning (6.1%), improper separation of placenta (4.7%), torsion of umbilical cord (4.5%), placental edema (4.3%), equine herpesvirus abortion (3.3%), bacteremia (3.2%), fetal diarrhea (2.7%), other placental disorders (total of 6.0%), and miscellaneous causes (1.6%). A definitive diagnosis was not established in 16.9% of the cases submitted. Streptococcus zooepidemicus, Escherichia coli, Leptospira spp., and a nocardioform actinomycete were organisms most fre-

quently associated with bacterial placentitis, and Aspergillus spp. was the fungus most often noted in mycotic placentitis. No viral placentitis was noticed in this series. Dystocia-perinatal asphyxia was mostly associated with large foals, maiden mares, unattended deliveries, and malpresentations. The results of this study indicate that in central Kentucky, the noninfectious causes of equine reproductive loss outnumber the infectious causes by an approximate ratio of 2:1, placental disorders are slightly more prevalent than non-placental disorders, Leptospira spp. and a nocardioform actinomycete are 2 new important abortifacient bacteria in the mare, the occurrence of contracted foal syndrome is unusually frequent, the incidence of twin abortion has sharply declined, and torsion of the umbilical cord is an important cause of abortion in the mare.[30]

Observations on 2,000 pregnancies revealed that 175 (8.7%) equine abortions occurred over a 4-year period. The peaks of abortion were at mid-gestation (20-32 weeks) and at late gestation (37-44 weeks). Abortion was higher in mares bred to donkey (10.4%) than in those bred to horse stallion (7.8%). Maximum abortions (80%) occurred in winter. Out of 175 equine abortions, 102 (58.3%) were due to infectious (bacterial, viral, fungal) causes, while 41.7% were due to noninfectious causes, viz. placentitis, malpresentation, twin pregnancy, foetal abnormality, toxaemia and trauma. Sixty-one abortions were grouped as due to unspecified noninfectious causes.[31]

Severe stress, such as colic, would appear to play a major part in late-term pregnancy loss.

The records of 105 pregnant mares and 105 non-pregnant horses with colic admitted to an equine hospital were reviewed. The 2 groups had similar types of colic and short-term survivability. Of the 105 pregnant mares, 31 were treated medically and 74 required surgical intervention. Thirty-three of the 105 mares died or were euthanatized. Thirteen (18%) of the 72 remaining mares aborted. Of 4 mares with severe medical cases, 2 died, 1 aborted, and 1 aborted and died. Of 27 horses with medical cases that required less intensive treatment, none died and 2 aborted. Of the 74 horses that required surgery, 45 survived to termination of pregnancy (foaling or abortion); 36 of these mares (80%) had a live foal. The type of surgical lesion had no effect on pregnancy outcome. Stage of gestation at initial examination, duration of anesthesia, or intraoperative hypoxia or hypotension had no effect on pregnancy outcome. However, when hypoxia occurred during colic surgery in the last 60 days of pregnancy, the mares either aborted or delivered severely compromised foals that did not survive.[32]

Stresses early in pregnancy associated with transport[33] or rectal palpation for pregnancy diagnosis[34] apparently have little or no effect on fetal loss.

Incidence of early embryonic death (EED) and associated changes in serum cortisol, progesterone and plasma ascorbic acid (AA) in transported mares were investigated. Mares were transported for 472 km (9 h) during either d 16 to 22 (T-3 wk, n = 15) or d 32 to 38 (T-5 wk, n = 15) of gestation. Blood samples were drawn from control, non-transported mares (NT-3 wk, NT-5wk, n = 24) and transported mares pre-trip, midtrip, and at 0, 12, 24, 48 and 72 h post-transport and daily for the next 2 wk. Incidence of EED between transported and non-transported mares was not different (P > .05). Serum cortisol in all transported mares increased (P < .05) relative to pre-trip values at midtrip and 0 h post-transport. Relative to NT mares, serum cortisol was higher (P < .05) at midtrip in T-3 wk mares and 0 h post-transport in T-5 wk mares. Serum progesterone in all T mares increased (P less than .05) at midtrip relative to pre-trip values and was higher (P < .05) in T-3 wk mares than in NT-3 wk mares at midtrip and 0 h post-transport. Post-transport decreases (P < .05) in concentrations of progesterone were observed in mares that aborted. Plasma AA in transported mares increased (P < .05) at midtrip in T-5 wk mares and decreased (P < .05) relative to pre-trip values at 24 and 48 h post-transport (T-3 wk and T-5 wk mares, respectively.[33]

Placentitis

There is little doubt that placentitis is an emerging disease in intensively managed broodmare farms.[35] It is possible that our sophisticated management procedures have led to more mares becoming pregnant, mares that without intense management may have struggled to become pregnant, thus creating a group of mares either susceptible to or more likely to be affected by placentitis.

Placentitis may be recognized by vulval discharge, premature lactation, or spontaneous abortion. Ultrasonography has been useful in examining the placenta at the region of the cervical star (Figure 57-3).

Feto-placental infection caused by microorganisms was the most common cause of death of fetuses, stillborn foals, and foals that died within 24 hrs after birth in central Kentucky. Pathologically, three types of placentitis were seen: ascending, diffuse, and focal mucoid. The pathogenesis in each form is believed to be different and each is associated with certain types of causative bacteria or fungi. Ascending placentitis was the most common type of placentitis prior to the 1998 foaling season in Kentucky. This form is thought to be the result of microorganisms gaining access to the cervical portion of the placenta during gestation by spread from the lower reproductive tract through the cervix. Streptococci and E. coli were the most commonly isolated bacteria. Diffuse or multifocal placentitis was less commonly diagnosed and is associated with hematogenous spread of microorganisms to the uterus of the mare with subsequent infection of the placenta. This form was associated with infection by bacteria in the genera Leptospira, Salmonella, Histoplasma, and Candida. Focal mucoid placentitis is also known as nocardioform placentitis. Nocardioform placentitis has emerged as the most commonly diagnosed type of placentitis over the last two foaling seasons and is characterized by unique pathology and distinct bacteria. At present the pathogenesis of this form is unknown. Diagnosis of placenti-

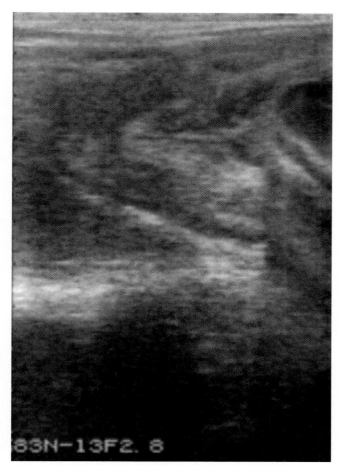

Figure 57-3 Placentitis. Note extreme thickening of the combined placenta.

tis during gestation is often difficult. Most mares show no outward signs of infection. Some mares will undergo premature mammary development with lactation and, occasionally, a vaginal discharge is present. Transrectal and transabdominal ultrasound examinations are useful in arriving at a diagnosis if placentitis is suspected. Various treatment modalities have been utilized in an attempt to maintain gestation for as long as possible to enhance foal viability. Placentitis results in several outcomes. In addition to abortions and stillbirths, the mare may produce small, weak foals or normal foals. The small, weak neonates represent a special management and medical challenge. These individuals have an increased risk of sepsis and orthopedic problems requiring extensive care.[36]

Placentitis is a common cause of equine abortions. In a majority of cases, the route of infection is believed to be ascending through the cervix, and an area of the chorion adjacent to the cervical star shows characteristic pathology in aborting mares. This area is depleted of chorionic villi, thickened, discolored, and covered by fibronecrotic exudate. Mares with placentitis due to a hematogenous infection show multifocal pathology of the chorionic surface of the placenta. Clinical signs

include udder development, premature lactation, cervical softening, and vaginal discharge. Treatment is often unsuccessful once the mare has developed clinical signs. Ultrasonographic evaluation of the placenta in late gestational mares allows the clinician to detect preclinical signs of placentitis and premature separation, which then could be treated in its early stages. Transabdominal ultrasonography: Focal areas of utero-placental thickening and partial separation of the allantochorion from the endometrium in the uterine body and horns, can be observed by this approach. The combined thickness of the uterus and the placenta (CTUP) should not be more than 12 mm at any site. In addition to evaluating the placenta a biophysical profile of the fetus can be performed by a transabdominal approach. Transrectal ultrasonography: This approach provides an excellent image of the caudal portion of the allantochorion adjacent to the cervical star. Using transrectal ultrasonographic evaluation of the placenta, we have observed abnormal thickness and partial separation of the allantochorion from the endometrium in mares with clinical signs of placentitis. In advanced stages, the space between the uterus and the placenta is filled with hyperechoic fluid. Normal values of the CTUP in an area immediately cranially and ventrally of the cervix were determined to be: <8 mm between day 271 and 300; <10 mm between day 301 and 330; and <12 mm after day 330. Increased CTUP suggests placental failure and pending abortion. Treatment of placentitis should be aimed toward elimination of the infectious agents, reduction of the inflammatory response, and reduction of the increased myometrial contractility in response to the ongoing inflammation. Broad spectrum antibiotics, anti-inflammatories (flunixin meglumine, 1.1 mg/kg BID; phenylbutazone, 4 mg/kg BID) and tocolytics (Altrenogest; Clenbuterol), are recommended for treatment of placentitis. Pentoxyfylline (7.5 mg/kg p.o. BID) has been suggested to increase oxygenation of the placenta through an increased deformability of red blood cells.[37]

Mare Reproductive Loss Syndrome (MRLS)

Chapter 56 specifically discusses MRLS.

A brief description of the problem and the steps taken to elucidate the etiology are listed below.

During 2001, central Kentucky experienced acute transient epidemics of early and late fetal losses, pericarditis, and unilateral endophthalmitis, collectively referred to as mare reproductive loss syndrome (MRLS). A toxicokinetic/statistical analysis of experimental and field MRLS data was conducted using accelerated failure time (AFT) analysis of abortions following administration of Eastern tent caterpillars (ETCs; 100 or 50 g/day or 100 g of irradiated caterpillars/day) to late-term pregnant mares. In addition, 2001 late-term fetal loss field data were used in the analysis. Experimental data were fitted by AFT analysis at a high (P < .0001) significance. Times to first abortion ("lag time") and abortion rates were dose dependent. Lag times decreased and abortion rates increased exponentially with dose. Calculated dose

X response data curves allow interpretation of abortion data in terms of "intubated ETC equivalents." Analysis suggested that field exposure to ETCs in 2001 in central Kentucky commenced on approximately April 27, was initially equivalent to approximately 5 g of intubated ETCs/day, and increased to approximately 30 g/day at the outbreak peak. This analysis accounts for many aspects of the epidemiology, clinical presentations, and manifestations of MRLS. It allows quantitative interpretation of experimental and field MRLS data and has implications for the basic mechanisms underlying MRLS. The results support suggestions that MRLS is caused by exposure to or ingestion of ETCs. The results also show that high levels of ETC exposure produce intense, focused outbreaks of MRLS, closely linked in time and place to dispersing ETCs, as occurred in central Kentucky in 2001. With less intense exposure, lag time is longer and abortions tend to spread out over time and may occur out of phase with ETC exposure, obscuring both diagnosis of this syndrome and the role of the caterpillars.[38]

From the preceding abstract quotations it appears that infectious causes of abortion, twins, and stress constitute a major proportion of reported fetal demise late in pregnancy, and many poorly defined factors such as uterine environment and the hormonal milieu are involved earlier in pregnancy. A background on endocrinology of the mare during pregnancy may be useful in providing rational approaches to therapy.

ENDOCRINOLOGY OF PREGNANCY

In mares, *maternal recognition of pregnancy* associated with production of an immunosuppressive agent, a pregnancy specific protein called early pregnancy factor, may be as early as 48 hours after conception. Early pregnancy factor has been detected in mice, sheep, human beings, and mares, and may, in the future, aid in detection of pregnancy and EED. The second time of maternal recognition of pregnancy probably arises on or before day 5 or 6 after ovulation, as fertilized ova are transported from the oviduct through the uterotubule junction into the uterus by 5 or 6 days after ovulation but unfertilized oocytes generally are retained in the oviducts.[39-42] The third recognizable time for maternal recognition (or reinforcement) of pregnancy occurs between 12 and 16 days. During this time, the conceptus is extremely mobile and probably secretes an antiluteolytic substance that prevents release of $PGF_{2\alpha}$, thus maintaining the corpus luteum and preventing the mare from returning to estrus.

Two experiments were performed to determine the critical time at which the equine blastocyst must be present within the uterus of the mare to prevent regression of the corpus luteum, and thus establish the critical time for the maternal recognition of pregnancy. A non-surgical blastocyst collection technique was developed to study this relationship between the blastocyst and the maternal ovary. Results from these experiments demonstrated that the cyclic life-span of the corpus luteum is not affected by the presence of the blastocyst within the

mare's uterus until after Day 14 after ovulation. Luteal function was prolonged when blastocysts were removed on Day 15 or later. The critical period for the maternal recognition of pregnancy in the Pony mare appears to be confined to the period between Days 14 and 16 after ovulation.[43]

Two experiments were conducted to assess the effect of exogenous hormone treatment on uterine luminal prostaglandin F (PGF). In the first experiment ovariectomized pony mares received either corn oil (21 days, n = 3), estradiol valerate (21 days, n = 3), progesterone (21 days, n = 3) or estradiol valerate (7 days) followed by progesterone (14 days, n = 4). Progesterone-treated mares had higher (P < .01) uterine luminal PGF compared with all other groups, and no differences were detected between other treatment comparisons. In Experiment II, uterine fluid was collected from 4 ovariectomized horse mares before and after treatment with estradiol valerate (7 days) followed by progesterone (50 days). Pre-treatment uterine luminal PGF levels were lower (P < .001) than post-treatment levels (.03 vs 76.80 ng/ml). In a third experiment PGF was measured in uterine fluid of pony mares on days 8, 12, 14, 16, 18 and 20 of the estrous cycle and pregnancy. In nonpregnant mares a day effect (P less than .03) was observed in which uterine fluid PGF increased during the late luteal phase and declined thereafter. In contrast, no day effect was observed in pregnant animals and uterine luminal PGF was lower (P < .001) than in cycling animals. These studies indicate that exogenous progesterone administration results in a large increase in uterine luminal PGF, whereas pregnancy results in suppression. Taken collectively with previous work from our laboratory, these results suggest that while the endometrium of pregnant mares is capable of producing large amounts of PGF, the presence of a conceptus impedes its synthesis and/or release which allows for luteal maintenance.[44]

Comparisons of estrone, 17 beta-estradiol, and plasma progestin concentrations were made in uterine fluid and peripheral blood of nonpregnant and pregnant pony mares. Concentrations of these steroids were also measured within yolk sac fluid from blastocysts on days 12, 14, 16, and 18 of pregnancy to obtain more complete analyses of the uterine environment (uterine fluid plus yolk sac fluid) of early pregnancy. Thirty mares were randomly assigned to six treatment groups (n = 5/group), and uterine fluid and peripheral blood samples were obtained on days 8, 12, 14, 16, 18, and 20 post-ovulation. After a recovery period of one estrous cycle, mares were bred at their next estrus. Animals were hysterectomized on the same treatment day to which they had previously been assigned in the nonpregnant phase of this study. Using this design, uterine fluid and peripheral blood samples were collected from each mare on equivalent days of the estrous cycle and pregnancy. Significant differences in day trends were found between nonpregnant and pregnant animals for estrogens and progestins in both uterine fluid and peripheral plasma. Furthermore, these data demonstrate that large increases in estrogens occur after day 12 of pregnancy in uterine and yolk sac fluids, with estrone becoming the predominant estrogen by days 18 and 20 in yolk sac and uterine fluids, respectively. These changes were not detected in peripheral plasma, which indicates that changes occurring within the uterine environment are not discernible in the systemic circulation during early pregnancy. These results indicate that the large amounts of estrogens appearing in uterine fluids during early pregnancy are of conceptus origin and may be an important factor in regulating the environment in which the conceptus develop.[45]

The next piece of the puzzle was also provided by researchers in Florida.

Cycling pony mares were bred and used to test the effect of restricted conceptus mobility on luteal maintenance (i.e., maternal recognition of pregnancy). In Experiment 1, uterine horns were ligated to restrict conceptus mobility to one uterine horn, Group 1; one horn plus the uterine body, Group 2; or one horn, the body and approximately 80% of the second horn, Group 3. Pregnancies were monitored with real-time ultrasonography. Four of five mares in Group 1 and two of four mares in Group 2 returned to estrus (Day 16.0 +– 1.9 and 14.5 +– 0.7, respectively) and subsequently lost the embryonic vesicles (Day 17.2 +– 1.2 and 15.7 +– 0.7, respectively). None of the four mares in Group 3 lost the vesicles. There was a significant effect of the interaction of treatment (amount of uterus available to the conceptus) and day on plasma progesterone (P) concentration (p < 0.005). In Experiment 2, conceptus mobility was restricted to one uterine horn in two groups of mares, of which the second was treated with the synthetic progestin, Regumate (allyl trenbolone). In the first group, each of three mares lost the vesicle (Day 17.3 +– 4.3). In the second group, four of five mares maintained the pregnancies, indicating that pregnancy failure was due to the effects of declining P. These data indicate that restricted conceptus mobility results in luteolysis in the mare, and that the subsequent decline in P leads to embryonic death. This supports the notion that unrestricted mobility of the equine conceptus, allowing it to interact with most the uterine endometrium, is necessary for luteal maintenance and conceptus survival.[21]

These studies have important ramifications regarding the effects of different uterine environments on the ability of mares to maintain pregnancy; for example, in cases of uterine cysts that impair mobility and the possible therapeutic implications of progestagens.

Estrogens

A minor maternal (ovarian) production of estrogen occurs between days 35 and 60 but has little diagnostic significance. A major increase in plasma estrogen concentration occurs after day 60.[46] This increase comes from the fetal placental unit and, thus, is not affected by ovariectomy.

Plasma total (conjugated + unconjugated) oestrogens were measured from Day 0 to 100 of pregnancy and compared with the levels found during the oestrous cycle. From Day 0 to 35 of gestation, the concentrations were similar to those during dioestrus. An increase in total oestrogens between Days 35 and 40 was followed by a plateau of 3 ng/ml between Days 40 and 60 which was slightly higher than preovulatory concentrations. This first increase in total oestrogen level was produced by the ovaries since values were suppressed after ovariectomy; stimulation may be due indirectly to PMSG causing follicular growth. After Day 60, a second increase was detected and considered to be of feto-placental origin as the levels at this time were not suppressed after ovariectomy. By Day 85, oestrogen concentrations exceeded those detected in non-pregnant mares so that a direct measurement of total oestrogens in plasma by a simplified radioimmunoassay after Day 85 of gestation offers a reliable method of pregnancy diagnosis.[46]

Concentrations of estrogen in urine and serum peak at about day 210 of gestation[47] and are thought to come from fetal gonads, which are enlarged at this time. If fetal gonads are removed, plasma estrogen concentrations drop immediately to very low levels.[48] In general, estrogen detection in serum or urine has only limited value for pregnancy diagnosis since they become reliable only relatively late in pregnancy. Earlier it was not recommended to test for estrogens before 150 days of pregnancy, but more recently, measurement of estrone sulfate (conjugated) for diagnosis of pregnancy and evidence of a viable conceptus has been advocated after day 60 of pregnancy.[49] Fetal death results in an immediate decrease in estrone sulfate concentration.[49] If a mare in the second or third trimester of pregnancy begins to lactate, measurement of estrone sulfate may provide an index of fetal viability. This may be particularly useful when other tests of fetal viability such as ultrasonography and/or electrocardiographic monitoring are not available.

Biological, chemical, and immunologic tests are available for estrogen determination. *Biological tests*, such as increased nipple length in guinea pigs or induction of vaginal cytological findings typical of estrus in immature or ovariectomized mice, are rarely used. They have been replaced by chemical tests largely because of cost and time. *Chemical tests* for urinary estrogen rely on color changes and fluorescence in the presence of warm, concentrated sulfuric acid. *Radioimmunoassay* can be used for determination of plasma total estrogen (conjugated plus unconjugated)[46] concentration or urinary estrone conjugates. The method described for plasma analysis[46] requires enzymatic hydrolysis and extraction and may not reveal all estrone conjugates because the concentration of estrone sulfate is 1,000 times higher in the urine. Direct conjugated estrogen measurement on serum or milk has been described,[50] and differentiation between pregnancy and estrus was possible after approximately 50 days. In mares, an enzymatic determination of unconjugated estrogens in the faeces for pregnancy diagnosis has been described.[51] It was possible to confirm pregnancy after 120 days of gestation, and because this technique may be totally noninvasive to the mare, some benefits to the equine reproductive industry may be realized.

Immunoreactive urinary oestrogen conjugates were assessed in daily urine samples (~ 5 samples/week) collected from 8 Przewalski's mares maintained under semi free-ranging pasture conditions. The relative percentage contributions of immunoreactive urinary oestrogens during different reproductive states (oestrus, luteal phase, early, mid- and late gestation) were determined using high-pressure liquid chromatography. In general, conjugated forms of oestrone (oestrone sulphate and oestrone glucuronide) were the major excreted immunoreactive oestrogens in non-pregnant and pregnant Przewalski's mares. Variations in urinary oestrogen conjugates indicated that the onset of oestrous cyclicity coincided with increasing daylengths, and the non-conception oestrous cycle was 24.1 +− 0.7 days (n = 17) in duration. Most copulations (29/35, 82.9%) were observed between Day -4 and Day +1 from the preovulatory oestrogen conjugates peak (Day 0). Based on known copulation dates, the mean gestation length was 48.6 +− 0.4 weeks (range 47.3-50.3 weeks). During pregnancy, urinary excretion of oestrogen conjugates increased apprx 300-fold over levels in non-pregnant mares, reaching peak concentrations by Week +24 (51% of gestation). These results demonstrate that longitudinal reproductive events, including oestrous cyclicity and pregnancy, can be monitored precisely by evaluating urinary oestrogen conjugates in samples from Przewalski's mares maintained under semi-free-ranging conditions.[52]

Further studies on uses of estrogen analysis are presented below.

Serum and urinary estrone sulfate concentrations were determined in 7 pregnant mares before and after prostaglandin-induced abortion (n = 4) or surgical removal of the fetus (n = 3) to determine the source of estrogen during early pregnancy (gestation days [GD] 44 to 89). Estrone sulfate concentrations also were determined in serum samples (stored frozen for 2 years) from 3 mares that had been ovariectomized between GD 51 and 58. Estrone sulfate concentrations decreased in serum and urine after expulsion or removal of the fetus (urinary patterns were more definitive than were patterns for serum), whereas a transient decrease in serum estrone sulfate concentration was observed after ovariectomy. Seemingly, products of conception are the major source of estrone sulfate during early pregnancy, although there appears to be some ovarian contribution. Serum or urinary estrone sulfate measurements provide a simple and accurate test for fetal viability after GD 44 in the mare.[53]

The removal of one of twin embryos was attempted by infusion of 24% (w/v) saline into the gestation sac in 2 mares by laparotomy. The treatment was successful in one mare (Case 1) and the untreated embryo remained viable. However, neither foetus survived in the second mare (Case 2). Plasma oestrone sulphate (E1S) concentrations fell immediately after treatment in both mares but recovered to approximately 50% of pre-treatment levels in Case 1. In Case 2 plasma E1S concentrations declined steadily and were < 1 ng/ml within 6 days of treatment. These preliminary results suggest that the method may be useful for selective removal of one of twin embryos in mares. Furthermore, plasma E1S concentrations may be a useful indicator of embryonic viability.[54]

Two mares received PGF-2 alpha twice daily until abortion, and 2 mares received a combined treatment with oestradiol benzoate and oxytocin. The mares were about 150 days pregnant. The PG-treated animals aborted after 37 and 61 h, respectively, and the fetuses were expelled in intact fetal membranes. The other 2 mares aborted 13 and 27 h after the first oxytocin injection, respectively, and showed strong uterine contractions and expelled the fetuses in disrupted fetal membranes. Concentrations of 15-ketodihydro-PGF-2 alpha increased both after PG and oxytocin injections and in association with the abortion, but after the PG-induced abortion there was an immediate return to basal levels and after the oxytocin-induced abortion there was a large increase in the concentrations, indicating damage of the uterus. Progesterone and relaxin concentrations followed the placental function and decreased in association with the abortions. Oestrone sulphate values differed in the two groups; the oxytocin-treated animals showed a rapid decrease while the mares treated with PG showed first a marked increase and then a decrease. Concentrations of PMSG appeared to be unaffected by the abortions.[55]

We evaluated 2 rapid non-instrumented field tests for pregnancy on feral horses (Equus caballus) because previous techniques required sophisticated and expensive instrumentation that limited their usefulness to field researchers. The measurement of urinary estrone conjugates (E-1C) by an enzyme immunoassay and based on observable color changes was 100% accurate when compared with instrumented spectrophotometrically measured tests for E-1C. A non-instrumented "dipstick" enzyme immunoassay for equine chorionic gonadotropin-like (eCG) molecules was 83% accurate in diagnosing mare pregnancies when compared with the results of the instrumented test for E-1C. The decrease in accuracy using the non-instrumented eCG test resulted from a time period of 40-140 days when eCG was measurable, whereas E-1C elevation were measurable after day 35 of a mare's pregnancy. Our results indicate that it is possible to detect pregnancy in free-roaming horses under field conditions and without instrumented assays; such field tests provide opportunities to study fecundity and fetal loss in a variety of free-roaming animals.[56]

Plasma cortisol, oestrone sulphate and progestagens were measured in 22 stressed pregnant mares (gestation length 17-336 days) as indicators of fetal viability. Mares were bled every 12 h from time of admission, and plasma was stored at -70 degrees C until assayed. Four normal mares were bled twice weekly from Day 270 to parturition to provide baseline endocrine data. Cortisol and progestagen concentrations were measured by radioimmunoassay and oestrone sulphate was measured by enzyme immunoassay. Mares were grouped according to clinical diagnosis: surgical colic (Group 1, n = 11), medical colic (Group 2, n = 7), and uterine torsion (Group 3, n = 4). Of the 16 mares in Groups 1 and 2 that survived to discharge, 12 mares foaled normally and 4 aborted, 3 during hospitalization. Following surgical treatment of uterine torsion, 2 mares aborted and 2 mares carried foals to term. Plasma cortisol was greater than 30 ng/ml in 19 of the 22 stressed mares at presentation and was less than 30 ng/ml in normal *mares at all collections. Cortisol concentrations remained elevated in mares during post admission complications. The mean cortisol concentration of mares with colic that subsequently aborted was higher at presentation, but not statistically different, than levels of mares that did not abort (135+/– 35 ng/ml and 83 +/– 19 ng/ml, respectively; mean +/– s.e.m.). Progestagen concentrations in normal mares ranged from 2-25 ng/ml. Progesterone concentrations in subject mares that subsequently foaled did not differ from normal mares, whereas concentrations in aborting mares (n = 5) either dropped rapidly (n = 3) or were low at the time of admission and decreased to < 2 ng/ml (n = 2). Oestrone sulphate concentrations that ranged from 7-5000 ng/ml, decreased after foaling or abortion. However, the concentrations remained above 38 ng/ml (range, 38-480 ng/ml) in those mares (n = 7) sampled post foaling or post abortion. Our results show that mares with colic that subsequently aborted had higher mean plasma cortisol concentrations at admission than mares that carried foals until term. No single sample of the 3 hormones measured was a reliable indicator of abortion. Oestrone sulphate was not an accurate indicator of foetal viability during late pregnancy.*[57]

Pregnant Mare Serum Gonadotropin

Pregnant mare serum gonadotropin (also referred to as eCG-equine chorionic gonadotropin) is produced by fetal trophoblast cells that invade the maternal endometrium on days 35 through 38.[58] These cells form "endometrial cups" that are white, raised plaques that increase in size until day 60 of gestation. A maternal immunologic rejection against the endometrial cups results in a decrease in their size beginning around day 70 and continuing through day 120 when they are no longer functional. Plasma concentrations of PMSG parallel the growth and regression of endometrial cups and are first detected from days 35 through 40, peak between days 60 and 65, and decrease to low or nondetectable values between 120 and 150 days of gestation. The exact function of PMSG is undetermined and is the source of much controversy. Current popular theory is that PMSG is responsible for a luteinizing hormone-like activity that causes either ovulation and/or luteinization of follicles resulting in formation of secondary CL. Serum analysis for PMSG should be performed between days 40 and 120 of gestation. When abortion occurs after day 35, endometrial cups may persist for a short time, which means that (1) PMSG is still detectable and may be responsible for a false positive pregnancy diagnosis, and (2) these mares commonly fail to return to estrus. In addition, when mares are carrying a mule fetus, the immunologic rejection of the endometrial cups occurs much earlier and extremely low or nondetectable concentrations of PMSG exist despite the persistence of pregnancy. An interesting observation is the apparent abortigenic ability of hCG when given too early (<35 day) pregnancies.[59] It is interesting to speculate on the interactions of these gonadotropins, especially in light of new evidence that suggests that not only are the secondary corpora lutea (CL) forming in association with PMSG, but that the primary CL of pregnancy has a resurgence that is temporally associated with the beginning of PMSG production.[60]

> *The temporal association between the first detectable increase in concentrations of circulating progesterone and equine chorionic gonadotropin (eCG) was studied in pregnant mares. Blood samples were collected on days 15, 20 and 25-40 from pony mares (experiment 1; n = 11) and days 11-40 from horse mares (experiment 2; n = 10). Mares were ultrasonically examined daily to evaluate the primary corpus luteum (experiment 3; n = 2-6) and to detect the formation of secondary corpora lutea (experiments 1 and 2). Formation of secondary corpora lutea was not detected in any mare prior to day 40 in experiment 1, but was detected in one mare on day 38 and in two mares on day 39 in experiment 2. In both experiments 1 and 2, there was a significant main effect of day for circulating concentrations of progesterone and was attributable to decreased (P < 0.05) concentration between days 12 and 15 (experiment 2) and increased concentrations after day 32 (experiment 1) or day 34 (experiment 2). Progesterone concentrations were higher (P < 0.05) on days 38, 39, and 40 than on days 29, 31, and 32 in experiment 1 and higher (P < 0.05) on day 40 than on days 32, 33 and 34 in experiment 2. When progesterone concentration in experiment 2 were normalized to the day that eCG was first detected (mean, day 35), mean concentrations were lower (P < 0.05) before detection of eCG than on the second day after detection. The cross-sectional area of the ultrasonic image of the primary corpus luteum (experiment 3) was greater (P < 0.05) on days 39, 40, 41, and 42 than on days 30 and 33. The cross-sectional increases in area of the primary corpus luteum in experiment 3 closely paralleled the increases in progesterone concentration in experiments 1 and 2. Combined results of the 3 experiments supported the hypothesis that resurgence of primary corpus luteum occurs in pregnant mares between days 30 and 40 and that the resurgence is a response to release of eCG into the circulation. More specifically, the results indicated that, on the average, the resurgence of the primary corpus luteum in the mare began on day 35.*[60]

Biological tests rely on the effects of PMSG obtained from mare serum, upon the reproductive tract of laboratory animals (e.g., stimulation of rabbit ovaries [Friedman test], rat uterus, mouse uterus), and production of spermatozoa from male toads. A practical, inexpensive bioassay involves the subcutaneous injection of 0.5 to 1 ml of mare serum into immature, 21-day-old female mice. Saline-injected mice serve as controls. The presence of PMSG will cause enlargement and congestion of the mouse uterus compared with controls when examined at 72 hours. The sensitivity of the biological assays is, in general, good. However, there is little diagnostic application for these assays because of the expense and time involved and the excellent immunologic testing methods now available. Immunologic methods of pregnancy diagnosis generally rely on an antigen/antibody reaction. The antibody is produced by hyper-immunization of another animal such as a rabbit, with PMSG as the antigen. Some reported immunologic assay systems are the haemagglutination inhibition test (HI), mare immunologic pregnancy (MIP) test, radioimmunoassay (RIA), direct latex agglutination (DLA), and enzyme-linked immunosorbent assay (ELISA). In addition, a radioreceptor assay has been described. Serum from pregnant mares (diagnosed by ultrasonography) has been used to compare the efficacy of the MIP test, DLA assay, and ELISA.[61] None of the 7 samples from pregnant mares obtained on day 35 resulted in positive reactions with the HI or DLA assay, but 3 out of 7 (43%) were diagnosed positive using ELISA. On day 40, a greater ($P < 0.01$) number of mares were detected pregnant with ELISA (16/16, 100%) compared to HI (5/16, 31%) or DLA assay (6/16, 37%). Between days 45 and 100, there were no differences in efficacy among the 3 tests. At 50 days and later, efficacy of the 3 tests ranged from 90% to 100%. Sera collected from 10 nonpregnant mares were used as control samples. None of these samples resulted in positive reaction. The authors concluded that all 3 tests were simple, quick methods that could be used for detection of pregnancy in mares.[61] Although the DLA assay was the easiest to conduct, all 3 assay procedures could be performed in less than 2 hours, and the ELISA, because of increased sensitivity, could be used to detect pregnancy slightly earlier than the other 2 methods.

Progesterone

Progesterone is produced by the CL and functions to maintain pregnancy. The CL forms from luteinization of granulosa cells and theca interna cells from the wall of an ovulated follicle. The primary CL is formed from the follicle that released the oocyte that resulted in pregnancy. After fertilization and recognition of pregnancy, the primary CL is maintained beyond day 15 until at least days 140 through 180 and probably longer. Progesterone concentrations peak at approximately day 20, then decline slightly until days 40 through 45, at which time secondary CL formation occurs, resulting in an increase in progesterone measurements until days 80 to 90 of pregnancy. It is speculated that secondary CL form from follicles that are stimulated by 10-day cyclic pulses of follicle stimulating hormone (FSH) and that either ovulation and/or luteinisation is initiated by PMSG. Ovariectomy commonly will result in abortion before day 60, but not after day 80.[62,63] Pregnancy is maintained by progestins (progesterone-like compounds) produced by the placenta beginning around days 60 through 90, with increasing concentrations until parturition.

Pony mares were bilaterally ovariectomized at different stages of pregnancy between Days 25 and 210. Abortion or fetal resorption occurred within 2 to 6 days after operations in all 14 mares ovariectomized between Days 25 and 45 and after an interval of 10 to 15 days in 9 of 20 other ovariectomized between 50 and 70 days. All 12 mares ovariectomized on either 140 or 210 days carried their foals to normal term. The termination of early pregnancy was preceded by a loss of uterine tone and of a palpable uterine bulge. The mean length of gestation in all mares in which pregnancy was not interrupted by ovariectomy was not significantly different from that in a group of contemporary control mares.

Plasma progestagen concentrations dropped to less than 2 ng/ml after ovariectomy, whether or not pregnancy was maintained. Mares ovariectomized on Day 25 and injected with 100 mg progesterone daily for 10 or 20 days remained pregnant during treatment but showed a loss of uterine tone and the fetal bulge disappeared within 4 to 6 days after the end of treatment. Non-pregnant ovariectomized or intact seasonally anoestrous mares injected i.m. with 50 or 100 mg progesterone daily for 8 weeks showed changes in uterine tone, length and thickness similar to those occurring in mares during early pregnancy.[62]

When used to assess ovarian activity in mares, measurement of plasma progesterone concentration is more reliable than observation of estrual behavioral patterns. Progesterone concentrations between 4 and 9 ng/ml are found 5 to 10 days after ovulation. If pregnancy ensues, higher concentrations are observed during days 16 through 20 compared to mares destined to return to estrus. In one study, measurement of plasma progesterone concentration in nonpregnant and pregnant mares at 2 stages, postovulation days 13 through 17 and 18 through 22, was 3.08 and 0.77 ng/ml in nonpregnant mares and 7.72 and 6.34 ng/ml in pregnant mares, respectively. Regardless, some pregnant mares will have low progesterone measurements, and some diestrous mares (with a retained corpus luteum) will have high progesterone measurements similar to those in pregnant mares. There are numerous progestins. If the assay for progesterone is not highly specific, many other progestins including progesterone metabolites will be measured in the serum and milk, particularly after day 60 to 90 of gestation, when progestins from the fetal placental unit are produced. In general, RIA and ELISA are highly specific for progesterone, whereas competitive protein-binding assay will detect progestins as well. Since progesterone has been shown to play a key role in pregnancy maintenance, it is not surprising that progesterone administration to habitually aborting mares has become a fairly common practice. Generally, most of the pregnancy losses in mares occur during the first two months of gestation. In one study,[64] various doses and regimes of administering progesterone were evaluated for their efficacy in maintaining pregnancy in ovariectomized pregnant mares. Forty-eight light-horse mares were confirmed pregnant on day 29 or 30 and randomly assigned to one of six treatments: (1) noninjected controls, (2) subcutaneous injection of 250 mg of progesterone in oil every other day, (3) intramuscular injection of 500 mg of Repositol progesterone every four days, (4) intramuscular injection of 1000 mg of Repositol progesterone every four days, (5) 22 mg of Altrenogest daily, and (6) 44 mg of Altrenogest daily. Hormonal treatments began on day 29 or 30 and ended on day 100 of gestation. As expected, none of the control mares maintained pregnancy after ovariectomy. Progesterone in oil (250 mg) administered every other day was only marginal in maintaining pregnancy (5 of 8). Administration of Repositol progesterone (500 mg every four days) was ineffective in maintaining pregnancy (1 of 8). In contrast, all mares administered 1000 mg Repositol progesterone every four days maintained their pregnancy.

There appeared to be no difference between the 2 doses of Altrenogest in maintenance of pregnancy; 7 of 8 mares maintained pregnancy in each group.

Occasionally, mares experienced low levels of progesterone (<1 ng per ml) and still maintained pregnancy. Therefore, progesterone insufficiency should not be based on a single blood sample but should be based on 2 to 3 samples collected during a given week. In this study, mares that had greater than 4 ng of progesterone per ml of blood were less likely to abort than those mares with levels less than 4 ng per ml. The level of progesterone achieved by exogenous treatment is dependent upon the type of progesterone used and the frequency of administration. Aqueous progesterone is cleared extremely rapidly from the blood and, therefore, should not be recommended for pregnancy maintenance. Progesterone suspended in an oil base (sesame, safflower, corn oil, etc.) must be administered on a daily basis. Repositol progesterone was the most common form of progesterone available to the practitioner. This progesterone is suspended in a propylene glycol base and is cleared relatively slowly from the blood of the mare. Injections of Repositol progesterone should be given every 4 to 7 days. Altrenogest cannot be measured in the blood of the mare, and therefore its clearance from the blood stream is apparently unknown. However, daily administration is recommended. Based on current information, it appears that 1000 mg of Repositol progesterone administered every 4 to 7 days would maintain progesterone concentrations at optimal levels for pregnancy maintenance. If progesterone in oil is used, then 200 to 300 mg should be given daily. Altrenogest at a level of .044 mg per kg of body weight appears to be effective in maintaining pregnancy. More recently, we transferred embryos[65] into ovariectomized mares administered either 300 mg of progesterone in oil daily or 22 mg of Altrenogest orally on a daily basis. Fifteen of 20 embryos transferred into ovariectomized mares treated with injectable progesterone resulted in a pregnancy compared to 14 of 20 embryos transferred into ovariectomized mares administered Altrenogest.

Embryo transfer into ovariectomized steroid-treated mares was used as a model to evaluate various progestin/estradiol treatments and to determine the level of progesterone necessary for the maintenance of pregnancy in mares. Once a donor mare was in estrus and had a > 35 mm follicle, an ovariectomized recipient was selected and assigned to one of three groups: 1) 1 mg estradiol (E-2) was injected subcutaneously daily until the donor mare ovulated; on the day of the donor mare's ovulation, daily intramuscular injections of 300 mg progesterone (P4) were commenced and continued until the end of the experiment (Day 35); 2) E-2 and P4 treatments were identical except E-2 was continued daily until Day 20; and 3) the same E-2 treatment as Group 1, 0.044 mg Altrenogest per kilogram body weight were administered daily until Day 35. Embryos were recovered 7 d after the donor mare's ovulation and were transferred via surgical flank incision. Twenty additional embryos (controls) were transferred into intact recipients that ovulated 1 d before to 3 d after the donor. Pregnancy rates did not differ (P > 0.05) among groups at

Day 14 or 35. Pregnancy rates at Day 35 for mares administered injectable P4 (70%) were identical to those given Altrenogest. Overall, pregnancy rates for ovariectomized-progestin treated recipients (28 of 40, 70%) were similar (> 0.05) to that of intact mares (16 of 20, 80%). Dose of P4 was decreased in Groups 1 and 2 to 200 mg (Days 35 to 39), 100 mg (Days 40 to 44), 50 mg (Days 45 to 49) and 0 mg (> Day 50). Blood samples were collected once on Days 34, 35, 39, 40, 44, 45, 49 and 50 and assayed for P4. Dose of Altrenogest was decreased to 0.022, 0.011, 0.0055 and 0 mg per kilogram body weight at Days 35 to 39, 40 to 44, 45 to 49 and > 50. Number of mares in Groups 1 and 2 that lost their pregnancy while given 200, 100, 50 or 0 mg P4 was 0, 2, 8 and 4, respectively. Doses of 0.022, 0.011, 0.0055 and 0 mg Altrenogest per kilogram body weight resulted in 0, 6, 4 and 3 mares aborting. Fetal death did not occur until concentrations of P4 decreased below 2.56 ng/ml 24 h after injection.[65]

Apart from occasional enlargement of the clitoris, seen in neonatal fillies,[66] prolonged administration of Altrenogest has not resulted in any deleterious effects. Another form of progesterone administration reported is in microspheres.

Administration of progesterone in poly(d-,l-lactide) microspheres was used to maintain pregnancy in mares after luteolysis was induced by treatment with prostaglandin F-2alpha at day 14 of pregnancy. Mares were given vehicle only (control, n = 6) or 0.75 g (n = 7), 1.5 g (n = 8), or 2.25 g (n = 5) of microencapsulated progesterone at days 12 and 22 of pregnancy. Serum progesterone concentrations were determined daily, and pregnancy was evaluated by transrectal ultrasonography on alternate days. Significantly (P < 0.05) more mares given 1.5 or 2.25 g of progesterone (6 of 8 and 4 of 5 mares, respectively), but not those given 0.75 g (3 of 7 mares), maintained pregnancy through day 32, compared with control mares (0 of 6). Progesterone concentrations decreased significantly (P < 0.025) in all groups after administration of prostaglandin F-2alpha at day 14, and significant (P < 0.05) effects of time and treatment on progesterone concentrations were found between days 12 and 22, and 22 and 32. Although treatment with 1.5-g and 2.25-g doses of microencapsulated progesterone improved maintenance of pregnancy, compared with that of vehicle-treated controls, administration of 2.25 g of microencapsulated progesterone appeared to be most efficacious in maintenance of pregnancy during the study interval.[67]

Micro-encapsulation has advantages in efficacy and a reduced administration schedule.

THERAPEUTIC CONSIDERATIONS

Management

General
There are few, if any, treatments to consistently decrease incidence of EED, but artificial insemination can limit bacterial challenge to a mare's uterus, thus reducing

potential losses from endometritis. In addition, any new information on causes and treatment of endometritis should result in increased breeding efficiency. Strict adherence to repair of external conformation defects and thus a reduction in caudal reproductive tract contamination is important. Efficiently handling twin conceptuses (see Chapter 54), better management of placentitis, recognition of exposure factors for MRLS, and prevention of devastating outbreaks of viral abortion are now able to be routinely prevented with management and/or vaccination.[68] The transfer of embryos from mares with poor uterine-biopsy grades into normal recipient mares is recommended to provide an environment more conducive to pregnancy maintenance. Unfortunately, recovery of embryos from subfertile mares is low. Perhaps the changes most likely to result in a decrease in incidence of EED is improving management factors related to uterine environment, nutrition, environmental temperature, infectious diseases, and other stresses. It seems that most problems of the horse are management related. There are few diseases or problems that our imposed management practices have not influenced or created. Take the case of the habitually aborting mare. It is most likely she has persistent and chronic uterine inflammation or fibrosis. We probably created it by poor hygiene, lack of exercise, amalgamation of too many mares in a stressful environment, and lack of appropriate therapy at the time of breeding or later. The pregnancy rates and foaling rates are generally better on well-managed breeding farms despite the fact that there is absolutely no selection for reproductive efficiency, just speed or other performance related parameters. Our belief is that persistent, unidentified, or poorly treated chronic inflammatory conditions of the uterus are responsible for the majority of problems of EED and abortion.

Foal Heat Breeding

One of the most important management issues still neglected somewhat is the practice of foal heat breeding.

Many of our clients wish to breed mares on foal heat. The reasons are generally obvious. The gestation of the mare averages 340 days, but a significant number are longer. Most of us involved with commercial breeding farms recognize a financial penalty for foals born later than the normal accepted times. Without breeding at foal heat it may be hard to maintain a foaling interval of 365 days in some cases. In addition, clients with brood mares on farms sometimes are paying high boarding costs and place pressure on managers to get their mares pregnant and send them home as soon as possible. Sometimes farm mangers cannot resist the temptation to breed at foal heat—despite the potential problems—just because the mare is showing heat and their knowledge that foal heat mares ovulate quite quickly.

However, fertility has been reported lower in mares bred during the first postpartum ovulatory period compared with mares bred during subsequent cycles,[12] and EED has been reported higher for mares bred at this time.[12,16,19] This decreased fertility may be due to failure to eliminate microbes during uterine involution[12,16] or their introduction at breeding. In addition, presence of uterine fluid during estrus[69] and diestrus[70,71] has been

shown to reduce fertility of mares. A study[69] was conducted to evaluate 2 hypotheses: (1) uterine involution and fluid accumulation could be effectively monitored with ultrasonography and used to predict fertility of mares bred during the first postpartum ovulatory cycle, and (2) delaying ovulation with a progestin would result in improved pregnancy rates in mares bred during the first postpartum ovulatory period. The previously gravid horn was larger than the nongravid horn for a mean of 21 days (range 15 to 25) after parturition. Uterine involution was most obvious at the corpus cornual junction. When the results of 3 ultrasonographic scans were similar, over a 5-day period, the uterus was considered to be involuted. On the average, uterine involution was completed by day 23 (range 13 to 29). Quantity and quality of uterine fluid were not affected by progestin treatment. Number of mares with detectable uterine fluid decreased after day 5 postpartum. Uterine fluid generally decreased in quantity and improved in quality between day 3 and day 15. Fewer ($P < 0.005$) mares became pregnant when uterine fluid was present during the first postpartum ovulatory period (3 of 9, 33%) compared to when no fluid was detected (26 of 31, 84%). Mares with uterine fluid during breeding did not have appreciably larger uterine dimensions compared with those mares not having fluid. There was no relationship between uterine size on day of ovulation and pregnancy rate. Ovulations were delayed, and pregnancy rates improved in progestin-treated mares. More ($P < 0.05$) mares became pregnant (23/28, 82%) when they ovulated after day 15, in the first postpartum ovulatory period, than mares that ovulated before day 15 (6/12, 50%). Ultrasonography has been proven useful in detecting mares with postpartum uterine fluid. Further, it could be used to aid in determining whether a mare should be bred, treated, or not bred during the first postpartum ovulatory period. During estrus, uterine fluid may be spermicidal and/or an excellent medium to support bacterial proliferation. When fluid is present during diestrus, it may cause premature luteolysis or EED.[71] Quantity of uterine fluid during the first postpartum ovulatory period appeared to be related to stage of uterine involution and was reduced or eliminated by delaying the ovulatory period with progestins. Progestin treatment not only allowed time for elimination of uterine fluid before the first postpartum ovulation, but it also significantly delayed the first postpartum ovulation. Results of this study concurred with those of others in which it was concluded that progestin treatment delayed onset of the first postpartum ovulatory period but did not affect rate of uterine involution.[72-74] Long-term progestin administration to normal, cycling mares has not been shown to adversely affect fertility.[75] However, treatment with progestins will affect uterine defense mechanisms[76,77] and thus care is recommended before prolonged progestin treatment is administered to postpartum mares or mares susceptible to infection. Since there were decreased pregnancy rates associated with uterine fluid and increased pregnancy rates as ovulation was delayed, it was suggested that both techniques could be used to manipulate breeding strategies and improve pregnancy rates from normal mares bred during the first postpartum ovulatory period.

The approach used at the GVEH for management of foal heat breeding is listed below.

1. All mares are examined at day 2 to 4 postfoaling. By that time, if problems have occurred during foaling, they will be identified. We believe that this exam is critical if we are to prevent mares from becoming "problem broodmares." Each year we identify mares that, if inappropriately treated, could become long-term disasters. Approximately 5% of mares will have placental tags present (despite excellent staff management), and another 5% will have problems with metritis and uterine damage. Many (15%) will have delayed involution suggested by increased size of the uterus and volume of fluids present.

2. All mares are treated with an infusion of lactated ringers saline with antibiotics. We believe that this helps only the occasional mare, but more importantly we have invaded the mares' reproductive tract and the treatment is aimed at preventing iatrogenic contamination.

3. Mares with no abnormalities identified are scheduled to be reexamined on day 9 or 10 postfoaling. Mares will not be bred any earlier than day 10. On day 9 or 10, if the mare has ovulated, she is scheduled for $PGF_{2\alpha}$ administration in 6 days. If no uterine fluid is detected and uterine tone is good, the mare may be scheduled to be bred. If there is a question, the mare is treated and/or reexamined according to follicle size and presence or absence of uterine fluid. It would be rare for a foal-heat breed to take precedence over a non-foal-heat breed with a stallion with a busy book (>150 mares per season with natural service).

4. Great care is taken to avoid breeding mares with intra-luminal fluid accumulations.

5. There are 2 more guidelines that we adhere to. First, we only breed mares on foal heat that are young and reproductively healthy (i.e., <12 years old and with their first, second, or third foal). Second, mares that have been confined without exercise (i.e., lunging) due to foal problems, such as angular limb deformities, are not bred on foal heat regardless.

Hormones

Progestins

By far the most popular treatment to aid in pregnancy maintenance is the *supplementation of progesterone or progestins*. This occurs despite advice that there is no scientific evidence to support the use of such compounds.[13,78,79] Most studies suggest that primary luteal inadequacy is not likely a cause of decreased progesterone levels.[80]

Plasma progesterone concentrations were measured in 179 mares bled on alternate days commencing with a positive pregnancy diagnosis on Days 17 to 18 after ovulation and concluding on Days 42 to 45. During this period 17 mares (10 per cent) lost their pregnancies, 11 before Day 25. In 15 mares the timing of the pregnancy loss could be determined with adequate accuracy; in only one did a decline in progesterone precede the loss.

Thus pregnancy loss between Days 17 and 42 was rarely caused by a fall in plasma progesterone.[80]

The exception is failure of mares to maintain either a CL or pregnancy when induced to ovulate from either the early transition or anestrous.[81,82]

Two experiments were conducted using a 21-day GnRH analogue treatment regimen to induce ovulation in seasonally anovulatory mares. In Experiment 1, non-treated (n = 20) and treated (n = 83) mares were defined as having inactive ovaries (largest follicle < 15 mm) at the start of treatment. In Experiment 2, non-treated (n = 7) and treated (n = 10) mares were defined as having active ovaries (largest follicle 21 to 29 mm) at the start of treatment. Less mares ovulated that had inactive ovaries at the start of treatment compared to mares that had active ovaries (26% versus 70%). In mares that had inactive ovaries at the start of treatment, the pregnancy rate on Day 11 (ovulation = Day 0) was not different between treated (14/22; 64%) and non-treated (14/20; 70%) mares. However, the embryo-loss rate between Days 11 and 40 was significantly higher in treated (9/14; 64%) than in non-treated (1/14; 7%) mares. Losses tended to occur more frequently between Days 15 and 25. A significant decrease in progesterone on Day 15 in treated mares with embryo loss corresponded to the first day that embryo loss was detected. In mares that had active ovaries at the start of treatment, pregnancy rate, embryo-loss rate, and ovarian and hormonal end points were not significantly different between the treated and non-treated mares. The results indicated that hormonal capacity was reduced and embryo-loss rate was high following GnRH-induced ovulation in mares that had inactive ovaries at the start of treatment.[81]

Another report suggests that, although an apparent low incidence, we should continue to watch out for mares with low progesterone that occurs before obvious fetal demise.[83]

Characteristics of spontaneous embryonic loss in 21 mares were compared with those of 52 contemporary mares that maintained pregnancy. Embryonic losses were, in retrospect, grouped according to day of loss and length of the interovulatory interval, respectively, as follows: group 1, ≤ day 20 and < 30 days (n = 10); group 2, ≤ day 20 and > 30 days (n = 3); and group 3, > day 20 and > 30 days (n = 8); ovulation was day 0. Mean diameter of the embryonic vesicle in group 1 was smaller (P < 0.05) on days 12-18 than in the pregnancy- maintained group, but among the pregnancy-maintained group and the embryonic-loss groups, the mean individual growth rates of vesicles was similar (no significant difference). A more frequent (P < 0.05) location of the vesicles in the uterine body on day 13 in group 1 was due to a greater proportion of small vesicles and for day 18 was due to a greater incidence of fixation failure. Luteal regression occurred at the expected time in 77% of the mares with loss sooner than day 20. Low concentration of progesterone on days 12, 15 and 18, a detected decrease in diameter of the corpus luteum on days 15 and 18, and an interovulatory interval of ≤ 30 days indicated that luteolysis was not prevented by the *embryonic vesicle in group 1. However, in mares in group 2, the corpus luteum was maintained as indicated by luteal diameters, progesterone concentrations, and prolonged interovulatory intervals. Thus, luteal maintenance occurred in 23% of mares with embryonic loss at ≤ day 20. In group 3 (loss > day 20), circulating concentrations of progesterone were either maintained (four mares) after embryonic death (cessation of embryonic heartbeat) or appeared to decrease before death (two mares) or on the day of death (one mare). The decrease in progesterone on the day of death seemed to be associated with acute endometritis. In another mare, embryonic loss was associated with continuing low concentrations of progesterone, a flaccid uterus, an oversized embryonic vesicle, failure of development of an embryo proper and collapse of the large vesicle on day 42. The apparent drop in progesterone before embryonic death in two of eight mares with loss after day 20 could have been associated with primary luteal insufficiency.*[83]

Thus, although in many cases pregnant mares are probably unnecessarily treated with progestins, it appears to do no harm. An exception is mares that are chronically infected. Administration of either Altrenogest or natural progesterone to a chronically infected mare will enhance the infection process. The mare should first be scanned with ultrasound, cultured, and a uterine biopsy obtained in order to confirm that she is not harboring a uterine infection. Another exception is the use of compounds that are ineffective for the intended purpose. Studies at the GVEH were able to demonstrate failure of hydroxyprogesterone caproate to maintain pregnancy in ovariectomized mares.[84] Hydroxyprogesterone caproate is commonly used in many countries, and apparently it has not been critically studied. Despite lack of definitive studies on frequency of a primary luteal defect on EED or the relative contributions of stress, $PGF_{2\alpha}$ release associated with uterine inflammation, genetic abnormalities, or uterine infection, many veterinarians, breeding farm managers, and mare owners are convinced of the beneficial effect of supplemental progestagens. Perhaps inappropriate administration of therapeutic substances that lack scientific documentation of efficacy are an even bigger form of reproductive wastage due to cost and lack of specified effect.

Experimental animals were part of a herd of 95 mares in good body condition kept on pasture at the Goulburn Valley Equine Hospital and supplemented as necessary with lucerne hay and grain. Ultrasonography was used to assess follicular development, ovulation and to diagnose early pregnancy. Twenty five mares were inseminated with approximately 500×10^6 progressively motile spermatozoa when they showed oestrus in association with a follicle greater than 30 mm in diameter. Fifteen mares diagnosed pregnant at day 14 after ovulation that had ovulated only one follicle were divided into three groups of five and treated as follows: Group A; supplemented with 500 mg hydroxyprogesterone caproate administered IM every 7 days beginning on day 15 of pregnancy. Group B; supplemented with 500 mg hydroxyprogesterone caproate IM every other day beginning on day 15 of pregnancy. Group C; supplemented with

0.044 mg/kg of oral Altrenogest daily from 15 days of pregnancy. All mares were unilaterally ovariectomized by colpotomy to remove the primary CL of pregnancy on day 17. Serum was harvested from mares on days 14, 16, 18, and 20, and analysed for progesterone using a commercial radio immunoassay. Ultrasonography was performed daily to monitor pregnancy after ovariectomy, presence of endometrial folds (Grade 0-3) and time to the next ovulation on the contra lateral ovary. Pregnancy loss was diagnosed by absence of a previously recorded vesicle.

Plasma progesterone concentrations in all mares were less than 1ng/ml the day following ovariectomy and were extremely low or undetectable in the following days. There was no difference in progesterone concentrations between any of the groups either before or after ovariectomy. All mares treated with hydroxyprogesterone caproate (groups A and B) lost their pregnancies within 5 days of ovariectomy. Characteristics of impending loss were observation of vesicle mobility (n = 6) and the presence of endometrial folds (n = 10) as the remaining ovary developed one or more large follicles. Pregnancy loss in mares in groups A and B was accompanied by a relaxing cervix. There was no difference in time to pregnancy loss for mares in group A or B. All mares treated with Altrenogest (group C) maintained pregnancy until 30 days. At that time, the heart beat was not visible in 1 of the 5 pregnancies and the developing foetus and foetal fluids were slowly reabsorbed. The four remaining mares were maintained on Altrenogest until day 100. One mare aborted a 10-month-old foetus and subsequently, 3 mares produced normal foals. All mares in groups A and B returned to heat and ovulated within 11 days after ovariectomy. Secondary CL development occurred at the expected times in the mares that remained pregnant (group C). The ovariectomy was a safe and efficacious procedure, and no untoward sequelae were noted.

Hydroxyprogesterone caproate has been specifically advocated for use in pregnancy maintenance of mares (manufacturers recommendations). Despite lack of research data supporting the drug for this purpose, its use appears to be widespread. It was not the purpose of this study to examine whether or not supplementation of progestagens is a rational therapeutic approach; however, if mares are treated with hydroxyprogesterone caproate with the expectation of actually helping them maintain pregnancy, then great caution would appear to be warranted. Our experiment suggests that hydroxyprogesterone caproate is not capable of supporting pregnancy when administered around day 18. In addition common sense would indicate that it is not likely to be of any more use when administered at a later time in pregnancy. In this study the method of ovariectomy did not appear to influence pregnancy loss, as Altrenogest was successful in maintaining all pregnancies until day 30 and 4 of 5 pregnancies until well past the time when ovarian steroids are no longer necessary for pregnancy maintenance. It should be noted that mares administered hydroxyprogesterone caproate received either 4 times (group A) or 15 times (group B) the manufacturer recommended doses. Mares in group A received one and *mares in group B received two treatments before ovariectomy. Because mares in these groups aborted, developed follicles and displayed oestrus behaviour after ovariectomy, it is unlikely hydroxyprogesterone caproate had much binding to progesterone receptors in these mares or that time from first treatment to ovariectomy (2 days) was responsible for the drug's inability to maintain pregnancy. Current recommendations for hydroxyprogesterone caproate for pregnancy maintenance in mares were 500 mg every 2-4 weeks. Another point of interest in this study was the relatively quick time to pregnancy loss (mean; 3.1 days, range; 2-5 days) compared to previous studies using $PGF_{2\alpha}$ as the method of CL regression. The mean number of days to embryonic loss was greater for mares treated with $PGF_{2\alpha}$ on day 12 (6.8 days) than for mares ovariectomized on day 12 (3.0 days).[85]*

Perhaps these findings demonstrate the effect of immediate total progesterone withdrawal as distinct from a more gradual decline noted after PGF_2alpha release. In addition, in our study vesicle loss was always associated with a softening cervix and the presence of endometrial folds; however, mares did not ovulate for a mean of 7.8 days after unilateral ovariectomy (range 5-11 days). The results of this experiment suggest that pregnancy in mares with inadequate luteal function cannot be maintained with hydroxyprogesterone caproate at 4-15 times the recommended dose rate. However, pregnancy could be maintained by Altrenogest, and endogenous progesterone supplementation from secondary CL development is possible despite exogenous progestagen therapy.[84]

Another study from CSU recently reexamined the dose of progesterone necessary for pregnancy maintenance.[86]

Exogenous progestins are often given to pregnant mares, but many questions remain unanswered as to the relationship between concentrations of progesterone and embryo survival. Thus, embryos were collected 7 days after ovulation and transferred into either ovarian-intact recipients (I, n = 15) or ovariectomized recipients which were given 100 mg progesterone (L, n = 15) or 1,500 mg progesterone (H, n = 15) daily. Concentrations of progesterone were determined in all mares from days 0 to 13. Recipients were examined for pregnancy with ultrasonography during days 11 through 25. Between days 28 and 100, twelve ovarian-intact, pregnant recipients were monitored for follicular and luteal changes and bled for determination of progesterone concentrations for 4 days at 2-week intervals. Twelve ovariectomized pregnant recipients were taken off injectable progesterone days 25-30 and pregnancy maintained to day 100 with an oral progestin, Altrenogest. Concentrations of progesterone in these mares were determined every 3 days. Progesterone treatment had no effect on maintenance of pregnancy to day 100 or size of embryonic vesicle (P > 0.05). Levels of progesterone during days 1 to 13 were 1.3 to 3.0 ng/ml, >25 ng/ml and 7 to 9 ng/ml for groups L, H and I, respectively. Concentrations of endogenous progesterone in ovariectomized pregnant mares became >1 ng/ml by day 91 of gestation indicating placental progesterone secretion. Increased concen-

trations of progesterone from days 60 to 100, seen in ovarian-intact, pregnant mares, were primarily due to secretions from corpora lutea. There was, in fact, a correlation between the number of 2^0-CL and progesterone level (r^2=0.74). Initial formation of secondary CL's (2^0-CL) occurred from 28 to 51 days, with peak formation of 2^0-CL on days 55 to 70 of gestation.[86]

Finally, a further study was useful in demonstrating just how little ability many of the progestagens either recommended or used actually have.[87]

Twenty five mares diagnosed pregnant on day 14 after ovulation were divided into five groups of five and treated as follows:

Group A; Supplemented with 1000 mg medroxyprogesterone acetate administered IM every 7 days beginning on day 16 of pregnancy.

Group B; Supplemented with 500 mg hydroxyprogesterone hexanoate administered IM every 4 days beginning on day 16 of pregnancy.

Group C; Supplemented with 0.044 mg/kg of oral Altrenogest daily from 16 days of pregnancy.

Group D; Supplemented with five implants (total 15 mg) of norgestomet placed subcutaneously as a single treatment on day 16 of pregnancy.

Group E; Supplemented with 500 mg megesterol acetate orally every day beginning on day 16 of pregnancy.

All mares were injected IM with 5 mg of the prostaglandin to induce luteolysis of the primary CL on day 18 of pregnancy. Mares were bled daily and serum was subsequently analysed for progesterone using an amplified enzyme-linked immunoassay (AELIA), developed and validated for horse serum,[88] until either abortion occurred or mares were ≥ 24 days pregnant with a foetus and detectable heart beat.

Ultrasonography was performed daily to monitor pregnancy, presence of endometrial folds, time to the next ovulation and time to either pregnancy loss or recognition of the foetus within the vesicle and normal growth until day 30.

All 5 mares in each of Groups A, B, D and E aborted between 2 and 8 days after $PGF_{2\alpha}$ administration, whereas none of the mares in Group C given Altrenogest daily aborted. The number of mares that aborted on days 2, 3, 4, 5, 6, 7 and 8 post $PGF_{2\alpha}$ administration were 10, 3, 3, 2, 1, 0 and 1, respectively and the mean (± s. d.) time to pregnancy loss was 3.3 (± 1.7) days

Serum progesterone concentrations in all mares had fallen to less than 2 ng/ml the day following $PGF_{2\alpha}$ administration and they remained very low or undetectable on the following days.

All the mares in Groups A, B, D and E returned to oestrus and ovulated within 11 days after $PGF_{2\alpha}$ administration. The mean (± s.d.) time to ovulation was 9.2 ± 1.6 days.

The results of this experiment demonstrated convincingly that medroxyprogesterone acetate, hydroxyprogesterone hexanoate, norgestomet and megesterol acetate were unable to maintain pregnancy in mares between days 18 and 30 after ovulation in the absence of endogenous progesterone secreted by a viable CL. It is reason-

able to conclude from these findings that the progestagens used in this study are not likely to be of any more use when administered at a later time in pregnancy. Pregnancy in the mare can be maintained solely by placental sources of progestagens from around day 80-100 of gestation,[62,64,89,90] but prior to this time ovarian corpora lutea, both primary and accessory[13,64] are the only endogenous source of this vital hormone of pregnancy.

The progestagens chosen in this study are those commonly administered by equine veterinary clinicians either to prevent abortion or to modify undesirable behaviour in performance horses. The dose rates of progestagen administration were from manufacturer recommendations. It was not possible in this study to conclude whether abortion occurred as a result of insufficient progestagen binding to progesterone receptors or an insufficient progestagen dosage. Altrenogest was used as a positive control since it had been shown in a previous study to maintain pregnancy in ovariectomised mares.[91] This earlier trial also showed hydroxyprogesterone caproate was incapable of maintaining pregnancy in the ovariectomised animals which apparently led the same substance being renamed and repackaged under the name of hydroxyprogesterone hexanoate. This difference in nomenclature was not known at the time that the present experiment began.

Despite a lack of basic research or efficacy data to support the administration of these compounds for pregnancy maintenance in the mare, they are widely used for this purpose. Hydroxyprogesterone hexanoate has been specifically advocated for use in pregnancy maintenance of mares (manufacturers recommendations). We cannot understand how such blatant misrepresentation can go unchallenged, either professionally or legally.

We are now at least cognizant of a few progestagens that we can use. Progesterone at around 150 mg/day, Altrenogest at 22 mg/day, and microencapsulated progesterone spheres. Little data exist on supplementation later in pregnancy when the placenta is the only source of progestins.

A study examined progestins at this time and the effect of supplementation.[90]

Two experiments were conducted to determine when a placental source of progestin was sufficient for maintaining pregnancy in the mare. In the first study, embryos were transferred into ovariectomized mares and pregnancy was maintained with Altrenogest. Altrenogest treatment was terminated at either day 100 (n = 6) or day 150 (n = 6). Twelve ovarian-intact mares were assigned to a second experiment on day 100 of gestation. On day 160 of gestation, these mares were assigned to one of three treatments: 1) ovariectomy on day 160 and given Altrenogest to day 200 (n = 4); 2) ovariectomy on day 180 and given Altrenogest to day 250 (n = 4); or 3) ovariectomy on day 200 and given Altrenogest to day 300 (n = 4). Blood samples were collected every 2 weeks from all mares in both experiments from day 100 to parturition and assayed for concentrations of progestins. Pregnancy loss from day 100 to parturition was not different among groups in either experiment. Serum concentrations of progestins in ovary-intact mares were

greater (P < 0.05) than those in ovariectomized pregnant mares until day 130, after which they were similar. Serum concentrations of progestins in the ovariectomized pregnant mares rose gradually from day 100 until near parturition. Serum concentrations of progestins in the ovary-intact pregnant mares declined from day 100 to day 157, did not vary significantly from day 157 to day 245, then rose until near parturition. Serum concentrations of progestins tended to decrease the sixth day prior to parturition. From these data, it was concluded that even though the ovary is a significant source of circulating progestins until day 130 of pregnancy in the mare, the feto-placental unit produces sufficient progestins to maintain pregnancy by day 100 of gestation.[90]

Unfortunately this study and others have not been able to address the question of whether or not supplementation of the feto-placental unit would likely ever be required.

Supplementation of estrogens has been recommended[92] or suggested for further examination.[93]

Nishikawa[92] suggested the rationale behind supplementation was to prolong the life of the CL. He administered stilbestrol in either tablet or injectable form at a dose of 60 to 90 mg (injectable) or 144 to 200 mg (orally) over a 2 month period starting at the third or fourth month of gestation. Fifty-seven percent of supplemented animals had miscarried 1 to 5 times prior to the years in which the experiment was performed (1949-1954). Significantly fewer (P < 0.0001) treated animals aborted (19/576, 3.3%) compared to control animals (474/3,734, 12.7%). Nishikawa states "that the treatment with estrogen is definitely effective for preventing abortion in mares," and "the treatment was highly praised by farmers." Despite this convincing evidence, further studies have failed to find any effect of diethylstilbestrol on progesterone secretion.[94] The work of Pashen[95] suggests that we need to look further at the role of the fetal gonads in pregnancy maintenance and parturition.

The effects of fetal gonadectomy on steroid production and the maintenance of pregnancy in the mare were studied. Removal of the fetal gonads resulted in an immediate fall in maternal plasma concentrations of conjugated and unconjugated oestrogens whereas progestagen levels remained unchanged. Hormone profiles in mares carrying sham-operated fetuses remained similar to those in unoperated control mares. Plasma levels of 13,14-dihydro-15-oxo- PGF-2 alpha (PGFM) were much lower, and uterine contractions weaker, during labour in mares carrying gonadectomized foals than in control mares. Pregnancy was maintained until parturition at term in the mares carrying gonadectomized fetuses. However, 3 of the 4 gonadectomized foals were dysmature and died during or soon after birth. The biosynthetic pathways involved in the production of oestrogens by the feto-placental unit and the possible role of oestrogens in fetal development in the pregnant mare are discussed.[95]

Supplementation with GnRH

A slight increase in pregnancy rate per cycle and more importantly a decrease in EED per cycle has been demonstrated with the GnRH agonist Buserelin.[96]

Two trials involving 578 mares were performed to investigate the effect of a single intramuscular treatment of 40 mu g buserelin, an analog of gonadotrophin releasing hormone, on pregnancy rate in mares. All mares were bred by natural mating and were allocated into pairs. One mare in each pair was injected with buserelin either on Day 10 or 11 (Trial 1) or on Days 8 to 10 (Trial 2) after ovulation. Pregnancy status of mares was determined by transrectal ultrasonographic examination on Day 14 or 15 after the day of ovulation and was repeated between Days 28 and 30 of pregnancy. In Trial 1, buserelin treatment increased the pregnancy rate at Days 14 and 15 (72.5 vs 66.6%; P < 0.01). At the second pregnancy examination, pregnancy losses were lower in the treated group of mares (4.1 vs 7.4%; P < 0.05). In Trial 2, buserelin also improved the pregnancy rate (57.2 vs 53.5%; P < 0.05) at Days 14 and 15. Pregnancy losses between the first and second examinations were lower in the treated group of mares (6.5 vs 12.0%; P < 0.05). Buserelin increased pregnancy rates after breeding at the first estrus in both trials. In addition, buserelin treatment increased the pregnancy maintenance rate at Days 28 to 30.

This finding has potentially interesting ramifications but needs to be replicated by others. Further work by Newcombe[97] has strengthened the data.

We conducted a series of trials over a four-year period on a total of 2,346 mares, to determine the effect of a single dose of the GnRH analog buserelin (20 to 40 mug im or sc) on pregnancy rates when given between 8 and 12 days after service. Although there were some statistically significant improvements in pregnancy rates in individual trials, meta-analysis of the data overall showed significant improvements at all times examined, i.e. 13 to 16, 19 to 23, 28 to 31 and 38 to 42 days after service. These results indicate that treatment of mares with 20 to 40 mug buserelin between Days 8 and 12 significantly increases pregnancy rates by approximately 10 percentage points.[97]

In addition, another study has supported the hypothesis (although the pregnancy rates were quite low).[98] It is not currently understood why this therapy is beneficial. One possibility is that the GnRH may be luteotropic and thus stimulate the primary CL of pregnancy.

Other Considerations

Antibiotics
Our belief is that persistent, unidentified, or poorly treated chronic inflammatory conditions of the uterus are responsible for the majority of problems of EED and abortion. It is common to see uterine inflammation using ultrasonography in mares that have undergone early pregnancy loss and then are given prostaglandins to return them to estrus. Therapies aimed at reducing this inflammation, infection, and irritation are a primary goal in our practice. To this end mares with a history of recurrent pregnancy loss are biopsied wherever possible and if the primary problem is uterine inflammation, they are placed on broad spectrum antibiotics throughout preg-

nancy.[99] The results from our practice appear very encouraging. When pregnancy continues, antibiotics are administered for 5 consecutive days every month. As with many treatments of endometritis, there is *no experimental data* available to document the efficacy of such treatments. However, at the GVEH we have been using this approach for 14 years now and have little doubt that the number of mares maintaining pregnancy is much higher than those mares not treated.

A study was reported wherein potential cases of chronic uterine infection/inflammation were treated with antibiotics, monthly, during the entire pregnancy. Because not all EED and abortion is caused by bacterial infection/inflammation, it was not expected that all mares would maintain pregnancy. The population we chose to treat had all undergone either EED or abortion at least once in the last season prior to entering the trial.

At the conclusion of the study, 43 mares had entered the program, they had a mean age of 14.2 years, and had EED or abortion an average of 2.2 times in the preceding 3.4 years.

At the conclusion of the study 36 mares had become pregnant (84%). Of the 36 pregnant mares, 3 underwent EED (8.3%), 4 aborted (11.1%), and 29 had foals (80.6%).[100]

Please recognize that valid, significant scientific data may not be possible to obtain from these studies. In the study presented above there were no controls. Caution is advised in interpreting studies without contemporary controls.

A recent publication highlights well the effect of post-foaling irritation.[101]

Records of 1,009 pregnancies in 574 foaling, barren and maiden Thoroughbred mares on a single stud farm, over a period of 12 years were examined. The farm is situated in the eastern Cape Province of South Africa, at an elevation of 1800 m, and in an area of climatic extremes. Records of 604 pregnancies in 249 foaling Thoroughbred mares were examined. For these purposes, those pregnancies in which a mare conceived in the same breeding season during which she had foaled were considered as pregnancies in foaling mares. Pregnancy was confirmed by rectal palpation by a single experienced practitioner. Of the 604 pregnancies examined, conceptus attachment occurred in the horn opposite the previously gravid horn in 345 cases (57%), and in the previously gravid horn in 259 cases (43%; P < 0.005). Unobserved foetal loss after pregnancy diagnosis amounted to 30 (9%) in the former group, while in the latter group (pregnancy established in the postgravid horn) 46 pregnancies were lost (18%; P < 0.005). This study confirmed that conceptus attachment tends to occur in the uterine horn opposite the previously gravid horn in foaling Thoroughbred mares conceiving during the same season. A significantly higher incidence of foetal loss accompanied conceptus attachment in the postgravid horn. Of 242 pregnancies in 162 previously barren mares, 95 (39%) occurred in the left uterine horn and 147 (61%) in the right horn (P < 0.005). The incidence of pregnancy failure in this group was 7%. The side of attachment did not affect the rate of loss. Eval-

uation of the records of 163 maiden mares revealed that conceptus attachment occurred in the left uterine horn in 58 (36%) pregnancies and in the right horn in 105 (64%) pregnancies (P < 0.005), which is consistent with previously reported observations. Pregnancy failure was recorded in 4% of maiden mares. Side of attachment did not influence rate of loss in this group.[101]

Lastly, we would serve our clients best by trying to identify which mares are in a high risk category for abortion or EED rather than trying to diagnose what has made the mare lose the pregnancy.

Equine high-risk pregnancy can be caused by conditions of the fetus or placenta. Placental abnormalities are the most common cause of equine abortion. Conditions that lead to equine high-risk pregnancy can be caused by infectious agents, physical abnormalities, or the ingestion of toxins. The diagnosis of fetal and placental conditions can be very challenging, as clinical signs are often absent; the most common premonitory sign of fetal or placental disease is premature lactation. Most congenital abnormalities (arthrogryposis, hydrocephalus, and hydrops, etc) have no treatment. Therapy in these cases is directed at facilitating parturition to salvage the future breeding potential of the mare. Patients with some infectious causes of high-risk pregnancy, such as bacterial placentitis, can be successfully treated. Early recognition of the infection and aggressive antimicrobial therapy, in some cases, control the infection and prolong gestation until a viable fetus is born. Additional therapy for placentitis can include the use of non-steroidal anti-inflammatory drugs and supplemental progestins.[102]

In this regard fetal monitoring has been useful in identification of placental problems and to aid in decision processes based on probability of successful treatments.

Immune Stimulation

Finally, the report on immune stimulation[103] having an apparent benefit on the mare's reproductive tract resulted in us utilizing the therapy (Eqstim) during estrus and in early pregnancy. The aim has been to reduce acute inflammation.

Thirty-seven mares, barren for at least one year, were diagnosed to have endometrial inflammation by cytological examination and/or bacterial culture. Sixteen of these mares (the control group) were treated with prostaglandin and reevaluated cytologically within 10 days of behavioral estrus. Fifteen out of sixteen (15/16) (93.8%) remained positive for endometrial inflammation. Twenty-one mares (immunologically treated group) were treated with Propionibacterium acnes by injecting 1 ml per each 113.3 kilograms body weight intravenously on days 1, 3, and 7 following the diagnosis of endometrial inflammation. They also received prostaglandin. Twelve of the immunologically treated mates were examined cytologically as were the control mares. One of twelve examined (1/12) (08.3%) was positive cytologically for endometrial inflammation when examined within 10 days after behavioral estrus. The other nine mares in the treated group were bred on the first behavioral estrus following treatment. Nine of nine (9/9) were determined to be pregnant to 60 days gestation. The other treated mares were bred following the cytological evaluation. Eighteen of the twenty-one treated mares (18/21) (85 7%) were confirmed pregnant to 60 days gestation.[103]

Further work on another immuno-modulator (Equimune IV)[104] has given further confidence to this as an approach to pre- and postbreeding inflamtory problems in mares.

Endometrial mRNA expression of the pro-inflammatory cytokines interleukin-1beta (IL-1beta), interleukin-6 (IL-6), and tumor necrosis factor alpha (TNF-alpha) was assessed in mares resistant (RM) or susceptible (SM) to persistent post-breeding endometritis (PPBE). Eight RM and eight SM were selected based on reproductive records and functional tests out of a herd of 2000 light cross-type mares. Three experiments were done to study transcription patterns in (i) basal conditions; (ii) after artificial insemination (AI); and (iii) after administration of an immunomodulator at time of artificial insemination. Endometrial biopsies were taken during consecutive cycles: (i) at estrus, when follicles reached 35 mm and at diestrus (7 +/– 1 days after ovulation); (ii) at 24 h post-AI, with dead semen (estrus) and in diestrus; (iii) at 24 It after treatment with a Mycobacterium phlei cell-wall extract (MCWE) preparation and AII (with dead semen), and at diestrus. MRNA expression was quantitated by real time PCR. Under basal conditions, SM had significantly higher mRNA expression of all cytokines in estrus and of IL-1beta and TNF-alpha in diestrus, compared to RM. After AI, there were no differences between RM and SM in estrus; however, mRNA expression for all three pro-inflammatory cytokines was higher than under basal conditions. In diestrus, RM showed significantly lower IL-1beta and TNF-alpha mRNA expression than SM. When MCWE was administered at time of AI, no differences between cytokine induction from RM and SM were found. Globally, mRNA expression for all three cytokines correlated well among themselves when expression was high. The present study showed that (i) in basal conditions RM had lower mRNA expression of pro-inflammatory cytokines than SM with no effect of estrous cycle; (ii) AI upregulated mRNA expression for all three cytokines in both RM and SM, with persistence in diestrus in the latter; (iii) treatment with MCWE at time of AI downregulated mRNA expression of IL-1 with significant effects in SM which behaved like RM. Immunomodulation with MCWE could be of help in restoring homeostatic local inflammatory mechanisms, thus assisting in the prophylaxis of post-breeding endometritis in mares.[104]

When a mare has a history of habitually aborting or experiencing EED, the decision of whether to use immune stimulation, supplement or not supplement with progestins, or use antibiotics is largely at the discretion of the owners and managers. Many owners and mare or farm managers, having invested so much time and money in getting the mare pregnant, will feel compelled to supplement or treat regardless of the lack of documented efficacy and our advice.

References

1. Villahoz MD, Squires EL, Voss JL et al: Some observations on early embryonic death in mares. Theriogenology 1985; 23:915-924.
2. Ball BA, Little TV, Hillman RB et al: Pregnancy rates at days 2 and 14 and estimated embryonic loss rates prior to day 14 in normal and subfertile mares. Theriogenology 1986; 26:611-620.
3. Carnevale EM, Ginther OJ: Defective oocytes as a cause of subfertility in old mares. Biol Reprod Mono 1995; 1:209-214.
4. Day FT: Clinical and experimental observations on reproduction in the mare. J Agri Sci 1940; 30:244-261.
5. Kenney RM: Cyclic and pathologic changes of the mare endometrium as detected by biopsy, with a note on early embryonic death. J Am Vet Med Assoc 1978; 172:241-262.
6. Ginther OJ, Bergfelt DR, Leith GS et al: Embryonic loss in mares: incidence and ultrasonic morphology. Theriogenology 1985; 24:73-86.
7. Belonje PC, van Niekerk CH: A review of the influence of nutrition upon the oestrous cycle and early pregnancy in the mare. J Reprod Fertil 1975; (Suppl):167-169.
8. van Niekerk CH, Morgenthal JC: Fetal loss and the effect of stress on plasma progestagen levels in pregnant Thoroughbred mares. J Reprod Fertil 1982; 32(Suppl):453-457.
9. Swerczek TW: Early fetal death and infectious placental disease in the mare. Proc AAEP 1980; 173-179.
10. Brendemuehl JP, Boosinger TR, Pugh DG et al: Influence of endophyte-infected tall fescue on cyclicity, pregnancy rate and early embryonic loss in the mare. Theriogenology 1994; 42:489-500.
11. Moberg R. The occurrence of early embryonic death in the mare in relation to natural service and artificial insemination with fresh or deep-frozen semen. J Reprod Fertil 1975; (Suppl):537-539.
12. Merkt H, Gunzel AR: A survey of early pregnancy losses in West German thoroughbred mares. Equine Vet J 1979; 11:256-258.
13. Allen WR: Is your progesterone therapy really necessary? Equine Vet J 1984; 16:496-498.
14. Liu IK, Shivers CA: Antibodies to the zona pellucida in mares. J Reprod Fertil Suppl 1982; 32:309-313.
15. Shivers CA, Liu IK: Inhibition of sperm binding to porcine ova by antibodies to equine zonae pellucidae. J Reprod Fertil 1982; 32(Suppl):315-318.
16. Platt H: Aetiological aspects of abortion in the Thoroughbred mare. J Comp Pathol 1973; 83:199-205.
17. Ginther OJ: Mobility of the equine conceptus. Theriogenology 1983; 19:603-611.
18. Fiolka G, Kuller HJ, Lender S: Embryonic mortality of horse. Monatshefte Fuer Veterinaermedizin 1985; 40:835-838.
19. Lieux P: Comparative results of breeding on first and second post-foaling heat periods. Proc AAEP 1980; 129-132.
20. Bain AM: Foetal losses during pregnancy in the thoroughbred mare: a record of 2,562 pregnancies. N Z Vet J 1969; 17:155-158.
21. McDowell KJ, Sharp DC, Grubaugh W et al: Restricted conceptus mobility results in failure of pregnancy maintenance in mares. Biol Reprod Mono 1988; 39:340-348.
22. McKinnon AO, Squires EL: Morphologic assessment of the equine embryo. J Am Vet Med Assoc 1988; 192:401-406.
23. Carnevale EM, Ramirez RJ, Squires EL et al: Factors affecting pregnancy rates and early embryonic death after equine embryo transfer. Theriogenology 2000; 54:965-979.
24. Woods J, Bergfelt DR, Ginther OJ: Effects of time of insemination relative to ovulation on pregnancy rate and embryonic loss rate in mares. Equine Vet J 1990; 22:410-415.
25. Koskinen E, Lindeberg H, Kuntsi H et al: Fertility of mares after postovulatory insemination. Zentralbl Veterinarmed [A] 1990; 37:77-80.
26. Chevalier Clement F: Pregnancy loss in the mare. Anim Reprod Sci 1989; 20:231-244.
27. Acland HM: Abortion in mares. In McKinnon AO, Voss JL (eds). Equine Reproduction, Philadelphia, Lea & Febiger, pp 554-562, 1993.
28. Fontaine M, Collobertlaugier C, Tariel G: Abortion and stillbirth of infectious origin in the mare – a study of necropsy of aborted fetuses, premature and stillborn foals. Point Vet 1993; 25:79-84.
29. Giles RC, Donahue JM, Hong CB et al: Causes of abortion, stillbirth, and perinatal death in horses: 3, 527 cases(1986-1991). J Am Vet Med Assoc 1993; 203:1170-1175.
30. Hong CB, Donahue JM, Giles RC et al: Equine abortion and stillbirth in central Kentucky during 1988 and 1989 foaling seasons. J Vet Diagn Invest 1993; 5:560-566.
31. Garg DN, Manchanda VP: Prevalence and etiology of equine abortion. Indian J Anim Sci 1986; 56:730-735.
32. Santschi EM, Slone DE, Gronwall R et al: Types of colic and frequency of postcolic abortion in pregnant mares: 105 cases (1984-1988). J Am Vet Med Assoc 1991; 199:374-377.
33. Baucus KL, Ralston SL, Nockels CF et al: Effects of transportation on early embryonic death in mares. J Anim Sci 1990; 68:345-351.
34. Irwin CFP: Early pregnancy testing and its relationship to abortion. J Reprod Fertil 1975; 23(Suppl):485-488.
35. Donahue JM, Williams NM: Emergent causes of placentitis and abortion. Vet Clin N Am Equine Pract 2001; 16:443.
36. Zent WW, Williams NM, Donahue JM: Placentitis in central Kentucky broodmares. Pferdeheilkunde 1999; 15:630-632.
37. Troedsson MH: Ultrasonographic evaluation of the equine placenta. Pferdeheilkunde 2000; 17:583.
38. Sebastian M, Gantz MG, Tobin T et al: The mare reproductive loss syndrome and the eastern tent caterpillar: a toxicokinetic/statistical analysis with clinical, epidemiologic, and mechanistic implications. Vet Ther 2003; 4:324-339.
39. Betteridge KJ, Mitchell D: Direct evidence of retention of unfertilized ova in the oviduct of the mare. J Reprod Fertil 1974; 39:145-148.
40. Betteridge KJ, Eaglesome MD, Flood PF: Embryo transport through the mare's oviduct depends upon cleavage and is independent of the ipsilateral corpus luteum. J Reprod Fertil 1979; (Suppl):387-394.
41. Flood PF, Jong A, Betteridge KJ: The location of eggs retained in the oviducts of mares. J Reprod Fertil 1979; 57:291-294.
42. van Niekerk CH, Gerneke WH: Persistence and parthenogenic cleavage of tubal ova in the mare. Onderstepoort J Vet Res 1966; 31:195-232.
43. Hershman L, Douglas RH: The critical period for the maternal recognition of pregnancy in pony mares. J Reprod Fertil 1979; (Suppl):395-401.
44. Zavy MT, Vernon MW, Asquith RL et al: Effect of exogenous gonadal steroids and pregnancy on uterine luminal prostaglandin F in mares. Prostaglandins 1984; 27:311-320.
45. Zavy MT, Vernon MW, Sharp DC et al: Endocrine aspects of early pregnancy in pony mares: a comparison of uterine luminal and peripheral plasma levels of steroids during the estrous cycle and early pregnancy. Biomed Tech (Berlin) 1984; 115:214-219.
46. Terqui M, Palmer E: Oestrogen pattern during early pregnancy in the mare. J Reprod Fertil 1979; 27(Suppl):441-446.
47. Nett TM, Holtan DW, Estergreen VL: Oestrogens, LH, PMSG and prolactin in serum of pregnant mares. J Reprod Fertil 1975; 23(Suppl):457-462.

48. Raeside JI, Liptrap RM, Milne FJ. Relationship of fetal gonads to urinary estrogen excretion by the pregnant mare. Am J Vet Res 1973; 34:843-845.

49. Jeffcott LB, Hyland JH, Maclean AA et al: Changes in maternal hormone concentrations associated with induction of fetal death at day 45 of gestation in mares. J Reprod Fertil 1987; 35(Suppl):461-467.

50. Hyland JH, Wright PJ, Manning SJ: An investigation of the use of plasma oestrone sulphate concentrations for the diagnosis of pregnancy in mares. Aust Vet J 1984; 61:123.

51. Bamberg E, Choi HS, Mostl E et al: Enzymatic determination of unconjugated oestrogens in faeces for pregnancy diagnosis in mares. Equine Vet J 1984; 16:537-539.

52. Monfort SL, Arthur NP, Wildt DE: Monitoring ovarian function and pregnancy by evaluating excretion of urinary estrogen conjugates in semi-free-ranging Przewalski's horses (Equus przewalskii). J Reprod Fertil 1991; 91:155-164.

53. Kasman LH, Hughes JP, Stabenfeldt GH et al: Estrone sulfate concentrations as an indicator of fetal demise in horses. Am J Vet Res 1988; 49:184-187.

54. Hyland JH, Maclean AA, Robertson-Smith GR et al: Attempted conversion of twin to singleton pregnancy in two mares with associated changes in plasma oestrone sulphate concentrations. Aust Vet J 1985; 62:406-409.

55. Madej A, Kindahl H, Nydahl C et al: Hormonal changes associated with induced late abortions in the mare. J Reprod Fertil 1987; 35(Suppl):479-484.

56. Kirkpatrick JF, Lasley BL, Shideler SE et al: Non-instrumented immunoassay field tests for pregnancy detection in free-roaming feral horses. J Wildlife Manage 1993; 57:168-173.

57. Santschi EM, LeBlanc MM, Weston PG: Progestagen, oestrone sulphate and cortisol concentrations in pregnant-mares during medical and surgical disease. J Reprod Fertil 1991; 44(Suppl):627-634.

58. Allen WR: Hormonal control of early pregnancy in the mare. Vet Clin North Am [Large Anim Pract] 1980; 2:291-302.

59. Allen WE: Pregnancy failure induced by human chorionic gonadotrophin in pony mares. Vet Rec 1975; 96:88-90.

60. Bergfelt DR, Pierson RA, Ginther OJ: Resurgence of the primary corpus luteum during pregnancy in the mare. Anim Reprod Sci 1989; 21:261-270.

61. Squires EL, Voss JL, Villahoz MD: Immunological methods for pregnancy detection in mares. Proc AAEP 1983; 45-51.

62. Holtan DW, Squires EL, Lapin DR et al: Effect of ovariectomy on pregnancy in mares. J Reprod Fertil 1979; (Suppl):457-463.

63. Shideler RK, Squires EL, Voss JL et al: Exogenous progestin therapy for maintenance of pregnancy in ovariectomized mares. Proc AAEP 1981; 211-219.

64. Shideler RK, Squires EL, Voss JL et al: Progestagen therapy of ovariectomized pregnant mares. J Reprod Fertil 1982; 32(Suppl):459-464.

65. McKinnon AO, Squires EL, Carnevale EM et al: Ovariectomized steroid-treated mares as embryo transfer recipients and as a model to study the role of progestins in pregnancy maintenance. Theriogenology 1988; 29:1055-1064.

66. Naden J, Squires EL, Nett TM: Effect of maternal treatment with Altrenogest on age at puberty, hormone concentrations, pituitary response to exogenous GnRH, estrous cycle characteristics and fertility of fillies. J Reprod Fertil 1990; 88:185-196.

67. Ball BA, Wilker C, Daels PF et al: Use of progesterone in microspheres for maintenance of pregnancy in mares. Am J Vet Res 1992; 53:1294-1297.

68. Studdert MJ: Vaccination of foals and pregnant mares with Duvaxyn EHV1, 4 vaccine. Vaccine 2002; 20:992.

69. McKinnon AO, Squires EL, Harrison LA et al: Ultrasonographic studies on the reproductive tract of mares after parturition: effect of involution and uterine fluid on pregnancy rates in mares with normal and delayed first postpartum ovulatory cycles. J Am Vet Med Assoc 1988; 192:350-353.

70. McKinnon AO, Squires EL, Carnevale EM et al: Diagnostic ultrasonography of uterine pathology in the mare. Proc AAEP 1987; 605-622.

71. Adams GP, Kastelic JP, Bergfelt DR et al: Effect of uterine inflammation and ultrasonically-detected uterine pathology on fertility in the mare. J Reprod Fertil 1987; 35(Suppl):445-454.

72. Loy RG, Evans MJ, Pemstein R et al: Effects of injected ovarian steroids on reproductive patterns and performance in post-partum mares. J Reprod Fertil 1982; 32(Suppl):199-204.

73. Pope AM, Campbell DL, Davidson JP: Endometrial histology and post-partum mares treated with progesterone and synthetic GnRH (AY-24,031). J Reprod Fertil 1979; (Suppl):587-591.

74. Sexton PE, Bristol FM: Uterine involution in mares treated with progesterone and estradiol-17beta. J Am Vet Med Assoc 1985; 186:252-256.

75. Squires EL, Heesemann CP, Webel SK et al: Relationship of Altrenogest to ovarian activity, hormone concentrations and fertility of mares. J Anim Sci 1983; 56:901-910.

76. Evans MJ, Hamer JM, Gason LM et al: Clearance of bacteria and non-antigenic markers following intra-uterine inoculation into maiden mares: Effect of steroid hormone environment. Theriogenology 1986; 26:37-50.

77. Winter AJ: Microbial immunity in the reproductive tract. J Am Vet Med Assoc 1982; 181:1069-1073.

78. Allen WR: Progesterone and the pregnant mare: unanswered chestnuts [editorial;comment]. Equine Vet J 1993; 25:90-91.

79. Wilker C, Daels PF, Burns PJ et al: Progesterone therapy during early pregnancy in the mare. Proc AAEP 1991; 161-172.

80. Irvine CHG, Sutton P, Turner JE et al: Changes in plasma progesterone concentrations from days 17 to 42 of gestation in mares maintaining or losing pregnancy. Equine Vet J 1990; 22:104-106.

81. Bergfelt DR, Ginther OJ: Embryo loss following GnRH-induced ovulation in anovulatory mares. Theriogenology 1992; 38:33-43.

82. McCue PM, Troedsson MH, Liu IK et al: Follicular and endocrine responses of anoestrous mares to administration of native GnRH or a GnRH agonist. J Reprod Fertil Suppl 1991; 44:227-233.

83. Bergfelt DR, Woods JA, Ginther OJ: Role of the embryonic vesicle and progesterone in embryonic loss in mares. J Reprod Fertil 1992; 95:339-347.

84. McKinnon AO, Figueroa STD, Nobelius AM et al: Failure of hydroxyprogesterone caproate to maintain pregnancy in ovariectomized mares. Equine Vet J 1993; 25:158-160.

85. Ginther OJ: Embryonic loss in mares: nature of loss after experimental induction by ovariectomy or prostaglandin F-2alpha. Theriogenology 1985; 24:87-98.

86. Knowles JE, Squires EL, Shideler RK et al: Relationship of progesterone to early-pregnancy loss in mares. J Equine Vet Sci 1993; 13:528-533.

87. McKinnon AO, Lescun TB, Walker JH et al: The inability of some synthetic progestagens to maintain pregnancy in the mare. Equine Vet J 2000; 32:83-85.

88. Allen WR, Sanderson MW: The value of a rapid progesterone assay (AELIA) in equine stud veterinary medicine and management. Proc Bain-Fallon Mem Lect, Sydney 1987; 76.

89. Holtan DW, Squires EL, Ginther OJ: Effect of ovariectomy on pregnancy in mares. J Anim Sci 1975; 41:359.

90. Knowles JE, Squires EL, Shideler RK et al: Progestins in mid-pregnant to late-pregnant mares. J Equine Vet Sci 1994; 14:659-663.

91. McKinnon AO, Tarrida del Marmol Figueroa S, Nobelius AM et al: Failure of hydroxyprogesterone caproate to maintain pregnancy in ovariectomised mares. Equine Vet J 1993; 25:158-160.

92. Nishikawa Y: Studies on reproduction in horses: singularity and artificial control in reproductive phenomena. Tokyo: Japan Racing Association, 1959.

93. Varner DD, Blanchard TL, Brinsko SP: Estrogens, osytocin and ergot alkaloids – uses in reproductive management of mares. Proc AAEP 1988; 219-241.

94. Nett TM, Pickett BW: Effect of diethylstilboestrol on the relationship between LH, PMSG and progesterone during pregnancy in the mare. J Reprod Fertil 1979; (Suppl):465-470.

95. Pashen RL, Allen WR: The role of the fetal gonads and placenta in steroid production, maintenance of pregnancy and parturition in the mare. J Reprod Fertil 1979; (Suppl):499-509.

96. Pycock JF, Newcombe JR: The effect of the gonadotropin-releasing-hormone analog, Buserelin, administered in diestrus on pregnancy rates and pregnancy failure in mares. Theriogenology 1996; 46:1097-1101.

97. Newcombe JR, Martinez TA, Peters AR: The effect of the gonadotropin-releasing hormone analog, buserelin, on pregnancy rates in horse and pony mares. Theriogenology 2001; 55:1619-1631.

98. Unger C, Schneider F, Hoppen HO et al: Pregnancy rates in mares after application of gonadotropin releasing hormone analogue, Buserelin, in warmblood mares. Theriogenology 2002; 58:635-638.

99. McKinnon AO, Voss JL: Breeding the problem mare. In McKinnon AO, Voss JL (eds). Equine Reproduction, Philadelphia, London, Lea & Febiger, pp 368-378, 1993.

100. McKinnon AO: Why is my mare losing her pregnancy? Equine Research Seminar 1998. 119-144. University of Sydney, Post Graduate Foundation in Veterinary Science, Sydney. Equine Research Seminar 98.

101. Gilbert RO, Marlow CHB: A field study of patterns of unobserved foetal loss as determined by rectal palpation in foaling, barren and maiden thoroughbred mares. Equine Vet J 1992; 24:184-186.

102. Santschi EM, LeBlanc MM: Fetal and placental conditions that cause high-risk pregnancy in mares. Compend Cont Educ Pract Vet 1995; 17:710-721.

103. Zingher AC: Effects of immunostimulation with Propionibacterium-Acnes (Eqstim(R)) in mares cytologically positive for endometritis. J Equine Vet Sci 1996; 16:100-103.

104. Fumuso E, Gigure S, Wade J et al: Endometrial IL-1 beta, IL-6 and TNF-alpha, mRNA expression in mares resistant or susceptible to post-breeding endometritis – Effects of estrous cycle, artificial insemination and immunomodulation. Vet Immunol Immunopathol 2003; 96:31-41.

CHAPTER 58

Late Term Pregnancy Monitoring

VIRGINIA B. REEF

The equine biophysical profile was developed to help the clinician recognize and more accurately characterize the intrauterine problems in late-gestation mares that affect fetal well-being.[1,2] The information obtained is used to formulate a treatment plan designed to improve the outcome, thereby decreasing fetal morbidity and mortality.[1,2] The human biophysical profile has been routinely used to identify fetal and intrauterine conditions that predispose to fetal compromise, distress, or death in utero.[3,4] Five variables are included in the human biophysical profile: fetal breathing movements, gross body movements, fetal tone, reactive heart rate, and a 2-cm (minimum) pocket of amniotic fluid.[3,4] Each variable receives a score of 2 if the minimal criteria are met and 0 if they are not. To calculate the biophysical profile these scores are summed, resulting in a total score between 0 and 10 for each fetus. The biophysical profile is a measure of the well-being of the fetus, in particular the likelihood of acute or chronic fetal hypoxemia and asphyxia.[3,4] The biophysical profile score is highly correlated with perinatal mortality and morbidity in the human fetus.[3,4] A low score indicates fetal distress and the need for immediate intervention, whereas a high score is compatible with fetal well-being.[3,4] The biophysical profile is used in late-gestation pregnancies to help the obstetrician decide when to intervene (either by inducing parturition or performing a cesarean section) and has helped reduce the incidence of fetal death.

DEVELOPMENT OF THE EQUINE BIOPHYSICAL PROFILE

The equine biophysical profile was developed after examining a normal population of mares in late gestation and three populations of high-risk pregnant mares.[1,2,5,6] The normal population of late-gestation mares included normal pregnant mares who had ultrasonography performed in late gestation, no illness on admission, uneventful pregnancies, and normal foals. The high-risk pregnancies included all late-gestation pregnant mares who had ultrasonography performed and had an illness on admission, an abnormal parturition, and/or an abnormal foal. All fetuses were greater than 298 days' gestational age at the time of the last examination. Mares whose foal was delivered by cesarean section were excluded from these studies. Earlier work by Adams-Brendemuehl and Pipers[7-10] described the technique of transabdominal ultrasonography of the pregnant mare,

normal findings during gestation, and abnormalities detected in late gestation as well as earlier in gestation.

ULTRASONOGRAPHIC EXAMINATION

Patient Preparation

The mare's ventral abdomen is clipped with No. 40 surgical clipper blades from the xiphoid to the pubis and laterally to the level of the flank fold. The skin is then washed thoroughly with warm water and surgical scrub to free the skin of all the surface debris. Ultrasound coupling gel is then applied to the clipped area, and the ultrasonographic examination is performed. If image quality is poor, the ventral abdomen should be examined for areas that are poorly clipped or where surface debris remains on the skin. Applying warmed coupling gel may also help improve image quality. To perform the transcutaneous examination, unsedated mares are scanned from the ventral abdomen using a 2.5-, 3.0-, or 3.5-MHz transducer and a depth setting of 26 to 30 cm and a 5.0-, 6.0-, or 7.5-MHz transducer and a depth setting of 12 to 20 cm, as has been previously described.[1,2,5,8-10] The lowest frequency transducer with the largest displayed depth available should be used for the initial uteral, fetal fluid, and fetal examination. The highest frequency transducer available that obtains a good-quality image with the smallest depth setting that displays the uterus and allantochorion should be used for the uteroplacental evaluations. The transcutaneous evaluation of the uterus, fetal membranes, and fetus are also combined with a transrectal fetal evaluation evaluating the uterus, the fetal membranes, fetal parts, and fetal fluids imageable from the transrectal window.

Fetal Assessments

Fetal Numbers
Fetal numbers are assessed. The typical "cut-pie" appearance of the nonfetal horn should be visible.

Fetal Position
Fetal position within the uterus is determined relative to the long axis of the mare.

Fetal Aortic Diameter
Fetal aortic diameter is measured from the leading edge to leading edge in the ascending aorta, close to the heart.

Fetal aortic diameter is a reliable indicator of fetal size.[1,2,5,6]

Fetal Thoracic Diameter

Maximal fetal thoracic diameter is measured across the widest portion of the thorax at the level of the diaphragm (withers to girth if possible). This is a fairly good indicator of fetal size but less reliable than fetal aortic diameter.[1,2,5,6]

Fetal Breathing

The fetus is evaluated for the presence of breathing movements and their regularity. The excursions of the fetal ribs are assessed, and the diaphragm is evaluated for contractions. Fetal breathing should be evaluated for a minimum of 30 seconds in the absence of fetal movement.[2,6]

Fetal Cardiac Activity

Fetal heart rates and rhythm are obtained with M-mode echocardiography at rest and after fetal movement.[1,2,6] The M-mode cursor is passed through any portion of the fetal heart where cardiac motion is detected, and an instantaneous fetal heart rate is obtained. Fetal heart rate can be obtained with instantaneous M-mode echocardiography in moving fetuses in most instances and is an indication of the normal heart rate variability in response to fetal movement.

Fetal Activity

Fetal activity is graded (0 to 3)[1,2,5,6] as follows:

  0 No activity witnessed during the entire examination
  1 Moves ≤33% of the examination time
  2 Moves >33% but ≤66% of the examination time
  3 Moves >66% of the examination time

Fetal Tone

Fetal tone is assessed as present or absent. Fetal tone is absent if the fetus appears limp.[1,2,5,6]

Fetal Fluids

Maximal vertical amniotic and allantoic fluid pocket depths are measured in six areas (cranial, mid, and caudal on each side of the fetus). The character of allantoic and amniotic fluid is assessed (0 to 3)[1,2,5,6] as follows:

  0 No particles observed during the entire examination
  1 Few particles observed ≤33% of the time
  2 Moderate amount of particles; particles observed >33% but ≤66% of the examination time
  3 Clouds of particles; observed >66% of the time

Maternal Assessments

Uteroplacental Thickness

The thickness of the uteroplacental unit is measured in each of the six areas (cranial, mid, and caudal on each side of the fetus). Measurements should be made in areas where the fetus is not lying against the ventral portion of the uterus, compressing the membranes.[1,2,5,6] Both the maximal and minimal uteroplacental thickness should be obtained.[6] Measurements should not be made in the non-fetal horn.[1,2,5,6]

Uteroplacental Contact

The contact between the uterus and the placenta is evaluated throughout the imageable portions of the uterus, and disruptions in uteroplacental contact are noted and measured.[1,2,5,6]

NORMAL FINDINGS

Fetal Numbers and Presentation

Normal mares in late gestation should have a single active fetus in anterior presentation.[1,2] The fetal head should be visible from a transrectal window in late gestation but not from a transcutaneous window.[2,6] Earlier in gestation until approximately 9 months, the fetus may be in any position. The fetal head may normally be imaged from the transcutaneous window before 298 days of gestation (Figure 58-1).

Fetal Aortic and Thoracic Diameter

The diameter of the fetal aorta (mean = 22.8 ± 2.15 mm) is significantly correlated with neonatal foal weight ($P < 0.0008$, $r = 0.72$) and maternal prepartum weight ($P < 0.002$, $r = 0.86$) in the late gestation fetus.[1,2] The fetal aorta is recognized as the circular artery centrally located in the heart (Figure 58-2). Fetal aortic diameter and thoracic diameter increase gradually throughout gestation. There is a trend for the maximal thoracic diameter to be associated with neonatal foal weight. In the normal fetus the thoracic diameter is approximately 10 times the fetal aortic diameter. This relationship holds true throughout most of gestation.

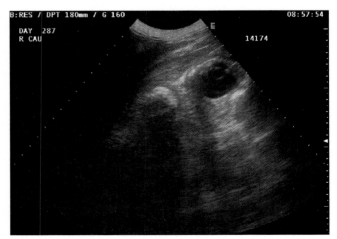

Figure 58-1 Transcutaneous sonogram of the fetal eye obtained at 287 days of gestation from the right caudal portion of the abdomen. Notice the anechoic lens surrounded by the echoic lens capsule within the fetal eye. This sonogram was obtained with a wide bandwidth 4.0-MHz convex linear array transducer imaging at 6.0 MHz and a displayed depth of 18 cm.

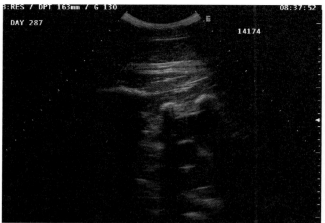

Figure 58-2 Transcutaneous sonogram of the fetal aorta within the fetal heart obtained at 287 days of gestation from the right side of the ventral abdomen. The fetal thorax is lying along the ventral aspect of the uterus, and the fetus is in an anterior presentation because caudal is to the left of the image. The fetal aorta is the anechoic circular structure in the center of the fetal thorax. This sonogram was obtained with a wide bandwidth 4.0-MHz convex linear array transducer imaging at 6.0 MHz with a displayed depth of 16.3 cm.

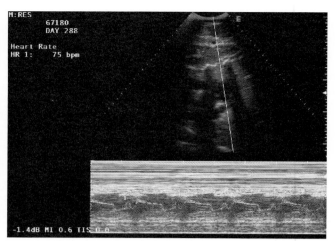

Figure 58-3 Transcutaneous sonogram of the fetal heart obtained at 288 days of gestation from the ventral abdomen near the mare's umbilicus. Notice the M-mode cursor bisecting the fetal heart, yielding the M-mode echocardiogram of the mitral valve within the fetal heart below. The fetal heart rate of 75 beats per minute was then calculated by placing a cursor at the same spot of the mitral valve at the same stage of the cardiac cycle on two consecutive beats. This sonogram was obtained with a wide bandwidth 4.0-MHz convex linear array transducer imaging at 6.0 MHz with a displayed depth of 21 cm.

Fetal Breathing and Cardiac Activity

There should be rhythmic fetal breathing present in late gestation, including movement of the ribs and contractions of the diaphragm.[6] The time of gestation at which fetal breathing movements first develop is currently unknown in the equine fetus. Normal late-term fetuses had a regular cardiac rhythm with a mean heart rate of 75 ± 7 beats per minute (Figure 58-3).[1,2,5,6] The fetal heart rate is associated with fetal gestational age and gradually decreases throughout gestation.[1,2,5,6] The equine fetal heart rate is slowest immediately before parturition. Fetal heart rate should increase with fetal activity.

Fetal Activity and Tone

The fetuses are normally active for approximately half of the normal ultrasonographic examination and have good fetal tone (fetal tone present).[1,2,5,6] This appears to be true throughout gestation.

Fetal Fluids

The maximal vertical depth of amniotic fluid surrounding the fetus in late gestation (7.9 ± 3.5 cm) is less than that of allantoic fluid (13.4 ± 4.4 cm), and few echogenic particles were detected in amniotic or allantoic fluid (Figure 58-4).[1,2,5] Fetal movement and transport of the mare stir up the particles. The particles in the amniotic fluid include cells shed from the fetal skin. Earlier in gestation there should be no echogenic particles detected in the fetal fluids. A hippomane is routinely detected in the allantoic fluid cavity of the late-gestation mare and is usually located near the withers of the fetus (Figure 58-5).

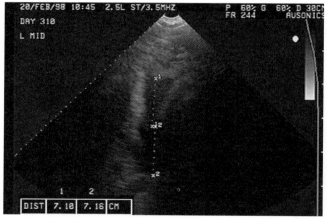

Figure 58-4 Transcutaneous sonogram of the fetal fluids obtained at 310 days of gestation from the left midventral portion of the mare's abdomen. The maximal vertical allantoic fluid depth is measured from the chorioallantois to the amnion (1×) and measures 7.10 cm, whereas the maximal vertical amniotic fluid depth is measured from the amnion to the fetus (2×) and measures 7.18 cm. This measurement is obtained in the fetal axilla, where the largest pocket of amniotic fluid is usually found. This sonogram was obtained with a wide bandwidth 2.5-MHz sector scanner transducer imaging at 3.5 MHz with a displayed depth of 30 cm.

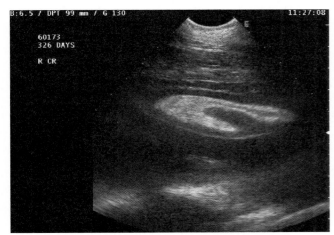

Figure 58-5 Transcutaneous sonogram of the hippomane in the allantoic fluid cavity obtained at 326 days of gestation from the right cranial portion of the ventral abdomen. Notice the hypoechoic and echoic concentric layering of the hippomane and its oval shape. This sonogram was obtained with a wide bandwidth 4.0-MHz convex linear array transducer imaging at 6.0 MHz with a displayed depth of 21 cm.

The hippomane moves freely within the allantoic fluid cavity with fetal movement.

Uteroplacental Thickness and Contact

The maximal uteroplacental thickness in late gestation is 1.15 ± 0.24 cm in the fetal horn (Figure 58-6).[1,2,5] This is true for the uteroplacental areas imaged transcutaneously, as well as those imaged transrectally.[11] Measurements in the tip of the nonfetal horn will be much thicker and should not be used. Earlier in gestation the combined thickness of the uteroplacental unit is less.[11] Uteroplacental thickness gradually increases with gestational age and should be no thicker than the gestational age of the fetus in mm plus 1 (e.g., at 5 months' gestation the combined uteroplacental thickness should not exceed 6 mm). Occasionally, small anechoic spaces are imaged between the uterus and placenta in normal pregnancies.

ABNORMAL FINDINGS

Fetal Numbers

Twins should be suspected if the nonfetal horn is not imaged in the late-gestation pregnant mare. The uterus should be carefully examined for two fetuses. A vertical membrane separating one fetus from the rest of the uterus represents the area of placental contact in a mare with twins.[2] The fetal thoraxes are the most recognizable structures of the fetuses (Figure 58-7). The fetal thoraxes should be carefully evaluated to determine if there is a fetal heart rate (fetal viability) and to determine if two different heart rates are present (common with twin pregnancies). Fetal heart rates should be measured with M-mode echocardiography, yielding an instantaneous

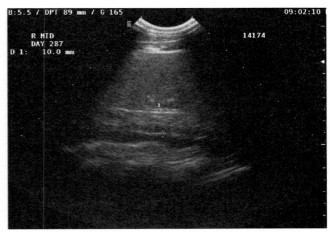

Figure 58-6 Transcutaneous sonogram of the uteroplacental unit obtained at 287 days of gestation. The normal uterus appears slightly more echoic than the allantochorion and together they measure 10 mm (1×). The fetus is lying immediately dorsal to the allantochorion with a small layer of hypoechoic allantoic fluid between the fetus and the placenta. This mare has a large area of heteroechoic fat immediately ventral to the uterus. This sonogram was obtained with a wide bandwidth 6.0-MHz microconvex linear array transducer imaging at 5.5 MHz with a displayed depth of 8.9 cm.

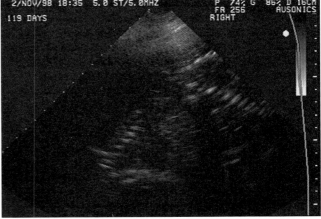

Figure 58-7 Transcutaneous sonogram of twin fetuses in utero obtained at 119 days of gestation. Notice the two triangular thoraxes separated by their adjacent hypoechoic placentas. This sonogram was obtained from the right caudal and ventral abdomen with a 5.0-MHz sector scanner transducer with a displayed depth of 16 cm.

fetal heart rate. If twins are present, the fetal thoraxes should be measured, and, if possible, the aortic diameter should be measured to determine fetal size. With most twin pregnancies there is a discrepancy in fetal size. Fetal mummies are difficult to diagnose because of their few readily identifiable parts and the lack of fetal fluids that surround them. The fetal thorax, identified as a hyperechoic triangular-shaped structure, may be the only iden-

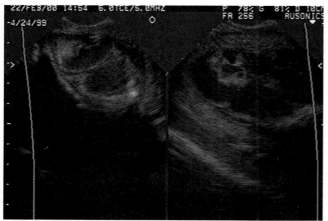

Figure 58-8 Transrectal sonogram of the eponychium on the bottom of the fetal foot obtained at 285 days of gestation. The right image is a long-axis view of the tissue on the bottom of the foot, and the left image is the corresponding short-axis image of the eponychium with the adjacent anechoic amniotic fluid. These sonograms were obtained using a 6.0-MHz wide bandwidth microconvex transducer imaging at 5.0 MHz using a displayed depth of 10 cm.

tifiable structure with mummification of the equine fetus. Be careful not to confuse the eponychium associated with the fetal foot for a mummified fetus (Figure 58-8).

Fetal Positioning

The positioning of the fetus(es) in utero is also helpful in confirming the presence of twins. Often the twins will be in different positions (one anterior and one posterior), making confirming the existence of twins easier. The detection of the fetal head in late gestation (≥ 298 days) is abnormal and may indicate an abnormal head position.[2,6] The fetuses with this sonographic finding in late gestation have all required assistance at the time of parturition because the head was back. With fetal death the fetus curls up on its long axis. The fetal head and neck are usually imaged along the ventral abdomen of the dead fetus.

Fetal Breathing

Irregularities in the breathing movements of the fetus are an indication of fetal stress in the late-gestation fetus. Absence of fetal breathing movements is a more severe indication of fetal stress and is probably associated with fetal hypoxia.[6]

Fetal Cardiac Activity

Fetal heart rate is too high if it is greater than 126 beats per minute for fetuses greater than 298 days of gestation. Fetal heart rate is too low if it is less than 57 beats per minute if gestational age is less than 330 days, less than 50 beats per minute if gestational age is 330 to 360 days, and less than 41 beats per minute if gestational age is greater than 360 days.[6] A range of fetal heart rates of less

than 5 beats per minute or greater than 150 beats per minute is abnormal.[6] Fetal cardiac arrhythmias are also abnormal.[1,2,5,6] Fetal heart rates that do not increase during periods of fetal activity are abnormal.

Fetal Aortic Diameter

Aortic diameter is predicted from the following regression equation:[1,2,5,6]

$$(Y = 0.00912*X + 12.46)$$

where

      Y = predicted aortic diameter
      X = the pregnant mare's weight in pounds
     * = multiplied by

A fetal aortic diameter with a standard error (5.038) 4 times larger or smaller than predicted is abnormal. Fetal aortic diameter of less than 18.5 mm in a late-term fetus is indicative of intrauterine growth retardation or twins.[1,2,5,6]

Fetal Thoracic Diameter

The maximal width of the fetal thorax is also an indicator of fetal size and is correlated with neonatal foal weight. A smaller-than-normal fetal thoracic diameter is also an indication of intrauterine growth retardation or twins.[1,2,5,6]

Fetal Activity

Any fetus that is inactive during the entire examination is considered abnormal, because this lack of movement was not detected in any normal fetuses.[1,2,5,6] Although quiet periods of up to 1 hour have been described in late-term equine fetuses with Doppler evaluations, this has not been seen in normal late-term fetuses with transcutaneous ultrasonography. Thus any periods of prolonged inactivity of the late-term equine fetus should be considered an indication of fetal stress and probable fetal hypoxia.

Fetal Tone

Lack of fetal tone is detectable as a limp fetus along the floor of the uterus in the ventral abdomen and is an indication of advanced fetal stress and severe fetal hypoxia.[1,2,5,6]

Fetal Fluids

The maximal vertical allantoic fluid depth in late gestation is abnormal if it is less than 47 mm or greater than 221 mm, and the maximal vertical amniotic fluid depth is abnormal if less than 8 mm or greater than 185 mm.[1,2,5,6] The lack of an adequate volume of fluid surrounding the fetus is associated with probable prolonged fetal hypoxia or the premature rupture of the fetal membranes. Excessive quantities of amniotic fluid may be associated with abnormalities of fetal swallowing. With

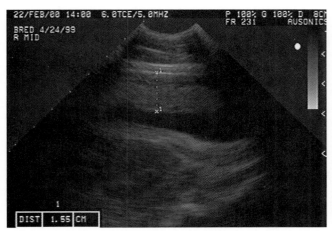

Figure 58-9 Sonogram of a thickened uteroplacental unit obtained at 285 days of gestation. Notice the thickened echoic allantochorion resulting in a combined uteroplacental thickness of 1.55 cm. Immediately dorsal to the thickened allantochorion is normal anechoic allantoic fluid and the fetus. This sonogram was obtained with a wide bandwidth 6.0-MHz microconvex linear array transducer imaging at 5.0 MHz with a displayed depth of 8 cm.

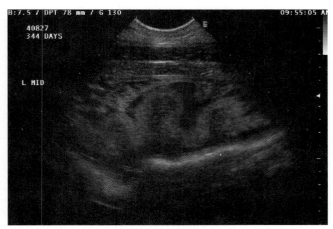

Figure 58-10 Transcutaneous sonogram of the uteroplacental unit obtained at 344 days of gestation. Notice the marked folding of the allantochorion with anechoic fluid between the uterus and the chorioallantois resulting in a combined uteroplacental thickness of 2.5 to 3.0 cm. This sonogram was obtained with a wide bandwidth 6.0-MHz microconvex linear array transducer imaging at 7.5 MHz with a displayed depth of 7.8 cm.

fetal death the fluids surrounding the fetus disappear as the fetus mummifies.

Both the amniotic and allantoic fluid may occasionally have clouds of particles detected, particularly after the mare ships to a referral institution or after fetal movement. Seeing clouds of particles throughout the examination is abnormal in late gestation. Large particulate debris in the amniotic fluid is indicative of fetal stress and may result in meconium staining of the fetus.

Uteroplacental Thickness

For the biophysical profile, the maximum uteroplacental thickness is abnormal if it is greater than 24 mm, and the minimal uteroplacental thickness is abnormal if it is less than 3.9 mm.[1,2,5,6] However, the mare should be treated for a probable placentitis if the uteroplacental thickness is greater than or equal to 15 mm in late gestation (Figure 58-9), as long as this measurement is not in the nonfetal horn. Significant uteroplacental thickening is consistent with placentitis or placental edema, whereas thinner-than-normal uteroplacental thickness indicates fibrosis and placental insufficiency. Placental folding outside of the nonfetal horn also occurs with placentitis and placental edema and is another indication of placental pathologic condition when detected in the fetal horn with placental thickening (Figure 58-10). Aggressive treatment of uteroplacental thickening caused by placentitis has resulted in improved outcomes, both in late gestation and in mares in which thickening of the uteroplacental unit has been detected in midgestation.[11]

Uteroplacental Disruption

Any large disruptions in uteroplacental contact are abnormal and indicative of premature placental separation

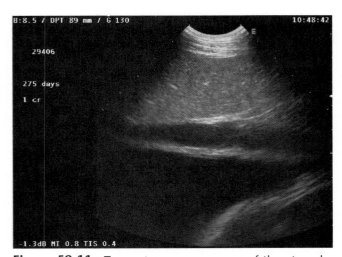

Figure 58-11 Transcutaneous sonogram of the uteroplacental unit obtained at 275 days of gestation from the left cranial portion of the abdomen. Notice the anechoic separation of the uterus and the placenta. This sonogram was obtained with a wide bandwidth 4.0-MHz convex linear array transducer imaging at 6.0 MHz with a displayed depth of 21 cm.

(Figure 58-11).[1,2,5,6] If these disruptions are extensive or progressive and the mare is in late gestation, induction of parturition may be indicated.

EQUINE BIOPHYSICAL PROFILE

The results from the normal pregnancies were compared with data obtained from fetuses of comparable gestational age from high-risk pregnancies to develop a biophysical profile specific for the equine fetus.[1,2,5,6] All fetuses that lacked breathing movements or had irregular breathing movements were abnormal. All fetuses that were inactive throughout the entire scan were abnormal at birth. All fetuses surrounded by decreased allantoic fluid quantities were abnormal at birth, with one exception. All fetuses with excessive amniotic fluid quantities were abnormal. All mares with large and progressive areas of placental separation delivered abnormal foals, with one exception. All mares with thickened uteroplacental units delivered abnormal foals, with one exception, and all mares with abnormally thin uteroplacental units delivered abnormal foals. The majority of foals with heart rate abnormalities were abnormal. There was a significant correlation between fetal aortic diameter and neonatal foal weight in these complicated pregnancies ($P < 0.0001$, $r = 0.85$). All small for gestational age fetuses were abnormal and were either twins or dysmature with intrauterine growth retardation.

Seven factors are included in the biophysical profile of the equine fetus (298 days' gestational age to term) that are indicative of fetal well-being, perinatal morbidity, and perinatal mortality.[1,2,5,6] The seven factors related to pregnancy outcome are fetal heart evaluation (heart rate, variation, and rhythm), fetal aortic diameter, fetal breathing movements, maximal fetal fluid depths, uteroplacental contact, uteroplacental thickness, and fetal activity. Although a low score was a definite indication of an impending negative outcome, a perfect score was not assurance of a positive outcome.[1,2,5,6] A score of 10 or less out of 14 is associated with the birth of an abnormal foal.[6]

Fetal distress is present when there is a decrease in any variable in the human biophysical profile. Decreased or absent fetal breathing movements, reactive heart rate, gross body movements, and/or fetal tone occur with acute hypoxia.[3,4] The disappearance of reactive fetal heart rate and fetal breathing are early manifestations of hypoxemia and acidemia, whereas the lack of fetal movement or fetal tone is associated with advanced hypoxemia, acidemia, and hypercapnea.[3,4] Decreased amniotic fluid depth indicates chronic fetal hypoxia in human beings.[3,4] Intrauterine growth retardation is assessed ultrasonographically in human fetuses but is not included in the human fetal biophysical profile.

Four of the seven factors that were related to outcome (fetal heart rate, fetal breathing, fetal movement, and fetal fluid quantities) are also incorporated in the human biophysical profile. The other three factors that were related to outcome in the equine fetus are fetal aortic diameter, uteroplacental contact, and uteroplacental thickness. These factors are most likely significant in the

equine late-gestation pregnancy and not in the human due to the differences in placentation between the species.

CONCLUSION

The equine biophysical profile, the signs of fetal distress, and the abnormal intrauterine conditions can be used to decide when and how to intervene in a high-risk pregnancy and in preparing for peripartum and postpartum complications.

References

1. Reef VB, Vaala WE, Worth LT et al: Transabdominal ultrasonographic assessment of fetal well-being during late gestation: a preliminary report on the development of an equine biophysical profile. Equine Vet J 1995; 28:200-208.
2. Reef VB: Fetal ultrasonography. In Reef VB (ed): Equine Diagnostic Ultrasound, Philadelphia, WB Saunders, 1998.
3. Manning FA, Harman CR, Menticoglou S et al: Assessment of fetal well-being with ultrasound. Obstet Gynecol Clin North Am 1991; 18:891-905.
4. Vintzileos AM, Fleming AD, Scorza WE et al: Relationship between fetal biophysical activities and umbilical cord blood gas values. Am J Obstet Gynecol 1991; 165:707-713.
5. Reef VB, Vaala WE, Worth L et al: Transabdominal ultrasonographic evaluation of the fetus and intrauterine environment in healthy mares during late gestation. Vet Radiol Ultrasound 1995; 36:533-541.
6. Worth L: Personal communication, Unpublished data, 2003.
7. Pipers FS, Zent W, Holder R et al: Ultrasonography as an adjunct to pregnancy assessments in the mare. J Am Vet Med Assoc 1984; 184:328-334.
8. Pipers FS, Adams-Brendemuehl CS: Techniques and applications of transabdominal ultrasonography in the pregnant mare. Am J Vet Med Assoc 1984; 185:766-771.
9. Adams-Brendemuehl CS, Pipers FS: Antepartum evaluations of the equine fetus. J Reprod Fertil Suppl 1987; 35:565-573.
10. Adams-Brendemuehl CS: Fetal assessment. In Koterba AM, Drummond WH, Kosch PC (eds): Equine Clinical Neonatology, Philadelphia, Lea & Febiger, 1990.
11. Troedsson MHT, Renaudin CD, Zent WW et al: Transrectal ultrasonography of the placenta in normal mares and mares with pending abortion: a field study. Proceedings of the 43rd Annual Convention of the American Association of Equine Practitioners, pp 256-258, 1997.
12. Sertich P, Reef VB, Oristaglio-Turner RM et al: Hydrops amnii in a mare. J Am Vet Med Assoc 1994; 204:1-2.
13. Renaudin CD, Troedsson MHT, Gillis CL et al: Ultrasonographic evaluation of the equine placenta by transrectal and transabdominal approach in the normal pregnant mare. Theriogenology 1997; 47:559-573.

CHAPTER 59

Dystocia and Fetotomy

GRANT S. FRAZER

TERMINOLOGY

In any discussion of obstetrics it is essential that there be a uniform appreciation of the terminology. *Dystocia* is defined as being abnormal or difficult labor—be it maternal (e.g., uterine torsion, pelvic anomaly, abdominal hernia) or fetal (size, presentation, position, posture) in origin.[1,2] While premature separation of the placenta ("red bag" delivery) meets this description, retention of the fetal membranes—an abnormality of stage III of labor—is not generally regarded as being a dystocia in the veterinary context. The terms *malpresented fetus* and *malpositioned fetus* are often used erroneously when the intent is to convey that the fetal head and/or neck—or one or more limbs—was not correctly aligned within the birth canal. It may be preferable to note that the fetus is maldisposed (*fetal maldisposition*) because this is an all-encompassing term that implies any combination of abnormalities—in presentation, position, and/or posture.[3] *Presentation* describes the orientation of the fetal spinal axis to that of the mare and also the portion of the fetus that enters the vaginal canal first (cranial or caudal longitudinal; ventrotransverse or dorsotransverse). Although the words *anterior* and *posterior* are still widely used in the veterinary literature, the correct Nomina Anatomica Veterinaria terms are *cranial* and *caudal*. *Position* describes the relationship of the fetal dorsum (longitudinal presentation) or head (transverse presentation) to the quadrants of the mare's pelvis (dorsosacral, right/left dorsoilial, dorsopubic; right/left cephaloilial). *Posture* pertains to the fetus itself and describes the relationship of the extremities (head, neck, limbs) to the foal's body. Postural abnormalities can be difficult to correct due to the remarkably long head, neck, and limbs of the foal. *Repulsion* describes the procedure whereby the fetus is repelled from the pelvic inlet such that the increased space in the uterus can be used to correct the maldisposition.[4] *Mutation* is an obstetrical term that is used to describe manipulation of the fetal extremities, together with correction of any positional abnormalities, such that assisted vaginal delivery can proceed. *Version* is the manual changing of the polarity of the fetus with reference to the mother. It is the manipulation that is employed when attempting to correct a transverse presentation. The head and forelimbs are repelled into the uterus, while the hindquarters are pulled into the pelvic canal.[4] Tocolytic agents (clenbuterol, isoxsuprine) inhibit myometrial contractions. These agents are administered by injection in many countries to relax the uterus and thus provide more space for obstetrical manipulations.[4,5]

THE PREPARTUM MARE

A ventral, edematous plaque of variable thickness (2 to 4 inches) may develop in late gestation. The increased weight of the gravid uterus affects lymphatic drainage and venous return from the ventral abdomen. This physiologic phenomenon must be differentiated from the painful inflammatory edema that is associated with impending—or actual—ventral body wall rupture (prepubic tendon, ventral hernia). In these cases the mare may be reluctant to move, the mammary secretions will often contain blood, and ultrasonography can demonstrate tearing and edema within the musculature. A canvas abdominal sling may provide sufficient support to permit some of these mares to carry the foal to term.[1]

Changes in the hormonal milieu during the last weeks and days of gestation result in physical changes in the mare—but the signs of impending parturition are quite variable between mares. Relaxation of the sacrosciatic ligaments may cause a discernible hollow to develop on either side of the tail head, especially in older mares. This change may not be evident in a well-muscled mare. Even when visible relaxation is not apparent, a palpable softening of the ligaments may be detected. Any elongation and relaxation of the vulva tends not to be noticeable until foaling is imminent. The most notable change is usually in the mammary gland. The pregnant mare's udder may start to increase in size during the last 4 to 6 weeks of gestation, and it generally becomes prominent within 2 weeks of foaling. The size of the udder is influenced by the parity of the mare, and some maiden mares will foal with minimal mammary changes. The onset of secretory activity is quite variable and cannot be used as a reliable indicator of impending parturition. Some mares may be observed to develop waxlike material on the teat orifices ("wax up") several days before foaling, whereas others may never develop these honey-colored beads of dried secretion on the teat orifices. The teats usually fill with colostrum 24 to 48 hours before foaling, but some mares may drip or "run" milk for several days before the onset of parturition. In these cases a substantial volume of colostrum may be lost, and plans should be made to supplement the foal's immunoglobulin intake. Electrolyte changes in mammary secretions can be used to predict "readiness for birth" if an observed parturition or a planned cesarean section (e.g., pelvic callus) has become necessary.[6-8] However, these electrolyte changes are not a reliable indicator of fetal maturity if a placental anomaly is present (e.g., placentitis, twins).

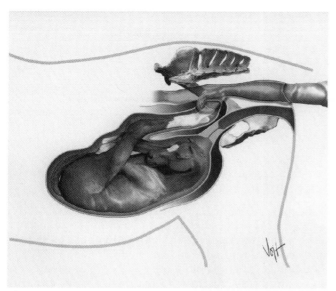

Figure 59-1 In late gestation the horn containing the hindlimbs comes to rest on the dorsal surface of the uterine body, with the tip of the horn directed towards the cervix. Although the forelimbs and neck are usually flexed, on some occasions the head or limbs may be extended. In some cases the hindlimbs may push the horn tip caudally such that the hooves come to lie over the fetal head.

By late gestation, the orientation of the uterine horns has changed dramatically, with the horn containing the hindlimbs coming to rest on the dorsal surface of the uterine body, with the tip of the horn directed towards the cervix.[9,10] Close to term the uterine body and gravid horn form what can be described as a U-shaped tube that tapers towards the tip. In some cases it is possible for the hindlimb hooves in the horn tip to be pushed so far caudally that they actually come to lie over the fetal head. Thus, when performing a per rectum evaluation of the pregnancy close to term, the fetal hooves that are palpable may sometimes be attached to the hindlimbs (Figure 59-1). Vigorous pistonlike thrusts of the hindlimbs, in association with elevation of the fetal rump, can result in the hooves being pushed well past the cervix into the rectogenital pouch.[9-11] This observation may explain the acute colic episodes that have been previously attributed to uterine dorsoretroflexion.[5] Although the gel-like pads on the fetal hooves may serve to protect the placenta and uterine wall from the vigorous activity of the hindlimbs, tears at the tip of the gravid horn can still occur during an unassisted foaling.[10,12-14]

A classic radiographic study demonstrated that the full-term equine fetus is lying in a dorsopubic position with the head, neck, and forelimbs flexed.[15] Although the caudal aspect of the fetus is in a dorsopubic position and intimately associated with the ventral uterine wall, the cranial portion has room to rotate within the uterine body itself. Recent ultrasonographic studies have shown that in a mare close to term (>330 days of gestation) the cranial aspect of the fetus may be in dorsopubic position approximately 60% of the time and in dorsoilial position during about 40% of observations. Although the fore-

limbs and neck are usually flexed (about 80%), on some occasions the head or limbs may be extended.[10,11] Thus palpation of the fetus cannot be used to detect impending dystocia (postural or positional complications) unless labor is already well advanced. However, if a transverse or caudal presentation is suspected, then a detailed transabdominal ultrasonographic evaluation is indicated to confirm the location of the fetal thorax and head. In both cases planned intervention may be warranted. In some cases transabdominal ultrasound may suggest that a fetus is transversely presented, yet the foal will be delivered normally. The so-called "body pregnancy" tends to cause abortion in the latter stages of gestation when the nutritional demands of the growing fetus are no longer being met. In these cases the placenta is underdeveloped and is characterized by the presence of short horns. It is this lack of development of a gravid horn that causes intrauterine fetal growth retardation and abortion due to placental insufficiency.[16,17]

Until recently it has been difficult to explain how 98.9% of foals are delivered in cranial presentation, with 1.0% being caudal, and only 0.1% being transverse.[3,18] A complex mechanism involving entrapment of the fetal hindlimbs within a uterine horn may be the answer. In early pregnancy, fetal rotation within the amniotic cavity and amniotic sac rotation within the allantoic cavity result in the characteristic twisting of the equine umbilical cord.[19-21] Between 5 and 7 months of gestation it appears that contraction of the horns serves to confine the allantoic fluid and fetus to the uterine body.[9-11,20,22] It has been theorized that neurologic signals within the maturing inner ear may orient the dorsum of the fetus with the concave slope of the ventral uterine wall and prompt it to lie with the cranial aspect elevated towards the cervix.[9-11,22,23] The acute angle between the horn and body by 7 months of gestation means that the fetus must be in dorsal recumbency before the hindlimbs can gain entry. After 9 months the hindlimbs remain enclosed within the uterine horn, and the hooves reach to the tip by the tenth month.[9-11,20,22] Although the fetus is then locked into a cranial presentation and dorsopubic position, it is possible for the entire pregnancy (uterus and fetus) to rotate approximately 90 degrees on the lower maternal abdominal wall. This occurs because any rotational movement of the caudal half of the fetus (pelvis and hindlimbs) by necessity will involve the close-fitting uterus. In extreme cases this rotation may progress into a clinical uterine torsion.[1,10,24]

NORMAL PARTURITION

The first stage of parturition is characterized by the development of coordinated uterine contractions. The increased uterine pressure pushes the chorioallantoic sac (in the region of the cervical star) against the hormonally relaxed cervix such that gradual dilation occurs. Mares vary in their display of symptoms that are consistent with the onset of first-stage labor. In some the increasing intensity of the uterine contractions may be manifest by restless behavior similar to that of mild colic. Patchy sweating often develops, and some mares expel colostrum. The mare may look at her flank, frequently lie down and get

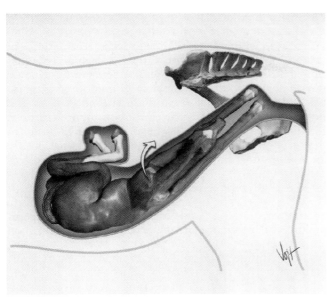

Figure 59-2 The fetus plays an active role in positioning itself for delivery. It must be healthy and viable to be able to make purposeful movements that rotate the cranial aspect through a dorsoilial position while the head and forelimbs are extended up into the birth canal.

up, stretch as if to urinate, and pass small amounts of feces.[4] In some mares a normal delivery may be preceded by one or more episodes of false labor. Although the fetus probably determines the day, the mare appears to be able to choose the hour for delivery. It is not uncommon for labor signs to abate if the mare is unduly disturbed by the external environment. Thus it is important that supervision of foaling mares be unobtrusive. Any untoward activity may lead to a stress response and suppression of uterine contractions—especially in nervous mares.

It has been proposed that the increasing uterine tone during stage I of parturition somehow stimulates the fetus to extend its head and forelimbs.[10] The fetus plays an active role in positioning itself for delivery and makes purposeful movements such that the cranial aspect rotates through a dorsoilial position as the head and forelimbs are extended up into the birth canal[15] (Figure 59-2). The characteristic side-to-side rolling each time the mare assumes lateral recumbency is thought to assist in positioning the foal correctly. Dystocia cases that involve a dorsopubic position with flexed extremities suggest that the fetus was compromised before the start of the parturient process. Such a fetus would not actively participate in the foaling process.[4,10,15,25] In some cases this may be indicative of advanced placentitis or fetal infection, and thus submission of tissue from a stillborn fetus and attendant membranes is recommended.[16] The neck and forelimbs will not normally be returned to a flexed posture once a viable fetus in stage I of delivery has actively extended them. However, fetlock flexion can develop if the hoof catches on the pelvic brim or on a fold of vaginal mucosa. Continued expulsive efforts from the mare can force the carpus to flex as well.[4] The onset of stage II is heralded by rupture of the chorioallantois

and discharge of the watery allantoic fluid. This occurs when the fetlocks—and sometimes the knees—are at the level of the external cervical opening.[10]

While the cranial aspect of the foal is passing through the birth canal, the hindlimbs remain locked within the uterine horn. The second stage of labor is characterized by strong abdominal contractions that provide the expulsive force necessary to expel the fetus. Preexisting defects in the abdominal musculature (prepubic tendon rupture, ventral hernia) adversely affect the mare's ability to mount sufficient intraabdominal pressure to expel the foal without assistance. These mares warrant close supervision because traction may need to be applied to the foal's forelimbs once stage II of labor has commenced.[1] Passage of the foal into the pelvic inlet initiates a reflex release of oxytocin from the posterior pituitary, thereby enhancing uterine contractility.[4] Most mares assume lateral recumbency once active straining commences, although it is not uncommon for the mare to get up once or twice during second stage labor. Appearance of one hoof within the translucent fluid-filled amnion at the vulva lips can be expected to occur within 5 minutes of rupture of the chorioallantois.[26] A dark yellowish green discoloration of the amnion and fluid is indicative of passage of meconium due to fetal stress. One forelimb should precede the other by several inches, such that the shoulders enter the pelvis successively. The measurement across the shoulders represents the widest portion of the foal. Thus the tendency for one limb to advance ahead of the other ensures that the cross-sectional diameter of the fetus at the shoulders is reduced. The soles of the hooves should be directed downward and the foal's head should be resting between the carpi, with the muzzle reaching the proximal metacarpus. By the time the nose reaches the vulva the cranial half of the torso has already rotated from a dorsopubic to a dorsoilial position. The foal's withers continue to rotate into a dorsosacral position as the head appears through the vulvar lips.[10] At this time the foal's shoulders have entered the pelvic canal.

Second stage labor in the mare is rapid, with the most forceful contractions occurring as the fetal thorax passes through the pelvic cavity. The amniotic sac may rupture during these expulsive efforts. However, the foal can be delivered with a portion of the sac wrapped around its head.[26] Although a viable foal should be able to free itself of the fetal membranes, foaling attendants should be instructed to free the foal's head promptly to avoid the possibility of suffocation. The fetal pelvis rotates through a dorsoilial position into a dorsosacral position, and the hindlimbs become extended as the fetal abdomen begins to pass through the vulvar lips. This occurs because at this point the stifles impinge upon the pelvic brim. The foal's rump remains closely apposed to the cranial dome of the uterine body as the contracting uterus and abdominal press combine to expel the foal. Thus at the time of the foal's delivery the cranial aspect of the uterine body is only about 12 inches from the cervix.[10] Forceful straining ceases once the foal's hips are delivered, and most mares will rest in lateral recumbency for several minutes. An active foal will extract its hindlimbs as it struggles to stand.

Most foals are delivered within 20 to 30 minutes after the chorioallantoic membrane ruptures. Primiparous

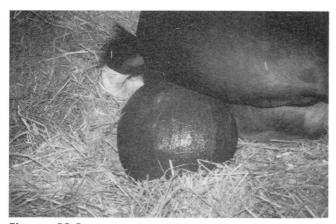

Figure 59-3 If the chorioallantois fails to rupture, the velvety red membrane appears at the vulvar lips ("red bag" delivery). Inevitably there has been premature separation of an excessive amount of the placental attachment. The fetus is likely to be deprived of oxygen, and thus immediate intervention is indicated. The protruding membrane should be manually ruptured and gentle traction applied to the limbs in conjunction with the mare's expulsive efforts.

dams generally require longer to expel the fetus than multiparous dams.[4,26] Delayed delivery (prolonged foaling time) increases the likelihood of fetal asphyxia or neonatal problems associated with hypoxia due to placental separation.[16,27] Often these losses occur in mares that were unattended at the time of foaling. The short, explosive birth process and the mare's tendency to foal at night increase the probability of unattended delivery.[27] Prepartum mares warrant close attention because careful monitoring of parturition may help to reduce the incidence of deaths attributable to neonatal asphyxia. A number of foaling monitors and video camera systems are available to alert personnel that foaling is imminent.[28] Attendants should suspect that the mare is experiencing obstetric problems if either the first or second stage of parturition is prolonged or not progressive. Occasionally the chorioallantois fails to rupture, and the velvety, red membrane ("red bag") appears at the vulvar lips (Figure 59-3). This is a common complication of induced parturition, and placental edema is a major problem in mares that have been exposed to endophyte-infected fescue hay or pasture.[29,30] In the latter scenario the pregnancy may be prolonged, and the mare is also likely to be agalactic. Premature separation of the placenta is an emergency situation because the foal is deprived of its maternal oxygen supply. Foaling attendants should be instructed to break the membrane and to provide gentle traction in unison with the mare's expulsive efforts. Although the foal should be delivered as quickly as possible, injudicious traction at this time can create a laceration in an incompletely dilated cervix.[2]

Experienced personnel can save many foals by early recognition of dystocias and by prompt intervention before serious complications arise. Signs that a mare may be experiencing difficulties include failure of any fetal parts or the amniotic membrane to appear at the vulvar lips within 5 minutes after rupture of the chorioallantois. If there is no evidence of strong contractions, and/or no progression in the delivery process within 10 minutes of rupture of the chorioallantois, then a vaginal examination is warranted. Other causes for concern are hooves upside-down or any abnormal combination of extremities appearing at the vulva (only one limb, hooves and nose in abnormal relationship, nose but not hooves, both forelimbs protruding but no head visible at the level of the carpi).[26] The most common impediments to delivery are malpostures of the long fetal extremities (head and neck, or limbs).[3,4,25] Failure to quickly identify a dystocia often results in the fetus becoming impacted in the birth canal by the mare's uterine contractions and strong abdominal straining. The secret to foal survival is a combination of experience and expediency. If farm personnel are experienced and referring veterinarians are well trained in dystocia management, prompt referral to a hospital in close proximity may permit delivery of a viable foal—even after an hour has elapsed since the chorioallantois ruptured.[31] It is probable that limited intervention causes less disruption of the fetal membranes and thus permits longer placental support of the fetus.

ASSESSMENT OF A DYSTOCIA CASE

The incidence of dystocia varies among breeds, with estimates ranging from 4% in Thoroughbreds to as much as 1 in 10 foalings in the heavily muscled Draft breeds. Hydrocephalus can occur in all breeds. Ponies are more likely to experience difficulties due to a large fetal skull that may resemble hydrocephaly in some cases.[3,32,33] Irrespective of the likelihood of being requested to provide obstetrical assistance to a mare, it is prudent for an equine practitioner to have a well-organized dystocia kit readily accessible for such occasions during the foaling season. Supplies necessary to provide cardiovascular and respiratory support to a compromised neonate should always be available. All equipment should be clean and preferably sterile. A nasogastric tube, pump, and bucket should be kept exclusively for delivering volume-expanding lubricant (e.g., carboxymethylcellulose) into the uterus. This is especially important in those countries (e.g., the United States) where injectable tocolytic agents (clenbuterol, isoxsuprine) are not available for obstetrical use.[4] Obstetrical chains, nylon ropes and handles are the basic requirements, and blunt eye hooks may occasionally be indicated.[2,4,34] A detorsion rod, an obstetrical snare, and a Kuhn's crutch repeller (with long nylon rope) can be useful in some instances—but require additional expertise.[4,35] These metal instruments can easily traumatize the reproductive tract and should be used with caution. Mechanical extractive devices can exert inordinate force and do not have a place in equine obstetrics. Fetotomy in the mare should be performed only by experienced obstetricians. Essential equipment includes a fetotome and threader (with brush), saw wire with handles, wire cutter, curved wire introducer, fetotomy (palm) knife, and a Krey hook.[36,37] Any prior obstetrical experience that has been obtained by managing bovine dystocias will be invaluable when a veterinarian is faced with the long extremities and forceful straining that inevitably complicate the resolution of equine obstetrical cases. A minimum of two people should be available to assist the obstetrician: one to hold the mare's head and at least one other individual to hold instruments and to assist with fetal delivery.

Dystocia in a mare should always be regarded as an emergency, especially if there is a possibility that the foal is still alive. Apart from potential loss of the foal, the mare's future fertility is often compromised, and some may even suffer fatal complications. Upon arrival the veterinarian should make a cursory assessment of the mare's general physical condition, noting in particular mucous membrane color and refill time (hemorrhage, shock).[2] A more complete examination may be indicated once attempts have been made to deliver a viable fetus. Time is the critical factor when managing an equine obstetrical case.[31] The perineal area should be inspected for the presence and nature of any vulvar discharge, the presence of fetal membranes, and to identify any fetal extremities. Excessive hemorrhage is indicative of soft tissue trauma. Moist fetal extremities may help to confirm that assistance was summoned promptly, whereas dry and swollen tissues are typical of more protracted cases. A malodorous discharge strongly suggests the presence of an emphysematous fetus, an uncommon occurrence that may be encountered in neglected cases.[4] Occasionally a foaling mare may present with a rectal prolapse, an everted bladder, or with loops of bowel (small intestine, colon) protruding from the vulvar lips.[2] While performing this external examination of the mare, the veterinarian should obtain the following information from the owner: age and parity number; expected foaling date; duration and intensity of labor signs; time since rupture of the chorioallantois; appearance of fetal membranes, limbs, or muzzle at vulvar lips; and whether any attempts at manual intervention have been made. It is not uncommon to be informed that the muzzle was present when an attempt was made to correct a simple limb malposture. Unfortunately these cases have often been complicated by a flexed head and neck posture before veterinary assistance is requested. Reports of fetal movement observed in the mare's flanks are often unreliable, and the mare's expulsive efforts can easily cause deceptive "movement" of exposed extremities in what is already a dead fetus.

The internal examination should be performed in a clean area with good footing and with sufficient room to ensure safety for all personnel involved. The use of rigid, closed-end stocks is contraindicated because of the propensity for parturient mares to become recumbent. However, adequate restraint is essential because the behavior of a mare in the second stage of labor is so unpredictable—and it can be violent. If used, the stocks should be open-ended with movable sides. Whenever possible, the initial examination should be performed on a standing mare in a large, well-bedded stall with nothing more than a twitch or lip chain for restraint. The person handling the mare should stand on the same side as the obstetrician and apply intermittent tension to the twitch or lip chain when instructed to do so. If the mare attempts to kick, the head should be pulled towards the handler such that the hindquarters will move away from the obstetrician. Although not essential, an initial rectal

examination may rule out the presence of a term uterine torsion, may determine the condition of the uterine wall (tears, spasm), and may provide useful information regarding the disposition of the fetus.[2,24] Before any vaginal examination the mare's tail should be wrapped and the perineal area thoroughly cleansed. The clinician's arms and hands should be scrubbed with disinfectant soap. The use of sterile sleeves is optional. The author routinely uses shoulder length rubber sleeves with surgical gloves attached. Although disposable plastic sleeves decrease tactile sensation, experienced obstetricians believe that the use of a sleeve reduces the amount of trauma inflicted upon the vaginal mucous membranes. Liberal application of lubricant is essential because the mare's vagina and cervix are easily traumatized, and future fertility can be jeopardized by the resultant adhesions and fibrosis. White petroleum jelly (Vaseline) is useful when performing the initial exploratory examination. If there is evidence of prior vaginal manipulations, it may be prudent to perform an abdominocentesis to ensure uterine integrity before instilling large volumes of liquid obstetrical lubricant.[14,38]

A rapid, thorough check should be made for lesions, lacerations, and contusions of the genital tract. The presence of any pelvic abnormalities that may impede passage of the fetus should be noted, the degree of cervical relaxation determined, and an assessment made as to whether or not the uterus is tightly contracted around the fetus. Although fetopelvic disproportion is uncommon in the mare, it can be a factor in some equine dystocias, especially those in primiparous mares.[16,27,39,40] The disposition of the fetus should be noted (presentation, position, and posture) and fetal viability determined.[2] Care should be exercised because an active fetal response to manipulations can easily complicate what was initially a simple dystocia. This is often the cause of the more extreme head and neck malpostures.[2,25,34] Placement of a rope snare behind the ears and into the mouth will ensure that the clinician always has control of the head. This will facilitate easy correction of a potentially life-threatening development such as lateral deviation of the head and neck if the fetus pulls away from the clinician's arm. Although tension on the head snare can force the mouth open, it is unlikely that the incisors will have broken the gum sufficiently to be of concern. Nevertheless, care should be taken to protect the uterus from the exposed incisors if retrieval becomes necessary. A mandibular snare will also suffice, but this should be used only to guide the head back into the pelvic canal. Excessive traction can easily cause a mandibular fracture.[4]

When obvious fetal movement is absent, limb withdrawal may be initiated in response to pinching of the coronary band. Slight digital pressure through the eyelid may arouse a response, as may stimulation of the tongue (swallowing). If the thorax can be reached, fetal heartbeat is definitive. In caudally presented cases, the digital and anal reflexes are useful as indicators of fetal viability.[2,4] Failure to elicit a response is not always an absolute confirmation of fetal death. When there is doubt about fetal viability, an ultrasonographic assessment of the fetal heart may be made with a 3.5-MHz transabdominal probe. If the fetus is in an abnormal position, the clinician should investigate the possibility of a term uterine torsion.[24] Once the cause of the dystocia has been determined, the obstetrician should ensure that the owner understands the various treatment options and costs and the inherent risks that may be associated with each approach. The prognosis for survival of both the mare and foal and the impact of the treatment options on the mare's future fertility should also be discussed. Sometimes the owner will place more value on the mare's nonreproductive attributes, whereas in other cases the mare's future fertility is of paramount importance. The economics of the case, the expertise of the clinician, and the proximity of hospital facilities are all factors to be considered when planning the best course of action to resolve a dystocia case.[2,31,34,36,41,42] Prolonged vaginal manipulations are contraindicated if future fertility is an objective. The mucous membranes are easily abraded and will inevitably heal with transluminal adhesions and fibrosis. Repeated insertion and removal of the obstetrician's arm not only traumatizes the vaginal canal and cervix, but also increases the bacterial load that is carried into the uterus. The clinician must be decisive, and if a brief manipulation is ineffective, then an alternate approach should be considered. One or two fetotomy cuts will often permit rapid, atraumatic extraction of a dead fetus, provided that the obstetrician is experienced in the technique.[36,37] Unfortunately, fetotomy is often used as a last resort when prolonged manipulations have failed to correct the problem, and extensive soft tissue trauma has already been inflicted. If a well-equipped veterinary hospital is close by, then immediate referral for general anesthesia, controlled vaginal delivery, or cesarean section may offer the best prospect for foal survival and the mare's subsequent fertility.[31,41]

CHEMICAL RESTRAINT

The choice of restraint will vary with the obstetrician and will be determined by such factors as the mare's demeanor, the complexity of the dystocia, and the expectation of fetal viability. If delivery of a live foal is anticipated, the clinician should consider the potential for altered placental perfusion and fetal cardiovascular compromise before administering any tranquilizers to the mare. Light sedation with acetylpromazine should have minimal effect on the foal. If extra restraint is required, xylazine is preferable to detomidine if the fetus is viable because its depressant effects are of much shorter duration. Neither xylazine nor detomidine should be used on its own to sedate a dystocia case because some apparently sedated mares can become hypersensitive over the hindquarters. A xylazine-acepromazine combination will provide good sedation in a quiet mare, but a xylazine-butorphanol combination may be preferable if extra sedation and analgesia is necessary. Reduced dosages should be used initially, especially in Draft breeds and miniatures that appear to respond more intensely to tranquilizers and sedative-hypnotic drugs than light breeds. Because opioid analgesics can cause some gastrointestinal stasis and impaction, it is especially important to administer mineral oil once the dystocia has been resolved if these agents have been used.[43,44]

The time involved in administering effective epidural anesthesia often makes this form of restraint impractical if a live foal is to be delivered. The majority of fetotomy procedures (one or two cuts) can be made on a standing mare, and in these cases, caudal epidural anesthesia may be used at the clinician's discretion. Although an epidural does not prevent the mare's myometrial contractions or the abdominal press, it will reduce vaginal sensitivity and thus suppresses the Ferguson reflex associated with vaginal manipulations.[4,43] If an epidural is used, a xylazine-lidocaine combination is recommended. A low dose is essential to avoid the complication of ataxia, especially if referral to a hospital is a possibility.[45] Myometrial contractions (uterine spasm) can be controlled by injectable tocolytic agents (isoxsuprine, clenbuterol) if they are available for veterinary use.[5] Although intravenous or intramuscular administration will cause rapid uterine relaxation, it is not known whether the oral formulations will achieve sufficient blood levels to provide the same effect on the parturient uterus.[46]

Short-term general anesthesia may be indicated when minor postural abnormalities are present, though maternal expulsive efforts make correction difficult, or when the attempts at correction have already exceeded 10 minutes. Although the uterus in an anesthetized mare will be relaxed, manipulations in lateral recumbency can still be difficult due to the increased abdominal pressure. The chances for successful resolution are enhanced if a hoist is available because the effects of gravity will greatly assist with fetal repulsion and manipulation. Hobbles should be placed on the hind pasterns and the mare's hindquarters briefly elevated some 2 to 3 feet from the floor. A xylazine-ketamine combination provides a smooth, short (10 to 15 minutes) duration general anaesthetic, but the addition of guaifenesin can provide an additional 10 to 20 minutes for fetal manipulation.[43] However, the mare should not remain in an elevated, dorsally recumbent position for very long. Apart from respiratory and cardiovascular compromise, hindlimb paresis can develop after prolonged suspension. Some of the mare's weight can be taken off the limbs by placing supportive pads under the hindquarters. If attempts at correction are successful, the mare should be lowered into lateral recumbency so that the foal can be extracted. In specialist equine hospitals that are located close to well-managed broodmare farms, the fetus is often still alive when the mare arrives. It is common practice to immediately anesthetize these mares and to maintain them with controlled ventilation and intravenous fluids.[31,47] By using the hind end elevation technique, almost three quarters of such cases can be resolved by controlled vaginal delivery. However, if the fetus is still alive and has not been delivered within 15 minutes, a cesarean section is performed. Under these optimal circumstances a 30% foal survival rate has been reported.[31,48,49]

FETAL MANIPULATION (MUTATION)

Often space limitations within the pelvic canal dictate that the fetus must be repelled deeply into the uterus before it is possible to manipulate the fetal body and especially the long extremities. Overzealous intervention is a major cause of uterine rupture. It may not be possible to achieve meaningful yet safe repulsion if the uterus is contracted down around the fetus.[4,14,38,50-56] Tocolytic agents are effective in relaxing a contracted uterus, but injectable formulations are not available in all countries.[4,5] Pumping warm obstetrical lubricant around the fetus will induce some uterine relaxation in most cases and may provide the extra space that is required to safely mutate the malposture.[2,34] However, it is imperative that the obstetrician first verifies that the uterus is intact, especially if there has been prior intervention by inexperienced personnel.[38] Most iatrogenic lacerations occur in the uterine body, whereas a rupture at the tip of the gravid horn is more likely to be caused by the thrusting activity of the fetal hindlimbs.[10,14] If a live fetus is found to be in an abnormal position (dorsopubic or dorsoilial), it may be possible to rotate it by applying lateral pressure over the shoulder. An active fetal response will often facilitate correction into a dorsosacral position. If the foal is dead, and the forelimbs are extended, it may be possible to mimic the normal rotational movements by combining torque with gentle traction on the obstetrical chains. Judicious use of a bovine detorsion rod can also facilitate this maneuver.[4] Correction of a malposture of the fetal extremities is the most common reason for intervention. Although attempts to extract a fetus with an uncorrected limb malposture pose a risk for both the fetus and mare, it is sometimes possible to be successful if the mare has a large pelvis and the fetus is very small or premature.[4] However, the cervix and vagina can easily be lacerated, and extreme pressures created by extraction attempts with an uncorrected malposture can cause fetal rib fractures and severe internal trauma. It should be noted that rib fractures and contusions can also occur during an unassisted delivery.[39,40] If the fetus is dead, many malposture cases can be rapidly resolved by one or two fetotomy cuts, provided that the clinician has the appropriate skills and equipment.[36,37,57] Poor technique and inappropriate fetotomy cuts often lead to infertility. The alternative is cesarean section.[31,41,49]

Once any malpositions and/or malpostures have been corrected, any traction must be applied with careful regard for both maternal and fetal well-being.[34] Often traction applied entirely by hand is all that is necessary, although obstetrical straps or chains may provide a better grip. If the chains are applied with a loop above the fetlock and a half hitch below the joint, the extractive force will be spread over a larger surface and this may decrease the possibility of a crush fracture. The eye of the chain or strap should be positioned on the dorsal aspect of the limbs.[4] Any traction that is applied to the head should be merely to correct a malposture and to direct passage thru the vaginal canal. A rope head snare (behind ears and into mouth) may be preferable to the use of eyehooks in foals since they are more susceptible to trauma than are calves. This is obviously not an issue if the foal is dead. However, tension on the head snare can force the mouth open, and thus care should be taken to protect the uterus if the incisors have erupted. A mandibular snare is sometimes useful on a viable foal, but it should be used merely to direct the head and not as a point of traction. Mandibular fractures can easily occur if excessive force is applied. If the mare is not anesthetized, any traction on the limbs should be applied as an adjunct to her expulsive efforts—*assisted* vaginal delivery. Traction should cease when the dam stops straining, thereby permitting rest and recovery. This approach is essential to ensure complete cervical dilation and to permit adequate dilation of the caudal reproductive tract, especially in primiparous mares.[34] Copious lubrication and slow traction, with continuous monitoring of cervical dilation, are essential when *controlled* vaginal delivery is performed on an anesthetized mare.[49] No more than two or three people (depending on size and strength) should apply traction to the fetus.[34] Excessive use of force may injure a viable foal and inflict maternal soft tissue trauma. Serious birth-related injuries in a foal may include fractured ribs, bruised costochondral junction of ribs, hemoarthrosis of shoulder joints, as well as internal hemorrhage and/or a ruptured viscus.[16,27,39,40]

Cranial (Anterior) Presentation

If the fetus is in an abnormal position (dorsoilial, dorsopubic), the obstetrician should always consider the possibility of a term uterine torsion.[5] Unlike the situation in the cow, spiraling of the vaginal wall is seldom detectable in mares. Palpation of the broad ligaments per rectum can confirm whether any significant displacement of the gravid uterus has occurred.[24] When a hand can be passed through the cervix, the fetal head or preferably the trunk should be grasped.[5] However, in most cases a uterine torsion is not present. It is not uncommon to encounter incomplete fetal rotation when an inexperienced foaling attendant prematurely summons veterinary assistance. Another possibility is that the foal has not been assisted in its positional changes by the normal rolling that accompanies the early phase of parturition in the mare. Uterine inertia due to subclinical hypocalcaemia may also play a role. If a live fetus is in an abnormal position (dorsopubic or dorsoilial), it may be possible to rotate it by applying lateral pressure over the shoulder. An active fetal response will often facilitate correction into a dorso-sacral position. If the foal is dead, and the forelimbs are extended, it may be possible to mimic the normal rotational movements by combining torque with gentle traction on the obstetrical chains. A cranially presented fetus, with forequarters in a dorsosacral position and with head and forelimbs extended, should require minimal traction to complete the delivery. It is important that one limb be advanced slightly ahead of the other. This ensures that the width of the fetus across the shoulders is reduced. Provided that there is adequate lubrication, most foals can be successfully delivered. However, if progress is not being made, then all traction should cease. The vaginal canal must be fully explored because there are three possible explanations that can be readily identified.[34] One scenario could be incomplete extension of a forelimb (elbow lock). The flexed shoulder and elbow joint causes increased depth and width of the fetus within the maternal pelvic inlet (Figure 59-4). This malposture should be immediately suspected if the fetal muzzle lies at the same level as the fetlocks instead of over the proximal metacarpal bones.[4,34] If both forelimbs are equally advanced into the

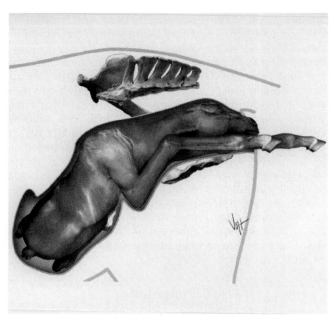

Figure 59-4 One forelimb should precede the other such that the shoulders enter the pelvis successively. The foal's head should be resting between the carpi, with the muzzle reaching the proximal metacarpus. Incomplete extension of a forelimb (elbow lock) should be suspected if labor is not progressing and the fetal muzzle lies at the same level as the fetlocks.

vaginal canal, there is a high risk of impaction of the fetal elbows on the pelvic brim. Palpation will reveal that the fetal olecranon is caught against the pubis. Correction involves repelling the fetal trunk while dorsomedial traction is applied to the affected forelimb. This will raise the elbow up over the floor of the pelvic inlet and permit full extension.[54]

Another explanation, *absolute* fetopelvic disproportion (fetal oversize), is not as common in mares as it is in cattle.[4,25,31] The shape of the mare's pelvis and the more elongated equine fetus tend to facilitate ease of delivery in most cases.[4,25] The size of the uterus (breed variation) plays a much greater role in determining ultimate fetal size than does the stature of the stallion.[58,59] Despite this, owners will often express concern about fetal oversize if the foal has been carried several weeks past the expected due date. Although this is a major concern with prolonged gestation in cattle, it is seldom an issue in overdue mares.[4] In fact, some cases of prolonged gestation in mares may involve a smaller-than-normal, dysmature fetus.[28] However, *relative* fetopelvic disproportion may be a significant factor in primiparous mares, and obstetric assistance (traction) is required much more often in these younger animals.[3,16,27,32,39] Foals from primiparous mares are more likely to sustain thoracic trauma compared with foals from pluriparous mares.[39] Approximately 30% of referral hospital dystocia cases are in primiparous mares, and these younger mares were disproportionately represented in a report on dystocia and neonatal asphyxia from the central Kentucky area.[16,18,25-27,39] Apart from fetal issues (malposition, malposture), dystocia in primiparous

mares may be further complicated by a tight vaginovestibular sphincter. This will predispose such cases to lacerations and rectovaginal tears.[39] If copious lubrication and gentle traction do not facilitate delivery, then cesarean section or partial fetotomy are the only alternatives. In experienced hands, a transverse section of the lumbar vertebrae followed by bisection of the pelvis will usually permit extraction of a large fetus.[5] The individual performing the fetotomy cut should be instructed to use long rather than short strokes. This spreads the wear on the wire and makes breakages less likely. The obstetrician should ensure that the head of the fetotome remains positioned correctly at all times.

The third explanation is a ventrovertical presentation with hip flexion and impaction of one or both hindlimbs. It has been suggested that this could be a variant of a ventrotransverse presentation where the cranial aspect of the fetus has become dislodged and entered the vaginal canal.[4] The mechanics of this malposture cause the fetal hindlimbs (hooves) to push against the pelvic brim whenever traction is applied to the forelimbs.[3,4,34] The dystocia is characterized by partial delivery of the anterior aspect of the fetus, followed by unproductive straining whereby the delivery fails to progress despite the mare's vigorous expulsive efforts. The cervix is easily damaged by the impacted limb during these expulsive efforts. Thus, the integrity of the ventral aspect of the cervix should be ascertained prior to rebreeding. Severe trauma can be inflicted on the mare if this hindlimb malposture is not recognized and inappropriate amounts of traction are applied.[4] It is essential that all traction is stopped if progress is not being made even though the forelimbs, head, and thorax are all correctly aligned. Correction of this malposture is contingent upon the fetus being repelled enough to permit the obstetrician's fingers to sweep the floor of the pelvic inlet. This is not always possible, especially if the fetus has been forcefully impacted in the birth caul. There may be either bilateral ("dog-sitting" posture) or unilateral ("hurdling" posture) hip flexion (Figure 59-5). The unilateral posture is more common.[25] In extreme cases the hindlimb may actually extend under the fetus and up into the vagina.[25] Although the hindlimb may be successfully repelled if the fetus is alive, it is a difficult procedure and is associated with some risk of uterine laceration. Limitations of arm length often preclude grasping the hindlimb. Sometimes merely rotating the fetus will dislodge the trapped hoof. One technique that is not without risk is to use a snare or threaded crutch repeller to loop around the pastern.[4] A long cord with a knot in one end is pulled through one eye of a Kuhn's crutch. The free end is passed through the other eye and the resulting loop placed over the trapped hoof. Tension is maintained on the long cord as the crutch repeller is advanced up the limb and seated against the pastern/fetlock. If used judiciously, the instrument may serve to repel the hoof away from the pelvic brim.[35,60] Although not an ideal "obstetrical" instrument, some practitioners have used a twitch to facilitate limb repulsion and delivery of a viable foal.

When the fetus is dead, repulsion attempts should not be performed on a standing mare. In these cases the repelled fetal hindlimb often will remain flexed instead of

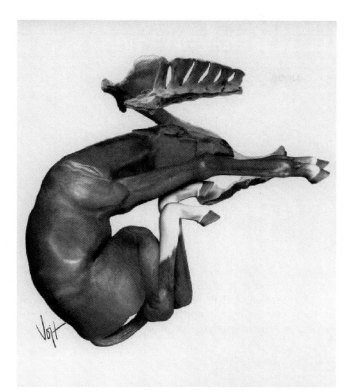

Figure 59-5 It is important to stop all traction if progress is not being made even though the forelimbs, head, and thorax are all correctly aligned. The floor of the pelvic inlet should be examined to determine if either bilateral ("dog-sitting" posture) or unilateral ("hurdling" posture) hip flexion are present. The mechanics of these malpostures cause the fetal hindlimbs (hooves) to push against the pelvic brim whenever traction is applied to the forelimbs.

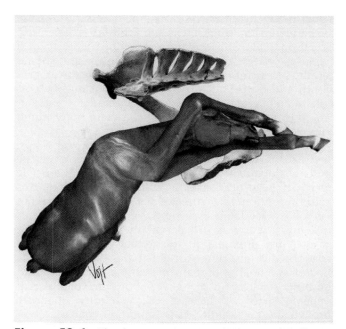

Figure 59-6 The foot-nape posture increases the diameter across the fetal chest, and the elbow may be lodged against the pubis. The mare's straining can cause the fetal hoof to lacerate the vaginal roof, and in extreme cases it may perforate completely through into the rectum (rectovaginal fistula). Further straining can tear through the caudal rectovaginal shelf and anal sphincter (third-degree perineal laceration).

returning to its normal position. There is an extreme risk that the hoof will then puncture the ventral uterine wall as the foal is being extracted.[36,37] Thus it is recommended that general anesthesia and hoisting of the hindquarters be employed to reduce the risk of ventral uterine rupture.[61] In experienced hands partial fetotomy is a viable alternative to cesarean section.[4,36,37,57,61] An initial cut transects the fetal trunk. If the hindquarters are repelled so that the hindlimbs can be accessed, there is potential for a uterine laceration from the exposed vertebral stump. Extreme caution is indicated.[4,61] A safer approach may be to bisect the pelvis, provided that the wire can be passed over the tail head and threaded down between the hindlimbs.[4,37] A surgical alternative to a complete cesarean section involves manipulation of the hindlimb through a ventral midline incision. An assistant may be able to extract the fetus through the vagina once the hindlimb has been grasped from within. If successful, this technique will reduce the potential for peritoneal contamination that can be associated with cesarean section.[60] If a cesarean section is to be performed, it is common practice to cut through the foal's vertebral column, and remove the fetal portion that is protruding through the vulvar lips. Thus only the retained hindquarters and trunk are subsequently removed through the surgical site.

If a foot-nape posture is present, one or both of the forelimbs will be displaced over the foal's head and pushed against the vaginal roof (Figure 59-6). The abnormal posture increases the diameter across the fetal chest, and the elbows may be lodged against the pubis.[4] This malposture is corrected by repelling the fetus into the uterus, lifting the limbs off the neck, and placing them in a lateral position. The head is then raised while at the same time obstetrical chains are used to apply ventromedial traction to the limbs until they come to lie under the head. Once the malposture has been corrected, fetal extraction can usually proceed quite uneventfully.[4,34] This relatively simple malposture can cause significant trauma to the vagina and perineum if it is not corrected immediately. Incorrect placement of the fetal hooves can cause severe trauma to the distal aspect of the birth canal. This is especially likely in maiden mares that do not have sufficient laxity in their vaginal and vestibular tissues to permit passage of a misplaced limb. The mare's straining can cause the fetal hoof to lacerate the vaginal roof, and in extreme cases it may perforate completely through into the rectum. This rectovaginal fistula may be all that occurs if the foal withdraws its hoof from the rectum before delivery. However, if the mare's strong expulsive efforts force the trapped limb caudally, it will dissect through the rectovaginal shelf and may even rupture through the anal sphincter. The resulting cloaca-like opening is known as a third-degree perineal laceration.[62-64] If a live foal is found to have a limb lodged in the rectum (fistula), it may not be possible to repel it in all cases.

Under these circumstances it may be necessary to incise the perineum and surgically create a third-degree perineal laceration. This will facilitate expeditious delivery of a viable neonate. Appropriate postpartum care should permit successful reconstruction of the perineal area within 4 to 6 weeks.[65] If the foal is dead, it may be possible to amputate the trapped limb with a fetotome, but care must be taken to ensure that the sharp bony stump does not create further trauma.

If one or both limbs are not visible at the vulvar lips, then either a unilateral or bilateral carpal flexion may be present. The affected limb is often lodged in the pelvic inlet.[34] If head/neck flexion is also present then this malposture should be corrected before the carpal flexion is resolved (see later discussion). Repulsion of the fetus back into the uterus will permit the flexed limb to be grasped just proximal to the fetlock. By rotating the wrist, the carpus can be rotated dorsolaterally while the flexed fetlock is brought medially and caudally into the birth canal.[4] This maneuver allows maximal use of available space by moving the extremity obliquely through the pelvic inlet. It is important that the clinician's hand be cupped over the bottom of the fetal hoof at all times while attempts are made to straighten the limb. Failure to do so may result in injury to the reproductive tract. Application of an obstetrical chain or rope snare to the pastern may be a useful aid because controlled traction can be applied externally while the internal hand manipulates the distal limb and then covers and guides the hoof.[4,34] Because most carpal flexions are relatively easy to correct manually, the obstetrician should be cognizant of the possibility of contracted tendons when difficulties are encountered. Flexural deformities are considered to be the most common congenital anomaly of foals.[16,18,27,33,36,37,57] Limb contractures are generally bilateral, with the forelimbs being affected more often than the hindlimbs, although it is not uncommon for all four limbs to be involved.[16,18,27,31,33] Severely affected limbs cannot be straightened, and needless trauma can be inflicted on the genital tract by prolonged attempts to manually correct this malposture.

If the mare has been in dystocia for some time, the amount of uterine contraction may prevent meaningful repulsion of the fetus. The fetus is invariably dead in such cases, and a relatively simple fetotomy cut at the level of the distal row of carpal bones can permit atraumatic extraction within minutes.[3,37,57] One channel of the fetotome is threaded, and the free end of the wire is attached to a curved wire introducer. The wire is passed around the affected carpus and then threaded down the empty channel of the fetotome. The head of the instrument is held firmly against the distal carpal joint to complete the cut (Figure 59-7). The distal radius remains as an anchor point for the obstetrical chain. A common error is to make the cut above or below the carpal joint.[36] A high cut will leave no anchor point for the chain, and a high or low cut creates a sharp stump of bone that can easily lacerate the uterus and/or vagina (Figure 59-8). The amputated distal limb should always be removed from the uterus before the fetus is extracted. Care should be taken to extend the proximal limb fully before applying

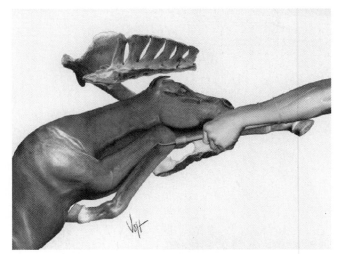

Figure 59-7 Uterine contraction may prevent the meaningful repulsion that is necessary to provide space for successful mutation. If the fetus is dead, a relatively simple fetotomy cut can rapidly and atraumatically resolve a dystocia due to a "flexed carpal" posture.

traction. This will ensure that an elbow lock does not prevent fetal extraction.

Malpostures involving the head and neck often occur when a viable foal pulls back from vaginal manipulations that are intended to correct a minor postural problem. If the muzzle engages the uterine wall or floor of the pelvic inlet, the mare's forceful expulsive efforts can drive the head and neck ventrally, or laterally along the thorax, while the forelimbs are pushed further into the vaginal canal (Figure 59-9). A rope head snare (behind ears and into mouth) that is applied before manipulating the limbs can facilitate head retrieval if a malposture does develop. The clinician should remember that any tension on the head snare can force the mouth open, and thus care must be taken to protect the uterus if the incisors are erupted and retrieval becomes necessary. Head and neck malpostures are very difficult to correct because the long neck often makes it impossible to reach the foal's head once this type of dystocia has occurred. The long nose and muzzle are an added complication.[4,34] In some especially difficult cases the displaced head will be rotated axially at the atlantooccipital joint such that the fetal mandibles are uppermost.[4] Prolonged, unrewarding manipulations can easily jeopardize the mare's future fertility. As with contracted tendons, it is essential that the practitioner consider the possibility of a "wry neck" when attempting to correct a displaced head and neck.[16,18,27] This congenital curvature of the cervical vertebrae is not amenable to correction by mutation, and needless trauma can be inflicted on the genital tract by unrewarding attempts to achieve the impossible. Inexperienced clinicians should consider referral as soon as a head and neck malposture is diagnosed.[34] In fact, reflection of the fetal head and neck is the most common reason for referring a dystocia case to a veterinary hospital.[3,18,25,31]

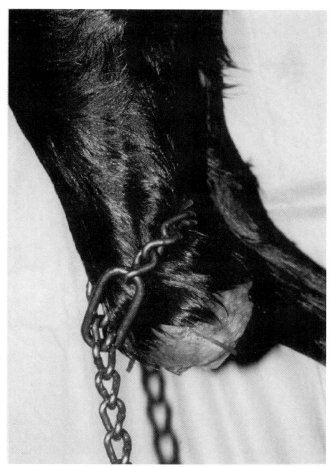

Figure 59-8 A carpal flexion fetotomy cut should be made at the level of the distal row of carpal bones. A common error is to make the cut above or below the carpal joint. A high cut will leave no anchor point for the obstetric chain, and a high or low cut creates a sharp stump of bone that can easily lacerate the uterus and/or vagina.

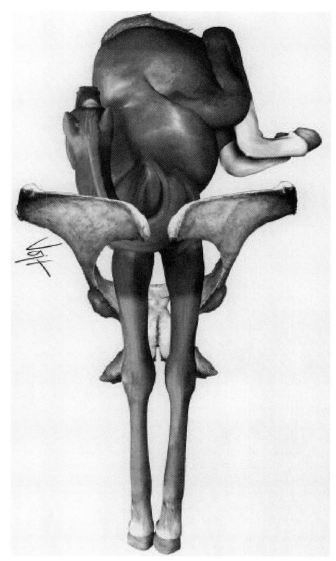

Figure 59-9 Head and neck malpostures are very difficult to correct because the long neck often makes it impossible to reach the foal's head. The length of the head and muzzle are an added complication. Thus these malpostures are the most common reason for referring a dystocia case to a veterinary hospital.

If the fingers can reach the foal's muzzle, it may be possible to exert traction on the corner of the mouth while moving the wrist to apply opposing pressure against the side of the head. Some obstetricians suggest applying a clamp (with a retrieving cord attached) to an ear so that the head can be retracted enough to permit placement of a mandibular snare. While application of a snare can be a useful method for correcting a lateral head and neck malposture, minimal tension should be applied to the mandible because it is relatively easy to cause a fracture. Gentle traction may be applied to the snare while the internal hand repels the rest of the head and neck. Attempts to grasp the orbital grooves should be made with caution if the foal is alive because pressure on the eyeball may provoke evasive movements that exacerbate the malposture. Eye hooks can easily cause damage to the foal's eye and thus should be used with caution on a live fetus.[4,18] If a portion of the head cannot be grasped, it may be possible to use an obstetrical chain looped around the neck to pull the head within reach. This should be done

with caution so that the muzzle is not forced against the uterine wall with such pressure that a rupture results.

Another technique that requires extreme caution is the use of a Kuhn's crutch.[4,35] In a manner similar to that previously described for correction of a "dog-sitting" posture, the long cord is fixed to one eye of the crutch. The free end is attached to a curved introducer that is passed over the neck and retrieved ventrally. The cord is withdrawn, untied from the introducer, and then passed through the other eye of the Kuhn's crutch. The free end of the long cord must be held firmly with the crutch handle. Moderate tension is maintained on the cord as the crutch is advanced along the lateral aspect of the neck towards the head.[4,35] If applied correctly, the loop around the foal's

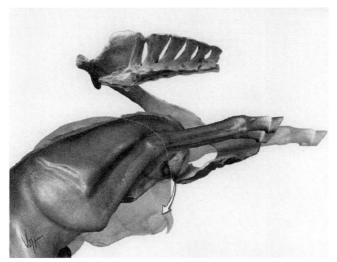

Figure 59-10   Ventral deviation of the head is relatively easy to correct if the long fetal nose is just below the pelvic brim (vertex or poll posture). In more severe cases the neck is tucked down between the forelimbs (nape posture), and in extreme cases the mandible rests against the sternum.

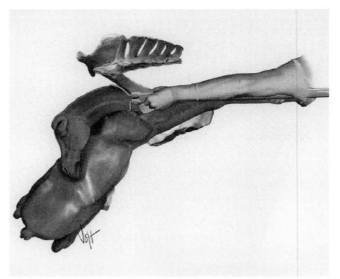

Figure 59-11   If a fetus with head and neck malposture is dead, then a relatively simple fetotomy cut can permit atraumatic extraction. The threaded fetatome is held against the curvature in the neck while the cut is made. A Krey hook attached to the vertebrae is useful to extract the severed head and neck. The vaginal canal should be protected by a hand covering the exposed vertebrae during fetal extraction.

neck will prevent the Kuhn's crutch from slipping off the neck and possibly rupturing the uterus. The advantage of the crutch is that there should be sufficient space for an arm to repel the fetal body while gentle traction on the crutch is used to draw the long head caudally. Once the hand can grasp the muzzle, it should protect the uterine wall while guiding the head into a normal posture for delivery. If the fetus is dead, a pair of forceps (with retrieving cord attached) can be attached to the skin of the neck in an attempt to pull the head caudally. Irrespective of the method chosen, correction of a lateral neck flexion can be extremely difficult. Factors influencing the likelihood of success include uterine tonicity, clinician arm length and skill, and the presence or absence of torticollis and facial scoliosis.[4,16,18,27,34]

Ventral deviation of the head is relatively easy to correct if the long fetal nose is just below the brim of the pelvis (vertex or poll posture). The head should be rotated laterally in an arc before attempting to bring the muzzle up over the pelvic brim. In more severe cases the neck is tucked down between the forelimbs (nape posture), and in extreme cases the mandible rests against the sternum (Figure 59-10). A mandibular snare may be useful to apply gentle traction to the head while the poll is repelled. Excessive tension on the snare can easily fracture the mandible. The fetus may have to be repelled deeply into the uterus to provide sufficient space to correct extreme ventral malposture. This may not be possible unless one or both forelimbs are placed in a carpal flexion, and pushed back into the uterus. A retrieving rope loop or obstetrical chain should be attached to the pastern to facilitate replacement of the limb once the neck flexion has been corrected. It is generally much easier to manipulate the head and neck when the forelimbs are not engaged in the pelvic canal. In a dystocia where there is head and neck flexion occurring concurrently with bilateral carpal flexion, it is imperative that the neck

flexion be corrected before the limbs are extended into the vaginal canal. This type of dystocia typically occurs if the fetus has died before or early in stage I of labor. Cesarean section or fetotomy are indicated if attempts to reposition the head and neck in a timely manner are unsuccessful.[4,36,37,49,57]

If a fetus with head and neck malposture is dead when the veterinarian arrives, then a relatively simple fetotomy cut can resolve these cases quite atraumatically.[18] The author believes that this approach is preferable to prolonged—and often unsuccessful—attempts at manual correction of this extremely difficult malposture.[36] Prolonged manipulations are contraindicated in the mare. The vaginal tissues are easily traumatized and invariably will heal with adhesions and fibrosis. It must be emphasized that inexperienced clinicians should not attempt fetotomy in the mare; prompt referral for cesarean section may be best for all concerned. When removing the head and neck, the wire is threaded as previously described for carpal flexion. If the fetus is tightly impacted in the birth canal, it may be difficult to pass the wire introducer between the flexed head and neck. If the fetotome can be successfully threaded, it should be held close to the curvature in the neck while the cut is made (Figure 59-11). A Krey hook attached to the vertebrae is useful to extract the severed head and neck. The hook is then attached to the vertebral stump of the fetus, and, along with traction on the forelimbs, extraction is readily achieved.[36,37] The vaginal canal should be protected by a hand covering the exposed vertebrae during the extraction. When the flexed neck cannot be reached, or it is too tightly flexed to pass the wire introducer, it may be possible to amputate the opposite forelimb. The head of the prethreaded fetotome

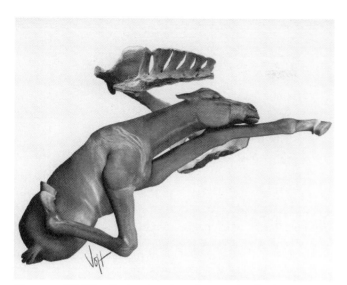

Figure 59-12 If the head and one forelimb protrude through the vulvar lips, then a unilateral carpal or shoulder flexion ("swimming" posture) should be suspected. The long extremities make correction of shoulder flexion malpostures difficult and time-consuming. The head and neck must be repelled back into the uterus to gain access to the retained limb. This is seldom easy to achieve.

is guided up the lateral aspect of the forelimb, and the wire loop is seated in the axilla. The fetotome is then advanced further into the uterus such that the head is positioned dorsocaudal to the scapula. An obstetric chain attaches the fetlock to the fetotome and holds the forelimb in extension. A correctly performed fetotomy cut will dissect up through the muscular attachments, thereby severing the entire forelimb from the chest wall. Often a dorsal remnant of the scapula will remain. This can easily lacerate the cervix and should be removed with a palm knife before the fetus is extracted.[4,36,37] A dangerous complication occurs if the fetotome is permitted to move caudally during the cutting procedure. The misplaced cut will most likely occur through the proximal humerus, creating an extremely sharp bone stump, and leaving the width of the shoulder joint intact. If the procedure is performed correctly, the extra space in the pelvic canal permits the fetus to be pulled further into the birth canal. Often this then permits the retained head to be reached and manipulated into correct alignment for delivery. Failing this, a second cut should be made through the now accessible flexed neck.

Shoulder flexion posture may be unilateral ("swimming" posture), (Figure 59-12) with head and one forelimb presented, or bilateral ("diving" posture), where only the fetal head protrudes through the vulvar lips (Figure 59-13).[4,18,25,34] An immediate cesarean section may be preferable if the foal is alive because the long forelimbs make manual correction of these malpostures difficult and time-consuming. The head and neck must be repelled back into the uterus to gain access to the retained limb(s), and this is seldom easy to achieve.[4] A soft rope snare should be placed on the fetal head so that it can be readily

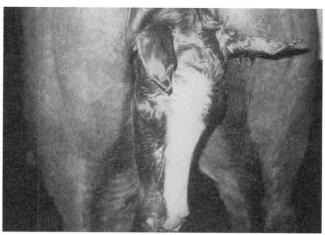

Figure 59-13 If bilateral shoulder flexion ("diving" posture) is present, then only the head will be protruding through the vulvar lips. An immediate cesarean section may be indicated if the foal is alive.

retrieved once the shoulder flexion has been corrected. If the limb can be reached, the mutation is performed in two stages. A carpal flexion is created by locating the retained humerus and working down to the distal radius. The limb is then pulled caudally and medially as the fetal body is repelled. If a rope loop can be passed around the radius, the external hand can apply traction on the distal extremity while the internal hand repels the fetus by applying pressure to the shoulder. Once the flexed carpus has been hooked over the brim of the pelvis, it can be extended as described previously. It must be remembered that it is not always possible to repel the head sufficiently to gain access to the retained forelimb. In these cases cesarean section may be the only option for delivery of a live foal. While attempts to extract a fetus with an uncorrected limb malposture pose a risk for both the fetus and mare, it is sometimes possible to be successful if the mare has a large pelvis and if the fetus is very small or premature.[4] However, the cervix and vagina can easily be lacerated, and extreme pressures created by extraction attempts with an uncorrected malposture can cause fetal rib fractures and severe internal trauma. Before attempting an uncorrected delivery the clinician must ensure that carpal flexion is not present, that fetal oversize is not an issue, and that copious lubrication has been applied. If the fetus is dead, a fetotomy cut to remove the head with as much neck as can be reached may provide sufficient room to correct the malposture.[4,36,37,57] This approach is definitely indicated if the mare is presented with only the dead foal's head protruding through the vulvar lips. Although extremely rare, bilateral amelia of the forelimbs will cause a "head only" delivery (Figure 59-14).

If a shoulder flexion cannot be manually corrected, an experienced obstetrician may be able to remove the retained limb *in utero* by performing a fetotomy cut. A palm knife is used to make a deep incision medial to the dorsal border of the scapula. It is essential that a long cord be attached to the palm knife so that it can be easily retrieved if the finger ring slips off. The curved wire intro-

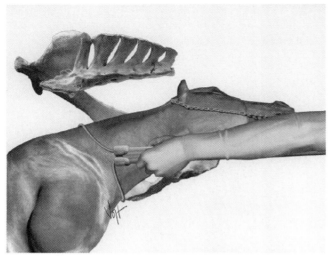

Figure 59-14 If a fetus with bilateral shoulder flexion is dead, then an experienced obstetrician may be able to perform a fetotomy cut. Removal of the head with as much neck as possible often provides sufficient space for an arm to correct the malposture. An obstetric chain anchors the head to the fetatome and holds the neck in extension while the cut is made. If the cut is successful, a hand should cover the exposed vertebral stump during fetal extraction.

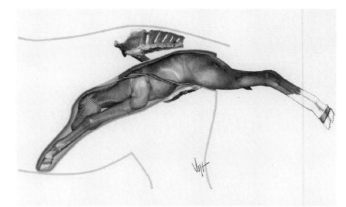

Figure 59-15 In caudal presentation there is an increased risk of fetal hypoxia due to compression of the umbilical cord under the fetal thorax. Premature rupture of the umbilical cord while the head is still retained within the uterine lumen can also cause fetal death.

ducer is passed down between the retained limb and chest wall and retrieved ventrally. The head of the threaded fetotome is positioned medial to the shoulder joint, and the wire loop is seated in the dorsal incision. In this instance the direction of the fetotomy cut will be down through the muscular attachments that hold the scapula to the thorax.[4,36,37] Correct positioning of the head of the fetotome and the wire loop is essential. If the wire slips out of the dorsal incision, an erroneous cut most likely will be made through the proximal portion of the retained humerus, creating an extremely sharp bone stump and leaving the width of the shoulder joint intact.

Caudal (Posterior) Presentation

If the soles of the hooves are facing upwards one of two abnormalities should be suspected. Either the foal is in caudal presentation or a fetus in cranial presentation has failed to rotate as it extended the forelimbs. Palpation of the hocks somewhere in the vaginal canal will confirm the diagnosis. There is only one joint (fetlock) between the hoof and the hock, whereas a forelimb has two joints (fetlock, carpus) between the hoof and the elbow.[4] In caudal presentation there is an increased risk of fetal hypoxia due to compression of the umbilical cord under the fetal thorax (Figure 59-15). Likewise, premature rupture of the umbilical cord while the fetal head is still retained within the uterine lumen can also cause fetal death.[34] Gentle traction on the hindlimbs in conjunction with the mare's expulsive efforts may facilitate delivery. Caudal presentation predisposes the mare to dystocia because the synchronized rotation of the fetal body and

extension of the extremities that has been described for cranial presentation often does not occur.[10,15] In many cases the abnormally presented fetus will be in a dorsoilial position.[18,25] Although only about 1% of foals are presented caudally, this malpresentation may account for 14% to 16% of referral hospital dystocia cases because any postural abnormalities of the long limbs create a major complication.[3,18,25,31] Typically both hindlimbs are involved in the malposture, suggesting that the etiology is associated with a failure of the normal extension mechanism.[3,18,25] Both bilateral hock and hip flexion cases are extremely difficult to correct under field conditions due to space limitations within the birth canal.

Hock flexion malposture accounts for about one quarter of referred caudal presentation cases.[3,18,25] The flexed hocks are palpable either at the pelvic inlet or impacted more caudally in the vaginal canal. These, and bilateral hip flexion ("breech") malpostures, can be extremely difficult to correct because it may not be possible to safely repel the fetus far enough cranially to permit manipulation of the retained limbs. Tocolytic drugs are extremely useful in these cases. Expansion of the uterus with large volumes of lubricant may also facilitate manipulations. Although a Kuhn's crutch can be used to repel the fetal rump, the instrument can easily perforate the uterus if it slips off the fetus. Anchoring one of the forks in the fetal anus/rectum may reduce the likelihood of this mishap. An assistant's arm may also suffice. However, there are safety issues when an assistant and clinician are working this closely in a standing mare. Certainly a well lubricated assistant's arm can provide meaningful fetal repulsion in an anesthetized mare that has the hindquarters elevated. The obstetrician is then able to focus on manipulating the retained limbs.

Straightening a flexed hock entails considerable risk because the hock is invariably forced against the dorsal uterine wall. In cases where the uterus is contracted there is a real possibility of creating a laceration or perforation.

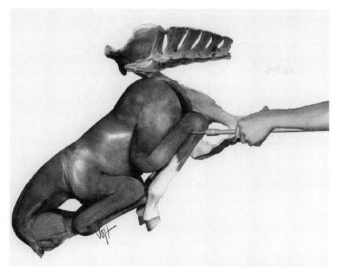

Figure 59-16 Correcting a "flexed hock" malposture entails considerable risk of uterine rupture because the hock is invariably forced against the dorsal uterine wall. If the fetus is dead, it may be safer to correct this dystocia by fetotomy. The cut is made through the distal row of tarsal bones such that an obstetric chain can be fixed above the os calcis to provide a point of traction.

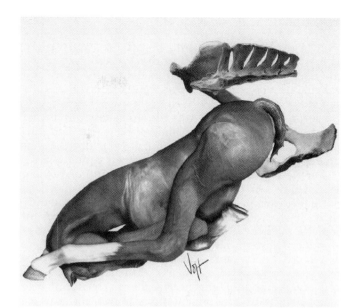

Figure 59-17 Manipulations involved in attempting to correct a bilateral hip flexion ("breech" posture) are especially time-consuming because the limbs are displaced under the fetal body. A bilateral hock flexion must be created before the limbs can be extended. Cesarean section will usually provide the best prognosis for fetal survival and future fertility.

The metatarsus is grasped and the fetus repelled into the uterus while the hock is pushed dorsolaterally. The procedure for medially and obliquely moving the extremity into the birth canal is similar to that previously described for correction of a carpal flexion.[4] An obstetrical chain or strap can be used to apply medial traction to the distal limb. It is important that the hoof be cupped in the hand as it is guided into the pelvic canal. If the foal is dead, and the obstetrician is experienced, it may be safer to correct a flexed hock dystocia by fetotomy.[4,36,37,49,57] The procedure is essentially the same as that described for amputation of a flexed carpus, with the cut being made through the lower row of tarsal bones (Figure 59-16). The comments about the adverse effects of a high or low carpal cut apply to the tarsal joint as well. Once the distal limb has been removed, an obstetric rope or chain can be fixed above the os calcis to provide a point of traction. The fetal body must still be repelled to permit the stifles to be extended up into the pelvic canal.

Approximately half of referred caudal presentation cases are breech (bilateral hip flexion posture). Even under ideal hospital conditions the manipulations involved in attempting to correct a bilateral hip flexion (breech) posture are especially time-consuming because the limbs are displaced under the fetal body (Figure 59-17). Cesarean section will usually provide the best prognosis for fetal viability and future fertility in these cases.[3,18,25,37] The comments for managing a hock flexion apply because, if mutation is attempted, the bilateral hip flexion must first be converted into a bilateral flexed hock posture.[4,34] The distal tibia is grasped and pulled caudodorsally until the hock is in a flexed posture. A rope or

obstetrical chain looped around the limb can help to retrieve the hock.[4] If successful, it is important to remember to flex both hocks before attempting to straighten either limb. If one limb is extended into the vaginal canal while the other hip remains flexed, the fetal body will move back into the pelvic canal, and this will make it extremely difficult to access the retained limb.[28] If the fetus is dead and cesarean section is not an option, the author recommends attempting to convert the bilateral hip flexion into a hock flexion posture, followed by correction with two fetotomy cuts through the distal row of tarsal bones. Provided that the clinician is experienced in the use of a fetotome, this may be safer and cause less trauma than attempting to straighten the limbs. Attempts to correct a bilateral hip flexion by fetotomy, without first creating a bilateral hock flexion, are often unrewarding due to difficulty in correctly placing the fetotomy wire.[37,57] It may not be possible to grasp the wire from below even if it can be passed over the fetal rump and down between the retained limb and body wall. If the wire can be retrieved, it is threaded down the other fetotome channel and the head of the instrument is placed firmly against the perineum on the side of the tail opposite the limb being amputated. The goal is to make a diagonal cut through the pelvis. This removes the entire hindlimb and the caudal aspect of the pelvis that includes the acetabulum.[4] Once the amputated limb has been removed from the pelvic cavity, there may be sufficient space to correct the remaining malposture and extract the fetus.

Transverse Presentation

Only about 1 in 1000 foals will be presented transversely. This is the culmination of a bicornual gestation in which the fetus was tightly packed into the uterine body and variable portions of both horns. Neither horn is as fully expanded as would be expected in a normal pregnancy.[3,10] However, the net effect of this abnormal gestation is that overall placental surface area may be increased, and thus the foals are often larger than normal—a factor to be considered if an attempt at vaginal delivery is contemplated. Under less-than-ideal management conditions these mares may not be recognized as being in labor. The normal vaginal pressure stimuli are not present, and only weak, if any, abdominal straining occurs.[4,18] Successful resolution of these dystocia cases requires a significant amount of obstetrical experience. This explains why these extremely rare presentations account for 10% to 16% of referral hospital dystocia cases.[18,25] If the fetus is alive, the delivery method of choice is cesarean section.[49] The majority of transverse presentations are ventrotransverse (Figure 59-18), with the abdomen and limbs of the fetus presented towards the birth canal.[3,18,25] Although the widespread adoption of ultrasonography has markedly reduced the likelihood of a twin birth, this possibility must always be explored when more than two limbs are present in the birth canal.[16,27]

In some instances it may be possible to repel the head and forequarters of the fetus while extending the two hindlimbs into the pelvic canal (version). If the manipulations are successful, the transverse presentation is thus converted into a caudal presentation for vaginal delivery.[3]

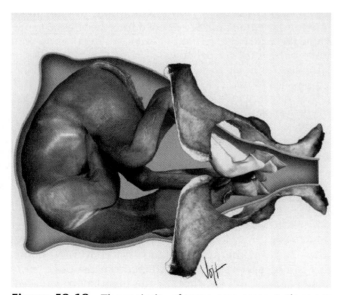

Figure 59-18 The majority of transverse presentations are ventrotransverse with the abdomen and all four limbs of the fetus presented towards the birth canal. If the fetus is alive, the delivery method of choice is by cesarean section. Successful mutation of these cases requires a significant amount of obstetric experience. In some instances it may be possible to repel the head and forequarters of the fetus while extending the hindlimbs into the pelvic canal. Fetotomy is seldom indicated due to the necessity for several cuts.

The likelihood of successfully resolving one of these cases is improved if the mare has been anesthetized and the hindquarters elevated.[34] However, extreme caution should be used during any manipulations because transverse fetal presentations are associated with a markedly increased incidence of fetal malformations. This is likely to be a consequence of restricted fetal movement in utero.[4] In approximately one third of cases attempts at correction may be complicated by the presence of flexural limb deformities, angular limb deformity, and vertebral deformity such as wry neck.[18] Dorsotransverse presentations, with the spinal column of the fetus presented towards the birth canal, are very rare. These cases warrant an immediate referral for cesarean section, even if the foal is dead.[3,18,25] Although an experienced obstetrician may be able to deliver a transversely presented fetus by multiple fetotomy cuts, the owner should be advised that this will be a difficult and time-consuming procedure. There is a high risk of trauma that most likely will impede the mare's future fertility.[34,36,37,57]

Fetal Anomalies

Apart from the "contracted foal syndrome" (limb contractures, scoliosis, and/or torticollis), fetal anomalies that have been reported in the horse include hydrocephalus, anencephaly, meningoencephalocele, microphthalmia, craniofacial malformations (wry nose), cleft palate, umbilical hernia, diaphragmatic hernia, cardiac anomalies, epitheliogenesis imperfecta, dystrophic chondropathy, scoliosis, and hydronephrosis.[16,33] In most cases these congenital anomalies are not related to hereditary factors and do not cause dystocia.[33] A very large umbilical hernia will usually cause evisceration of the fetus during parturition. Although these cases will present like a schistosomus reflexus birth in cattle (viscera protruding through the vulvar lips), the equine fetus does not appear to develop the dorsoretroflexion of the vertebral column that characterizes the ruminant condition.[2,4,16,33,66,67] Hydrocephalus is an occasional cause of equine dystocia, especially in pony breeds.[3,18,33] The condition occurs when increased intracranial pressure causes the bones of the skull to enlarge, sometimes almost doubling the size of the head.[18] The skull is often very thin, and many affected foals can be delivered after incising the soft portion of the skull with a finger knife, allowing the skull to collapse.[4] The trunk of the hydrocephalic fetus is generally smaller than normal and seldom interferes with delivery.[34] If the enlarged cranium is densely ossified, then a fetotomy cut may be necessary to reduce the size of the head.[4,36,37,57] This may be performed by looping the wire behind the ears and holding the fetotome between the eyes. Alternately, if the head is turned back, the wire loop may be placed in the mouth and the head of the fetotome held at the base of the skull. In both scenarios it is important to place a hand over the cut surface to protect the vaginal canal during extraction.

CONCLUSION

The third stage of parturition involves expulsion of the fetal membranes and is regarded as being normal if completed within 30 minutes to 3 hours.[4,65] Owners should be advised to seek veterinary assistance if passage of the membranes is delayed. Metritis and laminitis are common sequelae of membrane retention. In an attempt to reduce the incidence of membrane retention the author routinely employs the Burns technique after resolving a dystocia case.[12,68] This involves distending the chorioallantois with saline and then tying off the opening. A low dose of oxytocin (10 to 20 IU) is then administered, and most mares will pass the entire chorioallantoic sac within 30 minutes.[65] Although many of these cases may well pass the membranes unaided, it is recognized that obstetrical procedures predispose the mare to membrane retention.[69] The advantage of encouraging rapid passage of the entire chorioallantoic sac, with any introduced contaminants contained within, warrants the minimal effort involved in employing this technique. The fetal membranes should be examined as a matter of routine to ensure that they have been passed intact and to check for any placental anomalies that may forewarn of impending problems in the neonate. Abdominal discomfort in the postpartum mare may be due to uterine contractions, especially if the mare has been treated with oxytocin to promote passage of the fetal membranes. Other causes of abdominal pain should not be discounted, including rupture of the uterine artery. An abdominocentesis can provide useful prognostic information in the immediate postpartum period.[12,38] Variable amounts of perineal swelling are not uncommon after a dystocia, and the associated discomfort may contribute to fecal impaction. Routine administration of mineral oil can ease fecal passage in mares that have experienced a dystocia.

References

1. Frazer GS, Embertson R, Perkins NR: Complications of late gestation in the mare. Equine Vet Educ 1997; 9:306-311.
2. Frazer GS, Perkins NR, Embertson RM: Normal parturition and evaluation of the mare in dystocia. Equine Vet Educ 1999; 11:41-46.
3. Vandeplassche M: Dystocia. In McKinnon AO, Voss J (eds): Equine Reproduction, pp 578-587, Philadelphia, Lea & Febiger, 1993.
4. Roberts SJ: Veterinary Obstetrics and Genital Diseases (Theriogenology), 3rd edition, Woodstock, Vt, 1986.
5. Vandeplassche M: Prepartum complications and dystocia. In Robinson N (ed): Current Therapy in Equine Medicine 2, pp 537-542, Philadelphia, WB Saunders, 1987.
6. Ley WB, Bowen JM, Purswell BJ et al: The sensitivity, specificity and predictive value of measuring calcium carbonate in mare's prepartum mammary secretion. Theriogenology 1993; 40:189-198.
7. Ousey JC, Delclaux M, Rossdale PD: Evaluation of three strip tests for measuring electrolytes in mares' prepartum mammary secretions and for predicting parturition. Equine Vet J 1989; 21:196-200.
8. Paccamonti DL: Milk electrolytes and induction of parturition. Pferdeheilkunde 2001; 17:616-618.
9. Ginther OJ, Williams D, Curren S: Equine fetal kinetics: entry and retention of fetal hind limbs in a uterine horn. Theriogenology 1994; 41:795-807.
10. Ginther OJ: Equine pregnancy: physical interactions between the uterus and conceptus. Proceedings of the 44th Annual Convention of the American Association of Equine Practitioners, pp 73-104, 1998.
11. Ginther OJ: Equine physical utero-fetal interactions: a challenge and wonder for the practitioner. J Equine Vet Sci 1994; 14:313-318.
12. Frazer GS: Postpartum complications in the mare. Part 1. Conditions affecting the uterus. Equine Vet Educ 2003; 5:45-54.
13. Dascanio JJ, Ball BA, Hendrickson DA: Uterine tear without a corresponding placental lesion in a mare. J Am Vet Med Assoc 1993; 202:419-420.
14. Sutter WW, Hopper S, Embertson RM et al: Diagnosis and surgical treatment of uterine lacerations in mares (33 cases). Proceedings of the 49th Annual Convention of the American Association of Equine Practitioners, pp 357-359, 2003.
15. Jeffcott LB, Rossdale P: A radiographic study of the fetus in late pregnancy and during foaling. J Reprod Fertil Suppl 1979; 27:563-569.
16. Giles RC, Donahue JM, Hong CB et al: Causes of abortion, stillbirth, and perinatal death in horses: 3,527 cases (1986-1991). J Am Vet Med Assoc 1993; 203:1170-1175.
17. Whitwell KE: Investigations into fetal and neonatal losses in the horse. Vet Clin North Am 1980; 2:313-331.
18. Vandeplassche ML: The pathogenesis of dystocia and fetal malformation in the horse. J Reprod Fertil Suppl 1987; 35:547-552.
19. Vandeplassche M, Lauwers H: The twisted umbilical cord: an expression of kinesis of the equine fetus? Anim Reprod Sci 1986; 10:163-175.
20. Ginther OJ: Equine fetal kinetics: allantoic-fluid shifts and uterine-horn closures. Theriogenology 1993; 40:241-256.
21. Williams NM: Umbilical cord torsion. Equine Dis Q 2002; 10:3-4.
22. Ginther OJ, Griffin PG: Equine fetal kinetics: presentation and location. Theriogenology 1993; 40:1-11.
23. Curren S, Ginther OJ: Ultrasonic fetal gender diagnosis during months 5 to 11 in mares. Theriogenology 1993; 40:1127-1135.
24. Frazer GS: Uterine torsion. In Robinson N (ed): Current Therapy in Equine Medicine 5, pp 311-315, Philadelphia, WB Saunders, 2003.
25. Frazer GS, Perkins NR, Blanchard TL et al: Prevalence of fetal maldispositions in equine referral hospital dystocias. Equine Vet J 1997; 29:111-116.
26. Ginther OJ, Williams D: On-the-farm incidence and nature of equine dystocias. J Equine Vet Sci 1996; 16:159-164.
27. Hong CB, Donahoe JM, Giles RC et al: Equine abortion and stillbirth in central Kentucky during 1988 and 1989 foaling seasons. J Vet Diagn Invest 1993; 5:560-566.
28. Hillman RB: Dystocia management at the farm. Periparturient Mare and Neonate Symposium, pp 65-71, San Antonio, Tex, Society for Theriogenology, 2000.
29. Macpherson ML, Chaffin MK, Carroll GL et al: Three methods of oxytocin-induced parturition and their effects on foals. J Am Vet Med Assoc 1997; 210:799-803.
30. Brendemeuhl JP: Fescue and agalactia: pathophysiology, diagnosis and management. Periparturient Mare and Neonate Symposium, pp 25-32, San Antonio, Tex, Society for Theriogenology, 2000.
31. Byron C, Embertson RM, Bernard WV et al: Dystocia in a referral hospital setting: approach and results. Equine Vet J 2002; 35:82-85.
32. Vandeplassche M: Selected topics in equine obstetrics. Proceedings of the 38th Annual Convention of the American Association of Equine Practitioners, pp 623-628, 1992.
33. Crowe MW, Swerczek TW: Equine congenital defects. Am J Vet Res 1985; 46:353-358.

34. Frazer GS, Perkins NR, Embertson RM: Correction of equine dystocia. Equine Vet Educ 1999; 11:48-53.

35. Arthur G, Noakes D, Pearson H et al: Veterinary Reproduction and Obstetrics, 7th edition, London, WB Saunders, 1996.

36. Frazer GS: Fetotomy technique in the mare. Equine Vet Educ 2001; 13:195-203.

37. Bierschwal CJ, deBois C: The Technique of Fetotomy in Large Animals, Bonner Springs, Kan, VM Publishing, 1972.

38. Frazer GS, Burba D, Paccamonti D et al: The effects of parturition and peripartum complications on the peritoneal fluid composition of mares. Theriogenology 1997; 48:919-931.

39. Jean D, Laverty S, Halley J et al: Thoracic trauma in newborn foals. Equine Vet J 1999; 31:149-152.

40. Schambourg M, Laverty S, Mullim S et al: Thoracic trauma in foals: post mortem findings. Equine Vet J 2003; 35:78-81.

41. Freeman DE, Hungerford LL, Schaeffer D et al: Caesarean section and other methods for assisted delivery: comparison of effects on mare mortality and complications. Equine Vet J 1999; 31:203-207.

42. Emberstson R: Dystocia and caesarean sections: the importance of duration and good judgment. Equine Vet J 1999; 31:179-180.

43. LeBlanc MM: Sedation and anesthesia of the parturient mare. Periparturient Mare and Neonate Symposium, pp 59-64, San Antonio, Tex, Society for Theriogenology, 2000.

44. Luukkanen L, Katila T, Koskinen E: Some effects of multiple administration of detomidine during the last trimester of equine pregnancy. Equine Vet J 1997; 29:400-402.

45. Grubb TL, Reibold TW, Huber MJ: Comparison of lidocaine, xylazine, and xylazine/lidocaine for caudal epidural analgesia in horses. J Am Vet Med Assoc 1992; 201:1187-1190.

46. Card CE, Wood MR: Effects of acute administration of clenbuterol on uterine tone and equine fetal and maternal heart rates. Biol Reprod 1995; 1:7-11.

47. Taylor PM: Anaesthesia for pregnant animals. Equine Vet J Suppl 1997; 24:1-6.

48. Embertson RM, Bernard WV, Hance SR et al: Hospital approach to dystocia in the mare. Proceedings of the 41st Annual Convention of the American Association of Equine Practitioners, pp 13-14, 1995.

49. Embertson RM: The indications and surgical techniques for cesarean section in the mare. Equine Vet Educ 1992; 4:31-36.

50. Zent WW: Postpartum complications. In Robinson N (ed): Current Therapy in Equine Medicine 2, pp 544-547, Philadelphia, WB Saunders, 1987.

51. Pascoe J, Pascoe R: Displacements, malpositions and miscellaneous injuries of the mare's urogenital tract. Vet Clin North Am 1988; 4:439.

52. Fisher AT, Phillips TN: Surgical repair of a ruptured uterus in five mares. Equine Vet J 1986; 18:153-155.

53. Rossdale PD: Differential diagnosis of postparturient hemorrhage in the mare. Equine Vet Educ 1994; 6:135-136.

54. Perkins NR, Frazer GS: Reproductive emergencies in the mare. Vet Clin North Am Equine Pract 1994; 10:643-670.

55. Hooper RN, Blanchard TL, Taylor TS: Identifying and treating uterine prolapse and invagination of the uterine horn. Vet Med 1991; 88:60.

56. Brooks DE, McCoy DJ, Martin GS: Uterine rupture as a postpartum complication in two mares. J Am Vet Med Assoc 1985; 187:1377-1379.

57. Frazer GS: Review of the use of fetotomy to resolve dystocia in the mare. Proceedings of the 43rd Annual Convention of the American Association of Equine Practitioners, pp 262-268, 1997.

58. Tischner M, Klimczak M: The development of Polish ponies born after embryo transfer to large recipients. Equine Vet J Suppl 1989; 8:62-63.

59. Wilsher S, Allen WR: The influence of maternal size, age and parity on placental and fetal development in the horse. In Katila T, Wade J (eds): Havemeyer Monograph, vol 3, New York, DR Havemeyer Foundation, 2000.

60. Hunt RJ: Obstetrics. In Robinson N (ed): Current Therapy in Equine Medicine 5, pp 319-322, Philadelphia, WB Saunders, 2003.

61. Baldwin JL, Cooper WL, Vanderwall DK: Dystocia due to anterior presentation with unilateral or bilateral hip flexion posture ("dog-sitting" presentation) in the mare: incidence, management, and outcomes. Proceedings of the 37th Annual Convention of the American Association of Equine Practitioners, pp 229-240, 1991.

62. Aanes WW: Surgical management of foaling injuries. Vet Clin N Am 1988; 4:417.

63. Trotter G: The vulva, vestibule, vagina, and cervix. In Auer JA, Stick JA (eds): Equine Surgery, 2nd edition, Philadelphia, WB Saunders, 1999.

64. Freeman D: Rectum and anus. In Auer JA, Stick JA (eds): Equine Surgery, 2nd edition, pp 286-293, Philadelphia, WB Saunders, 1999.

65. Frazer GS: Postpartum complications in the mare. Part 2. Fetal membrane retention and conditions of the gastrointestinal tract, bladder and vagina. Equine Vet Educ 2003; 5:118-128.

66. Bezeck DM, Frazer GS: Schistosomus reflexus in large animals. Compend Contin Educ Pract Vet 1994; 16:1393-1399.

67. Whitwell KE: Morphology and pathology of the equine umbilical cord. J Reprod Fertil Suppl 1975; 23:599-603.

68. Burns SJ, Judge NG, Martin FE et al: Management of retained placenta in mares. Proceedings of the 23rd Annual Convention of the American Association of Equine Practitioners, p 381, 1977.

69. Vandeplassche M: Aetiology, pathogenesis and treatment of retained placenta in the mare. Equine Vet Educ 1971; 3:144.

CHAPTER 60

Premature Lactation in Mares

MARGO L. MACPHERSON
JUSTIN T. HAYNA
MATS H. T. TROEDSSON

Premature lactation in the pregnant mare can be defined as development of the mammary gland or milk production, or both, a minimum of 2 weeks before parturition. This condition is a dreaded clinical sign for the equine practitioner because it often is associated with impending abortion. The most common causes of premature lactation are twin pregnancies and bacterial placentitis. Uterine body pregnancies also may manifest with premature lactation[1]; however, the incidence of uterine body pregnancies is substantially lower than that of twins or bacterial placentitis. Abortion due to other causes (viral, fungal, or functional) generally occurs earlier in gestation and is not associated with udder development. Differentiating among the causes of premature lactation poses a challenge to the veterinary practitioner. Methods for diagnosing and managing causes of premature lactation are reviewed in this chapter.

HISTORY AND CLINICAL SIGNS

A common clinical presentation for mares in late gestation with at-risk pregnancies is development of the mammary glands earlier than 2 weeks before parturition. In mares with a history of normal pregnancy, mammary development may begin between 2 and 4 weeks before parturition, with the predominant increase in mammary size occurring in the final 2 weeks of gestation. The normal mammary gland changes of pregnancy, however, are contingent on several factors, such as parity and photoperiod. Development of udders more commonly occurs earlier in multiparous mares than in nulliparous mares. Nulliparous, or "maiden," mares frequently show very little udder development until immediately before parturition. In some cases, mammary development in nulliparous mares can be so scant that use of this sign to predict parturition or impending abortion may be more difficult. Although development of the gland can be slower in nulliparous mares, gland size and function usually are sufficient by the time the foal is ready to suckle.

Photoperiod can affect the length of gestation,[2] thereby influencing mammary development relative to parturition. Without knowledge of the typical gestational length of a given mare, it may be difficult to know when appropriate gland development should begin. Fortunately, most mares have approximately the same gestation length from year to year, so interpreting mammary development based on gestation length is more reliable in these mares. The one caveat to use of this rule of thumb is that season can affect length of the gestational period in a given mare. Specifically, a mare with an average gestation length (i.e., 333 to 342 days)[3] during days with maximal light may have a longer gestational period during days with minimal amount of light. Therefore, obtaining accurate breeding and foaling history for a mare can be critical in differentiating normal from abnormal mammary gland development.

Precocious mammary development may or may not be accompanied by spontaneous milk release (i.e., "streaming"). This should be differentiated from both the dried serous exudates ("waxing") commonly seen on the teats of mares nearing parturition and the serous to slightly milky secretions that can be expressed from teats of nonpregnant and prepubertal animals ("witch's milk"). The ramifications of premature milk release are multiple. Of paramount importance, this clinical sign most commonly is associated with an abnormal pregnancy. In addition, premature milk release results in loss of important immunoglobulins, which can be detrimental to survival of a neonate.[4,5] If premature milk release is identified, diagnosis and treatment of the inciting cause should be performed immediately. If possible, milk can be passively collected as it streams from the udder (and then frozen).

Colostrum and milk quality should be monitored at the time of delivery to ensure that immunoglobulin content is adequate. Colostrum quality can be evaluated using a colostrometer (Lane Manufacturing, Denver, Colorado)[6] or wine refractometer (Bellingham & Stanley, Kent, England).[7] Colostral specific gravity is measured using a colostrometer. Specific gravity of equine colostrum has been shown to have high correlation with immunoglobulin content (i.e., >3000 mg/dl with specific gravity >1.06).[8] An additional simple method for evaluating colostral quality involves measuring total proteins using a refractometer specific for sugar or alcohol.[7] Such refractometers have the necessary range of refraction to facilitate accurate measurement of colostral proteins. A reading of more than 23% sugar or 16° alcohol is consistent with good-quality (>60 g/L) colostrum.[7] Before use of either a colostrometer or a refractometer, both the equipment and the colostrum sample should be at room temperature to ensure an accurate reading.

Vulvar discharge sometimes is present in mares with abnormal pregnancy. Vulvar discharge and precocious mammary development typically occur together, but each symptom can be present independently. Bacterial placentitis is the most frequent cause of vulvar discharge. Vaginitis or abortion due to other causes (viral or fungal) also may cause vulvar discharge, although less frequently. If vulvar discharge is present, a swab for bacterial identification and antimicrobial sensitivities should be obtained. A direct swab from the discharge is useful for screening purposes. An additional swab of discharge noted in the cranial vagina or at the external cervical os also should be obtained. These samples may provide a more definitive identification of a specific organism if obtained under aseptic conditions. Taking swabs from the cervical lumen or uterus is contraindicated because of the potential to penetrate the cervix, with accompanying risk of disrupting the pregnancy.

Ventral abdominal edema occasionally accompanies premature lactation in mares with high-risk pregnancies. This clinical sign is very nonspecific and must be differentiated from abdominal enlargement associated with normal pregnancy or other gestational abnormalities such as partial rupture of the prepubic tendon, abdominal wall herniation, or equine infectious anemia.

Aberrations in systemic parameters (temperature, heart rate, respiratory rate, gut sounds) are not typically associated with premature lactation. Mares progressing in second-stage labor may experience elevated heart rates, but this finding is not consistent (ML Macpherson, unpublished data).

DIAGNOSIS

Transrectal Ultrasonographic Evaluation

Transrectal ultrasonography in late gestation is useful primarily for evaluating placental integrity at the cervical star, fetal fluid character, and limited evaluation of the fetus (i.e., activity, orbit diameter). Examination for twin pregnancies in late gestation using transrectal ultrasonography is highly unreliable—in direct contrast with the proven usefulness of this modality early in gestation, allowing prompt diagnosis and management of twin pregnancies.[9]

In late gestation, transrectal ultrasonography of the caudal allantochorion provides an excellent image of the placenta close to the cervical star.[10] This region is affected most frequently in cases of ascending placentitis. In the normal pregnant mare, the area visualized in the region of the cervical star is the combined uterine and placental (chorioallantoic) unit. Renaudin and co-workers[10,11] developed the technique for evaluation of the combined thickness of the uterus and placenta (CTUP) and established normal values in light horse mares throughout gestation. To perform the procedure, any fecal material is evacuated from the mare's rectum. The reproductive tract should be manipulated minimally to avoid stimulating the fetus. A 5- or 7.5-MHz linear transducer is placed in the rectum and positioned 5 cm cranial to the cervical-placental junction. The transducer is moved laterally until the large uterine vessel (possibly the middle branch of the uterine artery) is visible at the ventral aspect of the uterine body.[10] The CTUP is measured between the uterine vessel and the allantoic fluid (Figure 60-1). A minimum of three measurements should be obtained and averaged.

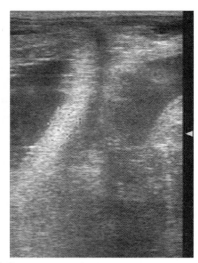

Figure 60-1 Transrectal ultrasound measurement of the combined thickness of the uterus and placenta (CTUP).

It is important to obtain all CTUP measurements from the ventral aspect of the uterine body, because physiologic edema of the dorsal aspect of the allantochorion has been noted in normal pregnant mares during the last month of gestation.[10] This finding may be misdiagnosed as pathologic thickening of the fetal membranes. In addition, the clinician should be sure that the amniotic membrane is not adjacent to the allantochorion, because this may result in a falsely increased CTUP. Conversely, fetal pressure on the caudal uterus can falsely decrease the CTUP. Care should be exercised to obtain measures when the fetus is not in the pelvic canal. Normal values for CTUP have been established.[10] Increases in CTUP of greater than 8 mm between days 271 and 300, greater than 10 mm between days 301 and 330, and greater than 12 mm after day 330 have been associated with placental failure and impending abortion.[12] Transrectal ultrasonographic examination is useful for identifying other abnormal conditions, including accumulation of purulent material (hyperechoic) between the uterus and the placenta (Figure 60-2). Measurements in such cases are meaningless because they will no longer reflect the true dimension of the combined unit and because evidence of accumulated purulent material is pathognomonic for placentitis.

Transabdominal Ultrasonographic Evaluation

Transabdominal ultrasonography is an excellent tool for evaluating the fetus and placenta in mares that are considered to be at risk for abortion during late gestation.[13-15] Fetal well-being can be assessed through transabdominal ultrasonographic evaluation of fetal heart rate, tone, activity, and size. Placental membrane integrity and thickness and fetal fluid character also are evaluated using this technique. Transabdominal ultrasonography also is the most accurate method to diagnose twins in late gestation.

Before the examination, proper preparation of the patient is important. Ideally, the mare's ventral abdomen

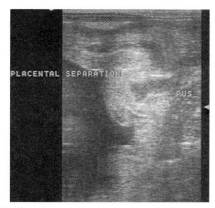

Figure 60-2 Placental separation and accumulation of purulent material at the cervical star area in a mare with ascending placentitis.

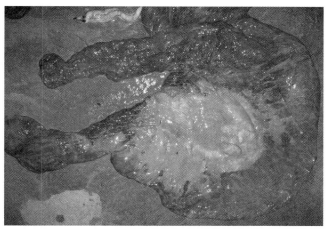

Figure 60-3 Placental lesions consistent with a *Nocardia*-form type of placentitis. Characteristics of this type of placentitis include a nonvillous area covered with a thick, mucoid exudate located at the juncture of the uterine body and pregnant horn.

is clipped from the mammary gland to the xiphoid process and up to the level of both stifles.[16] The area is cleansed of debris. Coupling gel or alcohol is applied. In cases in which clipping the ventral abdomen is not an option, thorough (and frequent) wetting of the abdomen with alcohol generally facilitates proper examination of the abdominal contents. Ultrasonographic examination of the equine abdomen is performed using a 2.5- or 3.5-MHz transducer with a depth setting of 20 to 30 cm.[13,14,16-18] Although a 5-MHz transducer can be used to measure fetal heart rates in late-gestation fetuses, the limited tissue penetration of this transducer type precludes its use for the thorough examination necessary to detect twins or perform complete fetal assessment. In most instances, a convex, curvilinear, or sector-scanner transducer is used for optimal depth penetration and image footprint.

All four quadrants of the abdomen are systematically examined; right cranial, right caudal, left cranial, and left caudal. The initial examination usually begins just cranial to the mare's mammary gland to ensure detection of a fetus as early as 90 days of gestation. The abdomen is scanned in a sagittal plane through all four quadrants because this is the most common orientation of the fetus (cranial or anterior position, sagittal plane) late in gestation.[16,17] Subsequent scanning in a transverse plane is necessary to image all aspects of the uterus and to confirm the number of fetuses.[19] Using this method, both the pregnant and the nonpregnant horns can be evaluated in their entirety and the fetal number determined.

In the normal pregnancy, the chorioallantois is intimately associated with the endometrium and cannot be easily identified as a separate structure. As with transrectal evaluation of the uteroplacental unit, mares with normal pregnancies should have a minimum CTUP of 7.1 ±1.6 mm and a maximum CTUP of 11.5 ± 2.4 mm.[13] Pregnancies with an increased CTUP have been associated with the delivery of abnormal foals.[13] This tool also is useful for identifying placental thickening and/or separation in mares with placentitis originating from a hematogenous infection. Additional findings in mares infected with *Nocardia*-form bacteria often include pla-

cental separation and purulent material at the base of the gravid horn and the junction of the uterine body[20] (Figure 60-3). The transabdominal approach is the most accurate means for diagnosing *Nocardia*-form placentitis. Transabdominal ultrasonography is not a useful tool for evaluating the caudal portion of the allantochorion (cervical star area), and evaluation of this area should be accomplished using transrectal ultrasonography as described.[10]

In addition to diagnosing placental disease, transabdominal ultrasonography is very useful for monitoring fetal health. Fetal parameters such as heart rate, size, activity, and tone can be assessed through a transabdominal approach. Locating a fetus is most easily achieved by identifying the fetal thorax. Confirmation of twins generally is made by identifying two fetal thoraces, with or without active heart beats. The fetal thorax is visualized as several linear hypoechoic shadows (intercostal spaces) interdigitated with linear hyperechoic ribs. The active fetal heart is easily identified at the cranialmost aspect of the fetal thorax, which is the end that narrows into the cervical spine. The average heart rate in a fetus at greater than 300 days of gestation is 75 ± 7 beats per minute.[13] Fetal heart rate slows by approximately 10 beats per minute after a gestational age of 330 days but can vary with activity levels. Heart rates can increase by 15 to 20 beats per minute during periods of activity.[16,17] Consistently low or high fetal heart rates are associated with fetal stress. Fetuses experiencing distress often become bradycardic initially and then become tachycardic in the terminal phase of life.[17,18]

Measurement of aortic diameter has been advocated as a method for determining fetal size.[13,16] This measure has been correlated with maternal weight, which is used to estimate fetal size. The aortic diameter is measured at the caudal border of the heart during systole. Although this is a useful tool, accurate measurement of aortic diameter can be challenging in the practical setting. Other means of determining fetal size include measurement of the thorax (using a transabdominal approach) biparietal diameter and/or fetal orbit diameter (using a transrectal approach).[16,21] The fetal thorax is measured from the spine to the sternum at the caudal aspect of the sternum.[16] Mean fetal thoracic measures in late gestation (range 298 to 356 days of gestation) are 183 ± 12 cm. Measures over a range of gestational ages currently are not available. Fetal thorax measures are most useful for comparing sizes of twins. Fetal eye size has been correlated with fetal age, rather than directly with fetal size.[21] Combined length and height measures of the fetal orbit (in millimeters) have a high correlation with fetal gestational age. As with any technique relying on measurements, variation can occur between operators and between examinations.

Fetal activity level and tone are easily determined during assessment of heart rate. Fetal activity can vary during the examination period, because fetuses have periods of sleep and wakefulness. In response to the ultrasound beam, the normal fetus commonly becomes very active during the examination period. Fetal activity has been described on a scale of 0 to 3.[13,16] A grade of 0 indicates no fetal movement over a minimum examination period of 30 minutes. A grade of 1 is assigned if minimal movement occurs ($\leq$33% of examination time), 2 if moderate activity is noted (33% to 66% of examination time) and 3 if the fetus is very active during the examination ($\geq$66% of the time). Fetal "tone" is a subjective term describing the viability of the fetus. A live fetus has excellent tone in that it actively flexes and extends the torso, neck, and limbs.[13,16] A fetus without tone most frequently will be found to be dead or in the terminal stage of life. An atonic fetus is flaccid and lies passively within the uterus and may be folded in on itself. Clearly identifying the atonic fetus can be difficult, because features such as the heart beat may be absent and traditional anatomic landmarks often may be obscured by the limbs of the flaccid fetus.

Serial examinations should be conducted to verify fetal well-being or distress. Once-daily transabdominal ultrasonographic assessments commonly are performed in high-risk mares. Fetuses experiencing distress often are evaluated several times a day to assess heart rate and activity level, particularly to determine if fetal distress is significant enough to prompt intervention such as induction of parturition. Only in rare cases would a mare suffering from ascending placentitis be considered a good candidate for induced parturition. More often, measures are instituted to encourage pregnancy maintenance, with the goal of precocious fetal maturation if preterm delivery is not preventable.

TREATMENT OPTIONS

Twin Pregnancies

Twin pregnancies are best managed by early detection and elimination of one embryonic vesicle using the manual crush technique. Delay in identification of a twin pregnancy until late in gestation poses a significant problem. Although some mares may successfully deliver live twins, a majority of mares will lose one or both pregnancies in the latter third of gestation.[22] Those mares that abort twins late in gestation (>250 days) or give birth to twins at term are at increased risk for dystocia. Methods for managing twin pregnancies are discussed Chapter 54.

Placentitis

Central to treatment of any disease is adequate understanding of its pathophysiology. Placentitis in mares commonly is caused by bacteria ascending through the vagina.[20,23,24] The bacterial pathogens most frequently implicated in equine placentitis are *Streptococcus equi* subspecies *zooepidemicus*, *Escherichia coli*, *Klebsiella pneumoniae*, and *Pseudomonas aeruginosa*.[25] Although bacterial infection initiates disease, recent work from an experimental model of ascending placentitis in pony mares showed that premature delivery may occur secondary to inflammation of the chorion, rather than as a consequence of fetal infection.[26,27] These inflammatory processes lead to prostaglandin production (PGE_2 and $PGF_{2\alpha}$) and stimulation of myometrial contractility, thus resulting in preterm delivery.[28,29] Therefore, therapies directed at resolving microbial invasion and inflammation and limiting uterine contractions probably are needed to effectively combat placental infections.

To date, treatment strategies for placentitis in mares are mostly empirical. Protocols frequently include combinations of antimicrobial agents (penicillin, gentamicin, trimethoprim-sulfa, and ceftiofur), anti-inflammatory drugs (flunixin meglumine, pentoxifylline), and agents to promote uterine quiescence (progestins, isoxsuprine, tocolytics). Early studies examined the ability of commonly used antimicrobial agents to penetrate equine fetal membranes.[30,31] In one study,[30] 11 normal pregnant mares were administered potassium penicillin, gentamicin, and trimethoprim-sulfadiazine. Samples of amniotic fluid, allantoic fluid, and mare and foal serum were obtained. Trimethoprim-sulfa was identified in amniotic and allantoic fluid, penicillin was detected in one allantoic sample, and gentamicin was not detected in fetal fluids. Only trimethoprim-sulfadiazine was present in serum of foals born to treated mares.

Florida workers[32] used in vivo microdialysis as a more sensitive means to identify potassium penicillin and gentamicin sulfate in allantoic fluid and serum of normal pony mares and mares with experimentally induced placentitis. Penicillin and gentamicin were detected in allantoic fluid, albeit at lower concentrations than those in serum of normal and infected mares. Both antibiotics remained above detectable limits for longer periods in allantoic fluid versus serum. Concentrations of penicillin in allantoic fluid achieved the minimum inhibitory concentration (MIC) against *S. equi* subspecies *zooepidemicus*. Gentamicin concentrations in allantoic fluid were adequate for effectiveness against *E. coli* or *K. pneumoniae*. Using microdialysis-based sampling methodology, flunixin meglumine was not detected in allantoic fluid of pony mares. Flunixin meglumine is highly protein bound, which may have prevented passage of the drug across the microdialysis sampling system. Results from this study regarding fetal viability were inconclusive because of the short treatment time (7 days) and limited number of subjects.

Recent data[33] using the same microdialysis technology have shown that trimethoprim-sulfamethoxazole and pentoxifylline also penetrate placental membranes and are detectable in allantoic fluid. Allantoic concentrations of both drugs were similar in nontreated and in treated mares with experimentally induced placentitis. As indicated by reported MIC values against *S. equi* subspecies *zooepidemicus*, the levels of trimethoprim-sulfamethoxazole achieved in allantoic fluid are sufficient to elicit an antibiotic effect for up to 4 hours after each treatment. Work under way (J. Graczyk, personal communication, 2005) has shown that trimethoprim-sulfamethoxazole and pentoxifylline also are present in fetal and placental tissues from infected, treated mares. Furthermore, mares treated from the onset of clinical signs of placentitis (after experimental infection) tended to carry foals longer than did untreated, infected control mares. The cumulative findings from these studies confirm the passage of penicillin, gentamicin, trimethoprim-sulfamethoxazole, and pentoxifylline across the blood-placental barrier and into the fetal fluids. These data provide a basis for therapeutic choices in treating mares placentitis in mares.

The pharmacokinetics or effects of several agents administered to mares with placentitis are still unknown, including widely used progestins. Progestins play an important role in inhibiting uterine smooth muscle gap junction formation until parturition is initiated.[34] Mares treated with progestins after prostaglandin-induced abortion (98 to 153 days of gestation) carried pregnancies to term, whereas control mares aborted.[35] Prostaglandin secretion was inhibited in treated mares. The effects of progestin therapy in late-gestation mares have not been critically evaluated. Recent work in women[36,37] has shown that progestin therapy lowers the incidence of preterm labor; therefore, this drug warrants further study on use in mares.

Other drugs commonly used to prevent uterine contractility in mares include isoxsuprine and clenbuterol. Isoxsuprine and clenbuterol have known smooth muscle relaxant properties, including effects on the uterus.[38] French workers reported[39] the efficacy of clenbuterol for preventing labor in 29 late-gestation normal mares. Mares with mammary secretion electrolyte changes suggestive of impending parturition were treated with clenbuterol (varying doses) or saline, once daily at 2200 hours, until parturition. No differences were detected between groups for length of gestation, number of treatments, or time to foaling after the last dose was administered. The authors concluded that clenbuterol was not effective in preventing the onset of myometrial contractions in normal-foaling mares at term. Treated mares in this study actually foaled earlier in the evening than did untreated mares. Side effects noted after treatment with clenbuterol included cardiovascular abnormalities and, in one instance, dystocia. Tocolytics, including these agents, most commonly are used to forestall preterm labor in women for approximately 48 hours. This time frame allows administration of glucocorticoids, which in turn promote fetal maturation.[40] Long-term use of tocolytic

agents in women has fallen out of favor because of significant side effects of these drugs. The lack of clear effect of tocolytic drugs for forestalling preterm labor in mares, combined with possible side effects, fails to support the use of these drugs in high-risk pregnant mares.

The perfect "recipe" for treating equine placentitis remains elusive. The use of combination therapy composed of an antimicrobial agent, anti-inflammatory agent, and uterine relaxant or tocolytic is the most promising solution to this difficult veterinary problem. Combination therapy has been supported with results from a large retrospective clinical trial from central Kentucky. Using clinical data, Troedsson and Zent (personal communication, 2003) examined records of 477 mares over 6 years to determine the effectiveness of treatment for placentitis. Fifteen mares were diagnosed with placentitis as indicated by increased thickness of the uteroplacental unit on transrectal ultrasound evaluation, placental separation and/or vulvar discharge, and udder development. Mares were given a combination of systemic antibiotics (e.g., trimethoprim plus a sulfa drug, or ceftiofur or penicillin plus gentamicin), pentoxifylline, altrenogest flunixin meglumine, and/or phenylbutazone. Antibiotic treatment was continued until abortion or delivery of a foal. Twelve of 15 (84%) treated mares carried their foals to term, and 11 of 15 (73%) gave birth to live foals. Liveborn foals also had birth weights similar to those of their normal counterparts, whereas dead or euthanized foals had significantly lower birth weights. Information from this study lends support for a placentitis protocol directed at reducing microbial invasion, inflammation, and uterine activity.

CONCLUSIONS

Premature lactation often is a clinical sign indicating a serious threat to late-term pregnancy. Identification of the cause of premature lactation, with rapid institution of appropriate treatment, can be critical to the viability of both mare and fetus. Tools such as transabdominal and transrectal ultrasonography provide diagnostic information that can dictate therapeutic directions. Therapies are directed at remedying the inciting cause of premature lactation.

References

1. Blanchard TL, Varner DD, Schumacher J et al: Manual of Equine Reproduction, 2nd ed. St. Louis, Mosby, 2003.
2. Hodge SL, Kreider JL, Potter GD et al: Influence of photoperiod on the pregnant and post partum mare. Am J Vet Res 1982; 10:1752.
3. Rossdale PD, Ricketts SW: Equine Stud Farm Medicine, 2nd ed. Philadelphia, Lea & Febiger, 1980.
4. Jeffcott LB: Passive immunity and its transfer with special reference to the horse. Biol Rev 1972; 47:439.
5. McGuire TC, Poppie MJ, Banks KL: Hypogammaglobulinemia predisposing to infection in foals. J Am Vet Med Assoc 1977; 166:71.
6. Leblanc MM, Tran T, Baldwin JL, Pritchard EL: Factors that influence passive transfer of immunoglobulins in foals. J Am Vet Med Assoc 1992; 200:179.

7. Chavatte P, Clement F, Cash R, J-F Gronget: Field determination of colostrum quality by using a novel, practical method. Proceedings of the 44th Annual Convention of the American Association of Equine Practitioners, pp 206-209, 1998.

8. Leblanc MM, McLaurin BI, Boswell R: Relationships among serum immunoglobulin concentration in foals, colostral specific-gravity, and colostral immunoglobulin concentration. J Am Vet Med Assoc 1986; 189:57.

9. Chevalier F, Palmer E: Ultrasonic echography in the mare. J Reprod Fertil Suppl 1982; 32:423.

10. Renaudin CD, Troedsson MHT, Gillis CL et al: Ultrasonographic evaluation of the equine placenta by transrectal and transabdominal approach in the normal pregnant mare. Theriogenology 1997; 47:559.

11. Renaudin CD, Troedsson MHT, Gillis CL: Transrectal ultrasonographic evaluation of the normal equine placenta. Equine Vet Educ 1999; 11:75.

12. Renaudin CD, Liu IKM, Troedsson MHT, Schrenzel MD: Transrectal ultrasonographic diagnosis of ascending placentitis in the mare: a report of two cases. Equine Vet Educ 1999; 11:69.

13. Reef VB, Vaala WE, Worth LT et al: Ultrasonographic assessment of fetal well-being during late gestation: development of an equine biophysical profile. Equine Vet J 1996; 28:200.

14. Adams-Brendemuehl C, Pipers FS: Antepartum evaluation of the equine fetus. J Reprod Fertil Suppl 1987; 35:565.

15. Vaala WE, Sertich PL: Management strategies for mares at risk for periparturient complications. Vet Clin North Am Equine Pract 1994; 10:237.

16. Reef VB, Vaala WE, Worth LT et al: Ultrasonographic evaluation of the fetus and intrauterine environment in healthy mares during late-gestation. Vet Radiol Ultrasound 1995; 36:533.

17. Pipers FS, Adamsbrendemuehl CS: Techniques and applications of trans-abdominal ultrasonography in the pregnant mare. J Am Vet Med Assoc 1984; 185:766.

18. Pipers FS, Zent W, Holder R, Asbury A: Ultrasonography as an adjunct to pregnancy assessments in the mare. J Am Vet Med Assoc 1984; 184:328.

19. Reef VB, Sertich PL, Turner RMO: Equine Diagnostic Ultrasound. Philadelphia, WB Saunders, 1998.

20. Hong CB, Donahue JM, Giles RC et al: Etiology and pathology of equine placentitis. J Vet Diagn Invest 1993; 5:56.

21. McKinnon AO, Voss JL, Squires EL, Carnevale EM: Diagnostic ultrasonography. In McKinnon AO, Voss JL (eds): Equine Reproduction. Philadelphia, Lea & Febiger, pp 266-302, 1993.

22. Jeffcott LB, Whitwell KE: Twinning as a cause of fetal and neonatal loss in thoroughbred mare. J Comp Pathol 1973; 83:91.

23. Platt H: Infection of the horse fetus. J Reprod Fertil Suppl 1975; 23:605.

24. Whitwell K: Equine Infectious Diseases V. Lexington, Ky, University of Kentucky Press, 1988.

25. Acland HM: Abortion. In McKinnon AO, Voss JL (eds): Equine Reproduction. Philadelphia, Lea & Febiger, pp 554-561, 1993.

26. Leblanc MM, Giguere S, Brauer K et al: Premature delivery in ascending placentitis is associated with increased expression of placental cytokines and allantoic fluid prostaglandins E-2 and F-2 alpha. Theriogenology 2002; 58:841.

27. Mays MBC, Leblanc MM, Paccamonti D: Route of fetal infection in a model of ascending placentitis. Theriogenology 2002; 58:791.

28. Pollard JK, Mitchell MD: Intrauterine infection and the effects of inflammatory mediators on prostaglandin production by myometrial cells from pregnant women. Am J Obstet Gynecol 1996; 174:682.

29. Dudley DJ, Trautman MS: Infection, inflammation, and contractions—the role of cytokines in the pathophysiology of preterm labor. Semin Reprod Endocrinol 1994; 12:263.

30. Sertich PL, Vaala WE: Concentrations of antibiotics in mares, foals and fetal fluids after antibiotic administration in late pregnancy. Proceedings of the 38th Annual Convention of the American Association of Equine Practitioners, pp 727-736, 1992.

31. Santschi EM, Papich MG: Pharmacokinetics of gentamicin in mares in late pregnancy and early lactation. J Vet Pharmacol Ther 2000; 23:359.

32. Murchie TA, Macpherson ML, Leblanc MM et al: A microdialysis model to detect drugs in the allantoic fluid of pregnant pony mares. Proceedings of the 49th Annual Convention of the American Association of Equine Practitioners, pp 118-119, 2003.

33. Rebello SA, Macpherson ML, Murchie TA et al: The detection of placental drug transfer in equine allantoic fluid. Theriogenology 2005; 64:776-777.

34. Garfield RE, Kannan MB, Daniel ME: Gap junction formation in the myometrium: control by estrogens, progesterone and prostaglandins. Am J Physiol 1980; 238:C81.

35. Daels PF, Besognet B, Hansen B et al : Effect of progesterone on prostaglandin F-2 alpha secretion and outcome of pregnancy during cloprostenol-induced abortion in mares. Am J Vet Res 1996; 57:1331.

36. da Fonseca EB, Bittar RE, Carvalho MHB, Zugaib M: Prophylactic administration of progesterone by vaginal suppository to reduce the incidence of spontaneous preterm birth in women at increased risk: a randomized placebo-controlled double-blind study. Am J Obstet Gynecol 2003; 188:419.

37. Meis PJ, Klebanoff M, Thom E et al: Prevention of recurrent preterm delivery by 17 alpha-hydroxyprogesterone caproate. N Engl J Med 2003; 348:2379.

38. Plumb DC: Veterinary Drug Handbook, 3rd ed. Ames, Iowa, Iowa State University Press, 1999.

39. Palmer E, Chavette-Palmer P, Duchamp G, Levy I: Lack of effect of clenbuterol for delaying parturition in late pregnant mares. Theriogenology 2002; 58:797.

40. Goldenberg RL: The management of preterm labor. Obstet Gynecol 2002; 100:1020.

CHAPTER 61

Mastitis

BETH A. ALBRECHT

Mastitis is an inflammation of the mammary gland that occurs infrequently in the mare. The low incidence of mastitis in mares has been attributed to the small capacity and the protected location of the equine udder. Mastitis may affect mares of any age and reproductive state. Cases of mastitis have been reported in fillies as young as 1 day[1] and mares as old as 24 years of age.[2] The incidence of mastitis is similar in nonlactating and lactating mares. Mares are affected by four types of mastitis based on etiology: bacterial, mycotic, verminous, and avocado toxicity–associated mastitis.

MAMMARY GLAND ANATOMY

The two mammary glands of the mare are encased within the udder. The udder is located beneath the cranial portion of the pelvis and the caudal portion of the abdominal floor and is partially protected by the pelvic limbs. Covering the udder is a thin, sparsely haired, well-pigmented skin that is endowed with sweat and sebaceous glands.[3] Grossly, the udder is divided into right and left halves by an external longitudinal intermammary groove,[3] and at the base of each half is one laterally flattened teat. Each half of the udder contains one mamma. Each mamma is composed of lobes that are subdivided into lobules and secretory alveoli. Milk produced in the secretory alveoli passes into interlobular ducts[4] that empty into lobar ducts and finally into a gland cistern. Each gland cistern drains a single mammary gland lobe. Milk passes from the gland cistern into the teat cistern and finally into the papillary duct (Figure 61-1). The papillary duct opens to the exterior via an ostium located in a depression at the apex of each teat. Two or three ostia are present in each teat, and each ostium represents the opening of a separate lactiferous duct system.[3] The number and unique arrangement of teat ostia complicate treatment of mammary gland conditions.

Mammary development in the mare varies with reproductive status of the animal. The equine udder is smallest in the nulliparous mare and increases in size to a capacity of approximately 2 L[5] in the lactating mare. Both the protected location and the small size of the udder minimize the incidence of mammary gland pathologic conditions in the mare.

BACTERIAL MASTITIS

The most common type of mastitis affecting mares is bacterial. Mares with bacterial mastitis will often have an insect sting, injury, or laceration of the teat or udder on the affected side and will present with a swollen, firm udder that is warm and/or painful to palpation (Box 6.2-1).[2] One or both mammae may be affected. Other signs may include ventral edema extending from the udder cranially and/or caudally and unilateral or bilateral hindlimb lameness ipsilateral to the affected mamma. Systemic signs may be present or absent and will vary between mares and causes. Common systemic signs include pyrexia, lethargy, and depression. Less commonly mares present with anorexia, sweating, elevated pulse and respiratory rates,[6] neutrophilia, and/or hyperfibrinogenemia.[2] The affected mammary gland will produce secretions that vary in consistency from milky to thick (Table 61-1). Mammary secretions from affected glands will vary in appearance (see Table 61-1) from a yellow to yellowish-brown or yellowish-gray in color[6,7] and may contain blood and/or flocculent material.[7,8] The mammary secretions should be evaluated to determine the type and severity of the mastitis.

Mammary secretions from a suspect mare should be collected for pathogen isolation and cytologic evaluation. Before sample collection, the teat should be cleaned with a dry gauze sponge and several streams of fluid should be stripped from the teat to reduce contaminants.[9] A 2- to 3-ml sample is then collected into a sterile container for analysis. Both pathogen isolation from and cytologic evaluation of the mammary secretions may be used to confirm the diagnosis of mastitis.

Less common techniques used to confirm the presence of mastitis include the California Mastitis Test or ultrasonography of the udder.[10] The California Mastitis Test is commonly used for dairy cattle but rarely used in horses. Ultrasonography of the udder allows one to distinguish between mastitis and other mammary gland lesions such as mammary gland abscesses and tumors (Box 61-2). Although both techniques can be useful, identification of the pathogen and cytologic evaluation of the mammary secretions are the preferred methods for diagnostic confirmation of mastitis.

Several bacterial species have been isolated from mammary gland secretions of affected mares (Table 61-2). Of these organisms, *Streptococcus* sp. account for over half of the observed cases of equine mastitis, and the most common isolate is *S. zooepidemicus*. Other commonly isolated organisms are *Escherichia coli*, *Klebsiella* sp., *Staphylococcus* sp., and *Corynebacterium* sp. Several other bacterial species have been reported, but these are infrequently observed (see Table 61-2). Most cases of equine bacterial mastitis are caused by a single organism.

Table   **61-1**

Characteristics of Mammary Gland Secretions

Characteristic	Colostrum	Milk	Mammary Involution	Mastitis
Color	Yellow	White	White	Yellow to yellowish-brown/gray
Consistency	Thick	Thin	Thin to thick	Thin to thick
Blood/blood clots	Absent	Absent	Absent	Present/absent
Flocculent material/ cell debris	Present	Absent	Absent	Present/absent
Protein	Present, gives a homogenous background with trichrome stain	Present, gives a granular background with trichrome stain	Generally present	Present
pH		7.4		approximately 6.4
Neutrophils	Absent	Absent	Few present early in involution, degenerate present in late involution	Present
Macrophages	Absent	Absent	Present late in involution	Present/absent
Bacteria/fungi	Absent	Absent	Absent	Present/absent
Nematodes (eggs, larvae, or adult)	Absent	May contain *Strongyloides westeri* larvae (>3 days post partum)[18]	Absent	Present/absent

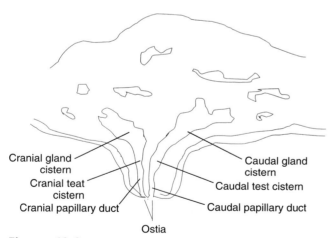

Figure 61-1 Normal anatomy of the equine udder and mammary gland.

Cranial gland cistern
Cranial teat cistern
Cranial papillary duct
Caudal gland cistern
Caudal test cistern
Caudal papillary duct
Ostia

Box   **61-1**

Common Clinical Signs of Mastitis

Swollen udder
Udder painful to touch
Elevated temperature of udder
Ventral edema
Hindlimb lameness

Box   **61-2**

Differential Diagnoses for Equine Mastitis

Normal periparturient mammary development
Normal mammary gland involution
Mammary gland abscess
Acute mastitis
Chronic mastitis
Mammary gland tumor
Mammary granulomas
Mammary gland induration

However, multiple organisms are cultured in approximately 5% of the cases examined.

Bacterial mastitis may be treated with systemic and/or intramammary antibiotics and supportive care (Box 61-3). Systemic administration of antibiotics is the easier and safer method of treatment. Systemic antibiotic therapy may include penicillin and gentamicin or trimethoprim/sulfadiazine initially and should be changed to an appropriate antibiotic once the organism and its antibiotic sensitivity have been determined. Failure to perform

Table 61-2

Bacterial Isolates from Equine Mastitis

Organisms	Percent of Isolates*	References
Actinobacillus sp.	2.8	McCue and Wilson,[2] Carmalt et al[19]
A. lignieresii	0.9[†]	Carmalt et al[19]
A. suis	1.9[‡]	McCue and Wilson[2]
Actinomycetes sp.	0.9[†]	Delorme and Hamelin[1]
Bacillus sp.	0.9	Albrecht and Samper[20]
Corynebacterium sp.	3.7	Addo et al,[7] Albrecht and Samper,[20] Seahorn et al[21]
C. ovis	0.9	Addo et al[7]
C. pseudotuberculosis	0.9	Albrecht and Samper,[20] Seahorn et al[21]
Enterobacter sp.	1.9	McCue and Wilson,[2] Albrecht and Samper[20]
E. aerogenes	0.9	McCue and Wilson[2]
E. agglomerans	0.9[†]	Albrecht and Samper[20]
Erwinia sp.	0.9	Bostedt et al[22]
Escherichia sp.	5.6	Delorme and Hamelin,[1] McCue and Wilson,[2] Albrecht and Samper,[20] Bostedt et al[22]
E. coli	5.6	Delorme and Hamelin,[1] McCue and Wilson,[2] Albrecht and Samper,[20] Bostedt et al[22]
Klebsiella sp.	4.6	McCue and Wilson,[2] Albrecht and Samper,[20] Bostedt et al[22]
K. pneumoniae	1.9	McCue and Wilson[2]
Micrococcus sp.	0.9	Bostedt et al[22]
Neisseria sp.	2.8	Bostedt et al[22]
Pasteurella sp.	0.9	McCue and Wilson[2]
P. ureae	0.9	McCue and Wilson[2]
Pseudomonas sp.	1.9	McCue and Wilson,[2] Roberts[8]
P. aeruginosa	1.9	McCue and Wilson,[2] Roberts[8]
Staphylococcus sp.	5.6	Delorme and Hamelin,[1] McCue and Wilson,[2] Bostedt et al,[22] Prentice,[23] Freeman et al[24]
S. aureus	0.9	Freeman et al[24]
Streptococcus sp.	53.7	McCue and Wilson,[2] Al-Graibawi et al,[5] Reese and Lock,[6] Albrecht and Samper,[20] Bostedt et al,[22] Prentice,[23] Freeman et al,[24] Strong,[25] Leadon and Gibbons[26]
S. agalactiae	0.9	McCue and Wilson[2]
S. dysgalactia	0.9	Bostedt et al[22]
S. equi	0.9	Prentice[23]
S. viridans	0.9	McCue and Wilson[2]
S. zooepidemicus	10.2	McCue and Wilson,[2] Al-Graibawi et al,[5] Albrecht and Samper,[20] Freeman et al[24]
Unidentified organism[§]	35.2	Delorme and Hamelin,[1] McCue and Wilson,[2] Albrecht and Samper,[20] Bostedt et al,[22] Freeman et al,[24] Bocquet et al[27]

*Values are percentage of total cases of mastitis examined. Multiple organisms were isolated in some cases.
[†]Equid less than or equal to 1 year.
[‡]Organism was identified from mammary secretions in two additional cases; however, a diagnosis of mastitis was not made.[28]
[§]No organism was cultured, or no attempt was made to identify the etiologic agent.

antibiotic sensitivity may result in chronic mastitis. If intramammary infusion of antibiotics is used, it is critical that all teat canals of the affected mamma receive antibiotics because two to three papillary ducts empty at the apex of each teat (see Figure 61-1). Care should be exercised when using intramammary infusions of antibiotics because mares with mastitis are often very painful and uncooperative. Intramammary antibiotic preparations for lactating cattle may be used. However, the teat canals of mares are generally smaller than those of dairy cattle, and care should be taken to avoid injuring the teat. Systemic and intramammary antibiotics may be used in combination; however, systemic administration of antibiotics that partition into the mammary gland provides the simplest approach to treatment of bacterial mastitis.

Supportive therapy should include frequent milking of the affected mammary gland. In addition, hydrotherapy and hot packs may be beneficial. If the mare has a foal,

Box   **61-3**

Mastitis Therapy

Frequent milking
Systemic antimicrobial
Intramammary antimicrobial
Hydrotherapy
Hot packs

she may not allow the foal to nurse. Therefore the foal should be monitored to ensure adequate nutrient intake and be provided supplemental feeding if necessary. Administration of a nonsteroidal antiinflammatory drug such as flunixin meglumine will improve the mare's level of comfort. The prognosis for mares with bacterial mastitis is good to excellent, and most mares will respond to therapy within 3 to 5 days and recover within 2 weeks. The mare's response to therapy should be monitored to prevent development of chronic mastitis.

MYCOTIC MASTITIS

Mycotic mastitis is a less common type of mastitis in mares. Mares with mycotic mastitis will present with clinical signs similar to those with bacterial mastitis. A clinical sign that may help in distinguishing between mycotic and bacterial mastitis is the consistency of the mammary secretions. Mammary secretions from a gland affected with mycotic mastitis may appear clear yellow and gelatinous with strands of cloudy material.[11] Cytologic examination of the mammary secretions may reveal fungal hyphae, allowing for the diagnosis of mycotic mastitis. Two species of fungi, *Aspergillus* sp. and *Coccidioides immitis*, have been reported as etiologic agents of mycotic mastitis.[1,11] Both *Aspergillus* sp. and *C. immitis* are more often associated with pulmonary disease than mastitis in Equidae, and mastitis may be a sequela to a mycotic pulmonary disease. *C. immitis* may remain latent for up to 15 years in a horse and during periods of stress, old age, pregnancy, malnutrition, or chronic pulmonary disease may become reactivated.[11] Therapy guidelines for mycotic mastitis are the same as for bacterial mastitis (see Box 61-3). The etiologic agent should be identified and an appropriate antimycotic agent selected. The antimycotic drug itraconazole is known to distribute into tissues with a high fat content and into milk and has been used at a dose of 3 mg/kg body weight[12] to treat cases of respiratory disease caused by *Coccidioides* sp. and *Aspergillus* sp. in horses. The efficacy of itraconazole therapy for equine mastitis has not been established, and prolonged administration may be required. The prognosis for a mare with mycotic mastitis is fair to good.

VERMINOUS MASTITIS

One case of verminous mastitis has been reported in the mare.[13] The affected mammary glands of the mare contained adult females, larvae, and eggs of a *Cephalobus* sp.

at necropsy. Members of the genus *Cephalobus* are soil-dwelling nematodes and in this case likely entered the mammary gland percutaneously. Levamisole therapy was attempted in this case but with limited success. Currently there is no recommended therapy for this type of mastitis.

Other parasites that may infect the equine mammary gland include *Strongyloides westeri*, *Halicephalobus deletrix*, *Draschia megastoma*, *Habronema muscae*, and *Habronema microstoma*.[13] However, currently none of these organisms have been identified as etiologic agents of equine mastitis.

AVOCADO TOXICITY–ASSOCIATED MASTITIS

Mastitis has also been associated with avocado (*Persea americana*) toxicity in horses.[14] Consumption of the leaves and/or fruit of *Persea americana* results in the release of the toxin, (Z,Z)-1-(acetyloxy)-2-hydroxy-12,15-heneicosadien-4-one (persin).[15] The toxin induces coagulative necrosis of the secretory acinar epithelium within the mammary gland of goats[16,17] and mice[15] and is likely to cause similar lesions in the equine mammary gland. In addition to mastitis, Equidae with avocado toxicity will show signs of mild colic; edema of the lips, tongue, mouth, head, neck, and ventral abdomen; depression; and in severe cases respiratory distress.[14] Mares with avocado toxicity–associated mastitis will recover without treatment within 2 weeks if the source of avocados is removed.[14] If the mare has severe respiratory distress and swelling of the head, administration of tripelennamine hydrochloride (1 mg/kg, IM) and flunixin meglumine (1.1 to 1.4 mg/kg IV) may be indicated.[14] The prognosis for mares with avocado toxicity–associated mastitis is good. However, if the damage to the mammary gland secretory epithelium is severe, scarring and adipose deposition will occur[15] and may reduce subsequent milk production. Avocado toxicity–associated mastitis has been documented in Australia and may be more common than reported.

SEQUELAE TO MASTITIS

Sequelae to mastitis are rare in mares and are most often due to failure to select an appropriate therapeutic agent and monitor the efficacy of the therapy. The most significant problems are chronic mastitis and mammary granulomas due to treatment failure. If mastitis is not treated, mammary gland induration may occur in response to chronic inflammation. This will not impair fertility, but an appropriate adoptive mare or milk replacer will be necessary for foals from this type of mare. In severe cases of chronic mastitis, mammary gland amputation may be necessary. Sequelae to mastitis can be avoided if an appropriate therapeutic regimen is selected.

References

1. Delorme JY, Hamelin A: Trois cas de mammites chez des pouliches nouveau-nees. Pratique Veterinaire Equine 1994; 26:276-278.

2. McCue PM, Wilson WD: Equine mastitis: a review of 28 cases. Equine Vet J 1989; 21:351-353.

3. Kainer RA: Reproductive organs of the mare. In McKinnon AO, Voss JL (eds): Equine Reproduction, 1st edition, Philadelphia, Lea & Febiger, 1993.

4. Baldwin RL, Miller PS: Mammary gland development and lactation. In Cupps PT (ed): Reproduction in Domestic Animals, 4th edition, New York, Academic Press, 1991.

5. Al-Graibawi MAA, Sharma VK, Ali SI: Mastitis in a mare. Vet Rec 1984; 115:383-383.

6. Reese GL, Lock TF: Streptococcal mastitis in a mare. J Am Vet Med Assoc 1978; 173:83-84.

7. Addo PB, Wilcox GE, Taussig R: Mastitis in a mare caused by *C. ovis*. Vet Rec 1974; 95:193-193.

8. Roberts MC: Pseudomonas aeruginosa mastitis in a dry non-pregnant pony mare. Equine Vet J 1986; 18:146-147.

9. Freeman KP: Cytological evaluation of the equine mammary gland. Equine Vet Educ 1993; 5:212-213.

10. Waldridge BM, Ward TA: Ultrasound examination of the equine mammary gland. Equine Pract 1999; 21:10-13.

11. Walker RL, Johnson BJ, Jones KL et al: *Coccidioides immitis* mastitis in a mare. J Vet Diagn Invest 1993; 5:446-448.

12. Plumb DC: Veterinary Drug Handbook, 4th edition, Ames, Iowa State Press, 2002.

13. Greiner EC, Calderwood-Mays MB, Smart GC et al: Verminous mastitis in a mare caused by a free-living nematode. J Parasitol 1991; 77:320-322.

14. McKenzie RA, Brown OP: Avocado (*Persea americana*) poisoning of horses. Aust Vet J 1991; 68:77-78.

15. Oelrichs PB, Ng JC, Seawright AA et al: Isolation and identification of a compound from avocado (*Persea americana*) leaves which causes necrosis of the acinar epithelium of the lactating mammary gland and the myocardium. Nat Toxins 1995; 3:344-349.

16. Craigmill AL, Eide RN, Schultz TA et al: Toxicity of avocado (*Persea americana* [Guatemalan var.]) leaves: review and preliminary report. Vet Hum Toxicol 1984; 26:381-384.

17. Craigmill AL, Seawright AA, Mattila T et al: Pathological changes in the mammary gland and biochemical changes in milk of the goat following oral dosing with leaf of the avocado (*Persea americana*). Aust Vet J 1989; 66:206-211.

18. Enigk K, Dey-Hazra A, Batke J: The clinical significance and treatment of milk-borne *Strongyloides westeri* of foals. DTW Dtsch Tierarztl Wochenschr 1974; 81:605-607.

19. Carmalt JL, Baptiste KE, Chirino-Trejo JM: *Actinobacillus lignieresii* infection in two horses. J Am Vet Med Assoc 1998; 215:826-828.

20. Albrecht BA, Samper JC: Unpublished, 2003.

21. Seahorn TL, Hall G, Brumbaugh GW et al: Mammary adenocarcinoma in four mares. J Am Vet Med Assoc 1992; 200:1675-1677.

22. Bostedt H, Lehmann B, Peip D: Zur Problematik der Mastitis bei Stuten. Tierärztl Prax 1988; 16:367-371.

23. Prentice MWM: Mastitis in the mare. 1974; Vet Rec 94:380-380.

24. Freeman KP, Roszel JF, Slusher SH et al: Cytologic features of equine mammary fluids: normal and abnormal. Comp Cont Educ Pract Vet 1988; 10:1090-1099.

25. Strong MG: Mastitis in the mare. Vet Rec 1974; 94:526-526.

26. Leadon DP, Gibbons PT: The putative association of α haemolytic streptococci with maternal mastitis and neonatal septicaemia. Equine Vet J Suppl 1988; 5:44-45.

27. Bocquet J, Rey J-D, Lequertier J: Traitement des mammites de la jument par la penethacilline. Bulletin Mensuel de la Sociâetâe Vâetâerinaire Pratique de France 1975; 59:281-290.

28. Jang SS, Biberstein EL, Hirsh DC: *Actinobacillus suis*-like organisms in horses. Am J Vet Res 1987; 48:1036-1038.

CHAPTER 62

Normal Prefoaling Mammary Secretions

WILLIAM B. LEY
G. REED HOLYOAK

Normal gestational length can vary widely in the mare. The majority of mares foal during "non-business" hours for most horse owners, as well as veterinarians. Thus many sleepless nights can be spent waiting up for the mare to foal. A 24-hour distribution of spontaneous foaling times for over 1,100 mares is depicted in Figure 62-1.[1] Physical signs of the mare's approaching readiness for foaling include a gestation length of greater than 320 days, udder enlargement with the presence of colostrum or milk in the teats, waxing on teat ends, and relaxation around the tail head, buttocks, and lips of the vulva. Although helpful, none of these signs is extremely accurate as a means of predicting when the mare will actually foal.

Studies of prefoaling milk (mammary secretion) electrolyte changes have demonstrated an association with the mare's approaching readiness to foal.[2-11] These electrolyte changes, especially with regard to calcium, have also been related to the development of maturity of the foal in the uterus and its subsequent survivability (i.e., viability) following a normal delivery.[4,8,10,12,13]

Prefoaling mammary secretion electrolytes are related to fetal readiness for birth.[4] Calcium carbonate ($CaCO_3$) content of such samples has been shown to be both sensitive and specific.[10] The predictive value of a positive test (PVPT) (defined as the first occurrence when $CaCO_3 \geq 200$ ppm) was determined to be 97.2%, for normal pregnant mares foaling spontaneously within 72 hours. Mares with placentitis and other causes of precocious lactation, however, have early elevation of mammary secretion calcium.[14] Before 310 days' gestation, elevated milk calcium levels indicate placental abnormality and not fetal maturity.

It has been suggested that the inversion of sodium and potassium concentrations in prefoaling mammary secretion does not occur in mares experiencing placentitis and may be a better indicator of in utero fetal maturation.[15] However, no published reports could be found to support this hypothesis other than the very early work of Peaker et al and Ousey et al.[2,4] These both used normal, spontaneously foaling mares for their investigations. We repeated this work (a) to evaluate prefoaling mammary secretion sodium and potassium concentrations and (b) to document the time of their relative inversion before foaling in normal mares. A consistent pattern could not be demonstrated[16]; 5 of 14 mares foaled normally, delivering live, healthy foals, and none demonstrated a sodium to potassium electrolyte inversion on any sample collected daily or twice daily from 7 to 10 days before spontaneous parturition. In a more recent work, it was reported that concentrations of potassium, calcium, citrate, and lactose increased and concentration of sodium decreased as foaling approached but that variation between mares was large.[11] These authors concluded that the use of prepartum equine mammary secretion electrolyte concentrations for prediction of time of foaling is unreliable due to the large variation in both absolute and change in electrolyte concentrations between mares. This is absolutely correct. None of these methods has yet been shown to predict time of foaling. Ley et al[10] stated that prefoaling mammary secretion $CaCO_3$ testing is a helpful prognostic tool to indicate the mare's approaching readiness for birth and a method to predict when the mare is not likely to foal within 24 hours when the $CaCO_3$ is less than 200 ppm. Ousey et al[4] suggested by their results that fetal maturity may be related to electrolyte concentration in mammary secretion and that an ionic score greater than or equal to 35 may indicate that induction would be successful in terms of maturity of the newborn foal. Leadon et al[3] stated that calcium concentrations of the mammary secretions proved useful in predicting full term and also in assessment of the chances of foal survival in prematurely induced parturition. Ousey et al[9] in a later report stated that mammary secretion electrolyte testing before foaling was not particularly accurate in predicting time of parturition, although it was a reliable means of indicating when it was not necessary to attend prepartum mares at night. It is reasonable to agree with Douglas et al[11] that these tests do not predict foaling time. Very few investigations have actually claimed that they do. Prefoaling mammary secretion electrolyte testing methods are simply a means to evaluate in utero fetal maturation and the approaching readiness for birth.

The FoalWatch test kit (CHEMetrics, Inc., Calverton, Va.) has been used extensively over many years by the authors and has proven useful in the routine management of mares in the prepartum period. Its intended use is to assist in determining when the fetus is likely mature in utero and the mare is approaching readiness for spontaneous foaling. This is based upon the ability of the kit to detect changes in the prefoaling mammary secretion (milk) $CaCO_3$ level. It is a tool that, when used in an appropriate manner, will allow one to attend the mare's

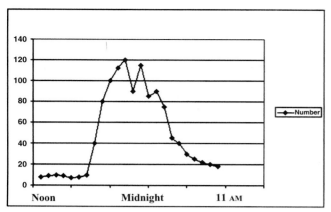

Figure 62-1 The distribution in a 24-hour period of spontaneous foaling times for over 1,100 mares. (Modified from Bain AM, Howey WP: Observations on the time of foaling in Thoroughbred mares in Australia. J Reprod Fertil Suppl 1975; 23:545)

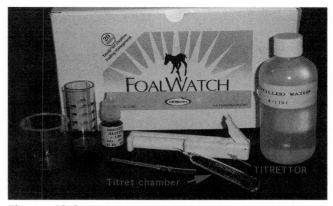

Figure 62-2 The FoalWatch test kit used to measure prefoaling mammary secretion calcium carbonate. The kit contains 20 vacuum-chambered titret ampules, the Titrettor apparatus, flexible tubing tips for the titrets, a sample collecting cup, a mixing cup for dilution of the sample, distilled water, indicator dye solution, and complete instructions.

foaling without an excessive number of sleepless nights. Alternatively, it can be used as a tool for accurately assessing when elective induction of parturition may safely be attempted. The advantages of this methodology include its accuracy and repeatability compared with other test kits or test strips available on the market, its ease of use, its quantitative (numerical) determination of the $CaCO_3$ level in each sample of prefoaling milk tested, and its economy.

WHEN TO BEGIN TESTING THE MARE

Begin sampling udder secretions and testing the recovered fluid approximately 10 to 14 days in advance of the mare's expected foaling date, calculated as 335 to 340 days from the last known breeding date. In mares with an unknown breeding date, testing should begin as soon as some udder enlargement is noted and a small amount of secretion can be obtained from the teats without undue effort. It is best to keep a close check on udder development on a daily basis and practice massage of the mare's udder and teats to allow her to get used to being handled in this area. Once-a-day sampling is sufficient until values of $CaCO_3$ are greater than or equal to 100 ppm. Thereafter, twice-daily sampling is recommended. More accurate assessment of the mare's readiness to foal will be from daily late afternoon to early evening sampling. Because a few mares will foal in the daytime (see Figure 62-1), a morning sample should not be neglected and is highly advisable when $CaCO_3$ values first are greater than or equal to 125 ppm.

TESTING PROCEDURE

Wipe the udder and teats with a clean, dry, soft paper towel before attempting to collect a sample. This reduces the amount of skin debris and dirt that might contaminate the sample, although such contamination will not alter the test result to any appreciable extent. This step is strongly recommended if the mare has been out in the

weather and is wet. The hands of the person doing the sampling also should be clean and dry. Two to 5 ml of prefoaling mammary secretion should be obtained per mare. It should be collected in a clean manner by gently stripping a small amount from each teat, using thumb and index or middle finger, into a clean plastic test tube or other sampling cup. The cup or test tube can be reused if it is thoroughly rinsed with distilled water and then dried between uses.

The sample should then be taken to a clean, dry, and warm area for testing. A syringe is used to draw up exactly 1.5 ml of the sample. The measured sample is placed into a mixing vial, and exactly 9.0 ml of distilled water is added. This dilution (i.e., ratio of 1 part mammary secretion to 6 parts distilled water) of the prefoaling milk sample is important because it adjusts the calcium level within the milk to an appropriate range for testing. This must be carefully and accurately performed at all times. After the dilution is completed, 1 to 2 drops of an indicator dye solution supplied in the test kit is added to the diluted sample. The instructions supplied with the kit should be followed as described in the product insert. Attach the flexible end of the valve assembly over the tapered tip of the glass titret so that it fits snugly. Lift the control bar of the Titrettor, and insert the assembled titret into the body of the Titrettor (Figure 62-2). Hold the Titrettor with the flexible pipet tip in the solution for testing, and press the control bar gently to break the prescored tip of the glass titret tip. (NOTE: Because the titret is sealed under vacuum, the fluid inside may be agitated when the tip snaps.) With the tip of the sample pipe immersed in the diluted solution, press the control bar firmly, but briefly, to pull in a small amount of fluid. The fluid in the glass titret chamber will initially turn orange to pink. Press the control bar again briefly to allow another small amount of sample to be drawn into the tube. After each sample is drawn into the glass titret chamber, rock or invert the entire Titrettor apparatus to mix the fluid contents. Watch for the color to change from orangish-pink to blue. At the transition stage, you may first note a slight grayish discoloration, or the solution in the chamber might appear to be colorless. Repeat aspiration of small aliquots until the desired color change is detected and remains without reverting to pink. Invert the glass titret chamber, and read the titret scale at the stable color change. If bubbles are present in the solution at this point, stand the titret upright for a few minutes and read the scale again. There may be a slight alteration in the actual value once the bubbles have disappeared. Base the final reading of the actual value on the bubble-free titret, estimated to the nearest premarked line on the scale. The scale units on the glass titret are calibrated to parts per million (ppm) of $CaCO_3$.

INTERPRETATION OF RESULTS

When the prefoaling mammary secretion $CaCO_3$ level first equals or exceeds 200 ppm, there is a 51% probability that spontaneous foaling will occur within the next 24 hours, an 84% probability that foaling will occur within 48 hours, and a 97% probability that foaling will occur within 72 hours.[10] The majority of mares foal within a short period of time when a value of 300 to 500 ppm $CaCO_3$ is obtained. But not all mares can be expected to reach these higher values. For mares that have not yet reached 200 ppm, there is a 99% probability that foaling will not occur within the next 24-hour period. This test does not predict the actual foaling time of the mare tested, and therefore expectations and claims that it does must be refuted.

As with many biologic systems, variations are to be expected; few diagnostic tests have the ability to be completely accurate and reliable with regard to predictive value in all situations. This test is an aid to foaling management programs and is not intended to guarantee successful warning of impending foaling in all mares. It does, however, increase the likelihood that fewer sleepless nights will be spent waiting up for the mare to foal, especially for inexperienced owners and foaling attendants.

INTERFERENCES OR COMPLICATIONS

Some mares are resentful of being milked, especially if they are maiden mares. Standing to the left side of the mare and facing her tail, press the left shoulder firmly against the middle of the mare's chest or midabdominal region, reach with the right hand first under her belly near the umbilicus, and rub gently and progressively toward the udder. Several attempts might be needed to reassure the mare that no harm is intended. With the collecting cup in the left hand, gently squeeze the base of one teat with right thumb and index or middle finger. Make this a pleasurable experience for the mare (i.e., offer her some grain while collecting the sample). The more comfortable the mare is with her prefoaling mammary secretions being collected, the greater the likelihood that she will accept her new foal attempting to suckle.

It is not unusual for maiden mares to fail to develop much of an udder before foaling, in which case one's ability to obtain a sample for testing will be greatly hampered. The "first milk" or colostrum is typically a very thick, honey-colored, sticky secretion. This is an appropriate sample to collect and test because calcium levels will be detectable just as with more "normal"-appearing milk.

Mares that have been exposed during the last 60 to 90 days of gestation to fescue grass, specifically the Kentucky-31 variety, infested by the endophyte *Acremonium coenophialum* may suffer from the toxin(s) that are produced within the grass.[17] Such mares very often fail to develop normal udder mass and function before foaling (e.g., agalactia). Without a sample for testing, this methodology will be of little help to evaluate approaching readiness for birth.

Because calcium contributes to the hardness of water, every precaution should be taken to rinse all reusable items thoroughly with distilled water before drying. Use only distilled water supplied in the kit or purchased from local grocery or drug stores for all sample dilutions in the testing procedure.

Obtaining the small sample volume that is required for testing on a once to twice daily basis for the 10 to 14 days' duration before foaling does not deprive the foal of any significant amount of colostrum or its immunoglobulin content. Many foals have been monitored during the research and development of this methodology, and in no case was a failure of passive transfer attributable to the sampling of prefoaling mammary secretions. In like manner, the quality of the mare's colostrum and its content of immunoglobulins was not affected. Mares that are prone to "running milk" before foaling will do so whether they have been sampled for testing or not. Such mares are still at risk of losing too much colostrum before foaling and should be managed accordingly.

The procedure of prefoaling mammary secretion sampling slightly increases the risk of mastitis development. This is true for any animal when milking is performed by hand, especially if precautions are not taken to wipe the skin and teat surfaces clean and dry them before obtaining the sample. If clumps of cellular debris or pink to red discoloration in the milk sample obtained from the mare is noted, proper diagnostic work-up and treatment is warranted (i.e., culture and cytologic examination).

Repeated sampling of well over 300 pregnant mares during their last 10 to 30 days of gestation has been considered by these authors to be an innocuous procedure. There have been no alterations in normal mare behavior or prefoaling activities. Premature parturition was not attributed to the testing procedure in the mares included in the evaluation of this method. Likewise, prolonged gestations were not observed. It is cautioned that premature or precocious lactation, inappropriate to an individual mare's gestational length and/or expected foaling date, may be attributable to placentitis and the potential for premature parturition of a septic neonate.[14,15]

TROUBLESHOOTING

It is not unusual for some mares to reach 100 to 175 ppm $CaCO_3$ and remain at that level for several days before proceeding up to 200 ppm or above (Figure 62-3). Variations occur between mares and even within the same mare from year to year. Patience and careful monitoring

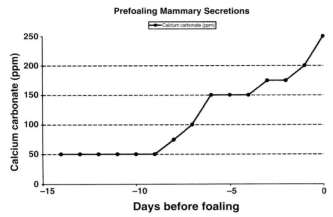

Figure 62-3 The calcium carbonate values for one mare as measured by the FoalWatch test kit plotted against days before spontaneous foaling. Day 0 is the day of foaling. Note the rise in values from day −10 to day −6, a plateau for several days, and then the final rise at day −1.

on a once to twice daily schedule are a must. A dramatic rise or significant change in value over a 12- to 24-hour interval, especially if the value is greater than or equal to 250 ppm, indicates that the mare is approaching readiness for birth. It does not predict that she is going to foal within any specific period of time.

Occasionally a value will drop from the previous day's sampling; this is not a cause for alarm. Repeat the test, and be certain that the dilution technique was accurate. Carefully draw small increments of the diluted sample, inverting the Titrettor several times between each aspiration, reading the scale with each repetition, and observing the color change. Initial color of the diluted sample once the indicator dye has been added will vary from early in the mare's testing period to later when she is closer to foaling. Early samples will appear more orange in color, later samples will appear a rose-pink to reddish purple. This is a normal variation and is not a cause for concern with regard to accuracy of the result.

CLINICAL USE AND APPLICATION

Prefoaling mammary secretion $CaCO_3$ testing has been used extensively by these authors for over 10 years and has proven useful in the routine management of foaling mares. Its intended use is to assist with the determination as to when the fetus is maturing in utero and the mare is approaching readiness to foal based upon changes in the prefoaling mammary secretion (milk) $CaCO_3$ level. It is a clinical tool that will aid the determination of when to attend the mare's foaling without an excessive number of sleepless nights. Alternatively, it can be used as a tool for accurately assessing when elective induction of parturition may safely be considered.

There are several protocols for induction of parturition in the mare that vary in action and time of onset to delivery. The three main methods reported for induction of foaling are oxytocin, prostaglandin $F_{2\alpha}$, and dexamethasone.[13,18-21] Oxytocin is generally considered the drug of

choice for inducing parturition in the mare.[19] It is associated with a rapid effect. Foaling usually occurs within 15 to 90 minutes of its administration. Various doses and routes of administration of oxytocin have been used to induce foaling. A dose of 2.5 to 5 IU will cause a slower progression toward delivery,[19,21,22] whereas 100 IU will initiate a more rapid delivery response.[19] Oxytocin can be given by subcutaneous (SQ), intramuscular (IM), and intravenous (IV) routes. One disadvantage of oxytocin is that it can override the physiologic events responsible for normal parturition without consideration for fetal maturity.[4] High doses of oxytocin can increase the incidence of perineal tears, uterine rupture, fetal cerebral vascular accident, fetal hypoxia, and premature placental separation.[19]

All mares that were induced to foal under our supervision had met the minimum criteria defined above. Their tails were wrapped, perineum washed with soap and water, and placed in stalls bedded with clean straw. In most mares, a prefoaling evaluation was performed using transabdominal ultrasonography to observe fetal activity, allantoic and amniotic fluid echogenicity and volume, and to obtain a fetal cardiac rate. Some mares additionally received prefoaling manual vaginal examination to determine relaxation of the cervix, but not all mares received this before initiation of induction. We have used the following method for induction of foaling: fenprostalene at 0.5 mg (Syntex Animal Health, Division of Syntex Agrsiness, Inc., Palo Alto, Calif.) administered SQ, followed in 2 hours with low-dose oxytocin (2.5 to 5.0 IU, IV, at 15- to 20-minute intervals until initiation of stage 2 labor). Our total dose of oxytocin does not exceed 20 IU. Withdrawal of fenprostalene from the veterinary market necessitated its elimination from our induction protocol. Currently we use only oxytocin at 2.5 to 5.0 IU per dose at 20-minute intervals to effect stage 2. Premature placental separation (PPS) was noted in 10% of mares.[21] This was immediately recognized and treated without undue complication to the viability of the foals during their neonatal periods. Dystocia rate was 5% with most related to retention of one forelimb at the carpus or shoulder or presentation of the poll (i.e., nose down). All dystocias were recognized early and corrective manipulations performed easily and rapidly, resulting in delivery of healthy foals. No foals or mares were lost as the result of the induction procedure.

Macpherson et al[23] evaluated three methods of oxytocin used to induce foaling in the mare. Three protocols for induction were compared: (a) 75 IU oxytocin by single IM injection, (b) 15 IU oxytocin by IM injection at 15-minute intervals for a maximum of five injections (e.g., 95 IU oxytocin total) or until rupture of the chorioallantois occurred, and (c) 75 IU oxytocin diluted in 1 L of physiologic saline administered by IV injection at 1 IU/min until rupture of the chorioallantois. The incidence of PPS was 38% (e.g., 6 mares experiencing PPS out of 16 total mares induced to foal) in their study. In our experience, using a decidedly smaller dose (i.e., 2.5 to 5.0 IU oxytocin by IV injection at 15- to 20-minute intervals until rupture of the chorioallantois or a total of 20 IU oxytocin), incidence of PPS was much reduced.

We have found the technique as described here to be a useful instructional tool for veterinary students.

Table   **62-1**

Comparison of Spontaneously Foaling Mares Versus Mares Induced to Foal Using Oxytocin*

Parameter	Induced Foalings	Spontaneous Foalings
Number of mares	7	13
Median foaling time	2 PM	11 PM
Range in foaling times	1 PM to 4 PM	2 PM to 7 AM
Mean dose oxytocin administered	10 IU	0 IU
Attended deliveries	7/7	12/13
Assisted deliveries[†]	3/7	1/12
Premature placental separations	1/7	0/12
Parturient trauma[‡]	0/7	1/13
End of stage 3 by 4 hours postpartum	7/7	12/13
Foal survival at 24 hours	7/7	13/13
Effective passive transfer rate	7/7	13/13
Foal morbidity at 24 hours	0/7	1/13

*All mares had prefoaling mammary secretion calcium carbonate testing performed.
[†]These mares were used for instructional purposes; we may have been overly cautious regarding the true clinical need for assistance or intervention.
[‡]One mare that foaled unattended had a third-degree perineal laceration.

Table 62-1 includes our data from the 2002 foaling season comparing two groups of mares, both monitored by prefoaling mammary secretion $CaCO_3$ testing, as well as all of the other signs of impending parturition. Seven mares were induced to foal using low-dose oxytocin as described above, and 13 mares were allowed to foal spontaneously. From a clinical standpoint we would not induce a mare without knowing her pattern of mammary secretion $CaCO_3$ for at least the previous 12 and preferably 24 to 48 hours. The induction protocol itself is safe and predictable. Our immediate attendance ensures all foaling difficulties are quickly recognized and corrected before any threat to life of mare or foal. Induction during routine working hours also ensures that support personnel are (or should be) readily available should additional, more intensive measures be necessary (e.g., anesthesia, cesarean section, neonatal intensive care). We have not found these to be necessary in any but a very few circumstances. Whether similar support measures would have been required given a spontaneous foaling (compared with induced) is a matter of conjecture. We believe in retrospect that they would have been.

SUMMARY

The clinical test of measuring and monitoring prefoaling mammary secretion electrolytes does not predict the actual foaling time of the mare and should not be expected to. As with many biologic systems, variations can and will occur. Few clinical tests consistently, accurately, and reliably predict future events. In the hands of clients, prefoaling mammary secretion monitoring gives them something more active to do than "just watch," and it gets them closer to the mare in more ways than one. The testing procedure discussed here, along with all other signs of the mare's approaching readiness for birth, gives the clinician the ability to effectively evaluate in utero fetal maturation response. Furthermore, it provides data upon which an informed decision may be made as to when it may be appropriate to induce foaling in as safe and effective a manner as possible.

References

1. Bain AM, Howey WP: Observations on the time of foaling in Thoroughbred mares in Australia. J Reprod Fertil Suppl 1975; 23:545.
2. Peaker M, Rossdale PD, Forsyth IA et al: Changes in mammary development and the composition of secretion during late pregnancy in the mare. J Reprod Fertil Suppl 1979; 27:555.
3. Leadon D, Jeffcott L, Rossdale P: Mammary secretions in normal spontaneous and induced premature parturition in the mare. Equine Vet J 1984; 16:256.
4. Ousey JC, Dudan F, Rossdale PD: Preliminary studies of mammary secretions in the mare to assess foetal readiness for birth. Equine Vet J 1984; 16:259.
5. Cash RSG, Ousey JC, Rossdale PD: Rapid strip test method to assist management of foaling mares. Equine Vet J 1985; 17:61.
6. Brook D: Evaluation of a new test kit for estimating the foaling time in the mare. Equine Pract 1987; 9:34.
7. Kubiak JR, Evans JW: Predicting time of parturition. Equine Vet Data 1987; 7:350.
8. Ley WB, Hoffman JL, Meacham TN et al: Daytime foaling management of the mare. Part 1. Pre-foaling mammary secretions testing. J Equine Vet Sci 1989; 9:88.
9. Ousey JC, Delclaux M, Rossdale PD: Evaluation of three strip tests for measuring electrolytes in mares' prepartum mammary secretions and for predicting parturition. Equine Vet J 1989; 21:196.
10. Ley WB, Bowen JM, Purswell BJ et al: The sensitivity, specificity and predictive value of measuring the calcium carbonate in mares' prepartum mammary secretions. Theriogenology 1993; 40:189.

11. Douglas CGB, Perkins NR, Stafford KJ et al: Prediction of foaling using mammary secretion constituents. N Z Vet J 2002; 50:99.

12. Ley WB: Pre-foaling management of the mare and induction of parturition. In Robinson NE (ed): Current Therapy in Equine Medicine, 3rd edition, Philadelphia, WB Saunders, 1992.

13. Ley WB, Hoffman JL, Crisman MV et al: Daytime foaling management of the mare. Part 1. Induction of parturition. J Equine Vet Sci 1989; 9:95.

14. Rossdale PD, Ousey JC, Cottrill CM et al: Effects of placental pathology on maternal plasma progestagen and mammary secretion calcium concentrations and on neonatal adrenocortical function in the horse. J Reprod Fertil Suppl 1991; 44:579.

15. Santschi EM, LeBlanc MM, Matthews PM et al: Evaluation of equine high-risk pregnancy. Compend Contin Educ Pract Vet 1994; 16:80.

16. Ley WB: Unpublished data.

17. Brendemuehl JP: Reproductive aspects of fescue toxicosis. In Robinson NE (ed): Current Therapy in Equine Medicine, 4th edition, Philadelphia, WB Saunders, 1997.

18. Carleton CL, Threlfall WR: Induction of parturition in the mare. In Morrow DA (ed): Current Therapy in Theriogenology, 2nd edition, Philadelphia, WB Saunders, 1986.

19. Hillman RB: Induction of parturition. In Robinson NE (ed): Current Therapy in Equine Medicine, 2nd edition, Philadelphia, WB Saunders, 1987.

20. LeBlanc MM: Induction of parturition in the mare: assessment of fetal readiness for birth. In Koterba AM, Drummond WH, Kosch PC (eds): Equine Clinical Neonatology, Philadelphia, Lea and Febiger, 1990.

21. Ley WB, Parker NA, Bowen JM et al: How we induce the normal mare to foal. Proceedings of the 44th Annual Convention of the American Association of Equine Practitioners, p 194, 1998.

22. Pashen RL: Low doses of oxytocin can induce foaling at term. Equine Vet J 1980; 12:85-87.

23. Macpherson ML, Chaffin KM, Carroll GL et al: Three methods for oxytocin-induced parturition: effects on the neonatal foal. Proceedings of the 42nd Annual Convention of the American Association of Equine Practitioners, p 150, 1996.

CHAPTER 63

Colostrum

THERESA BURNS

In normal equine pregnancy, the foal is born functionally agammaglobulinemic. Antibodies that protect the neonate from disease must be obtained from the colostrum. Successful passive transfer requires the following: the mare produces colostrum with adequate immunoglobulin levels, the colostrum is available in the immediate postfoaling period, and the foal ingests and absorbs the immunoglobulins in a timely manner. Failure of any of these steps results in inadequate passive transfer, which, if not recognized and treated urgently, may lead to septicemia and foal death.

COLOSTRUM PRODUCTION

The transfer of immunoglobulins from the maternal circulation to the mammary gland is termed colostrogenesis. In mares the concentration of immunoglobulins in the mammary gland increases in the last 10 days before foaling.[1] This appears to be an active process because immunoglobulin concentrations are higher in colostrum than in maternal serum. The hormonal influences on colostrogenesis in the mare are not well understood. During the period of colostrogenesis, serum progesterone and prolactin increase. Mares exposed to ergopeptides that have abnormally low progesterone and prolactin fail to develop udders or produce normal mammary secretion.[2] At parturition, serum progesterone falls and serum prolactin increases dramatically, possibly due to loss of opioid-induced suppression.[3] These changes may initiate the transition from colostrum to milk production. By 24 hours post partum, immunoglobulin levels in colostrum have decreased fortyfold.[4]

COLOSTRUM CONTENT

Colostrum contains immunoglobulins, maternal immune cells, and cytokines. In the mare, IgG is the major immunoglobulin class in colostrum, with approximately 60% isotype IgGb, 25% isotype IgGa, and 15% isotype IgG(T).[4] Normal colostrum has greater than 3000 mg/dl of IgG, with excellent quality colostrum having IgG levels greater than 6000 mg/dl.[5,6] Stimulation of the maternal immune system by intramuscular injection of levamisole or 1,3/1,6 glucan significantly increases colostral immunoglobulin levels.[7] Intramuscular vaccination of mares in the last trimester of pregnancy against rotavirus, *Streptococcus equi*, tetanus, and influenza increases colostral immunoglobulin levels against these pathogens.[8,9] During late pregnancy, mares should be housed on the farm where they will foal to stimulate colostral antibodies to local pathogens.

Colostrum contains more than 1 million cells per milliliter, including macrophages, lymphocytes, neutrophils, and epithelial cells. Other factors, including complement, lactoferrin, epidermal growth factor, interferon-γ, and insulin-like growth factor, are also present. In the mare the importance of the nonimmunoglobulin portions of colostrum has not been studied; however, they likely act both locally in the gut and systemically as modulators of the neonatal immune system.

COLOSTRUM QUALITY

Colostral IgG level can be estimated in the field by measuring specific gravity using a colostrometer[6] (Equine Colostrometer, Jorgenson Laboratories, Loveland, Colo.). The colostrometer consists of a graduated scale attached to a specimen chamber floated in a Plexiglas water-filled column. To measure specific gravity, the mare is milked and the specimen chamber is carefully filled with 15 ml of colostrum, sealed, and floated in the column. Colostrum with a specific gravity of 1.060 contains IgG levels of approximately 3000 mg/dl, whereas a specific gravity of 1.080 is approximately 6000 mg/dl. Care must be taken to use distilled water near 24° C for flotation, to fill the specimen chamber completely with colostrum, and to dry or rinse the chamber with alcohol after cleaning to remove water.

Colostral IgG level may also be estimated in the field using sugar or alcohol refractometers.[5] One drop of colostrum is placed on the refractometer, and the refraction angle is read. Measurements indicating colostrum with IgG levels greater than 6000 mg/dl are 16% and 23% for the alcohol and sugar refractometer, respectively.

A glutaraldehyde clot test is commercially available that allows semiquantitative analysis of colostral immunoglobulin levels (Gamma check C, Veterinary Dynamics, Templeton, Calif.). This test is based on the ability of glutaraldehyde to cross-link with proteins such as gamma globulins and fibrinogen to form a solid clot. Dilute colostrum is added to a test tube preloaded with glutaraldehyde. Clotting of the sample within 10 minutes is indicative of colostral IgG greater than 3800 mg/dl.

MAXIMIZING PASSIVE TRANSFER

Maximal absorption of colostral antibodies occurs within 6 hours after birth. By 24 hours after birth, gut absorption of intact macromolecules is minimal. Serum from all foals should be evaluated for adequate antibody levels at 12 to 24 hours of age.

If a foal is unable to nurse, colostrum should be administered by nasogastric tube as soon as possible after birth. Approximately 1 g IgG/kg body weight of colostrum is required to raise foal serum immunoglobulins above 400 mg/dl. For a 45-kg foal fed average colostrum with an immunoglobulin concentration of 3500 mg/dl, approximately 1.5 L is required to obtain serum immunoglobulin concentration of at least 400 mg/dl. This should be fed in doses of 250 to 300 ml every 1 to 2 hours. Placement of a small-gauge, indwelling nasogastric catheter will not prevent nursing and can be used for colostrum administration. Conditions such as prematurity, hypothermia, perinatal hypoxia, or diarrhea will reduce antibody absorption from the gut. In compromised foals, colostral volume per feeding must be reduced to avoid gastrointestinal upset. Plasma transfusion in addition to small volume oral administration may be required to ensure adequate antibody levels. In septic foals, colostral antibodies are quickly consumed, and plasma transfusions are often necessary despite adequate passive transfer. Although systemic antibody absorption is minimal in foals over 18 hours, there may be some local gastrointestinal protective effects of colostrum supplementation.

Colostral IgG levels in mares over 15 years of age should be evaluated because of declining quality associated with aging.[6] Mares that drip or stream mammary secretions before foaling lose colostral immunoglobulins. Secretions can be collected, evaluated for immunoglobulin concentration, and stored for administration to the foal at birth. Premature lactation is an indicator of placental and fetal pathologic conditions, so a complete high-risk pregnancy evaluation is warranted.

Foals without access to good-quality maternal colostrum may be given donor mare colostrum. This is obtained from mares with colostral immunoglobulin levels greater than 7000 mg/dl. After adequate initial nursing by the foal, approximately 250 ml of colostrum can be milked from the mare, filtered, labeled, and frozen in leakproof containers. Immunoglobulin levels in frozen colostrum are stable for at least 18 months. Slow thawing in warm water minimizes damage to immunoglobulins. Colostrum from mares with a history of neonatal isoerythrolysis should not be collected. Bovine colostrum has been shown to increase foal serum immunoglobulin levels and is tolerated by foals. However, antibodies are not specific against equine pathogens, and foals are not well protected against infection.[10,11] Caprine colostrum may be an alternative to bovine colostrum because does are often vaccinated against clostridial diseases, including tetanus.

References

1. Peaker M et al: Changes in mammary development and the composition of secretion during late pregnancy in the mare. J Reprod Fertil Suppl 1979; 27:555-561.
2. Ireland FA et al: Effects of bromocriptine and perphenazine on prolactin and progesterone concentrations in pregnant pony mares during late gestation. J Reprod Fertil 1991; 92:179-186.
3. Aurich C, Aurich JE, Parvizi N: Opioidergic inhibition of luteinising hormone and prolactin release changes during pregnancy in pony mares. J Endocrinol 2001; 169:511-518.
4. Sheoran AS et al: Immunoglobulin isotypes in sera and nasal mucosal secretions and their neonatal transfer and distribution in horses. Am J Vet Res 2000; 61(9):1099-1105.
5. Chavatte P et al: Field determination of colostrum quality by using a novel, practical method. Proceedings of the 44th Annual Convention of the American Association of Equine Practitioners, pp 206-209, 1988.
6. LeBlanc MM, McLaurin BI, Boswell R: Relationship among serum immunoglobulin concentration in foals, colostral specific gravity, and colostral immunoglobulin concentration. J Am Vet Med Assoc 1986; 189(1):57-60.
7. Krakowski L et al: The effect of non-specific immunostimulation of pregnant mares with 1,3/1,6 glucan and levamisole on the immunoglobulin levels in colostrum, selected indices of non-specific cellular and humoral immunity in foals in the neonatal period. Vet Immunol Immunopathol 1999; 68(1):1-11.
8. Wilson WD et al: Passive transfer of maternal immunoglobulin isotype antibodies against tetanus and influenza and their effect on the response of foals to vaccination. Equine Vet J 2001; 33(7):644-650.
9. Sheoran AS et al: Prepartum equine rotavirus vaccination inducing strong specific IgG in mammary secretions. Vet Rec 2000; 146:672-673.
10. Lavoie JP et al: Absorption of bovine colostral immunoglobulins G and M in newborn foals. Am J Vet Res 1989; 50(9):1598-1603.
11. Holmes MA, Lunn DP: A study of bovine and equine immunoglobulin levels of ponies fed bovine colostrum. Equine Vet J 1992; 23(2):116-118.

SECTION VIII

The Post-Foaling Mare

CHAPTER 64

The Postpartum Breeding Mare

WALTER W. ZENT

Broodmare practice is production medicine, and in order to be successful it should be approached in that manner whether breeding 1 mare or 1000. With this in mind, the management of the postpartum mare becomes critical. In the 1980s Dr. Robert Loy[1] showed that to keep mares from drifting toward the end of the calendar the herd must average 25 days from foaling to conception. This is a very difficult goal to maintain, and it takes very aggressive management of all mares but particularly the postpartum mare. Aggressive management does not mean that farm managers must breed every mare on foal heat or even short cycle every mare that is not bred; it means that managers must be actively engaged in the aggressive management of these mares so that the mare is bred at the earliest opportunity that will provide her with an optimal chance for conception.

The postpartum mare must be carefully evaluated before a management scheme is developed. In central Kentucky most mares are examined at 7 or 8 days post partum. It is important that the mare be examined thoroughly, starting with her external genitalia, vagina, cervix, uterus, and ovaries.

Her vulval lips are examined for tears and bruising. Lacerations of the vestibule are common, particularly in young mares or in mares that present particularly large foals. These lesions are caused by the stretching of the vulva and vestibule and can be rather severe. They will usually heal spontaneously without any treatment; sometimes, however, an abscess can form in the tissue and dissect ventrally and break out below and lateral to the vulva lips. As severe as some of these tears appear, this author has never seen them cause an ongoing problem. A speculum examination of the vagina and cervix must be carefully done. The vagina must be examined for lacerations and the pooling of urine. The cervix is examined for color, inflammation, and lacerations. If the cervix and vagina are inflamed, it is advisable to culture the mare and perform cytologic studies to make sure that the mare does not have an infection. After the external genitalia, vagina, and cervix are examined, a detailed examination of the uterus and ovaries should be done.

The examination of the uterus and ovaries should be started by carefully palpating the mare. The ovaries and uterus should be examined for size and position; any possible abnormality can then be noted and examined later by ultrasonographic examination. It is the author's opinion that fewer problems are missed if a thorough palpation is done before an ultrasonographic examination because the examiner will know what he or she is looking for with ultrasonography and do a more complete examination. A hematoma, enlarged uterus, abnormal bowel location, and ovarian tumors can all be diagnosed first by palpation and than confirmed with the ultrasound machine. Ultrasonography can also find abnormalities that are difficult or impossible to diagnose simply by palpating. Ovarian hematoma, uterine fluid, and large uterine cysts are all easy to diagnose with ultrasonography but difficult with palpation alone. After the mare has been carefully examined, a decision can be made as to how best to manage her to give her the earliest possible chance to conceive.

The criteria used for the evaluation of the eligibility of a mare to be bred on foal heat must consider all of the results of the initial examination. Mares with vulval bruising or lacerations of the vestibule are generally not bred on foal heat. The color and condition of the cervix must be evaluated; mares with severely bruised or inflamed cervixes are usually passed. If the mucus seen in and around the cervix is cloudy, the mare is not bred and a cytologic examination and culture are performed to establish the presence and extent of the inflammation and, if infected, what organism is involved. Most postfoaling endometritis and cervicitis are caused by a beta streptococcus; these infections are usually transient and many times will resolve on their own without any therapy. If a cervical laceration is suspected, a digital examination must be performed to evaluate the severity of the laceration. If a significant deficit evolving the entire length of the cervix is present, surgery may be required. Cervical damage is usually a reason to pass the foal heat and in most cases allow the mare to return to estrus naturally. It is often advisable to palpate the damaged cervix occasionally to prevent any adhesions that may develop between the cervix and the vaginal wall. Cervical damage can be a very serious complication to foaling and will frequently occur even without a dystocia if the mare foals too quickly without adequate cervical dilation.

After the visual examination a rectal and ultrasonographic examination should be performed even if it has already been determined that the mare will not be eligible to be bred on foal heat. The rectal examination should first be done to get the reproductive tract in proper position for ultrasonography and also to examine the ovaries, judge the size of the uterus, and feel for a hematoma or other possible abnormalities. After that examination has been performed, ultrasonography can be used to visualize the uterine lumen, uterine wall, and ovaries. The lumen of the uterus should be visualized to determine the presence of free fluid. If a significant amount of fluid is seen, the mare should not be bred on foal heat, and in most instances culture and cytologic examination should be performed to be sure that no infection is present. If the mare is not infected, she would be a candidate to be short cycled with prostaglandin. If the mare is infected, then she should be treated appropriately.

After it has been determined that the mare is suitable to be bred on foal heat, she must be examined to find the appropriate time for mating. In the author's opinion foal-heat mares should not be bred before the tenth day post foaling. If a mare ovulates before 10 days, it is better to wait and short cycle her 6 days post ovulation. The conception rate in mares bred less than 10 days post foaling is very low, and on a herd basis more time will be gained by waiting than rushing the early ovulators in hopes of getting the occasional mare in foal. It is very helpful if the mares are well teased. How long and well the mare shows is a great help to the veterinarian who is doing the selection of a breeding date. Most mares cycle at 9 or 10 days from foaling, but certainly not all do; it is normal for some mares not to show heat until 12 or 13 days post foaling or later.

Mares should have their vulva closed as soon as practical after foaling. If the mare has been opened for foaling, she will need to be sutured. If she was not opened, she may not need Caslick's procedure. It is best not to do Caslick's operation immediately after foaling or even in the first few days. Mares that may have a minor uterine artery hemorrhage may bleed if their blood pressure is raised by the twitch or the epinephrine that is in the local anesthetic. There have been cases of mares hemorrhaging and dying as they are being sutured. Caslick's operation should not be attempted if the vulval lips are infected because of tears or the raw edges as a result of the mare being opened for foaling. It is best to let the tissue completely quiet down before suturing is attempted because frequently the suture line will dehisce when there is too much inflammation in the tissue and the surgery must be repeated. If the surgery is done properly, mares can usually be sutured before they are bred without having the stallion tear them out. Many Thoroughbred mares must have a vulvoplasty before they will conceive because their vulva conformation is so poor that their reproductive tract will remain contaminated until this procedure is done. The author routinely examines mares on day 4

post foaling to evaluate their need to be stitched. About 60% of the mares that need to be sutured can be done at this time; the others will have to wait until the inflammation subsides before the procedure can be done.

Mares that are to be bred on foal heat should then be teased and examined to determine when they should be bred. Again, it is important to wait until the tenth day or later before they are bred. If they ovulate before day 10, results are usually better if they are allowed to go out of heat and then short cycled. Mares that are healthy enough to be bred should be scheduled and bred when appropriate. In several studies mares that are selectively bred on foal heat perform as well as mares that are bred at a later time. These same studies show that there is no significant difference in the fetal loss of mares bred on foal heat when compared with mares bred at a later time.

If mares are not bred on foal heat, then they can be managed by allowing them to return to estrus on their own or they may be given prostaglandin at 5 or 6 days post ovulation to allow them to return to heat earlier. If the mare is to be short cycled, she must be examined before the prostaglandin is given. The author believes that mares should always be palpated before they are given prostaglandin; this is important so that the behavior of the mare can be predicted. Palpation will give management an idea of how quick the mare will return to estrus. If there is a midcycle follicle present on the ovary, then the mare may come in heat very quickly or even ovulate before she shows signs of estrus. If management does not know that the follicle is present, it is easy to miss the heat and ovulation.

Another technique that some people have used to aid in foal-heat breeding is to delay the onset of foal heat with the use of progesterone and estradiol to block follicular development. If this technique is to be used, the protocol is to treat the mare for 3 or 4 days with 150 mg of progesterone and 10 mg of estradiol-17β. The treatment must begin in the first 24 hours after foaling, or it will not work properly. In the author's opinion it should be started within the first 6 hours after foaling for the best results. If started later than 24 hours, the mare's natural drive to have a foal heat will override the treatment and she will ovulate in spite of the therapy. This will delay the mare's natural follicular development for as many days as the veterinarian treats her, and in this manner the management can be sure that the mare will ovulate 10 days or later post partum. In several trials this therapy has worked very well.

Management of mares during the postpartum period should be done aggressively, but the author does not agree with the indiscriminate treatment of mares just because they have had a foal. Some clinicians have advocated the routine treatment of mares with antibiotics or other therapies; these should not be administered indiscriminately. The routine douching of foaling mares has also been advocated by some clinicians. Although the author believes strongly in flushing to remove fluid and debris from postpartum mares that have a problem, the procedure is not appropriate for every mare. The author does not believe that it has much effect on the conception rate on foal heat, and it may actually introduce problems that were not present before. In one study of

100 mares, 50% were flushed on day 4 post partum and the others were not. All mares were bred on foal heat unless some other problem was discovered. The results of this study showed that the most important factor affecting foal-heat conception was the length of time from parturition until breeding or ovulation, and the flushing appeared to have no effect. This is not to say that when a mare has a postpartum complication that douching is not indicated, just not routinely on every normal mare.

Breeding mares as soon as possible after foaling is important to the overall maintenance of a well-performing herd of mares. The proper use of foal heat is an essential part of this management. The aggressive use of every opportunity to expose mares to semen is valuable to keep the time interval between foaling and con-ception as short as possible. In the author's opinion the aggressive use of every heat period that is available is the most efficient and least expensive way to manage brood-mares. The management of a band of broodmares is just as much production medicine as the management of a herd of beef or dairy cattle, and even the causal breeder of pet horses will benefit from an aggressive approach to managing reproductive performance. It is less expensive, less time consuming, and much less frustrating than just letting nature take its course.

Reference

1. Loy RG: Characteristics of postpartum reproduction in mares Vet Clin North Am Large Anim Pract 1980; 2(2):345-359.

CHAPTER 65

Prefoaling and Postfoaling Complications

MELINDA STORY

COLIC IN THE PERIPARTURIENT MARE

Abdominal pain following delivery of a foal is normal in most mares. Uterine contractions that persist after foaling and expulsion of fetal membranes may be accompanied by some degree of discomfort, occasional rolling, and mild signs of distress. Judgment of the severity of postpartum pain is important so that more serious causes are not overlooked.[1] When examining periparturient mares showing signs of abdominal pain there are a number of complications to consider; these include rupture of the cecum or colon, colonic torsion and ischemic necrosis of the small colon[2] as well as uterine torsion, rupture of the urinary bladder and internal hemorrhage from rupture of the utero-ovarian or middle uterine artery.[2] In one study looking at postpartum death in mares, gastrointestinal disorders were the second most common cause, the majority being from perforation of the cecum.[3] Although many mares may eat less on their own as parturition nears,[4] one management technique that may reduce the incidence of gastrointestinal rupture is the reduction of roughage intake in the last few days prepartum.[5]

Broodmares late in gestation and after parturition appear to be at greater risk of large colon torsion than other horses.[6] This is likely due to the stretched abdominal musculature, which permits greater movement of the colon. The large late-gestational uterus may induce repositioning of the colon or partially obstruct the right ventral colon, leading to gas retention and eventually to torsion.[7]

Segmental ischemic necrosis of the descending colon can occur with rectal prolapse in which more than 30 cm of the rectum is prolapsed. Any condition causing tenesmus, including parturition, with or without dystocia, can lead to prolapse.[7] Some mares may suffer mesocolon tears without rectal prolapse. These cases are difficult to distinguish from the mild pain associated with uterine involution.[8] There is extensive collateral blood supply to the small colon; if the injured segment is limited, there may be sufficient blood supply to maintain intestinal viability. However, the compromised area may undergo fibrosis with subsequent narrowing of the lumen, which predisposes the horses to small colon impactions.[7] Exploratory celiotomy is recommended in cases of suspected mesocolon rupture. Although a left flank approach is possible,[2] the recommended approach is ventral midline[7] in order to fully evaluate the lesion and to allow resection and anastomosis of the small colon, if indicated.

If the lesion is inaccessible, a permanent colostomy may be indicated.[7]

Due to the wide range and devastating results of gastrointestinal complications that may occur in periparturient mares, careful assessment is essential. A complete physical examination, rectal palpation, transabdominal ultrasound, complete blood count, and abdominocentesis should all be considered for late-gestation through postpartum mares displaying persistent signs of colic.

PERIPARTURIENT HEMORRHAGE

Rupture of a Major Vessel

Clinical Signs and Diagnosis

The middle uterine, utero-ovarian, and external iliac arteries are the major vessels that supply blood to the uterus. Though any of these may rupture, uterine artery rupture is most common.[9,10] The vessel may rupture at any point in its course; however, the middle third is the usual site.[9] In a study of postpartum deaths, almost 40% were due to uterine artery rupture.[3] Incidence and severity of angiosis in endometrial vessels increases with the number of previous pregnancies and age.[11] Long-standing changes in the elastic and collagen fibers may predispose to rupture. These changes have been described as senile degenerative changes.[9] A correlation of low serum copper levels with artery rupture has been documented,[12] and low copper may account for vessel fragility in aged mares.[13] There appears to be a predilection for the right-side uterine vessel rupture.[3,14] This may be because the cecum displaces the uterus to the left, which places increased tension on the vessels in the right broad ligament. This condition may occur in dystocia, as well as routine deliveries.[3,4] Although hemorrhage may occur before, during, or after parturition, the first 24 hours postpartum is the most common time frame.[15]

Heart rate and mucus membrane color should be monitored in mares with dystocia. Though the mucus membrane color may not initially change, eventually the membranes will become pale and blanched. Mares may be very tachycardic with heart rates up to 140 beats per minute. Clinical signs may proceed very quickly. The mare may be found dead or moribund during or after birth.[16] If the blood is contained within the broad ligament, the bleed may be self-limiting as a hematoma develops within the broad ligament. These mares may be trembling and show signs of pain, likely due to stretching of the broad ligament.[3,15] Although rectal palpation can confirm a diagnosis of a hematoma developing in the broad ligament, this is often very painful to the mare and may be enough to cause fatal elevation of the mare's blood pressure.[16] The total protein and packed cell volume will likely not change immediately due to a relative loss of erythrocytes and plasma. Splenic contraction may also temporarily increase the hematocrit.[17] Abdominal ultrasound examination and abdominocentesis are of diagnostic value to confirm that hemorrhage has occurred.[16] Treatment of these mares may include conservative management or more aggressive medical therapy for shock, and it is up to the clinician to decide which approach to take based on the circumstances at hand. Surgical exploration to attempt repair of the vessel is contraindicated.

Treatment

Conservative management includes stall rest in a quiet, dark area with minimal disturbance. It is often best to leave the foal in the stall to keep the mare as quiet as possible.[17] Sedatives should be used with caution (especially acetylpromazine) because they may exacerbate hypovolemic shock.[15,16] The goal of conservative therapy is to reduce arterial pressure and encourage platelet-fibrin plug formation to seal the rent in the vessel wall.[16]

Although aggressive intravenous fluid volume replacement will elevate the blood pressure, in some instances it may be warranted and has proven successful to save valuable mares.[3,16,17] Initial emergency therapy should include 2 to 3 L hypertonic saline followed by 10 to 20 L lactated Ringer's solution over a period of 2 to 4 hours. An alternative to hypertonic saline would be the use of colloids such as plasma or hetastarch.[17] Supplemental oxygen via nasal insufflation at 5 to 10 L/min may also be initiated during the resuscitative period.[16] If the hematocrit continues to drop to less than 15%, whole blood transfusions (6 to 8 L over several hours) may be necessary.[17]

In addition to fluid volume replacement, flunixin meglumine (1.1 mg/kg) should be administered to reduce the inflammatory cascade, as well as to improve the comfort level of the mare.[16] Low-dose oxytocin (10 to 20 IU) may be useful to promote uterine involution. This may decrease the weight of the uterus and the tension on the ligaments, as well as decreasing the blood supply to the uterus.[16,18] Higher doses may induce a colic episode that could turn into fatal hemorrhage and should be avoided. If the mare survives the initial hemorrhagic crisis, broad-spectrum antibiotics are indicated to protect the mare from multiorgan failure that may be secondary to ischemic/reperfusion damage,[17] as well as to prevent infection of the hematoma.[19]

Aminocaproic acid is an antifibrinolytic amino acid used in human medicine. The drug binds reversibly to plasminogen and therefore blocks the binding of plasminogen to fibrin and its activation and transformation to plasmin. Through this mechanism, there is inhibition of tissue fibrinolysis and a stabilization of clots.[20] Conjugated estrogens can shorten prolonged bleeding times in humans; however, there is no documentation of the effect of these drugs in horses. The mechanism of conjugated estrogens on the bleeding time is unknown.[20] There is a delayed onset of action, though the duration of effect in humans is 10 to 15 days. The conjugated estrogens are useful for long-lasting hemostasis but may not be of benefit in the acute hemorrhagic crisis. Anecdotal reports suggest that a single intravenous dose of naloxone (8 mg) may be efficacious in reducing hemorrhage. However, data have been extrapolated from small animals, and evidence of effect in horses is lacking.[4,15,17] Historically, 10% buffered formalin given intravenously was considered to aid hemostasis. Recent studies were not able to prove any effect of formalin on coagulation parameters or bleeding times in normal horses.[21] Because of the lack of evidence of efficacy in horses, these drugs should be used with caution.

Prognosis

In the acute phase, prognosis for life is guarded. If the mare survives initially, she should be housed in a quiet, low-stress environment for 3 to 4 weeks.[10] Future pregnancies should be considered to be high risk, and the owners must be advised that repeat bleeding episodes may occur.[14]

UTERINE TORSION

Uterine torsion is an infrequent cause of equine dystocia, estimated at 5% to 10% of all serious equine obstetric problems.[22] The underlying cause of uterine torsion is unknown; however, vigorous fetal movement, sudden falls, and a large fetus in a small volume of fluid have been proposed as contributing factors.[23] Uterine torsion in the mare occurs less frequently than in the cow; however, there is a greater degree of difficulty in resolving the torsion, and the survival rate is lower in horses.[24]

Mares with torsions commonly present with signs of colic, with a duration of 6 hours to several days[25]; however, there are reports of chronic torsions of 2 to 8 weeks' duration.[26,27] The stage of gestation may range from 7 months to term, though in one report most were at 9.6 months.[28]

Clinical signs are the result of abdominal pain and include restlessness, sweating, anorexia, frequent urination, sawhorse stance, looking at the flank, and kicking at the abdomen.[15] Rectal temperature and heart and respiratory rates are typically within normal ranges or only slightly elevated.[29]

Diagnosis

Diagnosis of uterine torsion is based on physical examination and rectal palpation findings. In contrast to the cow, equine uterine torsions rarely involve the cervix; therefore vaginal examination is often not diagnostically helpful.[15] Upon rectal palpation, the broad ligaments are tense and spiraling in the direction of the torsion. Some authors believe the torsion is more common in a clockwise direction,[24] whereas others believe there is no difference in occurrence.[25] In the case of a clockwise torsion, the right uterine ligament is strongly stretched and runs immediately downward under the uterine body. The left ligament runs from its origin, over the body of the uterus to the right of the abdomen. Palpation of the ovaries may aid in identifying the broad ligaments. Any mare in the third trimester that is showing signs of colic should be palpated for uterine torsion. Depending on the stage of pregnancy and the degree and site of the torsion, there may be some constriction of the small colon, which could impede the ability of the palpator to perform a complete rectal examination.[28,29] In these cases the viability of the fetus, the integrity of the uterus, or the direction of the torsion may be difficult to determine.[28] Treatment should be initiated immediately upon diagnosis of uterine torsion to increase the chances for fetal and maternal survival.[23]

Treatment

Nonsurgical

If the mare is term and the cervix is dilated, manual detorsion through the cervix may be attempted. This usually is possible only if the torsion is less than 270 degrees.[29] A well-lubricated arm may be passed into the uterus to grasp the foal ventrolaterally and rock the fetus back and forth until the fetus and uterus roll into correct position.[23] Following correction of the torsion, the mare should begin second-stage labor; however, this may be delayed due to vascular congestion and edema and reduced uterine contractility.[29] In some cases of advanced pregnancy, a torsion may go unrecognized and an assisted delivery is attempted. If this occurs, there is a high incidence of uterine rupture and subsequent maternal death due to hemorrhage or peritonitis.[24,29]

If the mare is preterm, has a closed cervix, or the vagina or cervix is involved in the torsion, an alternate method of correction is recommended. Rolling an anesthetized mare can be used to correct a uterine torsion in the last trimester of pregnancy; however, it is not recommended near term because of the increased risk of uterine rupture.[30] The mare can be placed under general anesthesia and in lateral recumbency toward the side to which the torsion is directed. The mare is rolled quickly in the direction of the torsion in an attempt for the body to "catch up to" the uterus.[30] The object is to hold the uterus in place while the body is turned around the uterine axis. For example, if a torsion is clockwise, the mare is placed in right lateral recumbency and the mare is turned in a clockwise direction. In some cases, additional pressure may need to be applied either by ballottement of the mare's abdomen or by placing a wooden plank over the uterus and applying pressure while the rest of the mare's body is rolled. If a plank is needed to stabilize the fetus during rolling, one end is placed over the mare's upper paralumbar region, while a person kneels on it. The other end of the plank is directed to the ground off the back of the mare. The mare is rolled more slowly if this technique is used to reduce the risk of uterine rupture.[29] Although this procedure may be successful in some cases, some authors feel there is an increased risk of placental detachment, abortion, or fetal and/or maternal death after rolling.[22,25]

Surgical

Surgical management via a flank laparotomy is the most commonly recommended approach for tractable mares with no evidence of uterine rupture.[22,25] The flank incision is made on the same side as the direction of the torsion. It is easier to lift and push the uterus rather than to pull it into position. This method may decrease the chance of perforation of the uterus.[28] If the direction of the torsion is unknown, the incision is made on the left side.[14,28] The mare is placed in stocks and sedated. Epidural analgesia may also be helpful in the intraoperative and postoperative periods. The paralumbar fossa is clipped and aseptically prepared for surgery. The skin and abdominal muscles are desensitized by local infiltration of 2% lidocaine in a vertical line or inverted "L." A vertical flank incision is made, and either a grid (preterm mares) or a modified grid (term mares) approach is made into the abdomen.[23,25] The direction of the torsion may be confirmed by intraabdominal palpation of the uterus and broad ligaments and by palpating the dorsal surface of the uterine body forward from the cervix. The torsion is corrected by placing the forearm under the uterus or by gently grasping the fetal hocks. The uterus is rocked back and forth to gain momentum until it rocks into place. It is important to remember that the uterus may be friable, and overzealous attempts at correction may result in tearing of the uterus.[24] If this cannot be achieved, a larger incision may be made to allow the opposite hand to push against the dorsum of the uterus. Alternatively, a second incision on the opposite side of the mare may be made to allow access for a second surgeon. Correction of the uterine torsion is confirmed by palpation of the broad ligaments and the dorsal surface of the uterus beginning at the cervix. Fetal viability is assessed by stimulating the foal to move. It is important to carefully palpate the remainder of the abdominal cavity to ensure that other viscera are not displaced or incarcerated. The peritoneum is not routinely closed. The muscle layers are individually closed with No. 2 polyglactin 910 and the skin with nonabsorbable monofilament suture.[28,29]

If the torsion cannot be reduced with a flank approach, a ventral midline approach under general anesthesia may be necessary. This approach has the advantage of being able to inspect for the presence of uterine tears, hemorrhage, edema, and necrosis. In addition, a ventral midline approach is suggested in mares with suspicion of gastrointestinal involvement, a suspected uterine rupture, or a dead foal in the presence of a closed cervix.[25,28]

Once a torsion has been corrected, there is still concern for blood supply of the uterus, which may have been strangulated long enough to cause thrombosis.[24] If there is not gastrointestinal involvement, the fetus is alive, and the uterine wall is not severely congested and edematous, the prognosis for maternal survival and birth of a normal, live foal are good.[22] In another survey, survival of mares with uterine torsion treated surgically was reported as 73%.[25] Complications associated with correction may include premature placental separation, uterine wall necrosis, peritonitis, partial or complete dehiscence of the incision, endotoxic shock, and recurrence of a torsion during the same pregnancy.[29] Surgical or nonsurgical correction of the torsion does not adversely affect the mare for future pregnancies unless a cesarean section is performed.[25]

Mares treated with a celiotomy, flank or ventral midline, should be confined to stall rest for 4 weeks followed by small paddock turnout for another 4 weeks to allow the incision to heal, as well as to ensure careful monitoring of the impending foaling. Systemic support with fluid therapy, antibiotics, and antiinflammatory medications may be needed depending on the condition of the mare.

UTERINE RUPTURE

Diagnosis

Uterine rupture is a complication that may be associated with fetotomy, excessive manipulation during a dystocia, fetal malposition, uterine torsion, uterine lavage, or with a seemingly normal delivery.[4,31,32] There is also one report of uterine rupture secondary to hydramnios in a mare.[33] Complications that may be associated with uterine rupture include visceral herniation, peritonitis, hemorrhage, shock, and death.[28] When a uterine rupture has occurred, there may be damage to the endometrium, myometrium, or the tear may be full thickness. The most common site for uterine rupture to occur is at the dorsal aspect of the uterus.[34] Immediate diagnosis of a uterine tear may be difficult. Palpation of a mare after foaling may or may not reveal that a tear has occurred. Likewise, evaluation of the placenta may not indicate that uterine rupture has occurred.[35]

Diapedesis of red blood cells and peritoneal contamination may occur with partial-thickness tears.[34] If a full-thickness tear or rupture has occurred, there will likely be contamination of the abdominal fluid and an increase in white blood cell counts. Abdominocentesis may be of benefit for a diagnosis and is indicated in any mare that has abdominal pain after foaling, especially after dystocia or fetotomy.[34] Laparoscopy may be of diagnostic and potentially therapeutic benefit as well. The ability to visualize the tear and judge the extent of the damage may aid the clinician in making a therapeutic plan and having a better understanding of the prognosis.[36]

Treatment

Nonsurgical
Medical management may be successful in cases where the tear is small, occurring on the dorsal aspect of the uterus, if there is minimal continued hemorrhage, and when uterine therapy in the immediate postpartum stage is not indicated.[15] Therapy is aimed at treating circulatory shock and peritonitis. These mares may be cross-tied to decrease the risk of abdominal herniation through the uterine tear.[15]

Surgical
Surgical repair via a ventral midline celiotomy is the recommended treatment for large tears or if there is continued uterine hemorrhage, visceral herniation, and in those mares that do not respond to medical management.[15] Advantages of a ventral midline approach include the ability to fully evaluate both uterine horns and the body of the uterus, visualization of the gastrointestinal tract for concomitant damage, and the ability to lavage the abdominal cavity.[31] A flank approach may also be attempted if the tear can be localized to one horn before surgery.[31] Prolapsing the uterus to repair it in the stand-

ing mare has been described[37]; however, this is generally reserved for cases where economics prohibit general anesthesia.

If a ventral midline approach has been selected, the mare is induced under general anesthesia and the ventral midline is sterilely prepared for surgery. A caudal ventral midline approach is made into the abdomen to allow the uterus to be exteriorized, as well as enabling the surgeon to carefully explore the abdomen for damage to gastrointestinal viscera.[38] The tear is identified and the edges debrided as necessary. A continuous hemostatic suture to appose the endometrium to the subserosal myometrium may be necessary to control hemorrhage.[28] Care should be taken to ensure that the chorioallantois is detached from the uterine wall for a distance of 3 cm from the tear to ensure that it is not incorporated into the repair.[38] A two-layer inverting pattern with No. 2 absorbable suture is recommended for closure of the tear. The area should be thoroughly cleansed with sterile fluid and moistened laparotomy sponges. The abdominal cavity is lavaged with warm sterile saline that is removed with suction. Some authors recommend the placement of a peritoneal suction drain to allow for subsequent abdominal lavage.[28] Antibiotics may be infused into the abdominal cavity before routine three-layer closure.[38]

Postoperative therapy should include broad-spectrum antibiotics, nonsteroidal antiinflammatory medications, and heparin therapy to reduce the chance of adhesions, which may impair future reproductive status.[34] Oxytocin may also be included in the therapy to improve uterine involution. In addition, some mares may need intravenous fluid therapy and intensive supportive care, depending on the degree of peritonitis and the presence of circulatory shock.[34] The length of time of administration of these medications is determined by the degree of tissue trauma and contamination noted at surgery and by how quickly the mare responds to supportive care. These mares may also have some degree of small colon bruising and postoperative ileus. Measures to ensure adequate water intake and gradual reintroduction of grain and hay should be considered. Green grass and bran mashes with mineral oil may be offered to help return normal gastrointestinal motility.[38] Stall rest with hand-walking should be maintained for 4 weeks, followed by an additional 4 weeks of stall rest with small paddock turnout while the ventral body wall gains strength.

Prognosis
Prognosis depends on the size of the tear, as well as the degree of abdominal contamination. In one study, prognosis for life as well as breeding soundness was also related to how quickly the mares were referred for surgical correction of the tear and if uterine lavage had been previously initiated.[31] The possibility and timing of subsequent breeding will depend on the healing of the uterine defect and resolution of any uterine infection.[28]

UTERINE PROLAPSE

The mare's uterus is suspended cranially and laterally by the broad ligaments. The cranial attachment makes uterine prolapse less likely in horses than in the cow.[4]

Uterine prolapse can occur after a normal delivery; however, it is more commonly associated with abortion (especially at 8 to 10 months' gestation), prolonged parturition, dystocia, retained placenta, and old age.[28] The prolapse may not occur for several hours after fetal delivery.[39] The prolapse may be complicated by retained fetal membranes, uterine rupture, bladder eversion or prolapse, or intestinal herniation.[28] Affected mares often display signs of colic, straining, and shock, especially if there has been excessive bleeding from a damaged endometrium or uterine artery rupture due to the weight of the uterus.[28] It is important to initially assess the cardiovascular status of the mare so that supportive care can be initiated as indicated.

Treatment

In order to allow further evaluation and replacement of the uterus, sedation and analgesia with alpha-2 medications and butorphanol tartrate are indicated. In addition, epidural anesthesia and in some cases general anesthesia are necessary to reduce straining.[28,38] The uterus should be thoroughly lavaged with a dilute germicidal solution such as povidone-iodine. Fetal membranes that detach easily should be removed and the uterus examined for lacerations or devitalized tissue. Uterine rents should be debrided and repaired with absorbable suture.[28] In some instances the uterus may be gangrenous and require amputation; this is considered a heroic measure with a poor prognosis.[24]

After the uterus has been cleansed, sterile lubrication can be liberally applied and an assistant should elevate the uterus on a towel or board in order to use gravity to help with reduction. The cervix and vaginal walls can be gently replaced into the vaginal vault. The remainder of the uterus is gently kneaded with the palm of the hand, in order to avoid rupture of the compromised tissue with fingers, into the vagina and through the cervix.[28] In cases where the uterus is quite edematous, it may be necessary to compress the tissue with a bandage before trying to replace it.[28]

Failure to fully reduce both the gravid and nongravid horns may result in continued tenesmus and recurrence of the prolapse.[28] If needed, 5 to 10 L of sterile fluid may be infused into the uterus to aid in full reduction; this fluid then needs to be siphoned out to avoid additional straining. Administration of 10 to 20 units oxytocin may also help with uterine involution, though consideration must be given to the possible sequela of colic and continued straining.[28] Vulvar retention sutures or a Caslick's procedure may be indicted in some cases depending on the conformation of the mare and the amount of edema present.[15,28]

Careful monitoring for signs of circulatory compromise, intestinal involvement, and normal uterine position and involution must be considered. Supportive therapy, including intravenous fluids, broad-spectrum antibiotics, antiinflammatory medications, tetanus prophylaxis, and intrauterine therapy, should be initiated. Oral administration of fecal softeners such as mineral oil may also be indicated to reduce straining for 3 to 5 days following replacement of the uterus.[28] Rectal prolapse has

occasionally been associated with uterine prolapse. Generally, once the uterus is replaced, the weight of the uterus maintains the rectum in normal position as well. If the rectum continues to prolapse, a purse-string suture for 24 to 48 hours may be indicated. The purse string should be placed to allow for fecal passage (three fingers) and the horse closely monitored for signs of tenesmus.[28]

Prognosis

Overall, subsequent fertility has been reported to be good, though it likely depends on the degree of endometrial damage incurred at the time of prolapse.[18] Before rebreeding, it is recommended to culture and perform a biopsy of the uterus, and subsequent foalings should be closely supervised, though recurrence of uterine prolapse is uncommon.[28]

BLADDER PROLAPSE, EVERSION, AND RUPTURE

Bladder Prolapse

Prolapse of the bladder may follow a rupture in the floor of the vagina and may occur during or after parturition.[40] As the bladder protrudes, the urethra becomes obstructed, which prevents micturition, and subsequently the bladder distends with urine. The bladder may need to be punctured with a needle to allow drainage; it may then be reduced and the rupture in the vaginal floor repaired.[40]

Bladder Eversion

Eversion of the bladder through the urethra may also occur during parturition and is the more common scenario in the horse.[24] With eversion, urine dripping from the ureters is noted. The bladder needs to be evaluated for lacerations, then manually reduced through the urethral sphincter. Following reduction, a purse-string suture placed around a Foley catheter is the treatment of choice.[41] In addition to sedation, correction will be enhanced using epidural anesthesia to reduce straining.

Bladder Rupture

Rupture of the urinary bladder has been reported most commonly in male foals.[42] Although uncommon, cystorrhexis has also been reported in the adult horse associated with parturition.[43-45] In one study the estimated incidence was 1 in 10,000 births.[44] Bladder rupture may or may not be associated with dystocia. It has been suggested that bladder rupture may occur due to direct laceration during a dystocia or it may subsequently rupture if significant bruising occurred during parturition. Another possibility is that the foal may eliminate the outlet of maternal intravesicular pressure via the urethra. During parturition there is substantially increased intraabdominal pressure, which could cause the urinary bladder to rupture.[45]

Clinical signs of bladder rupture may include anorexia, tachypnea, mild signs of colic, pollakiuria to anuria, and progressive abdominal distension.[43-45] Metabolic changes will be similar to those observed in foals with ruptured bladder. These changes may include dehydration, azotemia, hyperkalemia, hyponatremia, and hypochloremia.[43,45] Definitive diagnosis of ruptured bladder may be made with the aid of abdominocentesis to evaluate for uroperitoneum and creatinine levels. Peritoneal creatinine concentrations two times that of plasma is considered diagnostic.[46] Also helpful with diagnosis is the use of sterile solutions of methylene blue or fluorescein instilled into the bladder with reevaluation of the abdominal fluid looking for these substances.[41] Cystoscopy may also be used for a definitive diagnosis, as well as to evaluate the extent and location of the rupture in order to then determine surgical accessibility.[45]

Treatment

Nonsurgical. Conservative management in economically limited cases may be attempted. Management includes supportive care, peritoneal lavage, and maintenance of a passive catheter with a one-way valve to allow adequate drainage of the bladder. Healing of the bladder by second intention may take 2 to 3 weeks. Continuous drainage of the peritoneal cavity with concurrent intravenous replacement is necessary to correct the metabolic disturbances.[47] Fluid support with 0.9% sterile saline should be used to stabilize the hyperkalemic, hyponatremic patient.[41,45] In addition, broad-spectrum antibiotics and antiinflammatory medications are indicated.

Surgical. The preferred method for treatment of a ruptured bladder is surgical repair via a caudal ventral midline approach. After entrance to the peritoneal cavity, fluid should be obtained for bacterial culture. The bladder is exposed, the laceration identified, and the wound edges debrided.[41] A double-layer inverting closure using absorbable, synthetic suture material is recommended. The bladder mucosa should be avoided in the closure to decrease the potential for cystic calculi formation.[48] Routine three-layer closure of the abdominal wall, subcutaneous tissues, and skin follow exploration of the gastrointestinal tract for any other foaling-related injuries.

If the bladder laceration is within the bladder neck, a caudal ventral midline approach may not allow surgical access. A standing approach through a urethral sphincterotomy has been described.[44] With caudal epidural anesthesia, the urethra and external urethral sphincter are incised. The surgeon may then reach into the bladder and evert it into the vagina where the laceration may be repaired. The bladder is then replaced and the urethral incision closed.[44] There has also been one report of repair of a bladder rupture through an atonic urethral sphincter that allowed the passage of the surgeon's hand and single-layer closure of the defect.[43] The risk is high for penetration of bowel if closure is attempted with this route because of the blind nature of the procedure, and it is therefore not recommended.

PERINEAL LACERATIONS/ RECTOVAGINAL FISTULAS

Please refer to Chapter 24 for coverage of this topic.

References

1. Asbury AC: The reproduction system. In Mansmann RA, McAllister ES, Pratt PW (eds): Equine Medicine and Surgery, Santa Barbara, Calif, American Veterinary Publications, 1982.
2. Livesey MA, Keller SD: Segmental ischemic necrosis following mesocolic rupture in postparturient mares. Comp Cont Educ Pract Vet 1986; 8:763-768.
3. Dwyer R: Postpartum deaths of mares. Equine Dis Q 1993; 2:5.
4. Zent WW: Postpartum complications. In Robinson NE (ed): Current Therapy in Equine Medicine 2, Philadelphia, WB Saunders, 1987.
5. LeBlanc MM: Diseases with physical causes. In Colahan PT, Mayhew IG, Merritt AM et al (eds): Equine Medicine and Surgery, Goleta, Calif, American Veterinary Publications, 1991.
6. Harrison IW: Equine large intestinal volvulus: a review of 124 cases. Vet Surg 1988; 17:77.
7. Dart AJ, Dowling BA, Hodgson DR: Large intestine. In Auer JA, Stick JA (eds): Equine Surgery, Philadelphia, WB Saunders, 1999.
8. Dart AJ, Pascoe JR, Snyder JR: Mesenteric tear of the descending (small) colon as a postpartum complication in two mares. J Am Vet Med Assoc 1991; 199:1612.
9. Rooney JR: Ruptured aneurysm of the uterine artery. Mod Vet Pract 1979; 60:316.
10. Threlfall WR, Immegart HM: Diseases of the reproductive tract. In Reed SM, Bayly WM (eds): Equine Internal Medicine, Philadelphia, WB Saunders, 1998.
11. Gruninger B, Schoon HA, Schoon D et al: Incidence and morphology of endometrial angiopathies in mares in relationship to age and parity. J Comp Pathol 1998; 119:293.
12. Lofstedt RM: Miscellaneous diseases of pregnancy and parturition. In McKinnon AO, Voss JL (eds): Equine Reproduction, Philadelphia, Lea & Febiger, 1993.
13. Stowe HD: Effects of age and impending parturition upon serum copper of thoroughbred mares. J Nutr 1968; 95:179.
14. Pascoe RR: Rupture of the utero-ovarian or middle uterine artery in the mare at or near parturition. Vet Rec 1979; 104:77.
15. Perkins NR, Frazer GS: Reproductive emergencies in the mare. Vet Clin North Am Equine Pract 1994; 10:643.
16. Frazer GS: Post partum complications in the mare. Part 1: Conditions affecting the uterus. Equine Vet Educ 2003; 15:36-44.
17. Sprayberry KA: Hemorrhage and hemorrhagic shock. Proceedings of the Bluegrass Equine Medicine and Critical Care Symposium, Lexington, Ky, Hagyard, Davidson and McGee, 1999.
18. Rossdale P: Abnormal conditions associated with birth. Postgraduate Committee in Vet Sci 1983; 65:97.
19. Vivrette SL: Parturition and postpartum complications. In Robinson NE (ed): Current Therapy in Equine Medicine, 4th ed., Philadelphia, WB Saunders, 1997.
20. Mannucci PM: Hemostatic drugs. New Engl J Med 1998; 339:245.
21. Taylor EL, Sellon DC, Wardrop KJ et al: Effects of intravenous administration of formaldehyde on platelet and coagulation variables in healthy horses. Am J Vet Res 2000; 61:1191.
22. Vandeplassche M, Spincemaille J, Bouters R et al: Some aspects of equine obstetrics. Equine Vet J 1972; 4:105.
23. Taylor T, Blanchard T, Varner D: Management of dystocia in mares: uterine torsion and cesarean section. Comp Cont Educ Pract Vet 1989; 11:1265.
24. Vaughan JT: Surgery of the equine reproductive system. In Morrow DA (ed): Current Therapy in Theriogenology, Diag-

nosis, Treatment, and Prevention of Reproductive Diseases in Animals, Philadelphia, WB Saunders, 1980.

25. Pascoe RR, Meagher DM, Wheat JD: Surgical management of uterine torsion in the mare: a review of 26 cases. J Am Vet Med Assoc 1981; 179:351.

26. Doyle AJ, Freeman DE, Sauberli DS et al: Clinical signs and treatment of chronic uterine torsion in two mares. J Am Vet Med Assoc 2002; 220:349.

27. Barber SM: Complications of chronic uterine torsion in a mare. Can Vet J 1995; 36:102.

28. Pascoe RR, Pascoe JR: Displacements, malpositions, and miscellaneous injuries of the mare's urogenital tract. Vet Clin North Am Equine Pract 1988; 4:439.

29. Vasey JR: Uterine torsion. In McKinnon AO, Voss JL (eds): Equine Reproduction, Philadelphia, Lea & Febiger, 1993.

30. Wichtel JJ, Reinertson EL, Clark TL: Non-surgical treatment of uterine torsion in seven mares. J Am Vet Med Assoc 1988; 193:337.

31. Fischer AT, Phillips TN: Surgical repair of a ruptured uterus in five mares. Equine Vet J 1986; 18:153.

32. Patel J, Lofstedt RM: Uterine rupture in a mare. J Am Vet Med Assoc 1986; 189:806.

33. Honnas CM, Spensley MS, Laverty S et al: Hydramnios causing uterine rupture in a mare. J Am Vet Med Assoc 1988; 193:334.

34. McCoy DJ, Martin GS: Uterine rupture as a postpartum complication in two mares. J Am Vet Med Assoc 1985; 187:1377.

35. Dascanio JJ, Ball BA, Hendrickson DA: Uterine tear without a corresponding placental lesion in a mare. J Am Vet Med Assoc 1993; 202:419.

36. Hassel DM, Ragle CA: Laparoscopic diagnosis and conservative treatment of uterine tear in a mare. J Am Vet Med Assoc 1994; 205:1531.

37. Snoeck MA: Uterine rupture in a pony. Tijdschr Diergeneeskd 1962; 87:1035.

38. Trotter GW, Embertson RM: The uterus and ovaries. In Auer JA, Stick JA (eds): Equine Surgery, Philadelphia, WB Saunders, 1999.

39. Roberts SJ: Injuries and diseases of the puerperal period. In Veterinary Obstetrics and Genital Diseases (Theriogenology), 3rd ed., Woodstock, Vt, 1986.

40. Arthur GH: Injuries and disease incidental to parturition. In Arthur GH, Noakes DE, Pearson H (eds): Veterinary Reproduction and Obstetrics, London, Bailliere Tindall, 1989.

41. Lillich JD, DeBowes RM: Bladder. In Auer JA, Stick JA (eds): Equine Surgery, Philadelphia, WB Saunders, 1999.

42. Brown CM, Collier MA: Bladder diseases. In Robinson NE (ed): Current Therapy in Equine Medicine, Philadelphia, WB Saunders, 1983.

43. Jones PA, Sertich PS, Johnston JK: Uroperitoneum associated with ruptured urinary bladder in a postpartum mare. Aust Vet J 1996; 74:354.

44. Higuchi T, Nanao Y, Senba H: Repair of urinary bladder rupture through urethrotomy and urethral sphincterotomy in four postpartum mares. Vet Surg 2002; 31:344.

45. Nyrop KA, DeBowes RM, Cox JH et al: Rupture of the urinary bladder in two post-parturient mares. Comp Cont Educ Pract Vet 1984; 6:S510.

46. Behr MJ, Hackett RP, Bentinck-Smith J et al: Metabolic abnormalities associated with rupture of the urinary bladder in neonatal foals. J Am Vet Med Assoc 1981; 178:263.

47. Beck C, Dart AJ, McClintock SA et al: Traumatic rupture of the urinary bladder in a horse. Aust Vet J 1996; 73:154.

48. Kaminski JM, Katz AR, Woodward SC: Urinary bladder calculus formation on sutures in rabbits, cats and dogs. Surg Gynecol Obstet 1978; 146:353.

CHAPTER 66

Postparturient Abnormalities

TERRY L. BLANCHARD
MARGO L. MACPHERSON

Postpartum abnormalities vary from minor conditions, requiring no treatment, to more severe life-threatening conditions that require prompt diagnosis and treatment to preserve the life and breeding potential of the mare. This chapter reviews the more common postparturient abnormalities that may occur in the mare.

RETAINED PLACENTA

The fetal membranes are usually expelled 30 minutes to 3 hours after parturition and are considered to be retained if they are not expelled within 3 hours after birth of the foal. The percentage of postparturient mares with retained fetal membranes is reported to range from 2% to 10%.[1,2]

The probability of retained placenta increases after dystocia, probably as a result of trauma to the uterus and myometrial exhaustion.[2,3] Disturbance of the normal uterine contractions at parturition[4] also might make retained placenta more likely. Retention has been reported to be more likely if severe placentitis was present, particularly if adhesion formation has occurred between the endometrium and chorion, or if infection has extended into the myometrium causing myometrial degeneration.[1] Placental retention is more common in the nongravid uterine horn, perhaps because of a progressive increase in the degree of placental folding and attachment from the gravid horn to the nongravid horn.[2] Retention of a portion of the placenta is also more likely to occur in the nongravid than gravid uterine horn because the chorioallantoic membrane is thinner, which predisposes to easier tearing.

Disturbed uterine contractions might result from fetomaternal endocrine dysfunction, inadequate release of oxytocin, or inadequate response of the myometrium to oxytocin. The role of oxytocin in placental expulsion is attested to by prompt placental expulsion after oxytocin-induced parturition and by the failure of some mares with retained placenta to exhibit the characteristic abdominal discomfort typically associated with uterine contraction and placental expulsion in the early postpartum period.[2,5]

With retained fetal membranes, a variable portion of the placenta may be exposed through the vulvar opening. The veterinarian may also be alerted to the possibility of retained placenta when no placenta is found after foaling. Aseptic intrauterine examination may reveal the presence of the placenta within the uterine cavity. Alternatively, part of the placenta may remain in the uterus and continue to initiate mild straining or colic after most of the placenta has been removed. For this reason the fetal membranes should be examined to ensure that they are complete and that no portion remains in the uterus. Retention of portions of the placenta other than just the tip in the previously nongravid horn is also possible, so thorough examination of both surfaces of the expelled chorioallantois is necessary to detect less obvious missing portions. To facilitate examination, the expelled placenta can be filled with water. If the placenta is trampled, it can be impossible to determine whether remnants remain in the uterus.[6]

Sequelae of retained placenta vary from none[7] (particularly if mares are well managed and promptly treated) to the development of metritis, septicemia, toxemia, laminitis, and death.[2,6] Uterine involution is often delayed even if mares do not develop these sequelae.[8,9] Retained placenta with serious sequela is reportedly more common in Draft horses than in light breeds of mares such as Thoroughbreds or Standardbreds.[10,11] Mares with retained placenta after dystocia are at greater risk of developing toxic metritis and laminitis.[3] Severe toxic metritis and laminitis after dystocia are believed to result from delayed uterine involution, increased autolysis of the placenta, and severe bacterial infection.[1] In patients with septic/toxic metritis after dystocia and retained placenta, the uterine wall becomes thin and friable or even necrotic. Absorption of bacteria and bacterial toxins probably follows loss of endometrial integrity and precipitates the peripheral vascular changes that lead to laminitis.[12,13]

Various treatments for retained placenta in mares have been advocated. Oxytocin therapy (alone or in conjunction with other treatments) is the most common and apparently the most beneficial form of management.[2,7] Recommended doses range from 10 to 60 units (smaller doses are typically given intravenously, whereas larger doses are given subcutaneously or intramuscularly) and can be repeated every few hours if the placenta is not passed.[1] The authors prefer to inject 5 to 20 units intramuscularly to promote more physiologic (peristaltic-like) uterine contractions. Clinical signs of abdominal discomfort occur within a few minutes of injection and are usually followed by straining. Discomfort is more pronounced with large doses and might result from intense and perhaps spasmodic uterine contractions. If abdominal discomfort is pronounced yet repeated dosing is deemed necessary, reducing the dose administered to as few as 5 units injected intramuscularly may likewise reduce abdominal discomfort to a more manageable level.

A less intense response may occur during slow intravenous drip of 30 to 60 units of oxytocin in 1 or 2 L of normal saline over a 30 to 60 minute period.[2] The main disadvantage of administering a slow intravenous drip is the time involved and the need to administer the oxytocin using an intravenous catheter and fluid line. Anecdotal reports from many practitioners would suggest success rates achieved with one treatment of oxytocin may be superior with this method of administration. One precautionary note is that uterine prolapse can occasionally occur following oxytocin therapy, so care should be taken to observe for this potential complication.

If not expelled shortly after injection of oxytocin, the placenta sometimes is expelled 1 or 2 hours later. The placenta can sometimes be extracted by applying gentle traction to the portion protruding from the patient's vulva. Vandeplassche[2] reports that vigorous manual attempts to remove the placenta can damage the uterus, including causing hemorrhage within the myometrium, so attempts to manually separate the placenta must be gentle. Twisting the portion of placenta that extends beyond the vulvar lips with one hand (some practitioners will wrap the protruding membranes around a sweat scraper to facilitate twisting), while simultaneously working the fingers of the other hand (within the uterus) between the placenta and uterine wall, is a technique used by some practitioners for manual separation. The authors caution that if the placenta seems to be tightly attached, manual attempts should cease and medical treatments relied on.

Mares that have undergone severe dystocia or that have aborted are less likely to respond to oxytocin therapy alone.[6] If the chorioallantois is intact, distension of the chorioallantoic cavity with 9 to 12 L of warm water or saline solution is an effective treatment of retained placenta. The opening of the chorioallantois is closed to contain the fluid. Stretch receptors are activated when the chorioallantois and uterus are distended, followed by endogenous release of oxytocin and separation of the chorionic villi from the endometrial crypts. Escaping fluid is forced back into the retained portion of the placenta until separation is complete and the placenta is expelled (usually 5 to 30 minutes). This treatment protocol reportedly results in more complete villous and microcarcuncular separation and can be used in conjunction with exogenous oxytocin therapy.[14]

Mares undergoing cesarean section frequently retain their placentas.[1] Retained fetal membranes have been reported to occur in approximately 30% of mares following cesarean section if the foal is dead and in 50% of cases when the foal is alive.[15] Furthermore, it is not uncommon for mares to retain their placentas for up to 3 to 5 days or more following cesarean section or severe dystocia.[3] Mares that retain their placentas for periods greater than 12 hours, including those following cesarean section, require aggressive therapeutic measures to prevent life-threatening sequelae such as septic metritis and laminitis.

Other treatments that can be combined with oxytocin therapy include systemic and local antibiotics, fluid therapy, uterine lavage, exercise (unless laminitis is present), and institution of prophylactic measures to prevent laminitis (e.g., systemic administration of cyclooxygenase inhibitors, application of foot pads). Continuing intrauterine treatment after the fetal membranes have passed is controversial; such treatment is particularly questionable if contamination of the reproductive tract was minimal and placental passage after treatment was prompt.[6] However, for placental retention beyond 24 hours post partum, the authors generally continue treatment (including daily uterine lavage) for 2 to 3 days after the placenta is expelled to ensure placental remnants are removed and any uterine infection is brought under control.

The rationale for uterine lavage in mares that are at risk of developing metritis is to remove debris and bacteria from the uterus in order to reduce contamination and create a less favorable environment for bacterial growth. Purulent material and cellular debris that bind to and inactivate many antibiotics are also removed by uterine lavage. After disinfection of the perineal and vulvar areas, a sterilized or disinfected nasogastric tube is passed into the uterus. The hand is cupped around the end of the tube to prevent the uterus and any remaining placenta from being siphoned into its end. The uterus is gently lavaged with warm (40° to 42°C), sterile, physiologic saline (administered via a sterile or disinfected stomach pump) in 3- to 6-L flushes until the effluent is relatively clear. For on-farm treatments, sufficient volume of sterile fluids may not be available. When this is the case, the authors commonly prepare 2 to 3 gallons of lavage solution in a disinfected bucket by adding 34 g NaCl and 20 ml povidone-iodine solution to each gallon of warm tap water. As discussed above, uterine lavage can be repeated on successive days until the initial effluent is free of purulent material and tissue debris.[6]

If there is concern that the patient might develop septic or toxic metritis and laminitis, systemic and intrauterine antimicrobial therapy are indicated. Intrauterine antimicrobials are administered after evacuation of lavage fluid. Because antimicrobial agents infused into the uterus seldom achieve acceptable levels anywhere except in the uterine lumen and endometrium, relatively high antibiotic doses are administered systemically to prevent or control the development of septicemia from uterine infection that might involve tissue deeper than the endometrium. The agents chosen should be compatible and should have broad-spectrum activity because a wide variety of organisms has been recovered from the postpartum uterus. The antimicrobial regimen must be effective against anaerobic bacteria (e.g., *Bacteroides* spp., *Clostridia* spp.) and endotoxin-producing organisms (e.g., *Escherichia coli*).[3] Antimicrobial agents effective against aerobic bacteria that are commonly employed include trimethoprim sulfadiazine (15 to 30 mg/kg PO twice daily) or penicillin G (22,000 mg/kg IV 4 times daily) plus gentamicin (6.6 mg/kg IV once daily). Metronidazole (15 to 25 mg/kg PO 4 times daily) is typically the drug of choice when treating anaerobic infections.

If there is evidence of toxemia (e.g., neutropenia with toxic neutrophils in the peripheral circulation, elevated heart and respiratory rates, altered mucous membrane perfusion, or other circulatory disturbance), cyclooxygenase inhibitors such as flunixin meglumine should be administered. Cyclooxygenase inhibitors have been shown to attenuate or prevent the circulatory disturbances associated with experimentally induced endotoxemia. Flunixin meglumine therapy is continued until there is no more danger of endotoxemia. The agent is usually given intravenously at a reduced dosage (0.025 mg/kg 3 times daily) in order to avoid potential adverse side effects.[6] Other drugs advocated for this purpose include phenylbutazone (2 to 4 mg/kg PO or IV twice daily), dimethyl sulfoxide (1 g/kg IV; 10% solution in 5% dextrose), hyperimmune plasma (2 to 10 ml/kg IV), and polymyxin B (6000 units/kg IV twice daily).[16]

Acute laminitis is a medical emergency, and treatment should commence as soon as possible. Many therapeutic regimens have been recommended for the treatment of laminitis. Current equine medicine textbooks should be referred to for discussion of various treatments for laminitis.

UTERINE PROLAPSE

The uterus of the mare rarely prolapses. Uterine prolapse is more likely to occur immediately after parturition but sometimes occurs several days later. Conditions causing strong tenesmus (e.g., vaginal trauma) combined with uterine atony will predispose to uterine prolapse.[1,17,18] The condition has been reported to be more common after dystocia when fetal membranes are retained.[19]

Only one uterine horn may be prolapsed, or the uterine body may constitute the major portion of the exposed uterus. Uterine prolapse may be complicated by rupture of internal uterine vessels, shock, or incarceration and ischemia of viscera, leading to death.[1,20,21] In addition, damage to the prolapsed uterus may predispose to development of tetanus.

Treatment of uterine prolapse is first directed at controlling straining, either by administration of sedatives, caudal epidural anesthetic, or general anesthetic.[1] If no clinical signs are present that suggest compromised circulatory capacity, a tranquilizer or sedative can be administered. If the mare is tractable and not showing signs of severe abdominal pain or shock, the authors also recommend administering an epidural anesthetic. A local anesthetic, such as 2% lidocaine (1.0 to 1.25 ml/100 kg), can be slowly administered into the epidural (first coccygeal) space to reduce abdominal straining.[22] An overdose may cause the mare to become ataxic or even fall. Alternatively, 0.17 mg/kg xylazine, as much as is required to 10 ml with 0.9% sterile NaCl, can be administered into the epidural space. Epidural injection with xylazine has been recommended to provide analgesia without hindlimb ataxia.[23] The authors typically use a combination of xylazine (0.6 ml, 30 mg), Carbocaine (2.4 ml), and sterile 0.9% NaCl (5 ml) for epidural injection in most light breeds of mares (body weight approximately 454 to 545 kg). This combination appears to provide good analgesia without causing ataxia or hindlimb weakness. If the mare is intractable yet shows no signs of circulatory shock, general anesthesia can be induced. When inhalation anesthetic is not available, short-acting intravenous anesthetic agents can be used (e.g., 1.1 mg/kg xylazine IV, followed by 2.2 mg/kg ketamine hydrochloride IV—once sedative effects of xylazine are apparent). Duration of anesthesia can usually be safely extended for short periods with intravenous administration of 1 L of 5% guaifenesin containing 1000 mg ketamine hydrochloride and 500 mg xylazine, which is dripped at a rate of 2.75 ml/kg/hr, or slowly to effect. When general anesthetic is used, it is advantageous to place the mare on a slight incline (30 degrees from horizontal) with its head downward; the incline should not be so great as to compromise respiratory function. With the mare in such a position, the uterus should be relatively easy to replace.[22]

In mares kept standing (after wrapping the tail and cleansing the perineal area), the uterus is lifted to the pelvic level in an attempt to restore circulation, reduce congestion, and decrease traction on ovarian and uterine ligaments that cause pain. Elevating the uterus also permits the bladder to resume its normal position, facilitates release of intestine incarcerated within the prolapsed uterus, and reduces the chance vessels in the broad ligaments will rupture.[1] If bowel is entrapped in the prolapsed uterus, ischemic damage to the bowel may have occurred that could warrant evaluation and treatment after performing a ventral midline celiotomy.[21] If the urinary bladder is distended, catheterization may be required before uterine replacement.[22] If the bladder cannot be catheterized, urine can be aspirated from the bladder through a large-bore needle.[24] The uterus is gently cleaned with a disinfectant soap, carefully removing any loosely attached placenta. If placenta is firmly attached, excess free placenta is removed to better enable replacement of the uterus and to decrease likelihood of persistent traction from the heavy placenta that might cause recurrence of the prolapse. Bleeding vessels should be clamped and ligated. Complete uterine tears should be sutured, bringing serosal surfaces into contact. Application of petrolatum jelly to the endometrial surface is useful for protection against lacerations during massage and replacement.[22] Placing the uterus inside two or three plastic garbage bags has been advocated to reduce risk of puncturing or lacerating the uterus during replacement. The garbage bags are removed as the uterus is pushed inside the vagina.[25]

To avoid reprolapse, the uterus must be completely replaced. The uterus, including both uterine horns, is gently kneaded per vaginam into its normal position. Gently filling the uterus with warm water may be helpful in ensuring complete replacement of uterine horns. Excess fluid is then siphoned off through a stomach tube.[22] Walking or jogging the mare down a gentle slope has been advocated to aid in full repositioning of the uterus.[26] Following replacement of the uterus, palpation of the genital tract per rectum is performed to ensure the uterus and ovaries have been returned to their proper position. Intrauterine antibiotics are given to control infection. Small doses (10 to 20 units IM q2-4h) of oxytocin are administered in an attempt to stimulate uterine contractions and thus reduce the chance of recurrence of the prolapse. Mares with uterine atony due to hypocalcemia (i.e., serum ionized calcium below 5.0 mg/dl) may benefit from slow intravenous administration of 100 to 300 ml of 20% calcium borogluconate mixed in 5 L lactated Ringer's solution. The heart should be auscultated periodically as calcium is given, and administration of calcium should cease if the heart rate or rhythm changes. Placing the mare in cross ties for 1 or 2 days has been advocated to reduce the chance of recurrence. A soothing, emollient salve can be placed in the vagina if vaginal lacerations are present. Suturing the vulva will also prevent pneumovagina and speed resolution of vaginal irritation, which might stimulate further straining. Broad-spectrum antibiotics are administered systemically to control infection. Other treatment is as described for metritis, and tetanus prophylaxis is required.[22] The mare should be monitored for evidence of internal hemorrhage, which can occur after uterine replacement.[24]

INVAGINATION OF UTERINE HORN

An invaginated uterine horn is suspected when a mare has mild colic unresponsive to analgesics. The invagination is sometimes associated with a placenta that remains attached to the tip of the uterine horn, causing partial inversion as a result of traction. Palpation per rectum usually reveals a short, blunted uterine horn and tense mesovarium. Intrauterine examination will reveal the dome-shaped, inverted tip of the horn projecting into the uterine lumen. The placenta may be incarcerated in the intussuscepted horn.[22] Rarely, in advanced cases, a reddish-black discharge will be associated with necrosis of the inverted uterus,[1] which might lead to peritonitis if unattended.[24]

Treatment involves replacement of the uterine horn to its normal position, which may require manual removal of the placenta. The mare is sedated to control straining. To manually separate the placenta, the placenta is carefully twisted at the vulvar opening while simultaneously attempting to manually separate the chorion from the endometrium.[22] This manipulation must be gentle to prevent damaging the uterus, which causes placental tags to remain attached to the endometrium.[27] The portion of the placenta protruding from the vagina should be severed if manual separation cannot be accomplished safely. Removing the free placenta reduces the weight pulling on the tip of the uterine horn, permitting it to return to its normal position. The invaginated portion of the uterine horn is gently kneaded inward to its normal position. If the examiner's arms are too short to reach or fully correct the invagination, a clean bottle can be inserted into the affected horn and used to gently push against the invaginated horn to aid in its reduction. Infusion of 1 to 2 gallons of warm, sterile saline solution (or other suitable lavage solution) has also been used to facilitate complete replacement of the inverted uterine horn. Aftercare is as described for uterine prolapse and metritis. If a portion of the placenta was left within the uterus, daily uterine lavage and intrauterine treatment is necessary until the portion of the placenta left within the uterus is expelled.[22]

On occasion, a mildly invaginated uterine horn will be noted in a mare with no untoward clinical signs. Such invaginations may not require treatment, but may persist for a few days postpartum. When an invaginated uterine horn is noted incidentally in a postpartum mare that has expelled her placenta and is not showing signs of discomfort, monitoring the extent of the invagination by palpation per rectum at daily intervals until the condition corrects itself may be all that is required.

UTERINE RUPTURE

Rupture of the uterus occurs predominantly during parturition either spontaneously (due to unknown cause) or secondary to dystocia. Many ruptures are acquired during fetal manipulation to correct dystocia.[1] A number of uterine ruptures are found in mares that seem to deliver the foal and expel the placenta normally. Common locations for uterine ruptures include the dorsal aspect of the uterine body and the tip of the previously gravid uterine horn. A tear in the portion of the expelled placenta that occupied the tip of the previously gravid horn may be noticed, sometimes with thrombosis and hemorrhage apparent in placental vessels viewed through the allantoic surface (suggesting bleeding occurred before placental detachment). These "spontaneous" uterine ruptures might result from the vigorous hindlimb extension that occurs when the fetal stifles finally engage the maternal pelvis during delivery (i.e., the hindlimbs rapidly straighten while they are still encased in the gravid uterine horn).[28] Rarely, in term mares that have not delivered, the fetus may be found free in the abdominal cavity, particularly if uterine torsion was present.[29] Preparturient uterine rupture due to hydramnios has also been described.[30] The uterus may also rupture during overly vigorous treatment in the postparturient period (e.g., during uterine lavage), particularly if the uterine wall was previously damaged or is friable.[31,32]

Although preparturient uterine rupture is extremely rare, it should be considered in prepartum mares with signs of depression or abdominal pain. The presence of uterine rupture should also be suspected if hemorrhagic vaginal discharge containing large blood clots is present.[31-33] The mare may or may not show signs of colic but rapidly becomes depressed if uterine rupture is not treated. Although exsanguination is uncommon, blood loss may be sufficient to result in anemia (packed cell volume [PCV] < 22%) and pale mucous membranes, and occasionally the mare will exhibit additional signs of hemorrhagic shock (profuse sweating, cold extremities, rapid pulse and respiratory rates) for the first hour or two after fetal delivery.[32] On occasion, viscera may herniate through the uterine rent and be found in the vagina or beyond the vulvar opening.[34]

Dorsal uterine tears can sometimes be identified per rectum as irregularities or an opening of the surface of the uterus.[32] Signs of discomfort may be elicited during palpation of the rupture.[31] If more than 1 to 2 days have elapsed since the uterus was torn, the uterus and abdominal viscera may feel tacky or roughened due to fibrinous adhesions/peritonitis. Careful palpation of the internal surface of the uterus per vaginam is more likely to result in location of the rupture. However, the large size of the postpartum uterus usually makes evaluation of the entire endometrial surface impossible. Furthermore, the postpartum endometrial folds are enlarged and edematous, which may also make it difficult to identify a uterine tear. A partial-thickness tear is palpated as a separation in the uterine wall, sometimes with a thickened edge that does not extend through all uterine layers. A full-thickness tear permits a finger or hand to be passed into the abdomen, allowing direct palpation of abdominal viscera. The presence of bowel or omentum in the uterine lumen or birth canal indicates a full-thickness tear.[32]

Abdominocentesis provides evidence for intraabdominal hemorrhage, even with some partial-thickness tears when diapedesis and peritoneal contamination occur. An undetected, full-thickness uterine tear culminates in septic degenerative peritonitis (i.e., peritoneal fluid will have a high white blood cell [WBC] count with many degenerate neutrophils, intracellular and extracellular bacteria, protein > 3 mg/dl, and erythrophagocytosis and hemosiderin in macrophages).[32]

The mare's response to treatment for uterine rupture depends primarily on how soon postpartum the condition is diagnosed and treatment is begun. Survival rate can reach 90% in mares treated within the first 24 hours after foaling but declines steadily thereafter. If evidence of circulatory compromise or dehydration is present, immediate treatment is instituted. Intravenous administration of a balanced electrolyte solution is usually adequate to restore circulatory volume. Intravenous administration of hypertonic saline, colloidal expansion products, or whole blood are seldom necessary in mares seen within the first 12 to 24 hours of foaling. Flunixin meglumine (0.25 to 0.5 mg/kg IV 3 times daily) can be administered to control pain and protect against effects of endotoxin. Systemic administration of broad-spectrum antibiotics (e.g., as listed for metritis) should begin early in the course of treatment.[32]

The best treatment for salvaging both the life and breeding potential of the mare is laparotomy and surgical repair of the uterine rupture.[32,35] This is best accomplished using a ventral midline approach with the mare under general anesthesia (refer to surgical texts for procedures). Following primary uterine closure, oxytocin is administered intramuscularly to stimulate uterine contraction and is repeated as necessary in the postsurgical recovery period. The abdominal cavity should be lavaged to remove bacteria and their enzymes. An abdominal drain should be sutured in place to allow the abdomen to be lavaged twice daily for 2 to 3 days with 5 to 10 L of warm lactated Ringer's solution. Other methods have been described for closure of the uterine tear, including prolapsing the uterus to allow suturing, and blind suturing of the tear per vaginam.[32]

If the mare's general condition makes her a poor anesthetic risk or financial constraints prevent surgery, conservative treatment is used. Conservative treatment consists of administering 1 to 3 mg ergonovine maleate intramuscularly (to contract smooth muscle in the uterus and uterine vessels) or oxytocin (if ergonovine is unavailable) every 2 to 4 hours, systemic administration of broad-spectrum antibiotics and flunixin meglumine, and intravenous replacement of fluids and electrolytes. Abdominal lavage can be performed to reduce contamination. Conservative treatment is most likely to be successful with small, dorsally located uterine tears, but the risk of fatal peritonitis developing is great.[1,32] Furthermore, mares that survive the peritonitis associated with conservatively treating a uterine tear may suffer reduced fertility as a consequence of adhesion formation in the abdomen and/or uterus.

Following either primary closure of the uterine tear or conservative treatment, the uterus should be massaged per rectum at 3- to 5-day intervals to break down forming adhesions. Tetanus prophylaxis is also indicated.[32]

INTERNAL HEMORRHAGE

Rupture of major utero-ovarian or uterine vessels (usually an artery), within the broad ligament, sometimes occurs at parturition or shortly thereafter. Rarely, a large vessel ruptures before parturition. External iliac artery rupture occurs less frequently.[1,36,37] Right utero-ovarian or middle uterine artery rupture occurs more commonly than left.[36,37] Age-related (i.e., mares greater than 10 years of age) degenerative changes in vascular walls, including aneurysm formation, are thought to predispose to vascular rupture.[36] Thrombosis and vascular rupture may also occur with uterine prolapse or torsion.[1] It has been postulated that increased blood flow and vessel diameter with exaggerated tortuosity occur with successive pregnancies, resulting in an increased load on vascular walls that contributes to damage. Subsequent uterine contractions and fetal movements, particularly during parturition, might then induce vascular rupture.[1]

After delivery of the foal and expulsion of the placenta, the affected mare appears uncomfortable (i.e., the mare is apprehensive, lies down, looks at her flank, and then rises and stands in one position for a prolonged time, shifting weight from one limb to the other). Inappetence is common.[38] In some cases the affected mare shows signs of severe, unrelenting colic.[1] Profuse sweating and evidence of hemorrhagic shock (pale mucous membranes, low PCV, increased pulse and respiratory rate, weakness and prostration) become evident. The heart rate may exceed 100 beats per minute in mares with severe hemorrhage. Rupture of the broad ligament with hemorrhage into the abdomen usually leads to rapid collapse and death.[1,38]

The colic associated with distension of the broad ligament may mistakenly be assumed to be that commonly associated with postparturient uterine contractions and expulsion of the placenta.[39] Alternatively, the mare may fail to show signs of pain, with hemorrhage being controlled within the broad ligament. A hematoma, usually 20 to 30 cm in diameter, may be detected in the broad ligament of the uterus during routine prebreeding examination of mares in which hemorrhage has been restricted to this area.[38] The mare that ruptures the broad ligament several days after foaling due to hemorrhage into a preexisting hematoma often dies suddenly.[37]

Palpation of the uterus and broad ligaments per rectum may or may not elicit signs of pain.[26,38] Transrectal ultrasonographic examination will often reveal clotting blood in the hematoma that appears echolucent in comparison with the rest of the uterus, with echogenic material being dispersed throughout the clot.[38] Some authors recommend avoiding per rectum examinations in the early postpartum period in mares suspected of having uterine hematomas because the added excitement/pain might exacerbate bleeding. Instead, they suggest transabdominal ultrasound examination (to detect swirling cellular elements within a hypoechoic medium, typical of intraabdominal bleeding), abdominocentesis, and hematologic analysis are sufficient to make a diagnosis without overly exciting the mare.[24,40]

Treatment of severe hemorrhage associated with rupture of uterine, utero-ovarian, or iliac arteries is frequently unrewarding.[1,41] The mare should be confined in a darkened stall in an effort to prevent activity and excitement. Management should include attempts to minimize excitement associated with any treatments that might exacerbate bleeding, causing the broad ligament to burst and death to occur. Analgesics, such as flunixin meglumine (1.1 mg/kg IV) and butorphanol tartrate (0.02 to 0.04 mg/kg IV) may be administered to control pain associated with distension of the broad ligament. Corticosteroids (1 to 2 mg/kg prednisolone sodium succinate IV) can be administered for shock. Intravenous administration of fluids and other shock therapy are likely to be of no therapeutic benefit if severe intraabdominal hemorrhage is occurring, which rapidly leads to extravasation and death. Intraabdominal hemorrhage can be confirmed by abdominocentesis.[38]

Circulating volume fluid replacement, plasma expansion therapy, and sometimes whole blood transfusion may be of benefit when hemorrhage is contained within the broad ligament, or when intraabdominal bleeding is slow. Administration of 4 to 6 ml/kg hypertonic (7%) saline, followed by infusion of 10 to 20 L lactated Ringer's solution over a 2- to 4-hour period, will often help to support circulation. Alternatively, hetastarch can be administered (6 ml/kg) in place of hypertonic saline solution.[40] The mare's circulatory status should continually be evaluated to determine whether whole blood transfusion will be necessary. Changes in laboratory parameters (e.g., a PCV <15%, a hemoglobin concentration <5 mg/dl, and a plasma protein concentration <4 mg/dl) are indicative of marked blood loss and deficient oxygen-carrying capacity. The clinician should remember that when marked quantities of whole blood are lost, laboratory parameters supporting the need for transfusion often lag behind clinical signs of hypovolemic blood loss. Therefore when clinical signs of hypovolemic blood loss (e.g., tachycardia, weak pulse, pale mucous membranes, weakness, and depression) are present, whole blood transfusion should be strongly considered.[38] The reader is referred to current textbooks for guidelines for collection of blood from a suitable donor and for administering blood to the affected mare.

Naloxone hydrochloride has been advocated for treating rupture of the uterine or utero-ovarian artery in mares.[42] Endogenous opioids may be released in hemorrhagic shock, and naloxone, a narcotic antagonist, should block these effects. The rationale for this theory is predicated on the finding that the administration of naloxone attenuated some of the cardiovascular responses associated with experimentally induced shock in horses.[43] Thus naloxone has been proposed as having a potential therapeutic value for shock treatment. Apparently naloxone antagonizes the actions of endogenous opioids mobilized by pain or stress that are involved in the regulation of blood pressure by the central nervous system.[44] Naloxone

(0.2 mg/kg: 90 to 100 mg per adult full-sized horse, can be repeated) is administered intravenously as a bolus[40] to the mare that has already been placed in a darkened, quiet stall. Whether this treatment is superior to simply placing the mare in the same type of quiet environment, with or without the administration of other drugs, is unknown.

An antifibrinolytic drug, aminocaproic acid, has also been used in some veterinary practices to control hemorrhage (e.g., with ruptured uterine arteries or hemorrhaging uterine incision sites from cesarean sections). This drug inhibits factors that promote clot lysis, thereby reducing secondary hemorrhage, and may be effective at controlling bleeding even when hemorrhage is not associated with excessive fibrinolysis. A 20-g loading dose mixed in 6 L lactated Ringer's solution is administered intravenously, followed by 10 g administered in a similar manner every 6 hours for 36 to 48 hours.[40] Additional therapy for hemorrhagic shock can include pentoxifylline (7.5 mg/kg IV or PO). Pentoxifylline increases erythrocyte flexibility and may increase oxygen delivery to ischemic tissues.[45] Sprayberry [40] cautions that, when giving pentoxifylline intravenously, it must first be filtered and mixed in 500 ml saline before being administered slowly intravenously.

In the case of a postpartum hemorrhage, the authors do not generally recommend that the foal be separated from the mare unless it is necessary to protect the foal from inadvertent injury by the colicky mare. Most mares become highly agitated when separated from their foals, and any increased activity can elevate blood pressure and cause disruption of a blood clot. If it is necessary to remove the foal from the dam, steps should be taken to ensure that the foal's nutrient and passive immunity needs are met.

Hematomas that remain contained within the broad ligament regress gradually over a few to several weeks. Some hematomas may remain palpable as firm uterine enlargements for several months or occasionally longer. Uterine hematomas may be detected per rectum during prebreeding examination of mares in which no postpartum problems were suspected. Ultrasonographically the consolidating hematoma will appear more echolucent than the rest of the uterus, with echodensities being dispersed throughout the clot. The hematoma will become palpably more firm and progressively more echodense as fibrous tissue organizes.[38]

Some investigators suggest that there may be an increased likelihood of recurrence of vascular rupture with fatal hemorrhage at the subsequent parturition.[1,24,37] However, a number of practitioners from large breeding farms report that affected mares are generally fertile, once the hematomas regress sufficiently in size, and usually deliver foals without recurrence of hemorrhage. Mares with palpable hematomas in the broad ligament should not be rebred before the second postpartum estrus.[38]

TRAUMATIC INJURIES OF THE BIRTH CANAL

Minor contusions and lacerations of the caudal birth canal occur commonly during parturition in mares, particularly with dystocia. Vulvar swelling and discharge, which may be hemorrhagic, alerts one to the possibility of birth canal trauma in the postparturient mare. Hemorrhagic vulvar discharge may originate from lacerations in the birth canal or from internal uterine trauma (e.g., difficult delivery; forceful, premature removal of fetal membranes). Minor lacerations and trauma of the vulva, vestibule, and vagina are more common in maiden mares, especially following delivery by traction. However, they also occur in maiden and pluriparous mares having seemingly uncomplicated births. Failure to open a previously sutured vulva (Caslick's operation) before delivery can lead to laceration of the vulva and perineum. Passage of the foal through the birth canal when the cervix is not completely dilated will result in cervical laceration. A complication of a difficult fetotomy is laceration(s) of the vagina and/or cervix.[4,46,47]

Deep vaginal lacerations or vaginal rupture may become infected and develop into draining fistulous tracts or abscesses. Hemorrhage may be profuse if a large blood vessel in the cervix, vagina, or vulva is ruptured. Alternatively, hemorrhage may result in a perivaginal hematoma or bleeding within the abdomen if the ruptured blood vessel is located in the peritoneal cavity.[1] Hematomas arising from bleeding pudendal or vaginal arteries dissect along the fascial plane within the vaginal cavity, resulting in unilateral or bilateral vulvar swellings that may induce colicky signs.[24,48] Rectal and vaginal examinations will reveal if these ventrolateral swellings are confined within the pelvis or if they extend along fascial planes inward along the abdominal wall.

Recurrent bleeding episodes from subepithelial varicose veins located at the vestibulovaginal juncture occasionally occur. Compression of pelvic veins by the gravid uterus with repeated pregnancies has been postulated as a cause of the varicosities, which are thought to be more common in mares with a tipped vulva and sunken anus.[49] Although varicosities may hemorrhage following parturition, spontaneous regression is more commonly the rule.[46]

Forceful removal of fetal membranes may induce intrauterine hemorrhage.[27] Rupture of the endometrium, and less commonly the entire uterine wall, should be suspected when extensive hemorrhage from the vulva is recognized. Hemorrhagic vulvar discharge may persist in mares with an inverted uterine horn or following replacement of a prolapsed uterus. Life-threatening hemorrhage from lacerations of the birth canal is uncommon. The mare may become anemic but usually will survive.[1]

When profuse bleeding from the vulva follows delivery of a foal, an immediate attempt should be made to locate the source of hemorrhage. The mare should be placed in a stock if hemorrhage is not profuse but obvious tears of the perineal region or vulva are present, or if unusual amounts of blood (particularly when large clots are present) are being discharged from the vulva. The tail is wrapped and tied to the side, and the perineal area is scrubbed with an antiseptic soap and rinsed. The vulvar lips are parted to enable the vulvar and caudal vaginal area to be visualized. Abrasions and lacerations of the mucosa are readily apparent.[46] Lacerations of the vagina

and vulva are more common than ruptured blood vessels, and generally are located near the vulvovaginal border.[1] Profuse hemorrhage from a large vessel in the cervix, vagina, or vulva rarely occurs but is identifiable in most cases by visual examination. Locating the torn end of such a large vessel can be difficult because it may retract into tissue when it is severed.

Perivaginal hematoma is identifiable by fluxuant swelling beneath the vaginal mucosa. Large perivaginal hematomas may constrict the vaginal canal and are most commonly located ventrally or ventrolaterally within the pelvis.[46] These hematomas seldom protrude through the vulvar lips, but when they do, they may be mistaken for prolapse of the vagina or urinary bladder.[1]

Deep perineal lacerations that penetrate through to the rectum, creating a rectovaginal fistula or third-degree perineal laceration (i.e., the perineal body is torn completely through, resulting in communication between the caudal rectum and vestibulum/vagina), are obvious and are accompanied by considerable tissue swelling, often with feces in the vaginal vault. Infection of the uterus occurs as a result of contamination with fecal material. Treatment of perineal lacerations is the subject of a different chapter.

Following visual examination of the caudal vagina, a sterile, disposable speculum or spreading-type metal vaginal speculum (e.g., Caslick's speculum) is lubricated and inserted into the vagina. A light source is directed into the vaginal vault to facilitate viewing. Vaginal or cervical lacerations, particularly when the submucosa is penetrated, are usually visible when spreading-type specula are used for vaginoscopy. Vaginal lacerations are probed gently with the fingers to ascertain if a full-thickness breach is present.[46] Some cervical lacerations may not be apparent until cervical closure occurs following the first postpartum ovulation.[50]

If a cause for the bleeding is not identified, the hand should be well scrubbed and the fingers used to palpate the vagina, cervix, and uterus. Full-thickness lacerations of the cranial vagina may be intraperitoneal, making it possible for intestine to prolapse through the vaginal rent. Intrauterine palpation is performed in an attempt to locate lacerations of the endometrium. Lacerations of the uterine mucosa may sometimes be palpated in this manner if they are within reach of the examiner. If a laceration of the birth canal is not visualized or palpated in spite of significant amounts of blood being expelled from the uterus through the cervix, a laceration of the endometrium should be suspected. An accumulation of large blood clots that fill the uterine lumen would suggest extensive endometrial trauma is present.[46] Abdominocentesis should be performed to ensure that a full-thickness tear of the uterus is not present.[51] Hemorrhage from the vulva may be detected following uterine rupture, but more commonly the uterine tear is detected after peritonitis develops.[32] If the mare is not febrile and the analysis of peritoneal fluid reveals no evidence of septic peritonitis, no attempt is made to remove large, space-occupying blood clots to avoid reinitiating bleeding.[24,46] Prolapsed intestine usually is accompanied by avulsion of the mesentery, necessitating celiotomy and intestinal resection after the prolapse is replaced into the abdomen.

Vaginal lacerations should be sutured per vaginam to ensure prolapse will not recur.[46]

No treatment is indicated for superficial lacerations or abrasions of the vulvar, vestibular, vaginal, cervical, or uterine mucosa. The slight bleeding associated with these lacerations rarely causes acute anemia, and the mare usually survives. If profuse bleeding from a large blood vessel in the birth canal occurs, the severed end of the vessel should be clamped with a hemostat and ligated with an absorbable suture material such as No. 2 polyglycolic acid or No. 2 polyglactin 910.[46] Alternatively, the hemostat may be left clamped in place for 24 to 48 hours before it is removed.[1] If the bleeding vessel cannot be located for clamping, a tampon can be inserted into the vagina and left to apply pressure in an attempt to control hemorrhage. The tampon can be made by filling a 2- or 3-inch stockinette with cotton, tying the ends with umbilical tape, and liberally coating the surface of the stockinette with petroleum jelly. The petroleum jelly is added to prevent sticking of the stockinette to vaginal surfaces, and the tampon is removed in 24 to 48 hours after bleeding has stopped.[46]

Fresh lacerations that either are full thickness through the vaginal wall or extend through the submucosa should be sutured. The authors prefer to use a single layer of absorbable suture material, such as No. 2 polyglycolic acid or No. 2 coated polyglactin 910, in a continuous horizontal mattress pattern to invert the mucosa or vaginal tissue into the vaginal lumen. If the laceration is in the vagina or vestibule but does not extend through all tissue layers, these cavities are coated with an emollient antibiotic preparation (e.g., mix a warmed 1-lb can of lanolin with 71 g oxytetracycline powder and 80 mg dexamethasone) to reduce irritation, control local infection, and prevent transluminal adhesions from occurring. This medication should be applied every 1 to 2 days until mucosal healing has occurred. During application of the antimicrobial creme or ointment, any transluminal adhesions discovered should be broken. The forming adhesions are fibrinous strands at this time and are easy to separate or remove by the gloved hand. If necessary to control pain, acepromazine (0.04 mg/kg IV) or xylazine (0.2 to 0.4 mg/kg IV) and butorphanol (0.02 to 0.04 mg/kg IV) can be administered before medicating the vagina. Antibiotics are also administered systemically for 5 to 7 days (e.g., trimethoprim/sulfamethoxazole, 30 mg/kg PO twice daily) to control infection, and phenylbutazone (1 to 2 g IV or PO twice daily) or flunixin meglumine (0.25 to 0.50 mg/kg IV twice daily) can be administered for 3 to 5 days to relieve discomfort and control pain. Mineral oil (1 gallon) can be administered by nasogastric tube once daily until the stool is soft and as necessary to maintain this stool consistency for 1 week. Keeping the stool soft will reduce straining during defecation.[46]

Because pneumovagina can further irritate the mucosa and cause straining that aggravates the condition and delays healing, the dorsal portion of the vulva can be sutured (Caslick's operation) to control windsucking. The vulva is only sutured low enough to prevent pneumovagina, but not so low as to prevent insertion of the hand and arm so that local medication can still be applied. Vulvar sutures can be removed in 10 to 14 days if the vagina and vestibulum have healed sufficiently. Failure to promptly treat vaginal or vestibular lacerations can result in transluminal adhesions that will preclude breeding.[46]

Treatment for full-thickness vaginal tears is the same as for partial-thickness tears, but the vagina is not medicated by hand until healing is complete to minimize the chance of causing dehiscence of suture lines. In addition, mares with full-thickness vaginal tears should be monitored over the first few days postpartum by serial analyses of abdominal fluid. Development of septic peritonitis requires intensive treatment that includes systemic administration of broad-spectrum antibiotics and nonsteroidal antiinflammatory drugs (NSAIDs), fluid and electrolyte replacement, and peritoneal lavage.[46]

When severe trauma to the vagina occurs, usually with prolonged dystocia and particularly when the dystocia is relieved by a difficult fetotomy, necrotic vaginitis may follow. This condition is extremely painful to the mare, and the mare strains frequently, if not constantly, expelling foul-smelling effluent from the vulva. Furthermore, life-threatening sequelae such as septicemia, diarrhea, and laminitis can occur as a result of necrotic vaginitis. Placement of a catheter ($3^1/_2$ French, 22 inch) in the caudal epidural space may be warranted if straining and windsucking are excessive. After threading the catheter 4 to 6 inches cranially in the epidural space, the catheter end is capped with an injection port (as needed) device and is sutured to the skin over the pelvis. Small amounts of local anesthetic (e.g., 2% lidocaine, or 2% lidocaine plus xylazine) or a suitable narcotic (e.g., morphine) can be administered as necessary to control pain and straining while avoiding the risk of ataxia or the mare falling. The catheter can usually be removed in 2 to 4 days as healing progresses. An emollient antibiotic preparation should also be applied to the vagina twice daily, and the vulva can be partially sutured to aid in controlling pneumovagina. The risk of developing complete transvaginal adhesions is great, so local treatment should be continued for 2 to 4 weeks, gently breaking forming adhesions during application of ointment. The authors prefer to use an antibiotic preparation that tends to stick to epithelial surfaces and contains a corticosteroid (e.g., lanolin-oxytetracycline-dexamethasone preparation described above) in an attempt to discourage fibrous tissue formation. In some cases in which firm adhesions develop, surgical removal of the bands of fibrous tissue at a later date may be successful in restoring lumen patency. In addition to application of antimicrobial preparations, broad-spectrum antibiotics are administered systemically for 5 to 7 days (e.g., trimethoprim sulfamethoxazole, 30 mg/kg PO q12h) to control infection, and phenylbutazone (1 to 2 g IV q12h) or flunixin meglumine (0.25 to 0.50 mg/kg IV q8-12h) is administered for 3 to 4 days to control inflammation. Tetanus prophylaxis is also required.[46]

Dissecting tracts (fistulas) occasionally develop following extensive vaginal trauma with disruption of the vaginal wall. Suppuration may result in abscess formation within the pelvic area[52] and rarely may extend along connective tissue planes into the abdomen, along the pelvic floor, or even along medial surfaces of the thigh. To promote healing of vaginal dissecting tracts, daily flushing with dilute (2% to 5% v/v) povidone-iodine solution through a rubber urinary catheter placed in the fistulous tract is performed for up to 2 weeks or until healing occurs. If an abscess forms in the vagina, it is punctured at the caudal-most aspect to promote drainage (taking care to avoid the urethra) and flushed as described above for the fistulous tract.[46] Broad-spectrum antibiotics are administered systemically for 1 to 2 weeks.[46,52]

Cervical lacerations seldom cause prolonged bleeding. Local antimicrobial preparations can be applied for a few days if the laceration is prominent, but no attempt at surgical repair is made for at least 1 month. Once the reproductive tract is fully involuted and the mare is in diestrus (when the cervix should be completely closed), the cervix can be evaluated to determine if it is capable of closing. The authors have noted cervical tears early in the postpartum period in numerous foaling mares, particularly when located in the caudal portion of the cervix, that did not prevent the cervix from closing properly once involution was complete. If the cervix remains open during diestrus after uterine involution is complete, surgical repair of the cervix can be performed to ensure that it will be capable of closing and maintaining pregnancy.[46]

Intrapelvic perivaginal bleeding that results in perivaginal hematoma formation is not treated unless the hematoma is so large that the examiner fears vaginal stenosis may occur. Application of ice packs (crushed ice placed in a rectal sleeve and inserted into the vagina 2 to 3 times daily for 1 to 2 days) for 15 to 20 minutes may help to control swelling of vaginal hematomas that protrude through the vulvar lips if applied during the first few hours postpartum.[53] For smaller hematomas that do not protrude through the vulvar lips, the vulva is sutured to control pneumovagina that may develop with straining. Large hematomas can be drained 2 to 3 days postpartum, after clot formation has occurred. A sedative such as acepromazine maleate (0.04 to 0.08 mg/kg IV), xylazine hydrochloride (1.1 mg/kg IV), or detomidine hydrochloride (0.02 to 0.04 mg/kg IV) is administered, and local anesthetic is infused into the area to be punctured. A sterile 12- or 14-gauge needle, attached to intravenous drip tubing and a 60-ml syringe, is inserted into the fluxuant areas of the hematoma. Blood-tinged serum is aspirated from the hematoma to reduce its size as much as possible. Most vulvar or vaginal hematomas regress within 3 weeks postpartum. Large perivaginal hematomas regress slowly and usually remain palpable for several months as they become increasingly firm. If hematomas do not regress or do not become progressively more firm in texture, abscessation should be suspected. Abscessation can be confirmed by an aseptic tap (purulent material will be aspirated) and should be incised and drained as previously discussed. Large intrapelvic hematomas sometimes leave permanent lumps of scar tissue that are palpable ventrally in the pelvic area. Unless marked vaginal stenosis occurs, the ability to deliver a fetus per vaginam is not compromised.[46]

Lacerations of the endometrium can seldom be reached per vaginam for suturing. If lacerations are within reach of the examiner, particularly when they extend into the submucosa, a one-handed technique can be used to suture the laceration. A needle threaded with a long strand of No. 2 polyglycolic acid or No. 2 coated polyglactin is carried into the uterus and carefully guided through the edges of the laceration in an everting (into the uterine lumen) horizontal mattress pattern. If endometrial bleeding continues, 1 to 3 mg ergonovine maleate is administered intramuscularly to stimulate contraction of the myometrium and smooth musculature of bleeding vessels in an attempt to induce hemostasis. Ergonovine maleate is preferable to oxytocin because of its contractile effects on smooth muscle of blood vessels (it directly stimulates vascular smooth muscle),[54] and injections can be repeated at 3-hour intervals. If ergonovine maleate is not available, 20 to 40 units of oxytocin can be administered intramuscularly to stimulate uterine contraction in an effort to control uterine bleeding. Intramuscular administration of oxytocin is preferable to intravenous administration because of the longer duration of action (approximately 1 hour) following intramuscular injection.[55] Oxytocin injection can be repeated at 2- to 4-hour intervals if necessary.

The mare's circulatory status should be monitored to determine if fluid replacement, plasma expanders, or whole blood transfusion will be necessary (see above discussion). Large blood clots found occupying the lumen of the uterus should not be removed.[24,46] In the authors' experience, these large clots are either expelled or resorbed by approximately 1 week postpartum. Although the presence of large blood clots, once resorbed or expelled, are not reported to cause intrauterine problems,[1] the authors prefer to lavage the uterus with warm (37° to 40° C) lactated Ringer's solution to remove any remaining clots and distend the uterus to aid in breaking down any intraluminal adhesions that may be forming. The authors do not perform the uterine lavage until approximately 5 to 7 days postpartum to reduce the chances of reinitiating bleeding.[46]

Mares with lacerations of the birth canal or endometrium should be examined at approximately 3 to 4 weeks postpartum, before rebreeding. If transrectal ultrasonographic examination reveals the presence of uterine fluid, the endometrium should be cultured for bacteria and a biopsy specimen should be taken to determine whether endometritis is present.[56,57] Bacterial endometritis should be treated with broad-spectrum antimicrobial drugs selected on the basis of culture and sensitivity. Once uterine involution is complete and damage to the birth canal is healed, the mare can be rebred.

References

1. Roberts SJ: Veterinary Obstetrics and Genital Diseases, Theriogenology, 3rd edition, pp 251-262, 277-352, 355-359, 361-367, 373-390, Woodstock, Vt, SJ Roberts, 1986.
2. Vandeplassche M, Spincemaille J, Bouters R: Aetiology, pathogenesis and treatment of retained placenta in the mare. Equine Vet J 1971; 3:144-147.
3. Blanchard TL, Elmore RG, Varner DD et al: Dystocia, toxic metritis and laminitis in mares. Proceedings of the 33rd Annual Convention of the American Association of Equine Practitioners, pp 641-648, 1987.

4. Vandeplassche M, Spincemaille J, Bouters R et al: Some aspects of equine obstetrics. Equine Vet J 1972; 4:105-109.

5. Hillman RB: Induction of parturition in mares. J Reprod Fertil Suppl 1975; 23:641-644.

6. Blanchard TL, Varner DD, Scrutchfield WL et al: Management of dystocia in mares: retained placenta, metritis and laminitis. Comp Cont Educ Pract Vet 1990; 12:563-569.

7. Threlfall WR, Provencher R, Carleton CL: Retained fetal membranes in the mare. Proceedings of the 33rd Annual Convention of the American Association of Equine Practitioners, pp 649-656, 1987.

8. Gygax AP, Ganjam VK, Kenney RM: Clinical, microbiological, and histological changes associated with uterine involution in the mare. J Reprod Fertil Suppl 1979; 27:571-578.

9. Steiger K, Kersten F, Aupperle H et al: Puerperal involution in the mare: morphological studies in correlation with the course of birth. Theriogenology 2002; 58:783-786.

10. Rossdale PD, Ricketts SW: Equine Stud Farm Medicine, 2nd edition, pp 220-224, 249-250, 260-276, Philadelphia, Lea & Febiger, 1980.

11. Freeman DA, Frazer GS, Hosmer TA: The incidence of dystocia and postfoaling complications in Draft and light mares. Proceedings of the Annual Meeting of the Society for Theriogenology, p 141, 2000.

12. Blanchard TL, Elmore RG, Kinden DA et al: Effect of intrauterine infusion of *Escherichia coli* endotoxin in postpartum pony mares. Am J Vet Res 1985; 46:2157-2162.

13. Blanchard TL, Orsini JA, Garcia MC et al: Influence of dystocia on white blood cell and neutrophil counts in mares. Theriogenology 1986; 25:347-352.

14. Burns SJ, Judge NG, Martin JE et al: Management of retained placenta in mares. Proceedings of the 23rd Annual Convention of the American Association of Equine Practitioners, pp 381-390, 1977.

15. Stashak TS, Vandeplassche M: Cesarean section. In McKinnon AO, Voss JL (eds): Equine Reproduction, pp 437-443, Philadelphia, Lea & Febiger, 1993.

16. Troedsson MHT: Fetal membrane retention and toxic metritis. Proceedings of the Annual Meeting of the Society for Theriogenology, pp 113-118, 2000.

17. Vandeplassche M: Uterine prolapse in the mare. Vet Rec 1975; 97:19.

18. Brewer RL, Kliest GJ: Uterine prolapse in the mare. J Am Vet Med Assoc 1963; 142:1118.

19. Zent WW: Postpartum complications. In Robinson NE (ed): Current Therapy in Equine Medicine, pp 544-547, Philadelphia, WB Saunders, 1997.

20. Pascoe J, Pascoe R: Displacements, malpositions and miscellaneous injuries of the mare's urogenital tract. Vet Clin North Am 1988; 4:439.

21. Vivrette SL: Parturition and postpartum complications. In Robinson NE (ed): Current Therapy in Equine Medicine, pp 547-551, Philadelphia, WB Saunders, 1997.

22. Hooper RN, Blanchard TL, Taylor TS et al: Identifying and treating uterine prolapse and invagination of the uterine horn in the mare. Vet Med 1993; 88(1):60-65.

23. LeBlanc PH, Caron JP, Patterson JS et al: Epidural injection of xylazine for perineal analgesia in horses. J Am Vet Med Assoc 1988; 193:1405-1408.

24. Frazer GS: Post partum complications in the mare. Part 1. Conditions affecting the uterus. Equine Vet Educ 2003; 15(1):45-54.

25. Cooper WL: Personal communication, 1979.

26. Perkins NR, Frazer GS: Reproductive emergencies in the mare. Vet Clin North Am Equine Pract 1994; 10:643-670.

27. Vandeplassche M: Obstetrician's view of the physiology of equine parturition and dystocia. Equine Vet J 1980; 12:45-49.

28. Ginther OJ: Equine pregnancy: physical interactions between the uterus and conceptus. Proceedings of the 44th Annual Convention of the American Association of Equine Practitioners, pp 73-104, 1998.

29. Wheat JD, Meagher DM: Uterine torsion and rupture in mares. J Am Vet Med Assoc 1972; 160:881-885.

30. Honnas CM, Spensley MS, Laverty S et al: Hydramnios causing uterine rupture in a mare. J Am Vet Med Assoc 1988; 193:334-336.

31. Brooks DE, McCoy DJ, Martin GS: Uterine rupture as a postpartum complication in two mares. J Am Vet Med Assoc 1985; 187:1377-1378.

32. Hooper RN, Schumacher J, Sertich PL et al: Diagnosing and treating uterine rupture in the mare. Vet Med 1993; 88(3):263-270.

33. Patel J, Lofstedt RM: Uterine rupture in a mare. J Am Vet Med Assoc 1986; 189:806-807.

34. Ponting MF, David JS: A case of uterine rupture in a mare. Equine Vet J 1972; 4:149-150.

35. Fischer AT, Phillips TN: Surgical repair of a ruptured uterus in five mares. Equine Vet J 1986; 18:153-155.

36. Rooney JR: Internal hemorrhage related to gestation in the mare. Cornell Vet 1964; 51:11-17.

37. Pascoe RR: Rupture of the utero-ovarian or middle uterine artery in the mare at or near parturition. Vet Rec 1979; 104:77.

38. McCarthy PF, Hooper RN, Carter GK et al: Postparturient hemorrhage in the mare: managing ruptured arteries of the broad ligament. Vet Med 1994; 89:147-152.

39. Lofstedt RM: Miscellaneous diseases of pregnancy and parturition. In McKinnon AO, Voss JL (eds): Equine Reproduction, pp 596-603, Philadelphia, Lea & Febiger, 1993.

40. Sprayberry KA: Hemorrhage and hemorrhagic shock. Proceedings of the Annual Bluegrass Critical Care Symposium, pp 1-16, Lexington, Ky, 1999.

41. Asbury AC: The Reproductive system. In McAllister ES (ed): Equine Medicine and Surgery, 3rd edition, pp 1305-1367, Santa Barbara, Calif, American Veterinary Publications, 1982.

42. Byars TD: Coagulopathies in the horse. Proceedings of the Annual Meeting of the American College of Veterinary Internal Medicine, pp 110-112, Blacksburg, Va, 1985.

43. Weld JM, Kamerling SG, Combie JD et al: The effects of naloxone on endotoxic and hemorrhagic shock in horses. Res Commun Chem Pathol Pharmacol 1984; 44:227-238.

44. Jaffe JH, Marten WR: Opioid analgesics and antagonists. In Gilman AG et al (eds): The Pharmacological Basis of Therapeutics, 8th edition, pp 485-521, New York, Pergamon Press, 1990.

45. Wattanasirichaigoon S, Manconi MJ, Delude RL et al: Lisofylline ameliorates intestinal mucosal barrier dysfunction by ischemia and ischemia/reperfusion. Shock 1999; 11:269-275.

46. Hooper RN, Carter GK, Varner DD et al: Postparturient hemorrhage in the mare: managing lacerations of the birth canal and uterus. Vet Med 1994; 89:57-63.

47. Blanchard TL, Youngquist RS, Bierschwal C et al: Sequelae to percutaneous fetotomy in the mare. J Am Vet Med Assoc 1983; 182:1127.

48. Rossdale PD: Differential diagnosis of postparturient hemorrhage in the mare. Equine Vet Educ 1994; 6:135-136.

49. White RSS, Gerring EL, Jackson PGG et al: Persistent vaginal hemorrhage in five mares caused by varicose veins of the vaginal wall. Vet Rec 1984; 115:263-264.

50. Brown JS et al: Surgical repair of the lacerated cervix in the mare. Theriogenology 1984; 22:351-359.

51. Frazer GS, Burba D, Paccamonti D et al: The effects of parturition and peripartum complications on the peritoneal fluid composition in mares. Theriogenology 1997; 48:919-931.

52. Dwyer R: Postpartum deaths of mares. Equine Dis Q 1993; 2:5.
53. Sertich P: Personal communication, 2002.
54. Adams HR: Adrenergic and anti-adrenergic drugs. In McDonald LE, Boothe MH (eds): Veterinary Pharmacology and Therapeutics, 5th edition, pp 89-112, Ames, The Iowa State University Press, 1982.
55. Marnet PG et al: Effets de doses excessives doxytocine sur la contractilite uterine chez la brebis. Revue Med Vet 1985; 136:315-320.
56. Kenney RM: Cyclic and pathologic changes of the mare endometrium as detected by biopsy, with a note on early embryonic death. J Am Vet Med Assoc 1978; 172:241-262.
57. McKinnon AO, Squires EL, Harrison LA et al: Ultrasonographic studies on the reproductive tract of mares after parturition: effect of involution and uterine fluid on pregnancy rates in mares with normal and delayed first postpartum ovulatory cycles. J Am Vet Med Assoc 1988; 192:350-353.

Index

Page numbers followed by f indicate figures; t, tables;
b, boxes.